EQUINE INFECTIOUS DISEASES

EQUINE INFECTIOUS DISEASES

DEBRA C. SELLON, DVM, PhD, DACVIM
Professor, Equine Medicine
Department of Veterinary Clinical Sciences
College of Veterinary Medicine
Washington State University
Pullman, Washington

MAUREEN T. LONG, DVM, PhD, DACVIM
Associate Professor, Large Animal Medicine
College of Veterinary Medicine
University of Florida
Gainesville, Florida

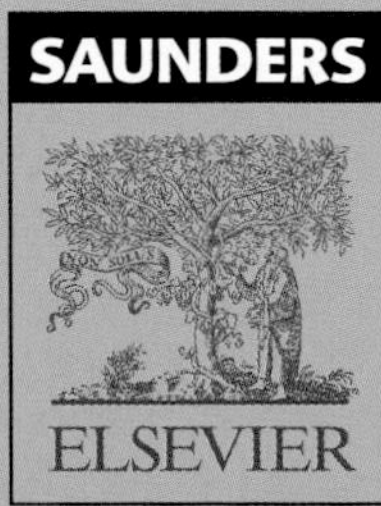

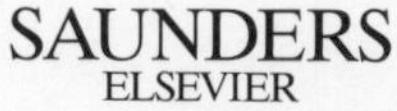

11830 Westline Industrial Drive
St. Louis, Missouri 63146

EQUINE INFECTIOUS DISEASES

ISBN-13: 978-1-4160-2406-4
ISBN-10: 1-4160-2406-9

Notice

Knowledge and best practice in this field are constantly changing. As new research and experience broaden our knowledge, changes in practice, treatment, and drug therapy may become necessary or appropriate. Readers are advised to check the most current information provided (i) on procedures featured or (ii) by the manufacturer of each product to be administered, to verify the recommended dose or formula, the method and duration of administration, and contraindications. It is the responsibility of the practitioner, relying on their own experience and knowledge of the patient, to make diagnoses, to determine dosages and the best treatment for each individual patient, and to take all appropriate safety precautions. To the fullest extent of the law, neither the Publisher nor the Authors assume any liability for any injury and/or damage to persons or property arising out or related to any use of the material contained in this book.

The Publisher

ISBN-13: 978-1-4160-2406-4
ISBN-10: 1-4160-2406-9

Publishing Director: Linda Duncan
Publisher: Penny Rudolph
Managing Editor: Jolynn Gower
Publishing Services Manager: Patricia Tannian
Senior Project Manager: Anne Altepeter
Design Coordinator: Teresa McBryan

Printed in China

Last digit is the print number: 9 8 7 6 5 4 3 2 1

Contributors

Marta Gonzalez Arguedas, DVM
Resident, Equine Medicine
Department of Veterinary Clinical Sciences
College of Veterinary Medicine
Washington State University
Pullman, Washington
Coronavirus Infections
Miscellaneous Gram-Positive Bacterial Infections

Udeni B. R. Balasuriya, BVSc, MS, PhD
Associate Professor of Virology
Veterinary Science
Maxwell H. Gluck Equine Research Center
University of Kentucky
Lexington, Kentucky
Equine Viral Arteritis

Joy L. Barbet, DVM, DACVD
Visiting Assistant Professor
Small Animal Clinical Sciences
Veterinary Medical Teaching Hospital
College of Veterinary Medicine
University of Florida
Gainesville, Florida
Ectoparasites of Horses

Michelle Henry Barton, DVM, PhD, DACVIM
Josiah Meigs Distinguished Teaching Professor
Large Animal Medicine
University of Georgia
Athens, Georgia
Endotoxemia

Alicia L. Bertone, DVM, PhD, DACVS
Endowed Chair of Equine Clinical Medicine and Surgery
Department of Veterinary Clinical Sciences
The Ohio State University
Columbus, Ohio
Infections of Muscle, Joint, and Bone

Thomas E. Besser, DVM, PhD
Professor
Department of Veterinary Microbiology and Pathology
College of Veterinary Medicine
Washington State University
Pullman, Washington
Salmonellosis

Corrie C. Brown, DVM, PhD, DACVP
Professor
Department of Veterinary Pathology
University of Georgia
Athens, Georgia
Recognition of Foreign Animal Diseases

Barbara A. Byrne, DVM, PhD, DACVIM
Assistant Professor
Pathology, Microbiology, and Immunology
School of Veterinary Medicine
University of California
Davis, California
Laboratory Diagnosis of Bacterial Infections
Laboratory Diagnosis of Fungal Diseases

Natalie Ann Carrillo, DVM
Lecturer
Large Animal Clinical Sciences
University of Florida
Gainesville, Florida
Candidiasis

Julie A. Cary, DVM, MS, DACVS
Clinical Instructor
Equine Surgery
Department of Veterinary Clinical Sciences
College of Veterinary Medicine
Washington State University
Pullman, Washington
Selected Boxes in Text

Carmen M. H. Colitz, DVM, PhD, DACVO
Assistant Professor
Veterinary Clinical Sciences
College of Veterinary Medicine
The Ohio State University
Columbus, Ohio
Ocular Infections

Elizabeth G. Davis, DVM, PhD, DACVIM
Assistant Professor
Equine Medicine
College of Veterinary Medicine
Kansas State University
Manhattan, Kansas
Respiratory Infections

Jennifer L. Davis, DVM, MS, DACVIM, DACVCP
Graduate Research Assistant
Molecular and Biomedical Sciences
College of Veterinary Medicine
North Carolina State University
Raleigh, North Carolina
Antimicrobial Therapy

Fabio Del Piero, DVM, PhD, DACVP
Associate Professor of Pathology
Pathobiology and Clinical Studies
University of Pennsylvania
Kennett Square, Pennsylvania
Rabies

Joseph A. DiPietro, DVM, DACVP, PhD
Institute of Agriculture
University of Tennessee
Knoxville, Tennessee
Cestodes

Thomas J. Divers, DVM, DACVIM, DACVECC
Clinical Sciences
College of Veterinary Medicine
Cornell Hospital for Animals
Cornell University
Ithaca, New York
Lyme Disease

Richard Drolet, DVM, MSc, DACVP
Department of Pathology and Microbiology
Faculty of Veterinary Medicine
University of Montreal
St-Hyacinthe, Quebec, Canada
Lawsonia intracellularis

Paulo C. Duarte, DVM, MPVM, PhD
Assistant Professor
Animal Population Health Institute
Department of Clinical Sciences
College of Veterinary Medicine and Biomedical Sciences
Colorado State University
Fort Collins, Colorado
Epidemiology of Equine Infectious Disease

J. P. Dubey, MVSc, PhD
United States Department of Agriculture
Agricultural Research Service
Animal Parasitic Diseases Laboratory
Animal and Natural Resources Institute, BARC
Beltsville, Maryland
Equine Protozoal Myeloencephalitis

Magdalena Dunowska, LW, PhD
Postdoctoral Fellow, Biosecurity Officer
James L. Voss Veterinary Medical Center
Colorado State University
Fort Collins, Colorado
Biosecurity

Roberta M. Dwyer, DVM, MS, DACVPM
Associate Professor
Department of Veterinary Science
Maxwell H. Gluck Equine Research Center
University of Kentucky
Lexington, Kentucky
Equine Rotavirus
Control of Infectious Disease Outbreaks

Cheryl L. Fite, DVM
Theriogenology Resident
Department of Veterinary Clinical Sciences
College of Veterinary Medicine
Washington State University
Pullman, Washington
Reproductive Tract Infections

Maria Julia Bevilaqua Felippe Flaminio, DVM, MS, PhD, DACVIM
Assistant Professor of Medicine
Clinical Sciences
Cornell University
Ithaca, New York
Immunotherapy

David E. Freeman, MVB, PhD, DACVS
Professor and Associate Chief of Staff
Large Animal Clinical Sciences
University of Florida
Gainesville, Florida
Respiratory Infections

Wolfgang Garten
Professor
Institute of Virology
University of Marburg
Marburg, Germany
Borna Disease

E. Paul J. Gibbs, BVSc, PhD, FRCVS
Professor of Virology
Infectious Diseases and Pathology
College of Veterinary Medicine
University of Florida
Gainesville, Florida
Equine Alphaviruses

Pamela E. Ginn, DVM, DACVP
Associate Professor
Infectious Diseases and Pathology
College of Veterinary Medicine
University of Florida
Gainesville, Florida
Skin Infections

Arthur Grabner
Professor
Faculty of Veterinary Medicine
University of Berlin
Berlin, Germany
Borna Disease

Ellis C. Greiner, PhD
Professor
Department of Pathobiology
Clinical Microbiology, Parasitology, and Serology Service
Veterinary Teaching Hospital
College of Veterinary Medicine
University of Florida
Gainesville, Florida
Laboratory Diagnosis of Parasitic Diseases

Amy M. Grooters, DVM, DACVIM
Associate Professor, Veterinary Clinical Sciences
Chief, Companion Animal Medicine
Veterinary Teaching Hospital
Louisiana State University
Baton Rouge, Louisiana
Pythiosis and Zygomycosis

Alan J. Guthrie, BVSc, BVSc (Hons), MMedVet, PhD
Director
Equine Research Center
Faculty of Veterinary Science
University of Pretoria
Pretoria, South Africa
African Horse Sickness

Joanne Hardy, DVM, PhD, DACVS, DACVECC
Clinical Associate Professor
Department of Large Animal Medicine and Surgery
Texas A & M University
College Station, Texas
Respiratory Infections

Christiane Herden, Dr Med Vet, DECVP
Institute of Pathology
University of Veterinary Medicine, Hannover
Hannover, Germany
Borna Disease

Sibylle Herzog, DVM, PhD
Research Associate
Faculty of Veterinary Medicine
Institute of Virology
Giessen, Germany
Borna Disease

Jill Higgins, DVM
Staff Veterinarian
Loomis Basin Equine Medical Center
Loomis, California
Coccidioidomycosis

Ashley E. Hill, DVM, MPVM, PhD
Assistant Professor
Department of Clinical Sciences
Colorado State University
Fort Collins, Colorado
Epidemiology of Equine Infectious Disease

Kenneth W. Hinchcliff, DVM, PhD, DACVIM
Professor
Department of Veterinary Clinical Sciences
The Ohio State University
Columbus, Ohio
Miscellaneous Viral Diseases

Melissa T. Hines, DVM, PhD, DACVIM
Associate Professor
Department of Veterinary Clinical Sciences
College of Veterinary Medicine
Washington State University
Pullman, Washington
Streptococcal Infections
Miscellaneous Gram-Positive Bacterial Infections
Rhodococcus equi
Leptospirosis

Merijo Eileen Jordan, DVM, MS
Veterinarian
Dorr Veterinary Clinic
Dorr, Michigan
Cestodes

Donald P. Knowles, DVM, PhD, DACVP
Department of Veterinary Microbiology and Pathology
College of Veterinary Medicine
Washington State University
Pullman, Washington
Equine Piroplasmosis

Catherine Kohn, VMD, DACVIM
Professor
Department of Veterinary Clinical Sciences
The Ohio State University
Columbus, Ohio
Aspergillosis
Miscellaneous Fungal Diseases

Michaela Kristula, DVM, MS
Associate Professor of Medicine
Clinical Studies
University of Pennsylvania
Philadelphia, Pennsylvania
Contagious Equine Metritis

Vanessa Kuonen, DVM, MS
Resident, Ophthalmology
Department of Veterinary Clinical Sciences
The Ohio State University
Columbia, Ohio
Ocular Infections

Gabriele A. Landolt, Dr Med Vet, MS, PhD, DACVIM
Assistant Professor
Department of Clinical Sciences
College of Veterinary Medicine and Biomedical Sciences
Colorado State University
Fort Collins, Colorado
Equine Influenza Infection

Jean-Pierre Lavoie, DVM, DACVIM
Professor
Department of Clinical Sciences
Faculty of Veterinary Medicine
University of Montreal
Montreal, Quebec, Canada
Lawsonia intracellularis

Dawn Logas, DVM, DACVD
Owner
Staff Dermatologist
Veterinary Dermatology Center
Maitland, Florida
Skin Infections

Katharina L. Lohmann, Dr Med Vet, PhD, DACVIM
Associate Professor
Large Animal Medicine
Western College of Veterinary Medicine
University of Saskatchewan
Saskatoon, Saskatchewan, Canada
Endotoxemia

D. Paul Lunn, BVSc, MS, PhD, MRCVS, DACVIM
Professor and Department Head
Department of Clinical Sciences
College of Veterinary Medicine and Biomedical Sciences
Colorado State University
Fort Collins, Colorado
Equine Influenza Infection

Robert J. MacKay, BVSc, PhD, DACVIM
Professor
Large Animal Clinical Sciences
College of Veterinary Medicine
University of Florida
Gainesville, Florida
Tetanus
Sporotrichosis

N. James MacLachlan, BVSc, PhD, DACVP
Professor
Pathology, Microbiology, and Immunology
University of California
Davis, California
Equine Viral Arteritis

John E. Madigan, DVM, MS, DACVIM
Professor and Associate Director
Large Animal Clinic
Department of Medicine and Epidemiology
University of California
Davis, California
Anaplasma phagocytophila
Neorickettsia risticii

Celia M. Marr, BVMS, MVM, PhD, DEIM, DECEIM, MRCVS
Hospital Clinician
Internal Medicine, Intensive Care, and Neonatology Service
Rossdales Equine Hospital
Newmarket, Suffolk
United Kingdom
Cardiovascular Infections

Rosanna Marsella, DVM, DACVD
Associate Professor, Dermatology
Small Animal Clinical Sciences
University of Florida
Gainesville, Florida
Dermatophilosis
Dermatophytosis

Brian J. McCluskey, DVM, MS, PhD, DACVPM
USDA, APHIS, Veterinary Services
National Surveillance Unit
Centers for Epidemiology and Animal Health
Fort Collins, Colorado
Vesicular Stomatitis

Robert H. Mealey, DVM, PhD, DACVIM
Assistant Professor
College of Veterinary Medicine
Department of Veterinary Microbiology and Pathology
Washington State University
Pullman, Washington
Equine Infectious Anemia

Paul S. Morley, DVM, PhD, DACVIM
Associate Professor, Epidemiology and Biosecurity
Director of Biosecurity
Animal Population Health Institute
Colorado State University
Fort Collins, Colorado
Epidemiology of Equine Infectious Disease
Biosecurity

J. Richard Newton, BVSc, MSc, PhD, DLSHTM, DECVPH, FRCVS
Head of Epidemiology
Epidemiology Unit
Centre for Prevention Medicine
Animal Health Trust
Newmarket, Suffolk
United Kingdom
Streptococcal Infections

Paul L. Nicoletti, DVM
Professor Emeritus
Pathobiology
University of Florida
Gainesville, Florida
Glanders
Brucellosis

Martin Krarup Nielsen, DVM
PhD student
Department of Large Animal Sciences
Royal Veterinary and Agricultural University
Frederiksberg C, Denmark
Nematodes

J. Lindsay Oaks, DVM, PhD, DACVIM
Assistant Professor
Washington Animal Disease Diagnostic Laboratory
Washington State University
Pullman, Washington
Laboratory Diagnosis of Viral Infections
Miscellaneous Gram-Positive Bacterial Infections
Mycobacterial Infections
Miscellaneous Anaerobic Infections

Demosthenes Pappagianis, MD, PhD
Professor
Medical Microbiology and Immunology
School of Medicine
University of California
Davis, California
Coccidioidomycosis

Mark G. Papich, DVM, MS
Professor of Clinical Pharmacology
Department of Molecular Biomedical Sciences
College of Veterinary Medicine
North Carolina State University
Raleigh, North Carolina
Antimicrobial Therapy

Simon F. Peek, BVSc, MRCVS, PhD, DACVIM
Clinical Associate Professor of Large Animal Internal Medicine
Department of Medical Sciences
University of Wisconsin
Madison, Wisconsin
Systemic Clostridial Infections

Nicola Pusterla, Dr Med Vet, Habil, FVH, DACVIM
Assistant Professor
Medicine and Epidemiology
School of Veterinary Medicine
University of California
Davis, California
Anaplasma ahagocytophila
Neorickettsia risticii
Immunoprophylaxis

Craig R. Reinemeyer, DVM, PhD
Adjunct Associate Professor
Department of Comparative Medicine
College of Veterinary Medicine
University of Tennessee
Knoxville, Tennessee

President
East Tennessee Clinical Research, Inc.
Knoxville, Tennessee
Nematodes

Juergen A. Richt, DVM, PhD
Associate Professor (Adjunct)
Iowa State University
Ames, Iowa
Veterinary Medicine Officer, Lead Scientist
Virus and Prion Diseases of Livestock Unit
National Animal Disease Center
Ames, Iowa
Borna Disease

Chantal M. Rothschild, DVM, DACVIM
Graduate Research Assistant
Department of Veterinary Microbiology and Pathology
College of Veterinary Medicine
Washington State University
Pullman, Washington
Equine Piroplasmosis

L. Chris Sanchez, DVM, PhD, DACVIM
Assistant Professor
Department of Large Animal Clinical Sciences
College of Veterinary Medicine
University of Florida
Gainesville, Florida
Gastrointestinal and Peritoneal Infections
Neonatal Septicemia

Kathy K. Seino, DVM, MS
Graduate Student
Large Animal Clinical Sciences
College of Veterinary Medicine
University of Florida
Gainesville, Florida
Central Nervous System Infections

Josh Slater, BVM&S, PhD, DECEIM, MRCVS
Professor of Equine Clinical Studies
Royal Veterinary College
London, United Kingdom
Equine Herpesviruses

Sharon J. Spier, DVM, PhD, DACVIM
Professor
Veterinary Medicine and Epidemiology
School of Veterinary Medicine
University of California
Davis, California
Miscellaneous Gram-Positive Bacterial Infections

Michael J. Studdert, BVSc, MVSc, PhD, DVSc, MACVSc, FASM
Professor
School of Veterinary Science
The University of Melbourne
Parkville, Victoria, Australia
Miscellaneous Viral Respiratory Diseases

W. Wesley Sutter, DVM, MS, DACVS
Staff Surgeon
Ocala Equine Hospital
Ocala, Florida
Infections of Muscle, Joint, and Bone

Corinne R. Sweeney, DVM, DACVIM
Professor of Medicine
Department of Clinical Sciences—New Bolton Center
University of Pennsylvania
Kennett Square, Pennsylvania
Streptococcal Infections

Ahmed Tibary, DMV, MS, PhD, DACT
Associate Professor
Veterinary Clinical Sciences
College of Veterinary Medicine
Washington State University
Pullman, Washington
Reproductive Tract Infections

Peter J. Timoney, MVB, MS, PhD, FRCVS
Chairman and Director
Veterinary Science
Gluck Equine Research Center
University of Kentucky
Lexington, Kentucky
Streptococcal Infections
Infectious Diseases and the International Movement of Horses

Hugh G. G. Townsend, BSc, DVM, MSc
Professor
Department of Large Animal Clinical Sciences
University of Saskatchewan
Saskatoon, Saskatchewan, Canada
Equine Influenza Infection

Josie L. Traub-Dargatz, DVM, MS, DACVIM
Professor
Equine Internal Medicine
Department of Clinical Sciences
James L. Voss Veterinary Teaching Hospital
Colorado State University
Fort Collins, Colorado
Salmonellosis
Biosecurity

David C. VanMetre, DVM, DACVIM
Associate Professor
Department of Clinical Sciences
Colorado State University
Fort Collins, Colorado
Biosecurity

J. Scott Weese, DVM, DVSc, DACVIM
Associate Professor
Clinical Studies
Ontario Veterinary College
Guelph, Ontario, Canada
Staphylococcal Infections
Enteric Clostridial Infections

Mary Beth Whitcomb, DVM
Lecturer
Veterinary Surgical and Radiological Sciences
School of Veterinary Medicine
University of California
Davis, California
Miscellaneous Gram-Positive Bacterial Infections

Pamela A. Wilkins, DVM, MS, PhD, DACVIM, DACVECC
Assistant Professor of Large Animal Medicine
Clinical Studies—New Bolton Center
University of Pennsylvania
Kennett Square, Pennsylvania
Rabies
Botulism

W. David Wilson, BVMS, MRCVS, PhD
Professor
Department of Medicine and Epidemiology (VM:VME)
Director of Large Animal Clinical Services
Verterinary Medical Teaching Hospital
School of Veterinary Medicine
University of California
Davis, California
Immunoprophylaxis

Dana N. Zimmel, DVM, DACVIM, ABVP (Equine Practice)
Assistant Professor
Large Animal Clinical Sciences
College of Veterinary Medicine
University of Florida
Gainesville, Florida
Urinary Tract Infections

To Jeff, Rance, and Ethan, in grateful appreciation of all they have done to support and encourage us in this and every endeavor of our lives

Preface

It is impossible to practice equine medicine and surgery without confronting the many faces of infectious disease and its impact on the health and well-being of our patients. Although this statement has been true since the earliest days of veterinary practice, the past few decades have seen an exponential increase in the rapidity of spread of infectious diseases in horses around the globe. This is nowhere more clearly explained than in the chapter on *Infetctious Diseases and the International Movement of Horses* by Dr. Peter J. Timoney, one of the premier equine infectious disease experts of our generation and current director of the Gluck Equine Research Center at the University of Kentucky in Lexington, Kentucky. With the increasing globalization of the equine industry and changing political realities of the world, equine veterinarians are finding themselves on the frontlines in an escalating battle against pathogens that have the potential to profoundly affect the health of our patients and the equine industry as a whole.

The germ of the idea for this book first infected our minds very early in our lives. We were eyewitnesses to the devastation of a brucellosis outbreak at a boarding facility at which horses were freely co-mingled with cattle. As young teenagers it was difficult to understand the necessity for euthanasia of outwardly healthy horses to safeguard the health and well-being of the majority of the animals on the farm. As veterinarians, we have seen others go through the same struggle as apparently healthy horses were euthanized because of a positive Coggins test. We have watched the economic hardships that ensue when a boarding stable or training establishment must be quarantined because of a disease outbreak. We have watched the struggles of large breeding farms that lose horses to strangles year after year despite impeccable management strategies and state-of-the-art vaccination schemes. In each of these professional situations we sought to find answers regarding the disease, its pathogenesis, and its control. However, answers were scattered in bits and pieces throughout the veterinary literature, making it nearly impossible for practitioners without access to state-of-the-art computer databases and with limited time for research to find those answers.

At some point, we became aware of an incredible text titled *Infectious Diseases of the Dog and Cat.* This beautiful text, edited by Dr. Craig Greene of the University of Georgia, summarizes current knowledge related to almost every infectious disease of dogs and cats. It describes the etiologic agent, outlines the important aspects of pathogenesis, presents the advantages and disadvantages of available diagnostic and therapeutic choices, and even explains the public health implications of each disease. This book clarified in our minds exactly what was needed for equine practitioners, infectious disease experts, and other individuals interested in equine health care. We extend our grateful appreciation to Dr. Greene and acknowledge the critical inspiration and many ways his book has shaped this text. Our goal is to provide anyone interested in equine health with a single source summary of the important aspects of equine infectious diseases that occur worldwide. The extensive references to the primary veterinary literature that are included on the accompanying CD-ROM will serve as a springboard to an even deeper understanding of the research manuscripts and clinical reports that have been the source for information contained in each chapter. A direct link to PubMed citations will enable users of the CD-ROM to click and access scientific abstracts of most references so that more extensive research is facilitated as needed by each reader.

ACKNOWLEDGMENTS

Without the input and hard work of innumerable individuals, this book would never have been completed. We thank each and every author who worked hard to provide us with just the type of information that was needed for this book and for being patient with the sometimes extensive editorial changes that we requested. We hope that each author is as proud to be associated with this book as we are.

We thank all the clinicians, researchers, and microbiologists who unselfishly shared photographs and images. Inclusion of the many illustrations truly makes this a unique veterinary text.

The staff at Elsevier—especially Jolynn Gower, Liz Fathman, and Anne Altepeter—have been extremely supportive and never wavered in their commitment to this project, even as it became apparent that we were going to be many, many pages over the initial estimate!

We hope that this book will be of value and service to the equine veterinarians and students whom we serve. If, in reading this text, each of you learns just a small fraction of the amount that we learned in the writing and editing, then our purpose will have been served.

Debra C. Sellon
Maureen T. Long

Contents

Section III
Bacterial and Rickettsial Diseases

Section IV
Fungal Diseases

Section V
Parasitic Diseases

Section VI
Prevention and Control of Infectious Diseases

SECTION • I
Clinical Problems

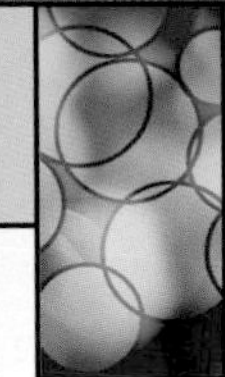

CHAPTER • 1

Respiratory Infections

EQUINE RESPIRATORY TRACT

Elizabeth G. Davis

Normal Respiratory Flora

Bacterial flora plays an important role in host health in a variety of tissues and organ systems, such as the skin, gastrointestinal tract, and urogenital system, as well as the respiratory system.[1] The upper airway of healthy horses contains many bacteria, including a variety of aerobic and anaerobic species. This flora competes with pathogenic species that, when present in large numbers, can colonize the epithelial surface. Normal equine respiratory flora includes *Streptococcus equi* subsp. *zooepidemicus, Pasteurella* spp., *Escherichia coli, Actinomyces* spp., and *Streptococcus* spp. Anaerobes predominate in the normal equine oral cavity and consist of several bacterial genera, including *Bacteroides fragilis, Fusobacterium* spp., *Eubacterium* spp., *Clostridium* spp., *Veillonella* spp., and *Megasphaera* spp.[2]

Typically, horses with infectious lower airway disease are infected with one of these bacteria, consistent with the concept that contamination of the lower respiratory tract originates from the upper airways. Aspiration can be the mechanism by which such contamination occurs, because head elevation and long-distance transport contribute to lower airway contamination and accumulation of mucus.[3-5] Contamination of the lower airway is common in apparently healthy horses, and many horses will have positive bacterial cultures when examined by tracheobronchial aspirate.

Pulmonary Defense Mechanisms

Endogenous pulmonary defense includes components of nonspecific and specific clearance mechanisms. Components of nonspecific clearance include anatomic barriers, mucosal lining, mucous secretions, and the mucociliary escalator. These nonspecific mechanisms are distinguished from specific immune effector molecules because they lack specificity and memory.

A major mediator of nonspecific clearance of debris and pathogens from the respiratory tract is the mucociliary escalator. The *mucociliary escalator* consists of a double layer of mucus that extends from the pharynx to the respiratory bronchioles. This mucous layer is propelled upward by the ciliated respiratory epithelium. Inhaled particles and debris are propelled in a proximal direction by a constant wave of upward movement by the cilia and mucus. The mucociliary system can become damaged by smoke inhalation and direct viral destruction.[6,7]

Influenza and herpesviruses replicate within and destroy ciliated epithelium, which requires approximately 21 days for regeneration. In addition, environment may play a role in clearance mechanisms because high ammonia concentration, such as that associated with a high degree of urine and fecal waste, will result in depressed ciliary motility.[8-10] Dehydration may also contribute to reduced pulmonary clearance because effective ciliary movement will be depressed with reduced fluidity of the mucous layer.

The major mediators of specific pulmonary clearance mechanisms are within the *bronchial-associated lymphoid tissue* (BALT). BALT exists within the submucosa of the segmental bronchi and terminal bronchioles. As with other lymphoid organs, BALT is an area where antigen-specific responses stimulate cell-mediated and humoral immune defense. B lymphocytes within BALT can switch to all classes of antibodies, although the predominant antibody produced in the upper respiratory tract is immunoglobulin A (IgA); immunoglobulin G (IgG) is secreted in greater quantities in the lower airways.[11] The advantage of upper respiratory secretion of IgA is the blockage of adherence of pathogens to the upper respiratory tract epithelium, a process referred to as *immune exclusion*. Memory is conferred by this arm of the immune system and thereby results in long-term protection from infectious disease.

The goal of immunization against pathogens is to produce high concentrations of antigen-specific responses that will confer resistance at the site of infectious challenge. A disadvantage of many intramuscular vaccines is that high levels of IgG are induced in circulation, with minimal levels of IgA produced at the mucosal surface. The intention of intranasally delivered vaccines is to induce local IgA production. The IgG production becomes essential when pathogens gain entrance to the lower airways. This antibody isotype is critical for opsonization and removal of bacteria and foreign material. Effective opsonization will result in effective phagocytosis and removal from the lower airways and pulmonary parenchyma. Some pathogens (e.g., herpesvirus) are capable of surviving and replicating within BALT, resulting in necrosis of lymphoid nodules. This contributes to a postviral state of immunocompromise in which the patient is susceptible to infection with secondary pathogens.

Below the level of the mucociliary escalator and the BALT, cellular responses are critical for immune protection of the equine host. The first phagocyte of importance is the *alveolar macrophage*, located in the terminal bronchioles and alveoli. The alveolar macrophage provides a bridge between innate and adaptive immune responses. Although these cells can ingest foreign material nonspecifically, they also serve as important antigen-presenting cells for T lymphocytes and development of adaptive immunity. Particles that are inhaled and reach the alveolar spaces are removed by local alveolar macrophages. Once they contain foreign material, these cells may be coughed up and swallowed, or they may move from the alveolar space and enter general circulation for ultimate clearance by the lymphatic system. The function of these cells depends on host status; long-distance transport or viral infection will destroy alveolar macrophages.[12]

Another important cell in the pulmonary system of horses is the *pulmonary intravascular macrophage* (PIM). These cells are important for removal of particulate matter (e.g., bacteria, toxins) from general circulation. Species that have PIMs include horses, pigs, ruminants, and cats. Mammalian species that do not have PIMs utilize hepatic Kupffer's cells and splenic macrophages for similar purposes. PIMs are critical for removal of bacteria or endotoxin on the first pass through the lungs, but they contribute to the inflammation induced after bacterial challenge.[13] Disadvantages of PIMs include the resultant inflammatory reaction that follows their activation. For example, phagocytosis of endotoxin is associated with pronounced inflammatory mediator release, microthrombus formation, neutrophilic influx, vasoconstriction, pulmonary edema, and endothelial damage that may lead to other systemic disorders. Species variation in sensitivity to endotoxin relates to the presence of PIMs, and intensified sensitivity to endotoxin is related to the number of PIMs in the pulmonary vasculature.

Epithelial protection of the respiratory tracts is provided not only by the mucosal lining and leukocytes within the submucosa, but also by mechanisms of the innate immune system. Antimicrobial peptides play an important role in innate immune protection in the pulmonary system of many species. Cathelicidin peptides have been identified in pulmonary equine neutrophils collected from heaves-affected individuals.[14] This class of antimicrobial peptide has been shown to play a role in pathogen clearance, having broad-spectrum activity against bacterial pathogens.[15] Other similar peptides are expressed in epithelial cells as well as within leukocyte subsets.[16,17]

Anatomic and Physiologic Considerations

The horse is an *obligate* nasal airway breather, which means that even under strenuous exercise, no air is obtained through the oral cavity or oropharynx. This consideration impacts the pathogenesis of equine infectious disease in two ways. First, contamination of the nasopharynx (and subsequently the lower airway) by bacteria within the oral cavity and oropharynx likely comes from prolonged changes in head placement (e.g., transport), fatigue of the pharynx of the horse (e.g., intense exercise), or changes in the local immunity of the nasopharynx (e.g., viral infection). Second, any change in the upper airway results in an immediate decrease in the exercise capacity of the horse. Thus any inflammatory condition, even as "innocuous" as lymphoid hyperplasia, may have a profound impact on performance and health of the lower respiratory tract.

The equine airway has a *monopodial* branching pattern, meaning that each branch gives rise to daughter branches. The respiratory tree is lined by mucous membrane and supported by lamina propria with cartilage and smooth muscle, depending on site. Ciliated cells and goblet cells (which produce mucus) line the bronchioles. The secretory cells change to Clara cells in the bronchioles. The alveoli are lined by a single layer of epithelial cells consisting of type I and type II pneumocytes. These cells are supported by a thin interstitium and a small amount of smooth muscle at each opening.

CLINICAL FINDINGS ASSOCIATED WITH INFECTIOUS RESPIRATORY DISEASE

In general, proper diagnosis of infectious respiratory disease depends on information gleaned from the history and physical examination, identification of abnormalities (problem list), and development of a diagnostic plan. Age and signalment and recent exposure to new arrivals may indicate viral respiratory disease. Long-distance travel before onset of respiratory signs indicates a horse is at high risk for pleuropneumonia. *Rhodococcus equi* occurs primarily in foals between 3 and 5 months of age.

Clinical signs of infectious respiratory disease may initially be nonspecific, including fever, depression, and possible anorexia. Signs referable to the respiratory system may include nasal discharge, cough, and tachypnea. Either upper or lower respiratory disease can cause these clinical signs. Respiratory stridor (usually upper respiratory tract disease) and respiratory distress (upper or lower respiratory tract disease) may also be present. Other nonspecific signs include epistaxis and cyanosis. With either acute viral infection or chronic lower airway disease, exercise intolerance is a feature. Weight loss may occur with chronic respiratory infection.

Physical examination should be thorough and include examination of all body systems. Normal respiratory rate of foals is between 20 and 40 breaths/min and in adults is between 12 and 24 breaths/min. Breathing should be slow and deliberate with no nostril flare. Auscultation of horses can be difficult because of the normally slow rate and character of breathing. Depth of breathing can be increased by performing a rebreathing examination with a plastic bag placed over the nares of the horse. Normal horses generally do not cough when encouraged to take a deep breath with rebreathing. Normal horses do not cough when the trachea is palpated. Concomitant percussion during auscultation may indicate a fluid line.

DIAGNOSTIC APPROACH TO INFECTIOUS RESPIRATORY DISEASE

Endoscopy may be used to confirm the presence of upper airway disease and to perform diagnostic tests such as transtracheal aspirate (TTA) or bronchoalveolar lavage (BAL). Diagnosis of rhinitis, pharyngeal lymphoid hyperplasia, guttural pouch disease, and retropharyngeal lymphadenopathy (presumably from *Streptococcus equi* subsp. *equi* infection; Fig. 1-1) may be facilitated by endoscopic examination. Radiographs of the sinuses are essential for identification of fluid or masses within sinuses, guttural pouches, and thorax. Diagnostic-quality thoracic radiography is difficult with most field equipment. Lower airway radiography is important for determining the type of pattern present but is not specific for

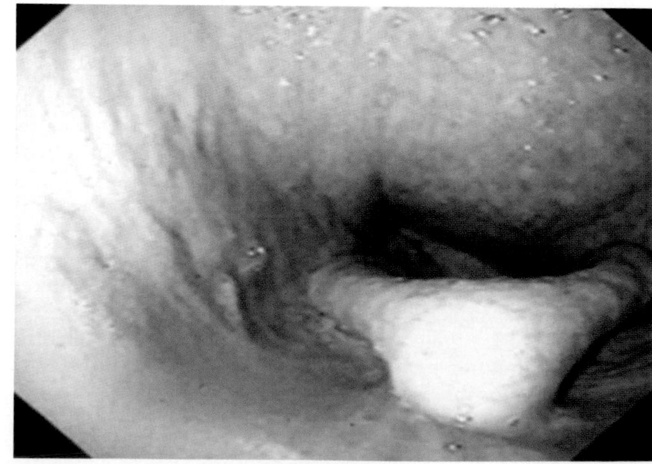

Fig. 1-1 Endoscopic view of upper airway of horse with severe pharyngeal compression associated with *Streptococcus equi* subsp. *equi* infection.

identification of any particular etiologic agents. Thoracic ultrasound is easily performed in the field, and although nonspecific for etiology, it is particularly useful to detect lower airway disease, including consolidation of the peripheral lung lobes and identification of pulmonary fluid. A 5.0-MHz linear probe (used for most rectal ultrasound examinations) will suffice for the majority of these examinations.

Ancillary diagnostic testing is critical for correct etiologic identification of potentially contagious pathogens. Nasopharyngeal or nasal passage swabs are particularly useful for diagnosis of viral respiratory tract disease. Polyester-tipped swabs are preferred because viruses may adhere to cotton fibers, decreasing the likelihood of isolating virus from the sample. The swabs should be placed in sterile viral transport medium and kept on ice until further analysis. Maintaining moisture with physiologic saline is an alternative for very-short-term transport. Swabs for viral isolation need to be only of standard length (6 inches); the only requirement is contact with the nasal mucosa. Viral swabs may be analyzed in three ways: viral culture, polymerase chain reaction (PCR), and antigen enzyme-linked immunosorbent assay (ELISA). Virus isolation and paired serum titers can be obtained to confirm the diagnosis of specific viral infections. Clinical signs of disease, local population, history, and vaccination status will influence the likelihood of viral infection.

Diagnosis of equine influenza is based on virus isolation, virus antigen detection, and paired serum testing (see Chapter 12). An ELISA test is commercially available for the detection of influenza virus particles in nasal secretions (Directigen FLU-A, BD Diagnostic Systems, Franklin Lakes, NJ). This potential stall-side test was not designed for equine use but has been validated for use in this species.[18]

Diagnosis of infection with equine herpesvirus (EHV)-1 and EHV-4 depends somewhat on disease manifestation (see Chapter 13). For example, diagnosis of infectious respiratory disease may be confirmed by PCR or culture of nasal swab samples (or buffy coat samples) or detection of increasing serum antibody titers to the virus. Virus isolation from a buffy coat smear, nasal swab, or postmortem tissues may provide important information. Additional diagnostic testing may include molecular characterization using the restriction endonuclease analysis of deoxyribonucleic acid (DNA) fragments. Cerebrospinal fluid (CSF) analysis should be performed in horses suspected of EHV myelopathy, often characterized by xanthochromia and albuminocytologic dissociation. Antibody titer analysis of CSF is of limited value for diagnosis of neurologic EHV disease because significant disruption of the blood-brain barrier has frequently occurred in affected horses.

Diagnosis of EHV-2 may be challenging because virus isolation does not provide consistently positive results. Paired serologic titers may provide suggestive information for establishing a diagnosis of upper respiratory disease in horses. PCR has also been used for diagnosis in horses.[19]

Definitive diagnosis of equine viral arteritis (EVA) infection is made on the basis of virus isolation from nasopharyngeal, vaginal or semen samples (see Chapter 14). PCR testing has improved sensitivity and specificity for detection of the virus in these samples. Acute and convalescent serum titers may provide additional information to facilitate confirmation of the EVA diagnosis in suspect cases. Gross examination of fetuses postmortem typically reveals edema, pleural effusion, and petechiation.

Equine rhinoviruses, such as equine rhinitis A virus (ERAV), are a cause of upper respiratory tract infection in horses (see Chapter 16). These infections can be more challenging to diagnose than other viral respiratory tract infections because seroprevalence can be high.[20] Of 28 cases where the rhinovirus was isolated from infected horses only six showed serologic evidence of viral exposure.[21] Therefore, when equine rhinitis B virus (ERBV) infection is a diagnostic differential, virus isolation is the preferred diagnostic test. Although a third rhinovirus, ERBV2, has been investigated as a possible etiologic agent of equine viral respiratory tract disease, its role remains unconfirmed.[22]

Culture of nasopharyngeal swabs or wash samples are useful for diagnosis of *Streptococcus equi* subsp. *equi* (strangles) infection in horses (see Chapter 28). Detection of *S. equi* DNA using the PCR test is also confirmatory for a respiratory infection secondary to *S. equi* infection. Carrier horses may be challenging to identify without endoscopic evaluation that includes examination of the guttural pouches. Culture and PCR of samples obtained from the guttural pouch of these horses are recommended. If both tests are negative, the horse is unlikely to be an *S. equi* carrier. PCR testing for *S. equi* is more sensitive than standard microbiologic culture techniques.[23]

Serology for diagnosis of equine respiratory viruses must be performed on paired sera obtained at least 2 to 4 weeks apart. A single paired serum titer is nondiagnostic and a waste of laboratory time and owner resources. Whenever possible, paired sera testing should be pursued and can be extremely useful if the index case is no longer shedding virus and for assessment of herd exposure. For herd testing, a minimum of 10% of the herd or group is necessary.

Communication with the appropriate diagnostic laboratory regarding differential diagnoses under consideration is recommended. Not all laboratories perform all types of diagnostic tests.

Fluid analysis of the trachea and lungs is often helpful in the diagnosis of lower airway disease. Transtracheal wash technique is discussed in more detail later in this chapter. Bronchoalveolar lavage is essential for analysis of the alveolar spaces; however, this technique is regional at best. Samples of both types may be submitted for cytologic evaluation, viral detection, and bacterial and fungal culture.

UPPER RESPIRATORY TRACT INFECTIONS

Rhinitis and Sinusitis

Nasal airways can be infected with a variety of viral, bacterial, fungal, and parasitic agents with resultant sinusitis or rhinitis. In this chapter, *rhinitis* in the horse is defined as infection of the nasal passage independent of the sinus. Infection may include the nasal concha but does not involve the conchal sinuses unless caused by viral agents. Specific viral agents include equine influenza virus, EHV-1 and EHV-4, equine rhinoviruses, and adenovirus.[20,22,24-29] Bacterial rhinitis is uncommon and usually occurs secondary to trauma or a foreign body. *Mycoplasma* spp. have been isolated at postmortem examination from horses with rhinitis.[7,21,29,30] A variety of mycotic agents, such as *Aspergillus* spp. (see Chapter 56), *Conidiobolus* spp. (usually *C. coronatus*) (see Chapter 55), and *Cryptococcus neoformans* (see Chapter 57), may cause rhinitis in horses.[31-34] The most common cause of parasitic rhinitis is myiasis resulting from *Habronema*, *Draschia* (see Chapter 62), and the Russian gadfly, *Rhinoestrus purpureus*.[35] Enzootic lymphangitis or glanders caused by *Burkholderia mallei* causes a specific granuloma within the sinus cavity (see Chapter 39).[36-42]

Horses with sinusitis most often have unilateral disease, unless the infection is viral or there is extensive involvement of the nasal septa. Most horses present with respiratory stridor and nasal discharge with diminished airflow.[24,26,28,29] Therapy usually involves surgical debridement, debulking of nasal granuloma, and local therapy for the specific agent.[28,43-45] Orally administered itraconazole has been described for treatment of recurrent nasal mycoses.[28,44] Although successful in this case, the pharmacokinetics of itraconazole are variable. Fluconazole may be a viable alternative. Detailed discussions of antifungal therapy in horses are presented in Chapters 56 and 71.

Sinonasal disease is very common in the horse. The horse has six pairs of sinuses, including the conchal sinuses, which exchange air with the nasal airway. The frontal sinuses may be affected with granulomatous masses (usually fungal or parasitic) or empyema (bacterial). The most common bacterial isolates are *Streptococcus* spp., with *S. equi* subsp. *zooepidemicus* and *S. equi* subsp. *equi* most frequently found. *Staphylococcus* spp. are the next most common isolates.[46-49] Mixed bacterial infections may occur. *Cryptococcus neoformans* and *Coccidioides immitis* also may cause granuloma formation within the paranasal sinuses[31-34] (see Chapter 51).

In a study of 277 horses with sinusitis, 24% had primary sinusitis with no history of predisposing trauma or dental infection.[49] Dental disease of the third to sixth maxillary cheek teeth was the most common predisposing factor for secondary sinusitis (22% of horses), followed by sinus cysts, neoplasia, progressive ethmoidal hematoma, trauma, mycotic infection, sinonasal polyps, and nasal epidermal inclusion cysts. Primary infection of a rostral maxillary cheek root infection was identified in only 4% of cases, although computed tomography (CT) evaluation was not used for diagnosis in many of these horses. Nasal discharge (most often unilateral but occasionally bilateral) and facial swelling were the most common clinical signs. Discharge can be mucopurulent to serosanguineous fluid with a foul smell. Clinical signs frequently persisted over several weeks (without other progressive systemic clinical signs). Other signs of frontal and maxillary sinus involvement included lacrimal discharge and exophthalmia.

Diagnostic techniques that may facilitate identification or characterization of sinusitis in horses include endoscopy, radiography, CT, and magnetic resonance imaging (MRI).[50-52] Endoscopy can detect changes in airway structure (84% of cases) and rule out ethmoidal hematoma.[48,49] Sinoscopy can also be performed through a space created in the skull by trephination in the standing horse.[26,31,48,49]

Radiography is essential for identification of fluid and masses within sinuses (Fig. 1-2). If there is no fluid, this modality is valuable for detection of tooth root abscess.[47,49-55] Usually the first molar is involved. CT and MRI are exceptionally valuable for detection of tooth root involvement and bony changes, which often involve the maxillary bone and facial crest.

Appropriate and effective treatment of sinusitis requires that underlying or predisposing conditions be accurately identified and treated, that debris be flushed from the sinus, and that associated infectious agents be properly identified. When fluid is present within a sinus, medical treatment with antibiotics alone is unlikely to be successful. Trephination and flushing or surgical debridement and drainage through a sinus flap are indicated.[28,44,45,48,56-59] Establishment of ventral drainage of the affected sinuses may be required. Local flushing is likely to be the most important component of therapy, although systemic antimicrobial therapy may be indicated for any horse with signs of osteomyelitis.

Prognosis is guarded for complete resolution of clinical signs, especially when apical dental disease is present. Frequently, tooth removal is indicated. Recurrence is most common with ethmoidal hematoma and neoplasia.[49]

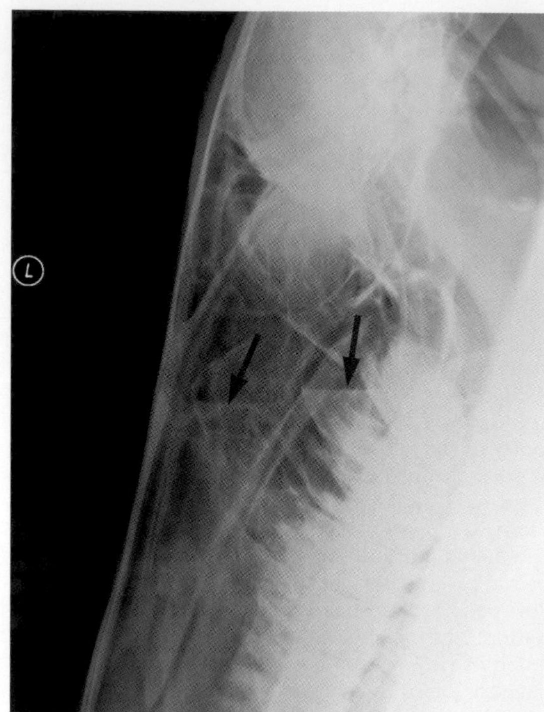

Fig. 1-2 Oblique radiograph of skull demonstrating fluid line in caudal maxillary sinus in horse presenting with chronic unilateral discharge. An air-fluid interface is demonstrated above the molars *(arrow)*. Purulent material was found on surgery in the maxillary sinus, consistent with empyema.

Lymphoid Pharyngeal Hyperplasia

Lymphoid pharyngeal hyperplasia is a common condition involving the upper respiratory tract of 2- and 3-year-old racehorses (Box 1-1 and Fig. 1-3). Most mild cases respond favorably to reduced athletic activity combined with systemic and topical antiinflammatory therapy. Dexamethasone can be administered at a dose of 0.02 to 0.05 mg/kg orally daily for 1 week, followed by half the original dose orally for 1 week, then the same dose orally every other day for an additional week. A throat spray of nitrofurazone, dexamethasone, and dimethyl sulfoxide is reported to be of benefit when administered topically.[56] Systemic immune modulation is reported to be effective for treatment of horses with lower airway inflammation and may also have some benefit in those with upper airway inflammation.[56,60,61] Occasionally, chronic disease occurs; reports have suggested that these horses may respond favorably to cautery of the dorsal roof of the pharynx.[62]

Organisms associated with a more prolonged course of pharyngeal hyperplasia include *S. equi* subsp. *equi*, equine influenza, EHV-1, EHV-2, and EHV-4. The condition is thought to result from chronic inflammation of the localized lymphoid tissues, particularly because these structures have a diffuse distribution within the mucosa in this species. Although some investigators have cultured the oropharynx of affected horses, no consistent etiologic agent has been identified. Normal inhabitants of the equine upper respiratory tract, such as *S. equi* subsp. *zooepidemicus*, *Bordetella bronchiseptica*, and *Moraxella* have been isolated; however, the direct association with lymphoid pharyngeal hyperplasia has not been determined. A grading system has been established for this condition; those horses with more severe inflammation have greater numbers of bacterial organisms isolated from their upper respiratory tract.[63]

Box • 1-1

Grading Scheme for Lymphoid Pharyngeal Hyperplasia

- *Grade 1:* Small number of white follicles scattered over dorsal pharyngeal wall. The follicles are small and inactive. This appearance is normal in horses of all ages.
- *Grade 2:* Many small, inactive white follicles over dorsal and lateral walls of pharynx to level of guttural pouches. Numerous follicles are larger, pink, edematous, and interspersed throughout.
- *Grade 3:* Many large, pink follicles and some shrunken white follicles distributed over dorsal and lateral walls of pharynx. In some individuals the follicles extend onto the dorsal surface of the soft palate and into the dorsal pharyngeal diverticula.
- *Grade 4:* More numerous pink and edematous follicles packed close together, covering entire pharynx, dorsal surface of soft palate, and epiglottis and lining guttural pouches. Large accumulations appear as polyps.

Modified from Raker CW: The nasopharynx. In Mansmann RA, McAllister ES, editors: *Equine medicine and surgery*, Santa Barbara, Calif, 1982, American Veterinary Publications.

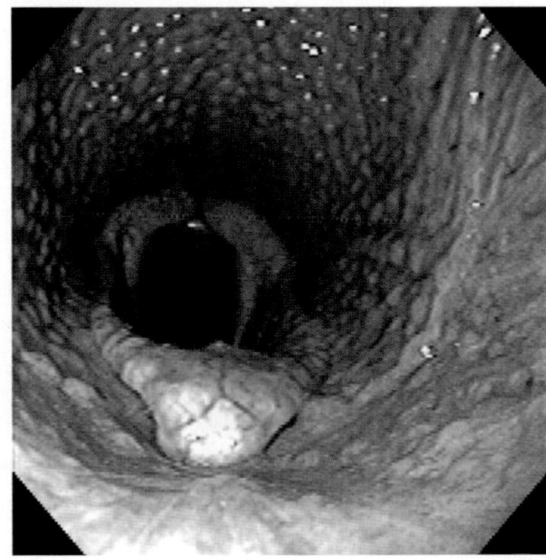

Fig. 1-3 Grade 3 lymphoid pharyngeal hyperplasia in 2-year old Thoroughbred colt (see Box 1-1).

Arytenoid Chondritis

Arytenoid chondritis is a progressive inflammatory condition of the arytenoid cartilages in adult horses, originating as an infectious condition. Most often, upper airway dysfunction is reflected in poor athletic performance and respiratory stridor. Diagnosis is based on upper airway endoscopy (Fig. 1-4). One manifestation of chondritis is the development of granulomas on the axial surface of the arytenoid cartilages. Clinical management of affected patients involves medical or surgical therapy. Although broad-spectrum antibiotic therapy has been attempted in many cases, it is rarely curative. Also of importance in the management of some horses with arytenoid chondritis is placement of a tracheostomy tube (Fig. 1-5).

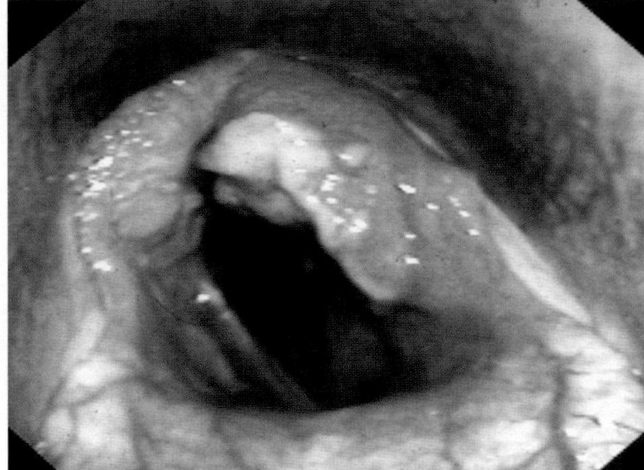

A

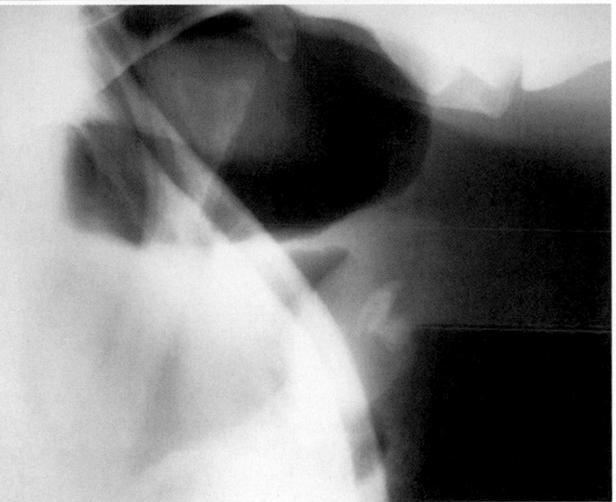

B

Fig. 1-4 Arytenoid chondritis as viewed in affected horse. **A,** Upper airway endoscopy showing severe inflammation and purulent exudate of affected arytenoid cartilage. **B,** Chronic inflammation resulted in mineralization of affected cartilaginous structures.

Several techniques are described for placement of a permanent tracheostomy.[6]

Viral Diseases

Equine influenza virus is classified as an orthomyxovirus with a single-stranded, segmented ribonucleic acid (RNA) genome[64] (see Chapter 12). Influenza viruses are classified on the basis of surface and internal protein antigens into three types: A, B, and C; only *type A* influenza is reported to infect horses. Major viral antigens include neuraminidase (NA) and hemagglutinin (HA). Two type A viral subtypes are known to cause disease in horses: H7N7 and H3N8.[64] The strain H7N7 was initially isolated in 1956 in Prague and designated A/equine/Prague/56. This H7N7 variant, termed *equine-1 influenza*, has not been isolated since 1980 and is believed to have disappeared from the equine population.[63] The H3N8 equine virus, called *equine-2 influenza*, was initially isolated in Miami in 1963 and designated A/equine/Miami/63.[65-67] Antigenic drift has subsequently resulted in many subtypes of variant equine-2 among horses, including A/equine/Fontainebleau/79, A/equine/Kentucky/81, A/equine/Saskatoon/90, and A/equine/Newmarket 2/93. Although antigenic *drift* has been observed for many years, antigenic *shift*,

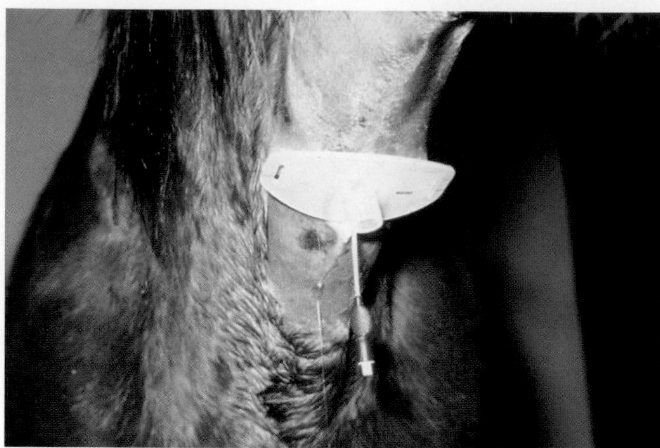

Fig. 1-5 Horse with upper airway obstruction presenting with severe dyspnea requiring placement of tracheostomy tube.

a larger-scale change in the antigenic nature of the equine influenza viruses, has not been documented to date.

Influenza is most common in horses commingled under stressful conditions, such as race training.[67] Infection occurs through inhalation of viral particles. The virus infects respiratory ciliated epithelium, leading to loss of the mucociliary escalator for pathogen and particle clearance. Therefore, viral infection predisposes affected individuals to secondary bacterial infection.

Clinical characteristics of equine influenza include a short incubation period of 1 to 3 days, high fever, depression, and paroxysmal coughing, which can be severe. Nasal discharge may begin as a serous fluid and change to a more mucopurulent character with disease progression and bacterial contamination. Submandibular lymphadenopathy is often associated with viral disease. Myositis, anorexia, and persistent cough may be signs associated with influenza infection. Immune status and previous vaccination will directly influence the course of disease; unvaccinated horses or those not previously exposed to the virus typically demonstrate the most severe clinical evidence of disease. Horses with influenza are at risk of secondary bacterial infection that may progress to bronchopneumonia and pleuropneumonia.

Equine herpesviruses are classified among the alpha (EHV-1, -3, and -4) and gamma (EHV-2 and EHV-5) herpesviruses (see Chapter 13). The viruses associated with respiratory disease of the greatest significance in the horse are EHV-1 and EHV-4. These α-herpesviruses are responsible for sporadic respiratory disease, abortion, and myeloencephalopathy. (EHV-4 is less likely to be associated with disease other than respiratory infection.) Fatal neonatal sepsis has been reported in association with EHV-4 infection, but EHV-1 is more often involved in this form of disease.[69,70] Because EHV is neurotropic, latency is possible and generally associated with the trigeminal nerve (cranial nerve V) ganglion or lymphocytes.[71] During times of severe stress or immune suppression, disease transmission is possible when latent virus is reactivated.

Clinical signs of disease associated with EHV typically include pyrexia, serous nasal discharge, and occasionally cough. In addition to respiratory disease, late-term abortion, neonatal sepsis, and myeloencephalopathy may also result from infection with EHV.[63,69-72]

Equine herpesvirus-2 (EHV-2), often referred to as *cytomegalovirus*, is a slow-replicating virus that typically results in self-limiting viral respiratory disease in young horses.[63] Many investigators question the role of this virus as a primary etiologic agent of fulminant respiratory disease in horses. EHV-2 has been recovered from both normal horses and young horses with clinical signs of respiratory tract disease.[73-76] Studies of seroprevalence and virus isolation reveal that young foals are often exposed to the virus. The virus could also be isolated from fluid collected by transtracheal aspirate of young horses with clinical respiratory tract disease, whereas it was rare to isolate the virus from tracheal fluid of clinically normal foals. Experimental inoculation of foals with EHV-2 results in chronic pharyngitis.[77] This organism may be a pathogen of concern in predisposing foals to bacterial pathogens such as *R. equi*.[73]

Although most often recognized for its association with the equine reproductive tract, *equine viral arteritis* (EVA) causes a mild to moderate respiratory disease (see Chapter 14). The virus is maintained in equine populations in carrier stallions because testosterone is required for persistence and maintenance of the virus in vivo. Carrier stallions maintain the virus within the ampulla and vas deferens. Clinical manifestations of EVA are similar to those of other viral respiratory tract diseases. Variations in the severity of clinical signs result from strain differences in virulence, pathogen dose, and host immune function. Incubation requires several days to 2 weeks, with a more rapid course of disease after venereal transmission. Clinical signs associated with respiratory tract infection include serous nasal discharge, submandibular lymphadenopathy, mild to moderate cough, and ventral edema. Most infections are self-limiting, although edema may be severe and respiratory distress evident. Abortion typically occurs within a month of exposure and disease development. Abortion may occur, although other clinical signs of EVA have not been observed. Neonatal foals infected with the virus demonstrate respiratory difficulty and rarely recover from viral infection.[78-80] Hematologic evidence of EVA includes leukopenia, characterized by a lymphopenia, and thrombocytopenia, which may be severe.

Equine rhinoviruses have been divided into two serogroups: equine rhinitis virus A and B (ERAV and ERBV) (see Chapter 16). ERAV is grouped in the *Aphthovirus* genus based on genotype and similarity with other members of this genus, such as foot-and-mouth virus, as well as the characteristic viremia and persistent shedding that occurs following infection with the virus.[19,27] ERBV is the sole member of the genus *Erbovirus*. A third serotype has been identified with the proposed classification in the erboviruses as ERBV2; currently this virus is referred to as P13/75 and is classified in the family *Picornaviridae*.[22] Clinical manifestations of disease typically include pyrexia, serous to seromucous nasal discharge, coughing, depression, anorexia, pharyngitis, and submandibular lymphadenopathy.[81] Mild lymphopenia and increased plasma fibrinogen concentrations have been reported in affected horses.

Strangles

Clinical disease in horses associated with *Streptococcus equi* subsp. *equi* infection (strangles) is most common in horses younger than 5 years, but very uncommon in young foals (<3 months) born to mares previously exposed to the organism (see Chapter 28). Natural infection results from direct contact with an infected or carrier individual that may have overt clinical disease or that has maintained the organism within the upper airway, most frequently the guttural pouch.[58] Transmission may also occur through fomites, such as on contaminated clothing or cleaning instruments.

Infection with *S. equi* primarily occurs through oral and nasal routes. Incubation from time of infection to manifestation of clinical signs varies from a few days to a few weeks and is influenced by pathogen virulence, dose of inoculum, and host immunity at the time of challenge. Some of the earliest clinical signs include fever, depression, and reduced appetite. Nasal discharge may initially be serous but with disease progression will become mucopurulent. Lymph node enlargement and abscess maturation generally require approximately 7 days to occur. Early in the course of infection, affected lymph nodes are sensitive to palpation and firm in nature. As rupture becomes imminent, a soft center develops, and a serous crust on the surface may be observed. Submandibular and retropharyngeal nodes are most often affected; edema may be severe, resulting in dysphagia and respiratory stridor. After rupture of abscess(es), swelling will diminish rapidly. Severe obstruction may necessitate that a tracheostomy be performed.

The most common hematologic abnormalities in *S. equi*–infected horses are leukocytosis caused by neutrophilia, hyperfibrinogenemia, and anemia of chronic disease. Definitive diagnosis is based on aerobic culture of nasal secretions, preferably obtained from the abscessed lymph nodes, the guttural pouch, or a nasopharyngeal wash.

Therapy

Specific recommendations for treatment of *S. equi* subsp. *equi* and acute viral respiratory tract disease of horses is discussed in detail in the relevant chapters of this text. Because of the severity of epithelial surface damage and the potential for secondary bacterial infection, all virally affected horses should be rested from race training during the course of disease and recovery. A significant cough may persist for weeks after onset of clinical signs of viral respiratory disease. A standard rule of thumb is to implement a week of rest from strenuous exercise for each day the horse demonstrates a fever. Recovery of the respiratory epithelium should be complete before reintroduction of strenuous exercise. During periods of high fever, depression, anorexia, and myalgia, nonsteroidal antiinflammatory therapy is recommended. If significant nasal discharge and fever are persistent, additional testing is warranted to rule out bacterial contamination.

LOWER RESPIRATORY TRACT INFECTIONS

Etiology and Epidemiology

Bacterial Pneumonia

Under normal conditions the equine lung contains only small numbers of potential bacterial or fungal pathogens; when present, they are considered transient contaminants. These bacteria are typically cleared by the normal defense mechanisms, as previously discussed. However, when the normal defense mechanisms are overwhelmed or pulmonary immune defense is impaired, proliferation of such contaminants may become pathogenic to the host. The most common source for contamination of the lower airways is aspiration of microorganisms from the upper respiratory tract. Gram-positive pathogens include *Streptococcus equi* subsp. *zooepidemicus*, *Staphylococcus aureus*, and *Streptococcus pneumoniae*. Gram-negative pathogens affecting the lower airways of horses include *Pasteurella*, *Actinobacillus* spp., *Escherichia coli*, *Klebsiella pneumoniae*, and *Bordetella bronchiseptica*. Anaerobic organisms that may infect the lower airways of horses include *Bacteroides fragilis*, *Peptostreptococcus anaerobius*, and *Fusobacterium* spp.

Miscellaneous Causes of Pneumonia

Infectious disease involving the lower respiratory tract is most often associated with bacterial infection, although fungal[32-34,82,83] and viral[71,84,85] pathogens are also potential invaders of the lower respiratory tract. Septic thrombophlebitis is considered a risk factor for metastatic spread of septic foci.[86] Some reports suggest that the presence of anaerobic organisms warrants a more guarded prognosis when cultured from horses with pleuropneumonia.[87] Polymicrobial infection may result from synergy among pathogens, particularly aerobes or facultative anaerobes and anaerobic organisms that favor survival of organisms that otherwise would not proliferate.

Pulmonary Abscess

Pulmonary abscess formation most often occurs in weanling-age foals in association with *Rhodococcus equi* infection (see Chapter 32). *Streptococcus equi* subsp. *zooepidemicus* is the organism most frequently cultured from the lungs of horses with generalized pneumonia and rarely results in abscess formation. Complications from *S. equi* subsp. *equi* infection include metastatic spread to various organs, including possible pulmonary abscess formation. Aspiration is another cause of focal pulmonary infection and abscessation. Aspiration pneumonia is a potential complication of esophageal obstruction or dysphagia in horses. Neonatal foals may develop dysphagia in association with hypoxic ischemic encephalopathy or nutritional muscular dystrophy, whereas adult horses may develop aspiration pneumonia after complete esophageal obstruction.

Pathogenesis

Bronchopneumonia occurs after colonization of the lower respiratory tract with bacteria. This colonization may occur after damage from viral infection or after an episode of impaired pulmonary clearance, as might occur after strenuous exercise or long-distance transport. Bacterial contamination of the lower airways may also lead to concurrent or subsequent pleuropneumonia or pulmonary abscess formation.

Primary viral respiratory tract infection predisposes adult horses to bacterial infection because of disruption of the surface epithelium, loss of the mucociliary elevator, and loss of surfactant production by type II pneumocytes. Pulmonary inflammation will lead to increased capillary permeability and pulmonary exudate; such an environment is conducive to the survival and replication of contaminating pathogens, particularly those that survive under conditions of low oxygen tension (anaerobes).

High-level performance horses may be predisposed to lower airway infection because alveolar macrophages are reduced in efficacy after strenuous exercise.[12] In addition, challenge is enhanced because horses in training are at greater risk for aspiration of pathogens and particulate matter. Horses used for performance activities often travel long distances, and persistent head elevation, as might occur in a trailered horse, reduces pulmonary clearance mechanisms within 6 to 12 hours.[3] Although many strategies have been used to enhance protection in such individuals, neither antibiotic therapy nor intermittent lowering of the head appears to reduce substantially the incidence of pulmonary infection.[87] Transportation for a distance greater than 500 miles in the preceding 2 weeks is an important risk factor for the development of pleuropneumonia in horses. Although uncommon, horses with severe gastrointestinal disease or those with pulmonary infection that remains unresponsive to antibiotic therapy may develop a pulmonary mycotic infection.[34] Diagnostic testing should be implemented to rule out fungal organisms as primary or secondary invaders.

Clinical Findings

Clinical findings in horses with pulmonary disease most often include depression, fever, and reduced food intake. Coughing is most frequently observed during physical exertion or with advanced disease. Horses with advanced disease may show respiratory distress as well as pronounced weight loss. Purulent nasal discharge with a fetid odor, evidence of thoracic pain, and epistaxis may occur in association with rupture of a pulmonary abscess. A sequela to severe disease may be laminitis; therefore, abnormal gait or intermittent recumbency may accompany evidence of pulmonary infection.

Diagnosis

Although clinical evidence may suggest pulmonary infection as the primary problem in equine patients, a thorough evaluation is warranted to ensure that all problems and diagnoses are appropriately managed. Physical examination should include careful auscultation to evaluate the patient for pulmonary air movement. If respiratory distress is observed, further manipulation for auscultation should not be performed. If pulmonary sounds are difficult to detect, however, a rebreathing bag may be applied to enhance the ability to detect air movement. When diminished pulmonary sounds are present, an ultrasound examination should be performed to determine if pleural fluid or pulmonary consolidation exists.

Hematologic findings consistent with bacterial infection include neutrophilic leukocytosis with a left shift, toxic changes in neutrophils, hyperglobulinemia, and hyperfibrinogenemia. Mild to moderate anemia may be associated with chronic disease.

Thoracic radiographs are useful to determine the extent and severity of pulmonary disease. Ultrasonographic examination will be helpful only for detection of peripheral parenchymal conditions or those associated with pleural effusions.

Sterile transtracheal aspirate samples should be obtained from the respiratory tract for culture and antimicrobial testing. Although endoscopy is a useful diagnostic test for horses with pulmonary disease, this usually is not the preferred method for collection of sterile samples for culture and sensitivity analysis. If *Pseudomonas* spp. are cultured from samples obtained by endoscopic transtracheal aspiration, results should be interpreted with caution because this organism is rarely a pathogen of the equine pulmonary system.

Therapy

Treatment of horses with historical, clinical, and hematologic evidence of pulmonary bacterial infection should include broad-spectrum antimicrobial therapy (pending sensitivity testing of isolates and implementation of more targeted antimicrobial therapy) and excellent supportive care. Although bacterial culture results are not available immediately on diagnosis of pulmonary infection, cytologic evaluation of pulmonary aspirates should give the clinician some indication of the type (Gram stain) and population (single vs. multiple classes of pathogens) of pathogens in the patient. Beta-lactam antibiotics combined with aminoglycosides provide good coverage for a variety of pathogens that may infect the lower airways of horses. Caution should be used in individuals that are debilitated or dehydrated.[71] Because of nephrotoxicity, aminoglycosides are contraindicated for use in patients at risk for renal impairment.

The prognosis for recovery from bacterial pneumonia is generally considered favorable for horses that have been managed appropriately in a timely fashion. Horses with severe disease that have not responded or incompletely respond to antimicrobial therapy may subsequently develop pleuropneumonia, which may worsen the prognosis for complete recovery and return to previous level of athletic function.

PNEUMONIAS

Pleuropneumonia

Etiology and Epidemiology

Pleuropneumonia is a condition in which infection associated with bronchopneumonia has spread to involve the pleura and the pleural space.[88] This disorder most often occurs in performance horses, frequently after long-distance transport.[63,71,89] Although apparently spontaneous cases of pleuropneumonia may occur in some horses, most affected horses have experienced one or more predisposing risk factors, such as long-distance transport, recent viral or bacterial respiratory tract disease, or a recent episode of general anesthesia.[87,90,91]

Most cases of equine pleuropneumonia result from bacterial infection, but reports also demonstrate that *Mycoplasma* spp.,[30] viral agents,[21] and mycotic agents[34] may be isolated, or the disease may occur as a complication of septic thrombophlebitis.[86] Rarely, pulmonary hydatidosis may be a cause of equine pleuropneumonia[92] (see Chapter 61). Bacterial pleuropneumonia can be associated with a single pathogen but more often results from a mixed infection that may include aerobic and anaerobic organisms.[87,91,93,94] The most important factor for the development of transport-associated pleuropneumonia is head position during long-distance transport.[87,89,95-97] The most compelling evidence for this claim is the observation that horses transported long distances without restraint of head position do not develop changes in lower airway cytologic findings. In contrast, horses without other stress had an estimated 75% increased likelihood of developing lower airway accumulation of bacteria and inflammatory debris after a minimum of 24 hours of head restraint.[3,87,88,91] High-intensity exercise in combination with long-distance transport further contributes to development of lower airway inflammation and impaired immune clearance mechanisms.[12]

Striving to prevent equine pleuropneumonia is important because the prognosis for return to previous level of athletic function may be guarded to poor in severe cases.[87,91] Complications associated with pleuropneumonia, such as laminitis and chronic abscess formation, may negatively influence the future athletic performance of affected individuals.[87]

Clinical Findings

Horses with pleuropneumonia may demonstrate a variety of clinical signs. However, disease should be suspected in horses with an appropriate history and that demonstrate lethargy, pyrexia, cough (may be a quiet cough because of pleural pain), nasal discharge (bilateral, may be bloody), shallow breathing pattern, increased laryngeal excursions, and painful, stilted gait. During the acute stages of the disease, horses are likely to have signs referable to pleurodynia. Pain may be demonstrated by pawing, reluctance to move, abducted elbows, stiff gait, guarded breathing pattern, or shallow respiration. Ballottement or percussion of the thorax typically reveals reduced air resonance and may elicit a painful grunt. Differential diagnoses for such cases include exertional rhabdomyolysis, laminitis, and colic.

Thoracic auscultation usually reveals abnormal pulmonary sounds. When pleural effusion is present, the most common finding is attenuation of audible bronchovesicular sounds over the ventral lung fields. In the dorsal lung fields, normal pulmonary sounds may be heard; more often, however, increased bronchovesicular sounds are heard, accompanied by crackles or wheezes. Before significant pleural fluid accumulation, abnormal pulmonary sounds may be heard diffusely.[98,99] With chronicity, friction rubs are common, reflecting fibrin accumulation along the parietal and visceral pleural surfaces.

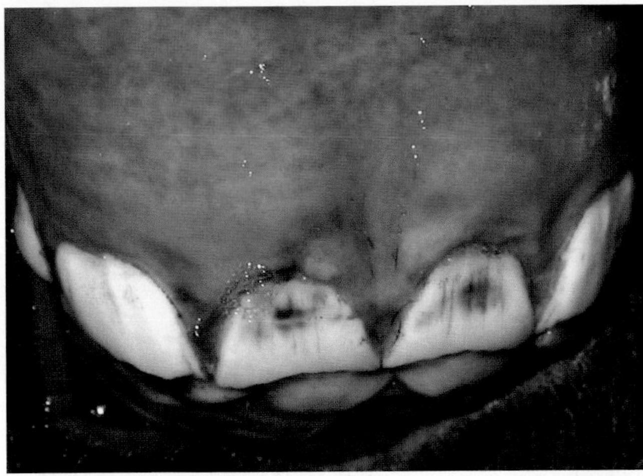

Fig. 1-6 Equine pleuropneumonia in yearling Thoroughbred gelding. Mucous membrane color was dark pink with severe injection of mucosal vessels and prominent toxic line visible surrounding the incisors.

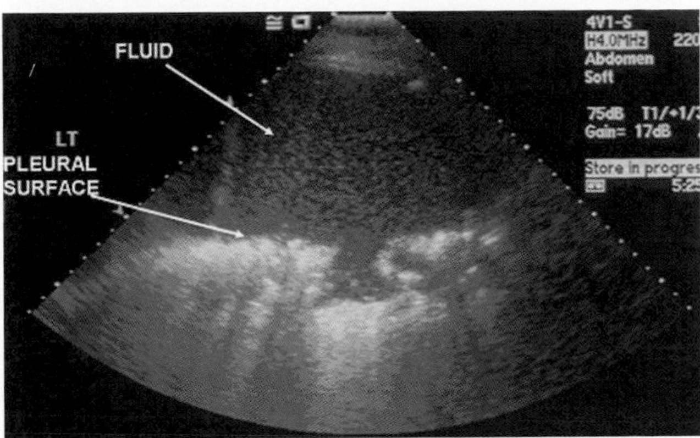

Fig. 1-7 Thoracic ultrasound using 5-MHz transducer showing significant pleural effusion and pulmonary consolidation in horse with pleuropneumonia.

Tachycardia and tachypnea are common findings in horses with pleuropneumonia. Jugular pulsation and severe respiratory distress may occur. Nasal discharge is often present and can vary from serous to mucopurulent to mucohemorrhagic in character. A fetid odor associated with nasal discharge, breath, or pleural fluid should increase the clinicians' suspicion of anaerobic infection. Mucous membrane color may be dark red to injected, depending on whether the horse is experiencing significant toxemia or ventilatory compromise (Fig. 1-6). Horses with subacute to chronic pleuropneumonia will often demonstrate weight loss, which may be dramatic.

Diagnosis

History and physical examination findings are often highly suggestive of pleuropneumonia. Definitive diagnosis is made on the basis of identification of septic fluid within the pleural space. Ultrasonographic examination (3.5- to 5.0-MHz transducer) will reveal evidence of pleural effusion.[63,71,100,101] Ultrasonographic examination is superior to radiography to confirm a diagnosis of pleuropneumonia because of fluid accumulation within the thoracic cavity (Fig. 1-7). Ultrasonography may also reveal evidence of pleural irregularities or changes within the pulmonary parenchyma, such as atelectasis, abscess formation, consolidation, and pulmonary hepatization.[101] "Comet tail" artifacts on pleural surfaces denote foci of inflammation or fibrosis on the visceral pleura.[71] The ultrasonographic character of pleural fluid in horses with pleuropneumonia may range from anechoic to hyperechoic, depending on the relative cellularity and fibrin accumulation. Evidence of bright gas echoes within the pleural fluid indicates anaerobic organisms within the pleural fluid. Other possible explanations for gas accumulation within the pleural space include previous thoracocentesis or severe parenchymal disease resulting in a bronchopleural fistula, with communication between the pleural space and conducting airways. Fibrin accumulation can be detected with ultrasound examination, typically visualized by strands or loculated cavitations. Familiarity with pleural ultrasonographic examination is important, because in some cases the pericardiodiaphragmatic ligament may be confused with fibrin accumulation.[101]

Thoracocentesis is required to determine specific characteristics of pleural fluid, such as leukocyte cell count and differential and total protein concentration. Fine-needle aspiration of parenchymal lesions may be indicated in horses with suspected pulmonary abscess formation. Samples of pleural fluid, pulmonary abscess aspirates, and transtracheal wash samples should be submitted for bacterial culture (aerobic and anaerobic) and sensitivity testing and cytologic analysis. Because pleuropneumonia in most horses begins as severe bronchopneumonia, culture of transtracheal wash samples is particularly important for identification of primary bacterial pathogens[71,88,90,98] (Fig. 1-8). Early in the course of disease, pleural fluid may be inflammatory but sterile, and an etiologic diagnosis would be missed if only pleural fluid samples were cultured. If the pleural sepsis results from a traumatic, penetrating wound, however, transtracheal wash analysis is not indicated, and the primary etiologic agents are best identified by culture and sensitivity testing of pleural fluid samples.[102]

Cytologic examination of pleural fluid is important diagnostically and may influence prognosis. Normal pleural fluid is an ultrafiltrate of plasma and is appropriately classified as a *transudate*. It is transparent, straw colored, and nonfetid. The total nucleated cell count should be less than 10,000 cells/μL and the protein concentration less than 2.5 g/dL. Differential analysis of normal pleural fluid reveals the majority of cells to be neutrophils, with few monocytes and mesothelial cells. Additional analysis may include measurement of glucose, lactate, and pH. Pleural fluid samples from horses with pleuropneumonia are usually acidic, with low glucose concentrations and increased lactate concentrations.[103,104] Pleural fluid glucose concentration is reported to be a reliable indicator of sepsis when concentrations are less than 2.22 mmol/L.[105]

Pneumothorax is a potential complication of pleuropneumonia, with a reported incidence of up to 43%.[106] Clinical evidence of pneumothorax may include dyspnea, tachypnea, loss of auscultable pulmonary sounds in the dorsal thorax, depression, anxiety, and cough. Radiography and ultrasonography are useful aids in the diagnosis of pneumothorax. When pneumothorax occurs as a complication to pleuropneumonia, it is usually unilateral. In general, horses with pneumothorax secondary to pleuropneumonia have a more guarded prognosis for recovery and survival as compared to horses with uncomplicated pleuropneumonia.[106]

Pleuropneumonia with secondary hemorrhagic pulmonary infarcts has been described in Thoroughbred racehorses shortly after a bout of strenuous exercise.[107] Affected horses showed evidence of acute respiratory distress with serosanguineous

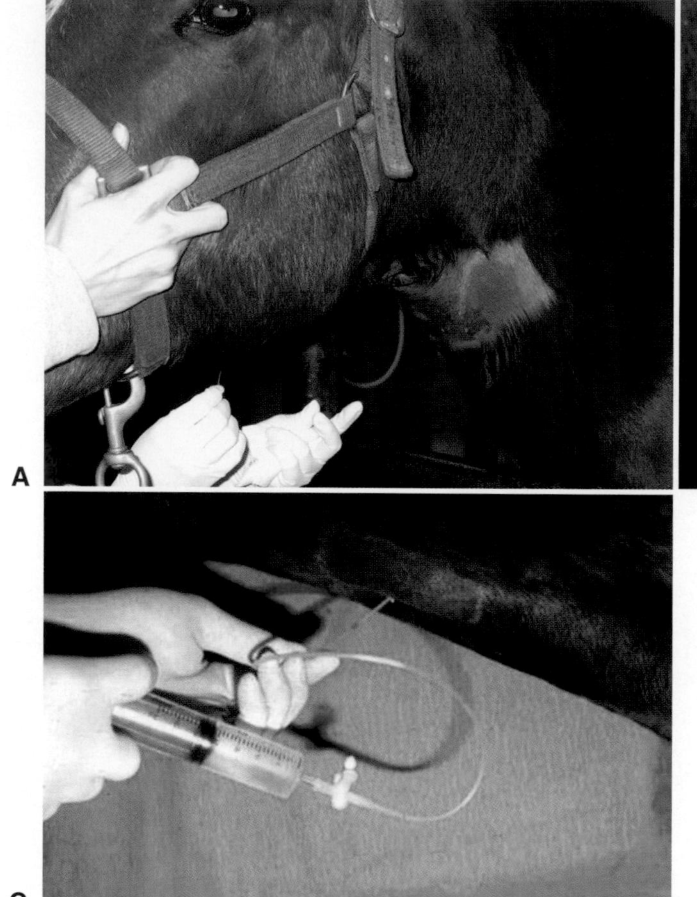
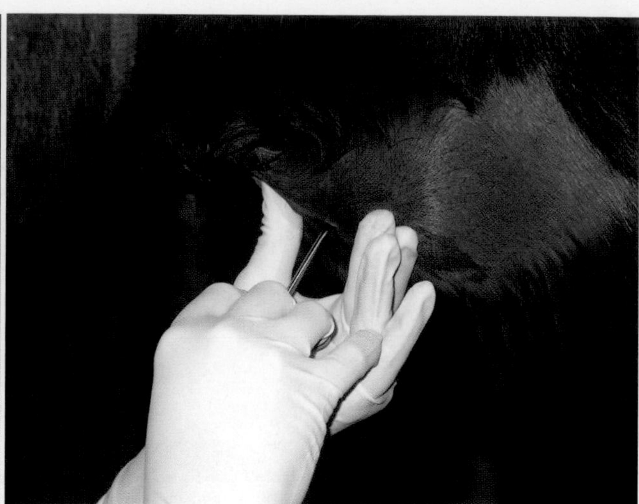

Fig. 1-8 Transtracheal wash analysis performed for collection of sterile aspirate from respiratory tract for bacterial culture and antimicrobial sensitivity testing. **A,** Hair clipped and sterile preparation performed in cranial one third of ventral cervical region. Local anesthetic and small stab incision are made over site of entrance to trachea. **B,** Trachea is penetrated with sterile trocar. **C,** Instillation with sterile isotonic fluid is followed by aspiration to collect sterile sample for culture analysis.

nasal discharge shortly after strenuous exercise. Thoracic radiography and ultrasound revealed evidence of pulmonary consolidation and pleural effusion in affected individuals; in contrast to many cases of pleuropneumonia, thoracocentesis revealed serosanguineous to hemorrhagic effusion. Although an underlying bacterial etiology was demonstrated in most affected horses, conventional management with antibiotic and antiinflammatory therapy was unsuccessful in resolving most cases. Therefore, although various manifestations of pleuropneumonia may occur, individuals with a history and clinical evidence of pulmonary infarction should receive a more guarded prognosis.[107]

Therapy

The primary goals of therapy in horses with pleuropneumonia include resolution of sepsis, clearance of effusion from the pleural space, and provision of excellent nursing care to avoid or manage the onset of complicating factors associated with the primary disease.

Antimicrobial therapy is generally aimed at broad-spectrum coverage for a wide variety of bacterial pathogens including gram-positive and gram-negative aerobes and anaerobic organisms.[99] Combination therapy with β-lactam (e.g., penicillin, 22,000 IU/kg body weight intravenously [IV] every 6 hours [q6h]) and aminoglycoside (e.g., gentamicin, 6.6 mg/kg IV q24h) antibiotics are the mainstay of antimicrobial therapy in horses with pleuropneumonia. Metronidazole (15-25 mg/kg q6-8h) is added to the treatment regimen if anaerobic infection is suspected. Identification of all bacterial species present is an important component of clinical diagnosis because the presence of obligate anaerobic organisms will influence patient prognosis.[87,91] Anaerobic organisms frequently isolated from horses with pleuropneumonia include *Bacteroides*, *Peptostreptococcus*, *Clostridium*, and *Fusobacterium* species (see Chapter 48). Although most of these anaerobic pathogens are sensitive to penicillin, some strains of *Bacteroides* are resistant to β-lactam therapy because of elaboration of β-lactamase enzymes that inactivate this class of antimicrobial. Metronidazole is a nitroimidazole antibiotic that is metabolized to its active form in the reducing environment produced exclusively by anaerobic organisms and is highly efficacious against this class of organisms.[108]

Supportive care for horses with pleuropneumonia frequently includes intravenous (IV) fluid therapy, especially during the acute stages of disease, when affected horses are typically depressed, anorectic, and dehydrated. Dehydration results from reduced voluntary fluid intake as well as a redistribution of fluid to the pleural space. IV fluid therapy aids in controlling pyrexia and maintaining secretions that can easily be removed by the mucociliary escalator rather than remaining inspissated within the pleural cavity. Nonsteroidal antiinflammatory therapy is indicated in the euhydrated patient to aid in management of pain, endotoxemia, and pyrexia associated with infection.[109]

Drainage of pleural fluid is required in patients with moderate to severe pleural fluid accumulation. Without appropriate removal, development of severe respiratory distress may ensue. If large volumes of pleural fluid exist within the pleural

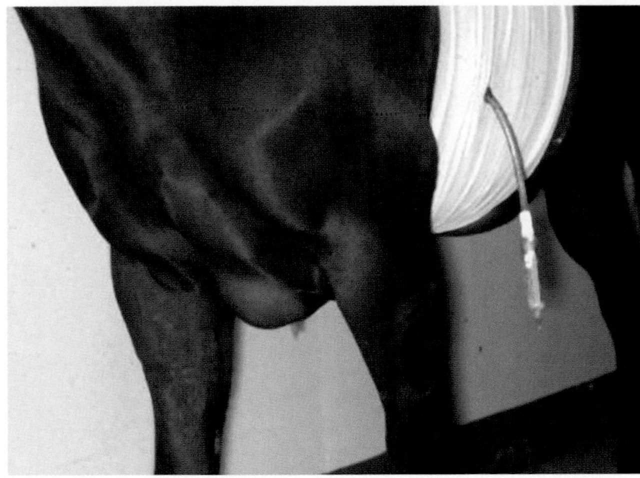

Fig. 1-9 Indwelling thoracic tube placed in Thoroughbred racehorse with pleuropneumonia.

space, antibiotic therapy alone will be unsuccessful at pathogen clearance.

Insertion of a teat cannula or female urinary (canine) catheter may be effective for removal of small amounts of fluid. In horses with accumulation of a large volume of fluid within the pleural space, indwelling thoracic tubes are indicated to maintain constant fluid removal. A one-way valve system is required on the end of such a tube to avoid the introduction of free air into the pleural space, or iatrogenic pneumothorax will occur.

Placement of the thoracic tube should be determined after ultrasonographic identification of the region of greatest fluid accumulation. Tube position should reflect the most ventral site of fluid accumulation. After the site has been selected and aseptically prepared, local anesthetic is generously infused from the skin surface to the pleural surface just cranial to the rib of interest. A stab incision large enough to allow for placement of the thoracic tube (24-32 French) is made using a #10 surgical blade. The tube is inserted into the incision site, and firm pressure is continued until a "pop" is felt, indicating the pleural space has been entered. Most horses will tolerate this procedure adequately with proper local anesthesia; in fractious animals, however, sedation may be required, with the clinician remembering that most patients are in critical condition and that heavy sedation may compromise their clinical stability. The thoracic tube should be introduced into the thoracic cavity to a depth of 7 to 9 cm, ensuring that the trocar needle remains in place, just penetrating the parietal pleura. The trocar is removed to check for fluid accumulation. A pair of Kelly forceps should be available because of the potential for air aspiration and subsequent pneumothorax as fluid is evacuated from the pleural space. After the initial fluid drainage is complete, the tube is sutured into place with a one-way stop valve on the end (e.g., Heimlich valve).

In many cases when the mediastinum remains incomplete, particularly in the early stages of disease, evacuation of one hemithorax will be successful in removal of fluid from the contralateral hemithorax (Fig. 1-9). Thoracic drainage tubes are left in place until significant fluid accumulation ceases, which may be days to weeks depending on the severity of disease. With chronic disease, fibrin accumulation will result in a complete mediastinum, which may necessitate bilateral thoracic drainage. In some horses, pleural lavage is indicated to aid in removal of inspissated material.

Surgical intervention is indicated in horses that do not recover after thoracic drainage through an indwelling tube.[110] A thoracotomy may be performed between rib spaces or may necessitate removal of a portion of rib. Surgical drainage is typically reserved for patients that have not fully recovered from pleural disease but are clinically stable. Description of the entire surgical procedure is beyond the scope of this discussion, but it should be performed over the area of chronic septic accumulation (identified by ultrasonographic examination). In some horses a surgical entry site needs to be reopened because of rapid closure, or bilateral procedures are required for horses with severe involvement of both hemithoraces.

Supportive care is focused on prevention of secondary complications, which may include pulmonary abscess formation, bronchopleural fistula, pneumothorax, cranial mediastinal abscess, restrictive pericarditis, laminitis, colic, antibiotic-associated colitis, and jugular vein thrombosis.[90,111]

The prognosis for horses with pleuropneumonia depends on the inciting pathogen and the duration of disease before seeking veterinary assistance. Infarctive pleuropneumonia, described earlier, is associated with an especially severe prognosis.

Interstitial Pneumonia

Interstitial pneumonia is a pulmonary condition that may affect horses of various age groups. Interestingly, adult horses with interstitial pneumonia are given a guarded to poor prognosis for recovery and survival,[71] whereas foals and weanlings provided with appropriate therapy and supportive care have a good prognosis for complete recovery.[112]

Etiology and Pathogenesis

Most cases of interstitial pneumonia are thought to result from a primary toxic or infectious insult, but at presentation, determining the exact etiology can be challenging.[112-115] Toxic pulmonary disease has been associated with ingestion of Crofton weed, pyrrolizidine alkaloids (*Crotolaria*, *Trichodesma*, and *Senecio*), perilla ketones, silicosis, and prolonged oxygen therapy. Hepatic metabolites of pyrrolizidine alkaloids cause cellular damage and death in the pulmonary endothelium.[114,116] Inhaled irritants or toxins may contribute to direct pulmonary damage, such as occurs after inhalation of smoke or agrichemicals.[117-119] Silicosis is a highly specific, chronic granulomatous pneumonia of horses and should be considered in horses with compatible clinical signs that originate from the Carmel Valley in California.[71]

The initial infectious or toxic agent causes alveolar damage, resulting in cell death and increased permeability at the level of the alveoli. Pulmonary congestion, interstitial edema, erythrocyte extravasation and alveolar edema occur during the exudative phase of the disease. Subsequently, alveolar infiltrates with inflammatory leukocytes and fibrin and increased permeability lead to fluid accumulation, impairing normal gas exchange mechanisms; hyaline membrane formation; and clinical respiratory distress. Acutely affected patients typically demonstrate respiratory distress, injected mucous membranes, and impaired pulmonary function. Subacute to chronic disease results in alveolar regeneration with alveolar type II pneumocyte proliferation to replace damaged type I pneumocytes. Fibroplasia leads to cellular proliferation and septal thickening, fibrosis, and ultimately, reduced pulmonary compliance.

Clinical Findings

Horses presenting with interstitial pneumonia are typically in severe respiratory distress, with labored breathing,

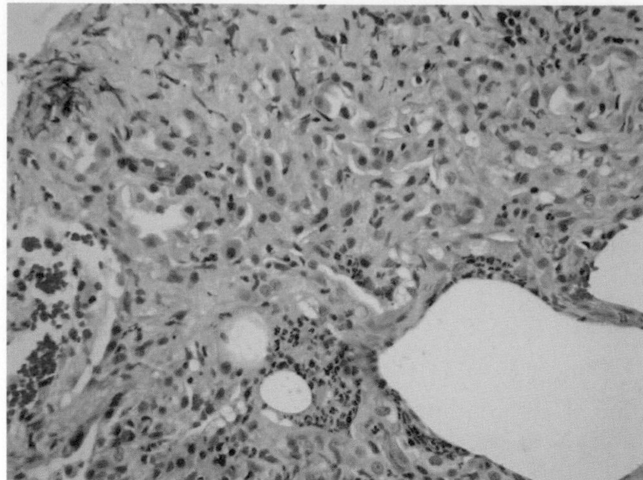

Fig. 1-10 Histopathology from middle-age horse diagnosed with interstitial pneumonia. Fibrosis and inflammation have resulted in loss of the normal parenchymal architecture; note loss of alveolar spaces for adequate gas exchange to occur.

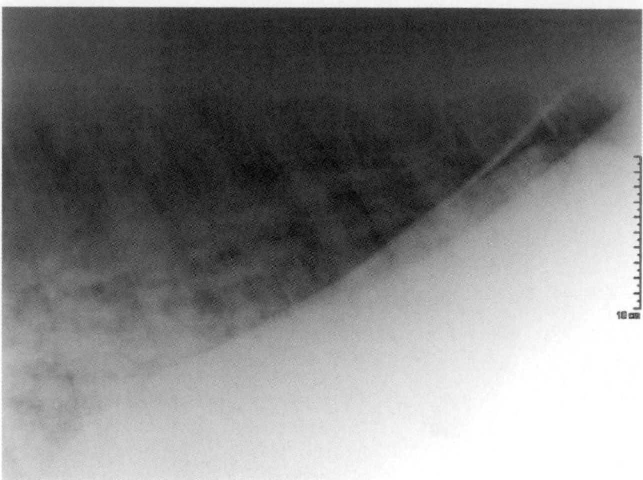

Fig. 1-11 Lateral thoracic radiograph of 20-year-old Appaloosa with severe interstitial pneumonia.

dark mucous membranes, poor pulse quality, and tachycardia. Some patients are mistakenly considered to have an obstructive disease such as heaves, but interstitial pneumonia is characterized by a restrictive rapid, shallow breathing pattern. Additional clinical features of disease include hypoxemia, a stress or inflammatory leukogram, hyperfibrinogenemia, and hypoxemia that may be severe. More chronic disease may be observed in mildly affected individuals with exercise intolerance and chronic cough.

Diagnosis

Definitive diagnosis of interstitial pneumonia in horses is based on histopathologic evaluation of a pulmonary biopsy (Fig. 1-10). Thoracic radiographs can be helpful in establishing a preliminary diagnosis of interstitial pneumonia. Two patterns of interstitial disease have been described in horses with interstitial pneumonia: discrete or diffuse nodules suggestive of neoplasia or mycotic disease and a diffuse increase in the radiographic interstitial pattern (Fig. 1-11). Serum titers may indicate recent exposure or infection with viral respiratory disease. Histopathologic evaluation of lung biopsies or specimens obtained postmortem will confirm the diagnosis of interstitial pneumonia. If silicosis remains a possibility, differential diagnosis is based on x-ray diffraction techniques on lung tissue preparations.[71]

Therapy

The prognosis for adult horses with interstitial pneumonia is guarded. In horses that present with mild to moderate disease, treatment should be aimed at improving oxygenation. Intranasal insufflation of oxygen is warranted for patients that are severely hypoxemic. Antiinflammatory therapy should initially include systemic corticosteroids (e.g., dexamethasone, 0.05-0.1 mg/kg IV daily), with transition to aerosolized corticosteroids (e.g., beclomethasone, 1500 μg intranasally two or three times daily)[120] as clinical improvement is observed. Corticosteroid therapy should be continued until clinical resolution is observed or no further improvement is noted with therapy. Prolonged corticosteroid therapy of several weeks to months should be anticipated because of the severity of lower airway inflammation associated with this condition. Bronchodilator therapy is indicated when severe bronchoconstriction exists. Beta-2-adrenergic receptor agonists are the drugs of choice for immediate bronchodilation and subsequent improvement of air movement to the lower airways (albuterol, 360-720 mg/kg q3-12h).[121,122] After initial stabilization, an additional therapeutic option is the use of a parasympatholytic agent (ipratropium, 360-470 μg/kg q6-12h)[123] combined with a β_2-adrenergic receptor agonist (albuterol). This combination (Combivent; 3M Pharmaceuticals and Boehringer Ingelheim, Canada) improves oxygen delivery to the lower airways, with the added advantage of an increased half-life, compared with β_2-adrenergic agonist therapy alone.

Prognosis

The prognosis for return to function is guarded for adult horses with interstitial pneumonia and favorable for foals that are managed appropriately. Supportive and antiinflammatory therapy may improve clinical status, but high-level athletic activity may be impaired.

Parasitic Pneumonia

Etiology

Parasitic pneumonia is a condition that may affect foals or adult horses. Parasites associated with this condition include *Parascaris equorum* larvae or the adults of *Dictyocaulus arnfeldi* (see Chapter 62). Clinically affected horses have obvious evidence of respiratory disease, including exercise intolerance and coughing that may be accompanied by nasal discharge, fever, and depression, particularly when secondary bacterial infection has occurred. *P. equorum* infection is most common in foals and weanlings, particularly those raised on breeding farms where the parasite resides in the environment and soil. *D. arnfeldi* infection may occur in horses of any age, but this parasite requires a donkey as a primary host to complete its life cycle.

Clinical Findings

Chronic coughing, mucoid to mucopurulent nasal discharge, respiratory distress, and poor overall body condition provide nonspecific evidence of parasitic disease in foals. Poor body condition and abnormal pulmonary sounds marked by increased bronchovesicular sounds, crackles, and wheezes are common findings on thoracic auscultation of horses with parasitic pneumonia. Poor body condition is a common finding because of intestinal involvement of parasitic infection. Colic may be a component of the history or may follow therapeutic anthelmintic treatment in severely affected individuals. Frequently the history also includes a poor response to appropriate antimicrobial therapy for suspected bronchopneumonia.

Diagnosis

Hematologic evaluation often reveals an inflammatory leukogram consisting of a mature neutrophilia, hyperfibrinogenemia, and hyperglobulinemia. In some patients, particularly early in the course of disease, hematologic evaluation may reveal few abnormalities. Hepatic parasitic migration *(P. equorum)* may result in mild to moderate hepatic enzyme elevation.[124] Thoracic radiography is a useful diagnostic test in affected individuals. A moderate to severe bronchointerstitial pattern is a common finding, whereas granuloma or abscess formation may be detected by radiographs in horses with advanced disease. Thoracic ultrasonographic examination will allow the clinician to detect the presence of pleural fluid or peripheral pulmonary consolidation.

Cytologic examination of a sterile tracheobronchial aspirate will often reveal abundant eosinophils (5%-50%, normal <2%); neutrophilic inflammation may be present concurrently, particularly with a secondary bacterial infection. Microorganisms are apparent with significant bacterial infection; culture is recommended to determine the presence of infection and to determine the antimicrobial sensitivity pattern for pathogens of concern. Fecal flotation is indicated to determine the presence of parasite ova being shed from the host. *D. arnfeldi* requires a donkey or mule host for life cycle completion; therefore, parasite eggs will only infrequently be detected in adult horses with lungworm infection. It is difficult to diagnose *P. equorum* infection on fecal flotation because tissue migration occurs during the prepatent period. Therefore, diagnosis is based on clinical signs, lack of evidence of bacterial infection, and tracheal wash cytology indicating eosinophilic pneumonitis. Response to therapy is supportive of the diagnosis, although antibiotic therapy may be required in combination with anthelmintic therapy.

Therapy

Severely hypoxemic patients may require oxygen insufflation. Severe pulmonary inflammation is induced by eosinophilic infiltrates necessitating bronchodilator and potentially aerosolized corticosteroid therapy (see previous recommendations on aerosol therapy). Oral anthelmintic agents used to treat *P. equorum* infection include fenbendazole at an initial low dose of 5 mg/kg. Careful monitoring for approximately 24 hours is recommended to observe the foal for evidence of deterioration or gastrointestinal distress. Laxative therapy may be required if gastrointestinal ascarid impaction is suspected. After the foal has received the low dose of fenbendazole without complication, the oral dose can be increased to 10 mg/kg daily and repeated for 5 days. This therapy is effective in killing adult and migrating larvae. Because this is a farm problem, other individuals on the same property of similar age should be managed appropriately, even if clinical evidence of disease is not apparent. Other anthelmintics used to treat *P. equorum* include pyrantel pamoate (6.6 mg/kg) and ivermectin (200 μg/kg). *D. arnfeldi* infection can be successfully treated with ivermectin (also 200 μg/kg), moxidectin (adult horses only, 400 μg/kg), thiabendazole (440, mg/kg/day twice), or levamisole (10 mg/kg).

Benzimidazole anthelmintic agents inhibit microtubule formation, which impairs the parasite's ability to move and ingest food. Energy metabolism is also impaired because of the inhibition of fumarate reductase.[4] Although many benzimidazoles are efficacious against intestinal larvae, they are not uniformly effective at killing migrating parasite larvae; however, at higher doses, fenbendazole is safe and effective at killing intestinal and tissue larvae. Anecdotal and personal observations suggest that this anthelmintic is highly efficacious, particularly when ivermectin resistance is suspected.

Pyrantel pamoate is an acetylcholine agonist that results in parasite paralysis.[125] At the recommended dose, this agent is effective at killing intestinal larvae, but not migrating larvae.[4,124] Avermectins are effective because of their ability to bind glutamate-gated chloride channels, and this class is effective against both *P. equorum* and *D. arnfeldi* adults and migrating larvae. Ivermectin has a reported efficacy of 76.9% for removal of intestinal *P. equorum* and 100% for removal of pneumonic larvae.[4,43] Overall, ivermectin and moxidectin have similar efficacy as effective anthelmintics in horses for many gastrointestinal parasites other than *Anoplocephala perfoliata*.[126] Based on these reports regarding anthelmintic efficacy, recommendations include combining therapeutic agents to maintain maximal efficacy. Initial treatment with fenbendazole (10 mg/kg PO daily for 5 days), followed in 14 days with an avermectin product at the appropriate dose, should clear the individual of both intestinal and pneumonic parasites.

Prognosis

Foals or adult horses with primary parasitic pneumonia and secondary bacterial infection will require concurrent antibiotic and anthelmintic therapy. The prognosis is excellent for recovery from parasitic pneumonitis. It is important to emphasize the need for complete deworming, including donkeys and mules, because they harbor the adult *Dictyocaulus* parasites that serve as a source for parasitic contamination to horses in the immediate environment.

GUTTURAL POUCH

David E. Freeman and Joanne Hardy

Guttural pouches are paired extensions of the eustachian tubes that connect the pharynx to the middle ear.[127] They are found in perissodactyls, such as equids, tapirs, some species of rhinoceros (except the white rhinoceros), some bats, a South American forest mouse, and hyraxes.[128-130]

Anatomy

The guttural pouches are separated from each other on the midline by the rectus capitis ventralis and the longus capitis muscles and the median septum.[127] Each pouch is in close contact rostrally with the basisphenoid bone; ventrally with the retropharyngeal lymph nodes, pharynx, and esophagus; caudally with the atlanto-occipital joint; laterally with the digastricus muscle and the parotid and mandibular salivary glands; and dorsally with the petrous part of the temporal bone, tympanic bulla, and auditory meatus. Each guttural pouch is divided ventrally into a medial and a lateral compartment by the stylohyoid bone, and it communicates with the pharynx through the pharyngeal orifice of the eustachian tube. The pharyngeal orifice is a funnel-shaped opening in the dorsolateral aspect of the pharynx that forms an oblique slit, rostral and ventral to the dorsal pharyngeal recess. The small end of the funnel opens into the guttural pouch. The medial lamina of each opening is composed of fibrocartilage directed in a rostroventral-to-caudodorsal direction. The capacity of guttural pouches in adult horses is 472 ± 12.4 mL, and the lateral compartment is approximately one third of the capacity of the medial compartment.[131]

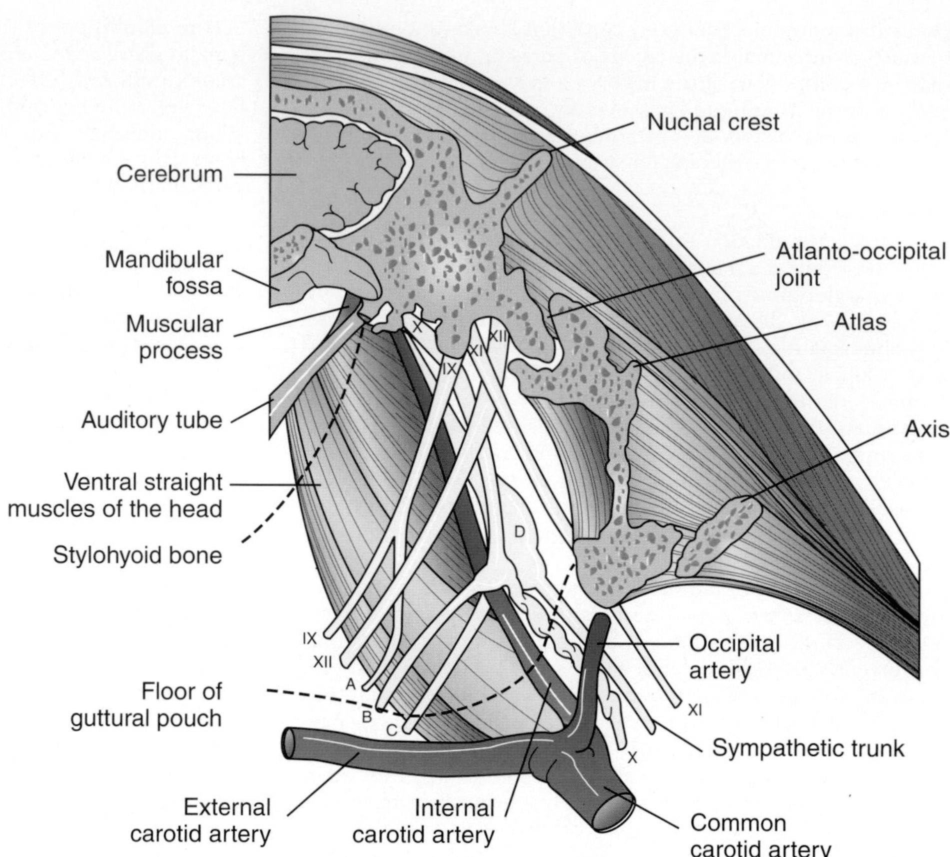

Fig. 1-12 Interior of medial compartment of left guttural pouch, viewed from lateral aspect in sagittal section of a horse's head. The section is cut through the styloid process of the petrous temporal bone on a line that divides the guttural pouch into medial and lateral compartments. *IX*, Glossopharyngeal nerve; *X*, vagus nerve; *XI*, accessory nerve; *XII*, hypoglossal nerve; *A*, pharyngeal branch of glossopharyngeal nerve; *B*, pharyngeal branch of vagus nerve; C, cranial laryngeal nerve; *D*, cranial cervical ganglion. (Redrawn from Freeman DE, Donawick WJ: *J Am Vet Med Assoc* 176:236, 1980.)

Pathogenesis

Clinical signs of important guttural pouch diseases are referable to injury of specific nerves and arteries in the guttural pouch and acoustic system. The internal carotid artery (ICA), cranial cervical ganglion, cervical sympathetic trunk, and the vagus, glossopharyngeal, hypoglossal, and spinal accessory nerves are all contained in a fold of mucous membrane along the caudal wall of the medial compartment[127] (Fig. 1-12). The cranial laryngeal nerve and the pharyngeal branch of the vagus nerve lie beneath the mucosa on the floor of the medial compartment. The external carotid artery (ECA) lies along the wall of the lateral compartment and gives off the caudal auricular artery and superficial temporal artery, and it continues as the maxillary artery (MA) along the roof of the guttural pouch. The facial nerve (cranial nerve [CN] VII) passes for a short distance over the caudodorsal aspect of the lateral compartment after it emerges from the stylomastoid foramen. The vestibulocochlear nerve (CN VIII) enters the internal acoustic meatus caudal to the facial nerve and divides into vestibular and cochlear branches that innervate components of the middle ear. CN VIII does not enter the guttural pouch but can become involved in guttural pouch diseases that affect the middle ear (e.g., temporohyoid osteoarthropathy). The mandibular nerve, a branch of the trigeminal nerve (CN V), emerges from the foramen lacerum, passes close to the muscular process of the petrous part of the temporal bone, and continues rostrally along the roof of the lateral compartment of the guttural pouch.

The guttural pouch is lined with pseudostratified ciliated epithelium containing goblet cells[127] in both adults and foals.[132] The guttural pouch mucosa has the ability to clear foreign substances, but this ability varies among different regions of the epithelium.[132] In a study on the distribution of various immunoglobulin (Ig) isotypes and subisotypes in the guttural pouch mucosa of healthy horses, IgGa was found in the guttural pouch mucosa, mucosal lymph nodules, and submucosal lymph nodules.[133] IgM was scattered in the mucosal lymph nodules and in the germinal centers of the submucosal lymph nodules. IgGc was recognized only in the submucosal lymph nodules, and IgA was detected in glandular epithelial cells and the surface layer of the mucosal epithelium.

Possible functions of the guttural pouches include pressure equilibration across the tympanic membrane, contribution to air warming, a resonating chamber for vocalization, and a flotation device.[134] A more recently proposed role is brain cooling, based on measurement of lower arterial temperatures in the cerebral side of the internal carotid artery compared with the cardiac side.[135,136] As shown by cadaver studies, opening of the pharyngeal orifice of the guttural pouch involves the levator and tensor veli palatini muscles and the pterygopharyngeus and palatopharyngeus muscles. Passive opening of the auditory tube involves a reduced tone in the stylopharyngeus and pterygopharyngeus muscles, accompanied by increased inspiratory pressure.[137] Although guttural pouch filling was previously reported to occur on expiration, the latter study demonstrated that filling occurs on inspiration.[137]

Clinical Examination

The guttural pouches are examined by external palpation, endoscopy, and radiography. Enlargement caused by empyema (purulent material in the pouches), but particularly by tympany (air engorgement), can be palpated externally. Guttural pouch endoscopy provides the most information regarding guttural pouch disease. Nonspecific evidence of guttural pouch disease, such as collapse of the pharynx and blood or pus draining from

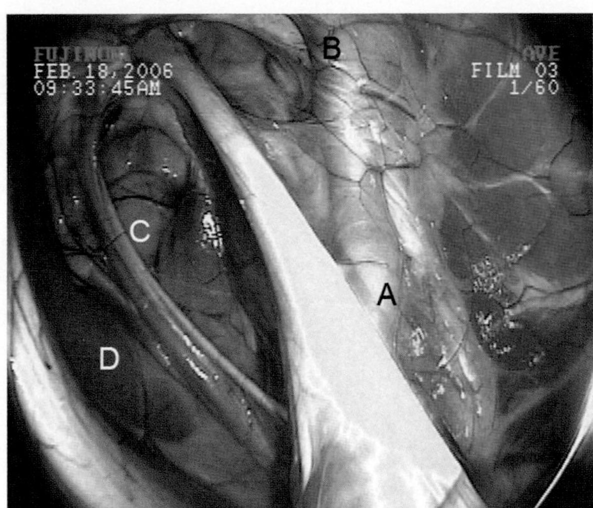

Fig. 1-13 Normal endoscopic anatomy of right guttural pouch. The narrow, pale structure that runs from dorsal to ventral is the stylohyoid bone that divides the caudoventral part into lateral (to left) and medial (to right) compartments. Sources of hemorrhage from guttural pouch: *A*, external carotid artery; *B*, maxillary artery; *C*, internal carotid artery; *D*, ventral straight muscles. (From Freeman DE, Hardy J: Guttural pouch. In Auer JA, Stick JA, editors: *Equine surgery*, ed 3, St Louis, 2006, Elsevier, p 592.)

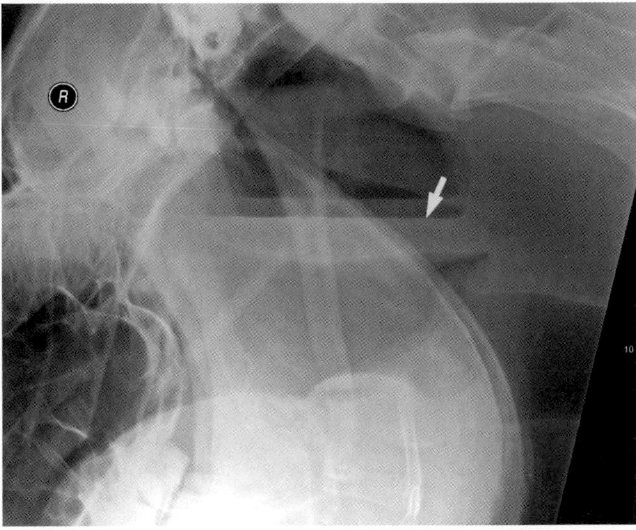

Fig. 1-14 Lateral radiographic view of horse's head revealing fluid accumulation in guttural pouches *(arrow)* caused by bilateral guttural pouch empyema.

the pharyngeal orifice, can be found on endoscopic examination of the pharynx. However, blood or pus from other respiratory sources may be aspirated into the guttural pouch opening and appear to drain from it, so that direct endoscopic examination of the pouches must be performed (Fig. 1-13). With the horse mildly sedated, the biopsy instrument is passed through the biopsy channel of the endoscope and used to guide the endoscope into the guttural pouch. The endoscope is placed so that the biopsy forceps is as close as possible to the lateral wall of the pharynx until successful insertion into the guttural pouch is achieved. Both pouches can be entered in this manner with the endoscope in the same nostril. Alternatively, the pharyngeal opening can be levered open with a Chamber's catheter to allow the endoscope to enter the pouches.

Lateral radiographic projections of the guttural pouches can demonstrate fluid lines, fractures and exostoses of the stylohyoid bone, radiopaque foreign bodies, and space-occupying masses[138] (Fig. 1-14). Air distention, as in tympany, can increase dimensions of the affected guttural pouch, sometimes beyond the second cervical vertebra. A dorsoventral or ventrodorsal projection is best used to image the stylohyoid bones and temporohyoid articulation. CT can provide an alternate imaging modality,[139-142] especially for imaging of the stylohyoid bone, inner ear, and petrous temporal bone in cases of temporohyoid osteoarthropathy.[142] Ultrasonography can be used to demonstrate soft tissue lesions in the guttural pouches, such as tumors[143] or muscle damage and associated submucosal hemorrhage.[144]

A percutaneous centesis technique through Viborg's triangle has been described for guttural pouch lavage and collection of samples for cytologic and microbiologic examinations.[145] The normal cytologic pattern is less than 5% neutrophils, a large proportion of ciliated columnar epithelial cells, a few nonciliated cuboidal epithelial cells, and less than 1% monocytes, lymphocytes, and eosinophils. The proportion of neutrophils is important, with less than 5% considered normal and greater than 25% considered abnormal. A high correlation exists between high cytologic score and presence of pathogenic bacteria such as *Streptococcus equi* subsp. *equi*.[146,147] The cytologic gradings and neutrophil concentrations of guttural pouch washings are increased in horses whose heads are restrained for more than 12 hours, as during long-distance transport. Washings from these horses are more likely to contain bacteria and yield potentially pathogenic bacteria.[148]

Empyema

Empyema of the guttural pouches is defined as the presence of purulent material (Fig. 1-15) or chondroids within one or both guttural pouches. Chondroids consist of inspissated purulent material, usually numerous individual round balls (Fig. 1-16). Empyema can affect horses of any age but usually occurs in young animals.

Etiology

Upper respiratory tract infections (especially those caused by *Streptococcus*), abscessation and rupture of retropharyngeal lymph nodes into the guttural pouch, infusion of irritant drugs, fracture of the stylohyoid bone, congenital or acquired stenosis of the pharyngeal orifice, and pharyngeal perforation by a nasogastric tube may cause empyema.[149,150] Persistence of guttural pouch infection in unsuspected long-term carriers could be responsible for recurrent outbreaks of strangles.[151]

Clinical Findings

Clinical signs of guttural pouch empyema include intermittent nasal discharge, swelling of adjacent lymph nodes, parotid swelling and pain, extended head carriage, excessive respiratory noise, and difficulties in swallowing and breathing. In rare cases, guttural pouch empyema can cause pharyngeal and laryngeal paresis.[152] In one study of 91 horses with guttural pouch empyema, 21% had chondroids, and the horses with chondroids were more likely to have retropharyngeal and pharyngeal swelling than those without this complication.[153] The number of chondroids present is variable, ranging from one to many, and both guttural pouches can be affected.

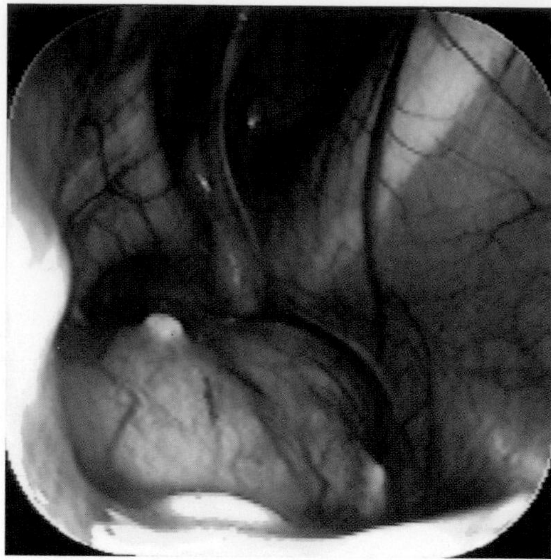

Fig. 1-15 Endoscopic view of interior of right guttural pouch of horse with enlargement and drainage from retropharyngeal lymph node on floor of medial compartment. Note purulent material on floor of the medial compartment. (From Freeman DE, Hardy J: Guttural pouch. In Auer JA, Stick JA, editors: *Equine surgery,* ed 3, St Louis, 2006, Elsevier, p 594.)

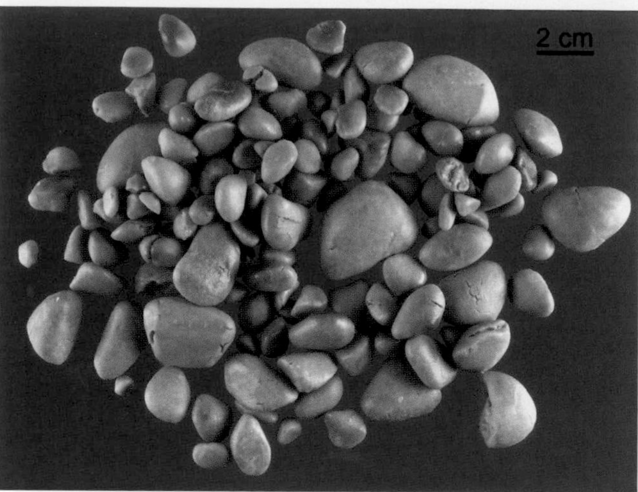

Fig. 1-16 Guttural pouch chondroids removed through modified Whitehouse approach. (From Freeman DE, Hardy J: Guttural pouch. In Auer JA, Stick JA, editors: *Equine surgery,* ed 3, St Louis, 2006, Elsevier, p 594.)

Duration of infection does not appear to correlate with development of chondroids.

Diagnosis

On endoscopic examination, a purulent discharge can be seen at the pharyngeal orifice of the affected side, with pharyngeal collapse in some horses. Fluid accompanied by masses seen within the guttural pouch on standing lateral radiographs suggests chondroids.[154] Fluid aspirates or saline washings can be obtained from the guttural pouch for culture and sensitivity testing; however, results should be interpreted with caution because microorganisms can be retrieved from the normal guttural pouch and upper respiratory tract. Horses that are carriers of, or infected with, *S. equi* subsp. *equi* in the guttural pouches can be identified by culture and PCR tests with repeated swabs[155] (see Chapter 28).

Medical Therapy

In acute cases, daily irrigation with physiologic saline solution is usually effective. An indwelling catheter, devised from polyethylene 240 tubing with heat-formed coils at one end, can be used for this purpose. Alternatively, a commercially available guttural pouch catheter (Cook Veterinary Projects, Bloomington, Ind; Mila International, Florence, Ky) or one made from a polypropylene canine urinary catheter can be used. Coiled catheters can be straightened to facilitate insertion by inserting a coaxial wire or by passage through a larger, curved catheter. The coiled end of the catheter is placed under endoscopic guidance within the pouch, and the free end is secured by a suture to the alar fold. A Foley catheter can also be used, but it should be advanced until the end is completely in the pouch because distention of the balloon within the pharyngeal opening could cause pressure necrosis. In larger horses, standard Foley catheters are not long enough to reach the guttural pouch. Alternatively, the pouch can be flushed through the biopsy channel of the endoscope, which has the advantage of delivery of the flush solution to areas coated with purulent material. After 7 to 10 days, irrigation should be interrupted briefly to assess the response, with the awareness that this treatment can cause some inflammation.

In horses that are severely dyspneic because of guttural pouch distention, a tracheotomy should be performed. If the response to medical treatment is poor or if the purulent material becomes inspissated or forms chondroids, surgical drainage of the guttural pouch should be considered (see later discussion). Chondroids can also be removed by maceration, followed by saline lavage or extraction by endoscopically guided grabbing forceps, a basket snare, or a memory-helical polyp retrieval basket (Cook, Bloomington, Ind).[155] Another technique involves repeated section of each mass by a diathermic snare (Olympus Optical, Irving, Texas) or a wire loop, with removal by suction, lavage, or extraction by basket-type endoscopic forceps (Gomco Equipment, Chemetron Medical Products, Buffalo, NY).[156] In one study, 44% of horses with chondroids were treated successfully by these noninvasive methods,[153] although removal by these methods can take a long time. If empyema is the result of occlusion of guttural pouch openings by adhesions, this occlusion may be relieved by blunt division through a surgical approach to the guttural pouch interior.[155] Chronic empyema of the guttural pouches, possibly unresponsive to medical therapy because of poor drainage through the pharyngeal ostia, can be successfully treated by using a laser to establish a permanent pharyngeal fistula into the guttural pouch.[157]

Response to medical treatment is usually satisfactory, and surgery is rarely indicated. Neurologic signs usually resolve once the infection is brought under control by medical or surgical treatment.

Surgical Therapy

Surgery of the guttural pouch through any approach should be a last resort because of risks of iatrogenic nerve damage. Identification of the guttural pouch lining and underlying nerves is difficult, especially in horses in which there is no distention, and can be facilitated by a lighted endoscope inserted into the medial compartment. A fixed structure, such as the stylohyoid bone, should be used as a guide for deep dissection. The mucosa should not be incised with sharp instruments, and retractors should be applied with care to avoid nerve damage. Because all approaches enter the pouch

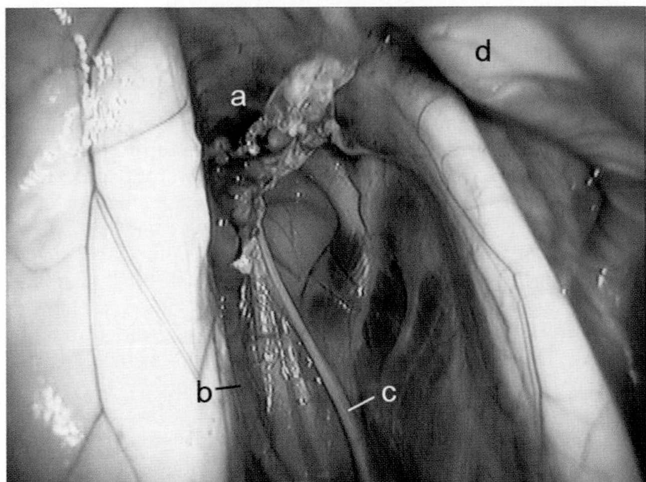

Fig. 1-17 Guttural pouch mycosis in typical location on roof of medial compartment (left guttural pouch), overlying internal carotid artery. *a,* Lesion; *b,* internal carotid artery; *c,* mucosal reflection that contains glossopharyngeal and hypoglossal nerves; *d,* maxillary artery lateral to stylohyoid bone. This small lesion did not cause epistaxis but did cause dysphagia that necessitated euthanasia. (From Freeman DE, Hardy J: Guttural pouch. In Auer JA, Stick JA, editors: *Equine surgery,* ed 3, St Louis, 2006, Elsevier, p 596.)

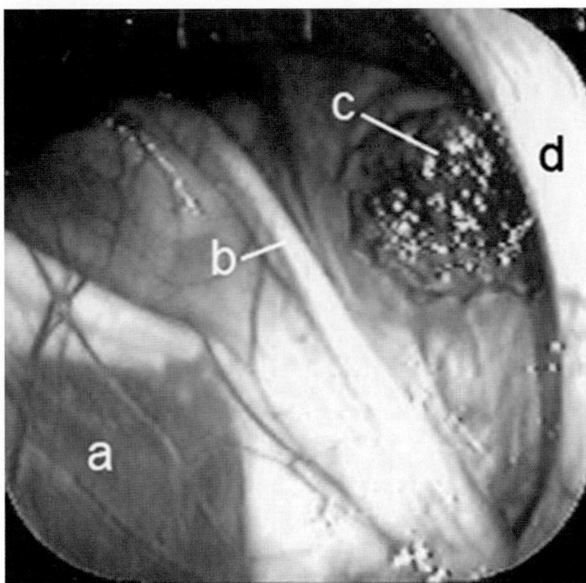

Fig. 1-18 Roof of left guttural pouch as viewed through retroflexion of endoscope. *a,* Insertion of ventral straight muscles of head; *b,* cartilaginous flap of eustachian tube; *c,* mycotic lesion on left maxillary artery; *d,* dorsal edge of stylohyoid bone. This approach provides an excellent view of these structures when the rostral end of the guttural pouch is obscured with hemorrhage. (From Freeman DE, Hardy J: Guttural pouch. In Auer JA, Stick JA, editors: *Equine surgery,* ed 3, St Louis, 2006, Elsevier, p 596.)

cavity in the same approximate area, none provides less risk of nerve damage than the others. Several approaches can be used to open the guttural pouch for removal of pus, mycotic plaques, and foreign bodies and to establish drainage. These include hyovertebrotomy, approach through Viborg's triangle (tendon of sternocephalicus muscle, linguofacial vein, vertical ramus of mandible), Whitehouse approach, and modified Whitehouse approach. Advantages of both Whitehouse approaches are direct access to the roof of the guttural pouch, digital access to the lateral compartment, excellent ventral drainage, and simultaneous access through the septum to both pouches. Although both approaches involve deep dissection, they do not appear to have a higher rate of complications than other approaches.

Open incisions in the guttural pouch are cleaned daily, and the guttural pouch cavity should be flushed daily with a nonirritating solution. Open incisions close spontaneously within 14 days, and the infection should also resolve within this time. Postoperative antibiotics can be given.

Guttural Pouch Mycosis

Etiology

Guttural pouch mycosis is usually unilateral, but rarely it may affect both pouches. There is no apparent age, gender, breed, or geographic predisposition to this disease. The cause of guttural pouch mycosis is unknown, although *Aspergillus* spp. can frequently be identified in the lesion. The typical lesion of guttural pouch mycosis is a diphtheritic membrane of variable size, composed of necrotic tissue, cell debris, a variety of bacteria, and fungal mycelia.[149] Aneurysm formation does not appear to precede or follow arterial invasion consistently and therefore is not essential to the pathogenesis of arterial rupture.

Clinical Findings

The most common clinical sign of guttural pouch mycosis is moderate to severe epistaxis, which is caused by fungal erosion of the ICA in most cases[158-161] (Fig. 1-17) and of the ECA and MA in approximately one third of cases[162,163] (Fig. 1-18). However, any branch of the ECA, such as the caudal auricular artery, can be affected. Several bouts of hemorrhage usually precede a fatal episode. Mucus and dark blood continue to drain from the nostril on the affected side for days after acute hemorrhage ceases.

The second most common clinical sign is dysphagia caused by damage to the pharyngeal branches of the vagus and glossopharyngeal nerves.[159] Aspiration pneumonia may develop in severe or protracted cases. Abnormal respiratory noise can arise from pharyngeal paresis or from laryngeal hemiplegia, which results from recurrent laryngeal nerve damage.[159] Horner's syndrome may develop from damage to the cranial cervical ganglion and postganglionic sympathetic fibers. The classic signs associated with this denervation are ptosis, miosis, and enophthalmos; patchy sweating; and congestion of the nasal mucosa. The reason equine sweat glands increase their activity when denervated is unclear.[164] Equine sweat gland myoepithelium is predominantly under α_2-adrenergic control, with additional α-adrenergic input from receptors. However, sweating after neurectomy may be caused by increased peripheral vasodilation, which increases blood flow and skin temperature. Ptosis is caused by a decreased tone of the superior tarsus muscle, and it is assessed by observing eyelash angles from a frontal view. Pupillary response to decreased sympathetic tone in horses is variable, and the maximal difference in pupil size is usually slight. Enophthalmos, which is the result of decreased smooth muscle retrobulbar tone and unopposed activity of the striated retractor bulbi muscle, is rarely obvious and usually evident as a slight protrusion of the nictitating membrane.[164]

Less common signs of guttural pouch mycosis are parotid pain, nasal discharge, abnormal head posture, head shyness, sweating and shivering, corneal ulcers, colic, blindness, locomotion disturbances, facial nerve paralysis, paralysis of the tongue, and septic arthritis of the atlanto-occipital joint.[158,159,165-168]

Diagnosis

Endoscopy is critical for diagnosis of guttural pouch mycosis and should be combined with the history and clinical signs. On endoscopic examination of a horse with epistaxis, blood can be seen draining from the pharyngeal orifice. In horses with dysphagia the roof of the pharynx can be collapsed, the soft palate can be displaced, and the nasopharynx may contain food material. The lesion appears as a white, tan, and black diphtheritic membrane on the roof of the affected guttural pouch, and its size can vary but bears no relationship to the severity of clinical signs. Part of the diphtheritic membrane can coat the stylohyoid bone and the bone can be thickened, but clinical signs usually do not develop from this change. Fistulas may form into the opposite guttural pouch and pharynx.[161] The presence of serum antibodies to *Aspergillus fumigatus* detected by ELISA cannot distinguish between horses with guttural pouch mycosis and healthy horses.[169]

Medical Therapy

The response to topical treatment is generally slow and inconsistent. Daily direct lavage through the endoscope can macerate the diphtheritic membrane, and the biopsy forceps or cytology brush of the endoscope can be used to detach it, provided any eroded artery was occluded beforehand. Topical povidone-iodine or thiabendazole, with or without dimethyl sulfoxide, has been used with mixed results.[161,162,165,170] Nystatin, natamycin, and miconazole have little activity against *Aspergillus*,[171] but amphotericin B is effective against this organism, although its use in the horse is limited by its toxicity.[172]

Successful treatment of dysphagia from guttural pouch mycosis has been reported with a combination of oral itraconazole (5 mg/kg) and topical enilconazole (60 mL of 33.3 mg/mL solution per daily flush) in one horse[170] and with topical enilconazole alone in another.[173] Itraconazole at 3 mg/kg twice a day in the feed can be effective against *Aspergillus* and other fungi in the nasal passage of horses, but treatment may be required for up to 4 or 5 months.[174] Bioavailability of another triazole antifungal agent, fluconazole, can be sufficiently high after oral and IV administration in horses to suggest a potential value in treatment of fungal infections.[175] The response to any treatment method that is measured solely by disappearance of the mycotic lesion should be interpreted with caution because spontaneous regression of the lesion over a variable time course is typical. Horses with blood loss should be treated with polyionic fluids and, if necessary, with blood transfusions, and horses with dysphagia should be fed by nasogastric tube or by esophagostomy and should receive nonsteroidal antiinflammatory drugs to reduce neuritis.

Surgical Therapy

The diphtheritic membrane can be detached by gentle swabbing and lavage through a modified Whitehouse approach. This treatment does not eliminate the risk of hemorrhage completely, and it does not slow or reverse progression of neurologic signs, but it does carry the risk of iatrogenic nerve damage and hemorrhage. In horses with epistaxis the affected artery should be identified by endoscopy and surgically occluded. Anecdotal but widely accepted evidence indicates that occlusion of the affected artery hastens spontaneous resolution of the mycotic lesion and thereby renders medical therapy unnecessary.[176]

In a horse with hemorrhage caused by guttural pouch mycosis, the involved artery or arteries should be occluded by one of the following procedures, or a combination, as soon as the diagnosis is made. The vessel to be occluded is determined by endoscopy. If accurate identification is impossible because landmarks are obscured by blood and diphtheritic membrane, all arteries in the pouch should be occluded.[163] Arteriography may be used to identify the affected vessel and to identify unusual anatomy. It is not required in all methods or in all cases; however, it does allow more precise and selective occlusion.[177]

In horses with guttural pouch mycosis, fatal or severe hemorrhage has followed ligation of the affected ICA and could be attributed to occlusion of the wrong vessel or to retrograde flow from the cerebral arterial circle (circle of Willis).[158,160,178,179] Complications likely occur because ligation of the ipsilateral common carotid artery in a horse bleeding from the ICA would increase flow in the affected artery and would be contraindicated.[180] However, the same procedure may provide some immediate benefit in horses bleeding from the ECA and its branches, although any such benefit could be temporary. Ligation of the affected ICA would decrease flow but not pressure, so bleeding could persist or recur. However, if access to definitive occlusion procedures is not immediate during a severe bleeding crisis, induction of general anesthesia to quiet the horse and ligation of the affected internal carotid artery could be attempted as a temporary measure.

Success with ICA ligation can be attributed to thrombosis distal to the ligature at some time after surgery.[158,160] To prevent backflow, an additional ligature has been placed distal to the mycotic infection;[179] however, this is difficult because the artery must be ligated deep within the guttural pouch, where it is likely to be obscured by the diphtheritic membrane. The site for ligation of the ICA is immediately distal to its origin, outside the guttural pouch, using a similar but more ventral approach to a hyovertebrotomy. The ICA is identified on the cardiac side of the occipital artery and deep to that vessel. In some horses, both arteries arise as a single trunk. If necessary, both ICAs can be ligated simultaneously without any apparent risk.[160,178]

The ECA can be ligated distal to the origin of the linguofacial trunk through an incision similar to that used for the ICA ligation but after extensive rostral dissection.[162] However, this procedure is generally unsuccessful because the ECA and MA have numerous collateral channels that allow retrograde flow to the affected segment.[127,163] Although ligation of the major palatine artery could prevent retrograde flow, a combination of this procedure with ligation of the ECA and ICA can cause ischemic optic neuropathy and permanent blindness.[181]

The *balloon catheter technique* allows immediate intravascular occlusion of the artery and prevents retrograde flow from the cerebral arterial circle.[161,182] Risk of retrograde flow is not diminished immediately by ligation alone, because this does not decrease blood pressure in the distal segment of artery.[183] Complications associated with this procedure are rare.[162,182] The catheter rarely penetrates the defect in the artery, and if it does, it can be withdrawn and redirected. Failure to prevent fatal hemorrhage in one case was caused by inadvertent catheterization and occlusion of an aberrant branch from the ICA, which left the affected segment of artery open to retrograde blood flow.[184] To prevent this mishap, approximately 6 cm of the ICA should be exposed to locate any aberrant branch. Such a branch should be ligated so that the catheter can be maintained in the ICA.[184]

Approximately 50% of horses with hemorrhage die from this complication,[159] but this risk can be eliminated or greatly reduced by occlusion procedures. These procedures must be performed as soon as possible after the first bout of hemorrhage to prevent subsequent bouts that could render the horse a poor candidate for anesthesia and surgery. Although the mycotic lesion disappears with time, neurologic signs can persist. Laryngeal hemiplegia is usually permanent, but recovery has been reported.[158] Some horses with dysphagia do eventually recover, but 6 to 18 months may be required and recovery may be incomplete.[158,159] Horses can recover from Horner's syndrome and facial nerve paralysis.

Balloon tip catheter occlusion has been fraught with failure because of inappropriate placement. Balloon occlusion of the MA is more effective than ligation. In addition, blindness associated with MA ligation (resulting in loss of flow to ophthalmic branch of MA) does not occur.[127,163,181,185] However, the owner should still be warned of the risk of blindness.

A detachable, self-sealing, latex balloon can be used to occlude the ICA successfully,[186] without the need for catheter removal, as required in some patients treated with the nondetachable balloons. Combined with angiography, the detachable system can also be used to occlude aberrant vessels that originate at a distance from the origin of the ICA.[187]

A *transarterial coil embolization technique* can selectively occlude the arterial segments involved in a mycotic lesion in horses with guttural pouch mycosis.[188-191] The coil embolization technique combines angiographic studies to image the affected vessels and identify any unusual vessels and sites of bleeding, followed by a selective embolization or occlusion of the affected vessels. Compared with the balloon catheter technique, transarterial coil embolization allows visualization of affected vessels throughout the procedure because it is performed under fluoroscopic guidance.[188] This is critical because aberrant vasculature has been described in horses with guttural pouch mycosis, and failure to identify and occlude such aberrant branches may result in fatal hemorrhage.[184,192] It is less invasive than the original balloon catheter procedures and requires shorter anesthesia and shorter hospitalization. Transarterial embolization can be performed during active bleeding. The surgical approach for all arteries in the guttural pouch is the common carotid artery exposed through a single incision. The disadvantages of this technique are the need for fluoroscopy (and the specialized equipment and expertise involved), positioning of the horse's head for fluoroscopy, and apparel and equipment for radiation shielding.

Temporohyoid Osteoarthropathy

Etiology

Temporohyoid osteoarthropathy is a progressive disease of the middle ear and components of the temporohyoid joint, such as the stylohyoid bone, the cartilaginous tympanohyoid, and squamous portion of the temporal bone. Horses of a wide age range and of any breed or either gender can be affected. The cause is thought to be an inner or a middle ear infection of hematogenous origin that spreads to the bones listed, causing them to thicken and the temporohyoid joint to fuse.[193] Other possible causes range from extension of otitis media/externa or guttural pouch infection to a nonseptic osteoarthritis.[193-197] Although guttural pouch mycosis can involve the same bony structures and temporohyoid articulation,[159] clinical signs of temporohyoid osteoarthropathy are rare with this disease.

Once the temporohyoid joint fuses and the associated bones thicken, forces generated by movement of the tongue and larynx during swallowing, vocalizing, combined head and neck movements, oral or dental examinations, and teeth floating may induce fractures of the petrous part of the temporal bone, resulting in facial nerve (CN VII) and vestibulocochlear nerve (CN VIII) dysfunction.[193-198] Severe new bone production and inflammation can damage the glossopharyngeal and vagus nerves where they leave the medulla caudal to the vestibulocochlear nerve.[127,199] After fracture of the petrous temporal bone, middle or inner ear infection could extend around the brain stem and involve additional cranial nerves and hindbrain structures.

Clinical Findings and Diagnosis

Early clinical signs include head tossing, ear rubbing, refusing to take the bit, refusing to position the head properly when under saddle, resistance to digital pressure around the base of the ears or on the basihyoid bone, and other nonspecific behavior changes. The disease can cause an acute onset of signs consistently referable to facial and vestibulocochlear nerve deficits, including asymmetric ataxia, head tilt with the poll to the affected side, and spontaneous nystagmus with the slow component to the affected side.[193] These signs can be revealed or exacerbated by blindfolding. Signs of facial nerve damage, including paresis or paralysis of the ear on the affected side, deviation of the upper lip away from the affected side, decreased tear production, and inability to close the eyes, are evident in most cases. Decreased tear production and inability to close the eyes may cause corneal ulcers, keratoconjunctivitis sicca, and exposure keratitis.[198,199] Dysphagia is rare but can result from damage to the glossopharyngeal and vagus nerves.[193]

Radiographs of the skull may depict proliferation and osteitis of the affected bones; however, endoscopy of the guttural pouch is in most cases a more sensitive method for detection of stylohyoid bone and temporohyoid joint involvement and thus for making the diagnosis[199] (Fig. 1-19). CT or MRI can precisely demonstrate bony and soft tissue changes in the middle and inner ear.[142]

Therapy

Medical treatment includes broad-spectrum antibiotics for infection, nonsteroidal antiinflammatory drugs to relieve pain and inflammation, and dimethyl sulfoxide to relieve inflammation.[193,201] Unilateral partial ostectomy of the stylohyoid bone has been used to create a pseudoarthrosis between the cut ends of the bone, which decreases the forces on the ankylosed temporohyoid and thereby prevents skull fractures[201] (Fig. 1-20). In this procedure, approximately 2 to 3 cm

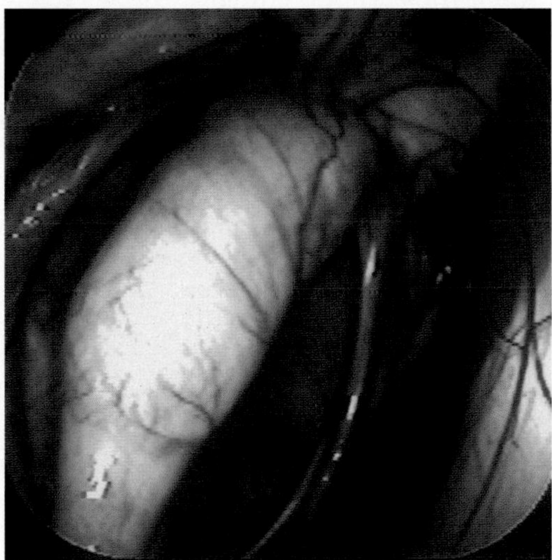

Fig. 1-19 Thickened stylohyoid bone with involvement of temporohyoid articulation in horse with clinical signs of damage to vestibulocochlear and facial nerves. (From Freeman DE, Hardy J: Guttural pouch. In Auer JA, Stick JA, editors: *Equine surgery,* ed 3, St Louis, 2006, Elsevier, p 599.)

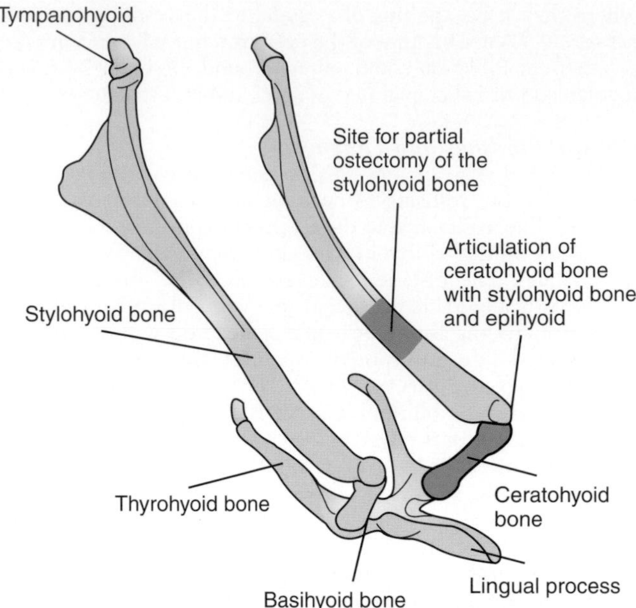

Fig. 1-20 Hyoid apparatus, showing sites for ostectomy procedures *(shaded)* for horses with temporohyoid osteoarthropathy. (From Freeman DE, Hardy J: Guttural pouch. In Auer JA, Stick JA, editors: *Equine surgery*, ed 3, St Louis, 2006, Elsevier, p 599.)

of the midbody of the stylohyoid bone is removed. Although this procedure appears to have merit as a prophylactic measure against more severe bone damage and associated neurologic consequences, it may cause transient dysphagia or injury to the hypoglossal nerve. When performed as a bilateral procedure, it causes permanent problems with prehension.[201]

An additional complication of partial ostectomy is regrowth of the stylohyoid bone approximately 6 months after surgical resection, with recurrence of clinical signs. Because of this complication, a ceratohyoidectomy has been recommended as a safer, easier, and more permanent surgical alternative.[199] Although the prognosis is good according to one report,[202] neurologic signs may persist,[200] especially if treatment is delayed. In general, the prognosis for stylohyoid arthropathy is dependent on the severity of clinical signs. Some degree of facial and vestibulocochlear nerve paresis can persist.[134] The corneal ulcers are difficult to treat, because there is an underlying problem with lid closure and tear production. A temporary tarsorrhaphy may help to manage the ocular complications until facial nerve function returns.

References

See the CD-ROM for a list of references linked to the abstract in PubMed.

Suggested Reading

Guttural Pouch

Alexander K, Baird JD, Dobson H, et al: What is your diagnosis? *J Am Vet Med Assoc* 220:297, 2002.

Bayly WM, Robertson JT: Epistaxis caused by foreign body penetration of a guttural pouch, *J Am Vet Med Assoc* 180: 1232, 1982.

Bentz BG, Dowd AL, Freeman DE: Treatment of guttural pouch empyema with acetylcysteine irrigation, *Equine Pract* 18:33, 1996.

Blazyczek I, Hamann H, Deegen E, et al: Retrospective analysis of 50 cases of guttural pouch tympany in foals, *Vet Rec* 154: 261, 2004.

Blazyczek I, Hamann H, Ohnesorge B, et al: Population genetic analysis of the heritability of guttural pouch tympany in Arabian purebred foals, *Dtsch Tierarztl Wochenschr* 110:417, 2003.

Blazyczek I, Hamann H, Ohnesorge B, et al: Guttural pouch tympany in German warmblood foals: influence of sex, inbreeding and blood proportions of founding breeds as well as estimation of heritability, *Berl Munch Tierarztl Wochenschr* 116:346, 2003.

Blazyczek I, Hamann H, Ohnesorge B, et al: Inheritance of guttural pouch tympany in the Arabian horse, *J Hered* 95: 195, 2004.

Darien BJ, Watrous BJ, Huber MJ, et al: What is your diagnosis? *J Am Vet Med Assoc* 198:1799, 1991.

Fintl C, Dixon PM: A review of five cases of parotid melanoma in the horse, *Equine Vet Educ*, 2001, p 43.

Greene HJ, O'Connor JP: Hemangioma of the guttural pouch of a 16-year-old Thoroughbred mare: clinical and pathological findings, *Vet Rec* 118:445, 1986.

Hance SR, Robertson JT, Bukowiecki CF: Cystic structures in the guttural pouch (auditory tube diverticulum) of two horses, *J Am Vet Med Assoc* 200:1981, 1992.

Harvey SC: Antiseptics and disinfectants; fungicides; ectoparasiticides. In Gilman A, Goodman LS, Rall TW, et al, editors: *Goodman and Gilman's the pharmacological basis of therapeutics*, New York, 1985, Macmillan.

May KA, Howard RD: Exercise intolerance secondary to parotid melanomas in a mare, *Equine Vet Educ*, 2001, p 246.

McConnico RS, Blas-Machado U, Cooper VL, et al: Bilateral squamous cell carcinoma of the guttural pouches and the left middle ear in a horse, *Equine Vet Educ*, 2001, p 225.

McCue PM, Freeman DE, Donawick WJ: Guttural pouch tympany: 15 cases (1977-1986), *J Am Vet Med Assoc* 194: 1761, 1989.

Merriam JG: Guttural pouch fibroma in a mare, *J Am Vet Med Assoc* 161:487, 1972.

Milne DW, Fessler JR: Tympanitis of the guttural pouch in a foal, *J Am Vet Med Assoc* 161:61, 1972.

Moulton JE, editor: *Tumors in domestic animals*, Los Angeles, 1978, University of California Press.

Raker CW: The nasopharynx. In Mannsmann RA, McAllister ES, editors: *Equine medicine and surgery*, ed 3, Santa Barbara, Calif, 1982, American Veterinary Publications.

Sullins KE: Endoscopic application of cutting current for upper respiratory surgery in the standing horse, *Proc Am Assoc Equine Pract* 36:439, 1990.

Tate LP, Blikslager AT, Little ED: Transendoscopic laser treatment of guttural pouch tympanites in eight foals, *Vet Surg* 24:367, 1995.

Tetens J, Tulleners EP, Ross MW, et al: Transendoscopic contact neodymium:yttrium aluminum garnet laser treatment of tympany of the auditory tube diverticulum in two foals, *J Am Vet Med Assoc* 204:1927, 1994.

Trigo RJ, Nickels FA: Squamous cell carcinoma of a horse's guttural pouch, *Mod Vet Pract* 62:456, 1981.

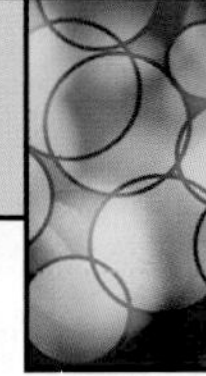

CHAPTER • 2

Cardiovascular Infections

Celia M. Marr

All components of the cardiovascular system, from cardiac tissues to blood vessels, are susceptible to infection. Fortunately, these conditions are relatively uncommon in the horse, but they can be devastating when they occur. Viral or bacterial infection can also act as a trigger for immune-mediated disorders, such as pericarditis and myocarditis. Fever is a common clinical feature of cardiovascular infections, and specific localizing signs will vary depending on the specific site of infection. In general, successful treatment relies on appropriate antimicrobial therapy. In many cases, however, systemic inflammatory response syndrome is a prominent feature, and supportive therapy is important and challenging in these severely compromised individuals.

INFECTIVE ENDOCARDITIS

Etiology and Pathogenesis

Infective endocarditis (IE) is an uncommon but frequently fatal disorder in horses. Endocardial lesions have been reported in association with Lyme borreliosis[1] and infection with *Shigella equirulis*.[2] However, review of clinical and pathologic reports of equine IE published since 1980 (34 cases),[3-18,29,31,32] together with an additional six cases seen at the author's clinic, has demonstrated that a range of microorganisms may be implicated in equine IE. *Actinobacillus equuli*,[3-5] *Pasteurella caballi*,[6] *Pasteurella/Actinobacillus* spp.,[7,8] *Pseudomonas* spp.,[9,10] *Escherichia coli*,[7,11] *Corynebacterium* spp.,[7] *Bacillus* spp.,[7] *Serratia marcescens*,[12] *Erysipelothrix rhusiopathiae*,[13] coagulase-positive *Staphylococcus* spp.,[14] α-hemolytic[7] and β-hemolytic[15] *Streptococcus* spp., and *Streptococcus equi* subsp. *equi*[16] are reported as causes of IE in horses, with no one organism emerging as distinctly more prevalent than the others. *Pasteurella/Actinobacillus* spp. (6 of 32 reported cases, 18.8%; 95% confidence intervals [CI] 5.2%-32.3%) and *Pseudomonas* spp. (3 of 32 cases, 9.4%; CI 0%-19.5%) occur more than once in this literature series, whereas the other organisms were each identified in one case only.

Rhodococcus equi was isolated from synovial and bony material removed surgically from a foal with septic osteoarthritis and mural IE, but blood culture from that foal yielded *Escherichia coli*.[11] A blood culture from a 14-year-old mixed-breed gelding with aortic IE in the author's clinic also yielded *R. equi*. That horse had no apparent immunosuppression or other reason to have become infected with *R. equi* and recovered after 6 weeks of treatment with trimethoprim-sulfonamide and rifampin. Although not a typical skin commensal, *R. equi* may have been a contaminant introduced during the blood collection. Fungal IE has been attributed to *Aspergillus* species in a horse with disseminated aspergillosis affecting the lungs, intestine, and peritoneal cavity, as well as the mitral valve and left ventricular wall.[17] In another report, *Candida* species affected the aortic valve and right atrial wall in an 11-year-old Thoroughbred.[9] In many cases of IE the causative microorganisms cannot be determined. Neither blood nor postmortem cultures allowed identification of a causative organism in 7 of 32 horses (22%; CI 7.6%-36.2%) in which culture was attempted.[7,9,18,19]

A combination of endothelial damage and bacteremia are prerequisites for the development of IE.[20,21] Preexisting heart disease is present in 42% to 98% of human IE patients, and 4% to 13% have congenital defects such as ventricular septal defect (VSD), with preexisting valvular regurgitation in most of the remaining patients.[22] Endothelial damage caused by the effects of high-velocity jets and turbulence leads to deposition of complexes of platelets and fibrin, which in turn are susceptible to colonization by bacteria or fungi during bacteremia or fungemia.[20,21] In horses the structures on the left side of the heart are most likely to be affected by IE, with the mitral valve affected slightly more often than the aortic valve, despite that preexisting valvular lesions are most likely to be present on the aortic valve[23] (Table 2-1). Mural endocarditis occurs less often in horses, possibly because an association between IE and VSD, which is an important predisposing factor in human IE, has not been identified in the horse, although this is a fairly common congenital abnormality in certain breeds, such as the Standardbred, Arabian,[24] and Welsh Mountain pony.[25]

The portal of entry of the causative microorganism is often not apparent. In humans, potential routes include dental infection and procedures, surgery, endoscopy, intravenous (IV) catheters, drug abuse, and infection of the skin, lungs, bowel, and urinary tract.[22] No established association exists between bacteremia and dental procedures in horses, but IE has occurred after repulsion of the first molar by trephination of the maxillary sinus in a case of endodontic infection caused by *Fusobacterium necrophorum*.[26] A 13-year-old mixed-breed mare at the author's clinic had concurrent temporohyoid osteoarthropathy and guttural pouch empyema from which β-hemolytic *Streptococcus* spp. were isolated, although blood culture was negative. Septic jugular thrombophlebitis is considered a risk factor for tricuspid IE in horses. Two of six reported cases of tricuspid IE[7] had recent jugular thrombophlebitis; a third case had an inactive thrombosis related to treatment for an unrelated condition 1 year earlier.[4] Permanent IV devices, such as transvenous pacing devices, are rarely used in horses but can predispose to IE.[27] IE has also been reported in foals with concurrent septicemia, umbilical infection,[7] and osteoarthritis,[11] but in most adult cases the route of infection remains unclear.

Once a critical mass of bacteria has been deposited on an area of damaged endothelium, vegetations consisting of platelets, fibrin, microorganisms, exopolysaccharides, inflammatory cells, and associated necrotic debris begin to develop.[28] Mitral and tricuspid vegetations typically occur on the atrial surface of the valve (Fig. 2-1), whereas aortic vegetations are more likely to develop on the ventricular surface. However, vegetations may occur on any endocardial surface, including the valve leaflets, ventricular or atrial endocardium, and the intimal surface

Table • 2-1

*Location of Lesions in 40 Cases of Infective Endocarditis**

LOCATION	NUMBER AFFECTED	PREVALENCE (%)	LOWER CONFIDENCE LIMIT (%)	UPPER CONFIDENCE LIMIT (%)
Cases with Single Site Involvement				
Mitral valve only	11	27.5	13.7	41.3
Aortic valve only	9	22.5	9.6	35.4
Tricuspid valve only	5	12.5	2.3	22.7
Pulmonic valve only	1	2.5	0	7.3
Mural: left atrium	11	27.5	0	7.3
Cases with Single or Multisite Involvement				
Mitral valve	21	52.5	37.0	68.0
Aortic valve	15	37.5	22.5	52.5
Tricuspid valve	8	20.0	7.6	32.4
Pulmonic valve	2	5.0	0	11.8
Mural sites	4	10.0	0.7	19.3
"Left heart" structures	26	65.0	50.2	79.8
"Right heart" structures	7	17.5	5.7	29.3
Both sides of heart	5	12.5	2.3	22.7

*With 34 cases from references 3-18, 29, 31, and 32, plus 6 cases from the author's clinic.

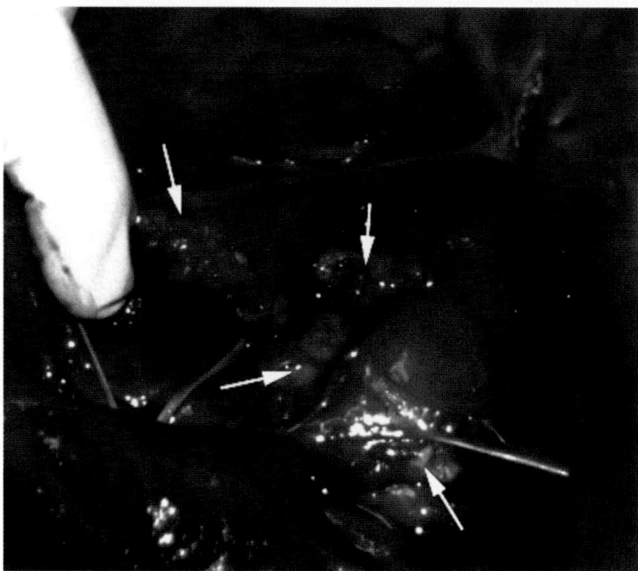

Fig. 2-1 Pathologic specimen from 8-year-old Thoroughbred stallion with infective endocarditis. Ventricular surfaces of tricuspid valve are normal, but vegetations *(arrows)* are visible protruding from the atrial aspect, at the line of closure. (Courtesy P Ramzan, Rossdale and Partners, Newmarket, Suffolk, UK.)

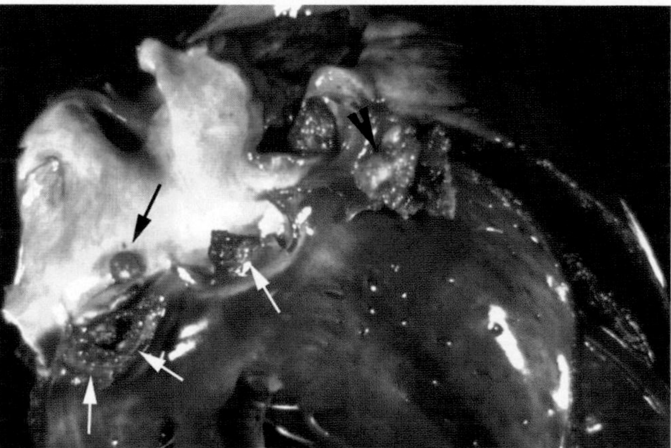

Fig. 2-2 Pathological specimen from 4-year-old Thoroughbred colt with infective endocarditis. Vegetations are attached to both the ventricular *(white arrows)* and the aortic *(black arrowhead)* aspects of the aortic valve. An additional small vegetation is attached to the intimal surface of the aorta *(black arrow)*. The tear in the left coronary cusp was created postmortem.

of the great vessels[28] (Figs. 2-2 and 2-3). Vegetations usually form at the line of valve closure.[21] "Kissing lesions" develop by spreading between adjacent cusps[21,28] (Fig. 2-4). IE can extend to involve adjacent structures, such as the chordae tendineae[7,12,29] and papillary muscles,[28] or can form myocardial abscesses through metastatic infection or direct extension.[8,30,31] Infected areas may perforate, leading to defects in the septum or aorta[31] or septic pericarditis.[28] Valve cusps[32] and chordae tendineae[7,12,29] can rupture, causing catastrophic regurgitation.

The hemodynamic consequences of IE involve the combined effects of regurgitation and the *systemic inflammatory response syndrome* (SIRS). Severe mitral regurgitation results in pulmonary hypertension and pulmonary congestion and may lead to right-sided heart failure.[33] In acute cases, there may be clinical and radiographic signs of pulmonary edema. Horses that survive the initial episode of acute mitral IE may develop signs of congestive heart failure (CHF), and resultant chronic pulmonary hypertension can lead to pulmonary artery rupture.[15]

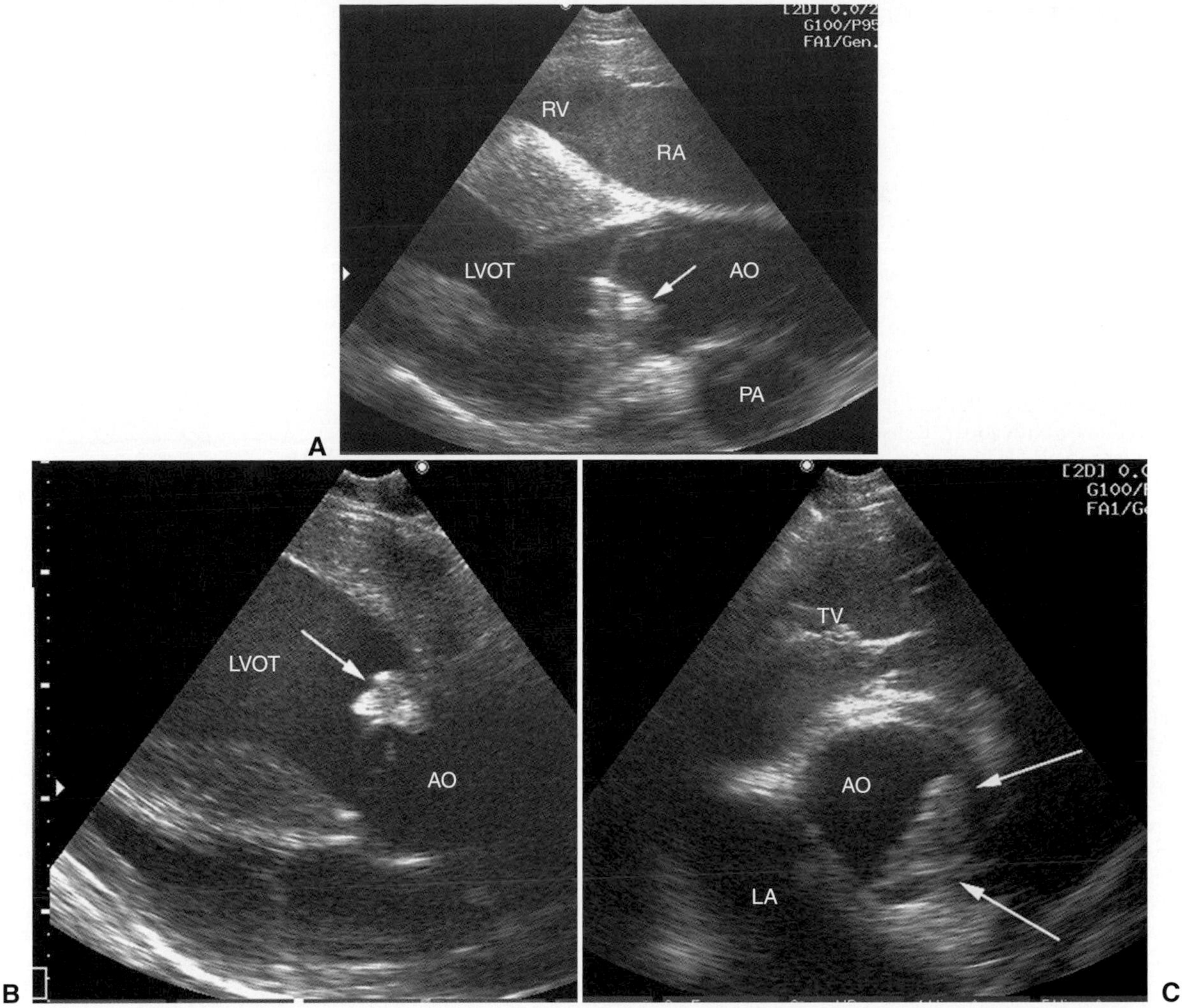

Fig. 2-3 Right (A) and left (B) long-axis echocardiograms of the left ventricular outflow tract *(LVOT)* and right short-axis (C) echocardiogram of the ascending aorta *(AO)* from 5-year-old Thoroughbred mare with infective endocarditis diagnosed 6 days earlier. Large, heterogenous vegetations *(arrows)* are attached to upper and lower aspects of the aortic valve and to the intimal surface of the aorta. *TV*, Tricuspid valve; *LA*, left atrium; *PA*, pulmonary artery; *RA*, right atrium; *RV*, right ventricle.

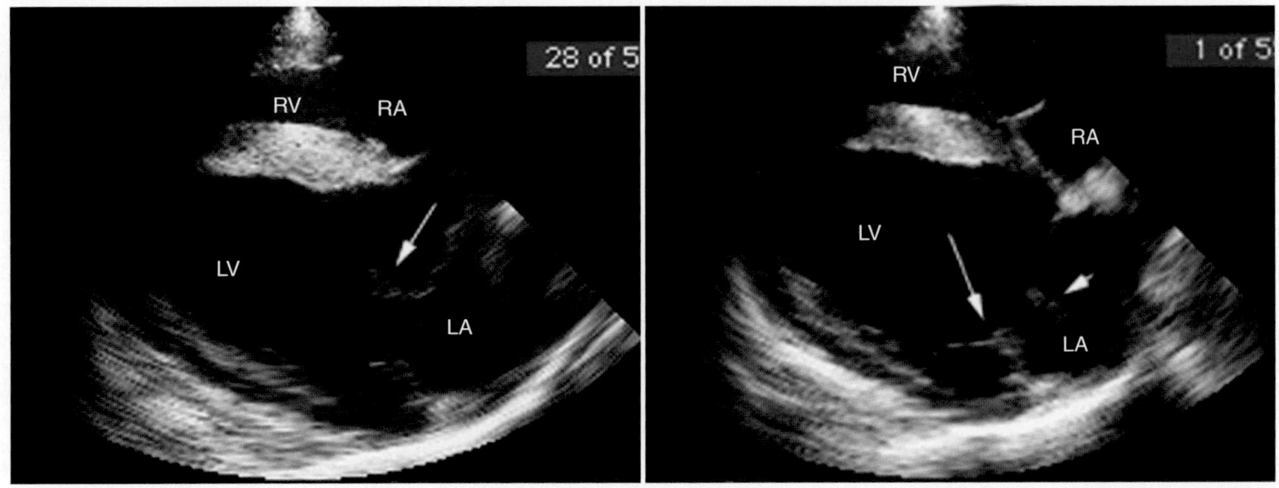

Fig. 2-4 Right long-axis echocardiograms from 8-year-old polo pony gelding with infective endocarditis diagnosed 2 days earlier. Vegetations *(arrows)* are visible on adjacent aspects of the septal and nonseptal cusps of the mitral valve, and rupture of a chorda tendinea is allowing a portion of the septal cusp *(arrowhead)* to prolapse into the left atrium *(LA)*. *RA*, Right atrium; *RV*, right ventricle; *LV*, left ventricle.

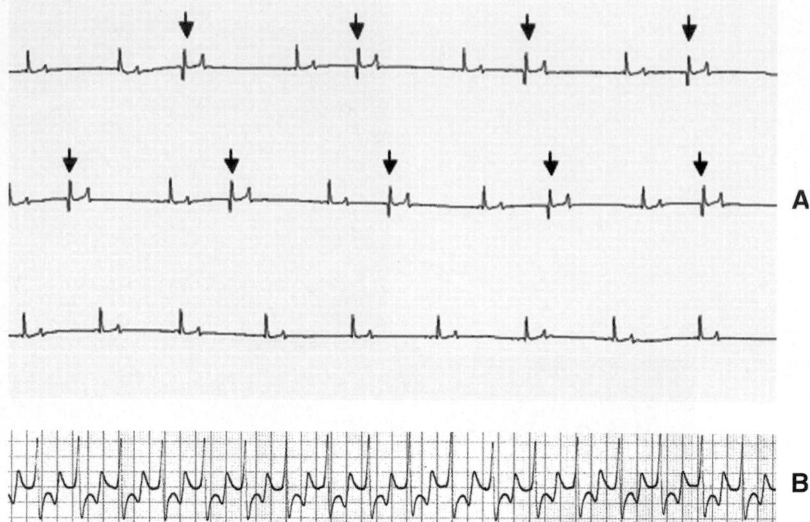

Fig. 2-5 A, Electrocardiogram (ECG) from 13-year-old mixed-breed mare with aortic infective endocarditis (IE) and concurrent myocarditis diagnosed 12 weeks earlier showing numerous isolated ventricular premature depolarizations. The mare's clinical status had improved considerably since this initial diagnosis, but she continued to have episodes of distress and weakness that were attributed to a paroxysmal ventricular arrhythmia (modified base-apex lead; see also Fig. 2-6). **B,** ECG from 5-year-old Thoroughbred mare with aortic IE diagnosed 6 days earlier showing an episode of monomorphic ventricular tachycardia that resolved after treatment with magnesium sulfate and lidocaine. One week later, 24-hour ambulatory ECG revealed normal sinus rhythm (base-apex lead; see also Fig. 2-3).

In general, aortic regurgitation appears to be better tolerated in horses than in humans, in whom severe hemodynamic collapse occurs more often with aortic IE or myocarditis than with mitral IE.[21] Nevertheless, in equine aortic IE, signs consistent with low cardiac output, left-sided heart failure, and CHF are reported.[19,31] Concurrent myocarditis or myocardial abscesses compromise myocardial function further, and arrhythmias are common (Fig. 2-5). Clearly, the more extensive the left-sided valvular pathology, the more severe are the hemodynamic consequences. Regurgitation caused by tricuspid IE is likely to have less direct hemodynamic impact,[7] although systemic venous and hepatic congestion can be expected.[10]

Regardless of the site of the vegetation, bacteremia is likely to induce SIRS and, consequently, distributive shock. The self-amplifying cascade of inflammatory mediators that is triggered in SIRS dysregulates hemodynamic control mechanisms. The pathogenesis of SIRS is described in Chapter 37. In brief, widespread vasodilation produces vascular blood pooling, decreased venous return, and decreased cardiac output.[34] This is exacerbated by a direct myocardial suppression, and when these changes are superimposed on mitral or aortic insufficiency, the situation worsens synergistically.[35]

Once IE is established, in addition to valvular pathology, local infection, bacteremia, and related hemodynamic consequences, embolic complications and immunologic events contribute to disease progression.[35,36] Myocarditis results from microabscesses, coronary vasculitis, immune complex deposition, and injury from microbial toxin production.[30] Myocardial infarcts,[8,9,29] coronary artery thrombosis,[6,8] and pulmonary artery thrombosis[2,6] may further compromise cardiac function. Embolic pneumonia occurs secondary to tricuspid IE.[4,10] Testicular, adrenal, and pancreatic infarcts have been described in a horse with aortic IE and a history of testicular torsion.[19] Renal infarcts are found in two thirds of humans who succumb to IE and were present in 8 of 28 horses (28.6%; CI 11.8%-45.3%) at postmortem examination.[5,7,9,19] All the equine cases of renal infarct involved IE in the left side of the heart; however, renal infarcts are occasionally associated with right-sided IE in humans, in whom the presumed source of emboli is thrombosed pulmonary vessels resulting from embolic pneumonia.[30]

Immunologically mediated glomerulonephritis, prerenal azotemia, and disseminated intravascular coagulation are also potential sequelae to IE.[4,10,30] The compromised individual with IE is at increased risk of developing acute tubular nephrosis in association with use of antimicrobials, such as the aminogylcosides.[30] Lameness and synovial effusion are common. Multifocal synovial distention is generally immunologic in origin;[6,12,15,18] however, septic embolism can lead to synovial sepsis, particularly in the digital sheath.[4,14] Various forms of neuropathology occur in approximately 30% of humans with IE, about half of whom have associated clinical signs and a high mortality rate.[37] These complications are relatively rare in horses, but their prevalence may be underreported (3 of 28 reported cases, 10.7%; CI 0%-22.25%) because of the lack of large, high-quality case series. Meningeal infarcts were described in two horses with IE, one of which had neurologic signs.[7] An additional horse with mitral and aortic IE developed unilateral blindness, optic neuritis, uveitis with endophthalmitis, and multifocal suppurative meningoencephalitis in association with *Actinobacillus equuli* infection.[5]

Clinical Findings

IE has been described in horses ranging from 2 months to 15 years of age, with a median age of 5 years and interquartile range of 10 months to 9 years. Thus, IE appears to be a disease of younger adults, although the demographics of the populations from which these cases were derived are unknown.[3-18,29,31,32] There is no apparent breed predisposition, but the ratio of males to females is 1.85:1, which is similar to that described in humans.[22] Fever is the most common presenting sign in horses with IE (Table 2-2).

Cardiac murmurs were present in all animals with left-sided involvement but in only three of six horses with tricuspid IE.[4,7,6] In the sole reported equine case of pulmonic IE, no murmur was detected.[4,7,14] Therefore, it is important to remember that absence of a cardiac murmur does not exclude a diagnosis of IE.[38] Murmurs are most likely to be absent in IE caused by a virulent microorganism that induces rapid, severe disease,[30] and interestingly, two of four equine reports include horses that died shortly after the onset of signs.[4,7] When present, the murmur of tricuspid regurgitation has its point of maximal intensity (PMI) over the right fourth intercostal space and is usually holosystolic. Mitral regurgitant murmurs are also holosystolic, with their PMI over the left fifth intercostal space. Aortic regurgitant murmurs are holodiastolic, with their PMI over the left fourth intercostal space, high in the axilla. Mitral IE and aortic IE are usually associated with very

Table • 2-2

*Major Clinical Findings in 35 Cases of Infective Endocarditis**

CLINICAL SIGN	NUMBER AFFECTED	PREVALENCE (%)	LOWER CONFIDENCE LIMIT (%)	UPPER CONFIDENCE LIMIT (%)
Fever and depression†	30	88.2	77.4	99.1
Cardiac murmur‡	28	87.5	76.0	99.0
Cardiac arrhythmia	11	31.4	16.0	46.8
Ventral edema	5	14.3	2.7	25.9
Lameness	9	25.7	11.2	40.2
Joint and/or tendon sheath distention	11	31.4	16.0	46.8
Weight loss	13	37.1	21.1	53.2
Respiratory signs	7	20.0	6.7	33.3

*With 29 cases from references 3-18, 29, 31, and 32, plus 6 from the author's clinic.
†Not reported = 1.
‡Not reported = 3.

loud murmurs that radiate over a wide area. Aortic IE murmurs, as with the murmur caused by severe degenerative aortic valve disease, typically have a squeaking or buzzing quality. A mitral regurgitant murmur with a honking quality should raise the suspicion of rupture of one or more chordae tendineae.

Additional signs of cardiovascular compromise that are not specific for IE include tachycardia, weak pulses, congested or pale mucous membranes, and petechiation. Affected horses are usually depressed, lethargic, anorexic, and weak.

Cardiac arrhythmias occur in approximately one third of horses with IE (Table 2-2). Ventricular arrhythmias may include isolated ventricular depolarizations or monomorphic or polymorphic ventricular tachycardias (Fig. 2-5). Episodic collapse or distress can be associated with arrhythmic episodes in both acute and chronic stages. Although no statistical association has been documented, horses with aortic IE appear to be most likely to develop ventricular arrhythmias. In humans, these are the patients most likely to develop coronary thrombosis and myocardial microabscess.[30] Supraventricular premature depolarizations[7,11,15] and atrial fibrillation[11] may occur, particularly in horses with mitral or left-sided atrial mural IE. Signs consistent with CHF, including ventral edema, pleural and peritoneal effusion, and venous congestion, may be detected on presentation or develop as disease progresses.

Lameness is a frequent presenting complaint for horses with IE (Table 2-2). This is often shifting in nature and may be associated with distention of one or more synovial structures.[6,12,15,18] IE should be considered as a potential source of hematogenous synovial sepsis.[4,14] Right-sided IE generally presents with clinical and radiographic signs relating to embolic pneumonia in humans.[38] Other clinical signs reported in horses with IE include ataxia or other neurologic abnormalities, blindness,[5] laminitis,[7] guttural pouch empyema, sinusitis,[26] umbilical infection,[29] and physitis.[11]

Diagnosis

Hematologic and blood biochemical abnormalities are not specific for IE but include leukocytosis (18 of 20 reported cases, 90%; CI 76.9%-100%), hyperfibrinogenemia (13 of 14 reported cases, 93%; CI 79.4%-100%), anemia (12 of 17 reported cases, 52.2%; CI 31.8%-72.6%), and less often, thrombocytopenia (1 of 13 reported cases, 7.1%; CI 0%-20.6%).[3-18,29,31,32] C-reactive protein (CRP), an acute-phase protein that increases in response to infection and inflammation, is considered particularly useful in diagnosis of IE in humans and is used to monitor therapy.[39] Suitable alternatives in the horse might be serum amyloid A and fibrinogen concentrations.[4] Increases in serum concentrations of creatinine and blood urea nitrogen warrant a guarded prognosis because they may indicate renal infarct.[7,19] Measurement of cardiac troponin I[40,41] and the cardiac isoenzyme of creatine kinase (CK-MB) can be useful in identifying myocardial lesions. Cardiac arrhythmias should be characterized; ambulatory electrocardiographic (ECG) monitoring may be useful in detecting paroxysmal arrhythmias that are not evident on a short rhythm strip.

The *Duke diagnostic criteria* for IE in humans, based on laboratory and echocardiographic findings, were developed to categorize patients as definite, possible, or rejected IE cases. *Major* criteria are (1) persistently positive blood cultures (the specific number of cultures required is defined by the specific organism in question) and (2) echocardiographic evidence of endocardial involvement. *Minor* criteria include (1) fever, (2) predisposition (e.g., preexisting heart condition), (3) vascular phenomenon (e.g., renal infarcts), (4) immunologic events (e.g., glomerulonephritis, positive rheumatoid factor), (5) positive blood cultures that fall short of the definitions of persistent bacteremia, and (6) suspicious but not definitive echocardiograms. Cases are *rejected* when (1) a firm alternative diagnosis is made, (2) the clinical signs resolve with antimicrobial therapy in 4 days or less, or (3) pathologic evidence is lacking at surgery or autopsy.[42] The Duke criteria are primarily a tool to allow comparison of patient groups in clinical research[30] but serve to emphasize the importance of blood culture and echocardiography in the diagnosis of IE. Echocardiography achieves improved sensitivity and equivalent specificity when these criteria are compared with older classification systems based on clinical and laboratory findings alone.[43-45] Similarly, in horses the majority of premortem diagnoses of IE are based on echocardiographic findings combined with laboratory findings.[5-8,10-12,14-16,18,31]

Blood culture is extremely important in the diagnostic evaluation of horses with IE because it may allow identification of a specific microorganism that will help define therapy. In IE there is continuous bacteremia, and therefore timing culture with fever spikes has no advantage. The optimal number of cultures is not known,[30] but at least three and ideally five blood samples obtained at hourly intervals using aseptic technique should be submitted. Prior antimicrobial therapy limits the likelihood of positive cultures.[20,43,46-48] Microorganisms were identified in 13 of 20 horses (68.4%; CI 47.5%-89.3%) when one to four cultures were submitted (median of two). In all cases, samples were obtained before antimicrobial therapy was initiated by the attending veterinarian, although almost all these horses had received antimicrobial medication before admission to the hospital where they were investigated. Passage of the blood sample through a device designed to remove antimicrobials before inoculation of blood onto culture media may enhance bacterial recovery rates. Cultures should be incubated for a minimum of 4 days before they are classified as negative because prior antimicrobial therapy may delay the growth of microorganisms.[20] Additional reasons for negative blood culture include extended course of illness, mural endocarditis, and infection with a fastidious microorganism or an obligate intracellular pathogen.[39]

The introduction of molecular techniques for the identification of microorganisms has lead to the recognition of a wide spectrum of causal organisms in culture-negative IE in humans,[49,50] and similar progress can be expected in veterinary medicine in the future. In such culture-negative infections, however, antimicrobial sensitivity testing is not possible, so the therapeutic advantage of identifying the specific causative organism is lost.[50]

Echocardiography has a pivotal role in the diagnosis of IE. The presence of an oscillating soft tissue mass attached to the valve cusps, endocardial surfaces of the cardiac chambers, or the intimal surface of the great vessels represents definitive evidence of a vegetation (see Figures 2-3 and 2-4). Many disease processes can cause thickening of the valve cusps, and it can be difficult to distinguish vegetations from other forms of nodular pathology. Recognition of oscillatory movement of a mass independent of movement of the valve confirms that it is a vegetation. In humans the use of transesophageal imaging provides superior resolution and has superior sensitivity to transthoracic echocardiography in detection of vegetations.[51] Currently, transesophageal imaging in horses is limited to a small number of veterinary hospitals and requires general anesthesia.[52] Because conventional transthoracic echocardiography requires transducers of relatively low frequency, vegetations may go undetected in some cases of equine IE.

Differentiating severe degenerative valvular disease from IE can be difficult. When severe nodular changes are detected in younger animals at low risk of severe degenerative valvular disease, particularly if the nodules are located on the low-pressure aspect of the valve (ventricular surface for aortic valve, atrial surfaces for mitral and tricuspid valves) and are accompanied by clinical and laboratory evidence of infection, a diagnosis of probable IE should be considered, with appropriate treatment instituted (at least until this diagnosis can be rejected after reaching an alternative diagnosis). In the early stages of the disease, vegetations tend to be fairly homogenous (see Figures 2-3 and 2-4), and as they become more organized, they become more echogenic and heterogenous. Additional structural changes may be visible, such as ruptured chordae tendineae, which cause portions of the valve (flail cusp) or chordae to prolapse into the atrium[33] (see Figure 2-4).

Doppler echocardiography allows identification of regurgitation and permits semiquantitation of its degree,[53] which is usually moderate to severe with IE (Fig. 2-6). Jet dimensions provide only a subjective impression of the degree of regurgitation, and these measurements are not very repeatable. Limitations are created by several factors; suboptimal image angulation leads to underestimation of jet size, particularly in the mitral valve, where regurgitant jets are often running at right angles to the image plane, and variation of the image plane is difficult because of anatomic constraints.[54] Additional Doppler echocardiographic findings indicative of

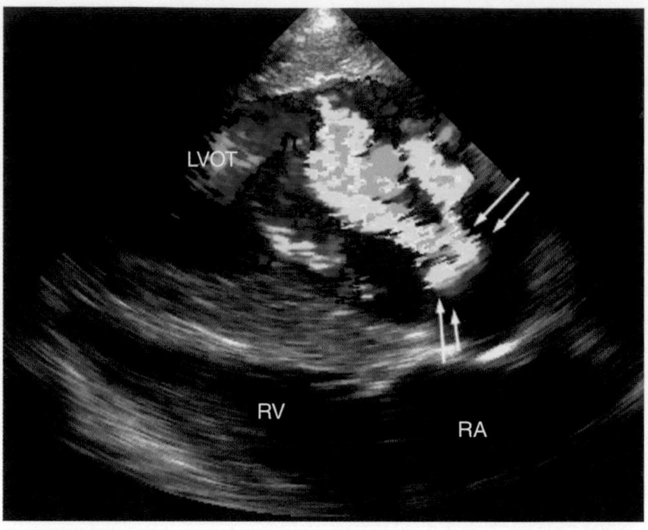

Fig. 2-6 Left long-axis color-flow Doppler echocardiogram from 13-year-old mixed-breed mare with aortic infective endocarditis and concurrent myocarditis of 12 weeks' duration. Two large (yellow and turquoise) jets of aortic regurgitation occupy most of the left ventricular outflow tract *(LVOT)*, and proximal flow convergence is present (between *arrows*). *RV*, Right ventricle; *RA*, right atrium. (See also Fig. 2-5.)

severe regurgitation include proximal flow convergence and velocity characteristics. Proximal flow convergence is recognized where nonturbulent, retrograde flow can be seen to speed up as it is approaching the regurgitant orifice, represented by bands of color on the proximal aspect of the regurgitating valve (Fig. 2-6). The velocity of flow across a regurgitant orifice or other intracardiac shunt is determined by the pressure difference between the two chambers in question.[54] With severe aortic regurgitation, flow early in diastole will have high velocity, but as left ventricular pressures rapidly increase resulting from the entry of the additional regurgitant volume, there will be a rapid deceleration of the regurgitant jet. In the presence of normal left atrial pressures that would be expected with mild mitral regurgitation, regurgitant flow between the left ventricle and left atrium is fast (usually greater than 5 ms^{-1}), whereas with severe regurgitation, the jet velocities are lower. However, accurate flow velocities also depend greatly on the operator, machine, and angle, and these velocities should be interpreted with extreme caution because they have not been validated as indices of severity of regurgitation in the horse. A useful rule of thumb is that if Doppler echocardiographic findings suggest that there is severe regurgitation, this is probably true. However, if Doppler echocardiography fails to demonstrate severe regurgitation in a horse in which clinical findings suggest otherwise, the clinician should remember that the Doppler echocardiographic findings may be misleading.

Two-dimensional and M-mode echocardiography are also useful in assessing the hemodynamic impact of valvular regurgitation.[33,55] In long-standing degenerative valve disease, the most accurate assessment of severity is gained by measurement of the diameter of the left ventricle, and these M-mode measurements correlate with heart failure score better than Doppler echocardiographic indices. Because IE is an *acute* severe condition, however, cardiac remodeling will not have occurred, and often the ventricular dimensions are normal despite the presence of severe regurgitation, although due to volume overload the ventricle may be hyperkinetic with

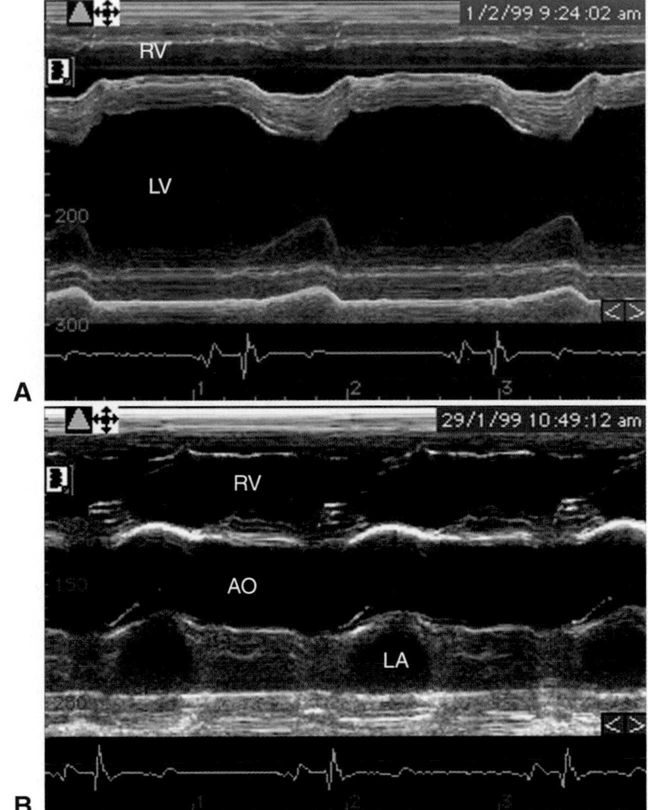

Fig. 2-7 M-mode echocardiograms from 8-year-old polo pony gelding with infective endocarditis diagnosed 2 days earlier. **A,** Ventricular image demonstrates that although there is no ventricular enlargement, the septal movement is exaggerated because the left ventricle is hyperkinetic. **B,** Left ventricular outflow image demonstrates flattening of the aortic root secondary to decreased cardiac output. *LV,* Left ventricle; *RV,* right ventricle; *AO,* aorta; *LA,* left atrium. (See also Figs. 2-4 and 2-8.)

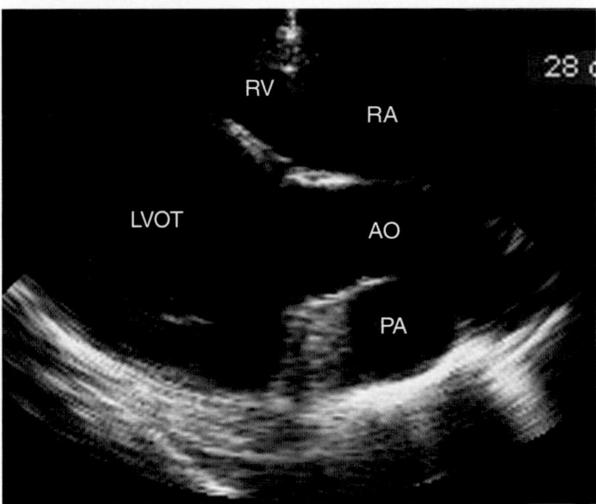

Fig. 2-8 Right long-axis echocardiogram of left ventricular outflow tract *(LVOT)* from 8-year-old polo pony gelding with infective endocarditis diagnosed 2 days previously. The pulmonary artery *(PA)* is dilated, and in this view it can be compared directly with the aorta *(AO)*. Note that measurements of the PA are made from the right inflow-outflow view. *RA,* Right atrium; *RV,* right ventricle. (See also Figs. 2-4 and 2-7.)

exaggerated movement of the septum and the free wall (Fig. 2-7). Fractional shortening* may be increased provided that myocardial function is maintained, but it may be decreased if there is concurrent myocardial failure. With reduced cardiac output, the diameter of the aortic root may be decreased and the movement of the aortic root depressed on M-mode echocardiography (Fig. 2-7). Dilation of the pulmonary artery is a sensitive indicator of pulmonary hypertension[33]; it can be identified by comparing the diameter of the pulmonary artery in a long-axis image of the right ventricular outflow tract with the diameter of the aorta in a long-axis image of the left ventricular outflow tract[56] (Fig. 2-8). In longstanding cases, signs of ventricular remodeling can be expected. As it enlarges, the left ventricle will typically take on a rounded or globoid shape at the apex, and M-mode measurements of the ventricular dimensions and septal-mitral E-point separation will increase.[33,55]

Therapy

The first goal of therapy is sterilization of the vegetations.[39,57] Successful treatment of IE requires bactericidal therapy over a prolonged period. It is extremely important to attempt to isolate the organism and determine antimicrobial sensitivity patterns if possible.[39] In the absence of specific culture results, broad-spectrum antimicrobial therapy should be instituted. Penicillin and gentamicin are the most common choices,* but previous reports have also described using ampicillin,[8] trimethoprim-sulfonamide,[3,7] metronidazole,[17] oxytetracycline,[6] ceftoxamine,[11] and rifampicin,[14] with no antimicrobial regimen emerging as superior to the others. Bactericidal drugs are preferable to bacteriostatic drugs in this life-threatening bacteremia.[39,58] It is difficult to predict the causative organism, although as noted previously, *Pasteurella* and *Actinobacillus* species represent about 20% of cases, and *Pseudomonas* spp. were isolated from about 10%. Consequently, penicillin with an aminoglycoside[57] or a fluoroquinolone such as enrofloxacin[58] can be predicted to have an appropriate spectrum of activity. Serum bactericidal titers can be used to monitor therapeutic efficacy. Serial dilutions of the patient's serum, collected at the end of dosing, are tested for their ability to inhibit growth of the bacteria previously isolated from the patient. Serum bactericidal titers of 1:16 or higher have been associated with successful outcomes in human IE.[57]

Drug efficacy may be compromised by poor penetration of the vegetation, high bacterial numbers and slow growth of deep-seated organisms.[57] The diffusion of antimicrobials within vegetations varies; ceftriaxone and penicillin generate a concentration gradient with decreasing levels towards the center, whereas others, such as fluoroquinolones, permeate the vegetation homogenously,[59] which, at least theoretically, should confer a therapeutic advantage. However, studies relating specifically to the pharmacokinetics and pharmacodynamics of common antimicrobials used in equine IE are lacking. Rifampin has excellent tissue penetration and should be effective against gram-positive organisms but should not be used in isolation because of concerns over the development of resistance. Rifampin also has potential to induce drug interactions with phenylbutazone and digoxin.[58] The clinician should

*Fractional shortening = LVIDd − LVIDs ÷ LVIDd where LVIDd = left ventricular internal dimension in diastole and LVIDs = left ventricular internal dimension in systole.

*References 4, 7, 11, 12, 14, 16, 17.

consider the possibility of concurrent renal pathology and prerenal azotemia and should use therapeutic drug monitoring with aminoglycosides to minimize the risk of renal toxicity.

Successful treatment of fungal IE has not been described in horses, although successful treatment of systemic candidiasis in foals with IV amphotericin B and oral fluconazole has been reported.[60] In humans, amphotericin B,[39] possibly combined with rifampin,[61] is used to treat IE caused by candidiasis. Fluconazole is less successful but avoids the nephrotoxic effects of amphotericin.[39]

Repeat blood cultures do not differentiate between complete and incomplete healing because vegetations may contain deep-seated organisms.[28] On the other hand, repeat cultures may be useful in identifying treatment failure.[57] In human medicine, serum concentrations of acute-phase CRP are used most often to monitor response to therapy and should begin to decrease within 24 hours of initiating effective therapy.[28] In horses, antimicrobial therapy should be continued until the white blood cell count, serum fibrinogen, and serum amyloid A concentrations have returned to normal. This may involve many weeks of treatment. After treatment is discontinued, these laboratory parameters as well as clinical signs (e.g., rectal temperature) should be evaluated frequently to ensure that any relapse can be detected early. The echocardiographic appearance of vegetations alters over time, becoming denser and more echogenic, but this does not necessarily provide any information on the sterility of the lesion.

Specific measures to combat SIRS are important in the early stages of therapy (see Chapter 37). All serum and plasma products containing antibodies to the lipopolysaccharide molecule, polymyxin B, pentoxifylline, flunixin meglumine, low-molecular-weight heparin, and aspirin are potentially useful.[34] However, renal function must be monitored carefully when polymixin B and nonsteroidal antiinflammatory drugs (NSAIDs) are used in patients that may have preexisting renal pathology.

Provision of cardiovascular support presents a particular problem in horses with IE. In conditions involving SIRS, high volumes of IV crystalloid and colloid fluids together with inotropic agents are advocated.[34] With severe regurgitation, however, increased preload and consequently increased stroke volume are likely to result in an increased regurgitant fraction, and therefore it is difficult to improve cardiac output with volume replacement.[35] In left-sided heart failure from other causes, vasodilators are used to support forward flow and cardiac output. The decrease in systemic vascular resistance (SVR) induced by SIRS may temporarily have a similar beneficial action in maintaining forward flow, and forward flow may decrease as SVR is restored when treating SIRS.[35] Drugs such as dopamine should be used cautiously because their beneficial effects in producing vasodilation of the renal, mesenteric, coronary, and intracerebral vasculature are present only when low doses (1-3 μg/kg/min) are used, whereas dopamine stimulates α-adrenoreceptors at higher doses, causing vasoconstriction. Similarly, because of its α-adrenoreceptor activity, norepinephrine is likely to be counterproductive in IE. The inotropic effects of dopamine and dobutamine mediated through β_1-adrenoreceptors are unlikely to be beneficial in many horses with IE. These drugs increase forward stroke volume by decreasing end-systolic volume; in acute mitral IE with normal left ventricular function, however, the afterload reduction created by the regurgitant pathway already allows for ejection to the point of minimum end-systolic volume.[35]

The arteriovenous dilator sodium nitroprusside along with diuretics is used to stabilize humans with left-sided IE, provided the arterial pressure is adequate for organ perfusion. Angiotensin-converting enzyme (ACE) inhibitors such as enalapril have a similar effect, and if arteriovenous dilation fails, the arterial dilator hydralazine is considered.[35] The pharmacokinetics of hydralazine have been established in the horse, with a dose of 0.5 mg/kg IV recommended.[62] Unfortunately, the oral bioavailability of enalapril in the horse is extremely low.[63] Sodium nitroprusside, hydralazine, and alternative ACE inhibitors have yet to be critically evaluated in equine patients with acute heart failure.[64] It is mandatory that the arterial pressure be monitored if such agents are employed. Furosemide is indicated if pulmonary edema is present and should be administered intravenously in the critically ill patient (1 mg/kg IV tid). Oral bioavailability is poor,[65] and the clinical response with oral administration is often disappointing.

Prognosis

The prognosis for equine IE is extremely guarded. Thirty-two of 40 horses (fatality rate 80%; CI 67.6%-92.4%) died or were euthanized (7 died, 19 euthanized, 6 not specified).[3-18,29,31,32] Even if the vegetation can be sterilized with antimicrobial therapy, unfortunately the structural damage to the heart valves is often so severe that CHF ensues. Clinical and laboratory signs of renal insufficiency and rupture of chordae tendineae warrant a poor prognosis.[29,30,33] Examination of the associations between survival and age, gender, affected cardiac sites, presence of arrhythmias, and clinical and laboratory findings has shown that horses with IE of the mitral valve, either alone or in combination with other sites, have an increased risk of not surviving (proportion of cases affecting mitral valve in nonsurvivors, 62.5%; in survivors, 12.5%; $p = 0.0174$; odds ratio 12.09; CI 1.27-106.9). No other factor was significantly associated with survival. This demonstrates that horses with mitral vegetations are less likely to survive, although clearly with such a small study group, the magnitude of the increased risk is difficult to quantify.

INFLAMMATORY VALVULITIS

Inflammatory valvulitis is an uncommon cause of valvular regurgitation in horses, occurring much less frequently than degenerative valvular disease.[66] Its pathologic features have not been documented rigorously, and detailed clinical descriptions are lacking. Early work on equine valvular pathology demonstrated inflammatory cell infiltrates in valvular lesions, and it was proposed at that time that this might represent a parallel condition to human rheumatic heart disease, but this hypothesis has not been explored critically. Acute rheumatic fever and its chronic sequela, rheumatic heart disease, remain a significant human health issue in developing countries.[67] The pathogenesis involves an exaggerated immune response to streptococcal epitopes in a susceptible host and probably involves molecular mimicry between epitopes on the pathogen and host tissues resulting from structural similarities between streptococcal M protein and myosin (α-helical, coiled molecules). Valvular tissue does not contain myosin, and the involvement of the valve results from the presence of laminin, which has a similar molecular structure to myosin and M protein.[67]

Inflammatory valvulitis is difficult to diagnose with certainty. It should be considered in horses with valvular regurgitation and echocardiographically visible valve thickening, for which the main alternative differential diagnoses are degenerative valvular disease, congenital valvular dysplasia, and IE. In particular, inflammatory valvulitis should be suspected in individuals with concurrent mild ventricular dysfunction when the regurgitation improves or resolves after a period of rest, with or without corticosteroid therapy, because the other forms of valvular disease are unlikely to respond in this way. It is important for the clinician required to offer a prognosis for horses presenting with cardiac murmurs of valvular regurgitation to remember that occasionally, valvular regurgitation may be reversible if caused by inflammatory valvulitis. Further studies are needed to define this condition and its pathogenesis, management, and prognosis.

MYOCARDITIS

Etiology and Pathogenesis

Infection with bacteria, viruses,[68] and fungi[66,69] can cause myocardial inflammation. Clinical signs consistent with myocarditis may also occur as sequelae to viral or bacterial respiratory infection.[66] However, detailed reports of such cases are rare, and specific information on the pathogenesis is minimal.

Clinical Findings

Horses with myocarditis can present with signs of varying severity depending on the extent of the pathology. With focal myocarditis, horses may display fairly mild signs (e.g., impaired performance) only on maximal exercise, whereas horses with generalized myocarditis will present with signs of acute heart failure (Fig. 2-9). In more severe cases, respiratory distress, weakness, ataxia, collapse, weak pulses, tachycardia, arrhythmias, cardiac murmurs, and pulmonary and ventral edema occur.

Diagnosis

All forms of cardiac arrhythmias can occur with both generalized and focal myocarditis. Ambulatory ECG monitoring is useful in identifying intermittent arrhythmias and assessing response to therapy. Radiotelemetric techniques are invaluable for identification of exercise-induced arrhythmias. Ventricular dilation and abnormal wall movement are the echocardiographic hallmarks of severe myocardial dysfunction. The ventricles may be subjectively enlarged with a globoid appearance at the apex (Fig. 2-10). Global myocardial dysfunction leads to reduction in movement of the ventricular walls (Fig. 2-11) and reduction in the fractional shortening. Focal myocardial disease may produce regional wall movement abnormalities, but often the echocardiogram is unremarkable. With ventricular dilation the septal-mitral E-point separation increases (Fig. 2-11, *B*), and reduced cardiac output leads to flattening of the aortic root on M-mode echocardiography, prolongation of the preejection period, and decreases in the left ventricular ejection periods.

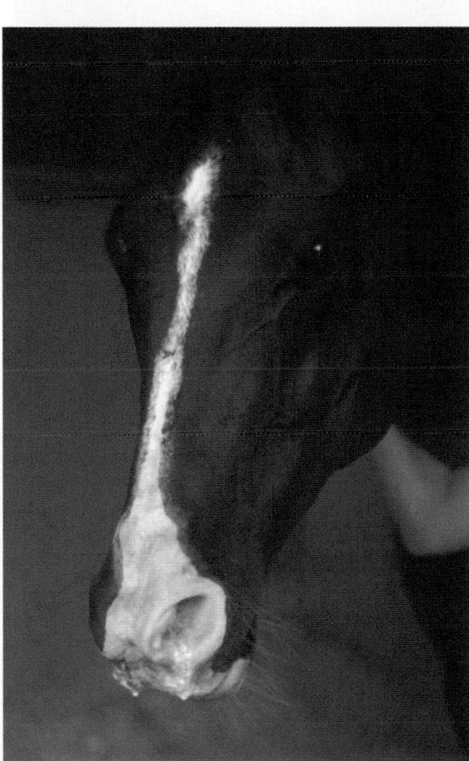

Fig. 2-9 Frothy nasal discharge, consistent with pulmonary edema, in 11-year-old Arabian mare with acute myocarditis.

Cardiac troponin I is considered the most specific biochemical marker of myocardial disease,[40,41] and increases in the serum concentration of CK-MB or lactate dehydrogenase (LDH) also suggest myocardial injury.[66] Marked increases in cardiac troponin I should prompt further investigations; however, minor increases are often encountered in biochemical profiles performed at the in-house laboratory at the author's clinic, and these horses rarely have any other evidence of myocardial disease when investigated with echocardiography or exercising and 24-hour ambulatory ECG monitoring. Evaluation of seven horses with myocardial pathology presenting to the author's clinic suggests that cardiac troponin I is not more sensitive than CK-MB for detection of myocardial disease in horses. Increases in CK-MB, but not in cardiac troponin I, were found in horses that had myocardial disease of more than 2 weeks' duration.* Further work is required to determine the sensitivity and specificity of biochemical markers of myocardial injury.

Therapy

Treatment of myocarditis has not been well defined. If an infective origin is suspected, broad-spectrum antimicrobials are indicated. With other forms of myocardial pathology, treatment with corticosteroids is often prescribed. Dobutamine (1-5 μg/kg/min) may improve cardiac output.[64] Furosemide may relieve pulmonary congestion, and digoxin has potentially beneficial positive inotropic effects and negative chronotropic effects. Digoxin can be associated with ventricular arrhythmias (or *dysrhythmias*), and phenytoin is recommended for treatment of digoxin-induced arrhythmias.[70] In the horse, supraventricular premature depolarizations are often prevented from reaching the ventricles by the action of the vagus nerve on the atrioventricular (AV) node, such that the ventricular rate remains fairly stable in their presence, rendering specific antidysrhythmic therapy unnecessary. Digoxin may be used concurrently to suppress conduction at the AV node if necessary. Ventricular arrhythmias are much more likely to require antidysrhythmic therapy. Accepted guidelines suggest that antidysrhythmics should be considered when the heart rate is rapid (>100 beats/min), the arrhythmia is polymorphic, and R-on-T phenomenon is present. However, the clinical status of the animal is the most important factor to consider, and the decision to use antidysrhythmic drugs should be based on the presence or absence of signs of low cardiac output (e.g., weakness, cold extremities, pallor, hypotension, azotemia). Procainamide, lidocaine, and quinidine gluconate are popular first choices for emergency treatment of unstable ventricular tachycardia. Magnesium sulfate is inexpensive and readily available and can be efficacious alone or in combination with other antidysrhythmic agents.[71] Phenytoin may be effective in cases refractory to therapy with other antidysrhythmics.[72] (See Table 2-3.)

Prognosis

The prognosis for myocarditis is variable. Horses with suspected focal myocarditis, manifested by cardiac arrhythmias

*Courtesy J. Sento and C. Marr (unpublished data).

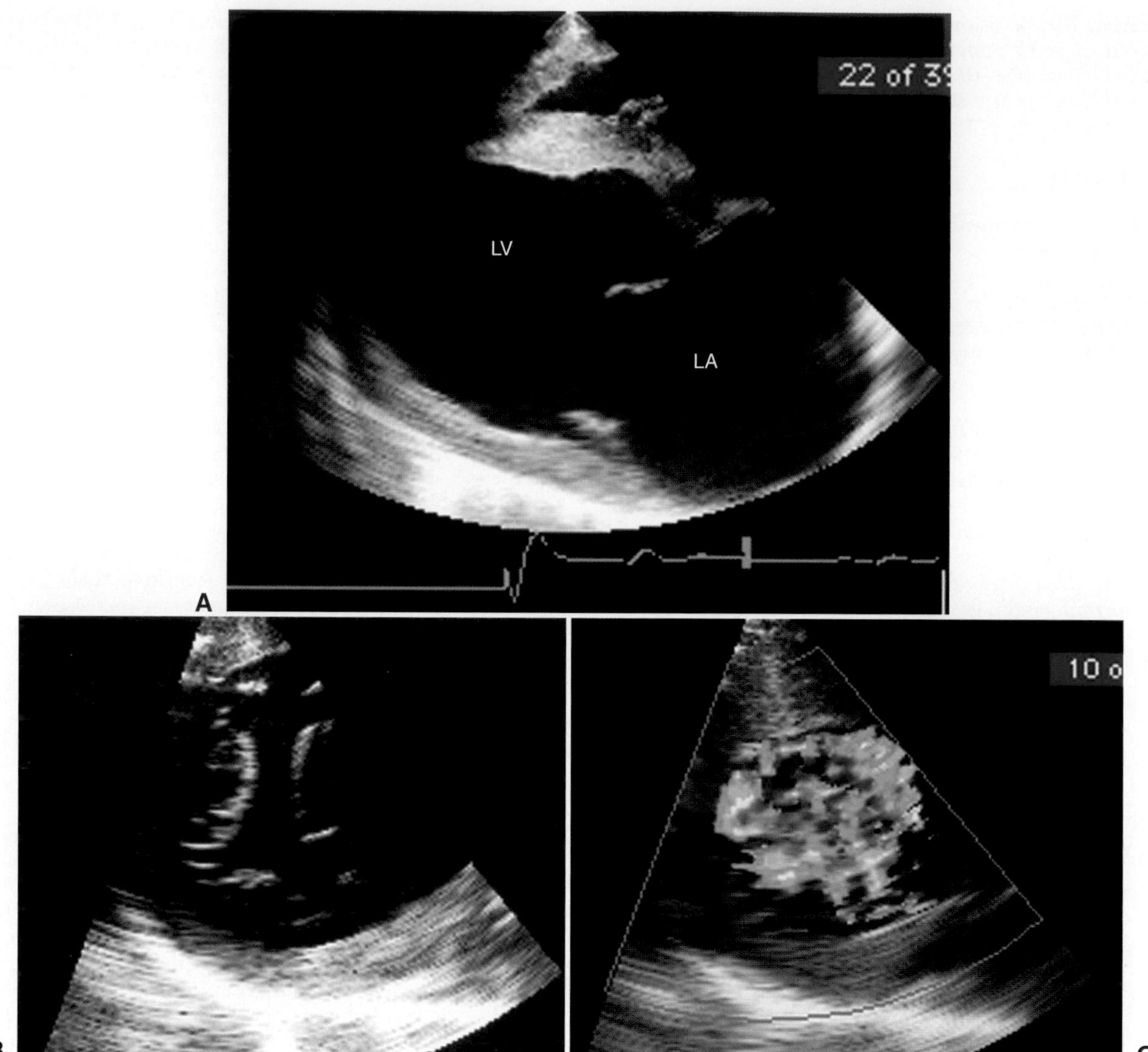

Fig. 2-10 Right long-axis echocardiogram of ventricles and atria **(A)** and left short-axis echocardiograms at level of mitral valve **(B)** and just above the mitral valve **(C)** from 7-year-old Thoroughbred gelding with myocarditis of unknown etiology. There is marked dilation of the left ventricle *(LV)* and left atrium *(LA)*. The mitral valve annulus is incompetent secondary to ventricular dilation *(B)*, and severe mitral regurgitation (green/yellow/turquoise) is evident on the color-flow Doppler image.

and poor performance, will usually have a good prognosis for life. Their athletic performance may be limited, however, and rider safety is an issue if persistent, exercise-induced arrhythmias are present. The prognosis for horses with generalized myocardial disease is poor.

PERICARDITIS

Etiology and Pathogenesis

Pericarditis can be effusive, noneffusive, or constrictive. *Effusive* pericarditis is most often fibrinous and neutrophilic in nature.[73-77] Much less often, nonfibrinous, eosinophilic and histocytic effusions have been described.[74] *Constrictive* pericarditis occurs when fibrin matures to fibrous tissue or when pericardial or myocardial injury results in fibrosis.[78] *Noneffusive* pericarditis is not well described in horses but should be considered in individuals presenting with signs consistent with pericardial disease in which no effusion is identified.[76] Rarely, pericarditis may be associated with *Mycoplasma felis* infection[79] and with trauma arising from external thoracic injury,[80] penetrating foreign bodies entering through the gastrointestinal tract,[81] and iatrogenic penetration during bone marrow aspiration.[82]

However, pericarditis appears to be of two major types: (1) *idiopathic* or immune-mediated infection and (2) *septic* pericarditis, caused by bacterial infection. Until recently, the vast majority of reported cases were classified as idiopathic. In humans, idiopathic pericarditis is viral in origin and is attributed to direct cytopathic effects, infiltration of tissues in which virus is evidenced by cytotoxic lymphocytes, and immune-mediated processes.[63] Similar mechanisms likely

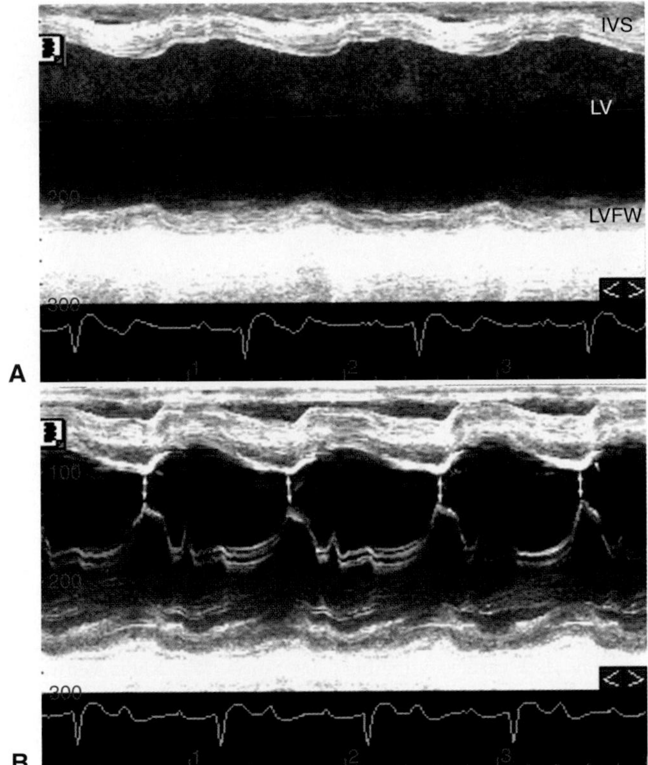

Fig. 2-11 M-mode echocardiograms at level of ventricles (A) and mitral valve (B) from 11-year-old Arabian mare with acute myocarditis. Movement of interventricular septum *(IVS)* and left ventricular free wall *(LVFW)* is greatly reduced, and there is increase in the septal-mitral E-point separation (*arrows* in *B*). *LV*, Left ventricle. (See also Fig. 2-9.)

occur in the horse. Horses with pericarditis often have a recent or current history of respiratory disease,[73,75,76] and rising titers to equine herpesvirus type 1 (EHV-1) have been observed on paired serology in 2 of 18 cases in one study.[76] Nevertheless, the evidence for a viral etiology, whether directly or through immune-mediated mechanisms, remains scant. Idiopathic pericarditis has also been observed as a sequela to pleuritis and peritonitis,[73,75,76] and occasionally there is evidence of concurrent immune-mediated disorders, such as vasculitis and hemolytic anemia.[76]

Bacterial infection is the other major cause of fibrinoeffusive and constrictive pericarditis. In an epidemic of equine pericarditis that occurred in association with early and late fetal losses in Kentucky (mare reproductive loss syndrome), bacteria were isolated from 13 of 32 pericarditis cases, with *Actinobacillus* spp. identified in 11 of 13 horses[77] and in three of four[83] and one of four[73] horses in other reports. *Escherichia coli, Enterococcus faecalis, Streptococcus equi subsp. zooepidemicus,*[77] *Streptococcus bovis,*[68] and *Corynebacterium pseudotuberculosis*[84] have been reported in individual cases, and β-hemolytic *Streptococcus* spp. were isolated in one of six[75] and 2 of 18 reported cases of equine pericarditis.[76] Of 85 cases reported in the literature since 1980, bacterial infection accounts for approximately one third of cases (27.1%; CI 17.6%-36.5%). *Actinobacillus* species are the most common isolate from pericardial fluid of horses with bacterial pericarditis (65.2%; CI 45.8%-84.7%).[68,73-88] *Actinobacillus* spp. are commensal bacteria of mucosal surfaces that appear to be pericardiotrophic in the horse. In the outbreak of pericarditis in Kentucky, exposure to Eastern tent caterpillars was the greatest risk factor for the development of pericarditis, and the temporal distribution of cases was consistent with a point-source epidemic.[89] Thus, some unidentified mechanism most likely led to a breakdown of mucosal barriers, facilitating opportunistic infection in these horses.[77]

The hemodynamic effects of effusive pericarditis depend on the volume of fluid within the pericardial sac and its rate of accumulation. Fibrin tends to accumulate in a villonodular arrangement on both inner surfaces of the pericardial sac (Fig. 2-12). Fluid and fibrin restrict diastolic filling of the

Table • **2-3**

Antidysrhythmic Agents Used In Horses

DRUG	INDICATIONS	DOSE*
Atropine	Bradycardia	0.005-0.01 mg/kg IV
Bretylium tosylate	Ventricular fibrillation	3-10 mg/kg IV
Digoxin	Supraventricular tachycardia	0.0022 mg/kg IV 0.011 mg/kg PO, q12h
Lidocaine	Ventricular tachycardia	0.25 mg/kg IV bolus, can repeat in 5-10 minutes
Magnesium sulfate	Ventricular tachycardia	0.004 mg/kg IV boluses, q5min intervals to 0.05 mg/kg
Phenytoin sodium	Ventricular and supraventricular tachycardia	20-22 mg/kg PO q12h for 3 or 4 doses followed by 10-15 mg/kg PO q12h
Procainamide	Ventricular and supraventricular tachycardia	1 mg/kg/min IV to 20 mg/kg
Propranolol	Ventricular and supraventricular tachycardia	0.03-2 mg/kg IV 25-35 mg/kg PO, q12h
Quinidine gluconate	Ventricular and supraventricular tachycardia	0.5-2.2 mg/kg bolus q10min to 12 mg/kg
Verapamil	Supraventricular tachycardia	0.025-0.05 mg/kg IV q30min to 0.2 mg/kg

**IV*, Intravenously, intravenous; *PO*, orally; *q12h*, every 12 hours.

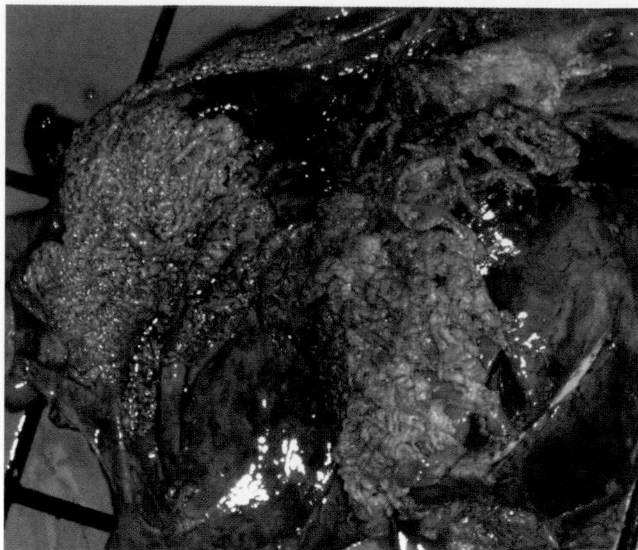

Fig. 2-12 Pathologic specimen from 14-year-old Thoroughbred gelding with septic fibrinoeffusive pericarditis of about 3 weeks' duration. Both the pericardial (left of image) and the epicardial (right of image) surface is covered with villonodular deposits of fibrin.

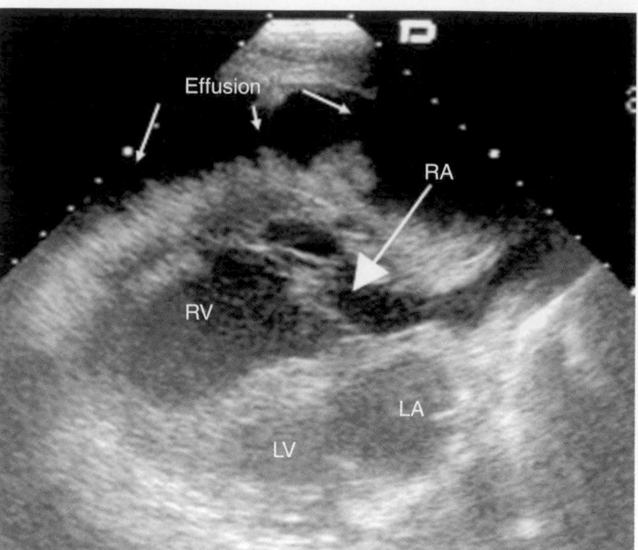

Fig. 2-13 Right parasternal long-axis echocardiogram from 2-week-old Thoroughbred colt foal with septic fibrinoeffusive pericarditis. Right atrium *(RA)* is collapsed from cardiac tamponade, and left cardiac chambers are small. *RV*, Right ventricle; *LV*, left ventricle; *LA*, left atrium. (See also Fig. 2-15.) (Courtesy Dr. Jan Bright, College of Veterinary Medicine and Biomedical Sciences, Colorado State University.)

heart and have the most impact on the low-pressure right side of the heart. With larger amount of fluid and fibrin, all cardiac chambers may be reduced in volume. Venous return is compromised, and diastolic myocardial perfusion and contractility are decreased, resulting in decreased stroke volume and cardiac output.[78] With constrictive pericarditis, the initial phase of diastolic filling is unimpeded, but when a critical diastolic volume is reached, filling ceases rapidly as the limit of the noncompliant pericardium is reached. Ventricular preload is decreased, leading to decreased stroke volume.[86] In both situations, there is a compensatory tachycardia to maintain cardiac output, and signs of right-sided failure predominate.

Clinical Findings

No specific breed predispositions for pericarditis have been identified. Younger horses may be at increased risk, although in the sole case-control study that has examined this risk factor, the study design may have biased this result.[89] Intact males were overrepresented and geldings underrepresented compared with the general hospital population in another study.[76] Common presenting complaints include fever, anorexia, and lethargy. Specific cardiovascular signs include tachycardia, weak peripheral arterial pulses, muffled heart sounds, cardiac murmurs, and pericardial friction rubs, which are usually biphasic or triphasic sounds that coincide with the heart rate and that may not become apparent until the pericardial effusion is removed. Pericarditis cannot be excluded in the absence of these signs, and horses often present with signs relating to concurrent respiratory disease. Right-sided heart failure is manifested by ventral edema, venous distention, and pleural and peritoneal effusions evident on ultrasonography.[73,75,78,86]

Diagnosis

Echocardiography

Echocardiography is the most important tool for diagnosis of pericarditis. Pericardial fluid creates an anechoic space between the parietal pericardium and the epicardial surface of the heart, and a subjective assessment of its volume can be made. Fibrin typically appears as tags of tissue that are slightly more echogenic than the myocardium (Fig. 2-13). Echocardiographic findings suggestive of cardiac tamponade include right atrial collapse, right ventricular early-diastolic collapse, overall decreases in chamber size, reduced fractional shortening, and decreased opening and slowing of the closure of the anterior leaflet of the mitral valve.[63]

The main alternative differential diagnoses for fluid within the pericardial sac are hemopericardium and neoplastic effusion; neither is typically associated with the accumulation of large amounts of fibrin. In *hemopericardium* the fluid is usually slightly echogenic, and diagnostic ultrasonography may reveal the source of hemorrhage, such as fractured ribs or a ruptured sinus of Valsalva aneurysm. Therefore, these structures should be examined carefully when fluid is detected within the pericardium. With *neoplastic effusion*, masses within the pericardial sac or heart may be visible, and cytologic characterization of the pericardial fluid may be diagnostic.

In constrictive pericarditis, pericardial thickening may or may not be evident. Characteristically, there is abrupt cessation of ventricular filling during early diastole, diastolic flattening of the left ventricular free–wall, and abnormal increases in tricuspid flow with abnormal decreases in mitral flow during inspiration.[78,86]

Electrocardiography, Thoracic Radiography, and Cardiac Catheterization

The most common ECG findings in horses with pericarditis are decreased QRS amplitude and electrical alternans (variations in amplitude).[74,75] Decreased QRS amplitude is caused by fluid damping and short-circuiting of the electrical signal (Fig. 2-14). This QRS decrease is not specific to pericarditis and can also be seen in horses with obesity, chronic respiratory disease, diaphragmatic hernia, and thoracic masses.[78]

Thoracic radiography adds little to the information obtained with echocardiography. Enlargement of the cardiac silhouette may be present (Fig. 2-15), but in many cases, pleural effusion obscures the heart.[74,86]

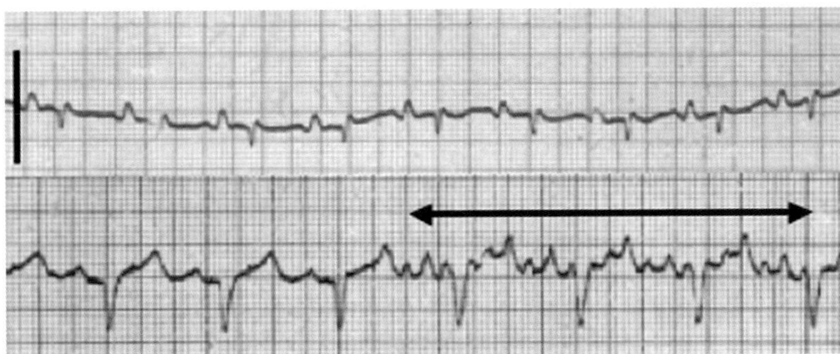

Fig. 2-14 Electrocardiograms from 18-month-old Standardbred filly with fibrinoeffusive idiopathic pericarditis. *Upper panel*, Small complexes that increase in size during pericardial drainage (*lower panel*, which has induced artifact resulting from muscle tremors [under *double arrow*]). Vertical bar indicates 1 mV; paper speed 25 ms^{-1}.

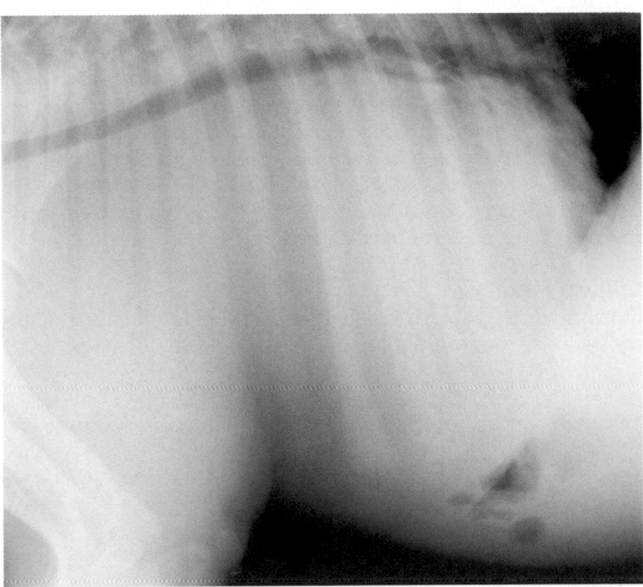

Fig. 2-15 Lateral thoracic radiograph from a 2-week-old Thoroughbred colt foal with septic fibrinoeffusive pericarditis. The cardiac silhouette is increased in size, with marked tracheal elevation. (See also Fig. 2-13.) (Courtesy Dr. Jan Bright, College of Veterinary Medicine and Biomedical Sciences, Colorado State University.)

Cardiac catheterization provides the definitive diagnosis of constrictive pericarditis. There is equalization of the right atrial and right ventricular pressures, and a dip-and-plateau configuration of the right ventricular pressure curve reflects the abrupt termination of diastolic filling when the limit of compliance of the pericardium is reached.[86]

Laboratory Investigations

Leukocytosis, neutrophilia, and hyperfibrinogenemia are common but nonspecific findings in pericarditis. Paired serology for influenza, equine herpesvirus, and equine viral arteritis may be useful. Renal function should be assessed because prerenal azotemia is often present.

Box 2-1 lists guidelines for collection of pericardial fluid. Pericardial fluid should contain less than 1500×10^6/L total nucleated cells and have a protein content less than 2.5 g/dL.[90] Samples of pericardial fluid should be submitted for bacteriologic culture, and culture of mycoplasmal species may also be useful. Ideally, culture should be performed before antimicrobial therapy is instituted. The diagnosis of septic pericarditis is based on the identification of increased

Box • 2-1

Technique for Pericardiocentesis

1. Location for pericardiocentesis
   - Left 4 to 6 intercostal spaces, approximately 6 cm ventral to point of shoulder.
   - Selection of site is facilitated by echocardiography.
2. Sedation for pericardiocentesis
   - May not be necessary depending on the horse's clinical status.
   - If necessary, use with caution; these drugs may exacerbate cardiovascular compromise.
3. Monitoring for pericardiocentesis
   - Monitor the cardiac rhythm for ventricular arrhythmias.
   - Have appropriate doses of procainamide, quinidine, or lidocaine at hand (see Table 2-3).
   - If ventricular arrhythmia occurs, the needle should be retracted immediately.
   - If ventricular arrhythmia persists, antidysrhythmic drugs are necessary (see Table 2-3).
4. Preparation of site
   - Clip and surgical scrub.
   - Infiltration of lidocaine in skin, subcutaneous layers, and intercostal muscles.
5. Selection of catheter and drain
   - For small sample collection: over-the-needle intravenous catheters (14 g, 15 cm) or blunt-ended teat cannulae.
   - For lavage: chest drains (16-24 French).
6. Insertion of catheter and drain
   - Stab incision.
   - Insert catheter and drain carefully using the minimum force while observing the ECG continuously.
   - Withdraw trocar promptly once pericardial sac has been penetrated.
   - Be prepared to seal the catheter with an artery forceps or similar instrument if air enters.
7. Maintenance of drain
   - Secure drain using purse-string suture.
   - After lavage, flush with a small volume of heparinized saline.
   - Seal drain with a clamp or sterile syringe.
   - Clean drain entry site twice daily.
   - Cover with gauze, tape, and bandage material to keep the site clean.

numbers of degenerative neutrophils, with or without cytologic evidence of bacteria. Idiopathic or immune-mediated pericarditis is characterized by the presence of increased numbers of well-preserved neutrophils. Monitoring glucose concentrations in the pericardial effusion may be helpful as an immediate assessment of sepsis. Glucose concentrations of less than 2.2 mmol/L (40 mg/dL) suggest sepsis, and concentrations greater than 3.3 mmol/L (60 mg/dL) probably indicate a sterile effusion.[79]

Therapy

Pericardial drainage and possibly lavage should be considered for horses with moderate to severe pericardial effusion.[76,85] Echocardiographic signs of cardiac tamponade, particularly marked right atrial collapse (see Fig. 2-13), should prompt emergency pericardiocentesis to restore cardiac function (see Box 2-1). During the procedure, ECG monitoring can identify ventricular arrhythmias and facilitate prompt treatment (see Fig. 2-14). After drainage, 1 to 2 L of 0.9% saline may be infused and left in place for 30 to 60 minutes before removal. Another liter of saline solution is then inserted and left in place until the next drainage-lavage cycle. Drainage-lavage may be repeated twice daily until the volume of fluid removed at the beginning of a drainage session is less than the amount infused at the end of the preceding session.[78]

Broad-spectrum antimicrobial therapy is indicated for horses with documented sepsis and while awaiting pericardial fluid cytology.[57] Antimicrobials are also often used prophylactically in horses with suspected nonseptic immune-mediated pericarditis.[76] Antimicrobial therapy is ideally based on pericardial fluid culture results, but these are often negative. Given the high prevalence of infection with *Actinobacillus* and *Streptococcus* species, appropriate empiric choices include penicillin and an aminoglycoside or cephalosporins. Experimental studies in dogs suggest that these drugs should penetrate the pericardium effectively.[57] Sodium penicillin G (10×10^6 units in a 420-kg mare)[76,85] and gentamicin (no dose reported)[75,78] can be instilled at the end of drainage as adjunctive antimicrobial therapy.

Corticosteroids have been advocated for treatment of idiopathic or immune-mediated pericarditis.[74,76] Decision making in these cases is complicated by the concern of possible active viral infection, but the majority of affected horses apparently are not viremic. Supportive therapy includes NSAIDs, and if the patient has prerenal azotemia, the cautious use of IV fluids is warranted. In this horse it is helpful to monitor central venous pressure so that fluid therapy can be closely titrated.

Prognosis

The prognosis for idiopathic or immune-mediated pericarditis appears to be very favorable.[74,76] Similarly, there are several reports of successful treatment of septic pericarditis using drainage or drainage-lavage techniques.[75,78,87] Constrictive pericarditis warrants a poor prognosis. A partial pericardiectomy technique has been reported but was ultimately unsuccessful because the pericardial fibrosis returned.[86] Chronic pericarditis has been associated with chronic lameness resulting from hypertrophic osteopathy in one horse.[88]

THROMBOPHLEBITIS

Etiology and Pathogenesis

Thrombophlebitis is defined as vein thrombosis accompanied by mural inflammation and is a common complication of IV catheterization.[91] The prevalence of jugular thrombosis in horses being treated for a variety of gastrointestinal (GI) diseases has ranged from 6% to 22%. Combining data from these studies suggests that the prevalence in this patient group is approximately 18% (CI 13.0%-22.8%).[92-94] Many proven and putative positive risk factors exist for thrombophlebitis. Use of home-produced fluid solutions, fever, diarrhea, and duration of IV treatment increase risk.[91] Foals and horses with colic or diarrhea are more likely to have bacteria isolated from catheters after removal.[95] Horses with GI disease are at risk of developing coagulopathies, which contributes to the propensity to develop jugular thrombophlebitis during treatment. Putative but unproven risk factors for thrombophlebitis include administration of antimicrobials and NSAIDs, which irritate the vascular endothelium; rapid IV fluid infusion rates; and standing with the head down for prolonged periods. These latter two factors may predispose to thrombophlebitis because they promote turbulent blood flow.[96]

Studies investigating catheter types and materials have lacked statistical power, but both catheter material and design are likely to be important. Flexible polyurethane over-the-wire catheters are assumed to have less risk than the more rigid polyurethane over-the-needle catheters, and Teflon or polytetrafluoroethylene catheters are likely to carry the greatest risk.[96] Jugular thrombophlebitis may be septic or nonseptic. Microorganisms most often isolated from the tips of IV catheters are coagulase-negative *Staphylococcus* spp., *Corynebacterium* spp., *Enterobacter* spp., and *Streptococcus* spp.[95]

Clinical Findings

Swelling or palpable thickening of the jugular vein is characteristic of thrombophlebitis. There may be variable degrees of

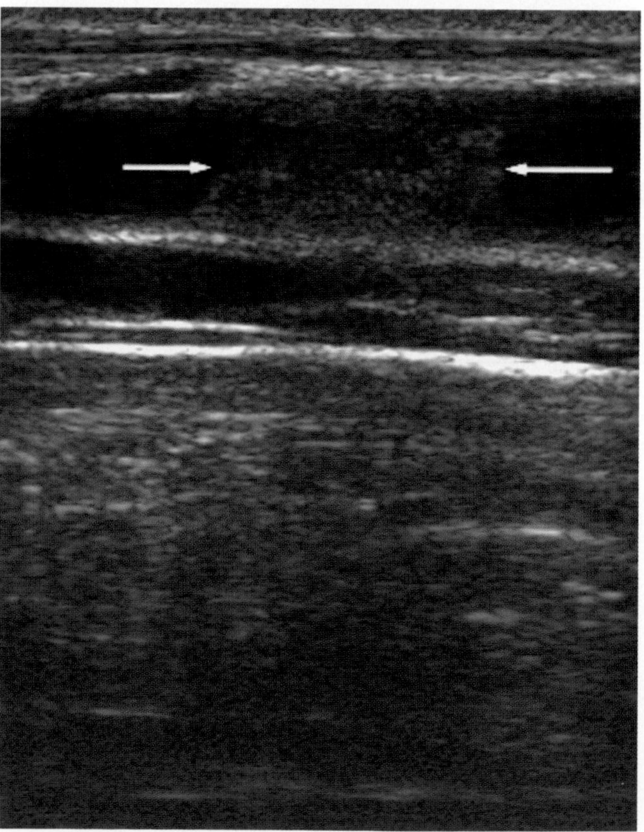

Fig. 2-16 Longitudinal ultrasonogram of jugular vein from 3-year-old Thoroughbred colt that developed jugular thrombosis after surgery to correct colon torsion. A small, homogenous, nonseptic thrombus is visible *(arrows)*.

perivenous swelling. Heat, pain, fever, and discharge from the site of venipuncture suggest sepsis. Acute-onset, severe thrombophlebitis may result in obstruction to venous drainage of the head, and swelling may occur in the supraorbital area, muzzle, and cheek on the affected side. Bilateral thrombosis may be associated with swelling of the tongue and airway obstruction. Chronic thrombophlebitis can lead to distention of the facial veins and discharging abscesses.

Diagnosis

Diagnostic Ultrasonography

Diagnostic ultrasonography is useful to characterize the nature and extent of thrombophlebitis. Nonseptic thrombi are usually uniformly echogenic and fairly small (Fig. 2-16). Septic thrombophlebitis has a heterogenous appearance, and in the early stages there may be numerous anechoic areas representing areas of fluid accumulation or necrosis (Fig. 2-17, *A*)

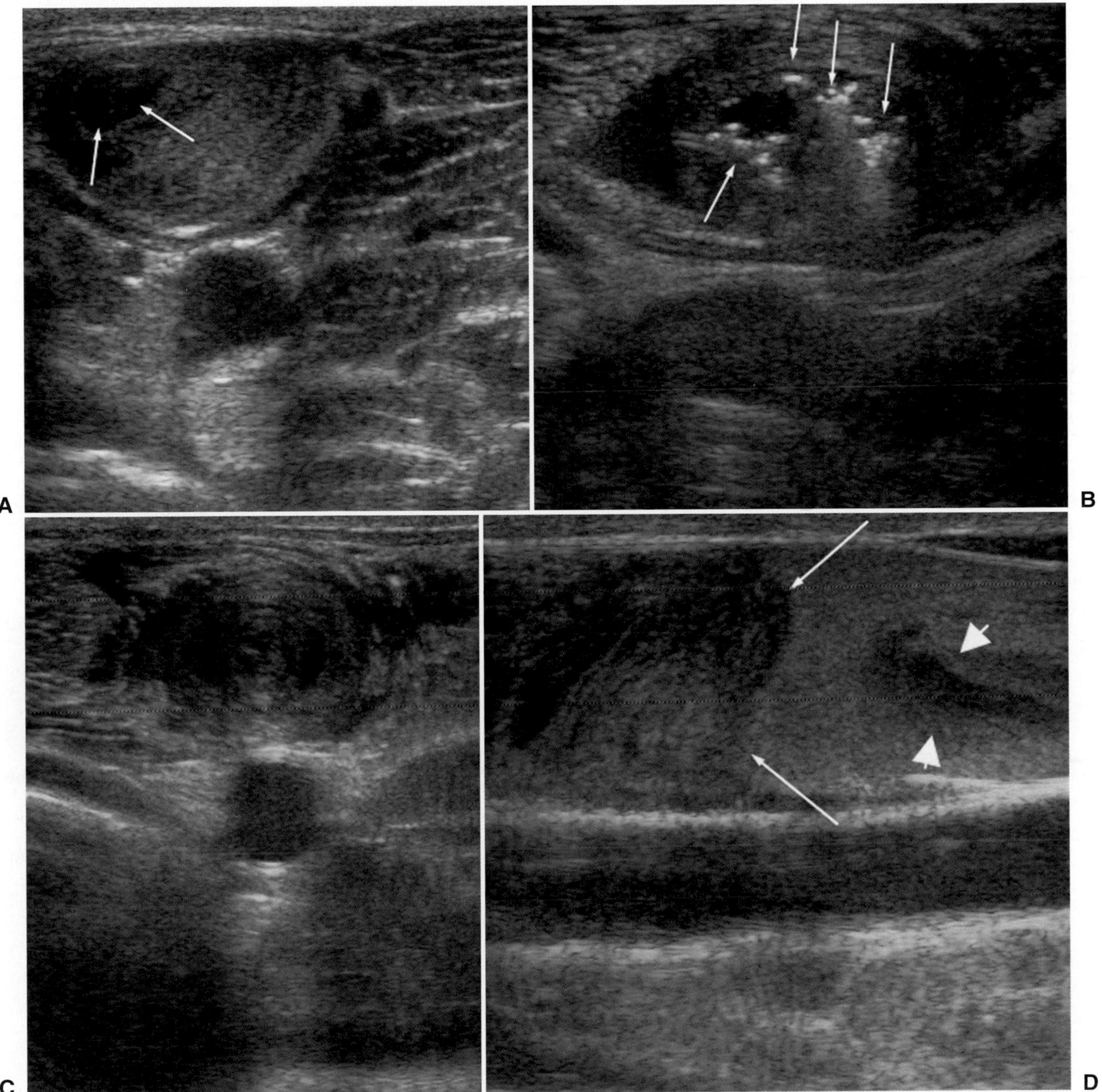

Fig. 2-17 Transverse (A, B, and C) and longitudinal (D) ultrasonograms of jugular vein from 5-month-old Thoroughbred filly that developed jugular thrombosis associated with colitis. An anechoic pocket (*arrows* in *A*) and echogenic gas echoes (*arrows* in *B*) are visible within a thrombus, confirming sepsis. The thrombus has an "onion ring" appearance in the transverse image *(C)*, and in the longitudinal image *(D)* the blood that is stationary proximal to the thrombus *(arrows)* is swirling and creating movement patterns within the vein *(arrowheads)*.

and hyperechoic areas with reverberation artifacts representing gas formation (Fig. 2-17, *B*). The thrombus will often have an onion-layer appearance on transverse images (Fig. 2-17, *C*). This layering is also evident on longitudinal images, reflecting the layers of platelets and fibrin that are deposited on the thrombus (Fig. 2-17, *D*). Variable degrees of thickening of the vessel wall are apparent. Perivenous swelling can readily be distinguished from thrombophlebitis, and perivascular edema typically has a honeycomb appearance. As thrombophlebitis resolves, the thrombus usually becomes more echogenic because of fibrosis and eventually contracts into irregular shapes as it shrinks away from the vessel wall (Fig. 2-18). Generally, it is possible to assess patency of the vein and visualize flow with conventional B mode images; however, color-flow Doppler imaging may depict this more elegantly (Fig. 2-18). Because jugular flow is sluggish and acute thrombi can be hypoechoic, in early thrombosis the blood may be more echogenic than the thrombus (see Fig. 2-17).

Laboratory Investigations

As in pericarditis, leukocytosis, neutrophilia, and hyperfibrinogenemia are common but nonspecific findings in septic thrombophlebitis. If disseminated intravascular coagulation (DIC) is suspected, platelet count, prothrombin time, activated partial thromboplastin time, fibrinolytic degradation products, and antithrombin III should be measured. Abnormality in four of five of these coagulation variables is considered indicative of DIC. The tips of catheters removed from an affected vein should be sterilely inserted into thioglycolate broth for bacterial culture. Blood cultures, swabs of discharging tracts at the catheter insertion site, and aspirates of fluid pockets obtained in a sterile manner may also be submitted for bacterial culture and antimicrobial sensitivity testing.

Therapy

Intravenous catheters should be removed at the first sign of potential problems. If possible, further IV therapy should be avoided. If continued IV therapy is needed and unilateral jugular thrombosis is present, it is prudent to place a catheter at an alternative site, such as the lateral thoracic or cephalic vein rather than the opposite jugular vein. Penicillin with an aminoglycoside, enrofloxacin, cephalosporins, and trimethoprim-sulfonamides are appropriate choices for antimicrobial therapy while awaiting results of microbiologic sensitivity testing. The presence of gas echoes may indicate anaerobic infection, and in these cases, metronidazole therapy should be considered. Generally, parenteral administration of antimicrobials is preferred in the acute stages of thrombophlebitis. Some horses with chronic septic thrombophlebitis require several weeks of antimicrobial therapy and oral administration of enrofloxacin, with or without metronidazole, or a combination of trimethoprim-sulfonamide and rifampin may be more practical. Horses with head swelling should be tied with the head elevated, ideally with the option of resting the head on straw bales or another suitable support. Oral aspirin (18 mg/kg every other day) and topical treatments, such as hot packing and application of dimethyl sulfoxide (DMSO) gel, may be helpful. Reconstructive surgery using saphenous vein grafts has been effective in horses with permanent thrombophlebitic stenosis.[97]

Prognosis

Jugular thrombophlebitis resolves uneventfully in most affected horses but can occasionally prolong treatment and delay hospital discharge for patients with primary GI disorders. Septic jugular thrombosis can be associated with a variety of serious complications (including IE)[7] temporary or permanent damage to the sympathetic and recurrent laryngeal

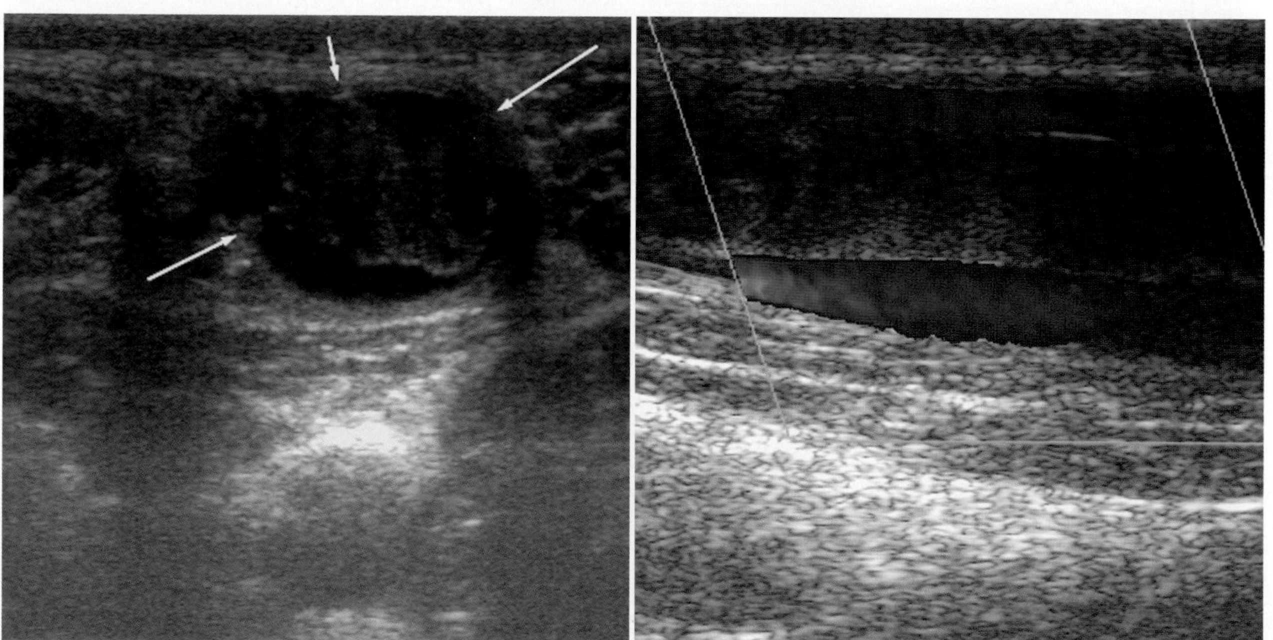

Fig. 2-18 Transverse (A) and longitudinal (B) ultrasonograms of jugular vein from 5-year-old Warmbred gelding that developed jugular thrombosis after severe colitis. Eight days after the onset of signs, as the thrombus begins to resolve, it contracts to an irregular shape with attachments to the vessel wall *(arrows)*. Color-flow Doppler imaging confirms that the vein is patent.

nerves, and upper airway edema that affects the horse's athletic performance. In most individuals, even with complete loss of the jugular vein, collateral circulation will develop to allow adequate venous drainage of the head.

Prevention

Thrombophlebitis can be minimized with (1) early identification and appropriate treatment of the coagulation disturbances associated with GI disease and SIRS (see Chapter 37); (2) careful selection, insertion, and use of IV catheters; (3) avoidance of homemade IV fluid solutions; (4) appropriate dilution of irritant drugs; and (5) avoidance of needlesticks in veins that are, or recently have been, catheterized. Catheters should be flushed frequently with heparinized saline (1 IU/mL) when not in continuous use, and Teflon over-the-needle catheters should be left in place for no more than 72 hours. Polyurethane over-the-needle catheters can be maintained for up to 5 days. Fluid lines should be changed every 24 hours in high-risk patients. It may be helpful to cover the catheter with bandage material in foals or horses that are frequently recumbent, although this is not done routinely in adult horses in most veterinary hospitals.[96]

ARTERIAL THROMBOSIS, ARTERITIS, AND AORTITIS

Horses with *aortoiliac thrombosis* are typically adults presenting for evaluation of hindlimb lameness, difficulty in breeding, or acute pain. Affected horses have cold extremities and reduced arterial pulses in the affected limbs. The condition can be diagnosed with ultrasonography or nuclear scintigraphy. The etiology is unknown but is not thought to involve infection.

Arterial thrombosis associated with sepsis is rare but has been documented in association with neonatal septicemia affecting the aortoiliac quadrification ("saddle thrombus");[98,99] in the digital,[100,101] metacarpal, and metatarsal arteries[101]; and in the major vessels of the metatarsal and metacarpal regions in older animals with enterocolitis.[101] In an additional case of brachial artery thrombosis in a foal with an atrial septal defect, it was suggested that the condition may have arisen following embolism from an atrial thrombus.[102] In septicemia and endotoxemia, abnormalities of hemostasis and fibrinolytic pathways may lead to arterial thrombosis. Thrombocytopenia and deficiencies in antithrombin III, caused by either excessive consumption or loss through the GI tract in protein-losing enteropathy, have been observed in affected patients.[100,101] Activation of procoagulants by endotoxin, dehydration, hypoxia, and acidosis may also contribute to the pathogenesis.[101] Clinical examination reveals that the affected limbs are cold, and there may be partial or complete sloughing of the hoof. Arterial thrombosis can be documented using Doppler ultrasonography, nuclear scintigraphy,[99] and contrast angiography.[102] Attempts to remove the thrombus by surgical embolectomy[102] and use of tissue plasminogen activator[99] and urokinase[100] have not yet produced successful results.

Cranial mesenteric arteritis is associated with migrating strongyle species. It has been documented in foals as young as 3 months.[103] As it migrates through the mesenteric arteries, *Strongylus vulgaris* induces thrombosis, inflammation, and intimal and adventitial fibrosis, and the accumulation of collagen leads to decreased arterial elasticity.[104] Affected animals present with recurrent or persistent colic, and a firm mass can sometimes be palpated at the mesenteric root. The condition is no longer common, presumably as a result of the widespread use of anthelmintics that are effective in reducing the burden of *S. vulgaris*. The diagnosis can be confirmed with transrectal ultrasonography[105]; typically a complex solid mass is visualized, representing fibrous tissue surrounding the mesenteric blood vessels (Fig. 2-19). Appropriate anthelmintic regimens should minimize the risk of cranial mesenteric arteritis (see Chapter 62).

Aortitis and *aortic root abscess* are rare conditions described in a horse with concurrent aortic valve IE[106] and also reported

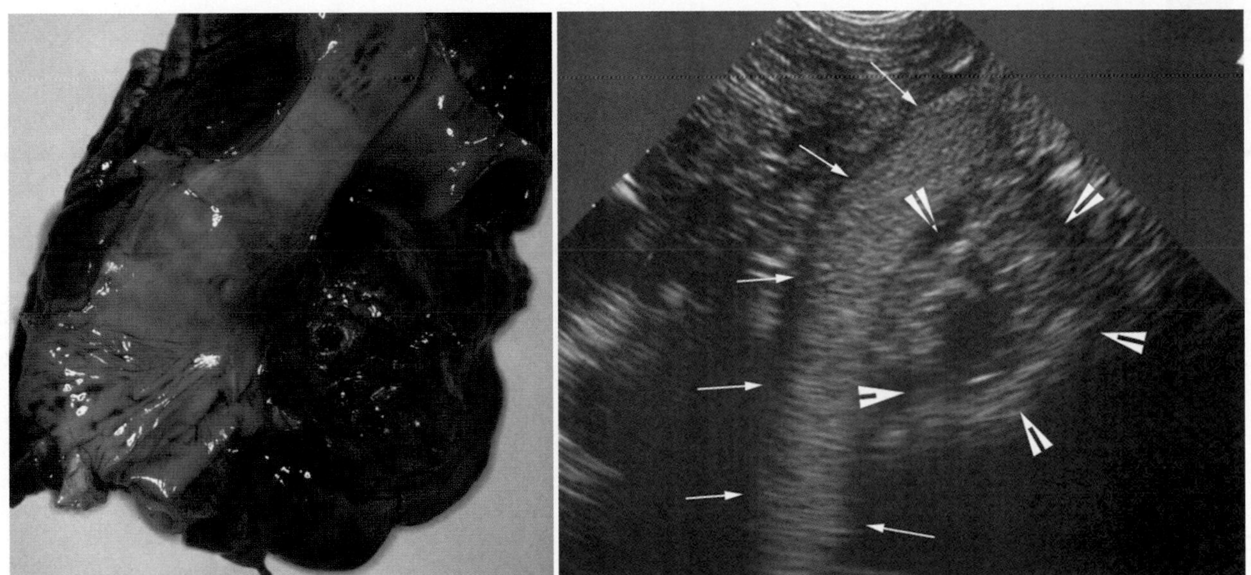

Fig. 2-19 A, Pathologic specimen from aged Connemara mare with pyrrolizidine alkaloid toxicity. A mass in the area of the mesenteric root was detected as an incidental finding. B, Transrectal abdominal ultrasonogram shows thick-walled blood vessels surrounded by fibrous tissue in longitudinal *(arrows)* and transverse *(arrowheads)* planes resulting from mesenteric arteritis.

as isolated conditions in a horse presenting with clinical signs similar to those of IE: fever, hindlimb swelling, lethargy, tachycardia, and a systolic murmur. The diagnosis was confirmed with echocardiography; blood culture yielded *Streptococcus* spp. Treatment with penicillin G and gentamicin was unsuccessful in this latter case.[107]

CARDIAC COMPLICATIONS IN SYSTEMIC INFLAMMATORY RESPONSE SYNDROME AND SEPTICEMIA

Cardiac Arrhythmias

Arrhythmias (or *dysrhythmias*) occurring secondary to other systemic diseases, particularly GI diseases accompanied by SIRS,[108,109] are encountered more frequently in horses than rhythm disturbances associated with primary myocardial pathology. In a group of 67 horses with duodenitis or proximal jejunitis, six (9%; CI 2.1%-15.8%) had arrhythmias, and ambulatory electrocardiograms (ECGs) obtained from 50 horses within 3 days of exploratory celiotomy demonstrated that 11 horses (22%; CI 10.5%-33.5%) developed isolated supraventricular premature depolarizations,[92] and eight horses (16%; CI 5.8%-26.2%) developed isolated ventricular premature depolarizations, including four (8%; CI 0.5%-15.5%) with idioventricular rhythms or paroxysmal monomorphic ventricular tachycardia. These arrhythmias are often self-limiting, requiring no specific treatment,[110,111] and often the arrhythmia is not recognized on physical examination. Occasionally, more clinically significant arrhythmias are encountered in critical care patients, and concurrent clinical signs of reduced cardiac output and marked tachycardia are recognized. Such arrhythmias can occur with other systemic diseases[109] and conditions associated with SIRS, such as IE and metritis (see Fig. 2-5).

In these horses, arrhythmogenesis is likely caused by multiple confounding factors, including the direct effects of endotoxin on the myocardium, autonomic imbalance resulting from GI distention, and metabolic, electrolyte, or acid-base imbalances.[108] Overall electrolyte balance is more important than isolated disturbances, although the electrolytes usually associated with arrhythmias are potassium, calcium, and magnesium.[92] With *potassium*, hyperkalemia leads to decreased P-wave amplitude and increased T-wave amplitude. Hypokalemia is associated with ventricular arrhythmias in humans[113] and horses[111] and has been implicated in the development of atrial fibrillation in horses.[112] *Calcium* principally affects the ST segment, and both hypocalcemia and hypercalcemia are associated with fatal ventricular arrhythmias.[112] *Magnesium* is an important cofactor in the sodium-potassium ATPase pump that regulates action potentials; hypomagnesemia is associated with ventricular arrhythmias.[113]

In addition to electrolyte imbalances at the intracellular or extracellular level, metabolic and acid-base disturbances and alterations of the autonomic nervous system play a role in the genesis of arrhythmias.[92] Addressing underlying and contributory factors are the main therapeutic goal. Strong evidence to support decisions on which specific antidysrhythmic agent to use in equine patients is lacking, and the decision to institute specific antidysrhythmic therapy is generally based on an assessment of whether it is likely that the arrhythmia will destabilize to a life-threatening state. Guidelines for treatment of arrhythmias are provided earlier in the section on myocarditis (see Table 2-3).

Cardiac Involvement in Multiple Organ Dysfunction

The distributive shock that occurs with endotoxemia and SIRS is principally caused by dysregulation of systemic vascular function and is accompanied by microthrombosis. However, a direct myocardial depressant mechanism may also come into play. Compared with measurement of cardiac output by thermodilution or lithium dilution techniques, echocardiography is not a particularly useful tool in critical care monitoring. However, horses and foals with endotoxemia or septicemia often have echocardiographic signs of global cardiac dysfunction, such as reduced fractional shortening, spontaneous contrast, and poor ventricular wall movement. Hypovolemic patients may have reduced cardiac chamber size, and in septicemic patients, mild pericardial effusions are fairly common. Thus, in addition to primary myocardial or pericardial diseases, endotoxemia and septicemia should be considered as major differential diagnoses when these echocardiographic findings are observed.

Mild fibrinous pericarditis, right atrial and ventricular enlargement, myocardial depression, and ventricular tachycardia have been observed in streptococcal toxic shock with multiple organ dysfunction in a horse.[114] Treatment of streptococcal shock consists of supportive care and symptomatic therapy. Maintaining adequate tissue perfusion with IV crystalloid and colloidal fluids and pressor agents is critical. Antimicrobial therapy is important and should be guided by the results of blood culture and antimicrobial sensitivity tests. In humans, fluoroquinolones are not recommended because these agents have a poor spectrum of activity against streptococci. Interestingly, in the single reported equine case, clinical deterioration was noted when initial treatment with ceftiofur, penicillin, and metronidazole was changed to enrofloxacin, although the microorganism that was identified on blood culture, *Streptococcus mitis*, was sensitive in vitro to enrofloxacin. Streptococcal toxic shock was previously associated specifically with *Streptococcus pyogenes* infection in humans, but it is now recognized in association with a wide range of *Streptococcus* spp. in both humans[115] and dogs.[116] In the last 20 years, this condition has been increasingly diagnosed in humans,[115] and streptococcal toxic shock may become more important in horses in the future.[114]

REFERENCES

See the CD-ROM for a list of references linked to the abstract in PubMed.

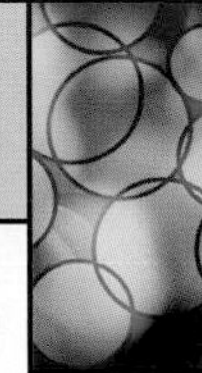

CHAPTER • 3

Gastrointestinal and Peritoneal Infections

L. Chris Sanchez

The common infectious diseases of the gastrointestinal (GI) tract and their pathogenesis are covered in detail individually in other chapters of this text. The primary goals of this chapter are to identify the normal microflora throughout the GI tract and briefly discuss an approach to the diagnosis and management of the primary clinical syndromes associated with these infectious processes.

ORAL CAVITY

Normal Flora

Most information regarding the normal flora of bacteria in the equine pharynx relates to upper respiratory tract infection and lower respiratory tract infection attributed to aspiration. Comparatively few studies have examined the normal flora of the equine oral cavity. Several aerobic and facultatively anaerobic organisms have been isolated from various locations throughout the pharynx, most notably *Streptococcus equi* subsp. *zooepidemicus*.[1,2] Anaerobic bacteria isolated from the normal equine pharyngeal tonsillar area include bacteria from the genera *Bacteroides*, *Eubacterium*, *Fusobacterium*, *Clostridium*, and *Veillonella*.[3]

Infectious Disorders

Unlike in small animals, infectious diseases of the oral cavity are relatively rare in horses. Primary problems with a possible infectious etiology include periodontitis and tooth root abscesses, pharyngitis, and dysphagia. Anaerobic organisms are frequently associated with tooth root abscesses.[4] Other infectious problems with potential impact on the oral cavity include infection from *Actinobacillus lignieresii*, the organism associated with swollen or "wooden" tongue[5,6] (Fig. 3-1); various fungal organisms such as *Candida* spp., which can cause thrush in foals (see Chapter 53); viral diseases such as vesicular stomatitis[7] (see Chapter 24); and infectious causes of dysphagia such as *Clostridium botulinum*[8,9] (botulism, see Chapter 46), equine protozoal myeloencephalitis (see Chapter 59), and West Nile virus (see Chapter 21).

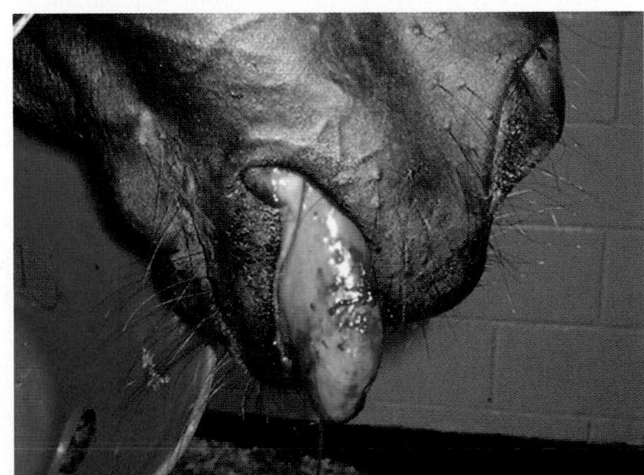

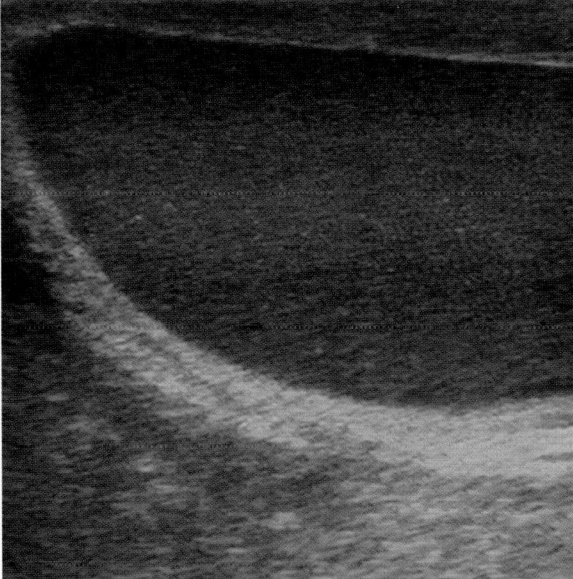

Fig. 3-1 **A,** Swollen tongue secondary to foreign body penetration. **B,** Ultrasound image demonstrating large abscess in the tongue. (Courtesy Dr. Steeve Giguere.)

ESOPHAGUS AND STOMACH

Normal Flora

The esophagus and stomach are not sterile environments. In one study, 2.8×10^9 total and 2×10^8 viable bacteria per gram of ingesta were recovered from the fundic region of normal ponies, with 1.9×10^9 total (but only 10×10^6 viable) bacteria/g recovered from the pyloric region.[10] In both regions, gram-positive organisms (rods and cocci) predominated, and very few cellulolytic bacteria (100-300/g) were isolated,[10] suggestive of the capacity for fermentation but minimal ability to utilize forage. Colonization of and attachment to the gastric squamous mucosa by several indigenous *Lactobacillus* spp. were recently described.[11]

Infectious Disorders

Infectious diseases of the esophagus mainly occur secondary to perforation and involve a mixed population of aerobic and anaerobic bacteria. Although polymerase chain reaction (PCR) fragments unique to gastric-dwelling *Helicobacter* spp.

have been identified in horses, an association between *H. pylori* and ulceration has not been established in adult horses or foals.[12,13] One case of emphysematous gastritis from *Clostridium perfringens* has been reported.[14]

SMALL INTESTINE

Normal Flora

Few studies have evaluated normal microbial populations in the equine small intestine. Total bacterial counts and proportion of gram-positive bacteria recovered from the ileum were similar to those seen in the stomach,[10] but viable bacteria numbered 3.6×10^7. In a study analyzing only anaerobic bacteria, increasing numbers of both culturable and proteolytic bacteria were identified in the duodenum, jejunum, and ileum.[15] Proteolytic bacteria composed a high proportion of the total bacteria in all regions, but accounted for almost all bacteria in the duodenum. Numbers of bacteria identified from the GI lumen outnumbered those recovered from the mucosa in all segments.[15]

Infectious Diarrhea in Foals

Most infectious causes of diarrhea in foals, unlike those in adult horses, affect the small intestine either alone or in combination with the large colon.

Bacterial Disorders

Clostridial organisms can act as primary pathogens in foals, causing disease in individual animals or as outbreaks on affected farms (see Chapter 44). *Clostridium perfringens* typically affects foals under 10 days of age. Types A and C are most often implicated, with type C resulting in more severe disease, hemorrhagic diarrhea, and higher mortality than type A.[16] Type A *C. perfringens* is typically isolated from the feces of normal foals, but the organism in general is more often isolated from foals with diarrhea.[17] A diagnosis is usually confirmed with the combination of clinical signs and culture of the organism from feces, preferably with genotyping of the obtained isolate. Observation of large, gram-positive rods on a fecal Gram stain should prompt the clinician to consider clostridial enteritis[16] (Fig. 3-2).

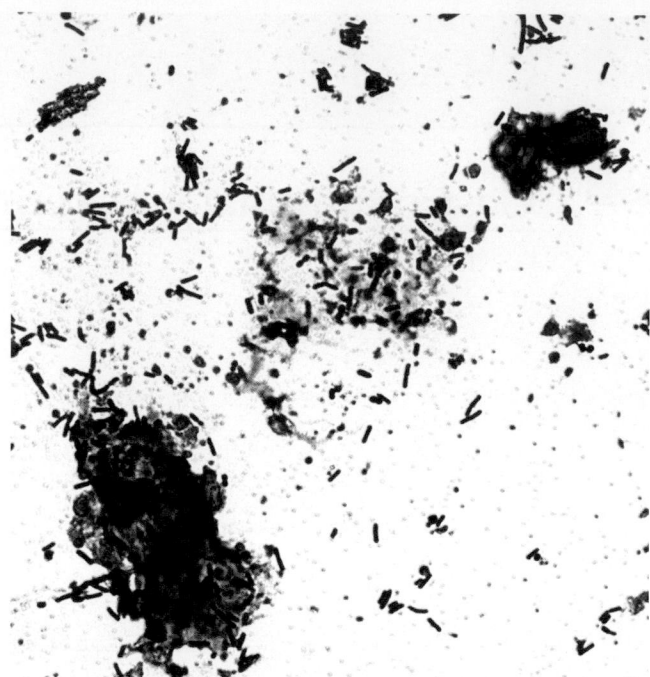

Fig. 3-2 Photomicrograph of Gram-stained feces of foal with *Clostridium difficile* enteritis. Note the numerous gram-positive rods. (Courtesy Dr. Michael Porter.)

Clostridium difficile has also been implicated as a cause of diarrhea in foals. Disease severity can vary from mild to hemorrhagic diarrhea. As with *C. perfringens*, *C. difficile* can be isolated from asymptomatic foals, and thus toxin detection in feces is useful for confirmation of a diagnosis.[18]

Commercial immunoassays are available for the detection of toxins A and B in feces as well as the enterotoxin of *C. perfringens* (CPE). Treatment is supportive, with the addition of directed antimicrobial therapy, typically with metronidazole. In some geographic locations, documented metronidazole resistance in *C. difficile* isolates has prompted therapy with vancomycin in select cases.[19]

The other predominant bacterial cause of enterocolitis in foals is *salmonellosis* (see Chapter 38). In addition to diarrhea, affected foals typically display clinical signs of sepsis. Diagnosis is confirmed by aerobic culture of blood and feces. Treatment is supportive and should include directed systemic antimicrobial therapy. Foals with systemic sepsis may develop diarrhea in association with their primary disease, with a reported incidence between 16% and 38%.[20-23] Although *Escherichia coli* is the most common etiologic agent associated with sepsis (see Chapter 6), it is not typically recognized as a primary cause of enteritis or enterocolitis in foals. There is an increased probability of diarrhea in foals with *Actinobacillus* sepsis compared with foals from which other organisms are isolated.[20]

Infection of older foals with *Lawsonia intracellularis*, an obligate intracellular pathogen, results in proliferative enteropathy[24-27] and should be considered in weanling-age foals with severe hypoproteinemia (see Chapter 36). Clinical signs include weight loss, ill thrift, depression, colic, peripheral edema, and variable fecal consistency, ranging from soft, normal stool to watery diarrhea. Protein loss can be severe. Diagnosis is based on clinical signs in combination with results of fecal PCR and serum antibody testing. Treatment includes supportive care, predominantly with colloid replacement, and directed antimicrobial therapy with erythromycin estolate and rifampin or chloramphenicol.[25,28]

Viral Disorders

The most common viral pathogen associated with diarrhea in foals is *rotavirus* (see Chapter 17). Typically, rotavirus affects foals between 5 and 35 days of age, with most foals at the younger end of this spectrum.[29] The most common and obvious clinical sign is diarrhea, and fecal consistency can vary greatly. Other signs relate to disease severity, including depression, anorexia, dehydration, and similar findings. The virus causes blunting of the small intestinal microvilli, with malabsorption and maldigestion. Diagnosis can be confirmed with fecal electron microscopy, which has a significant lag time, or commercial immunoassays, also performed on feces. Treatment is principally supportive, with extra emphasis placed on biosecurity protocols. Quaternary ammonium compounds are ineffective as disinfectant agents for equine rotavirus. The virus is extremely contagious, with morbidity approaching 100% in farm outbreaks. Prognosis is good with supportive care, and mortality is typically low in uncomplicated cases.

Other viral causes of diarrhea occur much less frequently and include coronavirus[30,31] and adenovirus[32,33] (see Chapters 18 and 16, respectively).

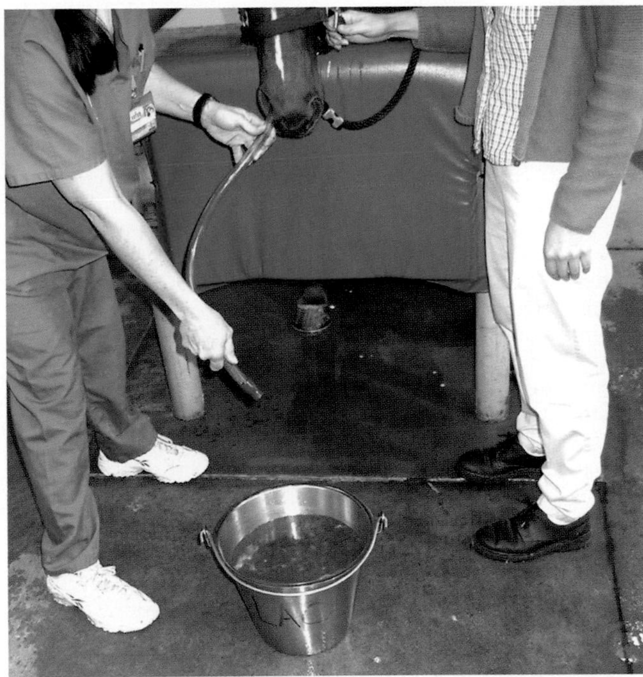

Fig. 3-3 Horse with duodenitis/proximal jejunitis (DPJ) with 20 to 30 liters of spontaneous reflux when nasogastric tube was placed.

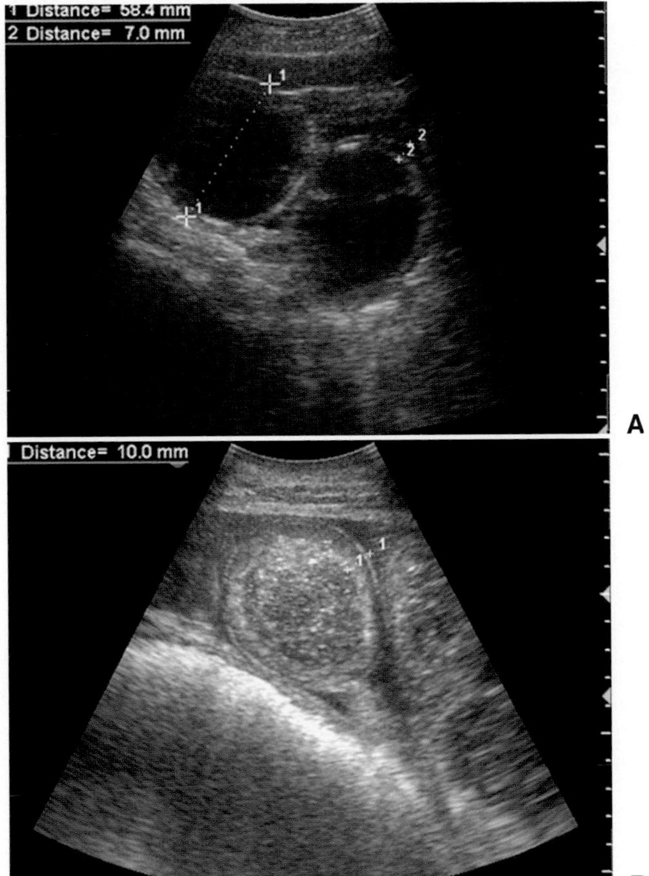

Fig. 3-4 Abdominal ultrasound images from horse with duodenitis/proximal jejunitis (DPJ). **A,** Dilated loops of small intestine. **B,** Thickened small intestine.

Protozoal Disorders

Cryptosporidium spp. are the major protozoal cause of diarrhea in foals (see Chapter 61).[17] These organisms are generally regarded as less significant relative to the major bacterial and viral diseases discussed previously.

Infectious Small Intestinal Disease in Adult Horses

Etiology and Pathogenesis

Proven infectious disorders of the small intestine of adult horses are rare. Horses do not appear predisposed to small intestinal bacterial overgrowth, which is common in dogs and humans. One equine disorder that has a suspected, but to this point unsubstantiated, infectious origin is *duodenitis/proximal jejunitis* (DPJ, also known as *anterior enteritis* or *proximal enteritis*), a syndrome of small intestinal inflammation characterized by copious quantities of gastric reflux (Fig. 3-3). In most affected horses, an underlying etiology cannot be determined and the syndrome of DPJ may include a wide variety of inflammatory small intestinal disorders resulting in a similar clinical presentation. In some horses, *Salmonella* spp. or *Clostridium* spp. are isolated from gastric reflux samples (see Chapters 38 and 44). Recently, toxigenic strains of *Clostridium difficile* were isolated from the reflux in five of five horses with DPJ and from none of six control horses with other causes of nasogastric reflux.[34] Mycotoxins of *Fusarium moniliforme* may also play a role in some cases of DPJ.[35]

Regardless of the initiating cause, intestinal inflammation results in changes in secretory activity and motility that contribute to a functional obstruction. Intestinal inflammation can change normal sensory-motor function, mucosal function, ion transport, and transepithelial permeability.

Clinical Findings

The most characteristic clinical signs in horses with DPJ include moderate to severe pain, which improves after gastric decompression; large volumes of gastric reflux; clinical signs of endotoxemia (see Chapter 37); and small intestinal distention evident on rectal palpation and ultrasonographic examination (Fig. 3-4).

Abnormal clinicopathologic findings in horses with DPJ can include hemoconcentration, neutropenia, acidemia, prerenal azotemia, hyponatremia, hypochloremia, hypokalemia, and increased hepatic enzyme activities.[36] Typically, peritoneal fluid has a mild to moderate increase in total nucleated cell count (TNCC, up to 20,000/μL), with a moderate to marked increase in total solids (up to 5 g/dL). However, the nucleated cell count may vary widely. These findings may help to differentiate horses with DPJ from horses with strangulating small intestinal disease, which tend to have higher numbers of red blood cells as well as a higher TNCC. However, the wide fluctuation in results obtained with these disorders may make differential diagnosis difficult in many horses, necessitating exploratory celiotomy.[37]

Therapy

Treatment of DPJ consists primarily of supportive care, with an emphasis on fluid therapy and gastric decompression. Particular care should be taken to administer maintenance fluid requirements and replace the fluid volume lost through gastric reflux. Therapy should also include nonsteroidal antiinflammatory therapy for analgesic and antiinflammatory effects, as long as renal function remains normal, and directed therapy to combat endotoxemia. If the affected horse's condition either deteriorates or fails to improve with medical therapy, surgical exploration can be considered.[38] Surgical exploration can offer manual decompression of the small intestine and rule out any physical obstruction. In protracted cases or in horses with increased serum triglyceride concentrations, intravenous (IV) parenteral nutritional support should be considered. Prokinetic therapy with erythromycin lactobionate, metoclopramide, bethanechol, or lidocaine may also be considered.[39,40]

With prompt medical therapy, horses with DPJ generally have a good prognosis for survival. Factors associated with a decreased risk of survival include increased peritoneal fluid protein concentration, increased anion gap,[41] and failure to respond to prokinetic therapy within 24 hours.[39] Potential complications of DPJ include laminitis, thrombophlebitis, peritonitis, adhesions, pharyngitis or esophagitis, and cardiac arrhythmias.

LARGE INTESTINE

Normal Flora

Much more is known about the resident microflora in the equine large intestine than the small intestine or the more orad portions of the GI tract. The cecum and colon have a large capacity and the capability for extensive fermentation by bacteria and protozoa. Total protozoal concentrations in the large intestine appear to increase in horses fed a diet high in forage, relative to a diet high in concentrate.[42] The colon has concentrations of both total and cellulolytic fungi more than 10 times greater than those found in the cecum.[42] At least two species of anaerobic phycomycetes capable of digesting plant cellulose and hemicellulose have been isolated from the equine cecum.[43] *Ruminococcus flavefaciens* has recently been identified as the predominant cellulolytic cecal bacterial species.[44] At least two types of spirochetes have been identified in the equine cecum.[45] Bacteriophages infecting spirochetes within the equine cecum[45] and bacteriophage-like particles have been demonstrated in various regions of the large intestine by electron microscopy.[46]

Acute Diarrhea in Adult Horses

Etiology

The principal infectious agents associated with colitis in horses include *Salmonella* spp. (see Chapter 38), *Neorickettsia risticii* (see Chapter 43; equine monocytic erlichiosis, Potomac horse fever), *Clostridium difficile*, and *Clostridium perfringens* (see Chapter 44). *Aeromonas* spp. are often isolated from horses with diarrhea, but their significance has not been fully determined. Parasites are not typically associated with acute diarrhea in adult horses, with the exception of larval cyathostomiasis in Europe and the northern part of the United States and Canada (see Chapter 62). The most common cause of outbreaks of colitis in horses is salmonellosis. Outbreaks of Potomac horse fever (PHF) and clostridial colitis are rare, although the latter may occur as a clustering of cases of foals or hospitalized horses. Because each of these agents is covered in depth in other chapters, this chapter focuses on a diagnostic and therapeutic approach to an individual horse presenting with acute diarrhea.

Diagnostic Approach

In all horses with acute diarrhea, a minimum database includes complete blood count (CBC) with fibrinogen and a biochemical profile. If available, venous blood gas analysis is desirable. Additional diagnostic tests to identify a specific etiologic agent can be performed on blood and feces. The clinician should remember the potential for co-infections within the same patient.

Diagnostic Tests on Whole Blood or Serum. Although an enzyme-linked immunosorbent assay (ELISA) has been described for diagnosis of *N. risticii* infection in horses, an immunofluorescent assay (IFA) for detection of specific antibody or polymerase chain reaction (PCR) assay for detection of organism is the preferred test. IFA utilizes serum, and PCR is performed on buffy coat or feces. Most laboratories that perform PCR use buffy coats isolated from standard ethylenediaminetetraacetic acid (EDTA)–treated whole-blood tubes. Infected horses develop high IFA titers (>1:640) within days of infection, often before clinical signs are apparent. Paired serum samples (acute and convalescent) should be collected within 5 to 7 days rather than the conventional interval of 2 to 4 weeks because infected horses rapidly develop high titers. It is generally believed that horses with PHF should have a titer of 1:80 or greater at the onset of signs; consequently, a negative titer indicates this disease is unlikely. Vaccination for PHF results in positive titers that usually disappear by 6 to 9 months. PCR offers the advantage of excellent sensitivity without the potential for interference from vaccination.[47,48]

Diagnostic Tests for Feces. Fresh fecal samples from horses with diarrhea should be submitted for aerobic culture, with a specific request for *Salmonella* spp. identification. These cultures require special media and antigens for serogroup identification and are readily available through most, if not all, commercial laboratories. Multiple cultures are preferable. Recovery of pathologic organisms can be difficult when feces are very watery, and thus the most productive cultures are performed on feces with at least some substance. Culture of a rectal mucosal biopsy sample may also improve the recovery rate.[49] PCR is reported to be a more sensitive method for detection of salmonella in feces.[50-53] The diagnostic significance of horses positive by PCR but negative by culture of multiple fecal samples remains to be determined. (Chapter 38 discusses *Salmonella* spp. diagnostic tests and their interpretation in detail.)

Anaerobic culture of feces should also be requested to facilitate detection of clostridial organisms. Strict anaerobic handling of the feces is critical to successful culture, especially for *Clostridium difficile*.[54] Recovery of *C. difficile* organisms is dramatically reduced after storage for 72 hours in aerobic conditions at 4°C.[54] Because clostridial organisms can be cultured from the feces of some normal horses, toxin detection is preferred for a diagnosis of clinically relevant disease. Commercial ELISA assays are available for detection of *C. difficile* toxins A and B, as well as the enterotoxin of *Clostridium perfringens* (CPE). Genotyping of *C. perfringens* isolates is also commercially available. Aerobic storage of fecal samples is unsuitable if samples are intended for culture of *C. difficile* because of the short length of time that organisms remain viable when stored under those conditions. However, toxins remain stable for at least 30 days when fecal samples are stored aerobically.[54] Many diagnostic laboratories will perform toxin testing, and some will provide packages including both culture and toxin analysis. (Chapter 44 discusses diagnosis of enteric clostridial infections in detail.)

Feces should be examined by sedimentation for sand and microscopically for increased fecal leukocytes. A Gram stain may be useful as an initial screen for clostridial organisms (long gram-positive rods). Cyathostome larvae are best detected by direct examination of feces (see Chapters 58 and 62).

Therapy

The primary goal of therapy for adult horses with diarrhea is restoration and maintenance of fluid, electrolyte, and acid-base balance. Specific pathogen-directed therapy may be indicated, depending on the etiologic agent identified. For many horses with acute colitis, initial IV fluid replacement is required because of tremendous volume losses. Typically, mild to moderate acidemia is corrected by restoration of plasma volume with an alkalinizing solution such as lactated Ringer's or Normosol-R. Sodium chloride solutions (0.9%) should be avoided because they can be acidifying and may worsen edema. In horses with severe dehydration, initial therapy with hypertonic saline may be used to restore circulatory volume, but must be followed by administration of isotonic fluids. Alternatively, hydroxyethyl starch (Hetastarch) can also be used for quick expansion of plasma volume while also inducing a rapid increase in colloid oncotic pressure.

Other goals of therapy include reducing inflammation, pain control, and limiting the effects of endotoxemia (see Chapter 37). Drugs used for theses purposes include nonsteroidal antiinflammatory drugs (NSAIDs), such as flunixin meglumine, which have analgesic, antiinflammatory, and antiendotoxemic properties.[55] As with other NSAIDs, the clinician must take care to avoid use of flunixin in horses with renal compromise, moderate to severe dehydration, NSAID toxicity, or right dorsal colitis. Adjunctive therapy with polymyxin B sulfate[56,57] and pentoxifylline[55,58,59] is suggested to combat the effects of endotoxemia.

Chronic Diarrhea in Adult Horses

Etiology

Chronic diarrhea is usually defined as diarrhea lasting longer than 4 weeks.[60] Fecal consistency can vary widely. Although many specific diseases can result in chronic diarrhea, identification of the inciting cause in a patient frequently remains elusive. Occasionally, problems of a non-GI nature, such as hepatic disease or abdominal abscessation, result in diarrhea. Infectious causes of chronic diarrhea include chronic salmonellosis (see Chapter 38) and parasitism with large or small strongyles (see Chapter 61). Recently, the spirochete *Brachyspira pilosicoli* was implicated in a herd outbreak of chronic diarrhea in weanling-age horses.[61] Noninfectious inflammatory causes of chronic diarrhea include granulomatous enteritis or colitis, neoplasia (predominantly lymphosarcoma), sand irritation, and right dorsal colitis (Fig. 3-5). Noninflammatory causes include a range of problems, with the common theme of disruption in the flora of the large intestine. This may or may not be related to a dietary disruption, and many affected horses have few other clinical signs. Regardless of the inciting cause, horses with chronic diarrhea remain very difficult to treat and have a guarded prognosis.

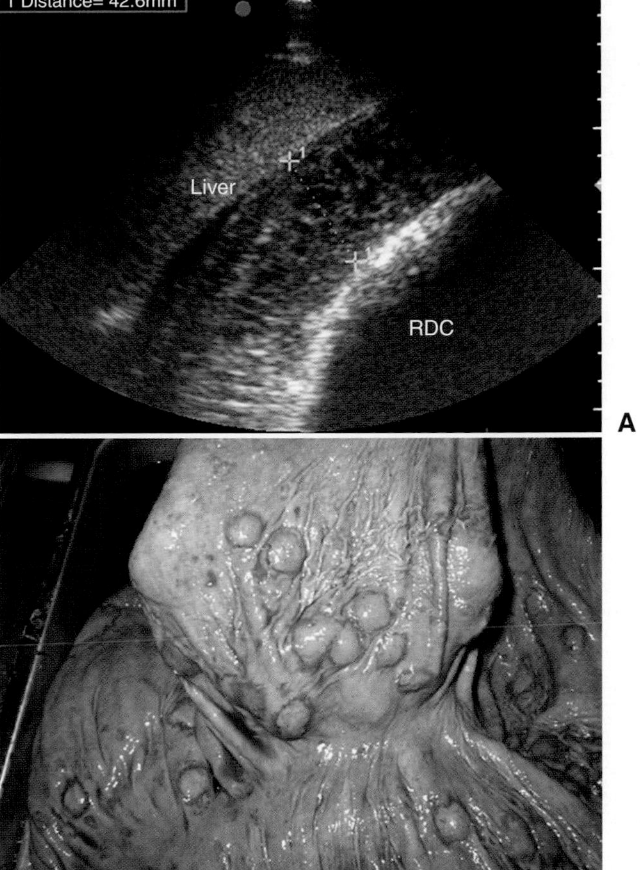

Fig. 3-5 A, Abdominal ultrasound image from aged pony with liver disease, low white blood cell count, and fever demonstrating greatly thickened right dorsal colon. **B,** Right dorsal colon of horse with thickened colon and actual granuloma formation in wall of intestine. (Courtesy Dr. Michael Porter.)

Diagnostic Approach

A minimum database for the individual horse with chronic diarrhea typically includes CBC with fibrinogen, serum biochemical profile, venous blood gas analysis, rectal examination, abdominal ultrasound, and analysis of peritoneal fluid. Results of all these diagnostic procedures are frequently normal, and further recommended analyses include a comprehensive fecal examination and rectal biopsy.

Comprehensive fecal analysis should include assessment for parasites (grossly and by fecal flotation or McMasters quantification), aerobic culture for *Salmonella* (five samples at a minimum 12-hour interval, as for acute diarrhea), water suspension for sand, unstained wet mount for protozoa and parasites, new methylene blue stain for fecal leukocytes, and Gram stain to determine the ratio of gram-positive to gram-negative bacterial flora.

Rectal biopsy is a simple, relatively noninvasive procedure.[62] Two samples should be obtained and submitted for culture *(Salmonella)* and histopathology. Histopathologic examination is most helpful for diagnosis of inflammatory and neoplastic bowel diseases.

Therapy

If a specific diagnosis is achieved, directed therapy should be initiated. (See individual chapters for a more detailed description of directed therapy based on the causative organism.) In all cases, free-choice access to fresh water is critical to maintenance of hydration. Many horses will consume balanced, isotonic electrolyte water, and such a solution should be offered in addition to fresh water. Alternatively, access to a salt or mineral block can serve as a substitute source of electrolyte replacement. Typical feeding recommendations include good-quality grass hay with limited legume hay and concentrate intake. Dietary changes alone are unlikely to provide a cure.

Nonspecific therapy for horses with chronic diarrhea may include transfaunation or administration of iodochlorhydroxyquin. Detailed descriptions of *transfaunation* procedures are sparse in the veterinary literature, as are reported benefits. Typically, cecal liquor is obtained either from an animal recently euthanized for non-GI reasons or from an animal implanted with a cecal cannula. Because these sources are rarely available in proximity to the affected animal, the procedure itself may be a fairly daunting task. After appropriate transfaunate is obtained, the clinician must decide whether to pretreat the recipient. Frequently, recipients are pretreated with acid-suppressing agents to enhance viability of transplanted bacteria and protozoa as they pass through the gastric environment. The efficacy of such treatment has not been validated in the horse. However, the potential value of transfaunation was recently highlighted during a herd outbreak possibly related to the spirochete *Brachyspira pilosicoli*.[61]

Iodochlorhydroxyquin, an 8-hydroxyquinolone derivative (also called clioquinol) originally recommended for treatment of trichomoniasis, has long been recommended for the treatment of chronic diarrhea.[63] Although chronic diarrhea in horses is more likely to result from disruption of the normal intestinal flora than from infection, some horses responded favorably to therapy. The response to treatment with iodochlorhydroxyquin is highly variable; it may worsen diarrhea in some horses. Therapy may result in improvement in fecal consistency, with reversion to diarrhea within a few days of discontinuing drug administration.[61]

Prognosis

Regardless of the inciting cause, if a horse has diarrhea for at least a month, the prognosis for complete recovery is guarded. The prognosis worsens with the duration of diarrhea.

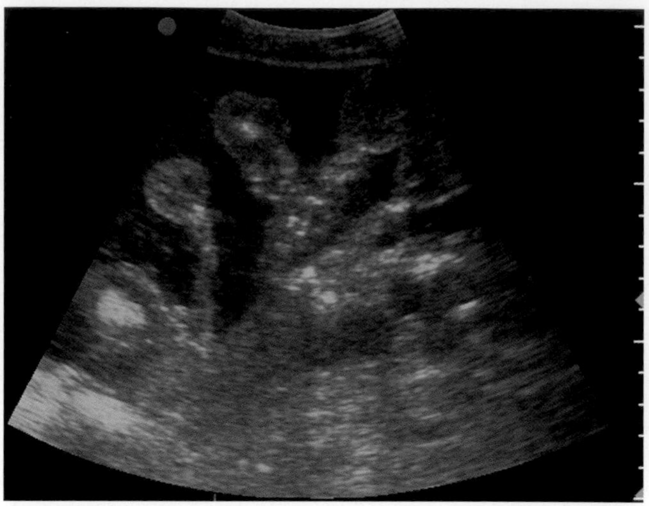

Fig. 3-6 Abdominal ultrasound image from a horse with septic peritonitis demonstrating increased quantities of hyperechoic fluid, with small intestine floating throughout the fluid (intestinal buds).

PERITONEAL INFECTIONS

Peritonitis refers to inflammation of the mesothelial lining of the peritoneal cavity and is typically caused by mechanical, chemical, or infectious insult to the parietal peritoneum. In addition to classification based on the causative insult, further classification may include onset (acute or chronic), distribution (localized or diffuse), origin (primary or secondary), and infectious nature (septic or aseptic). Acute, diffuse, septic peritonitis secondary to GI disease is the most common manifestation.[64]

Etiology and Clinical Findings

Most cases of peritonitis occur secondary to a GI event (e.g., perforation of any portion of GI tract), intestinal ischemia, DPJ, colitis, neoplasia, verminous arteritis, intestinal mural abscess, or other causes.[65,66] Iatrogenic causes include rectal tear, enterocentesis, castration, and abdominal surgery. Other causes include traumatic events (including uterine or vaginal perforation during foaling or breeding), mesenteric abscess (including those associated with *Streptococcus equi* subsp. *equi*), cholelithiasis, and others. Causes specific to the young foal include rupture of the urinary bladder or urachus, omphalitis or omphalophlebitis, sepsis, and *Rhodococcus equi* abscessation.

Organisms associated with GI rupture include a mixed population of gram-positive and gram-negative aerobic and anaerobic organisms, often with no clear predominance of one type. *Enterobacteriaceae*, *Streptococcus* spp., and *Staphylococcus* spp. are most often isolated from peritoneal fluid samples.[66,67] Common anaerobic isolates include *Bacteroides*, *Clostridium*, and *Bacillus* species. In foals, peritonitis is most frequently associated with *Streptococcus* and *R. equi* infections. Several case series describing peritonitis associated with *Actinobacillus equuli* have been reported.[68-70] Initial reports of *A. equuli* peritonitis originated solely in Australia, but one case was recently reported from the United Kingdom.[71]

Clinical signs of peritonitis in horses are variable and may include fever, depression, abdominal pain, diarrhea, and weight loss.[65] Depending on severity and localization, signs may also include those of endotoxemia and shock. Clinical signs in horses with *A. equuli* peritonitis include depression, inappetence, lethargy, and mild to moderate abdominal pain acutely or weight loss in a chronic form.[69,70] Postpartum mares with peritonitis secondary to a uterine perforation typically present with fever and depression, with or without abdominal pain.

Diagnosis

Definitive diagnosis of peritonitis is based upon an elevated TNCC in peritoneal fluid (>10,000 cells/μL). Culture of peritoneal fluid should be performed in all suspected cases, but this procedure has a low sensitivity, with only 9.5% to 32.5% of samples yielding positive growth.[65-67] Total cell count can be increased after enterocentesis, abdominal surgery, or open castration.[72-76] Thus, additional parameters must be considered in these populations. Abundant hypoechoic or variably echogenic peritoneal fluid (evident on abdominal ultrasound examination), fever, depression, and abdominal pain can all support the diagnosis (Fig. 3-6). A decrease in peritoneal fluid pH (<7.3) or glucose (<30 mg/dL) suggests the presence of septic peritonitis.[76] Peritoneal fluid cytology will typically reflect a septic process, with abnormalities ranging from the presence of bacteria or plant material to degenerate neutrophils (Fig. 3-7). If GI contents or plant material are evident, the clinician should take care to differentiate between GI rupture and enterocentesis. At sampling, alterations in TNCC and cytology should indicate peritonitis; enterocentesis can result in an elevated TNCC within 4 hours.[75] If a differentiation cannot be clearly made, a sample should be taken from an alternate location, preferably with ultrasound guidance. In postfoaling mares, the percentage of neutrophils in the peritoneal fluid can be increased for up to 7 days, but the total protein and TNCC should remain within normal limits.[77]

Therapy

Treatment of horses with peritonitis should begin with identification and correction of the underlying problem, if possible. If a GI source is suspected, an exploratory celiotomy is likely indicated. Supportive care is also critical to the treatment protocol.

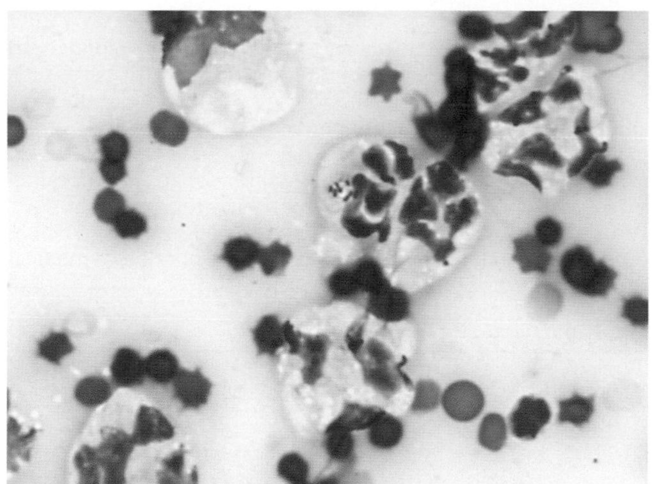

Fig. 3-7 Photomicrograph of peritoneal fluid from horse with septic peritonitis demonstrating toxic neutrophils with intracellular bacteria. (Courtesy Dr. Michael Porter.)

This should include correction of fluid deficits, acid-base and electrolyte imbalances, and colloid oncotic pressure. Anti-inflammatory and antiendotoxic therapies are also clearly of benefit (see Chapter 37). Additional analgesic and prokinetic drugs should be provided if necessary.

Antimicrobial therapy is critical to the management of septic peritonitis. Broad-spectrum coverage should be instituted pending results of peritoneal fluid culture and sensitivity. If positive results are obtained, therapy can be adjusted accordingly. A typical initial regimen includes penicillin, gentamicin, and metronidazole to cover gram-positive, gram-negative, and anaerobic spectrums, respectively. Because many *Bacteroides* species are resistant to β-lactam antimicrobials, metronidazole should be included in the antimicrobial therapy plan if anaerobic involvement is suspected. Enrofloxacin may replace gentamicin in the treatment regimen if warranted. The lipophilic nature of enrofloxacin can provide increased penetration into the peritoneal cavity. Neonatal foals with peritonitis should receive an antimicrobial regimen similar to that suggested for adults, although amikacin is frequently substituted for gentamicin because of increased sensitivity of commonly isolated organisms.[78] A combination of azithromycin or clarithromycin plus rifampin provides reasonable coverage for older foals or weanlings, because *Streptococcus* and *R. equi* are often associated with disease in these populations if a primary GI lesion is not suspected.[78] Although *A. equuli* is typically sensitive to either penicillin or trimethoprim-sulfonamide combinations, initial broad-spectrum coverage with penicillin and gentamicin is suggested pending culture results because of the resistance of some isolates.[70]

Abdominal drainage and lavage can help remove excess fluid, foreign materials, fibrin, and bacterial products from horses with peritonitis. Postoperative lavage decreases the incidence of experimentally induced abdominal adhesions in horses undergoing exploratory celiotomy[79] (Fig. 3-8). Open surgical exploration provides the most effective and thorough examination of all peritoneal surfaces and is recommended if GI perforation or ischemia is suspected, as well as in any other horses in which correction of a primary lesion is indicated. A ventral abdominal drain can either be placed at surgery or in the standing horse with sedation and local anesthesia. Techniques are described in detail elsewhere.[78,80]

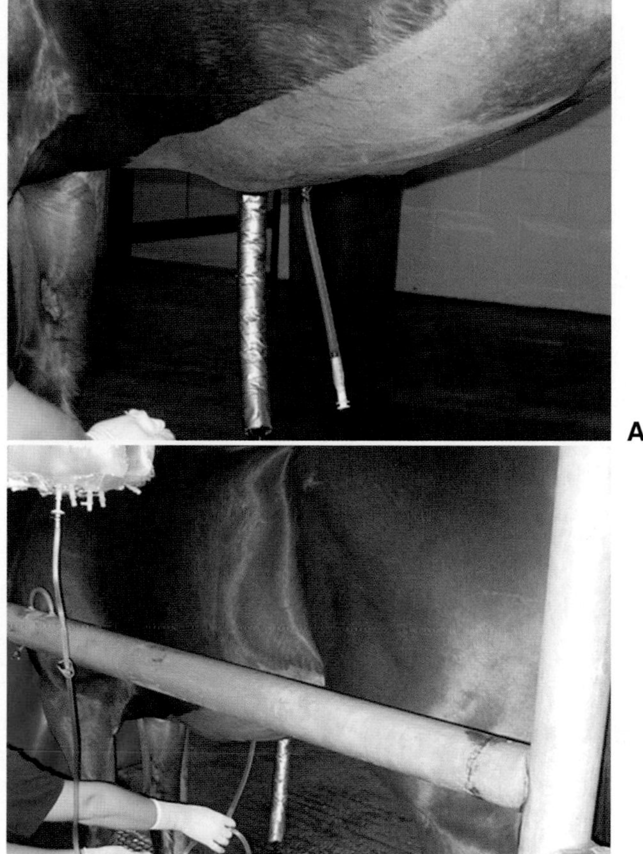

Fig. 3-8 **A,** Abdominal drain placement in most ventral point of abdomen in horse with septic peritonitis. **B,** Abdominal lavage system using the drain shown in *A*.

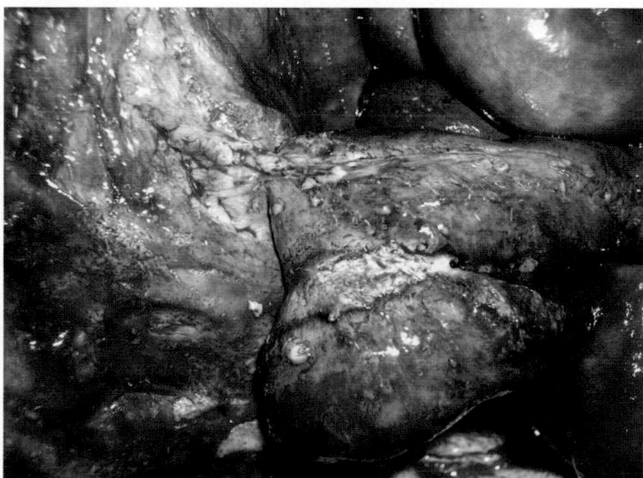

Fig. 3-9 Two-year-old horse with septic peritonitis and orchitis. The initiating cause was unknown; *Streptococcus equi* subsp. *zooepidemicus* was cultured from the abdomen of this horse.

Peritoneal lavage is typically performed by infusion of 10 to 20 liters of a balanced isotonic electrolyte solution (e.g., lactated Ringer's, Normosol-R) into the peritoneal cavity twice a day for 3 to 5 days, until the lavage solution becomes clear, or until the catheter becomes clogged with fibrin or omentum. Hypertonic solutions should be avoided because they may cause fluid shifts into the peritoneal cavity. The addition of povidone-iodine to a balanced solution should be avoided; concentrations as low as 3% may induce peritoneal inflammation.[81] Other agents, such as antibiotics and heparin, have also been suggested as components of peritoneal lavage solution, but data demonstrating their benefit are lacking. Active (or closed-suction) abdominal drains have also been advocated, with similar benefits and potential complications to other methods.[80] Lavage with a plain isotonic solution did not alter the pharmacokinetics of gentamicin administered systemically.[82]

Prognosis

The prognosis is grave for horses with peritonitis secondary to GI rupture. Reported survival rates for horses with peritonitis vary but can be as high as 59.7%[66] (Fig. 3-9). Some of the variability in reported survival percentages may be related to inclusion criteria, mainly whether or not horses with GI rupture were included. Septic peritonitis after abdominal surgery is reportedly associated with high mortality (56%).[66] Peritonitis associated with *A. equuli* carries a very favorable prognosis, and all horses in these reports responded to medical therapy, if attempted.[68-70]

REFERENCES

See the CD-ROM for a list of references linked to the abstract in PubMed.

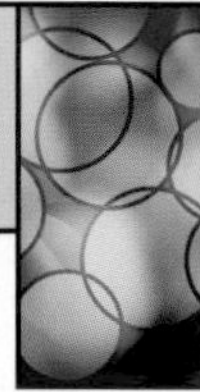

CHAPTER • 4

Central Nervous System Infections

Kathy K. Seino

Infections of the central nervous system (CNS) of horses, although uncommon, are some of the most devastating and frequently fatal diseases in horses. Diseases such as *equine protozoal myeloencephalitis* (EPM) and *West Nile virus encephalomyelitis* (WNE) have had a significant economic impact on the equine industry in recent years and stimulated investigations into preventive, diagnostic, and therapeutic alternatives for CNS infections in horses.

Viral, bacterial, rickettsial, protozoal, parasitic, and fungal pathogens may cause CNS infections in horses (Table 4-1). In small animals and in humans the causes of meningoencephalitis, in order of decreasing frequency, are viral, bacterial, protozoal, rickettsial, parasitic, and fungal, whereas in the horse the most frequently diagnosed CNS infections are probably of viral and protozoal origin.[1,2] In an Australian study, 30 of 450 horses with neurologic disease had an infectious or inflammatory disease, and 11 of these 30 had meningitis.[3] This study did not reflect the emergence of *West Nile virus* (WNV) in the United States in 1999 or account for CNS diseases that are present in North America, such as *Eastern equine encephalomyelitis* (EEE) or EPM.

Regardless of the type of etiologic agent involved, CNS infections require an accurate and rapid diagnosis and implementation of an appropriate course of treatment by the attending clinician. CNS infection should be suspected in horses with abnormal mentation, seizures, blindness, multiple cranial nerve abnormalities, and general proprioceptive deficits. Infections involving primarily the spinal cord may manifest as limb weakness, incoordination, and stiffness, with or without associated cerebral dysfunction. The reader is referred to chapters on individual diseases for detailed description and discussion of EPM (see Chapter 59), WNV (see Chapter 21), alphavirus encephalitides (see Chapter 20), rabies (see Chapter 19), equine herpesvirus myelopathy (see Chapter 13), *Streptococcus equi* subsp. *equi* (see Chapter 28), and *Anaplasma phagocytophilum* (see Chapter 42). This chapter provides an overview of CNS infection, pathogenesis, diagnosis, and treatment, with discussion of miscellaneous CNS infections not covered elsewhere in this text.

The appropriate term for infection and resultant inflammation of the CNS is determined by the specific area of the nervous system affected. Inflammation of the brain, meninges, spinal cord, and peripheral nerves is termed *encephalitis, meningitis, myelitis,* and *neuritis*, respectively. *Rhomboencephalitis* and *cerebellitis* refer to localized inflammation of the brain stem and cerebellum, respectively.[4,5] Frequently, more than one tissue or anatomic site may be affected. *Meningoencephalitis* is inflammation of the meninges and brain, and *meningoencephalomyelitis* is inflammation of the meninges, brain, and spinal cord. Inflammation of the brain and spinal cord, without meningeal involvement, is termed *myeloencephalitis*.

Infection of the CNS can also result in focal suppuration of the brain parenchyma or spinal cord and formation of abscesses. Localized areas of infection between the outermost meningeal layer (dura mater) and the skull and vertebral column are termed *epidural abscesses*. Inflammation between the outer two layers of the meninges (dura mater and arachnoid) is termed *subdural empyema*.[1]

NEUROANATOMY AND DISEASE

Brain and Meninges

Inside the protective barrier of the skull, the brain is surrounded by three layers of meninges: the outermost dura mater, or *pachymeninges*, and the *leptomeninges*, consisting of the inner

Table • 4-1

Equine Central Nervous System Pathogens

PATHOGEN	SELECT REFERENCES	PATHOGEN	SELECT REFERENCES
Viral		*Halicephalobus gingivalis*	93-95, 97, 98, 101, 103-109, 113, 114, 152
West Nile virus	15, 20, 22, 50, 115-119	*Draschia megastoma*	158
Western equine encephalomyelitis virus	121-129	*Trypanosoma evansi*	165-169
Eastern equine encephalomyelitis virus	122, 127, 129, 131-139	**Bacterial**	
Venezuelan equine encephalomyelitis virus	143, 144	*Escherichia coli*	9, 62
St. Louis virus	146	*Actinobacillus equuli*	62, 79
Murray Valley virus	149-151	*Streptococcus (equi, zooepidemicus, suis)*	7, 27, 62, 70, 174, 175
Louping ill virus	153-157	*Salmonella*	62, 63, 88
California group/snowshoe hare virus	159-164	*Pasteurella caballi*	11, 177-179
Main Drain virus	170	*Pseudomonas aeruginosa*	7
Semliki Forest virus	171	*Enterococcus*	8
Japanese encephalitis virus	172	*Actinomyces*	190, 191
Hendra virus	173	*Rhodococcus equi**	25, 79, 81, 82, 86, 89, 193
Nipah virus	173	*Brucella abortus**	89
Powassan virus	176	*Mycobacterium bovis**	11, 196-198
Aujeszky's disease virus	180	*Staphylococcus* spp.*	77
Equine herpesvirus type 1	41, 42, 181-187	*Actinobacillus lignieresii**	80
Equine infectious anemia virus	188, 189	*Klebsiella pneumoniae*, type 1	68
Rhabdovirus (rabies)	192	*Listeria monocytogenes*	36, 64
Kunjin virus	151, 194	**Protozoal**	
Borna virus	195	*Balamuthia mandrillaris*	111
Parasitic		*Sarcocystis neurona*	18, 48, 199-203
Setaria	120	**Fungal**	
Habronema	130	*Cryptococcus neoformans*	72-74
Hypoderma (lineatum, bovis, diana)	140-142	*Aspergillus niger, A. fumigatus**	75
Parastronglyus spp.	145	**Rickettsial**	
Strongylus vulgaris	130, 147, 148	Anaplasma phagocytophilum	204

*Denotes vertebral body osteomyelitis.

arachnoid membrane and pia mater (Fig. 4-1). The *pia mater* is adherent to the external surface of the brain and spinal cord, forming cuffs around penetrating vessels and merging with the ependymal lining of the fourth ventricle. Cerebrospinal fluid (CSF) occupies the subarachnoid space between the pia mater and arachnoid. Acute bacterial infections within the subarachnoid space typically begin with the leptomeninges of the brain and spinal cord and spread inward through the foramina of the fourth ventricle. Infections between the dura mater and arachnoid (subdural empyema) can spread over the entire cerebral hemisphere. The *dura mater* adheres to the periosteum of the skull and limits the spread of epidural abscesses (between the dura and skull), except where it invaginates into the cranial cavity to form four rigid septa: the falx cerebri, falx cerebelli, tentorium cerebelli, and diaphragma selli.[1]

The brain rests within the anterior, middle, and posterior *cranial fossae*, which are associated with the paranasal sinuses. The anterior fossa forms the roof of the frontal and ethmoidal sinuses. The *sella turcica* is located between the left and right middle fossa and forms the roof of the sphenoid sinuses. Infection in these paranasal sinuses can spread through the respective fossa centrally to the brain, resulting in epidural abscesses and subdural empyema. In the horse, these infections can be either bacterial or fungal.[6-10] Middle ear infections *(otits media)* within the petrous temporal bone may extend into the middle fossa to involve the temporal lobe of the brain or into the posterior fossa to involve the cerebellum or brain stem.[1,11]

Neuroanatomic localization of brain disease in the horse has been well described.[12-14] Briefly, infectious neurologic disease in the horse either is diffuse (e.g., viral or protozoal) or can have a single neuroanantomic signal (e.g., brain abscess). Neuroanatomic localization should be defined in terms of the five major regions of the CNS (and the cranial nerves): disease of the cerebrum, basal nuclei, rostral brain stem, caudal brain stem, and cerebellum.[14]

Seizure activity and moderate to severe *obtundation* are the most common signs of cerebral disease in the horse. Although the cortex controls conscious proprioception, this is difficult to localize to the cerebrum in the horse and in the absence of other clinical signs. Blindness occurs secondary to lesions in the

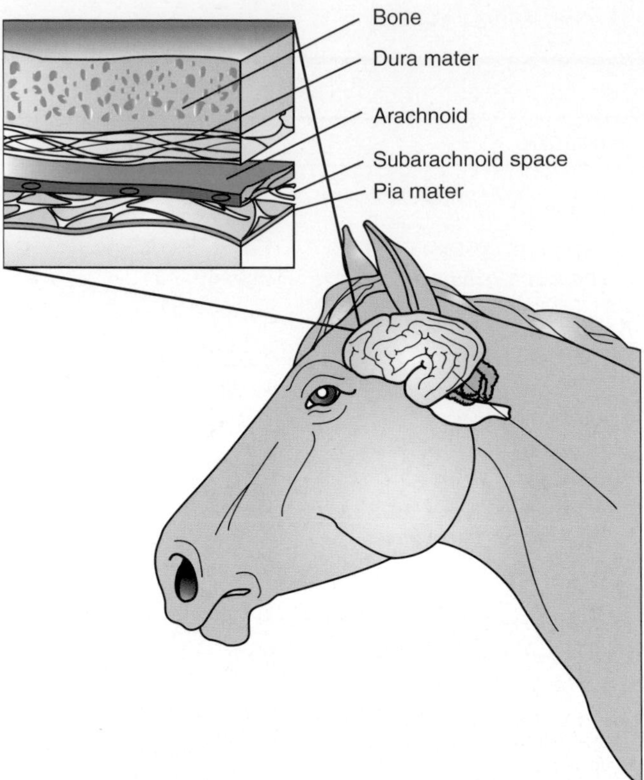

Fig. 4-1 Diagram of layers of meninges of the horse.

visual cortex. Cortical blindness presents as decreased normal reactions to visual cues, with normal pupillary light reflexes. A full ophthalmic examination is paramount to assessing cortical blindness. The most common clinical sign of focal disease of the basal nuclei is the inability to chew and form coordinated eating movements with the tongue, teeth, and oropharynx.[12-14] However, diffuse disease in this area involves the caudate nucleus, globus pallidus, putamen, and substantia nigra and should result in loss of coordination of movement. Extension to the reticular formation may result in abnormalities of the wake/sleep cycle.[15]

Clinical signs referable to lesions of the rostral brain stem can be differentiated on the basis of signs of abnormalities of cranial nerve (CN) II through CN IV. Vision, pupillary responses, and eyeball placement can be affected by disease in these areas. Postganglionic *Horner's syndrome* (ipsilateral ptosis, miosis, enophthalmos, and localized ipsilateral sweating) can occur if lesions are rostral to the foramen lacerum involving the sympathetic fibers as they course to the sphincter pupillae muscle (see Chapter 10).[12-14]

The hypothalamus, reticular formation, and pituitary gland are included within the diencephalon and mesencephalon of the brain stem. Hypothalamic and pituitary disease generally result in endocrine dyscrasia. The reticular formation is very important for arousal and coordination of motor function. Lesions associated with the caudal brain stem can be identified based on clinical signs indicating abnormalities of CN V through XII.

Cranial Nerves

All the cranial nerves exit through the meninges at the base of the brain and are susceptible to injury in horses with meningitis because of direct spread of infection or increased intracranial pressure. The clinical signs of multiple versus single cranial nerve abnormalities are important for ruling out specific etiologies.[12-14] For example, a weak horse with primary dysphagia and slow pupillary light responses has evidence of a multifocal or diffuse disease process such as botulism. Unilateral masseter atrophy consistent with CN V paralysis is a common finding in horses with clinical disease caused by *Sarcocystis neurona* infection.

Spinal Cord

The spinal cord has a central core of gray matter surrounded by the ascending and descending nerve tracts of the white matter. *Intramedullary lesions* (within the spinal cord) produce neuronal injury at one or more spinal cord segments and then expand laterally to involve motor and sensory nerve tracts. Clinical signs are observed caudal to the site of the spinal cord lesion because of damage to descending motor tracts.[12-14] Although clinical signs of spinal cord disease are most often bilateral in horses, severity is frequently asymmetric; a close examination will reveal that most intramedullary lesions, unless extremely focal, will have some degree of abnormality associated with the contralateral limb. On the other hand, *extramedullary lesions*, or lesions of the peripheral nerves, will involve a single limb. Peripheral or extramedullary lesions can produce signs of nerve root irritation. When a lesion is compressive on the spinal cord, from outward to inward, there is a stepwise loss of proprioception, then weakness. After onset of weakness, further compression results in loss of sensation, followed by loss of deep pain. A typical presentation for a horse with cervical vertebral myelopathy is a young, strong 2-year-old racehorse with spontaneous loss of balance.[16,17] Diffuse spinal cord disease is often observed in viral infections such as arbovirus infection, neurologic equine herpesvirus syndrome, rabies, and *Halicephalobus* infection, whereas multifocal, asymmetric disease is observed in horses with EPM.[18,19] West Nile virus can be highly variable, with either diffuse spinal signs or highly asymmetric clinical signs.[15,20-22]

Spread of infectious agents can be limited by neuroanatomic boundaries. The anatomic arrangements of the spinal meningeal layers (pia mater, arachnoid, and dura mater) are the same as described for the brain, and a plane of infection is possible between the arachnoid and dura. The spinal dura and periosteum diverge at the foramen magnum. At the level of the seventh cervical vertebra (C7), they are separated by a fat-filled epidural space that cannot prevent longitudinal spread of infection, and thus infection may extend over many segments.[1] In the horse the spinal cord ends as the cauda equina as the cord tapers into the conus medullaris, with distally coursing spinal nerve roots. Unlike in other species, the meninges end caudally between the second and third sacral vertebrae (S2 and S3) in the horse.[12,16] The cauda equina is a site associated with CNS inflammatory diseases and occasional peripheral neuritis.[23]

Vascularization

The blood supply to the CNS includes an extensive network of intercranial arterial and venous vessels fed by two sources, the basilar and internal carotid arteries, with multiple communications to the external circulatory vessels via the circle of Willis to ensure collateral circulation of the brain. The horse is distinct from other species because the internal carotid artery does not receive any blood from the maxillary artery. The details are beyond the scope of this review; however, some salient features are worth mentioning. The ophthalmic artery is a branch of the internal carotid artery, which is a branch of the main intercranial artery, the basilar artery. Therefore, CNS infection could result in septic emboli to the ophthalmic artery and consequent retinal lesions and loss of some visual fields. The middle cerebral artery has the greatest blood flow volume and is considered the area of greatest risk for septic embolization and mycotic aneurysms in the brain.[3] Brain infection most likely arises from infections with *Aspergillosis* and mucoracious fungi in lungs, uterus, and intestine[24] (see Chapters 56 and 57). In descending order of frequency, the internal carotid artery, external carotid artery, and maxillary arteries are the most common equine vessels to be affected with mycotic aneurysm and extracranial (guttural pouch) infection[1] (see Chapter 1).

Despite an extensive network of collateral circulation, three areas of the brain are supplied by only one or two vessels. Highly vulnerable to ischemic injury and abscess formation, these areas include (1) the middle and posterior cerebral arteries at the junction of the parietal, occipital, and temporal lobes; (2) the medial surface of the hemispheres of the cerebellum; and (3) cerebral white matter. No valves are present in the venous supply to the CNS, and the direction of flow may change with hemodynamic changes caused by pressure changes in the CSF and conditions such as cerebral edema. The anterior spinal cord is supplied by the cervical and intercostal arteries from the descending aorta and generally has a higher likelihood of infection than other parts of the spinal cord.[1,3] Data that support this have not been evaluated in the horse, although osteomyelitis of the cervical and thoracic spinal column may occur in foals.[25,26]

Blood-Brain Barrier and Cerebrospinal Fluid

The capillary system of the CNS is unique in that it consists of endothelial cells with tight junctions and no fenestrations, creating an effective *blood-brain barrier* (BBB).[1] The BBB is the primary protective barrier of the CNS and acts as a filter preventing access of large proteins, immunoglobulins, antigens, pathogens, and some antimicrobial agents (e.g., gentamicin, amphotericin B) to the brain.[1] Injury to the BBB by ischemic insult (e.g., septic emboli), vasculitis induced by inflammation, or increased levels of tumor necrosis factor alpha (TNF-α) can disrupt this protective barrier and predispose to CNS infection. Disruption of the BBB permits the entry of radiodense agents into the CNS for early visualization of abscesses on contrast magnetic resonance imaging (MRI) and computed tomography (CT) studies.[7,27] The blood supply to the pituitary gland, choroid plexus, and brain stem does not have tight junctions, and these areas are considered to exist outside the BBB.

Cerebrospinal fluid is an ultrafiltrate of plasma produced by active secretion from the choroid plexus in the lateral, third, and fourth ventricles and by diffusion across the meninges.[1,28-30] CSF protects and sustains the CNS.[31,32] It circulates outward through the ventricular foramina into the subarachnoid space and is reabsorbed over 3 to 4 hours through cells of the arachnoid villi along the superior sagittal sinuses. Blockage of the villi from inflammation, blood in the subarachnoid space, or occlusion of the superior sagittal or lateral sinuses prevents the reabsorption of CSF, and *communicating hydrocephalus* develops. *Obstructive hydrocephalus* results from blockage of CSF circulation at the ventricles caused by inflammation or compression of the ventricles, as might occur with abscess or hemorrhage. Unlike communicating hydrocephalus, redistribution of increased quantities of CSF and cerebral edema into the subarachnoid space is not possible in obstructive hydrocephalus, and there is increased likelihood of brain herniation and death.[1,32]

PATHOGENESIS

Entry of Pathogens

Most neurotropic viruses gain initial entry to the body through the bite of an infected mosquito or insect (e.g., arboviruses), the respiratory tract (e.g., herpesvirus), or the gastrointestinal (GI) tract. Dendritic cells or phagocytes at the site of initial infection transport virus to local lymph nodes, where it undergoes primary replication with subsequent viremia. Initial infection with bacterial or fungal organisms most often occurs through the respiratory, GI, reproductive, and urinary tracts.[2] Septic emboli from vegetative endocarditis are another potential source of bacteria or fungi for hematogenous spread to the CNS. Regardless of the initial route of infection, the majority of CNS pathogens probably enter the nervous system of the host by a hematogenous route.[1,2,5]

The exact mechanism by which pathogens cross the BBB and enter the CNS is uncertain for most viruses and bacteria, but several mechanisms have been proposed. Bacterial infections of the CNS frequently involve the meninges. A breakdown in the BBB due to ischemia of meningeal vessels secondary to emboli and inflammation may provide a route of access to the brain parenchyma with subsequent abscessation.[33-35] The initial systemic immune response to viral infection in the periphery results in release of cytokines, which stimulate increased expression of adhesion molecules on CNS endothelial cells and increased surveillance of the CNS by activated T cells.[5] Some viruses enter the CNS using these cells as a "Trojan horse." Other viruses use endothelial adhesion molecules to gain entry or induce release of TNF-α, with subsequent increased BBB permeability.[5] Intracellular pathogens, such as *Listeria monocytogenes* and rickettsial species, gain entry into the CNS by penetrating endothelial cells of the BBB or by traveling within phagocytes.[36]

Other than hematogenous spread, pathogens may access the CNS by direct invasion (trauma or iatrogenic introduction), spread from contiguous structures (e.g., paranasal sinuses, otitis media), or retrograde entry along nerve roots.[2,5,33,37] Despite the frequency of infections involving the equine head (e.g., sinusitis, tooth root abscesses, guttural pouch empyema), the number of CNS infections resulting from direct spread to the CNS appears to be low in horses.[37] Rabies virus gains entry to the CNS by retrograde axonal transport along peripheral nerves. Herpesvirus is thought to infect the peripheral trigeminal nerve during latent phases.[2] The potential for entry to the brain through the free nerve endings of the olfactory nerve in the nasal cavity has been proposed for rabies virus and arboviruses, especially *Venezuelan equine encephalitis* (VEE) virus, but has not been proved clinically.[38]

Immune Response of Central Nervous System

The response of the CNS to infection plays an important role in the pathogenesis of disease. In bacterial CNS infections, CSF concentrations of complement and immunoglobulin G (IgG) are low compared with concentrations in the peripheral circulation.[33] Complement and specific antibody are important for opsonization of bacteria, and a diminution of this function may be a critical factor in the pathogenesis of bacterial infections in the CNS. The presence of bacterial cell wall components in the CSF elicits the release of cytokines (e.g., interleukin-6 [IL-6], TNF-α, macrophage inflammatory protein [MIP-1a, -1b, –2]), which stimulate the entry of neutrophils, increased BBB permeability, and vasculitis; CNS edema; and inflammation of tissues surrounding the meninges.

The peak inflammatory response is observed 72 hours after the start of infection.[33] Degenerating leukocytes release toxins that stimulate vasospasm, local ischemia, and further tissue edema. Inflammation of the arachnoid villi where CSF is absorbed could result in communicating hydrocephalus; inflammation of the ependymal lining and ventricles where CSF is circulated may result in obstructive hydrocephalus. Initially there is redistribution of increased CSF and cerebral edema into the subarachnoid space with communicating hydrocephalus, but with severe edema and obstructive hydrocephalus, this redistribution is not possible. Within the confining structures of the skull, the increase in intracranial pressure may result in pressure necrosis of the brain parenchyma or death due to herniation of the cerebellum through the foramen magnum.[34] Vasogenic edema of the CNS is now viewed as a potentially fatal consequence of bacterial infection, and treatment of human patients with both antimicrobial and antiinflammatory medications has dramatically decreased the mortality associated with CNS infection.[38]

When infection occurs, the CNS must mount a controlled adaptive immune response that minimizes damage to brain cells.[5] Initially there is an innate immune response, with production of interferon-β (IFN-β), chemokines, and proinflammatory cytokines. These mediators activate microglia to express interleukin-1 (IL-1), TNF-α, and chemokines that stimulate increased expression of endothelial adhesion molecules (e.g., vascular cell adhesion molecule [VCAM-1], intracellular adhesion molecule [ICAM]). By 3 to 4 days after infection, peripheral inflammatory cells that were activated in secondary lymphoid tissues enter the CNS. Unlike in the periphery, nonlytic clearance of viruses and infected cells occurs in the CNS to prevent secondary damage to surrounding neurons and tissues. Viruses that remain latent in neurons are controlled by continued secretion of antibody, IFN-β, and IFN-γ by long-term lymphocytes.

As with bacterial CNS infections, control or elimination of viral infection in the CNS, without inducing unacceptable damage to neural tissue, requires a delicate balance of the CNS immune response. Induction of *apoptosis* (cell death) of neurons by microglia and stimulation of migration of T cells into the CNS are possible contributing factors to the neurodegeneration observed in degenerative diseases, such as Parkinson's and Alzheimer's disease.[39] Overexpression of C protein, important in the complement system, causes bystander neurodegeneration and oligodendrocyte damage.[40]

The immune response to equine herpesvirus type 1 (EHV-1) may be important in the pathogenesis of the neurologic form of this pathogen. Localization of EHV-1 in the CNS endothelium induces vasculitis. Subsequent CNS damage results from ischemia rather than direct neuronal insult; thus the disease is termed a "myeloencephalopathy" rather than "myeloencephalitis."[41] The exact pathogenesis of herpesvirus neurologic disease in horses remains unclear. The disease is sporadic and seems to be more common in horses with a previous history of exposure to this ubiquitous pathogen and in pregnant or lactating mares. Evidence of antigen-antibody complexes between EHV-1 antigen and EHV-4 antibody and decreased levels of complement activation have been observed in experimentally infected ponies.[42,43]

Other factors also play a role in the pathogenesis of viral infections. Nonsurvivors of *Japanese encephalitis virus* (JEV), a flavivirus infection, have increased levels of IL-6, interferon-α (IFN-α), and interleukin-8 (IL-8). Host genetic factors influencing production of these cytokines may be a factor.[44] Regardless of the immune response, viruses have developed strategies to facilitate evasion of the CNS immune response. For example, WNV may block the signaling pathway for IFN-α.[45]

Understanding of the host response to viral CNS infections is increasing and may explain the seemingly improper or inadequate immune response that allows the establishment of persistent infection. In human patients, certain types of vaccination or viral infection result in a multifocal inflammatory demyelinating process or *acute disseminated encephalomyelitis* (ADEM).[4] An immune-mediated attack against antigen in brain myelin appears to be the cause of ADEM. The poliomyelitis-like, acute flaccid paralysis observed in some people with West Nile encephalitis may be an example of ADEM.[46,47]

The old paradigm of the CNS as incapable of mounting an immune response to infection and being "immunologically privileged" has given way to the current recognition of the CNS as a specialized immune organ.[39] The innate and adaptive immune responses of the host play an important role in CNS infections. A better understanding of this role is important for ultimately developing novel therapeutic and preventive strategies.

CEREBOSPINAL FLUID CHARACTERISTICS

Collection Techniques

Cerebrospinal fluid may be obtained antemortem from two sites in horses: the *atlanto-occipital* (cerebellomedullary) *space* (Fig. 4-2) and the *lumbosacral* (LS) *space* (Fig. 4-3). The optimal site for sample collection is determined on the basis of the neuroanatomic localization of the suspected lesion and practical considerations regarding patient systemic health status and restraint options. In general, better diagnostic results are achieved if CSF is obtained from the site closest to the suspected lesion. The atlanto-occipital (AO) space is sampled under general anesthesia and may be preferable in nervous horses, horses undergoing anesthesia for another reason, or in horses with conformation preventing successful LS taps (LS subluxation). Conversely, a LS tap performed standing under sedation may be advantageous in an animal where recovery from general anesthesia is considered a risk because of the severity of neurologic disease.

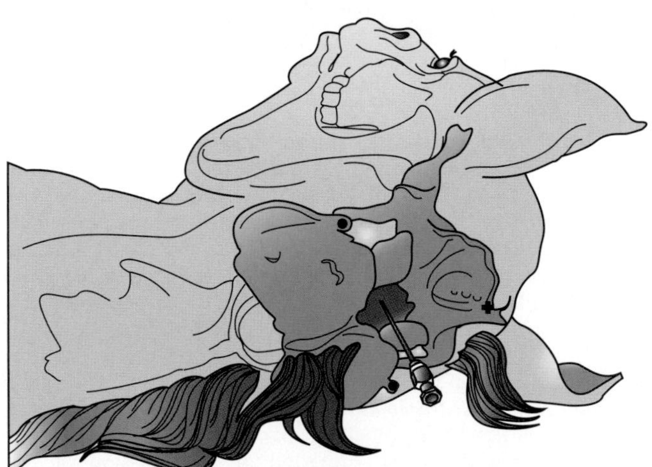

Fig. 4-2 Atlanto-occipital (AO) cerebrospinal fluid collection from recumbent horse. Spinal needle in position with stiletto removed. Palpable landmarks are the cranial borders of the atlas (•—•) and the external occipital protuberance (+) on the dorsal midline. (From Mayhew IG: *Cornell Vet* 65:500-511, 1975.)

Collection techniques for both AO and LS tap have been described in detail.[11,28,30] Briefly, *atlanto-occipital CSF collection* is performed with the horse under general anesthesia and lying in lateral recumbency. An area of the poll and neck (15-20 cm caudal to ears and 8-10 cm on either side of mane) is clipped and surgically prepped. The head is flexed so that the median axis of the head is at right angles to the median axis of the cervical vertebrae. A sterile 8.9-cm, 20-gauge spinal needle with stylet is inserted at the intersection of the cranial borders of the atlas and the external occipital protuberance along the dorsal midline. The needle should be parallel to the ground, perpendicular to the skin, and aimed toward the nose of the horse. The needle is gradually advanced until a "popping" sensation is felt with penetration of the AO membrane and cervical dura. The stylet is withdrawn, and the appearance of clear CSF at the hub indicates a successful procedure. If no CSF appears when the stylet is removed, the needle is rotated 90 degrees. If fluid is still not obtained, the stylet is replaced, and the needle is advanced carefully. The approximate depth of needle insertion for entry into the subarachnoid space is 5 to 8 cm. If the needle contacts bone at a depth of 2 to 5 cm, it should be withdrawn and repositioned appropriately. If blood appears at the hub of the needle when the stylet is removed and does not clear with CSF in 15 to 20 seconds, the stylet is replaced and the needle removed; a fresh needle is used for the next attempt. When CSF flows freely from the hub of the needle, the sample is collected by free flow or gentle aspiration into an appropriate tube. After the sample has been collected and the needle is withdrawn, the head of the horse is extended to a normal or slightly extended position to prevent leakage of CSF from the puncture site.[30]

Lumbosacral CSF collection in the horse is typically performed with the sedated horse standing as squarely as possible.[12,30] Landmarks for the LS site are the intersection of imaginary lines joining the caudal borders of the tuber coxae along the dorsal midline or at the highest point of the gluteal region of the horse. In addition to sedation, adequate restraint with a twitch and use of stocks are advisable. In response to penetration of the dura mater, sedated horses may show no reaction, or tail movement and slight flexion of the pelvic limbs, or violent kicking responses that can endanger the patient and the veterinarian. A 10 × 10-cm site is clipped and sterilely prepped. A 20-gauge, 15.2-cm spinal needle with stylet is inserted in a sterile manner and advanced carefully a few millimeters at a time. Care should be taken to keep the needle perpendicular to the dorsum and on midline. A "popping" sensation may be felt with penetration of the LS interarcuate ligament, dorsal dura mater, and arachnoid membrane. The stylet is removed to check for CSF at the hub. Gentle aspiration with a syringe may be necessary to initiate flow of spinal fluid. If no fluid is obtained, the needle (with the stylet replaced) is advanced to the floor of the vertebral canal and then withdrawn with slow rotation of the needle a millimeter at a time. A needle depth of 12 to 14 cm is usually required for successful CSF collection. Large-breed horses or obese horses may require longer needles. Queckenstedt's maneuver (bilateral occlusion of the jugular veins) may be performed by an assistant to increase intracranial and intraspinal pressure and facilitate CSF flow up the spinal needle. Rotation of the needle 90 degrees to remove occluding meningeal tissue and nerve roots from the needle point may also be helpful. Indirect aspiration with a syringe through an extension set connected to the spinal needle hub is recommended to minimize hemorrhage from excessive suction pressure and resultant occlusion of the needle with meninges. After adequate CSF is obtained, the stylet is replaced in the spinal needle, and the needle is removed. Collection of CSF from the LS space while the horse is in lateral recumbency (under general anesthesia or in a tetraplegic horse) is possible but is considered more difficult than in the standing horse. Attempts may be facilitated by elevating the upper pelvic limb so that the tuber coxae are perpendicular to the floor or by advancing the pelvic limbs cranially to flex the pelvis and LS joint.

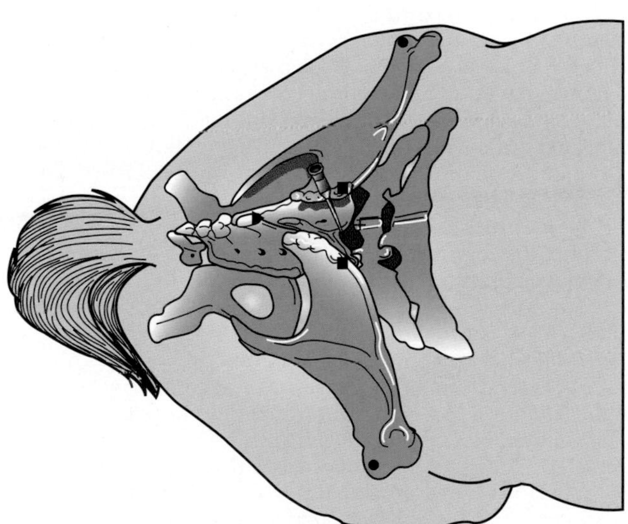

Fig. 4-3 Lumbosacral (LS) cerebrospinal fluid collection from standing horse. Spinal needle in position with stiletto removed. Palpable landmarks are the caudal borders of each tuber coxa (•—•), caudal edge of the spine of the sixth lumbar vertebra (L6) (+), cranial edge of the spine of the second sacral vertebra (S2) (▸), and cranial edge of each tuber sacrale (■—■). (From Mayhew IG: *Cornell Vet* 65:500-511, 1975.)

Both AO and LS collection techniques are regarded as safe procedures in the horse. A common complication is blood contamination of the sample with puncture of meningeal or spinal cord vessels. Initial blood contamination of CSF frequently clears after a few milliliters during collection; however, even microscopic amounts of blood in the CSF sample may result in false-positive results in testing for EPM in horses.[48] In humans, cerebellar herniation through the foramen magnum and herniation of the temporal cortex under the tentorium cerebelli are considered potential complications of CSF collection, especially in patients with increased intracerebral pressure, severe meningitis, or brain abscesses with deteriorating condition.[1] This complication has not been reported as a frequent sequela to CSF collection in horses. Evidence of extradural hemorrhage or formation of fibrous adhesions between the LS ligament and dorsal LS dura mater have been observed in experimental subjects postmortem. Penetration of the AO joint is another potential complication. Cellulitis and septic abscesses secondary to CSF collection in horses are rare.

Analysis

Analysis of the CSF may include measurement of CSF pressure and examination of sample cytology, total protein concentration, glucose concentration, biochemical alteration, turbidity, and color.[28,30] CSF pressure is measured by attachment of a manometer to the hub of the spinal needle before collection. Normal CSF pressure in the horse is approximately

300 mm H_2O (150-500 mm H_2O).[16,30,49] Increased opening pressure, when CSF is first obtained, may result from obstructive hydrocephalus. In addition to noninfectious congenital abnormalities, potential causes of obstruction include tumor, abscess, hemorrhage, and edema. An increased opening pressure that decreases by 20% to 50% after removal of 1 to 2 mL of CSF is indicative of an intracranial mass or spinal cord lesion cranial to the site of collection. Because CSF flows caudad from the ventricles of the brain, and because jugular compression causes increased blood volume in the cranial cavity with subsequent increases in CSF pressure, failure of the CSF pressure to increase in the LS site with bilateral jugular vein compression may indicate a compressive thoracic or cervical lesion.

Appearance

Normal CSF is clear and colorless and does not clot. *Xanthochromia* (yellow discoloration) of the CSF after centrifugation is caused by preexisting trauma, vasculitis, increased protein concentration (150 mg/dL), direct bilirubin leakage from high serum concentration, or breakdown of the BBB.[16,30,49] Xanthochromia with increased protein concentration is typical of equine encephalomyelopathy caused by vascular inflammation and increased BBB permeability.[42,43]

Clots may result from increased fibrinogen caused by inflammation. A CSF sample may appear turbid if there is an increase in quantity of white blood cells (>200 WBCs/μL), red blood cells (>400 RBCs/μL), or epidural fat cells, or if significant numbers of bacterial, fungal, or amebic organisms are present.

Cellular Evaluation

Cell counts and cytologic evaluation performed within 30 minutes of CSF collection are diagnostic. In normal horses and foals, less than 10 WBCs/μL is expected in the CSF. Cells are predominantly small (70%-90%) and large (10%-30%) mononuclear cells.[30,49] An initial neutrophilic pleocytosis followed by mononuclear pleocytosis is characteristic of EEE infections. However, CSF from horses with *Western equine encephalomyelitis* (WEE) and WNE is characterized by predominantly lymphocytic cells.[50] The increase in CSF nucleated cell count with viral infections is typically less (100-1000 cells/μL) than with bacterial meningitis. Eosinophilic pleocytosis with xanthochromia and increased protein concentration may be observed in CSF from horses with parasitic meningitis.[13,51] Infrequently, horses with parasitic meningitis can have a neutrophilic pleocytosis. Fungal organisms may be observed in the CSF of horses with fungal meningitis.[13] Although CSF analysis is useful to confirm the presence of an inflammatory process, to determine antibody titers to specific pathogens, and to monitor for therapeutic response, culture of viral or bacterial pathogens from CSF of horses with infectious neurologic disease is often difficult. Identification of viral etiologic agents in CSF is rare.[4]

Protein

Normal protein concentration in equine CSF ranges from 20 to 124 mg/dL and is typically higher in CSF obtained from the LS site (93.0 + 16.0 [65-124] mg/dL) than from the AO site (87.0 + 17.0 [59-118] mg/dL).[13,49,52] Differences in CSF protein between AO and LS samples that are greater than 25 mg/dL may indicate a lesion closer to the site of origin of the sample with greater CSF protein. CSF IgG and albumin concentrations may be determined by electrophoresis and radial immunodiffusion. These values are compared with serum IgG and albumin concentrations. An increase in the albumin quotient ([Alb CSF]/[Alb serum] × 100) is considered indicative of an increase in BBB permeability, as may be seen with equine herpesvirus myeloencephalopathy. An increase in the IgG index ([IgG CSF]/[IgG serum] × [Alb serum]/[Alb CSF]) may reflect intrathecal IgG production caused by inflammatory disease (e.g., EPM, meningitis, tumors, equine motor neuron disease).[52]

Biochemical Parameters

Increases in CSF creatine kinase (CK) are an unreliable indicator of neurologic disease in the horse and may be falsely elevated by contamination of the sample with epidural fat or dura during collection.[53-56] Lactic acid concentrations in the CSF may increase with some CNS diseases (e.g., EEE), head trauma, and brain abscesses.[13,52]

Immunologic Testing and Molecular Diagnostics

Detection of specific antibodies or antigens within the CSF may be helpful for the diagnosis of some viral, fungal, or rickettsial diseases. Use of polymerase chain reaction (PCR) for the diagnosis of viral encephalitis has become an important and sensitive tool.[4] Details of testing for specific diseases are presented in appropriate chapters.

GENERAL THERAPEUTIC CONSIDERATIONS

Antimicrobial Agents

Antimicrobial selection for treatment of horses with bacterial infections of the CNS is based on initial Gram stain, culture, and susceptibility results whenever possible.[57] Desirable antimicrobial traits include the ability to penetrate the CNS and predicted activity in the low-pH and high-protein environment of infected CSF.[35] Low-molecular-weight antimicrobial agents that are lipid soluble and have a degree of protein binding and ionization at physiologic pH are favored.[35,57] With inflammation, BBB permeability increases to allow penetration and accumulation of drugs that are normally actively transported out of the CNS (e.g., penicillin, cephalosporins).

To allow for maximum peak plasma concentrations, intravenous (IV) administration of antimicrobials is recommended initially. The rapid bactericidal killing needed for CNS infections in human patients requires drug concentrations that exceed the minimal bactericidal concentration by 10- to 20-fold.[33] Expected duration of therapy varies depending on the nature of the infection, but generally is 10 to 14 days.[33,57]

Antimicrobial agents with poor CNS penetration across the intact BBB include penicillins, cephalothin, cefazolin, ceftiofur, tetracycline, and aminoglycosides.[11,35,57] Good penetration is observed with fluoroquinolones, third-generation cephalosporins (e.g., cefotaxime, ceftazidine, ceftizoxine, ceftriaxone), sulfonamides, trimethoprim, pyrimethamine, doxycycline, chloramphenicol, rifampin, metronidazole, and macrolides. Enrofloxacin obtains therapeutic concentrations in the CSF for many gram-negative pathogens (e.g., *Escherichia coli*, *Salmonella*, *Actinobacillus*, *Klebsiella*) but is ineffective for treatment of most streptococcal and anaerobic pathogens. Its association with arthropathies in foals limits its use for treatment of neonatal bacterial meningitis. Potentiated sulfonamides (e.g., trimethoprim-sulfa combinations) are attractive therapeutic agents for CNS infections because they have a broad spectrum of activity, are inexpensive, and are administered orally, but unfortunately, antimicrobial resistance is common.

Third-generation cephalosporins are considered the antimicrobial of choice in human patients with bacterial CNS infection because of their activity against gram-negative bacteria, but these agents may be cost-prohibitive for use in horses. Although ceftiofur sodium is similar to true third-generation cephalosporins, it does not effectively cross the intact BBB in horses. Chloramphenicol is a bacteriostatic broad-spectrum antibiotic with activity against gram-positive, gram-negative, and anaerobic bacteria and is administered orally, but the associated human health risk (i.e., aplastic anemia) must be considered. Rifampin has activity against gram-positive and anaerobic bacteria and is distributed into the CSF, but it must be used in combination with other antimicrobials (e.g., erythromycin) because of the frequent development of bacterial resistance when used alone. Fluoroquinolones should not be used with rifampin because it is an inhibitor of ribonucleic acid (RNA) synthesis. Metronidazole is effective against anaerobic bacteria and is used in combination with third-generation cephalosporins for treatment of human patients with bacterial CNS infections.

Glucocorticoids, Osmotic Agents, and Diuretics

Increased intracranial pressure (ICP) caused by vasogenic edema or obstructive hydrocephalus is common in patients with bacterial CNS infections, and its control is critical for successful treatment of these patients.[35,57] The use of corticosteroids in patients with CNS infection is controversial because of their immunosuppressive effects; however, mortality was unaffected with corticosteroid administration to humans with brain abscesses.[58] Moreover, corticosteroids reverse the increased permeability of the BBB induced by inflammatory mediators (e.g., IL-6, TNF-α, prostaglandins, leukotrienes, IL-1). Administration of dexamethasone (0.25-0.75 mg/kg) to two horses successfully treated for intracranial abscesses was thought to be beneficial.[9]

Mannitol causes an osmotic shift of water into the vascular space, decreases blood viscosity, and increases cerebral blood flow and oxygen delivery.[9,57] The net result is vasoconstriction of the cerebral arterioles and a decrease in cerebral blood volume and ICP. A single dose of mannitol (0.15-2.5 g/kg IV) decreases ICP experimentally within 5 minutes, with peak effects at 10 to 40 minutes and lasting 90 to 120 minutes. Adequate hydration of the patient must be maintained.

The benefits of dimethyl sulfoxide (DMSO) for reduction of ICP are unclear, and most research has been performed in rodent models.[59] In one clinical trial, DMSO reduced ICP and improved clinical course of neurologic recovery. In another trial, continued therapy was necessary for maintenance of decreased ICP.[60] Objective studies regarding the efficacy of DMSO in horses for reducing ICP are lacking.[6,9]

Furosemide prolongs the effects of mannitol, but its effect as a sole agent for ICP reduction is inconsistent and delayed. Controlled ventilation to prevent hypercapnia and subsequent cerebral arteriolar vasodilation is advocated in human patients for the control of ICP.[1] Barbiturates reduce cerebral oxygen demand and are neuroprotective against brain injury.

Supportive Therapy

Properly trained nursing personnel and facilities equipped to handle horses with CNS dysfunction are essential because the size, strength, and severity of neurologic disease in some horses can render appropriate care extremely demanding and dangerous.[61] Rapid progression of disease is common in horses with CNS infections, necessitating the use of padded stalls and protective head gear, removal of shoes, and placement of leg wraps. Adequate bedding, periodic turning of the patient from side to side, or the use of slings to prevent formation of decubital ulcers is essential in the care of recumbent horses. Control of hyperthermia with ice water, alcohol baths, and fans may be indicated. Supportive care with IV fluids, parenteral nutrition, and electrolytes is necessary in an inappetent animal.

MISCELLANEOUS BACTERIAL INFECTIONS

Bacterial and Fungal Meningitis and Meningoencephalitis

Etiology

Bacterial meningitis most often occurs in septicemic foals, often caused by infection with *E. coli*, *Actinobacillus* spp., *Klebsiella* spp., *Streptococcus* spp., and *Staphylococcus* spp. (see Chapter 6). *Listeria* has been isolated from affected immunosuppressed foals (see Chapter 30).[8,62-66] Bacterial meningitis occurs rarely in older horses and may be caused by a variety of organisms.[37,67-71]

Clinical Findings

Early clinical signs of bacterial CNS infection include fever, stiff neck, obtundation, malaise, lethargy, anorexia, and photophobia.[6,11,33,61,72] The stiff neck (meningismus) is not caused by pain but rather by a reflex spasm of the neck muscles due to traction on inflamed cervical nerve roots. In human patients, meningismus is greatest with flexion and less with extension or rotation of the neck and is associated with involuntary flexion of the hip and knee (Brudzinski's sign). Hyperesthesia resulting in spasmodic extension of the legs with touching may also be observed in humans.

Extension of infection from the meninges into the brain parenchyma (meningoencephalitis) via blood supply through the Virchow-Robin spaces occurs rapidly and will manifest as multifocal or diffuse cortical disease. Forebrain disease is characterized by behavioral and mentation changes and may manifest as hyperexcitability, hyperesthesia, obtundation, and self-mutilation. Blindness, lack of menace, compulsive walking, circling, and anorexia may also be seen. Depressed consciousness, head tilt, loss of balance, ataxia, limb weakness, and cranial nerve deficits (e.g., facial paralysis, nystagmus, tongue paresis, pharyngeal paresis) indicate brain stem involvement. Cerebellar disorders are characterized by ataxia, intention tremor, and nystagmus. With increasing severity of disease, seizures and coma are likely.[11,61] In human patients, mycotic meningitis is often characterized by a chronic, slower onset of clinical signs than observed with bacterial meningitis.[34]

Clinical signs in foals may be more subtle because meningitis in the foal may be secondary to generalized sepsis.[66] Presentation in foals can vary from the ambulatory foal with increased body temperature and mild hyperesthesia to the fully recumbent and comatose foal. Foals may present with fever of unknown origin and increased irritability. Seizures are likely in foals with meningitis. Foals may or may not have abnormalities of blood work that support clinical signs; CSF analysis is mandatory to confirm meningitis in the foal.

In horses, fungal encephalitis caused by *Cryptococcus neoformans* (see Chapter 57) is associated with immunodeficiency and guttural pouch mycosis (see Chapter 1). Clinical signs are similar to those of bacterial meningitis. In the horse with guttural pouch involvement, signs associated with the primary disease may include epistaxis, dysphagia, laryngeal hemiplegia, facial paralysis, and mydriasis.[11,72-74] *Aspergillus niger* infection with mycotic vasculitis and right cerebral infarction was reported in one horse, associated with acute bacterial typhlocolitis[75] (see Chapter 56). The mare presented with a 10-day history of watery diarrhea, fever, increased heart rate, dehydration, dysphagia, and depression.

Diagnosis

As with any clinical problem, accurate diagnosis of CNS infection depends on obtaining a thorough history and a detailed physical examination of the patient. Neuroanatomic localization of the lesion in the CNS should be emphasized to facilitate development of an accurate list of differential diagnoses. Further diagnostic tests are chosen to support or eliminate specific differential diagnoses for that patient.

Bacterial meningitis should be suspected in a neonate with clinical signs and history of questionable immune status or concurrent septicemia.[66] A history of systemic infection, ethmoidal hematoma, otitis media, or guttural pouch empyema in adult horses with bacterial meningitis is common.[11,37] Diagnostic investigation to identify possible primary systemic infection is warranted in both adult horses and foals. Confirmation of a diagnosis of bacterial meningitis is usually obtained on the basis of clinical signs, CSF analysis, and imaging of the CNS.

Diagnostic evaluation is done to identify underlying systemic infection that may be associated with meningitis. This evaluation may include complete blood count (CBC), serum biochemical profile, urinalysis, thoracic or abdominal imaging, serology, and blood or urine culture, depending on the patient's clinical signs and presenting complaints. In foals, clinical signs may mirror metabolic encephalopathies associated with septicemia. CBC and serum biochemistry panel are warranted to rule out hypoglycemia, hyponatremia, and hepatic dysfunction.

Analysis of CSF is often invaluable for diagnosis of bacterial meningitis. In human patients, opening CSF pressures of 180 to 600 mm H_2O are reported. Increased white blood cell (WBC) count (100-10,000 cells/μL) with a predominantly neutrophilic profile and the presence of intracellular organisms are the hallmark of suppurative bacterial meningitis. A low WBC count with high numbers of bacteria is considered indicative of a poor prognosis. Decreased CSF glucose concentration, increased lactate concentration, and increased protein concentration are also observed in many patients.[33,34,49,52]

CT and MRI are standard in human medicine as aids in the diagnosis of bacterial meningitis and to rule out concurrent space-occupying lesions (e.g., neoplasia, intracranial abscesses)[33,34] (Fig. 4-4). As CT and MRI become more readily accessible to veterinarians, these scans may assume increasing importance as imaging modalities for diagnosis of horses with bacterial meningitis. Standard radiographic imaging of the skull or vertebral bodies may facilitate identification of predisposing conditions, such as fractures, vertebral body abscess, sinusitis, and otitis media.

Electroencephalography (EEG) is a sensitive tool for the diagnosis of intracranial disease in horses.[10] Abnormal electroencephalograms (EEGs) appear as high-voltage waves with discrete paroxysmal activity. The cold water test, with a 3- to 5-minute application of ice-cold water into the ear and monitoring for subsequent nystagmus, can help rule out central vestibular disease.[76]

Differential diagnoses for bacterial meningitis in foals include metabolic encephalopathies associated with septicemia, Tyzzer's disease, idiopathic epilepsy, cerebellar abiotrophy, intracranial abscesses, neonatal maladjustment syndrome, hydrocephalus, hydranencephaly, and hypoxia.[11] In adult horses, differential diagnoses for bacterial meningitis include mycotic meningitis and encephalitis, viral encephalitides, neoplasia, rabies, migrating parasites, metabolic derangement, hepatoencephalopathy, intracranial abscesses, leukoencephalomalacia, endotoxemia, botulism, tetanus, brain trauma, and intoxication with organophosphate, strychnine, metaldehyde, lead, arsenic, mercury, or bracken fern.

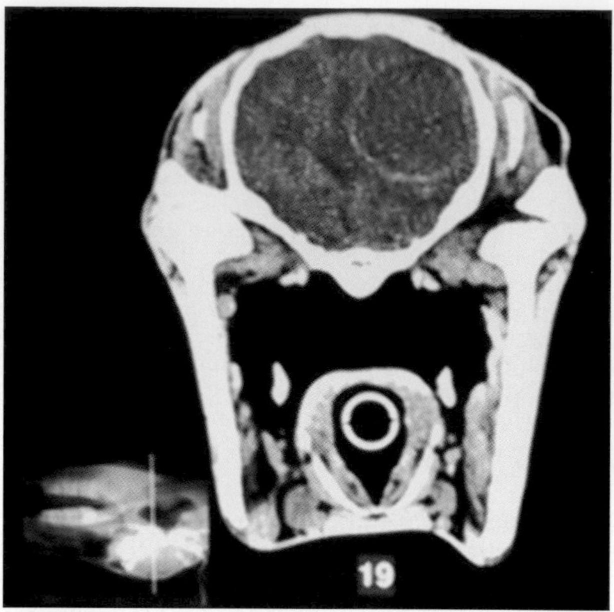

Fig. 4-4 Computed tomographic image of foal that presented with circling and blindness. Large abscess is visible in the foal's right hemisphere. This lesion was confirmed by surgical exploration and drainage. (Courtesy Dr. Rodney Belgrave.)

Postmortem findings are diagnostic in most horses with bacterial meningitis. Grossly congested, swollen, opalescent meninges with petechiation are observed. Histopathologic lesions include infiltration of the tissues with neutrophils and lymphocytes, choroiditis, bacterial colonies around blood vessels, and meningeal hemorrhage. In foals, evidence of septicemia and concurrent infection of the joints, umbilical cord, respiratory system, and GI system may be observed.[11] Culture of lesions will identify specific etiologic agents.

Therapy

Treatment of bacterial meningitis emphasizes elimination of bacterial pathogens and limiting the severe and often fatal consequences of the immune response within the CNS. Third-generation cephalosporins and metronidazole remain antibiotics of choice in human medicine, administered in combination with nonsteroidal antiinflammatory drugs (NSAIDs) and corticosteroids. The use of antiinflammatory medications with bactericidal drugs has reduced the mortality in children with bacterial meningitis from 30% to less than 5%.[38,57,77] Antimicrobials that do not induce cell lysis (e.g., imipenem) rather than traditional β-lactam antimicrobials have been recommended to reduce the amount of inflammatory bacterial debris created. Polymyxin B, which binds the lipid A portion of lipopolysaccharide; intracisternal injection of IgM antibody to lipid A; and intracisternal injection of anti-CD18 antibody to interfere with leukocyte migration into the CSF have also been suggested as novel therapeutic strategies for treatment of bacterial meningitis.[57] In human medicine there is growing concern about antimicrobial resistance. Resistant forms of *Streptococcus pneumoniae* have necessitated the use of third-generation cephalosporins with vancomycin.[38]

Methicillin-resistant *Staphylococcus aureus* (MSRA) was isolated in 3% of 163 patients (see Chapter 29).[77]

Prognosis for survival of horses with meningoencephalitis is fair to poor. Early diagnosis is critical, but vague clinical signs in horses early in the disease process often prevent timely medical care.[61]

Prevention

Although chemoprophylaxis with antibiotics is a mainstay in the prevention of bacterial meningitis caused by *Neisseria*, *S. pneumoniae*, and *Haemophilus influenzae* type B in certain human high-risk groups (e.g., infants, military recruits, workers) and in the prevention of infection of neonates during birth from carrier mothers of *Streptococcus agalactiae*, this type of treatment is not used in horses. Immunoprophylaxis with vaccination for *H. influenzae*, *S. pneumoniae*, and *Neisseria meningitidis* has been described for humans.[33-35,78] Vaccines against bacterial CNS pathogens are not available for horses.

Intracranial Abscesses

Etiology

Brain and spinal abscesses are rare in horses.[7,27] Evidence indicates that CNS infections may occur secondary to extension of infections involving other structures in the head (e.g., sinuses, otitis media, traumatic injury, tooth root abscesses).[37] *Rhodococcus equi* was isolated from an intracranial abscess and concurrent occipital osteomyelitis in a 3-month-old colt. The colt had presented for respiratory distress and a mild left-sided head tilt. The intracranial abscess was suspected to have resulted from dissemination of the pulmonary infection. *Streptococcus* spp. are a common isolate from brain abscesses in adult horses.[79] There is one report of iatrogenic spinal epidural abscess secondary to CSF aspiration.[80]

Clinical Findings

Horses with intracranial abscesses are often presented for evaluation of compulsive circling toward the side of the lesion, head pressing, fever, focal neurologic deficits, seizures, mentation change, papilledema, and ophthalmic tract deficits. Impaired vision has been frequently reported with brain abscesses in horses. Unilateral cortical abscesses result in loss of vision in the contralateral eye because of the high percentage of optic nerve fibers (85%) that cross at the optic chiasm in the horse compared with other species.[6] Although pituitary abscess is considered rare in horses because of the lack of defined rete mirabele vessels, six abscesses involving the pituitary were observed in four of five horses with intracranial abscesses.[37]

Diagnosis

Previous history of a severe purulent infection such as *Streptococcus equi* subsp. *equi* ("strangles") and other systemic bacterial infections (respiratory, gastrointestinal, reproductive, urinary, cardiovascular) are frequently reported in horses with intracranial abscesses.[6,9,27,37] Primary infections of the head (sinusitis, periocular lesions, dental disease, submandibular lymphadenopathy) without concomitant systemic disease are also considered risk factors. In horses, antemortem diagnosis of intracranial abscess is primarily made on the basis of clinical signs, neuroanatomic localization of the lesion, CSF analysis, ancillary diagnostic testing, and imaging of the brain and spinal cord. Human patients with suspected intracranial abscesses are empirically treated with antibiotics before ancillary testing with CT, MRI, and skull radiographs. Involvement of the pituitary gland may result in hyponatremia caused by inappropriate antidiuretic hormone secretion.[1]

CSF changes in horses with intracranial abscessation may be minimal and nonspecific. Increased protein concentration, decreased glucose concentration, and a mononuclear pleocytosis may be observed in affected horses.* Culture of the lesion itself through CT-guided stereotactic aspiration is preferred over culture of CSF for identification of a causative organism. Culture of a pathogen from the CSF of human patients with brain abscesses is successful in only 11% to 17% of cases, whereas culture of aspirates from intracranial lesions is 95% successful in untreated patients and 70% to 82.6% successful in patients treated with antibiotics before sample collection. Collection of CSF is contraindicated in neurologically unstable patients because of the risk of brain herniation.

Use of nuclear scintigraphy, CT, and MRI for imaging of the brain and spinal cord are routine for human patients with suspected CNS infection. Radiopharmaceuticals such as ^{99}Tc-hexmethylpropyleneamine oxime and ^{111}In-labeled leukocyte scintigraphy are useful for differentiation of abscesses from tumors. Labeled leukocytes accumulate in areas of active infection and inflammation.[58]

CT is considered superior to standard radiographs for anatomic visualization of brain abscesses. An intracranial abscess is seen as a hypodense area of avascular necrotic tissue and purulent discharge. With injection of iodinated contrast material, the hypodense area appears to be surrounded by an "enhanced ring," representing a region of hypercellularity and hypervascularity encapsulated by fibrous tissue (see Fig. 4-4). Surrounding the ring may be a hypodense area of brain edema.[9] Stereotactic CT-guided techniques are useful for direct aspiration of abscesses, with minimal damage to surrounding tissue.[58]

In humans, MRI is more sensitive and accurate than CT for the diagnosis of brain abscesses.[33,34,58] MRI is also more sensitive than CT for detection of cerebritis and cerebral edema, which frequently precede overt abscess formation.[58] With CT, small pathologic changes in the tissue are masked by "hardening artifacts," streaklike artifacts of low density caused by absorption of lower-energy photons in the x-ray beam by large radiodense structures. MR images are generated with T1-weighted, T2-weighted, proton density (PD)–weighted, and inversion recovery (IR)–weighted spin-echo sequences. Intracranial abscesses appear hypointense to isointense, with a hyperintense rim if there is capsule formation.[27] The contrast agent chelated gadolinium is excluded from the normal CNS. Its appearance in neural tissue after systemic injection indicates breakdown of the BBB.[7] The sensitivity of MRI has allowed clinicians to define four stages of intracranial abscess formation: early cerebritis (days 1-3), late cerebritis (days 4-9), early capsule formation (days 10-13), and late capsule formation (day 14 and onward). Initiation of treatment during the early stages of abscess formation before encapsulation of the lesion allows for better penetration of antibiotics and better prognosis for response to therapy.[58]

There are two reports of MRI for the diagnosis of intracranial abscesses in horses. In one horse, comparison of MRI and CT found that MRI demonstrated better spatial resolution and soft tissue contrast in delineating the surrounding tissue edema. MR findings of a chronic brain abscess in a 10-month-old filly correlated with the characteristics of a mature brain abscess and were confirmed by histopathologic changes.[7,27] Whether the advantages of MRI will improve the outcome for horses with brain abscesses remains to be determined because treatment was not pursued in all horses in these reports.

*References 6-9, 25, 27, 37, 77, 79-85.

Differential diagnostic considerations for intracranial abscesses in horses include otitis media, central vestibular disease, cholesterol granuloma, neoplasia, rabies, tetanus, EPM, equine herpesvirus myeloencephalopathy, polyneuritis equi, meningoencephalitis (viral, bacterial, fungal, protozoal), subdural empyema, aberrant parasite migration, intracranial hemorrhage, brain trauma, cerebral infarction, and intracarotid injection.[11]

Intracranial abscesses are usually obvious lesions if the brain is evaluated grossly during a postmortem examination. They are usually focal lesions of encephalomalacia with surrounding dense, fibrous connective tissue and dense aggregates of microglia.

Therapy

Long-term antimicrobial therapy and surgical intervention are recommended for treatment of horses with intracranial abscesses. Surgical intervention with craniotomy has been described in three horses.[6,9,37] In all three cases, poor response and/or progression of neurologic signs despite systemic antimicrobial therapy prompted surgical intervention. A 3-month-old colt that developed CNS infection after traumatic injury to the poll required two surgical procedures. The first was performed 7 days after hospitalization to culture and flush the fracture site, and the second was performed at day 20 for removal of a bone fragment and debridement of the matured abscess.[9]

Of the three horses with a reported successful outcome for treatment of brain abscesses, antimicrobial agents initially administered included crystalline penicillin or procaine penicillin intramuscularly (IM) with or without sulfa-trimethoprim.[6,9,37] Therapy was switched to procaine penicillin for 10 to 14 days, and then horses were discharged from the hospital with recommendations for treatment with sulfa-trimethoprim for 28 days. Cefazolin was infused into the craniotomy site in one affected horse.

Empiric therapy with antimicrobials is immediately instituted in all human patients with suspected intracranial abscesses.[58] Course of therapy is determined by whether the patient is a surgical candidate. Nonsurgical patients include those with stable neurologic condition, multiple abscesses, deep location of abscesses, abscesses in a sensitive area of the brain, concomitant meningitis or ependymitis, lesions less than 3 cm in size, and response to empiric antimicrobial therapy. Surgery is also contraindicated in patients with early cerebritis because of the risk of hemorrhage with aspiration. Surgery is considered in patients with rapidly deteriorating neurologic conditions (likely caused by increased intracranial pressure) or chronic encapsulated lesions that are nonresponsive to prolonged antimicrobial treatment. CT-guided stereotactic aspiration is the preferred technique; however, full-excision craniotomy may be necessary in rapidly deteriorating patients; patients with inaccessible lesions in the brain stem, thalamus, or basal ganglia; and lesions with gas abscesses. Fungal abscesses require direct infusion of antimicrobial drugs into the lesion because of the poor concentrations achieved by systemic administration of most drugs. Use of corticosteroids in patients with intracranial abscesses is controversial because it decreases antibiotic entry into the CNS and decreases collagen formation and glial response, but it may be indicated in rapidly deteriorating patients to reduce ICP.[58]

The veterinary literature suggests that the prognosis for horses with intracranial abscesses is poor. Of 13 affected horses, three horses were successfully treated, but one of the three succumbed to secondary laminitis.[8,9,15,30,31] Use of CT or MRI, long-term antimicrobial therapy, concomitant antiinflammatory therapy, and surgical intervention were common factors in the horses that survived.[30] In human patients, mortality associated with intracranial abscess is approximately 5%, with 10% to 58% having mild long-term neurologic deficits and 10% to 25% having posttherapy epilepsy. The success rate for treatment of intracranial infections in humans is likely the result of earlier presentation of the patient, rapid diagnosis and early surgical intervention with the use of CT and stereotactic drainage, and long-term antimicrobial therapy.[29]

Spinal Abscessation and Vertebral Osteomyelitis

Etiology and Epidemiology

Spinal abscesses are rare in horses.[3,11] Most reported cases originate from a preexisting vertebral osteomyelitis (more likely in foals) or diskospondylitis.[11] Common etiologic agents found in vertebral infections in foals include *Salmonella* spp., *Actinobacillus equuli*, *Escherichia coli*, *Streptococcus* spp., *Rhodococcus equi*, and *Klebsiella* spp.[11,25,86-88] Less common agents isolated from horses include *Mycobacterium avium*, *Actinobacillus lignieresii*, *Aspergillus* spp., *Eikenella corrodens*, and *Brucella* spp.[11,80,87,89,90] These bone infections are likely the result of hematogenous spread of the pathogen from primary systemic infection sites (lung, heart, GI) or probably secondary to septicemia in neonates.

The unique vascular anatomy of the vertebrae contributes to the pathogenesis of infection. The decreased blood flow of the tortuous metaphyseal arteries as they approach the vertebral physis creates an ideal environment for the embolization of septic thrombi. Furthermore, the metaphyseal vessels communicate with ventral vertebral plexus, which in turn drains into the post cava, the portal vein, and the pulmonary veins. The ventral vertebral plexus does not contain valves, and when blood flow reverses with an increase in abdominal or pleural pressure, regurgitated blood from infected sites in the body cavities showers the vertebrae and spinal cord with bacteria. As previously described, the posterior spinal cord blood supply is rarely involved in infections because it is supplied by an irregular portion of arterial plexuses, whereas the anterior spinal cord is supplied by the cervical and intercostal arteries from the descending aorta.[11]

Bone lesions may also develop from sequestra broken from fractured vertebrae. Injection of contaminated vaccines or drugs in the proximity of the spinal column is another potential route of infection. Septic arthritis of the AO joint resulting from extension of a mycotic guttural pouch lesion has been reported.[11] Spinal epidural infection secondary to epidural anesthesia is not considered a likely potential complication in horses.[91] There is one report of iatrogenic spinal epidural abscess secondary to CSF aspiration.[80]

Clinical Findings

Clinical signs depend on the anatomic area involved and the extent of infection. Horses with cervical spinal abscesses may appear stiff, may exhibit signs of neck pain, and may be reluctant to eat food from the ground. Additional signs may include pain, heat, swelling, and crepitus over the affected areas and associated signs of bacteremia (e.g., fever, depression, anorexia).[11,87,90] Neurologic deficits depend on the degree of spinal cord compression and inflammation and the area of the lesion. Hindlimb lameness, ataxia, weakness, paresis, cauda equine syndrome, and urinary incontinence have been described in horses with epidural abscesses, pelvic osteomyelitis, and sacral diskospondylitis.[11,54,81,82] If the infection is extensive and erodes through the dura mater, septic meningitis may develop. Extensive bone infection may also result in vertebral bone fracture and development of acute signs of spinal trauma.

Diagnosis

In horses, antemortem diagnosis of a spinal abscess is primarily made on the basis of clinical signs, neuroanatomic localization of the lesion, CSF analysis, ancillary diagnostic testing, and imaging of the spinal cord. Plain radiographs are considered the most diagnostic for spinal abscesses, with osteomyelitis manifesting as hyperlucency and increased bone density in the affected vertebrae (Fig. 4-5). Myelography may be used to define spinal cord compression further.[92] Nuclear scintigraphy (^{99m}Tc–methylene diphosphonate [MDP] and labeled leukocytes) may be beneficial when bone lesions are not well defined on plain-film radiography, as with extradural abscesses.[82] In foals, CT or MRI may be beneficial.

CBC in affected horses is often consistent with a chronic inflammatory focus and may include hyperfibrinogenemia, neutrophilia, monocytosis, nonresponsive anemia, and left shift. In neonates with inadequate colostral immunoglobulin transfer, plasma globulin levels may or may not be increased. CSF evaluation may not be as beneficial because most spinal abscesses do not infiltrate through the dura and into the pachymeninges. Normal or mild increases in protein concentration may be seen.[11,87,90] Diagnostic testing to evaluate underlying primary infection is indicated.

Therapy

As with intracranial abscesses, prolonged systemic antimicrobial therapy is indicated for the treatment of vertebral abscesses. Selection of a broad-spectrum antimicrobial is advocated but ideally should be based on results obtained from culture of the primary underlying systemic infection. Access to the vertebral lesion may be difficult because of the large epaxial muscles of the horse.[11] Surgical drainage and curettage of necrotic bone constituted successful therapy in one horse.[90] Use of NSAIDs may be beneficial to reduce inflammation and musculoskeletal pain. Use of a supportive fiberglass neck cast has been described to stabilize infected cervical vertebrae in smaller and compliant patients. Easier access to water and food by lifting the feed buckets may be beneficial for horses with neck pain.

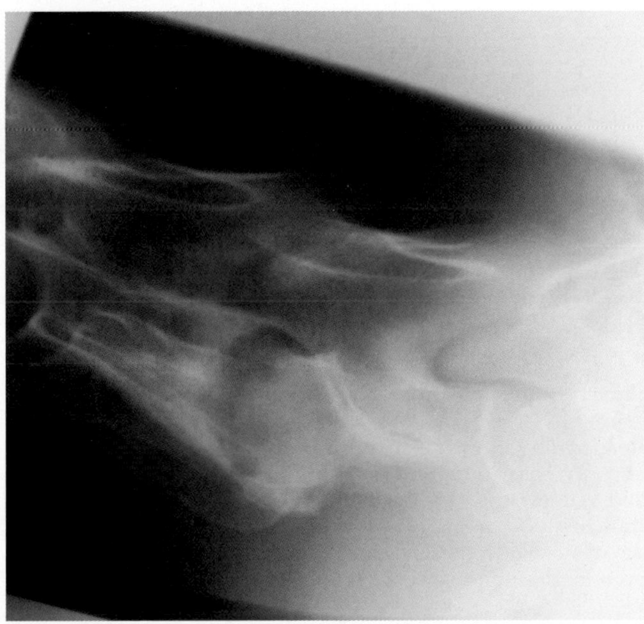

Fig. 4-5 Radiograph of distal cervical vertebra of horse with osteomyelitis (diskospondylitis) at C6-C7. Initial films demonstrated a large, lytic lesion. The horse recovered after long-term antibiotic therapy with mild residual spinal deficits. (Courtesy Dr. Steeve Giguere.)

As with intracranial abscesses, vertebral osteomyelitis and spinal cord abscesses are potentially life threatening, and prognosis is guarded.[11,87]

MISCELLANEOUS PARASITIC INFECTION

Maureen T. Long

Verminous encephalitis is rare in horses but does occur in the Midwest and Southeast United States. Specific causes to consider include *Strongylus vulgaris*, *Setaria* filariae, *Halicephalobus gingivalis*, *Draschia megastoma*, and *Hypoderma* (see Chapter 61). *Setaria* and *Strongylus* cause brain or spinal cord disease. Signs are ipsilateral and sudden, resulting from an infarctive process. *Halicephalobus* and *Hypoderma* usually are intracranial.

Halicephalobus gingivalis Encephalomyelitis

H. gingivalis, previously known as *Micronema deletrix* and *Halicephalobus deletrix*, causes sporadic brain infection in horses resulting from an aberrant infection. This parasite was identified and named in 1954.[93-95] Infection has been identified in humans as well.

Etiology and Epidemiology

Halicephalobus parasites are free-living nematodes of the order Rhabditida (family *Rhabditidae*) that normally reside in soil and humus.[95] In Florida, infection with *H. gingivalis* is anecdotally associated with a swampland environment, although stabled horses have developed the disease. Actual species characterization had been limited until recent molecular techniques were applied to analysis of this organism.[96] The nematode identified as *H. deletrix* is one of seven nematodes that belong to the *Halicephalobus* genus.

Recent genetic analysis demonstrates several different clades.[96] Isolates from clinical cases and from the environment are not aligned geographically, although there are differences among isolates from cases in Tennessee compared with California. Only one type of *Halicephalobus* is associated with mammalian infection; all other species have been obtained solely from environmental sampling.

The life cycle of *H. gingivalis* has not been completely determined; only females have been recovered from tissue sections.[93,94,97] Eggs and immature larvae are present in these infections, indicating an asexual reproductive cycle in tissues. Free-living male worms have been recovered from soil, indicating sexual reproduction does occur.

Pathogenesis

Disease in horses infected with *H. gingivalis* may affect the CNS and the renal, ocular, and reproductive tracts.[94,95,98,99] Little is known about the pathogenesis of this disease in horses. High numbers of organisms are observed in tissue sections. Regardless of infection site, the tissue burden of this organism is dense, and there is an extremely severe tissue reaction with suppurative inflammation and eosinophilic localization within tissue. Abscess and severe, fulminant pyogranulomatous disease is associated with infection.

Site of entry for the parasite is hypothesized to be through breaks in the skin or mucous membranes. Mammary, uterine, and renal infection has been reported independent of CNS infection.[99-101] In one horse with CNS infection, a large, oral granulomatous lesion was observed.[102] Breaks in urogenital mucosa may also provide an important pathway for invasion. Two stallions with renal infection, one with concurrent testicular involvement, have been described.[103] Vertical transmission may also occur in horses.[104] Localization to the kidney may occur through ascending infection, resulting in perirenal granulomas. These frequently coincide with CNS infection. Ocular and periocular infections have also been described in horses.[98,103]

Clinical Findings

Horses with CNS infection usually present with signs of fulminant encephalitis. Rarely, peripheral CNS infection has been described. Most horses have a rapid onset of progressive cerebral signs, with head pressing, coma, extensive loss of proprioception, recumbency, and death.[98,104,105] Onset can be insidious initially, but with cerebral and hindbrain infestation, signs rapidly progress. One horse has been described with cauda equina clinical signs consisting of ataxia, flaccid tail, fecal impaction, and urinary incontinence.[106] Parasitic granulomas were associated only with spinal nerve roots of the cauda equina.

Diagnosis

There is no specific antemortem test for diagnosis of *H. gingivalis* in horses. CBC is usually normal except for possibly an eosinophilia. Hypergammaglobulinemia has been described in the literature and associated with several clinical cases at the University of Florida. CSF that contains eosinophils is highly suggestive of a parasitic infection. CSF total nucleated cell count and total protein concentration are usually significantly increased. Very high numbers of nondegenerate and degenerate neutrophils have been observed cytologically in the CSF of affected horses.

CNS infection with *H. gingivalis* is usually confirmed by histopathology; however, renal involvement with perirenal granulomas is highly suspicious for *H. deletrix*.[93,96-99,101-103,105,107-112] Histopathologic identification of the parasite in tissues is the most common way in which the organism is diagnosed. In tissue section the parasite has a smooth, thin cuticle with what is called a "plymyarian-meromyarian" musculature, and the nematode body ends in a tapered tail. The pendocoelom and rhabditiform esophagus is composed of a corpus, isthmus, and bulb. The parasite has an intestinal tract lined by single, nucleated cuboidal cells. The ovary and uterus can be visualized as a "flexed" structure.

Therapy

Reports are limited on treatment of *H. gingivalis* infection.[107,113,114] A 12-year-old gelding with a granuloma in the orbit was successfully treated with oral ivermectin (0.55 mg/kg every 14 days) and surgical debulking. There was no evidence of infection in any other organ system. Although ivermectin is likely active against systemic infection, it is unlikely that CNS levels obtained after oral therapy are high enough to treat intracerebral *H. gingivalis*. High-dose treatment with fenbendazole in addition to ivermectin is indicated for neurologic disease caused by *H. gingivalis*, although the prognosis for survival is exceedingly poor.

Prevention and Control

Because limited information is available regarding the epidemiology of *H. gingivalis* infection, no specific control measures can be recommended. Good pasture management and restriction of horses from marsh or swamp environments are indicated.

REFERENCES

See the CD-ROM for a list of references linked to the abstract in PubMed.

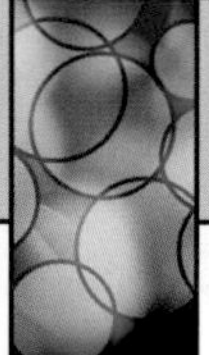

CHAPTER • 5

Infections of Muscle, Joint, and Bone

W. Wesley Sutter and Alicia L. Bertone

Musculoskeletal infections are a common clinical problem encountered in equine practice. Infections in the adult horse are often associated with trauma. Conversely, musculoskeletal infections in the foal are more likely to be of hematogenous origin. In both foals and adults, musculoskeletal infections are associated with significant morbidity and mortality. A rapid, accurate diagnosis and prompt initiation of appropriate therapy are important for a successful outcome.

MUSCLE INFECTIONS

Infectious myositis may be caused by bacteria, viruses, or parasites as either a primary or a secondary disease process. *Primary* infectious myositis occurs when inflammation is caused by active infection of muscle tissue with a pathogen. In *secondary* infectious myositis, muscle inflammation occurs as a response to current or past infection at other body sites, and viable pathogens are not usually present in the affected muscle tissue. Primary infectious myositis may result from direct inoculation of a pathogen (through the skin) or hematogenous localization to a single muscle or multiple muscle groups.

Primary Bacterial Myositis

Etiology

Bacterial infection occurring in association with trauma is the most common form of primary infectious myositis. *Streptococcus equi* subsp. *equi* (see Chapter 28), *Clostridium* spp. (see Chapter 45), and *Staphylococcus* spp. (see Chapter 29) are common bacterial isolates from these cases.[1] Mixed gram-negative and anaerobic bacterial muscle infection with abscessation can occur secondary to infection of deeper structures.[1,2] Many different bacterial agents can colonize muscle from a hematogenous route, including *S. equi* subsp. *equi* and *Clostridium* spp.[3-6] *Salmonella* can cause localized myonecrosis and infection secondary to septicemia in both adult horses and foals[7] (see Chapter 38).

Clinical Findings

In general, clinical signs of primary bacterial myositis reflect whether infection is generalized or localized. Presentation may vary depending on the type of organism and whether signs of systemic toxic insult are present. Clinical findings of localized infection include signs typical of impending or fully mature abscess formation, such as fever, pain (on palpation), edema, and localized swelling. Localized myositis may be insidious if deep muscular structures are involved. Mild to non–weight-bearing lameness can be the primary clinical sign. Injection site abscesses caused by non–toxin-producing organisms can present with moderately painful swelling and no other signs. Infections with organisms such as *S. equi* subsp. *equi*, *Corynebacterium pseudotuberculosis*, and *Staphylococcus aureus* can be accompanied by generalized edema, serum leakage, vasculitis, and cellulitis. Signs of systemic toxemia include red to injected mucous membranes, tachycardia, tachypnea, poor peripheral pulses, and reluctance to move.

Diagnosis

A diagnosis of primary bacterial myositis can be quite obvious if the lesion is localized; however, if generalized myositis or localized myositis without external swelling is present, identification of myositis, let alone infectious myositis, can be problematic. Detailed history of recent injections, trauma, travel, and other systemic complaints should be closely considered. A complete blood count (CBC) may reveal an inflammatory leukogram (neutrophilia with or without a left shift) and hyperfibrinogenemia. If chronic or viral infection is present, these tests may be normal. Increased serum creatine kinase (CK) and aspartate transaminase (AST) activities indicate muscle inflammation or necrosis. Muscle enzymes may not be significantly elevated when localized or occult infection exists.

For localized infection, ultrasound evaluation, radiography, and scintigraphy may assist diagnosis and interventional strategies. Even with an obvious abscess, ultrasound of affected muscle can facilitate evaluation of the extent of the lesion and assessment of response to therapy. Radiographs of the affected area may be indicated if skeletal involvement is suspected. Nuclear scintigraphy has been suggested to aid in localization of abscesses in muscle either by soft tissue phase imaging or by the use of radiolabeled autologous white blood cells.[8]

Diagnostic testing should include efforts to isolate or identify the causative agent. For localized infections, aspiration and culture of soft or fluid-filled swellings is recommended. Culture of samples obtained by deep swab of draining tracts is important. Both these techniques should be performed aseptically. Culture of fine-needle aspirates from swollen, inflamed muscles may yield inciting organisms such as *S. aureus* and *C. pseudotuberculosis*. Muscle biopsy may be indicated in some cases to confirm the presence of myositis and obtain diagnostic culture results. Aerobic, anaerobic, and fungal cultures should be requested when indicated. Identification of parasites is usually accomplished with histopathology. Serology can aid diagnosis of *C. pseudotuberculosis* (see Chapter 30). High *S. equi* subsp. *equi* titer may reflect recent exposure or active infection, if vaccination has not been recent.

Therapy

Therapy for infectious myositis depends on the etiologic agent, type of presentation (generalized or localized), and other organ involvement. For localized infection without systemic clinical signs, local drainage and flushing with isotonic solution are essential and may be the only indicated treatment. When there is evidence of cellulitis, systemic infection, or septicemia, antimicrobial and antiinflammatory therapy is indicated. Antimicrobial therapy should reflect culture and sensitivity results whenever possible. Initial therapy, before receipt of culture results, should be broad spectrum and, with life-threatening infection, administered parenterally.

Clostridial Myonecrosis

Etiology

Clostridial myonecrosis, gas gangrene, and *malignant edema* are all terms used to describe a rapidly progressing infection of muscle with *Clostridium* spp. resulting in severe myonecrosis[9] (see Chapter 45). Clostridial myonecrosis occurs most often after intramuscular (IM) or perivascular injections but may also be associated with traumatic puncture wounds. It may occur in horses after deep IM injection of a variety of substances, including flunixin meglumine, ivermectin, B-complex vitamins, vitamin E, selenium, synthetic prostaglandins, dipyrone, phenylbutazone, antihistamines, and vaccinations.[9,10] *Clostridium septicum* and *C. perfringens* are the species most often cultured from areas of myonecrosis in horses; however, other *Clostridium* spp., including *C. chauvoei*, *C. novyi*, and *C. fallax*, have also been isolated from affected horses.

The origin of the bacteria is unknown. Attempts to culture clostridial organisms from external sources have been unsuccessful. Some authors have hypothesized that spores are present in normal muscle, and that colonization occurs after IM injection with an irritating substance provides a suitable anaerobic environment for bacterial proliferation. Clostridial exotoxins play a central role in the massive myonecrosis associated with infection. These exotoxins directly affect the venous endothelium, creating intravascular platelet aggregation and leukostasis. Resultant decreases in tissue pH and oxygen tension impair immune defenses and create an ideal environment for clostridial growth.[11] Clostridial exotoxins can also have a significant systemic effect, causing shock and in some cases hemolytic anemia.[12,13]

Clinical Findings

Clinical signs of clostridial myonecrosis typically develop within 6 to 72 hours of IM injection.[10,14] Affected horses often show signs of shock and are painful, tachycardic, and dehydrated. It is not unusual for horses with clostridial myonecrosis to present for colic. Horses with cervical muscle infections may be lame in a thoracic limb and may have severe facial swelling. Palpable subcutaneous crepitus is considered a hallmark of this disease but may be absent early in the disease, especially if deep (gluteal) muscles are involved. Many horses will have localized swelling, heat, and sensitivity at the injection site; as the disease progresses, however, the skin may become cool and discolored. Any anatomic location used for IM injection can be affected; the cranial cervical muscle region may be affected in association with inadvertent perivascular injections. Clinicopathologic abnormalities are variable and may be consistent with shock. Increases in serum muscle enzyme activities may be seen, but rarely reflect the severity of the condition, most likely because of poor perfusion of the necrotic area.[15]

Historically, the prognosis for horses with clostridial myonecrosis has been considered to be guarded to poor.[9] More recently, a retrospective study of 37 horses with clostridial

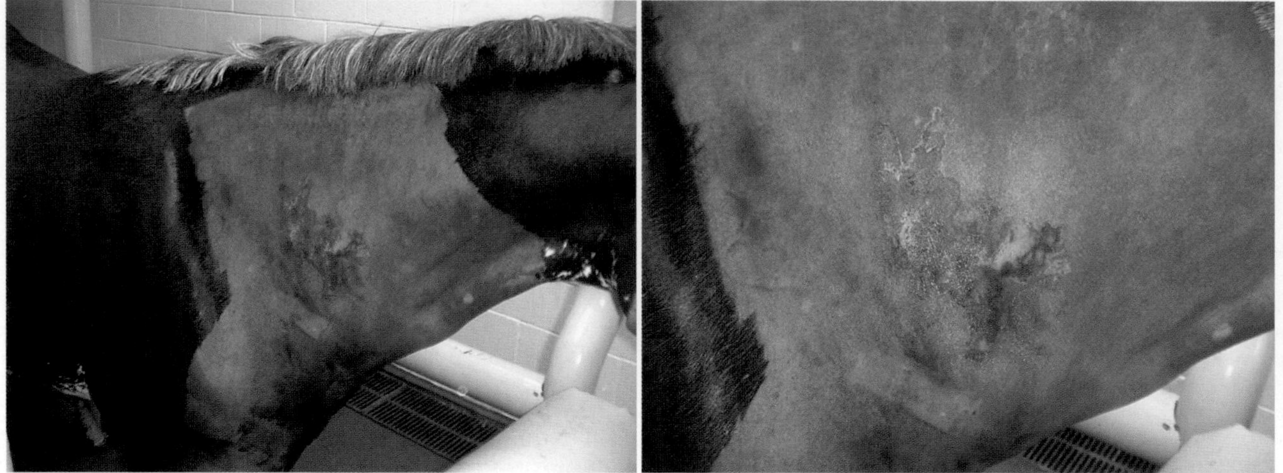

Fig. 5-1 A, Right caudal cervical region of horse with clostridial myonecrosis. B, Note the areas of demarcation of the skin in the affected area.

myonecrosis reported an overall survival rate of 73%.[10] Several factors appear to be important in the successful management of this disease. First, prompt diagnosis and early initiation of antimicrobial therapy (typically high doses of penicillin G) are very important. Second, the early use of fasciotomy and myotomy appears to improve prognosis. Both retrospective studies report a better prognosis with C. *perfringens* infections (19%-25% mortality) than with infection by other clostridial organisms, especially C. *septicum* (50%-85.7% mortality).[10]

Diagnosis

A history of recent IM injection with physical examination findings consistent with severe acute injection site infection is sufficient for a presumptive diagnosis of clostridial myonecrosis (Fig. 5-1). Ultrasound of the affected tissues may support the diagnosis, revealing fluid accumulation, gas, and changes in the muscular/fascial echotexture. Fluid aspirate cytology or muscle sample impression smear with Gram staining can immediately confirm the presence of numerous gram-positive rods characteristic of clostridial infection (Fig. 5-2). Fluid and/or muscle samples should be submitted for anaerobic cultures.

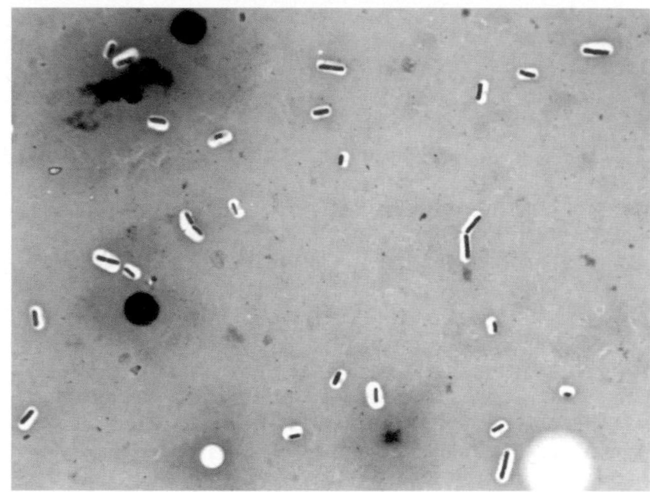

Fig. 5-2 Gram stain of fluid aspirate from horse with clostridial myositis. Multiple gram-positive rods are present.

Therapy

Prompt antimicrobial therapy is necessary for effective treatment of clostridial myonecrosis. High doses of potassium penicillin G, 44,000 IU/kg body weight intravenously (IV) every 4 to 6 hours (q4-6h), are usually recommended. However, clostridial organisms are generally susceptible to a number of antibiotics, including oxytetracycline, chloramphenicol, metronidazole, and rifampin. Evidence in a mouse model of C. *perfringens* myositis suggests that oxytetracycline, metronidazole, and rifampin therapy may be more effective than treatment with potassium penicillin G.[16] This is likely related to the ability of these antimicrobials to decrease toxin production. The ideal antimicrobial regimen would have potent bactericidal effects and decrease toxin production. In vitro, C. *perfringens* α-toxin production and survivability are high with penicillin G treatment, suggesting that this may not be the optimal antimicrobial choice. Tetracycline and chloramphenicol suppress toxin production but have limited effect on survivability. Rifampin and metronidazole have superior efficacy for suppression of both survivability and toxin production.[16] Therefore, combination therapy with penicillin G and either rifampin or metronidazole may be appropriate. However, a subsequent study using the mouse model of C. *perfringens* myositis showed decreased survivability with penicillin G and metronidazole combination treatment compared with metronidazole alone.[16] Currently, equine clinical data suggest that high doses of penicillin G are the first antibiotic choice for treatment of horses with clostridial myonecrosis.[10]

Myotomy and *fasciotomy* are important in the treatment of clostridial myonecrosis. These procedures allow drainage and debridement of necrotic areas, oxygenation of tissues, and some degree of disinfection. In at least one large retrospective study, myotomy and fasciotomy performed early in the course of disease were thought to result in decreased overall mortality.[10] These authors suggest that myotomy and fasciotomy should be performed as soon as possible, stressing the importance of performing a Gram stain on wound exudate at that time. Although there are no guidelines as to where and how many myotomy and fasciotomy incisions to make, starting in

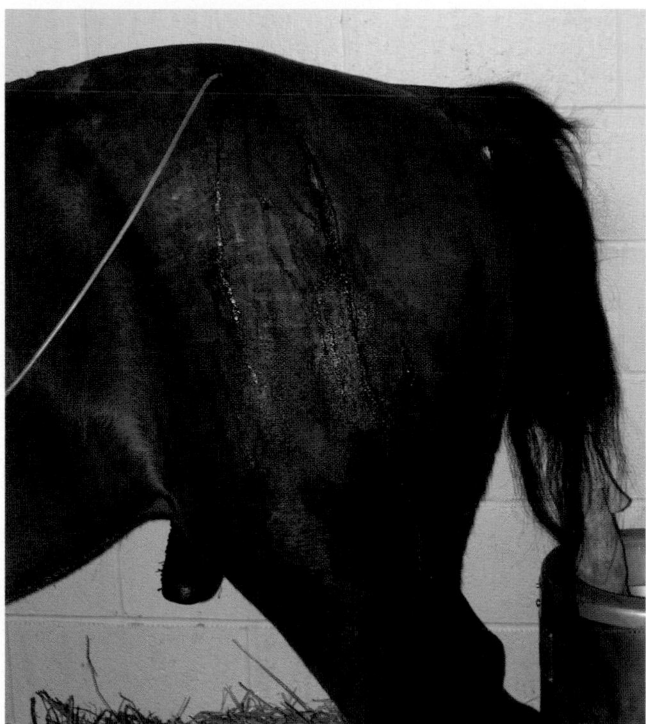

Fig. 5-3 Horse with multiple small fasciotomies and oxygen insufflation through proximal fasciotomy.

areas with palpable subcutaneous crepitus or severe muscle damage is prudent (Fig. 5-3).

Hyperbaric oxygen, if available, may be beneficial for treatment of horses with clostridial myonecrosis but should be used in conjunction with standard treatment protocols. In combination with penicillin G or metronidazole in mice, early hyperbaric oxygen treatment resulted in increased survival compared to treatment with antimicrobial therapy alone.[17]

General supportive care, including antiinflammatory medication, pain management, and appropriate fluid therapy, should be initiated. If horses are recumbent because of generalized muscle inflammation, use of a sling may minimize secondary muscle damage and decubital ulceration.

Primary Fungal Myositis

Etiology

Primary fungal myositis may occur after direct inoculation of the etiologic agent, as may occur with phycomycoses (see Chapter 55). Alternatively, hematogenous dissemination of systemic fungi may result in infectious myositis[18,19] (see Chapter 51).

Clinical Findings

Most fungal infections are localized and fairly obvious. Coccidioidomycosis may be localized or may have concomitant widespread systemic disease with infection of the lung and liver (see Chapter 51).

Diagnosis and Therapy

Diagnosis of localized fungal myositis is similar to that described for diagnosis of bacterial myositis. Diagnosis of specific systemic fungal infections is discussed in detail in the appropriate chapters. Treatment of fungal myositis may include local therapy, surgical excision of lesions, and local or systemic administration of antifungal drugs. Therapy for specific localized or systemic fungal infections is described in detail elsewhere in this text.

Primary Parasitic Myositis

Etiology

The most common causes of parasitic myositis include *Sarcocystis* spp.,[1,20,21] *Trichinella* spp.,[22-24] and *Trypanosoma evansi*.[25] Aberrant parasitic migrations from various nematodes can occur. Rarely, hydatidosis has been associated with infectious myositis.[26]

Clinical Findings

With parasitic myositis, horses usually have generalized muscle infection (unless there is a localized area of aberrant parasite migration). Trichinellosis in the horse is often occult. Affected horses have variable clinical signs, ranging from mild generalized stiffness to signs of severe generalized pain with reluctance to move. Horses with chronic parasitic infections, such as sarcocystosis or trypanosomiasis, may present with weight loss or ill thrift and moderate to severe muscle wasting. Horses with hydatid disease usually have widespread systemic infection of internal organs leading to chronic wasting.

Diagnosis and Therapy

Diagnosis of parasitic myositis is usually accomplished by biopsy and histopathologic examination of the affected muscle. Treatment of specific parasitic infections is discussed elsewhere in this text. The most important health risk for humans associated with equine muscle infection is related to consumption of parasitized horse meat.[21,23,27-31] Outbreaks of human trichinellosis occur fairly regularly in the countries of the European Union. Horse meat is screened for infected muscle in slaughter plants; however, it is advisable that preparation of human meals with horse meat follow appropriate guidelines for inactivation of *Trichinella* larvae in equine muscle before consumption.

Secondary Infectious Myositis

Etiology

Streptococcal infections and several viruses may contribute to development of secondary myositis in which viable infectious agents are not present in the affected muscle tissue.[3-6] Lesions are usually generalized, affecting several muscle groups. The primary infectious agent triggers myositis as an inflammatory or an immune-mediated process. *Streptococcus equi* subsp. *equi* is associated with two types of myositis in horses: *acute* severe myositis, characterized by infarction of muscle, and *chronic* generalized muscle wasting. Both manifestations of streptococcal myositis are thought to be immune-mediated disorders and are discussed in more detail in Chapter 28. Myositis may occur concomitant with, or as a sequela to, acute viral infection. Viral myositis has been demonstrated or postulated to occur secondary to infection with equine herpesvirus (see Chapter 13), equine influenza virus (see Chapter 12), and African horse sickness (see Chapter 15).

Clinical Findings

Horses with myositis secondary to systemic infection present with generalized stiffness and lameness. Most affected horses demonstrate reluctance to move, and laminitis is the most common differential diagnosis. Muscles may or may not be painful on palpation. Horses with muscle infarction or necrosis may have areas of localized edema and pain. When widespread, these horses can have signs of circulatory failure accompanied by poor peripheral perfusion.[32,33]

Diagnosis and Therapy

Diagnosis of secondary myositis is accomplished by muscle biopsy to demonstrate histopathologic lesions of immune-mediated or inflammatory myositis. The approach to diagnosis of a specific underlying systemic infection depends on the type of infection that is suspected. Diagnosis of *S. equi* subsp. *equi* infection is discussed in Chapter 28. Diagnosis of equine influenza, equine herpesvirus, and African horse sickness is discussed in Chapters 12, 13, and 15, respectively.

SYNOVIAL INFECTIONS

Septic arthritis and tenosynovitis are common clinical problems in horses with potentially devastating consequences. Mortality estimates vary between 15% and 50%.[34-38] In adult horses, these infections are most often caused by direct bacterial contamination of a synovial structure resulting from trauma or as a sequela to surgery or intrathecal injection. Hematogenous spread of infection is much rarer in adult horses but should not be overlooked as a differential diagnosis in the acutely lame horse. In foals, most synovial infections are of hematogenous origin. Failure of transfer of passive immunity, respiratory infection, and gastrointestinal infection should be considered as potential concurrent problems in foals diagnosed with septic synovial structures (see Chapter 6).

Etiology and Pathogenesis

Whether inoculation occurs from a wound, surgery, or injection, a similar sequence of events occurs after bacteria enter the joint. Colonization of the synovial membrane causes a severe inflammatory response. This results in the production of various inflammatory mediators, which are largely responsible for the clinical signs as well as damage to the synovial lining and joint. Therefore, treatment should include measures to control inflammation and eliminate bacterial infection.

A variety of bacteria may be isolated from synovial infections that are traumatic in origin. *Enterobacteriaceae* and anerobes are most frequently isolated. Horses that develop infection as a sequela to surgery or intrathecal injection are more likely to have staphylococcal infections.[34]

Historically, synovial infections in foals were postulated to originate from umbilical infections. It is now recognized that these infections may originate from other sources, including the respiratory and gastrointestinal tracts. Foals with poor transfer of passive immunity are predisposed to septic arthritis.[39] The pathogens most frequently isolated from foals with neonatal sepsis are also the bacteria most often isolated from joints of foals with septic arthritis (see Chapter 6). Young foals (<3 weeks) are more likely to have infection of multiple joints, whereas older foals (>4 weeks) generally have only one affected joint.[40] The most common bacterial organisms isolated from septic arthritis in foals are *Enterobacteriaceae,* most notably *Escherichia coli*. Other gram-negative organisms, such as *Salmonella* spp., are relatively common isolates. The most common gram-positive organisms isolated from foals with septic arthritis include *Staphylococcus, Streptococcus,* and *Rhodococcus equi*.[34]

Fungal infections of synovial structures are rare but should be considered, especially if a fungal organism is cultured from more than one site or more than one sample from the same site. Fungal infection of synovial structures may originate either hematogenously or by direct inoculation.[41]

Clinical Findings

The hallmark clinical sign of synovial infection in the appendicular skeleton of the horse is *severe lameness*. The onset and severity of clinical signs depend on the mode of contamination, degree of contamination, pathogenicity of the organism involved, amount of open drainage from the synovial structure, and previous treatment with intraarticular corticosteroids. Although clinical signs are evident within 24 hours of experimental inoculation of equine joints with bacteria,[42,43] the onset of clinical signs from "natural" infection appears to be slower. In one study, joint infections on average became apparent on day 8 after surgery, with a range of 1 to 25 days.[34] It is questionable whether all affected joints were inoculated at surgery.

In the authors' opinion, postoperative joint infections can be separated into two groups: (1) those showing clinical signs within 3 to 5 days, presumably inoculated at surgery, and (2) those showing clinical signs 2 to 4 weeks after surgery, presumably resulting from extension of superficial infection. Incomplete removal of sutures and extension of infection through the suture tracts after removal appear to be major contributing factors to delayed infection.

The onset of clinical signs of synovial infection after trauma is variable. Much of this variability may be explained by the degree of open drainage (horses with sealed synovial infections tend to be more lame), inflammation, and pain associated with tissue trauma, which may be indistinguishable from that caused by synovial infection, and by delayed recognition by owners or trainers. The onset of lameness and clinical signs of synovial infection after intrathecal injections is also somewhat variable, depending on the factors just listed as well as whether or not corticosteroids were administered. Tulamo et al.[43] showed that co-administration of corticosteroids with an infective dose of bacteria significantly delayed clinical signs and synovial fluid changes for up to 2 days. In two retrospective studies describing infection after intrathecal injection, the onset of clinical signs varied from 2.5 to 7 days.[34,38]

Synovial effusion, local edema, heat, and sensitivity to palpation are usually observed in horses with synovial infection. Experimental models of infection suggest that these signs may briefly precede clinical lameness.[42,43] Body temperature is usually increased in synovial sepsis,[43] but the lack of a fever does not rule out joint sepsis, especially in adult horses. Foals typically have higher fevers than adult horses. In one study, 45% of foals with septic arthritis had a body temperature 102° F (38.9° C) or higher.[34]

Diagnosis

Synovial Fluid Analysis

Synovial fluid analysis is necessary for the diagnosis of infection. Grossly, synovial fluid from an infected joint is serosanguineous and turbid (increased cellularity) with decreased viscosity resulting from decreased hyaluronic acid content. Samples from affected joints may contain visible fibrin and debris. The sample should be submitted for total and differential cell count, total protein measurement, and immediate culture. Most samples from infected synovial structures have a total white blood cell (WBC) count greater than 30,000 cells/μL (normal <1000/μL, predominantly mononuclear cells), a differential with 90% or more neutrophils, and a total protein concentration greater than 4.0 g/dL (normal <2.0 g/dL). A Gram stain should be performed; positive findings confirm the diagnosis and may guide antimicrobial therapy. A sample of synovial fluid should be cultured aerobically and anaerobically. The fluid should be cultured in a broth culture system designed for culturing body fluids[44] (see Chapter 27). Synovial biopsy and culture do not yield better results than culture of synovial fluid and are not recommended.[45]

Diagnostic Imaging

The primary goal of diagnostic imaging of synovial infections is to determine if the infection has extended into surrounding bone or resulted in cartilage damage. This information can be used as an adjunct to determine prognosis and modify treatment strategies if necessary. Radiographs should be obtained in most horses with synovial infections.

Septic osteitis or osteomyelitis may precede or follow septic arthritis. Septic epiphysitis and physitis must be ruled out in all foals with septic arthritis. Osteomyelitis and osteitis are less common with tendon sheath infections than with joint sepsis; however, the sesamoid bones may be affected.[46]

Articular bone destruction and joint collapse are not early findings in septic arthritis and indicate that the infection has been present for at least 2 to 3 weeks. Comparative views of the contralateral extremity may be necessary to recognize subtle changes. Advanced imaging techniques such as computed tomography (CT) and magnetic resonance imaging (MRI) can provide additional information regarding the extent of lesions, especially in horses with septic physitis.

Therapy

Synovial infections in horses are considered a medical emergency. Three basic tenets for treating bacterial infection of synovial structures should be observed: systemic antimicrobial therapy, local antimicrobial therapy, and lavage. It is prudent, if possible, to acquire a diagnostic synovial fluid sample before administration of antibiotics. Based on the gross appearance of the fluid, treatment can be initiated immediately. At a minimum, intraarticular antibiotics and broad-spectrum systemic intravenous (IV) antibiotics are indicated until culture and sensitivity results are received. Through-and-through needle lavage (or other lavage) should be done immediately in all joints in which the synovial fluid is grossly abnormal or has an increased total nucleated cell count, increased total protein concentration, and greater than 90% neutrophils (Fig. 5-4). Infected synovial structures with abundant fibrin or cellular debris require open arthrotomies and/or endoscopic debridement and lavage to improve removal of inflammatory debris.[47-49]

Historically, chlorhexidine, iodine, and dimethyl sulfoxide (DMSO) have been recommended in addition to lavage solutions in an attempt to increase antiinflammatory or antimicrobial efficacy. However, lavage with these additives may be deleterious to synovial structures at concentrations expected to be effective for killing bacteria or decreasing inflammation.[44,50-52] Therefore a balanced electrolyte solution without additives is recommended as the optimal lavage fluid.

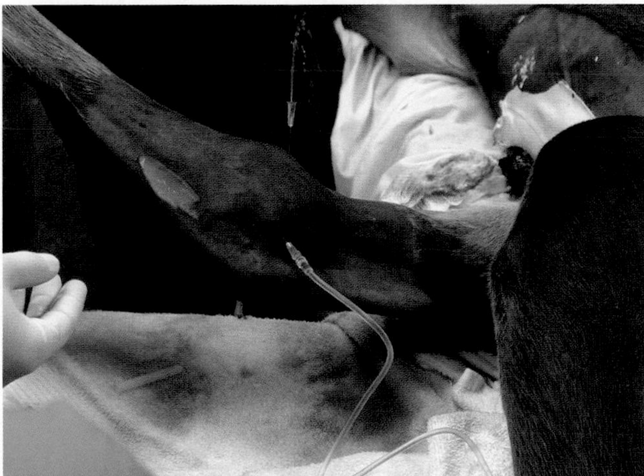

Fig. 5-4 Through-and-through lavage of tibiotarsal joint in foal with septic arthritis. (Courtesy Dr. Debra Sellon.)

The optimal frequency and duration of through-and-through lavage for treatment of septic arthritis is controversial. Some clinicians recommend that infected synovial structures be flushed daily for 3 days and the synovial fluid analyzed on the last day to determine if additional lavage is needed.[53] Lavage and intraarticular antibiotics tend to irritate the joint, and often the WBC count and total protein count will remain increased during this time. Therefore the clinical response to treatment (lameness, joint effusion, heat) should be strongly considered when determining the frequency and duration of joint lavage. A total WBC count less than 20,000 cells/μL is a reasonable goal and can be used as one of the indicators of when to discontinue joint lavage.

Closed suction drainage can also be used to treat infected synovial structures. Typically, a flat fenestrated silicone drain (Jackson-Pratt) is inserted within the joint and connected to a suction device that can be purchased commercially. Although clinical reports of this type of therapy are limited in horses,[54] repeated needle evacuation during the first 5 to 7 days of infection is used with success in humans.[55]

Initial Systemic Antimicrobial Therapy

Staphylococci are common bacterial isolates from synovial infections that occur after surgery or intrathecal injection. Amikacin and cefazolin remain the antibiotics of choice for treating these infections in horses. *Amikacin* is an excellent empiric choice for treatment of most synovial infections of horses.[56] Amikacin is expensive when used systemically in the adult horse but can be economical for local antibiotic therapy, as discussed next. One common strategy for treatment of synovial infections in horses is administration of broad-spectrum antimicrobials intravenously (e.g., potassium penicillin G and gentamicin) with local delivery of amikacin. A knowledge of hospital or regional antimicrobial sensitivity patterns can assist with decisions regarding initial antimicrobial selection. For example, gentamicin was effective in 85% of isolates in one study, providing a relatively high degree of confidence in its use.[56]

Synovial infections after trauma are often polymicrobial and caused by *Enterobacteriaceae* and anaerobes. Broad-spectrum antibiotics that include a reasonable anaerobic spectrum are indicated. Particular attention should be paid to wounds with gross fecal contamination or infected joints near the foot, such as the coffin or pastern joints. *Bacteroides fragilis* is typically resistant to penicillin G. The addition of oral metronidazole to the therapeutic plan should give appropriate coverage for this organism.[56]

After culture and sensitivity results are received, appropriate changes (if needed) in systemic antimicrobial therapy can be made (Table 5-1). The duration of treatment with systemic antibiotics varies depending on response to therapy. As a general guideline, the authors continue systemic antimicrobial treatment for a minimum of 2 weeks after amelioration of clinical signs. If osteomyelitis is present, the duration of therapy should be longer, often 4 to 8 weeks. Plasma fibrinogen concentrations can be monitored every 1 to 2 weeks and antimicrobial therapy discontinued after fibrinogen levels return to normal (usually <500 mg/dL).

Local Antimicrobial Therapy

The delivery of high concentrations of antimicrobial drugs directly into an infected synovial structure often results in rapid elimination of infection. Most local techniques result in little or no increase in serum concentrations of antibiotics and

Table • 5-1

Systemic Antibiotics Used to Treat Osteomyelitis and Septic Synovial Structures

DRUG	MANUFACTURER	SYSTEMIC DOSE*	OTHER USES†
Amikacin	Amiglyde (Fort Dodge)	*Adult:* 15 mg/kg IV q24h *Foal:* 21-25 mg/kg IV q24h	RP, IA, AIB
Ampicillin	Amp-equine (Pfizer)	20 mg/kg IV q6h	
Ceftriaxone	Rocephin (Roche Laboratories)	50 mg/kg IV q24h	RP, IA, AIB
Cefazolin	Ancef (Glaxco Smith-Kline)	10-20 mg/kg IV q6h	AIB
Ceftazidime	Fortaz (Glaxco Smith-Kline)	30-50 mg/kg IV q6-12h	RP, IA, AIB
Ceftiofur	Naxcel (Pharmacia & Upjohn)	2-8 mg/kg IV q6-24h	IA, AIB
Cefotaxime	Claforan (Aventis)	25 mg/kg IV q6h	
Chloramphenicol	Generic	50 mg/kg PO q6h	Human health risk
Doxycycline	Generic	10 mg/kg PO q12h	Variable oral absorption
Enrofloxacin	Baytril (Bayer Corp)	2.5-10 mg/kg IV q12-24h	Arthropathies (foals), tendon weakening or rupture
Erythromycin	Generic	20-30 mg/kg PO q8h	May cause hyperthermia and diarrhea
Fluconazole	Diflucan (Roerig)	5 mg/kg PO q24h	Susceptible fungal infections; AIB
Gentamicin	Gentocin (Schering-Plough)	6-7 mg/kg IV q24h	RP, IA, AIB
Imipenem-cilastatin	Primaxin (Merck)	10-20 mg/kg IV q6h	RP, IA, AIB
Metronidazole	Generic	15-25 mg/kg PO q6h	AIB
Oxytetracycline		8-10 mg/kg IV q12h	
Procaine penicillin G		22,000-40,000 IU/kg IM q12h	
Potassium penicillin G		10,000-40,000 IU/kg IV q4-6h	
Rifampin	Rifadin (Hoeschst Marion Roussel)	5-10 mg/kg PO q12h	Do not use alone
Ticarcillin/clavulanate	Timentin (Smith-Kline Beecham)	50 mg/kg IV q6h	Antipseudomonal
Trimethoprim-sulfa	Generic	20-30 mg/kg PO q12h (based on sulfa portion) 15-24 mg/kg IV q8-12h	
Vancomycin	Vancocin (Eli Lilly)	6 mg/kg IV q8h	AIB; use slow infusion

**IV*, Intravenously; *PO*, orally; *IM*, intramuscularly; *q24h*, every 24 hours.
†*RP*, Regional perfusion; *IA*, intraarticular; *AIB*, antibiotic-impregnated beads.

can be used safely in combination with appropriate systemic dosing. Several methods of local administration of antimicrobials are possible. The simplest technique is repeated intraarticular administration of antibiotics using a needle. Intravenous regional perfusion (Box 5-1 and Fig. 5-5), intraosseous regional perfusion (Box 5-2), constant-rate infusion pumps, and antimicrobial-impregnated beads (Box 5-3) may also be used to deliver antimicrobial drugs to tissues at a minimum inhibitory concentration (MIC) several orders of magnitude higher than that achievable by systemic administration.

Aminoglycosides are the most common class of antimicrobial agent used for direct intrasynovial injection. The ideal dose and frequency are dependent on the synovial fluid volume, pathogenic organism involved, and antimicrobial used. As a general guideline, 1 g of gentamicin will maintain a MIC effective against most microorganisms in the joint for 24 hours and in the surrounding bone for 8 hours.[57] Similarly, ceftiofur at a dose of 150 mg in the antebrachiocarpal joint will maintain sufficient bactericidal concentrations for 24 hours.[58]

Intravenous regional limb perfusion is performed by catheterizing a vessel (typically a vein) in the area of infection and applying a tourniquet above and below the region (see Box 5-1 and Fig. 5-5). Antimicrobials are perfused into the local area through the catheter. Typically, antimicrobial doses of one third and up to the systemic dose are diluted to a final volume of 30 to 60 mL and injected slowly. The tourniquet is maintained for 30 minutes. In infected areas, inflammation and vascular impairment may decrease the exposure of diseased tissue to systemic antimicrobials. Conceptually, with regional limb perfusion, the vascular system in the region is dilated, and increased vascular hydrostatic pressure and concentration gradient drive the antimicrobial into the soft tissue, resulting in high local concentrations that would be unachievable by nontoxic systemic doses. The most frequently used (reported) antimicrobials are the aminoglycosides[57,59-61]; however, the authors have successfully used third-generation cephalosporins for regional limb perfusion. With aminoglycoside regional IV perfusion, antimicrobial concentrations within the joint fluid are expected to be 5 to 50 times greater than that achievable with systemic IV administration[59] and remain above the MIC of most organisms for 24 hours.[57] Based on these data, the authors generally perform regional limb perfusions daily for the first 3 to 5 days or until a clinical response is evident.

Intraosseous regional limb perfusion is performed by inserting a cannulated screw into the medullary cavity of a long bone in proximity to the infected area (see Box 5-2). Importantly, the cannulated screw must be customized or purchased with an

Box • 5-1

Intravenous Regional Limb Perfusion*

- Aseptically prepare area over the blood vessels to be used for perfusion.
- Prepare appropriate dose of antimicrobial drugs, diluted in saline, to a final volume of 30 mL for lower limb perfusion or 60 mL for upper limb perfusion.
- Appropriate anesthesia or sedation should be administered, depending on whether the procedure is performed in the anesthetized or standing horse. If the procedure is to be performed standing, consider adding 10 mL of local anesthetic agent (e.g., lidocaine 2%) to the perfusate. Alternatively, appropriate regional nerve blocks may be performed.
- Apply tourniquets proximal and distal to the region to be perfused. Perfusion of regions including the fetlock and below does not require a distal tourniquet.
- Apply tourniquet proximal to the region to be perfused.
- Insert small-gauge, over-the-needle catheter or butterfly catheter into the appropriate blood vessel.
- Begin injection of the perfusate. The volume should be injected slowly over 5 to 10 minutes to avoid damage to small blood vessels. If the perfusion is performed standing, it is recommended to tape the extension set to the tourniquet to prevent movement of the horse and inadvertent removal of the catheter.
- During the injection, periodically aspirate with the syringe to confirm that the needle remains appropriately situated in the blood vessel.
- After completion of the regional perfusion, the catheter may be removed and a small pressure bandage placed over the vessel puncture site. Alternatively, the catheter may be left in place for the duration of the soaking time and the extension set secured to avoid backflow of blood.
- The tourniquet should be left in place for 20 to 25 minutes after completion of the injection.
- Treatment of a wound, lavage of a joint, and other therapies may be performed while the regional perfusion is "soaking."

Courtesy Dr. Julie Cary.
*Recommended antibiotics for regional limb perfusion in an adult horse: ceftiofur, 1g; amikacin, 500 mg; and gentamicin, 1g.

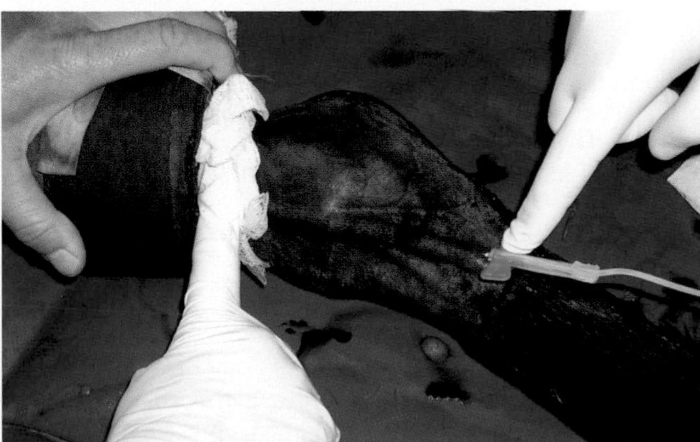

Fig. 5-5 Regional limb perfusion performed in foal with septic tibiotarsal joint. (Courtesy Dr. Debra Sellon.)

Box • 5-2

Intraosseous Regional Limb Perfusion

- Procure a 5.5 × 20—mm cannulated screw with a Luer-Lok attachment affixed to the screw.
- Alternatively, a standard extension set will fit snugly into a 4.0-mm drill hole, obviating the need for a cannulated screw.
- The procedure may be performed under general anesthesia or in the standing, sedated adult patient. The tourniquets and intraosseous perfusion tend to be painful. A regional perineural block is recommended in patients that will undergo cortical drilling while standing.
- Aseptically prepare the skin overlying the area in which the bone will be drilled. Ideally, select a metaphyseal region close to the region to be perfused.
- Prepare antibiotics and saline to a total volume of 25 to 30 mL for perfusion of the metacarpus or tarsus or 40 to 50 mL for perfusion of the radius or a larger long bone.
- Infuse local anesthetic into the soft tissues overlying the site in the bone to be cannulated (e.g., dorsolateral cortex of center of metacarpus).
- Make a 1-cm stab incision into the skin, subcutaneous tissue, and periosteum. Retract the tissues gently, and drill a unicortical hole 4 mm in diameter. The hole should be tapped to 5.5 mm in diameter.
- Place the cannulated screw with the Luer-Lok attachment into the predrilled and tapped hole.
- Apply tourniquets proximal and distal to the region to be perfused. Perfusion of regions including the fetlock and distal areas does not require a distal tourniquet.
- Attach the male end of the extension set to the Luer-Lok adapter, and infuse the antibiotics and saline over 5 minutes. Anesthetic solution such as 2% mepivacaine (5 mL) may also be injected to decrease discomfort associated with the procedure.
- Thirty minutes after completion of the antibiotic infusion, the tourniquet may be removed.
- The screw is removed under aseptic technique. The skin should be closed over the incision. Alternatively, a sterile bandage may be placed without closing the incision. The skin incision may be opened for successive treatments.
- At the completion of treatment regimen, the skin and subcutaneous tissues should be debrided and the incision closed.

Courtesy Dr. Julie Cary.

Box • 5-3

Antimicrobial-Impregnated Polymethylmethacrylate (PMMA) Beads

Items needed:
- Half-dose PMMA bone cement (Surgical Simplex P Radiopaque Bone Cement, Howmedica Osteonics, Mahwah, NJ). This package contains 20 g of sterile PMMA powder and 10 mL of sterile liquid that is 97.4% v/v methylmethacrylate.
- Mixing bowl (sterile) with spatula or mixing device
- Sterile gloves
- Sterile field (table cover or drape)
- Scissors (sterile)
- Antibiotics

Recommended antibiotic doses:
- Cefazolin, 1 g
- Amikacin, 1 g
- Imipenem, 500 mg

Procedure:
1. Using sterile technique, open packet with 20 g of sterile PMMA powder and empty into sterile bowl.
2. Add antimicrobials to dry powder. If antibiotics are in dry powder form, add them to the PMMA powder dry, without reconstitution.
3. Mix sterile PMMA powder and antimicrobials well.
4. Add 10 mL of liquid methylmethacrylate and mix until tacky and starting to set.
5. Immediately begin rolling portions of resultant mixture into small, cigar-shaped rods or small, round beads. After the mixture starts to set, only a brief time is available to change the shape of the beads. Therefore, several people with sterile gloves may be required to prepare all beads within the available time.
6. Beads are ready to use within 10 to 15 minutes.
7. Remaining beads may be sealed in sterilization pouches and gas-sterilized for later use.

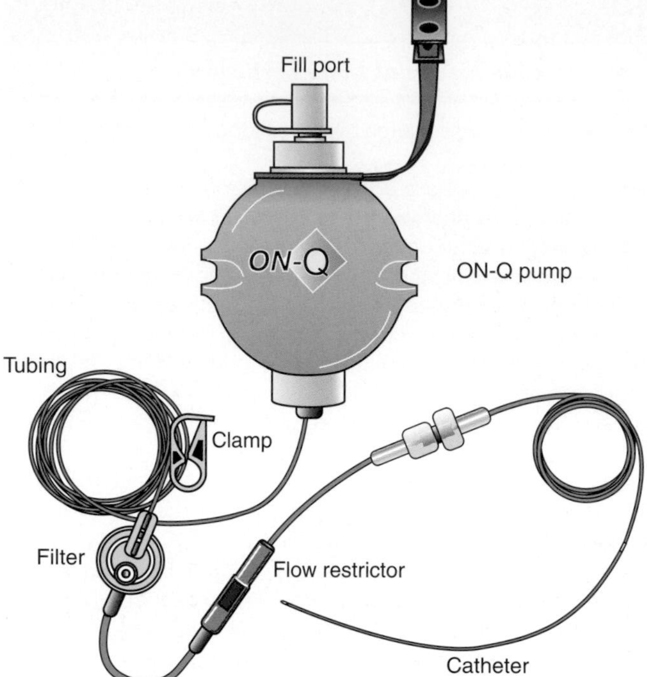

Fig. 5-6 Example of constant-rate infusion system (On-Q Painbuster) that can deliver antimicrobials and anesthetics to synovial structure. (Courtesy I-Flow Corp., Lake Forest, Calif.)

adapter that will fit an extension set for perfusion. As with IV regional limb perfusion, tourniquets are placed above and below the infected area. Antimicrobial solution (30- to 60-mL volume) is infused slowly through the cannulated screw at a dose similar to that previously described for IV regional limb perfusion. The tourniquets are maintained for a total time of 30 minutes. Experimentally, studies have shown that intraosseous perfusion results in lower synovial concentrations of antibiotic than does IV regional limb perfusion.[59] Increased technical difficulty (placing a bone screw) and a small risk of fracture are additional disadvantages to this technique.

Constant-rate infusion pumps and intrasynovial catheters may also be used to deliver high concentrations of antimicrobials and obviate the need for multiple needle punctures. Latex balloon infusion systems with calibrated delivery systems can deliver a constant volume of antimicrobial solution to the joint (Fig. 5-6). This results in very high antimicrobial concentrations within the joint. Lescun et al.[62,63] showed that by delivering 1 g of gentamicin every 8 hours to the tarsocrural joint, concentrations exceeding 100 times the MIC of most equine pathogens could be maintained for several days. They showed no significant effects on histologic scores of cartilage or synovium using this protocol for 5 days. In the authors' practice, these systems are routinely used to treat infected synovial structures. One advantage is the ability to add local analgesics in severely painful infections, although compatibility with the antimicrobial used should be investigated. Catheter placement also requires some planning. For example, catheters placed dorsally in the antebrachiocarpal, midcarpal, and pastern joints can become crushed as the animal ambulates. This can result in loss of catheter function or even foreign debris within the joint. The catheter should be placed in an area where it will not be subjected to crushing, such as the back of the joint or palmar or plantar pouches.

Intrasynovial use of antimicrobial-impregnated beads provides another method to deliver high concentrations of antimicrobials to synovial structures (see Box 5-3). Farnsworth et al.[64] showed that gentamicin-impregnated polymethylmethacrylate (PMMA) could be used intraarticularly. However, when PMMA beads were inserted into the tarsocrural joint of horses with diffuse synovitis, acute increases in synovial WBC count, prolonged increases in total protein concentration, superficial cartilage erosions, and in some cases marked capsular thickening resulted. Therefore, because of the associated inflammatory reaction, potential for mechanical abrasion of cartilage surfaces, necessity for removal (if nonabsorbable), and availability of superior methods, antimicrobial-impregnated beads may not be the best option.

The prognosis for septic arthritis is guarded to good with appropriate and timely therapy. Foals typically have a poorer prognosis than adult horses.[34] Multisystemic disease often accompanies septic arthritis in foals and significantly decreases their chance of survival.[65] A guarded to grave prognosis should be given for foals with multiple infected joints and concurrent osteomyelitis or multisystemic disease. Extension of infection into the surrounding bone, joint collapse, and protracted infection are strong indicators of a poor prognosis.

BONE INFECTION (SEPTIC OSTEOMYELITIS AND OSTEITIS)

Etiology and Pathogenesis

Infection of bone can be caused by direct trauma, hematogenous spread, extension of a contiguous focus of infection, or inoculation at surgery. One key conceptual difference is that hematogenous infections spread from the "inside out," whereas most other causes of osteomyelitis spread from the "outside in." The pathogenesis after trauma to bone involves acute inflammation of bone, with vascular engorgement, edema, cellular infiltration, and abscess formation. The associated increase in intramedullary pressure spreads pathogens throughout the bone cortex, with intracortical extension facilitated by the haversian systems and Volkmann's canals. With continued extension, the periosteal space may become involved.[66]

In foals, hematogenous spread of infection into the bone is a common cause of osteomyelitis.[67] Typically, the metaphyses of long bones are affected. In young animals, blood flow is slow and turbulent in the venous sinuses of the metaphyses near the site of endochondral ossification. Bacteria can become lodged at these sites and readily establish infection. In the neonatal foal the metaphyseal blood supply communicates with the epiphyseal blood supply via the transphyseal vessels. The epiphyseal blood supply communicates with the blood supply of the joint synovium.[68-70] This provides a direct route for infection from the joint to spread to the bone, or vice versa. As the animal ages, the epiphyseal and metaphyseal blood supplies become independent. In foals the transphyseal vessels start to regress at 14 days of age and disappear almost completely by 45 days of age.[71] Generally, this protects the epiphysis from infection,[72] and septic arthritis and septic physitis/epiphysitis are less likely to coexist in older foals.

In adult horses there is a paucity of information regarding the most likely etiologic agents of osteomyelitis. Retrospective studies suggest that most horses with traumatic osteomyelitis have mixed antimicrobial infections, with *Enterobacteriaceae*, β-hemolytic streptococci, and staphylococci being the most frequently isolated organisms.[34,73] Osteomyelitis after surgery is often caused by staphylococci, but mixed infections may also occur. In foals, *Enterobacteriaceae* are the most common organisms isolated from osteomyelitis. In older foals, *Rhodococcus equi* osteomyelitis should be considered as a differential diagnosis[74] (see Chapter 32). Mycotic or phycomycotic infections can be found in the bone in horses but are less common than bacterial infections (see Chapter 55).

Clinical Findings

The clinical signs of osteomyelitis are variable. Most horses with osteomyelitis of the limbs will present with moderate to marked lameness. Soft tissue swelling, heat, and sensitivity to palpation are almost always present and may be the only clinical signs of osteomyelitis involving the head. Exceptions are osteomyelitis involving bones heavily covered by muscle or hoof capsule. In these horses, lameness may be the only clinical sign. Laboratory findings are variable. Leukocytosis or hyperfibrinogenemia may be present but are certainly not diagnostic.

The most common sites of osteomyelitis in the foal are the distal tibial physes and the distal third metacarpal/tarsal physes.[75] Affected foals will generally present with marked lameness and palpable heat, pain, and swelling, which often can be distinguished from joint effusion if the joint is not involved. The swelling in affected foals may be soft and fluctuant, in contrast to swelling in affected adults, which usually is firm. This difference is caused by the relatively loosely attached periosteum and thin cortex in young animals, which allows suppuration and expansion.[72] In more proximal limb locations (e.g., proximal humerus, femur), swelling may not be obvious because of surrounding muscle mass.

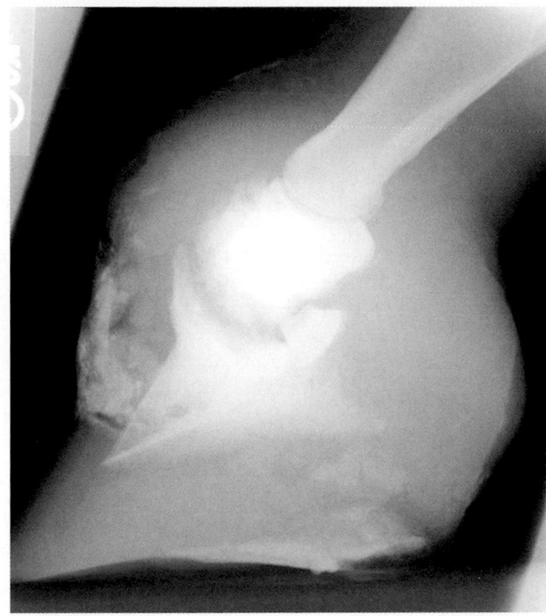

Fig. 5-7 Radiograph of severe osteomyelitis of coffin joint demonstrating sclerosis, lysis, and periosteal new bone production.

The most common sites of osteomyelitis in the adult horse are the metacarpal and metatarsal bones and the phalanges.[76] In these areas, lameness is a common clinical finding, whereas in the head and axial skeleton, painful soft tissue swelling with or without draining tracts may be the only clinical sign.

Diagnosis

Diagnosis of osteomyelitis and osteitis is usually confirmed by radiography. Lesions typically appear lytic, with varying degrees of sclerosis and periosteal new bone production (Fig. 5-7). Osseous sequestra are a relatively common feature of osteomyelitis in horses, especially in areas with minimal soft tissue covering. With periosteal damage or wound infection, the outer cortex of the bone is susceptible to ischemia and infection. If the bone becomes necrotic, it will separate from the parent bone, forming a sequestrum.

Radiographic changes require 30% to 50% bone density (mineralization) with at least 1 cm of affected area.[77] This may result in delayed recognition of lesions, especially early in the disease process. Radiographs of the contralateral limb can assist in detecting subtle changes, but it may take 10 to 14 days after injury or onset of clinical signs to see radiographic evidence of infection. Unfortunately, this can delay the diagnosis and therefore timely treatment of osteomyelitis.

In human patients, advanced imaging techniques such as nuclear scintigraphy, MRI, and CT are often used to improve the accuracy of diagnosis of osteomyelitis. These modalities are becoming more widely accessible to veterinarians and are being increasingly used for diagnosis of osteomyelitis in horses.

A three-phase scintigraphic scan with methylene diphosphonate (MDP) can aid in the diagnosis of equine osteomyelitis. Increased uptake of the radiopharmaceutical in all three phases (flow, pool, bone) is supportive of osteomyelitis. However, the diagnosis may be complicated by recent trauma, surgery, or orthopedic implants. These coexisting conditions significantly decrease the specificity (as low as 38% in human patients) of results.[78] WBC scans can be performed in horses using hexamethylpropyleneamine oxime (HMPAO)–labeled WBCs.[26,79] The main advantage to this technique is an increase in specificity for detection of osteomyelitis. False-negative scans are possible with chronic or partially treated osteomyelitis. In the future, newer techniques (e.g., ciprofloxacin labeling) may provide more accurate and less technically demanding methods to detect osteomyelitis.

CT provides high spatial as well as contrast resolution of bone and its surrounding tissue. It is best used for determining cortical changes associated with osteomyelitis and providing a three-dimensional image that can be used to guide surgical treatment or biopsy. In horses, complex joints such as the hock can be difficult to evaluate with plain radiography. CT is especially useful for localizing and characterizing these lesions.[80] The presence of metallic implants often precludes the use of CT because of beam-hardening artifact. Other limitations in the horse include the necessity for general anesthesia and gantry aperture limitations. In adult horses, CT is often limited to the distal extremities and head. Large horses may be difficult to image, except for lesions distal to the tarsus or carpus.

MRI is one of the most sensitive tools for diagnosis of osteomyelitis in human patients.[77] MRI can detect the differences between normal and abnormal bone from the differences in their density of water protons. Several clinically available imaging sequences and contrast agents can be used to increase the accuracy of detection. In the area of lesions, T1-weighted images will show low signal intensity (fluid is dark, fat is bright), and T2-weighted images will show increased signal intensity (fluid is bright, fat is dark). MRI will clearly define the extent of osteomyelitis lesions and provide information related to the chronicity of the infection. Images cannot be obtained from horses with ferrous implants. Nonferrous implants are routinely used in human patients and allow subsequent MRI. MRI shares some of the limitations of CT regarding aperture size and ability to image much of the adult equine skeleton. The increasing availability of equine MRI facilities will change the way veterinarians diagnose and treat osteomyelitis.

Ultrasound may be used to evaluate soft tissue swelling and is especially useful for detection of increased quantities of synovial fluid or abscesses in severely swollen or heavily muscled areas. Subperiosteal fluid or pus may be visible, which can support the clinical diagnosis of osteomyelitis. These fluid pockets can be aspirated for culture. Sequestra and foreign bodies may be detectable and aid in treatment planning or the decision for further diagnostic efforts. With experience, ultrasound can be used to detect early changes (not radiographically apparent) of osteomyelitis. A thin fluid layer immediately adjacent to the bone is usually detectable, and occasionally, periosteal lysis or proliferation may be observed.[81]

Biopsy, culture, and sensitivity are necessary to confirm septic osteomyelitis and to determine the best course of antimicrobial treatment. However, because many horses with osteomyelitis require surgical debridement, these diagnostic procedures are often done at treatment.

Therapy

The treatment of osteomyelitis can be involved and often requires intensive care best provided in a hospital environment. Many of these horses should be referred to veterinary hospitals where the appropriate diagnostic testing and necessary treatments are routinely performed.

Systemic antimicrobial treatment for osteomyelitis should be selected after consideration of the most likely pathogens. Whenever possible, the causative organism(s) should be identified and antimicrobial sensitivity patterns determined. Long-term antimicrobial therapy is often necessary, and adverse effects and economics should be considered. Initial empiric therapy in horses generally consists of broad-spectrum IV antimicrobials (e.g., combination of β-lactam and aminoglycoside antibiotic).

Oral antimicrobial options are limited but can be used effectively. Trimethoprim-sulfa (TMS) antimicrobials are often effective against β-hemolytic streptococcal infection; however, resistance is common, and use of TMS alone is questionable for treatment of most horses with osteomyelitis. Chloramphenicol is effective against many organisms typically isolated from equine osteomyelitis lesions; however, human health concerns and controversy over its oral absorption in horses tend to limit its use by many clinicians. In the authors' opinion, chloramphenicol remains one of the few clinically effective oral antibiotics for osteomyelitis that can be safely used long term. Rifampin in combination with a macrolide or azalide antimicrobial drug is often used to treat *Rhodococcus equi* infections (see Chapter 32). Additionally, the authors have used rifampin in combination with TMS or enrofloxacin to treat osteomyelitis. In human patients, rifampin is considered one of the most effective antistaphylococcal agents and is useful in eradicating intraleukocytic bacteria and penetrating the bacterial glycocalyx. Rifampin should not be used alone because resistance will quickly develop.[72] As a general rule, antimicrobial administration should be continued for several weeks after the resolution of clinical signs.

Unfortunately, by the time most cases of osteomyelitis in the horse are diagnosed, they have advanced beyond the point when systemic antimicrobial therapy alone is effective. Surgical debridement is indicated when nonviable tissue is present. Nonviable tissue can provide a continuous nidus of infection, leading to persistence or recrudescence of infection. Debridement removes debris, eliminates dead space, restores soft tissue integrity, encourages vascular supply, and thus encourages complete healing and resolution of infection.[72] Necrotic bone can be distinguished from healthy bone during curettage; healthy bone is much harder and bleeds. Bone should be debrided until healthy bleeding margins are obtained. Large defects in the bone may require cancellous bone grafts to restore structural integrity and promote healing.

Local antimicrobial delivery techniques described earlier, such as IV regional limb perfusion, interosseous perfusion, and antimicrobial-impregnated beads, are indicated for treatment of horses with osteomyelitis. Antimicrobial-impregnated beads made with PMMA may be especially useful for treatment of osteomyelitis because they can be implanted and left to deliver antimicrobials for an extended time. They can be prepared at surgery or stored for future use. Antimicrobial release from PMMA occurs in a bimodal manner. First, in a rapid phase, approximately 5% of the antimicrobial is released within the first 24 to 48 hours. A slow-release phase then provides bactericidal concentrations for the next few weeks to months.[82] Single agents or combinations of antimicrobials may be used. Several factors affect release of antimicrobials from PMMA beads, including heat stability and water solubility. Table 5-1 lists some common antimicrobials that effectively elute from PMMA. PMMA beads are nonabsorbable, and removal at a later date may be required. Tissue irritation often leads to some degree of fibrous tissue formation. In difficult osteomyelitis cases, the benefits of therapy with PMMA beads generally outweigh these disadvantages.

Plaster of Paris (POP) beads can also be used to deliver antimicrobials. POP beads have the advantage of being absorbable and have reported osteoinductive and osteoconductive properties. Disadvantages are that most of the antimicrobial is released in the first 48 hours (80% with gentamicin), they are unlikely to maintain concentrations above MIC for

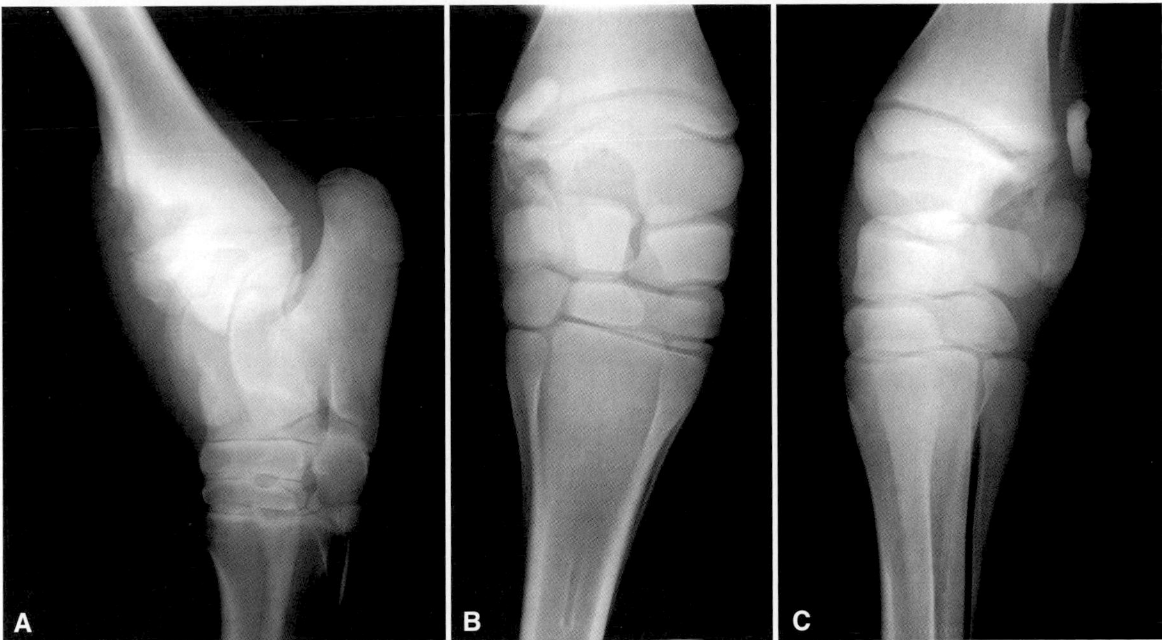

Fig. 5-8 A, Foal with infected distal tibial physis and metaphysis. B and C, Foal with infected epiphysis (lateral styloid process). The bone abscess was debrided and drained percutaneously and a PMMA bead left to deliver local antimicrobials.

longer than 2 weeks, and they require fabrication and gas sterilization in advance to implantation.[83] In the future, better carriers for antimicrobials will likely be available, providing better biocompatibility, longer release times, and enhancement of new bone production.

Foals with septic osteomyelitis involving the metaphysis, physis, and epiphysis are difficult to manage. The diagnosis is generally not evident until radiographic changes are apparent (Fig. 5-8). Typically, an area of soft tissue swelling with pus formation can be found at the affected site. This is usually adjacent to the affected side of the physis. The prognosis generally worsens after radiographic changes are evident. If elected, treatment should be aggressive. If osteomyelitis involves the physis and metaphysis, drainage should be established through the skin. Often, a curette can be used to open and debride the affected area of bone. Care should be taken to avoid excessive damage to the physis and surrounding bone when debriding. Implanted antibiotic-impregnated beads combined with regional perfusion techniques can be used for local antimicrobial therapy. Less frequently, osteomyelitis will involve the epiphysis. Infection of the adjacent joint is almost always present concurrently. Lesions may be debrided arthroscopically. However, every effort should be made to preserve the weight-bearing surface and structural integrity of the epiphysis. If peripheral, the lesion can be opened and debrided through the skin and joint capsule.

Infected orthopedic implants generally must be removed before infection can be resolved. Unfortunately, there is often a trade-off with necessary stability provided by the implants. In situations where it is not practical to remove the implant(s), efforts must be made to minimize extension of the infection and further destruction of the implant bone interface. Removal of implants not providing stability, all possible glycocalyx (bacterial slime), dead bone, and any other foreign material is necessary for host defenses to fight infection effectively.[84]

Many factors affect the prognosis for horses with osteomyelitis. Unfortunately, the body of knowledge regarding osteomyelitis largely consists of retrospective studies with relatively small case numbers, and information often must be extrapolated from other species. Duration of osteomyelitis is one of the most important factors affecting prognosis. Delays in diagnosis and referral are major factors contributing to treatment failure.

Horses with significant radiographic evidence of osteomyelitis have a guarded to poor prognosis and require aggressive surgical intervention. Extensive joint or other synovial structure involvement also has a significant negative impact on prognosis. Osteomyelitis in these locations complicates surgical treatment, and necessary debridement may result in loss of cartilage and joint congruity. Only in select joints such as the proximal interphalangeal joint, fetlock, carpus, or distal tarsal joints can arthrodesis or facilitated ankylosis be considered an option. In these cases, immobilization combined with debridement, bone graft, and potentially limited implants can result in salvage of the animal. Conversely, osteomyelitis in areas of the head, metacarpals and tarsals, and coffin bone can often be treated effectively with debridement and antimicrobial therapy. In general, if osteomyelitis is focal and surgically accessible, debridement may be curative, and often the joint infection will resolve after bone removal. The horse with diffuse, multifocal or surgically inaccessible osteomyelitis, particularly with concurrent joint infection, has a poor or guarded prognosis.

Supportive Care for Horses with Severe Lameness from Infection

The management of pain in acute and chronic equine musculoskeletal infections can be difficult. The physiologic consequences of severe pain are beyond the scope of this chapter. However, in the adult horse, support-limb laminitis is a major concern in all horses in which the unaffected limb bears the majority of the weight. Nonsteroidal antiinflammatory drugs (NSAIDs), primarily phenylbutazone, are indicated in almost all cases. Unfortunately, NSAIDs may be insufficient in controlling pain and promoting weight bearing on the injured limb. A simple method of providing additional analgesia is to use morphine (0.06-0.12 mg/kg IM q6h) with acepromazine (5-10 mg). Other options include regional nerve blocks, epidural anesthesia (hindlimb pain), fentanyl patches, lidocaine patches, and continuous-rate infusion of butorphanol. If an infusion pump or catheter is being used to deliver antimicrobials constantly and locally into the joint, mepivacaine or other local analgesic can be added if it is compatible. Systemic IV infusion of lidocaine (50 μg/kg/min) can be an effective analgesic agent.

Horses developing support-limb laminitis may exhibit a sudden increase in weight bearing on the injured limb or greater time spent in recumbency. Differentiating clinical improvement in the affected limb from the development of laminar pain in the support limb is critical. It is not unusual for pain from laminitis to supersede pain from severe infection. Careful monitoring of digital pulses and willingness to bear weight on the support limb is important. Providing adequate sole support, primarily in the heel region, appears to be beneficial for prevention and treatment of laminitis in some horses. This can be accomplished with soft bedding (ideally sand), foam pads taped to the bottom of the foot, or dental impression material molded to the sole. Systemic IV infusion of lidocaine (50 μg/kg/min) has some antiinflammatory properties that may be beneficial in management of pain associated with early support-limb laminitis.

Pain management to encourage weight bearing on the injured limb is important in foals. Increased loading of the support limb can create varus angular limb deformities and pain from physitis, whereas decreased weight bearing on the injured limb can result in limb contracture. These complications can occur within 1 to 2 weeks in foals and can become the limiting factor in recovery if the infection resolves. Support of the infected limb with bandages or splints may be necessary to encourage loading.

REFERENCES

See the CD-ROM for a list of references linked to the abstract in PubMed.

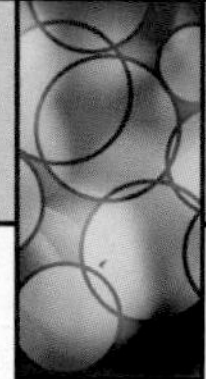

CHAPTER • 6

Neonatal Septicemia*

L. Chris Sanchez

Localized and systemic bacterial infections remain a leading cause of morbidity and mortality in the equine neonate despite recent advances in prevention and treatment.[1,2] Many factors can influence a foal's risk for the development of sepsis in the peripartum period. This chapter discusses those factors as well as causative organisms and therapeutic options. In addition, factors influencing prognosis and potential preventive strategies are addressed.

ETIOLOGY

Predisposing Factors and Routes of Infection

Many maternal and postnatal events can predispose an equine neonate to infection, including maternal illness, alterations in gestational length, partial or complete failure of passive transfer of immunity, poor sanitary conditions, and improper umbilical care. Maternal factors predisposing to neonatal sepsis include dystocia, premature placental separation, placentitis, and various other forms of maternal illness (e.g., colic). These problems were contributing factors in 24% of bacteremic foals in a recent study.[12] Many of these factors can be interrelated, with placentitis as a primary event and other problems such as premature placental separation occurring secondarily (see Chapter 8). In utero infection of the fetus caused by placentitis occurs typically by ascending infection and often results in premature delivery.[13] Because chronic placentitis in the mare often results in precocious fetal maturation, a premature foal born to such a mare likely has a greater chance of being septic but a higher probability of survival than a foal born at a similar gestational age to a mare without placentitis or other chronic stimulation.

Failure of passive transfer of immunoglobulin (FPT) is a major risk factor for equine neonatal sepsis. Because the foal is relatively immunonaive at the time of birth, postnatal transfer of immunoglobulin through ingestion and absorption of colostral antibodies is critical for prevention of foal infection. A number of studies have documented a close relationship between the concentration of foal serum immunoglobulin G (IgG) and incidence of disease.[14-17] Clearly, factors other than the magnitude of passive transfer also are involved in determining disease risk. The route and timing of transfer are likely relevant, along with the potential for bacterial challenge. Farm management is particularly important, including general cleanliness, stocking density, exposure to disease, maternal nutrition, and prepartum vaccination and deworming programs. One study has demonstrated that foals with partial FPT were at no greater risk of disease than those with adequate transfer on a well-managed Standardbred farm.[18]

Postnatal routes of infection include the umbilicus, gastrointestinal (GI) tract, and respiratory tract. Although the umbilicus has been traditionally regarded as an important site for bacterial pathogen entry into the foal, the role of the intestinal tract has been recently reevaluated.[19] It is suggested that too much emphasis is placed on the magnitude of colostral antibody transfer, rather than the *timing* of ingestion of colostrum. This concept was raised 30 years ago, when it was demonstrated that noninvasive *Escherichia coli* could

*Used with permission from Sanchez LC: Equine neonatal sepsis: medicine and surgery, *Vet Clin North Am Equine Pract* 21(2):273-293, 2005.

Table • 6-1

Summary of Reported Frequency of Bacterial Isolates

	STUDY							
	WILSON AND MADIGAN[30]	KOTERBA et al[28]	RAISIS et al[35]	MARSH AND PALMER[8]	STEWART et al[12]	HENSON AND BARTON[33]		
YEARS OF STUDY	**1978–1987**	**1982–1983**	**1989–1992**	**1991–1998**	**1993–2000**	**1986–1990**	**1991–1995**	**1996–2000**
Number of animals	47	27	24	155	101	—	250	—
Blood cultures only?*	No	Yes	No	Yes	Yes	—	No	—
Admission only?†	No	No	No	No	Yes	—	No	—
Isolates (%)‡								
Escherichia coli	30.6	56	50	18.7	39	59	29	26
Enterobacter spp.	3.5	3.7	12.5	12.3	14	18	8	9
Klebsiella spp.	12.9	7.4	—	3.9	11	16	15	7
Proteus spp.	—	3.7	4	—	1	—	—	—
Salmonella spp.	—	3.7	12.5	2.9	5	17	1	3
Actinobacillus spp.	18.8	7.4	12.5	8.9	30	11	8	7
Pasteurella spp.	—	3.7	—	1.5	—	—	—	—
Pseudomonas spp.	4.7	3.7	—	4.9	2	—	—	—
Enterococcus spp.	—	—	—	9.4	14	0	2	19
Streptococcus spp.	8.3	—	8	9.4	10	33	15	8
Staphylococcus spp.	3.5	3.7	—	9.8	3	7	8	15
Clostridium spp.	2.4	3.7	—	—	—	—	—	—
Acinetobacter spp.	—	—	—	4.9	—	—	—	—
Citrobacter spp.	4.7	—	—	—	—	—	—	—
All anaerobes	—	—	—	4.5	6	—	—	—
Other gram-negative bacteria	4.7	—	—	4.5	—	—	—	—
Other gram-positive bacteria	5.9	—	—	—	—	—	—	—

*Blood cultures only: whether samples analyzed were restricted to culture of blood only or if they included culture of blood or infected tissue collected at necropsy.
†Admission only: whether samples analyzed were restricted to those obtained on the date of a particular foal's admission to the hospital.
‡Data are expressed as a percentage of the total isolates from each study.

be absorbed by the intestine of neonatal piglets before gut closure.[20] In the pig and the lamb, the ability to absorb macromolecules is regulated by luminal content, and closure can be delayed for up to 5 days by deprivation of milk or colostrum. Conversely, the period before gut closure can be shortened by feeding a large volume of colostrum or milk shortly after birth.[21,22]

Less work has been performed in the foal, but several key details have been established. The foal does not fully discriminate between maternal IgG and other macromolecules, and absorption of macromolecules occurs through specialized cells by pinocytosis. The absorption of macromolecules peaks shortly after birth and declines to less than 1% by 20 hours.[23] Unlike other species, absorption of IgG does not appear to be Fc receptor mediated in the foal. The foal will selectively absorb IgG and immunoglobulin M (IgM) over IgA.[24] Unlike the piglet or the lamb, intestinal permeability to IgG cannot be delayed through withholding of macromolecules in the foal.[25] It is not known whether premature closure can be induced by the feeding of macromolecules immediately after birth.

Significant postnatal factors other than FPT that affect risk for neonatal sepsis include gestational age and environmental conditions. Foals with exceptionally short or long gestation are at increased risk for the development of sepsis.[26] Unsanitary environmental conditions can result in an increased bacterial load to the neonatal GI tract, especially during the initial period of udder seeking.

Causative Organisms

Retrospective studies have examined the most common organisms isolated from blood culture and necropsy specimens of septic foals (Table 6-1). Although gram-positive organisms predominated in the 1940s to 1950, *E. coli* has been the predominant organism isolated from septic foals in recent studies, regardless of clinic location or methodology.* Era and geographic location appear to play a major role in the significance of other pathogens. In Pennsylvania in the late 1990s, gram-positive bacteria (*Enterococcus*, *Streptococcus*, and *Staphylococcus* spp.) cumulatively played a major role in disease pathogenesis,[8] whereas *Actinobacillus* spp. accounted for approximately 30% of all isolates at Ohio State University in the late 1990s.[12] A Georgia study has reported a dramatic decrease in the percentage of *E. coli* isolates between 1986

*References 8, 12, 28, 30, 33, 35.

and 1990 and later 5-year sampling periods (1991–1995 and 1996–2000).[33] The organisms with increased prevalence over the same period were *Enterococcus* spp. and *Staphylococcus* spp. A study evaluating trends by decade (1980s and 1990s) in a Florida population found that *E. coli* remained the predominant isolate, percentages of gram-negative nonenteric and gram-positive organisms remained steady, the percentage of anaerobes increased, and the gram-negative, nonenteric organisms decreased.[36]

Systemic fungal infections also can occur in neonatal foals. The most frequently isolated organism is *Candida albicans*, a dimorphic fungus, although other organisms may play a similar role[37,38] (see Chapter 53). These infections are typically associated with prolonged hospitalization and invasive monitoring techniques[38] or immunodeficiency.[37] Prolonged antimicrobial therapy and the administration of parenteral nutrition have been suggested as risk factors for the development of candidiasis. A common clinical sign is fever unresponsive to antimicrobial therapy. Most foals with systemic candidiasis will develop *thrush* (white plaques on the lingual surface of the tongue) either concurrently or before showing clinical signs of systemic infection; thus a daily oral examination is recommended for all hospitalized foals. Antifungal therapy should be strongly considered in any presumed septic foal that develops thrush and is clearly indicated in any animal with a confirmed isolate.

PATHOGENESIS

Much of the clinical syndrome classically associated with equine neonatal sepsis is caused by a nonspecific inflammatory response to the infectious organism. Many terms have been used to describe this response and its associated syndromes and processes. A set of definitions was described in 1991 by the American College of Chest Physicians and the Society of Critical Care Medicine,[3] and a summary of this consensus report follows.

The *systemic inflammatory response syndrome* (SIRS) refers to a systemic inflammatory response, regardless of the inciting cause, which results in at least two of the following four clinical manifestations: (1) fever; (2) tachycardia; (3) tachypnea or hyperventilation; and (4) leukocytosis, leukopenia, or a relative increase of circulating immature neutrophils. When SIRS occurs in response to a confirmed infectious process, the process is termed *sepsis*. Infection refers to the invasion of normally sterile host tissue by microorganisms or to the inflammatory response generated in response to those organisms. The presence of viable bacteria in the blood is termed *bacteremia*, and the presence of other viable pathogens in the blood is described similarly (e.g., *viremia, fungemia*). When sepsis is associated with organ dysfunction, hypoperfusion, or hypotension, the event is termed *severe sepsis*. *Septic shock* is defined as sepsis-induced hypotension that persists despite adequate fluid therapy and is accompanied by hypoperfusion abnormalities or organ dysfunction.

Manifestations of organ dysfunction in the horse can include laminitis and coagulopathy in addition to renal, GI, hepatic cardiovascular, or pulmonary dysfunction.[4] The *multiple organ dysfunction syndrome* (MODS) describes the alteration of organ function in an acutely ill patient such that homeostasis cannot be maintained. MODS can occur either as a primary event (i.e., direct result of trauma) or secondary to a host response. Recently, a syndrome of immunosuppression caused by an exuberant systemic antiinflammatory response resulting in increased circulating levels of antiinflammatory mediators, leukocyte anergy, or increased susceptibility to infection has been termed the *compensatory antiinflammatory response syndrome* (CARS). If an individual fluctuates between episodes of SIRS and CARS, the term *mixed antiinflammatory response syndrome* (MARS) applies.[5]

Endotoxin plays a critical role in the pathogenesis of septic shock in gram-negative sepsis[6,7] and is particularly important in the foal, because the most frequently isolated organisms are gram-negative bacteria.[2,8] The pathogenesis of sepsis, endotoxemia, and the systemic inflammatory response has been reviewed extensively in both humans and horses and is covered in detail in Chapter 37.[3,9-11]

CLINICAL FINDINGS

Physical Examination Findings

The initial clinical signs of sepsis in foals can be vague and vary widely but frequently include depression, decreased or absent suckling from the mare, and lethargy, which may progress to recumbency. For those foals considered normal at any time before onset of illness, depression and anorexia are often the first clinical signs recognized. The examination of the foal should include an examination of the mare's udder to assess fill. Depressed foals will often stand with their head underneath the mare and can have dried milk on their foreheads. As a result of lack of suckling, dehydration and hypoglycemia become more significant problems as time progresses. Tachycardia and tachypnea are common but not always present. The mucous membranes often develop a bright or injected appearance, and the capillary refill time may be rapid. Rectal temperature may be normal or mildly increased, and sepsis should not be ruled out on the basis of a normal rectal temperature. Hypothermia can be associated with advanced sepsis or moderate to severe prematurity. Left untreated, these early signs will progress to septic shock, in which there is deterioration of the cardiovascular system (cyanosis, muddy mucous membranes, tachycardia, weak pulse, and peripheral shutdown) and often death.

In addition to the systemic parameters mentioned previously, septic foals may have additional localizing signs associated with specific foci of infection. Diarrhea is one of the most common early localizing signs in foals with sepsis and no other evidence of enteric pathogens. Occasionally, diarrhea may be the first clinical sign observed. Other localizing signs of sepsis include uveitis, seizures, joint effusion with or without lameness, lameness alone or in association with edema and pain over a physis, respiratory disease or distress, subcutaneous abscesses, patent urachus, and omphalitis. Importantly, many foals with umbilical remnant infection or abscessation often have normal external umbilical structures. Thus, ultrasonographic examination of the umbilical structures is recommended in any presumed septic foal.

Clinicopathologic Findings

Clinical signs and historical information alone often are sufficient for the clinician to develop a reasonable suspicion of neonatal sepsis. In addition to the physical examination findings, however, laboratory data may be helpful for diagnosis of early sepsis. Leukopenia, characterized by neutropenia, is the most common hematologic finding associated with acute sepsis. In one study, septic foals less than 1 week of age had a lower total white blood cell (WBC) count, both neutrophils and lymphocytes, and higher bands and monocytes than healthy, age-matched controls.[27] Premature or dysmature foals also will often have neutropenia in the absence of sepsis; however, septic foals typically have a degenerative left shift and evidence of toxicity (e.g., Döhle bodies, toxic granulation, vacuolization), whereas these findings are not typical of uncomplicated prematurity. In older septic foals (8-14 days) the total WBC count, neutrophils, and bands are higher than in age-matched controls.[27] A high fibrinogen concentration at or shortly after birth should raise the suspicion of in utero infection.[28]

Abnormal serum glucose concentrations are common in septic foals. Hypoglycemia is common initially, especially in foals less than 24 hours of age.[28] Although hypoglycemia is related predominantly to decreased intake, endotoxemia can contribute to hypoglycemia by decreasing hepatic gluconeogenesis and increasing peripheral glucose uptake. In the initial phase of treatment, the rate of glucose supplementation should be monitored carefully because many foals develop hyperglycemia in response to dextrose infusion. Other biochemical abnormalities common in septic foals include azotemia and hyperbilirubinemia.[2]

Common abnormalities found on arterial blood gas (ABG) analysis include acidemia and increased lactate concentrations. One early report demonstrated a high incidence of metabolic, respiratory, or mixed acidosis.[28] A recent report has indicated significant differences in arterial lactate concentration between foals with a positive versus negative blood culture, those that met the criteria for SIRS versus those that did not, and those that met the criteria for septic shock versus those that did not.[29] These differences were noted at admission and at 18 to 36 hours after admission for the blood culture and SIRS variables, but numbers precluded an analysis for the septic shock variable. Stewart et al.[12] have noted that foals with gram-negative enteric bacteremia were more likely to have an elevated arterial carbon dioxide tension ($Paco_2$) than other foals with bacteremia.

The coagulation and fibrinolytic systems of the septic newborn often are abnormal, with clinically relevant decreases in antithrombin III and increases in prothrombin time (PT), activated partial thromboplastin time (APTT), and fibrinogen and fibrin degradation products (FDPs).[27] A detectable plasma endotoxin concentration but not a positive blood culture result was significantly correlated with abnormal PT and APTT in this study; thus endotoxemia, not bacteremia, is likely associated with the development of coagulopathy in septic foals. Some patients may develop active hemorrhage or thrombosis, which can include thrombosis of major arteries, such as the aorta or iliac, femoral, or brachial artery (Fig. 6-1).

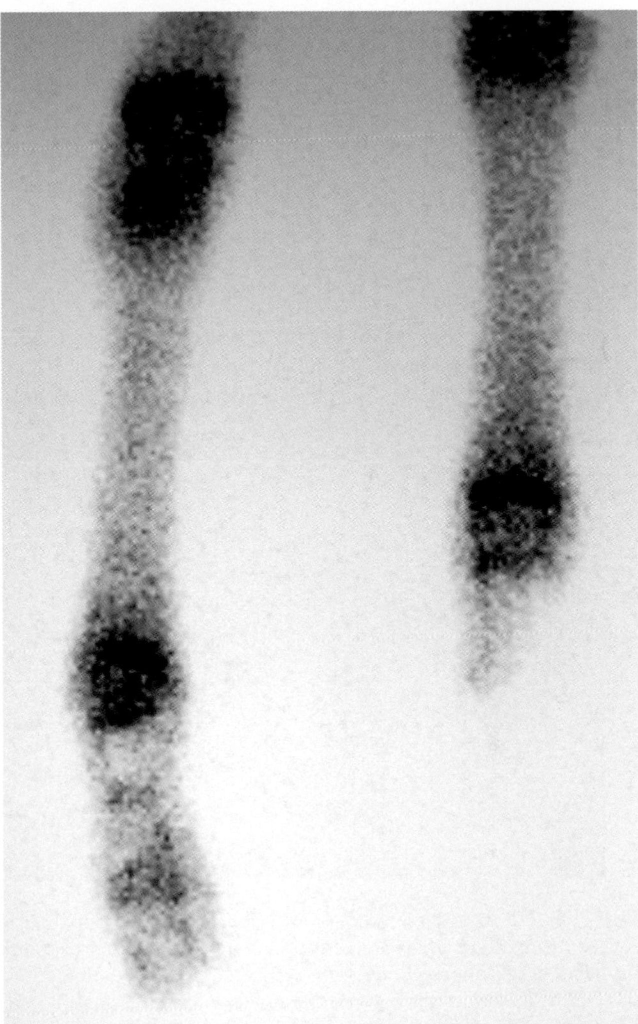

Fig. 6-1 Nuclear scintigraphy, soft tissue phase, of forelimbs of neonatal foal with septicemia. The left front foot was cold, with no palpable digital pulse. Note the lack of radioisotope accumulation distal to the pastern, indicating thrombosis of the arterial blood supply to the distal limb.

Focal or Localized Infection

Signs consistent with a secondary focus of infection, such as pneumonia, septic arthritis, osteomyelitis, omphalitis, and meningitis, also may occur in septic foals.

Respiratory Involvement

The lungs are a very common site of focal infection in the septic foal, with a reported incidence of pneumonia ranging from 28%[12] to 50%.[62] Respiratory rate and effort, thoracic auscultation, and rectal temperature often can alert the clinician to the possibility of pneumonia in a patient. Respiratory function is best assessed in septic foals with ABG analysis.[2,55] Thoracic radiographs provide an estimation of disease severity and distribution (Fig. 6-2). In addition to hematogenously acquired pneumonia, septic foals are at risk for aspiration of either meconium or milk, depending on their presentation. Directed antimicrobial therapy and the maintenance of an acceptable arterial oxygen tension (Pao_2) with intranasal oxygen insufflation are the most frequently administered forms of therapy. In those foals with severe hypercapnia in addition to hypoxemia, mechanical ventilation may be necessary.

Gastrointestinal Involvement

Diarrhea or enteritis also is common in septic foals, with a reported incidence of 16% to 38%.[12,26,62,63] In a study from Ohio State University, foals with *Actinobacillus* spp.–induced bacteremia were six times more likely to have diarrhea than those with other isolates.[12] With or without enteritis, septic foals also may display signs of ileus or colic. Most of these problems resolve with symptomatic treatment and systemic improvement. The clinician must carefully monitor fluid, electrolyte, and acid-base status in foals with diarrhea and replace ongoing losses. Options for analgesic therapy in colicky foals are somewhat limited; flunixin meglumine should be used cautiously because of the potential for gastric ulceration. Opiates such as butorphanol provide a reasonable short-term option for analgesia in such foals.

Umbilical Involvement

Omphalitis refers to infection of umbilical structures (Fig. 6-3). Umbilical remnant infections are considered to be a common source of continued bacterial shedding and have been

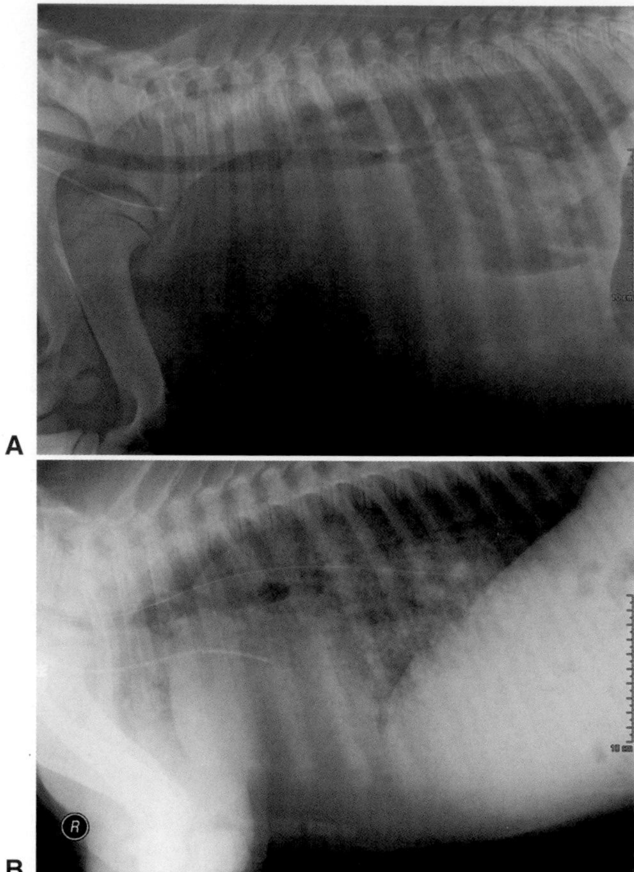

Fig. 6-2 **A,** Lateral radiographic view of 1-day-old foal with severe interstitial pneumonia, consistent with hematogenous infiltration of lung secondary to sepsis. **B,** Lateral radiographic view of thorax of neonatal foal with severe aspiration pneumonia. Note the more severe radiographic abnormalities within the cranioventral thorax compared with *A*.

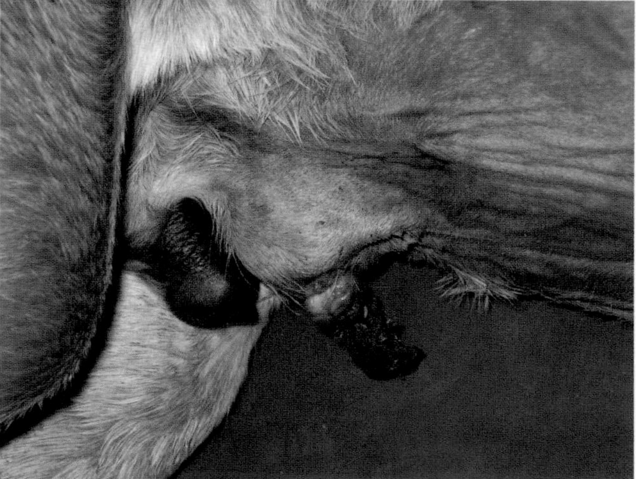

Fig. 6-3 Enlarged external umbilicus consistent with infection of urachus and vascular structures external to body wall. Ultrasonographic examination of the abdomen of this foal revealed enlargement of the internal urachus and umbilical arteries. The entire umbilicus was surgically resected.

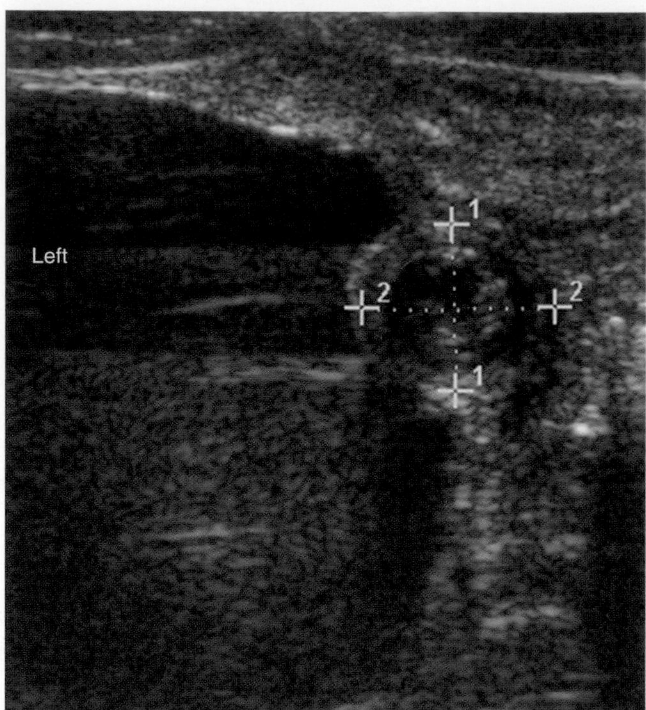

Fig. 6-4 Ultrasonogram of umbilical structures of foal. This image was obtained just cranial to the bladder and caudal to the umbilical stump and demonstrates dilation of the left umbilical artery with thickening of the arterial wall.

reported to occur in 13% of septic foals.[63] Ultrasonographic evaluation of these structures is critical because external signs (pain, heat, and swelling) are frequently absent (Fig. 6-4). Treatment options include long-term antibiotic therapy or surgical resection. Many septic foals will develop a *patent urachus* without involvement of other structures; the reported incidence in septic foals is 21%.[63] This problem will often resolve with continued antibiotic therapy, with or without topical therapy.

In one study, *uroperitoneum* was diagnosed in 2.5% of hospitalized neonates, and foals with uroperitoneum were less likely to survive if they had a positive versus negative sepsis score.[64] An interesting note from that study was that, presumably, septic foals receiving fluid therapy were typically older and less likely to have the classic electrolyte abnormalities associated with uroperitoneum. This suggests that the septic foals were diagnosed earlier, but the condition occurred later in life. Thus, ischemia and subsequent necrosis of the bladder or urachus may be the cause of uroperitoneum in the septic population. Because of these risks, routine ultrasonographic assessment of the umbilical structures is recommended for all hospitalized neonates in whom sepsis is either confirmed or suspected. The frequency of repeat ultrasound examinations depends on the individual foal's clinical progression.

Septic Arthritis and Osteomyelitis

Orthopedic infections are common in septic foals and represent one of the most important life-threatening and performance-limiting complications (Fig. 6-5). The reported incidence of *septic arthritis* ranges from 26% to 33%,[12,63,65] and that of *osteomyelitis* is 11% to 12%.[63,65] Clinical signs include lameness and joint effusion; thus daily palpation of every joint in all hospitalized neonates is imperative. Any sign of lameness

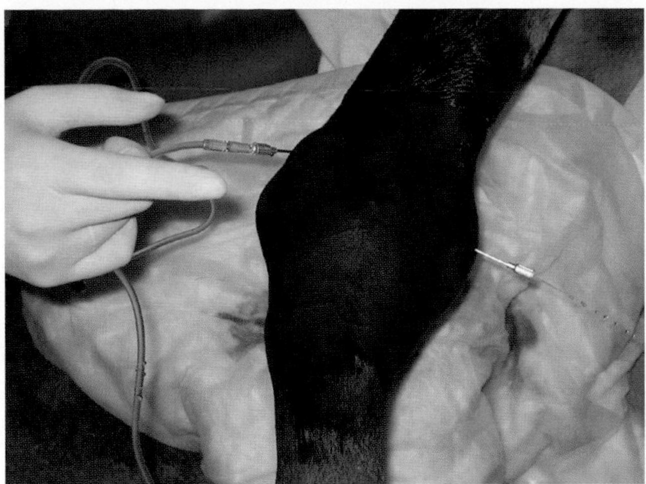

Fig. 6-5 Neonatal foal with septic arthritis of tibiotarsal joint. The foal is being treated by lavage of the affected joint. Fluid lavage with 1 L of lactated Ringer's solution was accomplished through 14-gauge, 1-inch needles. After the lavage, 250 mg of amikacin was injected into the joint before removal of the lavage needles.

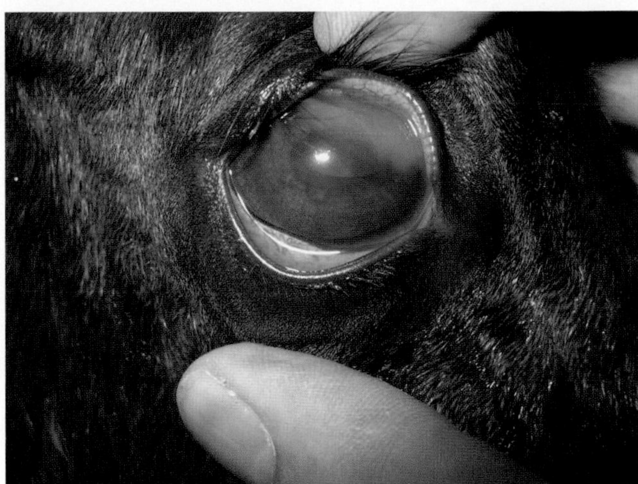

Fig. 6-6 Right eye of neonatal foal with septicemia. The corneal surface is stained with fluorescein dye, demonstrating a large ulcer with secondary miosis.

or joint effusion in a neonate should be considered septic until proved otherwise.

Bone infections normally occur at the epiphysis of long bones, the metaphyseal side of growth plates, costochondral junctions, and the articular facets of vertebral bodies. At the University of Florida, osteomyelitis or infectious synovitis occurred in 80% of foals, from which *Salmonella* spp. were isolated from blood cultures (Sanchez and Lester, unpublished observations, 2003). This was, by far, the most striking association between a particular isolate and a focus of infection. Chapter 5 discusses the diagnosis, treatment, and prognosis associated with orthopedic infections.

Meningitis

Meningitis is a rare but extremely serious complication of neonatal sepsis (see Chapter 4). Severe depression is common in foals with bacterial meningitis; however, this can be difficult to assess in a severely compromised, obtunded, or comatose foal. Other clinical signs may include seizures, head tilt, strabismus, nystagmus, and extensor rigidity, depending on the areas of the central nervous system (CNS) that are involved. Identification of neutrophilic pleocytosis in cerebrospinal fluid (CSF) usually provides a definitive diagnosis. Prognosis is poor to grave, but if therapy is attempted, third-generation cephalosporins (e.g., cefotaxime) have been recommended.[40] The major differential diagnosis for neurologic signs in a septic neonate is *hypoxic-ischemic encephalomyelopathy* (HIE). Typically, foals with HIE present within 24 to 48 hours after birth, whereas the age of foals with meningitis is more variable. Foals with gram-negative bacteremia are less likely to have seizures than those with other isolates.[12]

Ocular Involvement

The most common ocular complication in the septic foal is corneal ulceration (Fig. 6-6) (see Chapter 10). Ulceration can occur because of entropion in a dehydrated foal or, more often, because of trauma. Because foals do not always show clinical signs of corneal ulceration, a daily ophthalmic examination, including fluorescein staining, should be performed in all hospitalized foals. Another possible ophthalmic complication in septic neonatal foals is uveitis. When uveitis occurs, it is typically an ocular extension of the systemic disease process.

Coagulopathy

Disorders of coagulation can occur in septic foals, manifested clinically by either hemorrhage or thrombosis. The most common abnormality probably is jugular venous thrombosis at the site of an indwelling venous catheter. Other areas of thrombosis include the brachial artery, digital artery, metatarsal and metacarpal arteries, diffuse vascular thromboses throughout the distal limb, the aortic termination, the lungs, and the colon[27,66-69] (see Fig. 6-1).

DIAGNOSIS

A blood culture is the "gold standard" for the diagnosis of systemic bacterial infection (see Chapter 27). The identification of a causative organism allows for directed antimicrobial therapy. Samples for culture should be collected from a large vein (usually the jugular or cephalic, but other sites, e.g., saphenous vein, can be used as well) after surgical clip and aseptic preparation. The sample should be collected in a sterile syringe without anticoagulant and placed immediately into an appropriate medium, such as thioglycolate and tryptic soy broth (BBL Septi-Chek, Becton Dickinson, Sparks, Md). A fresh needle should be used for the instillation of blood into the culture medium. Sample collection from a venous catheter is acceptable, provided the procedure is performed directly from the catheter at the time of placement without compromising sterile technique. For foals that are receiving antimicrobial therapy before sample collection, an appropriate medium, such as tryptic soy broth with resins (BBL Septi-Chek), also is available and may improve microbial recovery. Regardless of the medium used, care should be taken to infuse the recommended volume of blood to promote optimum recovery.

Two considerations limit the usefulness of blood cultures for diagnosis of sepsis. First, positive results are not usually available for at least 48 hours. Second, false-negative results are common. Many foals with histologic evidence of sepsis at necropsy have historical evidence of a negative blood culture. This finding can result from a number of factors, including previous antimicrobial therapy and low circulating bacterial numbers. In one study, only 40% of *E. coli* infections were successfully identified by blood culture compared with necropsy culture.[30] Thus, additional means for identifying at-risk foals would be a valuable tool for the attending clinician.

The first scoring systems were adopted and modified in the 1980s, with a stated aim of predicting whether a foal would be septic before the return of blood culture results.[31,32] The modified "sepsis score" currently used in many hospitals is calculated based on a number of historical and physical findings and laboratory data and has a reported sensitivity and specificity of 92.8% and 85.9%, respectively.[32] The sepsis score has not been as accurate at other institutions. Recent data have shown a false-negative rate of 48% in blood culture–positive foals in Ohio.[12] In a study at the University of Georgia that examined foals with a sepsis score greater than 11, a positive blood culture, or greater than three foci of infection, 43 of 247 foals had a sepsis score less than 11 but at least one of the other criteria, and 46 of 250 had a sepsis score greater than 11 without either of the other criteria.[33] In a Virginia study,[32] the modified and original sepsis scores[31] each produced a positive predictive value of 84%, with negative predictive values of 55% and 53%,[34] respectively. Results from these studies stress the importance of regional and institutional variability in the accuracy of scoring systems.

The modified sepsis score was reevaluated recently at the University of Florida, the same geographic population from which it was originally generated, and obtained a similar sensitivity (89%) but lower specificity (67.5%) using positive blood culture alone as a gold standard, rather than including evidence of specific foci of infection at necropsy as well (Sanchez and Lester, unpublished observations, 2003). Because of the heavy weighting of historical information and related problems, moderately to severely premature foals often can have a positive sepsis score without a positive blood culture. However, because many of the maternal problems resulting in prematurity also can lead to systemic sepsis, this crossover is readily predictable. The problems with the clinical application of these scoring systems are their relatively low specificity and negative predictive value. Thus, although a "positive" score is supportive of sepsis in a suspected animal, a "negative" score alone should not be used to withhold antibiotic therapy from an at-risk foal. Similarly, the use of a positive score alone, without complementary culture results or necropsy findings, should be used cautiously to confirm a diagnosis of sepsis for retrospective studies.

THERAPY

Antimicrobial Therapy

Antibiotics provide the basis of therapy for septic foals. Initially, a broad-spectrum bactericidal approach must be used based on previous experience and costs. Antimicrobial therapy should begin immediately in any foal in which sepsis is suspected. Treatment should not be delayed pending blood culture results because sensitivity data typically require 3 to 4 days. Therapy can be altered if necessary when these data become available. A minimum therapeutic course of 2 weeks is recommended for bacteremic foals without localizing clinical signs. If localizing signs such as pneumonia or septic arthritis are present, a minimum course of therapy of 4 weeks is preferred.[26] Table 6-2 presents the recommended dosages for frequently used antimicrobials. Chapter 71 provides a detailed general discussion of antimicrobial therapy in horses.

Few published veterinary reports discuss antimicrobial sensitivity of organisms isolated from bacteremic neonatal foals. A common theme is that a lower percentage of gram-negative isolates are sensitive to gentamicin than to amikacin.[2,8,33,36,39] Paradis[2] has reported that 95% and 91% of gram-negative isolates were sensitive to amikacin and cefotaxime, respectively, whereas sensitivity to gentamicin and trimethoprim-sulfa was much lower. The same study found that the three antimicrobials to which staphylococcal organisms were most sensitive were cephalothin, tetracycline, and chloramphenicol, whereas streptococcal organisms were most sensitive to chloramphenicol, ampicillin, and penicillin. Wilson et al.[39] reported a cumulative sensitivity of all isolates from 33 foals as greater than 90% for imipenem, ciprofloxacin, ceftriaxone, and ceftazidime; 80% to 89% for amikacin and ceftizoxime; and only 70% to 79% for gentamicin and ceftiofur. Organisms such as *Enterobacter* spp., *Acinetobacter* spp., *Enterococcus* spp., and coagulase-positive *Staphylococcus* spp. have demonstrated substantial resistance.[8] *Enterobacter* spp. also demonstrated increasing resistance to amikacin, gentamicin, and trimethoprim-sulfa in another study.[36] Interestingly, a study from the University of Georgia revealed considerable gram-positive and gram-negative resistance to cefotaxime but no amikacin resistance for *Enterococcus* isolates.[33] The same study revealed an efficacy of at least 70% against all organisms for chloramphenicol or ceftiofur.

Table • **6-2**

Recommended Antimicrobial Dosages

AGENT	PREPARATION	ROUTE	FREQUENCY (hr)	DOSAGE (/kg)	REFERENCES
Amikacin	Sulfate	IV, IM	24	21-25 mg	75, 76
Gentamicin	Sulfate	IV, IM	24	6.6 mg	
Ampicillin	Sodium	IV, IM	6	25 mg	
Ampicillin	Trihydrate	IM	12	25 mg	
Penicillin G	Potassium	IV	6	22,000-40,000 IU	
Penicillin G	Procaine	IM	12-24	22,000 IU	
Cefotaxime	Sodium	IV	6	40 mg	40, 77
Ceftiofur	Sodium	IV, IM	12	2.2-4.4 mg	78

IM, Intramuscular; *IV*, intravenous.

Thus, based on available data, a recommended initial therapeutic approach involves combining amikacin or a third-generation cephalosporin with penicillin or ampicillin. The use of amikacin should be tempered in light of the foal's cardiovascular and renal status. If a foal is severely hypovolemic and azotemic, cephalosporin would be a safer initial choice. If amikacin is used, therapeutic drug monitoring is recommended to ensure appropriate dosing for each individual. An additional recommendation is to monitor creatinine levels serially every 2 to 3 days or perform serial urinalyses that include sediment examination to monitor for potential adverse renal effects. Cefotaxime is a good choice for foals with gram-negative meningitis[40] or those with unresponsive pneumonia.

Unfortunately, the range of oral antibiotics for use in horses is limited. Because of significant resistance, trimethoprim-sulfonamide combinations should not be used in septic foals without documented sensitivity, and then only as a long-term option after initial parenteral therapy. Aminobenzyl penicillins (amoxicillin and ampicillin) and first-generation cephalosporins (cefadroxyl and cephradine) have good bioavailability in young foals (in contrast to older foals and adult horses) but have a limited gram-positive spectrum of activity.[41-44] Cefpodoxime proxetil, a third-generation cephalosporin available for oral administration, was recently shown to be effective against 90% of *Klebsiella* spp., *Pasteurella* spp., and β-hemolytic streptococci.[45] An increase in the frequency of administration would likely increase the effectiveness of this drug against *E. coli*. Fluoroquinolones, such as enrofloxacin, have an excellent spectrum of activity against gram-negative and some gram-positive organisms but have been associated with arthropathy in foals.[46,47] Thus the use of these agents should be reserved for those cases with documented resistance to other antimicrobial agents and informed owner consent.

Antiendotoxin Therapy

Not surprisingly, many septic foals have detectable plasma endotoxin concentrations.[27] Recent in vitro work suggests that β-lactam antimicrobials may be more likely than aminoglycosides (alone or in combination with ampicillin) to induce endotoxemia and tumor necrosis factor-α activity during the treatment of *E. coli* sepsis.[7] Agents often used for the treatment of endotoxemia include flunixin meglumine, pentoxifylline, and polymyxin B sulfate.[48,49] None of these agents has been scientifically evaluated for the treatment of endotoxemia in foals; thus recommendations are extrapolated from work in vitro and in adult horses (see Chapter 37). Flunixin and polymyxin B are potentially nephrotoxic and thus should be used with caution. Flunixin meglumine also has the potential for causing gastric ulceration. Pentoxifylline may reduce mortality without adverse effects in septic neonates[50] but not adults.[51]

Antifungal Therapy

Antimicrobial agents for treatment of systemic candidiasis include fluconazole, itraconazole, miconazole, and amphotericin B.[38,52] Fungal sensitivity profiles, if available, may help direct therapy (see Chapters 49 and 56). The pharmacokinetic and pharmacodynamic activities of these drugs have not been established in foals. Amphotericin B has been administered intravenously (IV) at a range of 0.1 to 0.5 mg/kg once a day, starting therapy at the lower dose and increasing by 0.1-mg/kg increments per day.[38] Because this drug can cause potentially life-threatening nephrotoxicity, serum creatinine concentrations, urine production, and urinalysis should be monitored closely. Fluconazole has previously been administered orally at 4 to 10 mg/kg once daily. This agent is less expensive, easier to administer, and has fewer adverse effects. Miconazole has been administered at a dosage of 1 mg/kg IV every 8 hours.[38]

Cardiovascular Support

Fluid therapy is critical in foals with hypovolemia, acid-base disorders, septic shock, or hypotension. In-depth discussions of fluid therapy[53] and the use of inotropes and vasopressors[54] in the neonatal foal have been recently presented. These are two of the most important concepts in the initial treatment of sepsis, and the reader is directed to the cited references for additional information.

When a foal presents in septic shock, fluid resuscitation is critical. Initial choices typically include a combination of crystalloid (e.g., lactated Ringer's solution) and colloid (e.g., hydroxyethyl starch) preparations. Arterial or venous lactate concentration, systemic blood pressure, cardiac output, and central venous pressure can provide additional information regarding volume status and estimation of tissue perfusion.[55] Once normovolemia has been restored, neonates typically require approximately 100 mL/kg/day (5 L/day for 50-kg foal) to maintain adequate hydration.

Clinicopathologic variables to monitor continuously in septic foals include arterial or venous blood gases (depending on pulmonary status), electrolytes (especially sodium and potassium), and glucose. Physical parameters of importance include careful examination for the development of edema (conjunctiva, distal limbs, and other signs), urine output, vital signs, and temperature of the distal limbs. Derangements in any of the monitored parameters should be addressed as they arise to maintain optimal tissue perfusion.

Gastric Protectants

Although uncommon, sick foals may develop gastric ulcers, especially in the glandular region of the stomach. The use of prophylactic antacid therapy is controversial and depends on the preference of the clinician. The gastric pH in critically ill foals can differ greatly from that seen in healthy foals. Severely ill, predominantly recumbent patients frequently have alkaline gastric pH patterns.[56] In addition, sick foals capable of acid production respond more variably to IV ranitidine administration than their normal cohorts. Thus, glandular ulcer disease in sick neonates is likely not strictly an acid-related problem, and factors such as alterations in mucosal blood flow may contribute. In addition, gastric alkalinization can contribute to bacterial translocation.[57] Therapeutic options for acid suppression in the neonatal foal include omeprazole and ranitidine.[56,58,59] Sucralfate remains a possible alternative for ulcer prophylaxis, especially in foals receiving nonsteroidal antiinflammatory drugs. For a more complete discussion of this topic, the reader is directed to more recent reviews.[79]

Experimental Therapy

Although a variety of experimental therapies have shown promise for treatment of sepsis, few have resulted in reduced mortality in large-scale human clinical trials. Administration of recombinant activated protein C has consistently been associated with decreased mortality, especially in the most severely affected patients.[60] This agent, however, has been associated with significant adverse effects and is currently not a viable therapeutic option in foals. Although high-dose corticosteroid administration has been associated with increased mortality in septic patients, hydrocortisone administered at physiologic doses decreases mortality attributable to septic shock in human patients.[61]

PROGNOSIS

Survival rates for foals with neonatal sepsis have increased from the rate of 25% reported in the early 1980s.[28] More recent retrospective studies have reported short-term survival rates ranging from 45% to 55%.[12,33,63,70] Other investigators have reported survival rates ranging from 32%[27] to 72%.[35,62,71] Approximately 50% to 60% of all bacteremic foals admitted to the University of Florida neonatal unit survive to discharge (Sanchez and Lester, unpublished observations, 2003).

Several factors have been associated with survival in retrospective studies. Barton et al.[27] found that foals infected with gram-negative organisms are more likely to die than those with gram-positive infections. In a Texas study the duration of illness before admission was inversely related to survival, whereas the ability of a foal to stand on admission was positively correlated with survival.[63] A study of septic foals at the University of Georgia found that foals were more likely to survive if they had a sepsis score less than 11, a negative blood culture at admission, a serum glucose level of greater than 60 mg/dL, a body temperature greater than 100°F, a total CO_2 greater than 15 mmol/L, or a low or normal plasma fibrinogen concentration.[33] In the Florida study the prognosis worsened if multiple organisms were isolated from the blood or if multiple foci of infection were involved[12] (Sanchez and Lester, unpublished observations, 2003). In the Ohio State study, foals with multiple blood isolates had longer periods of hospitalization, but not decreased survival. Corley et al.[29] reported that a normal arterial lactate concentration at admission or 18 to 36 hours after admission was a good predictor of survival, whereas increased blood lactate concentrations were not a good predictor of nonsurvival.

Few studies have addressed the long-term survival and performance of neonatal intensive care unit (NICU) survivors, much less those specifically of septic foals. In a summary of septic Thoroughbred foals admitted to the University of Florida, approximately 75% of short-term survivors are registered, and approximately 50% start at least one race (Sanchez and Lester, unpublished observations, 2003). This observation is similar to that reported for overall NICU survivors, in which the percentage of starters was lower than the control population, but performance over a 2-year period was not different in those animals able to make at least two starts.[71] Similar findings have been reported for foals with neurologic disease and those with pneumonia caused by *Rhodococcus equi*.[72,73]

PREVENTION

Clearly, given the wide range of potentially devastating problems associated with sepsis, attempts to prevent disease are extremely important. Not surprisingly, methods of disease prevention address the documented risk factors and routes of infection discussed previously. The following suggestions constitute a basic guide for veterinarians and horse owners. Although many of the options presented make sense, none has been proved to reduce the incidence of sepsis. Thus the decision to implement some or all of these practices will depend on the individual farm situation.

Maintain Clean Environment

Although this is one of the most basic concepts in all of medicine, its importance cannot be overemphasized. Foaling stalls should be thoroughly cleaned and disinfected between mares. For each inhabitant, the stall should be cleaned at least daily, if not twice daily, and plentiful clean, dry, fresh bedding should be provided for the mare and foal.

Reduce Potential Bacterial Load Introduced during Udder Seeking

The mare's hindquarters, perineum, and udder should be thoroughly cleaned with soap and water after foaling but before the foal's introduction.[19] The key feature to this step, which often is overlooked, is that the mare also must be dried. Drying should be performed just outside the stall, rather than in the stall, to prevent contamination of the foal's new environment, which is the point of the exercise. This step requires great commitment on the part of the farm because it is labor intensive.

Ensure Rapid Gastrointestinal Intake

The volume, quality, and timing of colostrum administration are all likely important factors for optimizing passive transfer of immunity. Ideally, foals should receive 6 to 8 ounces of good-quality colostrum as soon as they develop a strong suckle reflex. The risk of milk aspiration when untrained individuals attempt to bottle-feed a newborn, potentially weak foal must be considered. Colostrum administration through nasogastric tube is recommended for foals with a suboptimal or absent suckle reflex.

Ensure Adequate Passive Transfer of Immunoglobulin G

Traditionally, passive transfer of maternal IgG to the foal has been considered to be the most important factor in disease prevention. Although other factors clearly play a role, adequate IgG transfer should still be assessed and treated, if necessary. Assessment of blood immunoglobulin concentrations should be performed for all foals at 24 to 48 hours of age. Optimally, IgG concentration should exceed 800 mg/dL at this time. (See recent reviews of diagnosis and treatment of FPT in foals for further information.[80,81])

Ensure Appropriate Umbilical Care

No published studies in foals have critically evaluated the different preparations used for routine postpartum umbilical care. In human neonates, surprisingly few randomized, double-blind clinical trials have broached this issue. In a recent review of published studies, 4% chlorhexidine consistently reduced the risk of umbilical and periumbilical infections.[74] This concentration of chlorhexidine also is typically used for treatment of foals and thus appears to be a preferred alternative to the povidone-idodine solutions used previously.

REFERENCES

See the CD-ROM for a list of references linked to the abstract in PubMed.

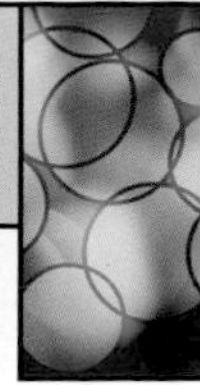

CHAPTER • 7

Skin Infections

Dawn Logas and Pamela E. Ginn

Skin infections, especially contagious dermatologic diseases, include some of the most common causes of equine skin disease. In one report, 25% of all dermatologic diagnoses made over a 21-year period were infectious in origin.[1] For the clinician, it is important to diagnose these conditions quickly to prevent spread to other horses and potentially their human companions. Many of these infectious agents are discussed in detail elsewhere in this book. The purpose of this chapter is to provide an overview that assists the clinician in differentiating, diagnosing, and treating conditions given the appropriate historical information, clinical presentation, and laboratory data.

GENERAL COMMENTS

A detailed history is an extremely important component of any dermatologic workup (Box 7-1). The age at time of onset, time of the year, presence of itching, and any other notable detail not generally observed during a short examination can assist physical diagnosis. Additional questioning should include whether any topical medications, home remedies, or systemic medications have been used. Response to medications (independent of season) and time to relapse (if a response occurred) are valuable pieces of information to assist diagnosis.

The environment is a causal or predisposing factor for many diseases of the skin. A detailed description or personal inspection of the environment is needed. Chronic exposure to moisture, such as wet bedding, constant rain, or muddy pastures, can contribute to the original condition and prevent response to therapy.

A basic physical examination should be performed on every patient that exhibits skin disease. Many infectious diseases of the skin reflect the underlying health, nutrition, and immune status of the horse. This can help differentiate primary from secondary conditions. In addition, it is important to determine if the skin lesions reflect the primary condition of the skin. Often the clinician's first examination is performed after many other therapies have been attempted. Primary lesions consist of pustules, papules, and macules. Most secondary lesions consist of crusts, scales, and alopecia. Noting the presence or absence of pruritus will rule out (or rule in) many diseases. It is important to note if the lesions occur singly or multiply. Determining what structures are involved should also be part of the physical diagnosis (in addition to confirmation by biopsy).

Dermatologists have a basic and straightforward diagnostic armamentarium that differentiates most diseases. Skin scrapings are essential for diagnosis of parasitic infections (see Chapter 64). Punch biopsies of skin are quick and inexpensive and can yield much needed information. Collection of a sterile biopsy for culture is necessary for bacterial and some fungal infections. When disease is global and long-standing, a wedge biopsy may yield more information regarding the primary etiology. Accurate histopathologic assessment with appropriate knowledge of equine-specific diseases is essential. For example, horses develop sarcoids frequently and fibrosarcomas rarely, and the two conditions are treated very differently (see Chapter 25). Special stains for bacteria and fungi should be pursued when appropriate.

Although many therapies for skin disease in the horse are palliative, etiology-specific treatment should be pursued rather than overuse of broad-spectrum antibiotics. Many primary conditions (e.g., autoimmune disease) have a suppurative component from secondary infection or a leukoclastic feature (e.g., purpura hemorrhagica). Understanding which conditions require antibiotics will save time and money and will be safer for equine patients and owners.

Box • 7-1

Questions for Dermatologic Problems

- Where and when did the lesion start?
- What was the initial appearance of the lesion?
- Which occurred first, pruritus or the lesion?
- Is the condition seasonal or nonseasonal?
- Are other animals or humans affected?
- Is the horse receiving drugs or feed supplements?
- Have any topical therapies been attempted?
- What does the horse eat, and have there been any dietary changes?
- Has the source of the feed been changed?
- Are horses stabled or pastured?

CRUSTING/SCALING DERMATOSES

Bacterial Etiologies

Crusting/scaling dermatoses affect primarily the epidermis and upper levels of the dermis and have many causes. Often these dermatoses start as small papules that quickly progress to crust and scale. In addition, clinical signs may include small papules, erosions, excoriations, alopecia, and varying degrees of pruritus (Boxes 7-2 and 7-3).

Bacterial folliculitis is most often caused by staphylococcal bacteria *(Staphylococcus aureus, S. intermedius, S. hyicus)*.[2,3] Other bacteria infrequently associated with folliculitis include *Streptococcus equi* subsp. *equi*, *Streptococcus equisimilis*, and *Corynebacterium pseudotuberculosis*.[4-6] **Dermatophilosis** is another bacterial crusting/scaling dermatosis in the horse (see Chapter 31).

Box • 7-2

Pruritic Crusting/Scaling Dermatoses

Noninfectious
- Chorioptic mange
- Sarcoptic mange
- Psoroptic mange
- Pediculosis
- Cutaneous onchocerciasis
- Culicoides hypersensitivity
- Atopy
- Food allergy

Infectious
- Dermatophytosis
- Dermatophilosis
- Staphylococcal folliculitis
- Corynebacterial folliculitis
- *Malassezia* dermatitis
- Besnoitiosis

Box • 7-3

Nonpruritic Crusting/Scaling Dermatoses

Noninfectious
- Trombiculiasis
- Idiopathic seborrhea
- Pemphigus foliaceus

Infectious
- Dermatophytosis
- Dermatophilosis
- Staphylococcal folliculitis
- Corynebacterial folliculitis
- *Malassezia* dermatitis
- Poxvirus

Clinical Findings

Most cases of folliculitis start in the spring or summer. The lesions start as small follicular papules that can develop into transient pustules that rupture to form crusted pustules (Fig. 7-1). Small foci of alopecia with scaling develop in areas of infected follicles, leading to a moth-eaten appearance of the hair coat. In severe cases, lesions may enlarge, ulcerate, and have a purulent or serosanguineous discharge. If complicated by furunculosis, nodules and fistulous tracts may be present. Papular lesions can be more painful than pruritic. Most of these lesions start in the tack areas and are associated with friction, high temperature and humidity, excessive sweating, poor grooming practices, and possibly biting insects. Horses also develop staphylococcal folliculitis of the caudal aspect of the pastern and fetlock, which is considered to be one of the causes of "grease heel." If left untreated, lesions of folliculitis may become widespread.

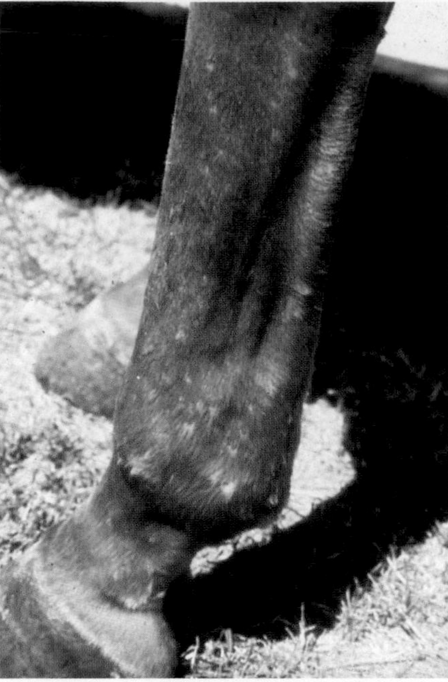

Fig. 7-1 Folliculitis of distal limb that cultured positive for *Staphylococcus* spp.

Diagnosis

Diagnosis is made by cytology of lesions (pustules, crusts), culture of lesions, and histopathology. Samples for culture are best obtained from fresh papules or pustules. If these are not available, the exudate from underneath a crust is acceptable. The histopathologic findings of bacterial folliculitis are characterized by epidermal acanthosis with variable degrees of folliculocentric neutrophilic pustules and serocellular crusting. Neutrophils fill the follicular lumens. Follicular distention with rupture and resultant pyogranulomatous dermatitis may be present. Bacteria may or may not be detected within the lesions.

Therapy

Treatment consists of systemic antibiotics, topical therapy, and improved grooming practices and attempts to eliminate other predisposing factors. Antibiotic selection should be based on results of culture and sensitivity testing. This is especially true now that methicillin-resistant *Staphylococcus aureus* (MRSA) infections that potentially can be transferred to horse personnel are being diagnosed more frequently in horses[7-9] (see Chapter 29). Antibiotic therapy should last at least 3 to 4 weeks, or 7 to 10 days beyond clinical cure. Topical therapy may consist of chlorhexidine or benzoyl peroxide shampoos. Benzoyl peroxide has the most antibacterial activity but may dry and bleach the coat. Therefore the frequency of topical application depends on the severity of disease and the topical agent used. For most cases, once-weekly to every-other-week application is adequate.

Prevention

Improved hygiene is required both for prompt resolution of infection and for prevention of recurrences. All blankets should be thoroughly cleaned with hot water and bleach. Tack should be kept as clean as possible. Cleaning of equipment should be continued on a routine basis. The horse should not be ridden while lesions are active. After the lesions have improved, the horse should be cooled properly and rinsed well after each ride. The horse should be bathed once or twice weekly in hot weather and should always have a clean saddle blanket each time it is ridden.

Fungal Etiologies

Dermatophytosis is a common cause of crusting and scaling (see Chapter 54). *Malassezia* has recently been associated with crusting/scaling dermatitis in the horse.[10] *Malassezia pachydermatis* is a lipophilic, nonmycelial, saprophytic yeast often found on normal and abnormal skin of various mammals, including the horse. A novel *Malassezia* species also inhabits normal horse skin. This organism has not been completely characterized but is closely related to *Malassezia sympodialis*. As in the dog and cat, *Malassezia* in the horse tends to be associated with other dermatologic diseases, including atopy, insect bite allergy, food allergy, and dermatophytosis.

Clinical Findings

Lesions consist of greasy to waxy crusts and scales with a foul odor. Pruritus ranges from negligible to severe. The lesions usually start in the intertriginous areas (axilla and groin) but can become generalized.

Diagnosis

Diagnosis is confirmed by finding numerous *Malassezia* organisms on skin surface cytology. Histopathologic changes of *Malassezia* dermatitis in the horse have not been specifically described. In other species, *Malassezia*-associated dermatitis is characterized by epidermal acanthosis and hyperkeratosis with parakeratotic crusts. Yeasts are detectable in high numbers within the keratin. Inflammation is mild and consists of mixed leukocytes within the dermis.

Therapy

Successful treatment includes management of predisposing conditions and specific antifungal therapy. Ketoconazole, miconazole, clotrimazole, and selenium sulfide all have good activity against *Malassezia*. These antifungal agents are available in a variety of mainly small animal shampoo, rinse, and cream preparations. Many are available in gallon containers and can be used on horses. The affected areas should be kept as dry as possible, as should the horse's environment.

Parasitic Etiologies

Besnoitiosis is a rare coccidian protozoal infection caused by *Besnoitia bennetti*[11] (see Chapter 61). It has been reported throughout the world in both wild and domestic animals. The definitive host for some species of *Besnoitia* is the domestic cat. Sporulated oocysts shed in the feces of the definitive host release sporozoites when ingested by susceptible intermediate hosts, such as the horse. Parasitic replication and migration throughout the connective tissues of the intermediate host leads to parasitic cyst formation in many tissues. Numerous cysts can be found in the dermis and subcutaneous tissues.

Clinical Findings

Lesions start as small papules in glabrous areas. These papules spread to cover the entire ventrum, perineum, and face and may become generalized. The nasal, oral, and pharyngeal mucosa may also be affected. As the lesions mature they become thick and crusted. Alopecia and pruritus are common and affected horses may be febrile, depressed, and weak.

Diagnosis

Diagnosis of besnoitiosis is made by biopsy. Histopathologically, the dermis and subcutis contain many large (300-650 μ), round, thick-walled cysts filled with protozoal bradyzoites. There is a perivascular mononuclear infiltrate and marked epidermal hyperplasia with hyperkeratosis. Cysts are actually hypertrophied fibroblasts.

Therapy

Successful treatment of besnoitiosis has not been reported in the horse, although trimethoprim-sulfamethoxazole was effective in a miniature donkey.[11]

Viral Etiologies

Poxvirus

Poxvirus infections in horses are rare and have several forms. Poxviruses have been associated with some cases of exudative dermatitis of the flexor aspects of the hind pasterns (another possible cause of "grease heel"). A mucocutaneous form of poxviral infection affects the muzzle and buccal cavity and can spread to the face and other parts of the body. A third type of equine poxvirus infection is *equine papular dermatitis*, seen in the United States and Australia.

Clinical Findings. Horses develop firm papules up to 0.5 cm in diameter. Lesions begin on the lateral neck, shoulders, and thorax, and eventually become generalized. Equine papular dermatitis is highly contagious and spread by direct contact and fomites. In Kenya, a generalized poxviral disease called *Uasin Gishu disease* is characterized by generalized papules that become large papillomatous proliferations over time.

Diagnosis. Histopathologically, the lesions of Uasin Gishu disease are identical to those of molluscum contagiosum. Lesions of poxvirus infection begin as erythematous macules that quickly become papular, leading to a transient vesicular stage that gives rise to a pustule and then a crust. Healing with scar formation is typical. In haired areas a fine, powdery scale may form. Histopathologic changes vary with stage of the lesion. The cells of the epidermal stratum spinosum often show cytoplasmic swelling, leading to keratinocyte rupture and vesicle formation. The dermis is edematous with variable degrees of perivascular mononuclear cell and neutrophil infiltration. Neutrophils migrate into the epidermis to form pustules, which rupture to form crusts. The epidermis becomes extremely hyperplastic. Intracytoplasmic inclusions typical of poxvirus infection may be evident. Affected horses may show various systemic signs, including pyrexia, lameness, ptyalism, and depression. The symptoms are self-limiting and last 20 to 30 days.

Molluscum Contagiosum

Etiology. Molluscum contagiosum is a rare proliferative poxviral disease in horses caused by a molluscipoxvirus.[13] The disease is mildly contagious between horses, and transmission occurs by direct skin-to-skin contact and indirect contact with fomites.

Clinical Findings. The clinical and histopathologic changes of molluscum contagiosum are identical to those seen in horses with Uasin Gishu disease. However, the causative agent of equine molluscum contagiosum cannot be grown in culture, whereas the agent of Uasin Gishu can be cultured. Lesions usually begin in one area, such as the chest or neck, then become widespread, with affected animals having hundreds of lesions. Lesions start as papules that become hyperplastic with thick crusts and horny projections.

Diagnosis. Diagnosis of molluscum contagiosum is made by biopsy and is characteristic of the disease. Discrete foci of endophytic epidermal hyperplasia form pear-shaped lobules in the superficial dermis. Keratinocytes are greatly swollen and contain large intracytoplasmic inclusions known as "molluscum bodies." Affected keratinocytes slough through a pore that forms in the stratum corneum and enlarges to become a central crater. The dermis is not inflamed.

Therapy

Treatment of poxvirus infections consist of supportive care and prevention of secondary bacterial infections. Topical therapy with antibacterial shampoos, clean blankets, and dry stalls all help to prevent secondary infection. No reported treatment, including an autogenous bacterin, has been successful for treatment of molluscum contagiosum. Horses may remain covered with hundreds of lesions for several months to years. In some cases, many of the lesions will regress over time, although the regression of all lesions has not been reported. Occasionally, horses will have small numbers of incidental and self-limiting lesions.

PAPULONODULAR DERMATOSES

Papulonodular dermatoses have deeper lesions that extend into the lower layers of the dermis (Box 7-4). These lesions consist of multiple or large papules to nodules that may ulcerate, drain, and crust over.

Bacterial Etiology, Diagnosis, and Treatment

Bacterial furunculosis is merely a progression of folliculitis. The most prominent lesions are often seen in the saddle region and include furuncles, draining tracts, and ulcerations. Diagnosis, histopathologic findings, and treatment are the same as discussed for folliculitis. Antibiotic choice should always be based on culture and sensitivity results, and systemic antibiotic therapy should continue for at least 6 to 8 weeks instead of 3 to 4 weeks. If only a few lesions are present, 2% mupirocin ointment can be tried instead of systemic antibiotic therapy.

Box • 7-4

Papulonodular Dermatoses

Noninfectious
- Fly bites
- Collagenolytic granuloma
- Tick bite granuloma
- Hypodermiasis (warbles)
- Demodectic mange
- Axillary nodular necrosis
- Straw itch mites
- Unilateral papular dermatosis

Infectious
- Poxviruses
  - Equine molluscum contagiosum
- Papillomaviruses
- Bacterial furunculosis
  - Staphylococcal
  - Streptococcal
  - Corynebacterial
- Leishmaniasis

Papillomavirus

Papillomatosis in the horse is caused by several different DNA papovaviruses (see Chapter 25). Lesions begin as small, smooth, white to gray papules that grow into pedunculated lesions with multiple frondlike keratin projections. Diagnosis is made by histopathology; viral papillomas are characterized by an exophytic, extremely hyperkeratotic and hyperplastic epidermis supported by thin dermal cores. The keratinocytes of the spinous and granular layers have ballooning degeneration and may have intranuclear, pale, basophilic viral inclusion bodies. The stratum granulosum has large and irregularly shaped keratohyaline granules.

Leishmaniasis

Etiology

Leishmania, an intracellular protozoal parasite of the mononuclear phagocyte system, can cause papulonodular skin disease in horses.[14] Cutaneous leishmaniasis in horses is seen primarily in South America but has been reported in horses residing in the United States. Endemic foci of leishmaniasis exist in Texas, Oklahoma, and Ohio. The majority of cases reported in the United States have been in the dog. Leishmaniasis is caused by *Leishmania braziliensis braziliensis*, a protozoal parasite transmitted by the sandfly. Lesions consist of papules and nodules that become ulcerated and crusted. Common locations for lesions include the muzzle, pinnae, scrotum, neck, and legs.

Diagnosis

Histopathology is usually diagnostic for leishmaniasis, and lesions consist of a superficial and deep granulomatous dermatitis. Inflammation can be diffuse or organized as distinct granulomas (Fig. 7-2). *Leishmania* amastigotes can be identified within macrophages, giant cells, or occasionally within endothelial cells or fibroblasts or free in the interstitium.

Therapy

Few reports of treatment of leishmaniasis in horses have been published. One horse was successfully treated with sodium stibogluconate. This drug is specific for the treatment of leishmaniasis and is a systemic therapy. Many potential adverse effects are associated with this medication, including pain with intravenous injection. Arrhythmias occur in people, and

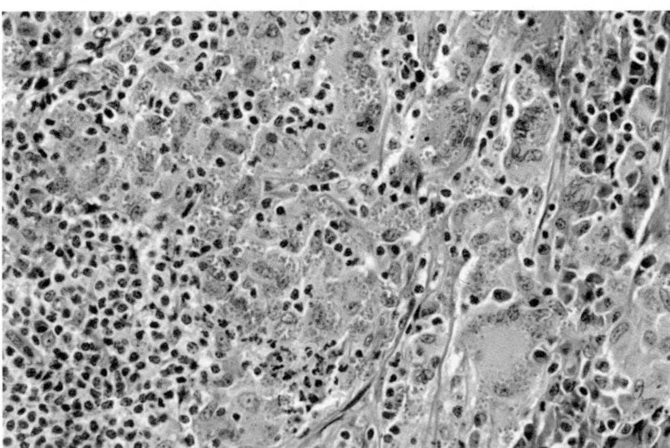

Fig. 7-2 *Leishmania* infection in horse. Changes consist of granuloma containing giant cells.

the drug is contraindicated in pregnant women and patients with renal disease.

LARGE NODULAR/MASS DERMATOSES

Etiology

Nodular/mass dermatoses form a single mass lesion or several large nodular lesions grouped together and have many different etiologies (Box 7-5). These lesions affect primarily the deep dermis and subcutaneous tissue. Eventually, the underlying muscle tissue may also be involved. The overlying epidermis may be completely normal or may contain multiple draining tracts and ulcers.

Subcutaneous bacterial abscesses in the horse can be caused by any bacterium that is inadvertently inoculated into the skin or subcutaneous tissue. *Staphylococcus aureus* in particular but also other staphylococcal species are frequently cultured from these lesions (see Chapter 29). *Streptococcus* spp. (see Chapter 28), *Actinomyces* spp., *Nocardia* spp. (see Chapter 30), *Pseudomonas aeruginosa*, and *Mycobacterium* spp. (see Chapter 33) have been reported less frequently. *Corynebacterium pseudotuberculosis* causes particularly deep-seated abscesses (see Chapter 30). The typical presentation is a solitary, large abscess on the ventral chest, although multiple lesions anywhere on the body can be seen. Insect bites have been proposed as the means by which *C. pseudotuberculosis* is inoculated into the subcutaneous tissue.

Subcutaneous mycoses in the horse can be caused by a myriad of ubiquitous soil saprophytes that are inadvertently inoculated into viable tissue. Eumycotic fungi such as *Pseudallescheria boydii* form granules or grains in the tissue.[15] These are normally solitary lesions that may or may not have draining tracts. The grains in the exudate may be dark or white depending on the particular fungus involved. *Phaeohyphomycotic* fungi form pigmented hyphae in tissue but not granules. These fungi normally form multiple, nonulcerative nodules. *Zygomycotic* fungal infections are characterized by nonpigmented, poorly staining hyphae in the tissue. These fungi usually cause solitary, ulcerative, granulomatous masses (see Chapter 55). *Sporothrix schenckii*, a dimorphic fungus (see Chapter 52), and *Pythium insidiosum*, an oomycete (see Chapter 55), cause lesions similar to those just described.

Box • 7-5

Large Nodular Dermatoses/Mass Lesions

Noninfectious
- Cutaneous habronemiasis
- Primary screwworm
- Blowfly
- Squamous cell carcinoma
- Sarcoid
- Mast cell tumor

Infectious
- Bacterial
  - *Staphylococcus*
  - *Corynebacterium* (pigeon breast)
  - *Nocardia*
  - Actinomycetes
  - Mycobacteria
  - Glanders
- Fungal
  - Eumycotic mycetomas
  - Phaeohyphomycosis
  - Zygomycosis
  - Sporotrichosis
- Oomycetes
  - Pythiosis

Diagnosis

Diagnosis is made by cytologic examination with culture and sensitivity testing of the exudate. If the abscess does not mature, open, and drain, histopathology and tissue culture may be needed to make the diagnosis. Diagnosis and differentiation of subcutaneous fungal infections is best accomplished by histopathology with tissue culture and sensitivity. Most subcutaneous mycoses are characterized by a nodular to diffuse, granulomatous to pyogranulomatous, deep dermatitis and panniculitis (Fig. 7-3). Lymphocytes and plasma cells may be numerous, and microabscesses may be present. The fungal organism can usually be identified within the areas of inflammation. The overlying epidermis may be acanthotic or ulcerated.

Therapy

Treatment of bacterial subcutaneous infections is best accomplished by using heat or poultices to promote drainage. Once mature, the abscess should be surgically incised, drained, and lavaged. This therapeutic approach is much more effective than systemic antibiotic therapy. Systemic antibiotics should be reserved for cases in which the abscess does not mature or cannot be drained. Antibiotic selection should be based on culture and sensitivity results. Treatment of fungal infections consists mainly of complete surgical excision. These fungi are notoriously resistant to antifungal drugs. However, specific antifungal therapy may be beneficial in treatment of sporotrichosis (see Chapter 52).

PASTERN DERMATITIS

Equine pastern dermatitis (EPD) is an infectious disease of horses variously known as "scratches," "mud fever," "grease heel," and "cracked heels."[16-20] This disease is highly variable in terms of etiology, duration, and response to therapy (even during sequential outbreaks in the same horse). Etiologic agents

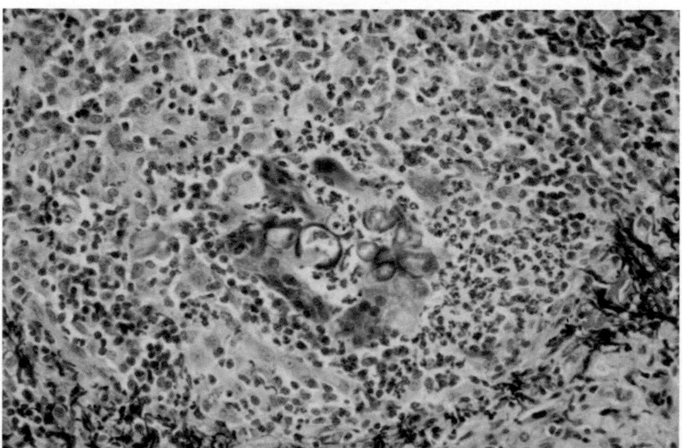

Fig. 7-3 Pyogranuloma with phaeohyphomycotic fungi.

responsible for EPD include *Staphylococcus aureus*, *Dermatophilus congolensis*, and *Chorioptes* mites.[17-20] A recent case reported in the literature described concurrent infection with intradermal spirochetes and *Pelodera strongyloides*.[16] This etiology may be similar to that of papillomatous digital dermatitis of cattle.

A severe form of pododermatitis, *verrucous pastern dermatitis*, has been described in Draft horses.[17,18] This disease may be staged based on severity and degree of histopathologic change. An increased risk of disease is associated with poor hygiene in the stable and poor quality of the pasture on which horses are managed. However, others have hypothesized an autoimmune etiology for this condition.

Clinical Features

EPD can affect any breed of horse, although it is most often described in Draft breeds. Feathering over the pasterns is a likely predisposing factor. This disease has no age or gender predilection but is reported more frequently in adult horses.[17-20] Dermatitis affects the caudal aspect of the pasterns, especially in the hindlimbs. The lesions occasionally spread dorsally and anteriorly, involving the front of the pastern and fetlock areas. The condition is frequently bilateral and symmetric, although a single limb may be affected in some horses. Lesions are most common on the nonpigmented areas of the pasterns. If left untreated, lesions coalesce and may produce large areas of ulceration and suppuration.

EPD is not usually associated with systemic clinical signs, and the general health of the animal is unaffected. If there is severe disease, secondary distal limb edema and fever may occur. Ultimately the disease can progress to severe ascending cellulitis. Lameness is variable and can be quite severe.

Diagnosis

Diagnosis of EPD is frequently made solely on the basis of clinical signs. If pustules are present, contents may be obtained for Gram stain of smears, bacterial culture, and antibiotic sensitivity testing. Punch biopsy, obtained with sterile technique, is the appropriate sample for culture. Pastern folliculitis should be differentiated from other causes of pastern dermatitis, especially allergic contact dermatitis, photosensitization, dermatophytosis, dermatophilosis, and idiopathic pastern dermatitis ("grease heel"). The lesions of grease heel are generally those of a diffuse inflammation rather than papules and pustules. The lesions of photosensitization are not limited to the posterior aspect of the pastern or fetlock regions and only involve areas that lack pigmentation.

Therapy

It may be necessary to heavily sedate or anesthetize an affected horse for initial therapy because lesions can be quite painful. The affected area(s) should be clipped and washed well with an antiseptic solution (e.g., povidone-iodine, benzoyl peroxide). Application of an astringent such as aluminum acetate solution (Domeboro, Bayer) may be helpful. An appropriate antimicrobial ointment is then applied twice daily. Systemic antibiotic therapy is rarely, if ever, indicated. In severely affected horses, therapy with injectable procaine penicillin may be considered. Broad-spectrum antibiotics or those with a predominantly gram-negative spectrum may be indicated based on culture results.

REFERENCES

See the CD-ROM for a list of references linked to the abstract in PubMed.

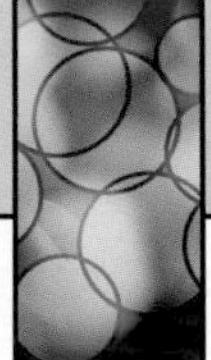

CHAPTER • 8

Reproductive Tract Infections

Ahmed Tibary and Cheryl L. Fite

Infections of the reproductive tract cause a myriad of clinical disorders manifesting primarily as infertility, abortion, and birth of septic foals. This chapter discusses the etiology, pathogenesis, clinical manifestations, treatment, and prevention of these diseases in the mare and stallion. Infectious processes of the reproductive tracts may be divided into *venereal* and *opportunistic*. The venereal diseases present important economic and regulatory issues and are reviewed separately in this chapter.

REPRODUCTIVE TRACT INFECTION IN NONPREGNANT MARES

Infection of the reproductive tract in the mare, especially endometritis, is the leading cause of infertility in horses and results in substantial annual losses. The female reproductive tract possesses a variety of mechanisms to protect itself against infection. These include physical barriers (vulva, vestibulovaginal sphincter, cervix), local immune mechanisms, and the physical ability to eliminate products of inflammation. Uterine infections, reported in 25% to 60% of barren mares,[24,111] become established when one or several of these natural defense mechanisms fail or become overwhelmed. Bacterial infections result in infertility, early embryonic loss, placentitis, birth of septic foals, and postpartum metritis. Salpingitis, cervicitis, and vaginitis may be part of the clinical presentation of acute or chronic reproductive tract infections in the mare.

Uterine Infections

Etiology

Infectious *endometritis* is a major cause of infertility and early pregnancy loss* and is estimated to affect 25% to 40% of

*References 23, 24, 107, 110, 111, 148, 149, 323, 326, 335.

broodmares.[109] These infections become established when normal defense mechanisms fail to clear potentially pathogenic organisms after they are introduced into the uterus.[282] The most common sources of uterine contamination include coitus, parturition, artificial insemination, and aseptic genital examination and manipulation.[149,381,385] Age, parity, number of barren years, and uterine biopsy grade influence likelihood of persistence of infection.[76,333]

The organisms most frequently isolated from mares with endometritis are *Streptococcus equi* subsp. *zooepidemicus, Escherichia coli, Pseudomonas aeruginosa,* and *Klebsiella pneumoniae*.[149,356,385] Infections caused by *P. aeruginosa* or *K. pneumoniae* are often considered venereal diseases because the organisms are often introduced during coitus, insemination with infected semen, or genital manipulations. *K. pneumoniae* capsule types 1, 2, and 5 are highly pathogenic.[307]

Commensal bacteria such as *Actinomyces pyogenes, Proteus* spp., and *Staphylococcus* spp. are occasionally isolated from mares with endometritis. They are considered likely to be the causative organisms of endometritis if the diagnosis is supported by cytologic or histopathologic evidence of concurrent inflammation. Alpha-hemolytic *Streptococcus, Enterobacter* spp., and *Staphylococcus epidermidis* are rarely causes of equine endometritis and should be considered simple contaminants.[79] *Corynebacterium* spp. and anaerobic bacteria such as *Bacteroides fragilis* may occasionally cause endometritis in horses.[6] Anaerobes are most often isolated from postpartum and foal-heat samples.[335] *Taylorella equigenitalis* is the causative agent of a highly contagious venereal metritis, *contagious equine metritis* (CEM) (see Chapter 41).

The pathogenicity of bacteria depends on their ability to adhere to the endometrium, preventing their removal by normal uterine clearance mechanisms. Adhesive proprieties of *S. equi* subsp. *zooepidemicus* are probably mediated by fibronectin-binding proteins and hyaluronic acid capsule.[130,199,232,433] Attachment of *K. pneumoniae* to endometrial cells is facilitated by pili and capsule.[129] Persistent colonization by *P. aeruginosa* is assisted by the secretion of an adhesive matrix that forms a biofilm.[291] These biochemical proprieties also are important in resistance of bacteria to opsonization, phagocytosis, and the action of antimicrobials.[96,113,284,433] Resistance to phagocytosis is often observed with *S. equi* subsp. *zooepidemicus* and *K. pneumoniae* and is probably mediated by antigenic variation, antiphagocytic M-like proteins, hyaluronic acid capsule, or polysaccharide and Fc receptors.[113,433] Bacterial toxins promote deterioration of complement and exacerbate uterine inflammation.[243]

Candida spp. and *Aspergillus* are the most common fungal organisms isolated from the uterus of mares with endometritis.[385] The incidence of fungal infection in mares with endometritis is estimated to vary between 0.1% and 5%.[99,100,120,318,444] Fungal organisms isolated from the equine uterus include *Aspergillus* spp., several *Candida* spp., *Cryptococcus neoformans, Fusarium* spp., *Hansenula anomala, Hansenula polymorpha*, several *Rhodotorula* spp., *Scedosporium apiospermum, Saccharomyces cerevisiae, Trichosporon beigelii,* and *Torulopsis candida*.*

Prolonged antibiotic therapy may be a predisposing factor for yeast overgrowth.[444] The use of antibiotic-containing semen extenders for artificial insemination may be partially responsible for the apparent increase in the number of mares with fungal endometritis (J. Aurich, personal communication). Transmission of fungal organisms from stallions has not been demonstrated, although fungi have been cultured from the urethra (*Mucor* spp.), fresh semen (*Absidia* spp.), and extended semen (*Candida* spp.) of stallions.[252]

Mycoplasma spp. have been isolated from the external genitalia and semen of clinically normal and infertile stallions, but their exact role in uterine infection is not well established.[273,367,448] In vitro, *Mycoplasma equigenitalium* produces a consistent cytopathic effect on the ciliated epithelium of the oviduct, with variable severity depending on strain.[31] *M. equigenitalium, M. subdolum,* and *Acholeplasma* spp. are associated with infertility, endometritis, vulvitis, and abortion in mares and with reduced fertility and balanoposthitis in stallions.[167,201,203,273] *M. equigenitalium* and *M. subdolum* were isolated from the genital tract of mares (5%-34%) and aborted equine fetuses (7%); however, the presence of mycoplasmas is not always correlated with reduced fertility.[30,167,201,203,273]

*References 82, 99, 100, 249, 279, 300, 444.

Pathogenesis

Physical Barriers. The uterine cavity is protected from ascending infection by several anatomic structures.[237] The first line of defense is provided by the seal of the normal *vulvar labia*. Evaluation of vulvar and perineal conformation should be included in all prebreeding examinations or evaluations for infertility. The vulva should be in a vertical position aligned with the anal opening (Fig. 8-1, *A*). The labia should be tight, with most of its length below the tuber ischii. The vulvar lips may become parted as a consequence of malformation caused by previous traumatic injuries or lesions (Fig. 8-1, *B*). In older multiparous mares, there is a tendency for extreme relaxation of the vulvar lips, particularly during estrus, as well as tilting of the dorsal aspect of the vulva caused by relaxation of the perineal body. In this situation the vulva becomes horizontal as it is pulled cranially over the tuber ischii (Fig. 8-1, C). These anatomic changes predispose the mare to *pneumovagina* (windsucking) and *pneumouterus*, ultimately causing urine to pool in the cranial vagina and contaminate the uterus when the cervix is open. Contamination with fecal material adds to the increased risk of infection.

The second physical barrier in the prevention of contamination of the vagina and eventually the uterus is the *vestibulovaginal sphincter*. In a normal mare the vestibulovaginal area remains sealed even when the vulvar labia are parted. Compromised vestibulovaginal sphincter function is suspected when air is sucked into the vagina or if the examiner is able to visualize the vaginal cavity directly after parting the vulvar lips. The vestibulovaginal sphincter may become compromised secondary to rectovaginal tears and other foaling injuries.

The third important anatomic barrier to infection is the *cervix*. The cervix is open during estrus, late gestation, and in the immediate postpartum period. However, compromised cervical function is observed in some mares, and this entity may remain open during anestrus and even diestrus. The most common cause of cervical incompetence is a cervical lesion consequent to dystocia.

A plan for treatment and prevention of uterine infection should include a plan to reestablish normal barrier function. Surgical procedures such as episioplasty, vestibulovaginoplasty, and rectovaginal tear repair should be considered if indicated.

Immunity and Uterine Defense. The concept that mares may be innately "resistant" or "susceptible" to uterine infection was introduced in the 1960s based on the ability of mares to clear experimentally induced or naturally acquired bacterial endometritis.[183,299] Young mares experimentally inoculated with *S. equi* subsp. *zooepidemicus* clear infection within a few

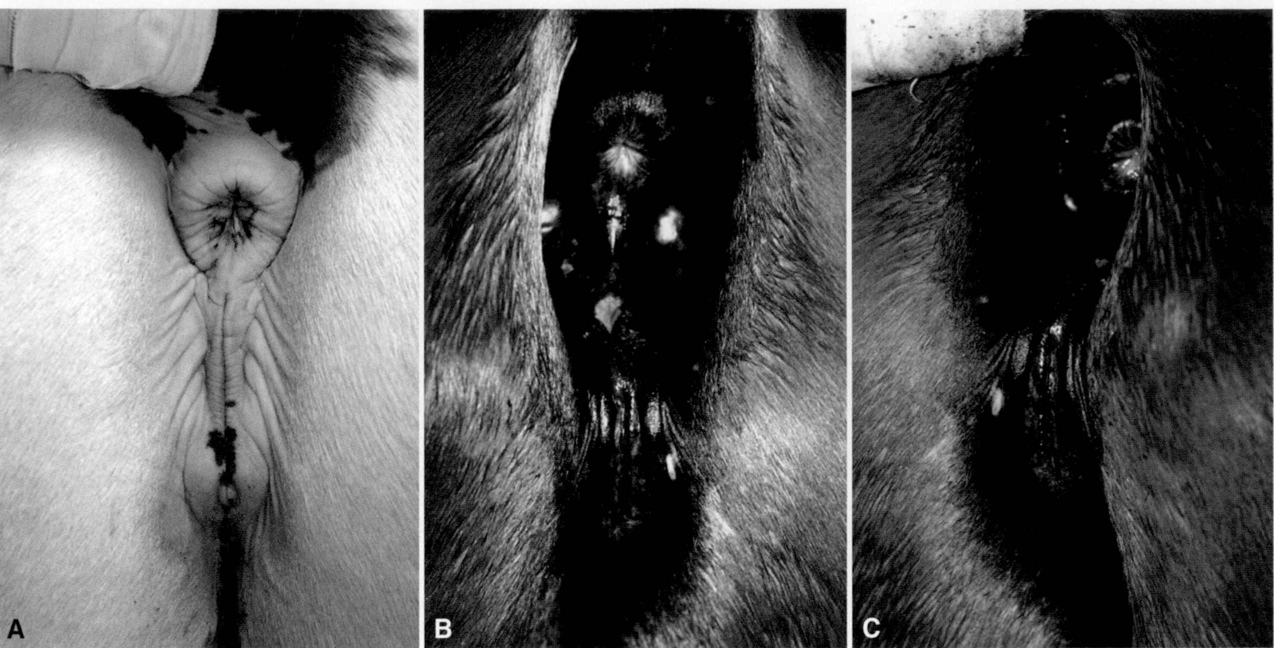

Fig. 8-1 A, Normal conformation of vulva in the mare. B, Abnormal conformation with parting of vulvar lips at dorsal commissure. C, Abnormal conformation with tilting of vulvar lips.

hours,[183] whereas barren mares inoculated with *S. equi* subsp. *zooepidemicus* and *P. aeruginosa* have a delayed elimination of bacteria.[299] These observations led to further investigation into uterine defense mechanisms to clarify the role of local immunity, neutrophil function, opsonization, and phagocytosis in the prevention and clearance of uterine infection.

Immunoglobulins. The predominant immunoglobulins in uterine secretions are IgG and IgA produced within the endometrium.[15,196,272,434-436,438] Uterine immunoglobulin concentration does not differ between mares susceptible and resistant to endometritis, suggesting that this is not a major factor in susceptibility to infection.* In fact, susceptible mares tend to have slightly higher concentrations of intrauterine immunoglobulins than do resistant mares, but susceptible mares are less efficient at opsonizing streptococci during acute infection.[15]

Neutrophils. Neutrophil chemotaxis is induced by bacteria, endotoxin, spermatozoa, semen extenders, and even sterile water and saline. A massive influx of neutrophils into the uterine lumen occurs in both susceptible and resistant mares[15,18] after local exposure to foreign proteins.[18,424,439,440] In some mares, this stimulation elicits a persistent inflammatory response after breeding that has been termed *persistent mating-induced endometritis* (PMIE). Neutrophils play an important role in this phenomenon, and their effects are exacerbated if bacteria are present.[254,391]

The events leading to PMIE are initiated by a local reaction to the primary antigen, with local production of inflammatory mediators, especially prostaglandin E_2 (PGE_2), and neutrophil influx.[372] Increased vascular permeability resulting from proinflammatory mediators exacerbates the neutrophil influx and leakage of serum proteins into the uterus, peaking as early as 4 hours after inoculation.

*References 15, 234, 272, 420, 434, 438.

This response is primarily mediated by inflammatory mediators such as leukotriene B_4 (LTB_4) and PGE_2.[43,422,424] Mares susceptible to PMIE have a higher expression of proinflammatory cytokines (interleukin-1 beta [IL-1β], IL-6, and tumor necrosis factor alpha [TNF-α]) during estrus and IL-1β and TNF-α during diestrus.[142] It is unclear whether chemotactic responsiveness differs between PMIE-susceptible mares and nonsusceptible mares.[235,236,419] A second influx of inflammatory fluid is seen 12 hours later. Resistant mares are able to eliminate most fluid by 12 hours in response to the effects of oxytocin and prostaglandin on the myometrium. Susceptible mares fail to eliminate fluid, often because of inherent endometrial or myometrial pathology that renders uterine contractions less efficient in uterine clearance.

The phagocytic activity of neutrophils is thought to be enhanced on entry into the uterine cavity.[419,422] Phagocytic activity is higher in ovariectomized mares treated with estrogens,[423] suggesting that neutrophil phagocytic activity may be highest during estrus. Phagocytic activity of circulating neutrophils is no different between susceptible and resistant mares; however, phagocytic activity and life span of uterine neutrophils are significantly reduced in susceptible mares.[16,83,422,446] Susceptible mares are more likely to have uterine clearance problems and accumulate more fluid, which may contribute to a reduction in the viability of neutrophils. Differences in neutrophil function between mares susceptible and resistant to endometritis have been demonstrated.[234-236]

Opsonizing activity in the uterus peaks 8 hours after inoculation with streptococci.[163] Studies using heat-treated uterine fluid suggest that complement is not a primary opsonizing factor in the uterus.[62,163] Complement is cleaved in uterine fluid, reducing its opsonizing ability within the uterine environment.[14,62] The uterine environment of endometritis susceptible mares seems to be hostile to complement.[18,62,219,422] In contrast, the opsonizing capacity of serum and degree of serum complement activity does not differ between susceptible

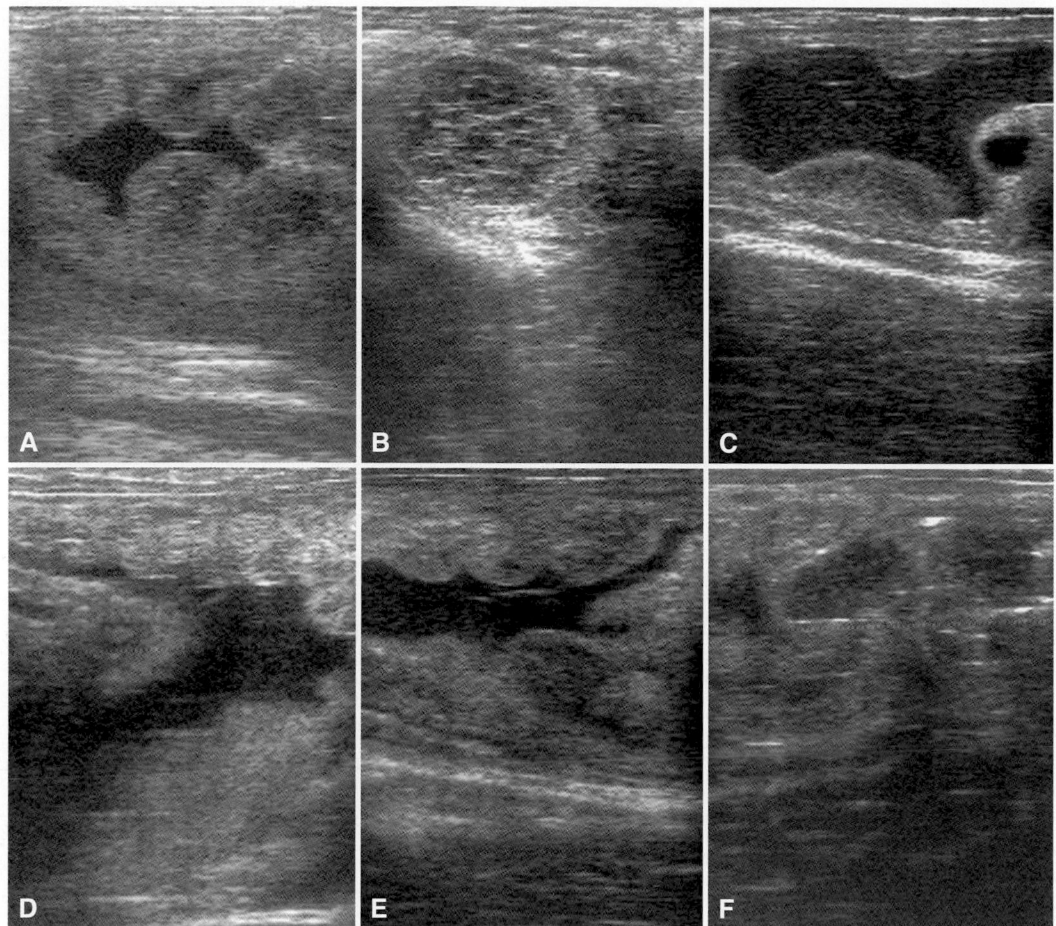

Fig. 8-2 Persistent mating-induced endometritis (PMIE). **A,** **C,** and **D,** Ultrasonograms of uterus at 6, 12, and 18 hours after insemination, respectively. **B,** Corpus hemorrhagicum. **E** and **F,** Uterus after initiation of oxytocin therapy.

and resistant mares.[14,18,44,62,416] These observations provide a rationale for the use of serum infusion for the treatment of endometritis.[14,292]

Physical Clearance of Infection. Physical clearance of pathogens and inflammatory debris from the uterus plays a major role in the prevention of persistent infection and is most effective during estrus.* Younger mares are able to eliminate both antigenic (*S. equi* subsp. *zooepidemicus*) and nonantigenic (microsphere) particles more quickly than older mares.[127] Mares susceptible to infectious endometritis are unable to eliminate bacteria from the uterus in the immediate postovulatory period.[222,397,398]

The effect of uterine pathology on susceptibility to endometritis has been demonstrated.[334] Gross anatomic changes, such as large pendulous uteri, defective myometrial activity, pendulant broad ligaments, and degenerative changes to the vascular and lymphatic drainage of the uterus, are also involved in delayed uterine clearance and the pathogenesis of endometritis.[194,224,228] Microscopic alteration of the endometrium (ulceration, degeneration, or lack of cilia) may be involved in failure of mucociliary clearance.[80,130,131,139,334]

*References 7, 74, 128, 192, 246, 278, 280-282, 395, 396, 418.

Myometrial contractions are less frequent and of shorter duration and intensity in susceptible mares,[337,399] perhaps because of increased fibrosis or biochemical factors affecting uterine contractility. Uterine contractions are reduced in the presence of nitrous oxide (NO), which is found in high concentration in susceptible mares.[7] The role of prostaglandin secretion in PMIE remains unclear despite numerous investigations, possibly reflecting variation in factors inherent to the endometrium that cannot be easily controlled in experimental studies.[28,70,71]

Diagnosis

Uterine infection may be suspected on the basis of a history of infertility, recurrent endometritis, mucopurulent vaginal discharge, predisposing anatomic features, early embryonic loss, or observation of fluid accumulation on examination of the uterus by ultrasonography. Clinical signs may include vaginal discharge. Confirmation of the diagnosis of uterine infection requires endometrial cytology and uterine culture. Uterine biopsy may be helpful in some cases.

Accumulation of large quantities of fluid during estrus or postbreeding is a good indication of mare susceptibility to endometritis (Fig. 8-2). Resistant mares eliminate mating-induced endometritis within 6 to 12 hours after breeding, whereas susceptible mares may retain variable amounts of

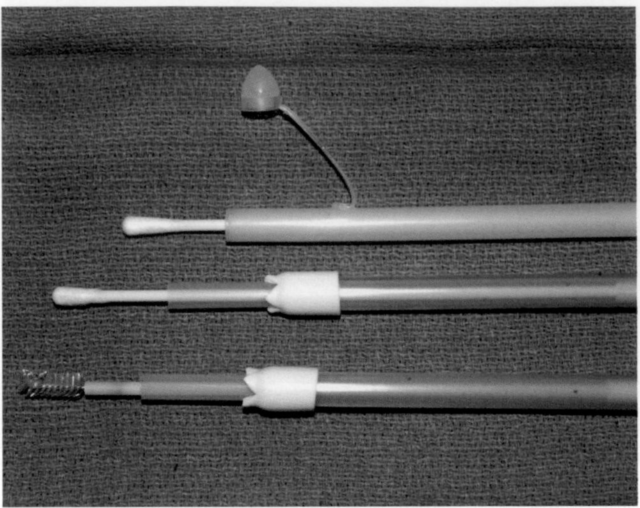

Fig. 8-3 *Top,* Single-guarded uterine swab with "pop-out" cap that can be used to collect material of endometrial cytology. *Middle,* Double-guarded swab for endometrial culture and cytology. *Bottom,* Double-guarded endometrial brush for cytology.

fluid for several days. Accumulation of fluid in the uterus is associated with decreased pregnancy rates. All mares should be evaluated 24 hours after breeding and treated if a pocket of fluid remains within the uterine cavity.[25,255,278,320] Mares with a history of infertility or that are known to be susceptible to endometritis should be evaluated or treated as early as 6 hours after breeding.[392]

Several methods for collection of uterine cytology samples have been described. These include the use of double-guarded swabs, uterine cytology brushes, and low-volume uterine flushes.[74] In the authors' opinion, uterine cytology brushes and small-volume uterine flushes provide the best specimens for endometrial cytology (Fig. 8-3). Swabs are often reliable if there is fluid in the uterus or if the swab is wetted with a sterile saline solution before sampling.

Interpretation of uterine cytology samples may be confusing because of the lack of standardized methodology for evaluation. The most common staining technique for uterine cytologic specimens is a rapid Wright-Giemsa stain (Diff-Quik). Interpretation is based on evaluation of the type of cells and organisms observed[74,75] (Fig. 8-4). Quantitative methods for the interpretation of equine endometrial cytology have been reviewed recently.[74] Diagnosis of endometritis may be based on the number of neutrophils per number of

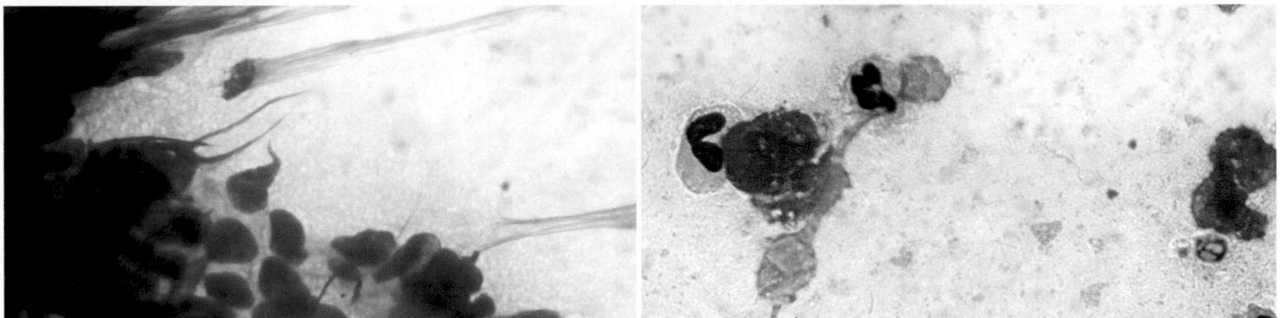

Fig. 8-4 Endometrial cytology stained with Diff-Quik. **A,** Normal endometrial cells. **B,** Slight inflammatory reaction. **C,** Mating-induced inflammation (note sperm cells). **D,** Severe infectious inflammation.

high-power microscopic fields, as a ratio of neutrophils to epithelial cells, or as a percentage of all cells. Endometrial cytology may provide an important clue to fungal infection. Cytology may be negative if infection is recent.[100]

Endometrial swabs should always be submitted for anaerobic and aerobic bacterial as well as fungal culture. Blood agar plating may be used in the initial fungal culture, but specific culture techniques are required for more precise diagnosis.[100]

Endometrial biopsy is an important and highly accurate method for the diagnosis of uterine inflammation. Special staining techniques, such as Gomori's methamine silver, are particularly helpful for the diagnosis of fungal endometritis.[140]

Interpretation of diagnostic results may be challenging at times. Bacteriologic culture and cytology from endometrial biopsy are most accurate (high sensitivity and positive predictive value) for diagnosis of endometritis. The sensitivity of bacteriologic culture from endometrial biopsy is 82%; diagnosis based on cytologic and bacteriologic examination of endometrial swabs has a sensitivity of 77% and 34%, respectively.[279]

Therapy

Treatment of equine endometritis may include local or systemic antimicrobial therapy, uterine lavage, plasma infusions, and colostrum infusion. Most treatment recommendations are made on the basis of clinical experience, with limited evidence for comparative efficacy within the veterinary literature. The authors most frequently recommend treatment of uterine infections with uterine lavage to remove debris and other products of inflammation that may reduce antimicrobial activity, followed by antimicrobial therapy for 5 to 7 days.

Uterine Lavage. The goal of uterine lavage is to "clean" the uterine cavity of organisms, dead neutrophils, cell debris, and products of inflammation before local antimicrobial therapy.[13,209,401] Uterine lavage may enhance uterine contractions and clearance as a result of transient irritation of the endometrium.[447] Uterine lavage is performed using warmed, balanced electrolyte solution (e.g., lactated Ringer's, physiologic saline) with or without added antiseptics. A new solution specifically formulated for flushing of the equine uterine (Equine Uterine Flush, AB Technology, Pullman, Wash) is adjusted to appropriate pH and osmotic pressure and contains surfactants to aid in the removal of organisms and debris. Uterine lavage is preferably performed using a large Foley catheter in the same manner as for embryo collection (Table 8-1).

The addition of antiseptics such as povidone-iodine or chlorhexidine to uterine lavage fluid is occasionally recommended for the treatment of equine endometritis. However, there is some concern about the effect of these antiseptics on neutrophil function. At high concentration, antiseptics may cause severe inflammation (necrosis) and irreversible damage to the endometrium, with evidence of discomfort at the time of infusion.[406] Povidone-iodine solution may be used at a concentration of 0.05% (5 mL of 10% povidone iodine solution in 1 L of balanced salt solution) to facilitate elimination of bacterial infection. Adverse reactions are observed in mares after infusion with solution at a concentration of 1% or more.[57] Uterine lavage with 0.05% solution of povidone-iodine solution 4 hours after breeding did not adversely affect pregnancy rates.[59] Use of chlorhexidine diacetate is contraindicated in mares.[17] Chlorhexidine gluconate may cause vulvar inflammation and vaginal straining at concentrations as low as 0.5% and endometrial inflammation at concentrations of 0.25%.[186]

Lavage with EDTA-TRIS (1.2 g NaEDTA and 6.05 g TRIS/L of H_2O, titrated to pH 8.0 with glacial acetic acid) 3 hours before infusion of antibiotic has been recommended for treatment of persistent uterine infection with *Pseudomonas* spp. Ethylenediaminetetraacetic acid (EDTA) is thought to bind Ca^{++} in bacterial cell walls, making cell walls permeable to antibiotics and bacteria more susceptible to bactericidal activity of antibiotics.[442]

Antimicrobials. The aim of local uterine infusion of antimicrobials is specifically to eliminate the causative organism[35,233,385] (Table 8-2). The choice of antibiotic is dictated by results of endometrial culture and sensitivity, predicted antimicrobial efficacy in the uterine environment, and consideration of possible adverse uterine effects. Nonbuffered or precipitating solutions should be avoided. *Streptococcus equi* subsp. *zooepidemicus* and *E. coli*, two of the most common bacterial causes of endometritis, are sensitive in vitro to amikacin and gentamicin.[356] The selection of antimicrobial for intrauterine infusion should take into account the pH and solubility of the drugs as well as the solution used for infusion. Some antibiotics, such as ceftiofur, will lose most of their activity if diluted in a saline solution.[332] The volume of infusion should be sufficient to treat the entire uterine cavity, usually between 60 and 120 mL. Aqueous solutions of sodium benzypenicillin, neomycin, polymixin, and furaltadone are generally safe and useful for treatment of horses with acute endometritis.[320,332] Aqueous solutions of penicillin, ampicillin, carbenicillin, ticarcillin, ticarcillin and clavulanic acid, kanamycin, and neomycin have also been recommended. Low-pH antimicrobials such as gentamicin and amikacin should be buffered with an equal volume of 7.5% sodium bicarbonate before infusion.[17,58,393]

Uterine infusion of enrofloxacin was an effective treatment for endometritis in 80% of 17 mares.[144] Antimicrobial concentrations in endometrial tissues were greater than the minimum inhibitory concentration (MIC) for most bacterial pathogens for up to 24 hours after intrauterine infusion of enrofloxacin at a dosage of 2.5 mg/kg.[143] Moderate endometrial inflammation was observed 24 hours after infusion but resolved progressively within 2 weeks.

Treatment of fungal endometritis requires large-volume uterine flushes followed by intrauterine therapy with antimycotic drugs for 7 to 10 days. Treatment for a longer duration may be required for some mares. The drugs most often used are polyene antimicrobial agents (e.g., amphotericin B, nystatin, natamycin), which alter membrane permeability, and imidazole derivatives (e.g., clotrimazole, econazole, ketoconazole, fluconazole, itraconazole), which interfere with nutrient exchange across the fungal cell wall and cell membrane.[99] The prognosis for fertility after treatment of fungal endometritis remains generally poor because of the histologic changes resulting from the chronic inflammation.[444]

Lufenuron, a benzoylphenyl urea derivative and inhibitor of chitin synthesis, used for flea control in dogs and cats, has been recommended for treatment of mares with *Candida parapsolosis*, *Candida paratropicalis*, and *Aspergillus fumigatus* uterine infections. The inhibition of fungal growth is thought to be caused by disruption of the chitin-rich cell wall that surrounds these organisms. Intrauterine lavage is performed with lufenuron (540 mg) suspended in 60 mL of sterile saline solution.[174]

Systemic antimicrobials (e.g., amikacin,[63] gentamicin,[297] ticarcillin,[366] procaine penicillin G, ampicillin, potentiated sulfonamides,[17] ceftiofur sodium[242]) have been used for the treatment of endometritis, but little is known about drug concentrations obtained within the endometrium or treatment efficacy after systemic administration. Systemic treatment

Table • 8-1

Guidelines for Uterine Flushing and High-Volume Uterine Lavage

UTERINE FLUSHING	HIGH-VOLUME LAVAGE (POSTPARTUM)
Indications	
Chronic endometritis, pyometra	Partial or total placental retention
Endometritis	Metritis
Persistent mating-induced endometritis	After obstetric manipulation/fetotomy
	After uterine prolapse
Equipment	
Silicone Foley long catheter (28 or 34 French, 100-mL cuff)	Stomach tube; make sure that tube has several side openings (1-1.5 cm in diameter).
Flushing bag (2.5 L)	Bucket
	Stomach pump
Mare Preparation	
Sedation if needed.	Often needed.
Wrap tail in plastic sleeve.	Wrap tail in plastic sleeve.
Palpation per rectum to evacuate feces.	Palpation per rectum to evacuate feces.
Clean perineal area and vulva.	Clean perineal area and vulva.
Place catheter using sterile sleeve and lubricate.	Place nasogastric tube deep into uterine cavity (within chorioallantoic cavity if placenta is retained).
Insert catheter into cervix and inflate balloon, making sure it is snug against anterior cervical os.	Protect orifices of tube by cuffing hand around it.
Fluid Choice	
Warm saline (least preferred)	Warm saline
Warm lactated Ringer's solution (LRS)	Warm distilled water + 34 g of table salt per liter
Proprietary fluid (e.g., Equine Uterine Flush lavage solution)	Warm LRS (may be too expensive)
	Warm tap water with 5 mL of 10% povidone-iodine solution and 8.5 g of table salt per liter
Fluid Delivery and Monitoring	
Gravity using flushing bags	Pumped directly into uterine cavity
Volume varies from 500 mL to 2 L	Up to 15 L (depends on size of uterus)
Palpate transrectally to make sure that both uterine horns are sufficiently distended before emptying.	Flush twice a day if mare retained placenta or mare is sick.
Repeat flushing until return is clear.	Repeat flushing daily as needed (until placenta is passed if retained).
Monitor fluid retained by ultrasonography or measuring fluid collected.	Monitor by transabdominal ultrasound.
Evacuation Help	
Before and after flushing: oxytocin (10-20 IU intramuscularly)	Retained placenta (20 IU oxytocin every 4 hours in first 12 hours)
Postbreeding flushing should be started no earlier than 4 hours after breeding.	Exercise mare.

has the advantage of preventing inadvertent recontamination of the uterus and repeated trauma to the vagina and cervix in mares. Ciprofloxacin (2.5 g/day) and probenecid (1 g/day) were recommended for systemic treatment of *Pseudomonas* infection.[393] Although an oral dose of ciprofloxacin of 0.5 mg/kg has been used by some practitioners,[61] pharmacokinetic studies have shown that bioavailability of the drug is not very high.[119] Fluoroquinolone antibiotics such as enrofloxacin and ciprofloxacin reach therapeutic concentrations in endometrial tissue after intravenous (IV) administration.[2,290] Endometrial concentrations of metronidazole were very low after systemic treatment for 4 days.[365]

Mannose Infusion. Development of resistance to multiple antibiotics has become an important issue in practice. The efficacy of specific sugar solutions in preventing bacterial adhesion to the endometrium has been investigated in vitro. Mannose solution significantly reduced adhesion of *E. coli, P. aeruginosa,*

Table • 8-2

Antimicrobials for Treatment of Endometritis in Mares

DRUG	DOSE*	COMMENTS
Gram-Positive Bacterial Infections		
Penicillin sodium of potassium salt	5 million units (U)	Very effective for streptococci; economical.
Ampicillin	1-3 g	Can be very irritating; use at high dilutions; sodium salt precipitates on endometrium that remains in uterus for prolonged period.
Carbenicillin	2-5 g	Reserved for persistent *Pseudomonas* (synergistic efficacy with aminoglycosides); usually given on alternate days with aminoglycosides; slightly irritating.
Gram-Negative Bacterial Infections		
Gentamicin sulfate	500-1000 mg	Highly effective; generally nonirritating when mixed with an equal volume of $NaHCO_3$ and diluted in saline.
Amikacin sulfate	2 g	Use for *Pseudomonas*, *Klebsiella*, and persistent gram-negative infections.
Kanamycin sulfate	1 g	Toxic to spermatozoa; do not use close to breeding.
Polymyxin B	1 million U	Particularly effective against *Pseudomonas*.
Neomycin sulfate	3-4 g	Use for sensitive *E. coli*; can be irritating; do not use near time of breeding.
Gram-Positive and Gram-Negative Bacterial Infections (broad spectrum)		
Cephazolin sodium	1 g	
Ticarcillin	1-3 g	Use for *Pseudomonas*; do not use for *Klebsiella*.
Ceftiofur sodium	1 g	Once daily either intramuscularly or by intrauterine infusion.
Fungal (Yeast) Infections		
Nystatin	0.5-2.5 million U	Primarily for yeast (e.g., *Candida albicans*) in the growing phase; insoluble, suspend in 100-250 mL sterile water and vigorously mix immediately before infusion.
Amphotericin B	100-200 mg	For infections with *Aspergillus, Candida, Mucor,* or *Histoplasma;* dilute in 100-250 mL sterile water, a relatively insoluble suspension.
Clotrimazole	500-700 mg	For yeast infections (*Candida* spp.); crushed tablets mixed with 40 mL sterile water.
Fluconazole	100 mg	For *Candida* spp. infections.
Miconazole	200 mg	Most efficacious for yeast infections (*Candida* spp.) and some resistant fungal infections; infuse once daily for up to 10 days; dilute in 40-60 mL sterile saline before infusion.

*All doses are for intrauterine infusion unless otherwise indicated.

and *S. equi* subsp. *zooepidemicus* to the endometrium. Inhibition of adhesion of *E. coli* was possible with a concentration as low as 0.4 mg/mL, whereas inhibition of *P. aeruginosa* adhesion required a concentration of 75 mg/mL; a concentration of 3.13 to 25 mg/mL caused significant inhibition of *S. equi subsp. zooepidemicus* adhesion. *N*-acetyl-D-galactosamine inhibited adhesion of *E. coli* and *P. aeruginosa* only. If these results are confirmed in vivo, lavage with mannose solution might be a good adjunct or alternative to antibiotic therapy of endometritis.[199]

Plasma Infusion. Intrauterine infusion of autogenous plasma (100 mL) anticoagulated with heparin or sodium citrate is suggested to enhance neutrophil function in endometritis-susceptible mares.[14,18] Some clinical trials showed significant benefit with this approach,[13,14,292] whereas others were unable to show enhanced bactericidal activity after plasma infusion.[3,91,401] Infusion of plasma with leukocytes may improve pregnancy rate compared with infusion of plasma alone.[257] The discrepancies between results may be caused by several factors, including the strain of bacteria and the amount and type of antibodies present in plasma. Infusion of serum from horses hyperimmunized against specific strains of *S. equi* subsp. *zooepidemicus* is reportedly more effective in increasing phagocytosis than the infusion of nonimmune serum.[421]

Colostrum Infusion. The goal of colostrum infusion is to enhance the local uterine defense mechanisms by increasing the concentration of immunoglobulins in the uterine cavity. This treatment is reported to be successful in uncontrolled studies.[104,106]

Prevention

Prevention of uterine infection is accomplished by decreasing the likelihood of contamination and by early recognition and treatment of PMIE. Contamination of the uterus can be prevented by correcting vulvar conformation and observing strict hygiene during breeding and genital manipulation. Susceptible mares should be monitored before breeding and bred using minimum-contamination breeding technique.[195] The purpose of this monitoring is to reduce the chance of contamination of the uterus by bacteria and to eliminate the products of the inflammatory reaction caused by semen.

The primary mechanism for prevention of fluid accumulation in the uterus is contraction of the uterine musculature in response to oxytocin. Oxytocin release is observed in mares after mating, teasing, genital manipulation, and infusion of fluid into the uterine cavity.[73,281,369] Oxytocin injection improves uterine defense by promoting uterine fluid evacuation.[11,218,227,320] Administration of 20 IU of oxytocin intramuscularly (IM) induces uterine contraction for up to 90 minutes.[246] Oxytocin administration to mares susceptible to PMIE at 4 hours after breeding aids in the elimination of excess fluid and improves fertility.[25,320,336] The standard dose for an average mare is 10 IU intravenously (IV) or 20 to 25 IU IM.[70-72,246,320,392] Large doses may decrease uterine contractions.[72,246] Oxytocin therapy may be repeated every 6 hours for 24 to 48 hours after breeding.[278,392] A 7% increase in pregnancy rate is reported with a single injection of oxytocin (25 IU IM) within 72 hours of breeding.[320] Oxytocin does not interfere with ovulation or gamete transport if administered no earlier than 4 hours after breeding.[55,278]

Prebreeding and postbreeding uterine lavage may be indicated in mares that tend to accumulate a substantial amount of fluid during estrus.[57,59,60,407]

Prostaglandin $F_{2\alpha}$ ($PGF_{2\alpha}$; 5-10 mg IM) or its analog, cloprostenol (250 μg IM), is recommended for the treatment of mares with PMIE because of their ecbolic proprieties.[55,220,278,396] Cloprostenol induces weaker but more sustained uterine contractions than oxytocin and is helpful when excessive uterine edema is present.[93] Repeated administration of cloprostenol should be avoided because it has been associated with transient reduction of circulating progesterone levels during diestrus.[55,278]

Prophylactic in utero administration of antibiotics to PMIE-susceptible mare after breeding has been suggested. A combination of oxytocin treatment and intrauterine infusion of broad-spectrum antibiotics increases pregnancy rates in susceptible mares.[4,320] However, such an approach may pose some risk of development of antimicrobial resistance.

Postpartum Metritis

Postpartum uterine infections are of particular importance because of their severity and effect on the general health of the mare. Septic postpartum metritis is often a result of nonhygienic manipulation during foaling, obstetric manipulations, and retained placenta. Mares with postpartum metritis may present with severe systemic complications of endotoxemia and laminitis. Treatment consisting of daily large-volume uterine flushes, systemic antimicrobial therapy, and appropriate therapy for endotoxemia and dehydration should be immediately initiated in affected mares.[112,138,298]

Other Infections of Nonpregnant Mares

Infectious *vaginitis* and *cervicitis* may occur as part of the uterine infection process or as a result of local irritation or laceration. Vaginal injuries secondary to breeding or parturition may lead to abscess formation and adhesions.[33,101,261,322,343]

Infectious inflammation of the ovaries *(oophoritis)* with abscessation and peritoneal adhesions may occur after abdominal surgery or peritonitis (Fig. 8-5). Oophoritis may also occur as a consequence of repeated transvaginal ultrasound-guided follicular aspiration.[47] Affected mares may present with abdominal pain, anorexia, fever of unknown origin, and weight loss. Transrectal ultrasonography may help in the diagnosis of these infections. Confirmation of the diagnosis and evaluation of the extent of the lesions may be achieved by laparoscopy. Ovariectomy is usually required for treatment of this condition.[164,321]

Salpingitis is rare in the mare but may result from ascending infection from the uterus after parturition.[164] Salpingitis has been described in mares with contagious equine metritis (CEM)[1] (see Chapter 41). Bilateral salpingitis results in sterility.

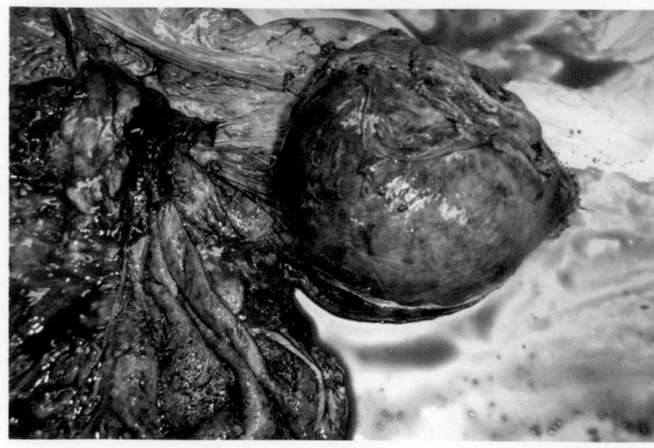

Fig. 8-5 Ovarian abscess and adhesions.

INFECTIOUS CAUSES OF ABORTION

Causes of equine abortion in several countries have been extensively reviewed (United Kingdom,[304,359,431] United States,[153,177,178,374-377] New Zealand and Australia,[22] France,[134,404] Egypt,[101] India[145]). One third to half of all equine abortions are estimated to be the result of infection.[359] Numerous organisms have been associated with infectious abortion, including viruses, bacteria, and fungi. The prevalence of each organism differs geographically. In England, equine herpes viral abortion predominates.[359] In France, 79% of infectious abortions are caused by bacteria and 21% by viruses.[134]

Bacterial Abortions and Placentitis

Placentitis is a significant cause of equine late-term abortion, premature delivery, and neonatal death. It is implicated as a cause of abortion in as many as 50% of all mares that abort.* Placentitis is diagnosed in approximately 157 cases of fetal loss each year in Kentucky (approximately 30% of all submitted fetuses).[445] It may be caused by a variety of bacterial, fungal, viral, and protozoal organisms.[304,305,316] Bacterial placentitis is most common; fungal placentitis is reported in fewer than 10% of horses with placentitis.[177,178,359]

Placentitis is generally classified as three types: ascending, diffuse, and focal mucoid.[445] With the exception of *Leptospira* spp., most bacterial or mycotic placentitis of mares is the result of an ascending infection.[248,374]

Ascendant Placentitis

Ascending placentitis is the most common type of placentitis in horses.[306,316,445] Bacteria isolated from the placenta are comparable to those isolated from the uterus of mares with endometritis.[175,331,445] *Streptococcus equi* subsp. *zooepidemicus*, *E. coli*, *Pseudomonas aeruginosa*, *Enterobacter* spp. and *Klebsiella pneumoniae* are the most frequent isolates.[89,175,316,375,431]

In a retrospective study of 954 cases of equine abortion, placentitis was recognized in 24.7% of all submissions.[178] A bacterial or fungal organism was isolated in 68.6% of placentitis cases, and 57.4% of cases yielded bacteria both from the placenta and the fetal organs. The most common

*References 153, 177, 178, 306, 359, 429, 445.

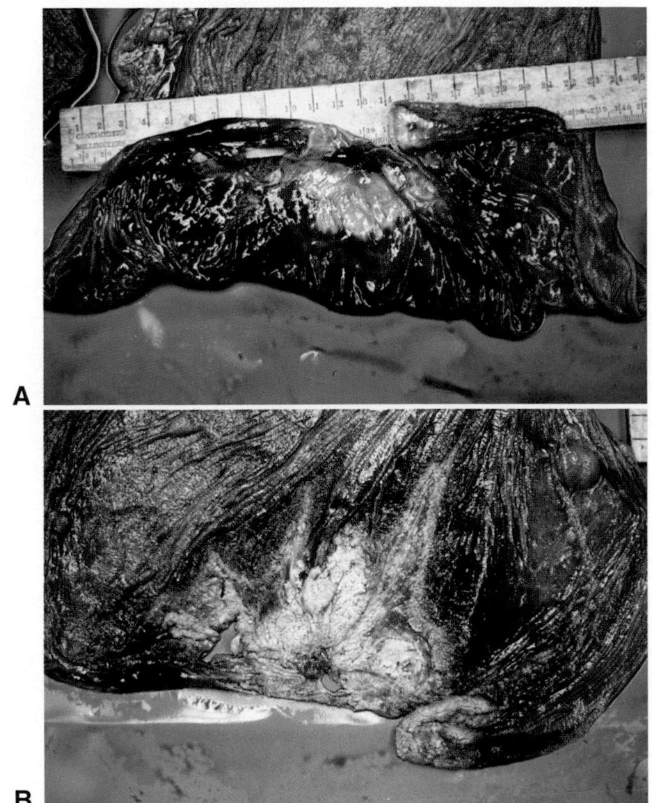

Fig. 8-6 Placenta showing severe ascendant placentitis. **A,** Allantoic surface. **B,** Chorionic surface.

microorganisms isolated include *S. equi* subsp. *zooepidemicus, E. coli, Leptospira* spp., nocardioform *Actinomyces, P. aeruginosa, Streptococcus equisimilis, Enterobacter agglomerans, K. pneumoniae,* α-hemolytic streptococci, *Staphylococcus aureus,* and *Actinobacillus* spp.[101,134] Other bacteria isolated include *Proteus mirabilis, Citrobacter diversus,* and fecal and environmental contaminants.[178] Abortions resulting from hematogenous infection with *Actinobacillus equuli*[425] and *Corynebacterium pseudotuberculosis* have been reported.[145,308]

There is a wide geographic variation in the frequency of specific bacterial and fungal isolates associated with equine placentitis and abortion. A high incidence of fungal placentitis is reported in England.[431] The incidence of mycotic placentitis varies from region to region because of climate and other environmental factors.[306,430] Emphysematous placentitis caused by clostridial infection was one of the top four causes of bacterial abortion in an early study.[316] There are numerous reports of *Enterobacter agglomerans* placentitis in horses.* The importance of anaerobic bacteria, *Mycoplasma* spp., *Chlamydia,* and rickettsial organisms in equine placentitis is uncertain.[108,319,335]

Except for placentitis caused by *Leptospira* spp. or the nocardioform actinomycetes, most equine placentitis occurs in two forms: (1) acute diffuse placentitis with infiltration of neutrophils in the intervillous spaces or (2) focal necrosis of the chorionic villi. Placentitis from abortions before midgestation are chronic, focal, or focally extensive at the cervical area and characterized by necrosis of chorionic villi, presence of eosinophilic material on the chorion, and infiltration of mononuclear inflammatory cells in the intervillous spaces, stroma of villi, chorion, allantois, and vascular layer. Lesions may be either acute or chronic.[178]

*References 101, 133, 134, 152, 210, 229, 261, 307, 322, 386.

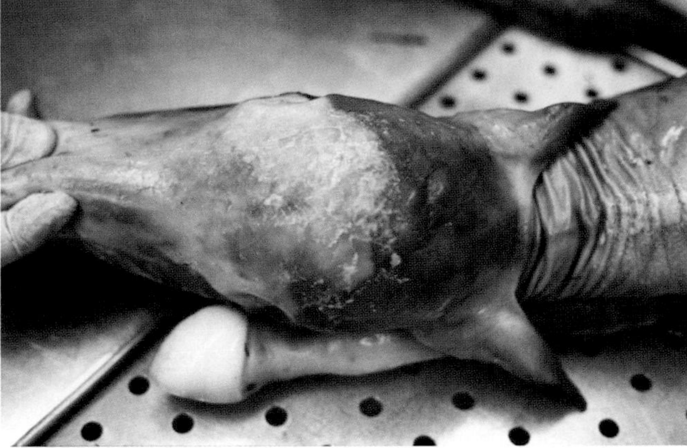

Fig. 8-7 *Escherichia coli* abortion. White mucoid exudate on fetal head surface.

Bacterial placentitis most often induces abortion between 6 and 9 months of gestation. Placentitis resulting from *E. coli* tends to cause later abortion and more stillbirths. Placentitis from *S. equi* subsp. *zooepidemicus* tends to be acute and focal or diffuse. In acute bacterial placentitis the fetus is generally expelled before 8 months of pregnancy. Acute or diffuse placentitis may not be easy to recognize on gross examination of the placenta. Histologic evaluation of the allantochorion may reveal bacterial emboli with necrosis of chorionic villi or infiltration of neutrophils in the intervillous space. Chronic or focal placentitis typically results in birth of premature or weak foals or late-term abortions. Lesions tend to be located at the cervical star, where discoloration and thickening are observed (Fig. 8-6).

Escherichia coli placentitis is usually acute in mares that abort before 7 months of gestation but is more likely to be chronic and focally extensive, involving the cervical star, in mares that abort after 9 months of gestation. Placental edema and the presence of a white mucoid exudate on the chorion and fetal surface are common findings after abortion caused by *E. coli* placentitis (Fig. 8-7).

Pseudomonas aeruginosa placentitis causes abortion between 6 and 9 months of gestation. It is usually acute and may be either focal or diffuse with a thickened and discolored cervical star. Histologically, the primary abnormality is ulceration of the chorion with infiltration of neutrophils in the villi, chorionic stroma, and vascular layer.

Lesions caused by infection with *Streptococcus equisimilis* are similar to those of *S. equi* subsp. *zooepidimicus*. Abortion occurs between 6 and 8 months of pregnancy.

Gross and histologic features of mycotic placentitis were described in detail by Hong et al.[178] Mycotic placentitis and abortion are most likely to occur in the late gestational period. Fungal organisms associated with equine abortion include *Aspergillus* spp.,[121,145,177,303] mucoraceous fungi, *Histoplasma caspulatum,*[153,345,373,374,445] *Candida* spp.,[249,355,445] *Mucor* spp.,[145] *Coccidioides* spp.,[215,250,371] and *Cryptococcus neoformans*.[34,300,341]

Focally extensive placentitis is usually observed at the cervical star and adjacent area as a thick, leathery area. Histologically, except for histoplasmosis and candidiasis, the fungi induce a chronic, extensive placentitis characterized by extensive necrosis of the chorionic villi, neovascularization in the chorionic stroma, infiltration of neutrophils, mononuclear cells, or mixed inflammatory cells in the villi and chorionic stroma, and presence of fungal hyphae in the necrotic debris. Adenomatous hyperplasia with or without squamous metaplasia of the chorionic epithelium are frequently observed.[178] *Histoplasma capsulatum* caused a multifocal granulomatous placentitis and abortion in one mare in the seventh month of gestation and three mares in the tenth month. Four newborn foals died from severe granulomatous pneumonia within a few days of birth, and a weanling Thoroughbred developed granulomatous pneumonia and lymphadenitis at 5 months of age.[330]

With *Candida* spp. infection, placentitis is generally diffuse, necrotizing, and proliferative with extracellular, yeastlike spores in the chorionic epithelium. Chronic, focally extensive placentitis is most common, with expulsion of foals late in gestation.[178]

Hematogenous Multifocal or Diffuse Placentitis

Multifocal or diffuse placentitis is less common than acute, focal placentitis and is usually a result of hematogenous spread of microorganisms to the uterus. This occurs with leptospirosis, salmonellosis, histoplasmosis, and candidiasis. A special focal mucoid form of placentitis, *nocardioform placentitis*, is emerging as common in several U.S. regions.[178]

Leptospira spp. Placentitis

Leptospira spp. placentitis is characterized by diffuse lesions secondary to hematogenous spread (see Chapter 34). Leptospirosis as a cause of placentitis seems to be more frequently diagnosed in Kentucky[115,116,178,445] than in other regions of the world,[411,431] probably because of specific regional characteristics and the difficulty in isolating or detecting the pathogen. An outbreak of leptospiral abortions has been described on a Thoroughbred farm in California after a flood.[198]

Most leptospiral abortions occur between 6 and 9 months of gestation. The affected placenta is thick, heavy, edematous, hemorrhagic, and occasionally covered with a brown mucoid material on the chorionic surface. Occasionally the affected placenta lacks detectable gross lesions. Green discoloration or cystic adenomatous hyperplasia of the allantois is observed in some cases. Fetal antibody against *Leptospira* spp. may be detected in foals by microagglutination test.[178] Spirochetes are present in large number in the placental sections. Several species of leptospire have been isolated from aborted equine fetuses (e.g., *L. pomona*, *L. grippotyphosa*, *L. interrogans* serovars *bratislava* and *pomona* type *kennewicki*, serovar *harjo* type *hardjoprajitno*).* High-titer agglutinating antibody (>1:6400) may be observed in mares, but interpretation of serologic tests remain difficult without confirmation of infection by culture and isolation. Antibiotic treatment for 5 days (penicillin G) has been reported to help prevent abortion during an outbreak.[198]

Nocardioform Placentitis

Nocardioform placentitis is a distinct type of equine placentitis first described in the United States in the late 1980s. Over the past 15 years an increasing number of cases of equine nocardioform placentitis have been diagnosed in Kentucky.[117,153,177,445]

Nocardioform actinomycetes induce a chronic placentitis that results in late-term abortion, stillbirth, or premature birth. The lesion is an extensive and severe exudative, mucopurulent, and necrotizing placentitis centered on the junction of the placental body and horns rather than the cervical pole.[178] Infection of the placenta is generally thought to be a sequela of the hematogenous spread of the microorganisms from a primary port of entry.[117,413] The fetus is often severely underdeveloped, with no remarkable gross or histologic lesions. The placental lesion is focally extensive (15-30 cm) and frequently located at the base of the uterine horns or at the junction between the body and horns of the placenta. The affected area is thickened, and its chorionic surface is covered with brown, necrotic, mucopurulent exudate and dotted with white or yellow granular structures. Underneath this mucoid material, the chorionic surface is reddish white, mottled, and roughened. Villous necrosis and adenomatous hyperplasia of the allantoic epithelium and hyperplasia with or without squamous metaplasia of the chorionic epithelium are frequently observed.[78,178]

Various groups of gram-positive, filamentous, branching bacteria have been implicated as etiologic agents in mares with nocardioform placentitis, including *Nocardia* spp., *Rhodococcus rubropertinctus*, and *Amycolatopsis* spp.[49,124,177,413] However, most severe infections of this type are caused by the actinomycete *Crossiella equi*.[118]

A nocardioform isolate from equine placental lesions in the United States was determined by phylogenetic analysis to be closely related to *Crossiella cryophila*, a member of the genus *Crossiella* described in 2001.[217] Subsequent polyphasic identification found that the isolates represent a new species of *Crossiella*, for which the name *C. equi* was proposed.[118] Polyphasic taxonomic studies on actinomycete strains isolated from equine placentas from horses in Kentucky and southern United States indicate that the isolates are members of the genus *Amycolatopsis*. It is proposed that these strains be classified as three novel species of the genus *Amycolatopsis* and named *Amycolatopsis kentuckyensis*, *Amycolatopsis lexingtonensis*, and *Amycolatopsis pretoriensis*.[213]

During the 2002 and 2003 foaling seasons, *Cellulosimicrobium (Cellumonas) cellulans* (formerly *Oerskovia xanthineolytica*) was isolated from fetal tissues or placentas from cases of equine abortion, premature birth, and term pregnancies in Kentucky. Significant pathologic findings included chronic placentitis and pyogranulomatous pneumonia. In addition, microscopic and macroscopic alterations in the allantochorion from four of seven cases of placentitis were similar to those caused by *Crossiella equi* and other nocardioform bacteria.[48]

Pathogenesis and Diagnosis of Placentitis

Because of the importance of placentitis in the pathogenesis of bacterial abortion, researchers at the University of Florida developed models for study of ascendant placentitis to gain insight into the pathogenesis of disease and provide a method to optimize diagnostic and treatment recommendations.[225,226,244,262,368] Bacterial infection of the chorioallantois induces an increase in expression of proinflammatory cytokines (IL-6 and IL-8) in placental tissue. Subsequent release of PGE_2 and $PGF_{2\alpha}$ into the allantoic fluid leads to premature delivery.[223,226,262] The premature delivery of the fetus is most likely caused by acceleration of the fetal maturation process induced by changes in placental function. The resulting endocrine changes lead to increased uterine contractures and intrauterine pressure, causing dilation and induction of labor. A premature increase in maternal plasma progestins may be an indication of accelerated fetal maturation or fetal stress. Foals may survive if they are near term (>305 days).[225,286,287]

Clinically, placentitis is suspected in mares with premature udder development or lactation and vaginal discharge. However, most mares with placentitis do not show any outward signs of infection.[225,445]

*References 32, 114-116, 153, 177, 198, 309-311, 353, 354, 378, 411, 445.

Placentitis may be diagnosed by transrectal and transabdominal ultrasound examination.[66,402,445] Measurement of the combined thickness of the uterus and placenta (CTUP) by transrectal ultrasonography is particularly helpful in the diagnosis and monitoring of ascendant placentitis.[193,327-329,390,394,400] The measurements are obtained 2.5 to 5 cm cranial to the cervical-placental junction using a 5- or 7.5-mHz linear transducer. The area measured should be on the ventral aspect of the uterine body just above the middle branch of the uterine artery (Fig. 8-8). Normal CTUP for light horses is less than 8 mm between 271 and 300 days of gestation, less than 10 mm between 301 and 330 days of gestation, and less than 12 mm from 330 days of gestation to term.[26,193,327,328,394] These measurements are slightly higher in Warmblood and Draft horses and lower in ponies.[26,66,193] Placental malfunction has been associated with CTUP of greater than 15 mm in horses and greater than 12 mm in ponies after 310 days of gestation.[66,225]

During ultrasonographic evaluation, other features of infectious placentitis may be identified. These include placental separation and accumulation of purulent hyperechoic heterogenous fluid between the endometrium and the placenta and increased echogenicity of fetal fluid. Increased echogenicity of fetal fluid is caused by meconium, inflammatory debris, and hemorrhage.[225]

Endocrinologic evaluation may also help in determining placental pathology and risk for abortion. The most important hormones evaluated are progestins, which are relatively stable during a normal pregnancy. A change in serum progestin concentration (increase or decrease) by more than 50% or a value that is constantly out of reference laboratory range signals placental pathology or fetal stress.[225,288]

After abortion or premature birth, most cases of chronic placentitis are easily recognized on gross examination, but microscopic histologic examination is important to determine the presence of acute placentitis[359] (Fig. 8-9). In acute placentitis the infection may be contained within the placenta, and the fetus is usually sterile. Some foals may be born alive with neonatal septicemia.[359]

Treatment of Placentitis

The ultimate goal in treatment of equine placentitis is to maintain gestation for as long as possible to enhance foal viability.[244,445] Treatment recommendations include tocolytic drugs to reduce uterine contraction, antiinflammatory drugs to block the production of cytokines and prostaglandins, and antimicrobial therapy to control growth of bacteria.[225,244]

Antimicrobial therapy should be based on culture and sensitivity patterns of bacteria isolated from vaginal discharge or cervical swabs. Pharmacologic studies have shown that potentiated sulfonamides, gentamicin, potassium penicillin, and ceftiofur can cross the placenta and reach MICs sufficient to control *S. equi* subsp. *zooepidemicus* for penicillin G (22,000 IU/kg every 6 hours [q6h] IV) and *E. coli* or *K. pneumoniae* for gentamicin (6.6 mg/kg q24h IV).[43,44,47]

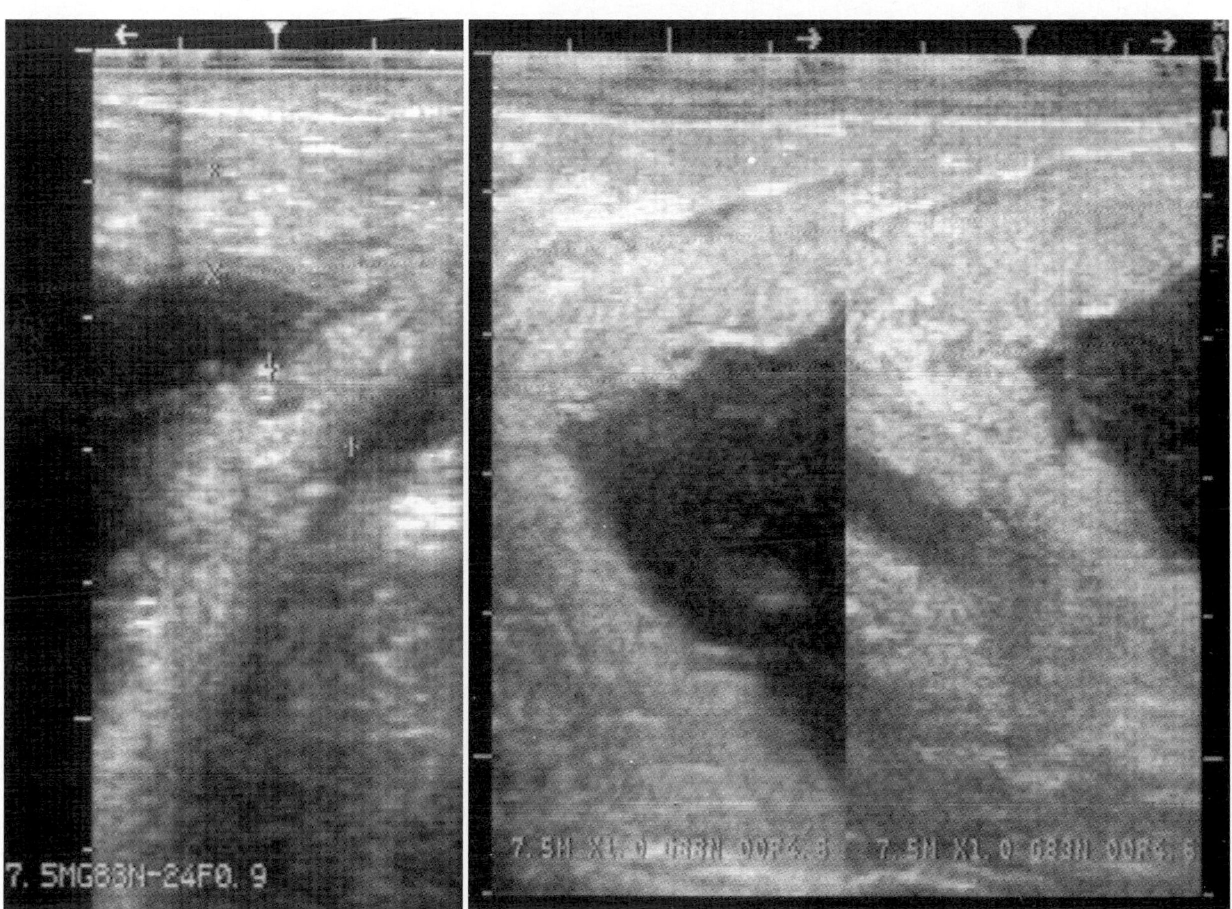

Fig. 8-8 Ultrasonogram showing area of measurement of combined uteroplacental thickness. **A,** Normal. **B,** Slightly thickened.

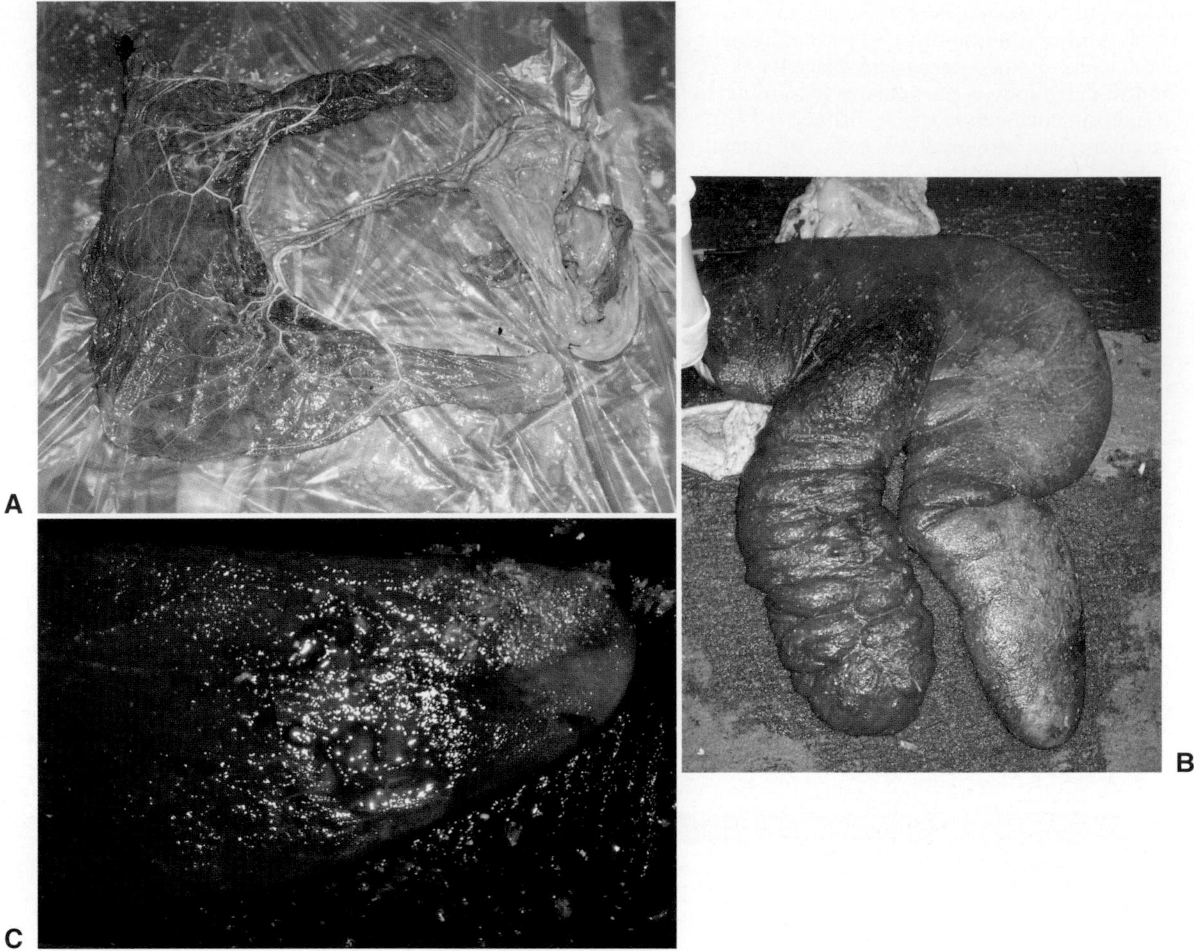

Fig. 8-9 Equine placenta. **A,** Normal allantochorionic membrane (fetal side). **B,** Normal allantochorion, uterine side (after distention with water). **C,** Necrotic changes in allantochorion caused by placentitis.

Trimethoprim-sulfamethoxazole (30 mg/kg q12h orally [PO]) presents an excellent choice for the treatment of placentitis caused by susceptible organisms because of its good uterine penetration.[225,344,352]

Antiinflammatory therapy is recommended for mares with placentitis to diminish the effects of proinflammatory cytokines and prostaglandins. The most frequently used medications are nonsteroidal antiinflammatory drugs (NSAIDs) such as flunixin meglumine (0.5-1.1 mg/kg twice daily PO or IV). Pentoxifylline has also been used to block the effects of endotoxin (8.5 mg/kg q12h), as discussed in Chapter 37.[223,225,244,275]

Induction of uterine quiescence is obtained by administration of progestins to interfere with upregulation of prostaglandin and oxytocin and reduce myometrial activity.[56] The oral synthetic progestin, altrenogest, is used at the label (0.044 mg/kg PO q12-24h) or two times the label (0.088 mg/kg PO q24h) dose.[445] Alternatively, progesterone in oil can be administered at 300 mg IM q24h.[225,244]

Diagnostic Approach for Equine Abortion

A precise diagnosis should be pursued in any case of abortion, premature birth, or birth of a compromised or septicemic foal. Diagnosis of the cause of abortion or in utero infection can be made in most cases with proper history, clinical observations, and collection and submission of all required samples. In one study, only 7.7% of equine abortions, stillbirths, or neonatal foal loss remained undiagnosed when the fetus, placenta, and serum from the dam were submitted.[359] The undiagnosed cases were associated with extensive damage to tissues by scavengers, as well as absence of placenta or early abortion. Samples from the dam should include serum and vaginal or uterine swab.

The importance of placental examination in the diagnosis of abortion, stillbirths, or premature births cannot be overemphasized. Normal and abnormal characteristics of the placenta and descriptions of proper examination of the equine placenta and its pathology have been described elsewhere.[285,346,428,429,437] Clients should be instructed to obtain the placenta for proper examination as soon as possible after each foaling. Weight of the placenta should be determined; normal placental weight is approximately 11% of the foal weight. The placenta is usually expelled inside out with the allantoic surface exposed (see Fig. 8-9). It should be gently cleaned of any bedding material, grass, or dirt with cold water, then laid out flat and all surfaces examined. The umbilical cord should be of normal length. The amniotic sac and chorionic surface (red velvety surface) is examined from the cervical star to the tips of the horns on all sides. Samples should be obtained from areas of grossly normal and abnormal placenta and submitted for histopathology, immunohistochemistry, and culture. Some morphologic characteristics of the placenta may allow immediate exclusion of infectious causes of abortion (e.g., umbilical cord torsion, body pregnancy, twin pregnancies). Chronic infectious inflammation is generally easy to detect because of the thick, leathery nature of the placenta. Lesions of placentitis appear tan or brown and thick and may have overlying tenacious, fibrinonecrotic exudate. Cytologic evaluation of a contact smear may reveal inflammatory cells and responsible organisms. Lesions of ascending placentitis are usually located on the cervical star, whereas diffuse hematogenous placentitis, as in leptospirosis, may cause diffuse lesions. Nocardioform placentitis has characteristic lesions on the cranial ventral uterine body.[382]

Although it is possible to perform fetal or neonatal necropsy in the field when necessary, it is preferred that the entire carcass be sent to a diagnostic laboratory if possible. If fetal necropsy is performed in the field, proper precautions should be taken to document lesions, prevent contamination, and obtain appropriate samples. Fetal blood samples as well as pleural and peritoneal fluids should be obtained. Tissue samples from any abnormal-appearing tissues and from all major organs (e.g. liver, lung, kidney, adrenal gland, placenta, heart, thymus, brain, spleen, small intestine) should be submitted for histopathologic evaluation.[382]

Viral Causes of Abortion

Equine Herpesvirus

Despite the widespread use of inactivated and live herpesvirus vaccines, equine herpesvirus (EHV) remains a common cause of equine abortion[9,123,296] (see Chapter 13). EHV-1 abortion storms continue to be reported in various areas of the world.* The principal mode of transmission from horse to horse is by direct contact with the virus through nasal secretions, reproductive tract discharge, placenta, or aborted fetuses. However, short-distance airborne spread of infection is possible.[9,154,155] Farm personnel, equipment, feed, and water may act as fomites to facilitate transmission.[9,296]

Some abortions are likely caused by reactivation of latent infection rather than primary exposure.[8,9] The most common cause of equine herpesvirus abortion is EHV-1, although EHV-4 has also been isolated from some equine abortion cases. Both viruses cause similar lesions in the liver and lung; evaluation of the spleen is particularly useful for identification of red pulp necrosis caused by EHV-4.[432] Regardless of which herpesvirus is involved, the pathogenesis of abortion is attributed to vascular necrosis.[9,46,50,361,363] Viral nucleic acid can be demonstrated in endothelial cells of endometrial arterioles, within endometrial glands, and within placental microcotyledonary infarctions.[296,360] Transplacental transfer of the virus may result in a virus-positive fetus, or severe endometrial vascular pathology (vasculitis and multifocal thrombosis) may result in abortion of a virus-negative fetus.[296,362] Abortion occurs most often during the last third of pregnancy. In utero infection near term may result in the birth of a live infected foal that usually dies a few days later.[296]

For confirmation of herpesvirus abortion, antigen detection in combination with virus isolation, immunochemistry, or polymerase chain reaction (PCR) on fetal lung, liver, spleen, and thymus is recommended. Virologic and serologic investigation of the mare is also recommended.[10,216,347]

*References 27, 165, 267, 296, 382, 408.

It is important to realize that EHV-1 abortion may occur despite regular vaccination. Causative factors include the mare's individual immunity, level of contamination, virulence of the viral strain, and the performance of available vaccine.[9,212] Therefore, for maximum protection, vaccination strategies should be combined with appropriate biosecurity measures to minimize the likelihood of exposure of pregnant mares to EHV.[9,135]

Vaccines for the control of respiratory diseases caused by EHV-1 have been available for several decades, and currently more than a dozen commercial vaccines are available throughout the world.[295,296] There are also several vaccines that claim protection against abortion caused by EHV-1. These vaccines should be administered according to the manufacturer's label instructions, usually at 5, 7, and 9 months of gestation.

Management practices that should be part of an EHV abortion prevention program include maintenance of small groups of horses segregated by age and by immune and physiologic status (pregnancy status and stage). Foaling mares should be segregated from the rest of the herd. Particular attention should be given to the risk of mixing equids from different species that may carry different susceptibility or strains of EHV.[9] The most important epidemiologic risk is posed by introduction of new horses onto the farm. If introduction of new animals cannot be avoided, a 21-day quarantine is recommended.

An outbreak of EHV mandates early diagnosis of infected animals and interruption of viral transmission using strict sanitary measures for movement of personnel and animals between stables and paddocks, as well as use of disinfectants. Particular attention should be given to disposal of or shipping of fetuses and placenta to appropriate diagnostic laboratories. Mating activities should preferably be halted during an active outbreak.[9]

Equine Viral Arteritis

Equine viral arteritis (EVA) is a venereal disease of horses that can result in abortion (see Chapter 14). Abortion storms have been reported as part of the clinical presentation of the disease.* Abortion rates can approach 60% in a naive population[387] as the result of direct impairment of placental function and severe fetal infection.[90,126,158] Diagnosis can be made by viral isolation, immunohistochemistry, PCR, or serology.[156,180,379] Aborted fetuses may show subcutaneous edema, petechial hemorrhages in the pleura and epicardium, and increases in pleural fluid. However, these changes are not necessarily present in all EVA abortion. Gross pathologic changes have also been reported in a few affected placentas, including placentitis and full-thickness necrosis. Other nonpathognomonic histopathologic lesions in the fetus may include vasculitis and perivasculitis in the heart, lung, and spleen; pneumonia and hemorrhage in alveoli; and inflammatory changes in the liver, spleen, and placenta. Control of the disease is based on vaccination.

Parasitic Causes of Abortion

Abortion in mares has been associated with a variety of protozoa, including *Trypanosoma evansi*,[357] *Trypanosoma equiperdum*,[86] *Babesia* spp.,[95,230,382] and *Neospora* spp.[302] However, there are no studies on the pathogenesis of abortion caused by these parasites.

Neospora caninum, an apicomplexan protozoan parasite, has been isolated from an aborted equine fetus in North Carolina[122] and in one fetus from Normandy in France.[317] However, great discrepancies exist between the prevalence of

*References 90, 92, 105, 125, 188, 283, 380, 387.

Neospora-positive horses, estimated at between 2% and 23% depending on location, and infected fetuses. Serologic surveys show 11.5% (n = 536) *Neospora*-positive horses in Alabama,[81] 23% (n = 296) in slaughtered North American horses,[122] 23% (n = 434) in France,[302] and 2% (n = 208) in horses from several locations in the United States.[409] Although not statistically significant, a higher prevalence of antibodies against *N. caninum* has been reported in mares with a history of reproductive failure than in mares with normal fertility.[258] Seroprevalence of antibodies to *Neospora* spp. is significantly higher in recently aborting mares in France compared with mares with no history of recent abortion. *N. caninum* deoxyribonucleic acid (DNA) was detected in three fetal brains, two fetal hearts, and one placenta.[302] The identification of *N. caninum* sequences in fetal tissues is interesting, but the role of *N. caninum* in equine reproductive failure and abortion can only be speculative at present and must be further evaluated.[301,302]

Other Infections Causing Abortion

Chlamydia

Genital chlamydiosis of horses is reported to result in mild chronic salpingitis,[263] decreased reproductive rates,[173,441] poor ejaculate quality,[412] and occasional abortion.[42,157,170,229]

Detection of chlamydial organisms in aborted equine fetuses ranges from 20% to 55%.[43,108,229] However, other infectious organisms were isolated from many of the same cases, and it was not possible to determine the primary cause of abortion. Chlamydial organisms that have been isolated from horses include *Chlamydophila pneumoniae*, equine biovar, associated with respiratory diseases, and *C. abortus* and *C. psittaci*, identified in equine abortion cases.[170]

In Hungary, chlamydiae were detected by immunohistochemistry and PCR in 83% of equine abortions, but they were not determined to be the primary cause of abortion.[380] The significance of chlamydial infection in equine abortion is contested by others. No chlamydial inclusions were found in a retrospective study of tissues from 142 aborted foals in Switzerland examined by immunohistochemistry. The same authors were unable to detect any *Chlamydia* organism (culture and PCR) from 49 aborted foals in northern Germany.[137]

Mycoplasma

The significance of acholeplasmas and mycoplasmas in equine abortion is undetermined. *Mycoplasma* has been isolated from the lung or liver of aborted equine fetuses.[166] Of 404 mares, mycoplasmas were cultured from the cervix of 5.2%.[200,202] *Mycoplasma bovigenitalium* was isolated from an aborted equine fetus.[214] Mycoplasmas were isolated from the placenta and stomach contents of an equine fetus aborted 35 days prematurely. The only gross pathologic lesions observed were darkening of the dorsal apical lobes of the lungs and a few necrotic patches 15 to 25 cm in diameter in the placenta.[273]

Other Infectious Organisms

Abortions have been associated with *Salmonella abortus equi* in horses* and donkeys,[176,245] *Shigella* spp.,[145] *Brucella abortus*,[97,313,338] and *Brucella suis*.[94] *Neorickettsia risticii* has also been identified as a cause of abortion in horses[102,103,238-240] (see Chapter 43). Abortion from *Aeromonas hydrophila*, a bacterium found in stagnant water, has been reported in a few horses.[136]

An unusual case of abortion in a 6-year-old mare has been associated with a spirochete *(Borrelia parkei–B. turicatae)* transmitted by ticks in California.[415] The 9-month-pregnant mare presented with a history of yellow vaginal discharge and did not respond to antimicrobial or antiinflammatory treatment. The spirochete was isolated from the fetus, suggesting transplacental transmission.

During the *mare reproductive loss syndrome* (MRLS) outbreak in Kentucky in 2000 and 2001, significant bacterial growth (*Actinobacillus* spp., α-streptococci) was a common feature in tissues of aborted fetuses.[69] This led some authors to hypothesize that the pathogenesis of MRLS implicated hematogenous spread to the fetoplacental unit of bacteria carried from the oral cavity and intestinal tract by the setae, or stiff bristlelike barbed hairs, of the exoskeleton of the Eastern tent caterpillar.[388]

*References 5, 134, 145, 176, 210, 404, 445.

REPRODUCTIVE TRACT INFECTION IN STALLIONS

Infectious Disease of Prepuce and Penis

Acute inflammation of the prepuce *(posthitis)* and inflammation of the penis *(balanitis)* may occur secondary to several infectious diseases. Balanoposthitis is most often caused by coital exanthema (EHV-3 infection), dourine, or parasitic infestation (e.g., *Onchocerca* spp., *Setaria* spp., habronemiasis).[383]

Preputial abscesses may occur subsequent to bacteremia (*Streptococcus equi* subsp. *equi* or *Corynebacterium pseudotuberculosis*). In some areas of the world, *C. pseudotuberculosis* abscesses may have a seasonal incidence that parallels the increase in arthropod (vector) population[64,208] (see Chapter 30). Factors such as a high concentration of horses and *Habronema* spp. infestation are predisposing factors for these abscesses.[268,325,383] Treatment is generally limited to medical or surgical management of the abscess because systemic antimicrobial therapy is often unsuccessful.[208]

Several infectious diseases may cause lesions on the penis, including dourine, coital exanthema, EVA, and equine infectious anemia. Nonspecific balanitis is generally caused by superinfection with bacteria or fungus.[383] Predisposing factors include increased accumulation of smegma or overzealous cleaning of the penis with disinfection. Excessive use of antiseptic solution may promote the destruction of the normal flora of the penile mucosa and the selection of some bacteria (e.g., *P. aeruginosa, K. pneumoniae*).[52] Treatment of nonspecific balanitis requires sexual rest and local application of antimicrobial ointment.

Coital exanthema (EHV-3) and dourine (see Chapter 61) are specific infectious processes that involve the penis and are discussed in the section on venereal diseases.

Cutaneous habronemiasis (summer sores) is characterized by granulomatous lesions caused by larvae of *Draschia megastoma, Habronema muscae*, and *Habronema microstoma*[98,383] (see Chapter 62). Habronemiasis is generally seasonal and parallels the fly population. These infections are often found in areas with high heat and humidity and in areas with high density of animals and poor sanitation. Occurrence of this diseases has declined with regular use of avermectin anthelmintics.[132,383] The larvae of gastrophils are carried by infested flies to the genital area and cause an inflammatory process with rapid development of a granulomatous lesion[98,348,427] (Fig. 8-10).

Diagnosis of habronemiasis is based on the location and characteristics of the lesions as well as the presence of predisposing factors (e.g. season, lack of sanitation). Lesions are generally observed at the level of the glans penis or urethral process. Yellow caseous masses composed primarily of eosinophils and larvae are present within the lesions. These lesions should be differentiated from sarcoids or squamous cell carcinoma.[270,271,276,383]

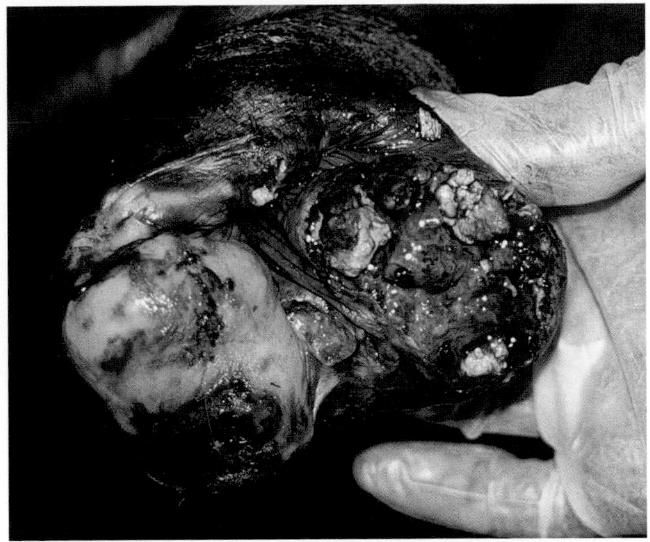

Fig. 8-10 Stallion penis with habronemiasis lesions.

Confirmation of the diagnosis is easily made with histopathologic evaluation of a biopsy of the lesion or by contact smears. Wright-stained smears may allow visualization of the larvae.[270,271,276] Slices of larvae may be seen surrounded by masses of eosinophils on histopathologic evaluation. Squamous cell carcinoma lesions may be complicated by larvae infestation because these lesions tend to attract flies.[270,271,276,383]

Treatment of habronemiasis consists of killing parasites, reducing the degree of inflammation, and treating the secondary bacterial infection. The drugs most often used for elimination of larvae are diethylcarbamazine, organophosphates, and ivermectin. Local and systemic treatment with an organophosphate compound has been advocated in the past but is controversial because of its toxicity.[348,349,427] Ivermectins (ivermectin, 0.2 mg/kg) remain the best choice for local and systemic treatment. The majority of larvae are killed within 1 week, and improvement of the lesions is generally observed within 1 to 5 weeks after treatment.[98,171,172] Treatment with a single oral dose of ivermectin (120 mg for a 570-kg horse) has been reported; about 15% to 20% of horses require a second treatment.[56] Old extensive lesions may require up to three treatments at 10-day intervals.[12] Chronic severe lesions may require surgical ablation.[132,269,370,383]

The inflammatory process may be reduced by treatment with diethylcarbamazine or corticosteroids. Ointment containing 30 mg of dexamethasone and 120 mg of nitrofurazone has been used to diminish the inflammatory reaction caused by dead larvae after ivermectin treatment. Prevention of habronemiasis should include protection of genital lesions with insect repellant,[53] regular cleaning of the external genitals, and regular use of ivermectins, especially during the peak of fly season.[383]

Infections of Testes and Epididymis

Orchitis

Orchitis may be caused by bacteria, viruses, or parasites. Bacterial orchitis and periorchitis are relatively rare in stallions.[29] Infection may be ascendant, secondary to trauma, or hematogenous.[29,54,383] Hematogenous infection with *S. equi* subsp. *zooepidermicus*, *S. equi* subsp. *equi*, *Actinobacillus equuli*, *Pseudomonas mallei*, *Salmonella abortus equi*, *Brucella abortus*, and *C. pseudotuberculosis* may occur.[29,54,383] Hematogenous infection with *Actinobacillus equuli* has been described in a 2-month-old colt presenting with acute abdominal pain, leukocytosis, and mature neutrophilia.[29] Infections caused by *Streptococcus* spp., *Staphylococcus* spp., and *E. coli* occur secondary to peritonitis.

Systemic clinical signs may include fever, abdominal pain, and poor libido. Local signs may include increased scrotal size, scrotal edema, and increased sensitivity of the scrotal area. Scrotal/testicular ultrasonography may identify areas of liquefaction of the testicular parenchyma or development of granulomatous lesions[314,383] (Fig. 8-11). Horses with chronic

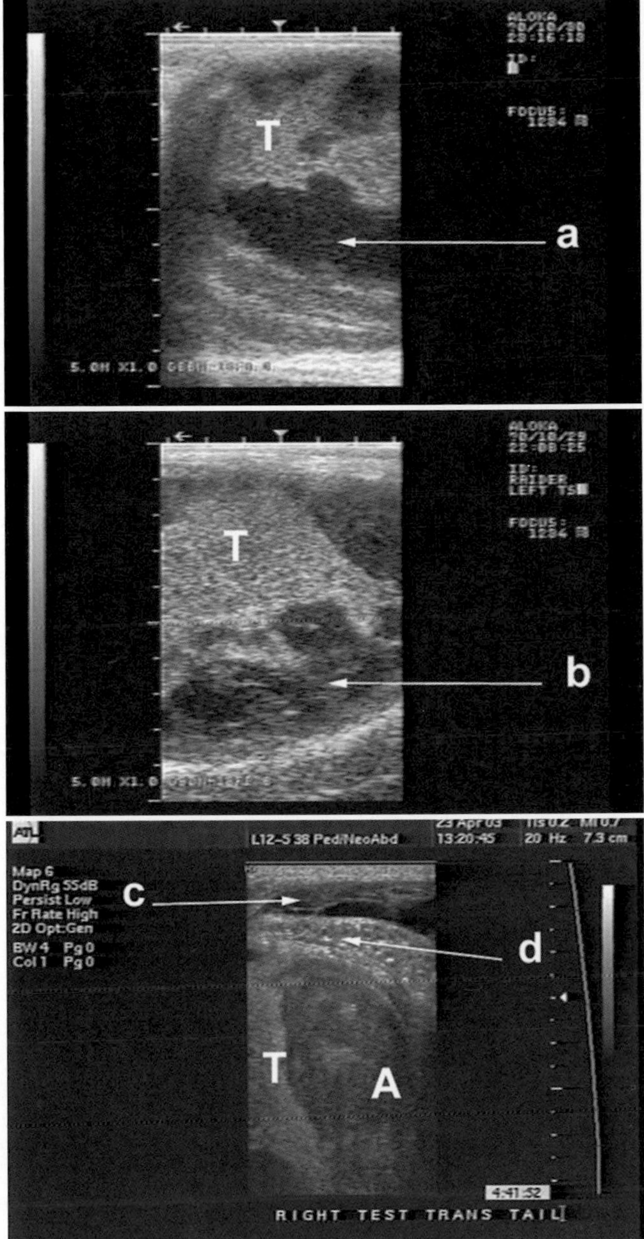

Fig. 8-11 Ultrasonogram of testicle of stallion with orchitis caused by *Corynebacterium pseudotuberculosis* infection. *T*, Testicular tissue; *a* and *b*, abscessed areas; *c*, thickened scrotum with fibrin; *d*, periorchitis; *A*, abscess in testicle.

orchitis may have adhesions between the tunica vaginalis and subcutaneous tissue, azoospermia, high numbers of neutrophils in the ejaculate, a high percentage of sperm abnormalities, and poor motility.[36,54,383]

Differential diagnosis should include all other causes of increased scrotal size, including inguinal hernia,[29] hematocoele,[38,161] hydrocoele,[383,384] testicular cord torsion,[191] spermatic artery thrombosis,[179,181] and testicular neoplasia.[77,383] Neutrophilia, fever, and hyperfibrogenemia without cardiovascular signs suggest orchitis rather that inguinal hernia with intestinal incarceration.[29]

Treatment of bacterial orchitis may be attempted with systemic antibiotics and NSAIDs, as well as local hydrotherapy, but is generally unrewarding. Unilateral infections are usually best managed by hemicastration. When bacterial orchitis responds to antimicrobial treatment, the affected testicle will progressively atrophy and become fibrotic.

Viral orchitis has been reported in some horses with equine infectious anemia, EVA, and influenza.[105,383] Orchitis has also been described in horses with granulocytic erhlichiosis.[159]

Parasitic orchitis may be caused by migratory larvae (larva migrans) of *Strongylus edentatus*.[45,259,260,277,358]

Epididymitis

Infections of the epididymis are rare in stallions and are generally accompanied by orchitis. Therefore the same bacteria and parasites associated with orchitis are associated with epididymitis in the stallion.* *Pseudomonas aeruginosa* is the most common isolate from bacterial epididymitis in stallions.[351]

Acute epididymitis is very painful and often accompanied by local swelling and fever. Colic signs may be present even in horses with chronic epididymitis. Periorchitis and peritesticular adhesions and sperm granulomas may develop following rupture of the epididymis. Systemic signs and palpable changes are often suggestive of the diagnosis. Azoospermia is possible. Ejaculates may show oligospermia, hypoasthenia, and increased numbers of decapitate sperm cells with increased numbers of neutrophils in the ejaculate.† Prognosis for fertility is poor in horses with bilateral epididymitis.

Infections of Accessory Glands

Infections of the stallion accessory sex glands are relatively rare.[37,410] *Seminal vesiculitis* is most common.[39,146,147,182,364] Bacterial isolates from stallions with seminal vesiculitis include *P. aeruginosa*, *K. pneumoniae*, *Streptococcus* spp., *Staphylococcus* spp., *Proteus vulgaris*, *Acinetobacter calcoaceticus*, and *Brucella abortus*.‡ Both ascendant routes, from the urinary system, and hematogenous routes of infection are possible. Seminal vesiculitis may be associated with infection of the ampullae of the ductus deferens (ampulitis).[39]

Clinical signs of seminal vesiculitis are variable. Chronic infection may occur without any systemic signs. Acute infection is characterized by pain during ejaculation or transrectal palpation. Seminal vesiculitis may be suspected in stallions with hemospermia or infertility.§ The ejaculate may appear brown or reddish in color and contain a high number of red blood cells and neutrophils.[39,41,141,364]

Diagnosis of seminal vesiculitis requires evaluation of the gland by transrectal ultrasonography and urethroscopy.[314,315,383] The inflamed seminal vesicle increases in size and becomes very soft and easily palpable. In some cases the gland may show

*References 168, 169, 207, 241, 389, 405.
†References 168, 169, 206, 351, 389, 405.
‡References 39, 40, 146, 162, 182, 184, 189, 205, 251, 364.
§References 39, 141, 251, 364, 383, 410.

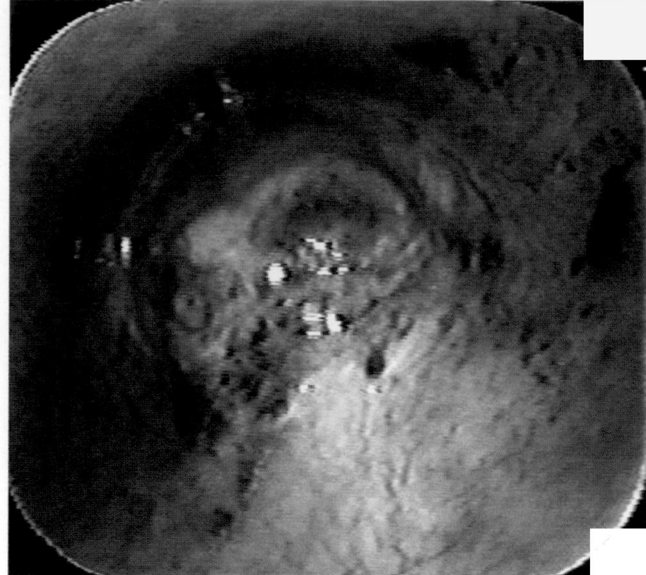

Fig. 8-12 Videoendoscopic view of inflamed colliculus seminalis.

lobulation and irregular contour.[141,251,253,410] On ultrasonography, the gland is two to three times the normal size, and its content is densely hyperechoic (normally anechoic).[251,253] Endoscopic examination of the colliculus seminalis may reveal localized inflammation[41,141,383,414] (Fig. 8-12). Chronic seminal vesiculitis may not show any changes on endoscopic examination.[39] The examination of the gland itself is possible with a small-diameter endoscope (Fig. 8-13). Culture and cytology of fluid obtained directly from the gland by endoscopic aspiration of the ejaculatory duct allow confirmation of the diagnosis.[383,410] Microbiologic evaluation may also be performed on samples obtained from preejaculate and postejaculate urethral swabs or sperm.[41]

Treatment of seminal vesiculitis is very difficult because the majority of antimicrobials cannot reach the gland in sufficient concentration.[39,41,141] Broad-spectrum antimicrobials with a high volume of distribution, such as trimethoprim-sulfonamide combinations, may be used systemically.[141] Enrofloxacin reportedly reaches adequate concentration in the seminal vesicles after parenteral administration.[41] Direct flushing and local infusion of antimicrobial drugs into the glands are the preferred method of treatment.[146,383] Local lavage with amikacin and oral treatment with trimethoprim-sulfonamide for 8 days have been successful for the treatment in a stallion with seminal vesiculitis from *Proteus vulgaris*.[146]

The use of minimum-contamination breeding technique may be indicated in difficult cases of seminal vesiculitis.[40,195] Infusion of an extender containing a specific antimicrobial into the uterus of a mare before breeding, combined with postbreeding uterine lavage, helps prolong the survival of semen and control bacterial growth.[39-41,57,59,60,221] If artificial insemination is an option, collection of the sperm-rich fraction and dilution with an extender containing the proper antimicrobial are indicated.

A radical treatment of seminal vesiculitis consisting of surgical excision of the affected glands has been described. However, such surgical technique is complicated and often leads to ejaculatory disorders.[205]

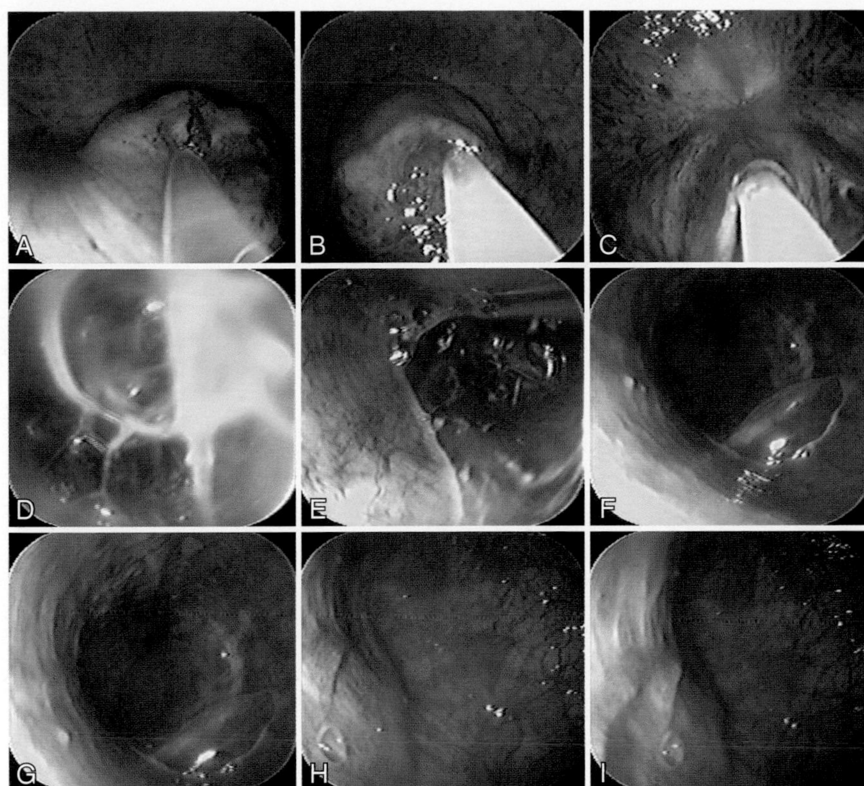

Fig. 8-13 Videoendoscopic catheterization of seminal vesicle (A, B, and C), seminal vesiculitis, and seminal vesicle before (D, E, and F) and after (G, H, and I) flushing.

EQUINE VENEREAL DISEASES

The most common equine venereal diseases are CEM (see Chapter 41), coital exanthema (see Chapter 13), EVA (see Chapter 14), and dourine (see Chapter 61). Some bacteria responsible for endometritis in the mares, such as *P. aeruginosa* and *K. pneumoniae,* are also considered venereal. Some of these diseases are subject to strict regulatory guidelines in several countries, and the veterinarian should be aware of the proper procedure for reporting positive or suspect cases.

Venereal Transmission of *P. aeruginosa* and *K. pneumoniae*

Pseudomonas aeruginosa and *Klebsiella pneumoniae* endometritis can be spread between horses by venereal transmission.* Bacteriologic studies should be routinely performed on recently introduced mares and stallions to prevent such infection. Culture is also indicated if there is an increased incidence of endometritis on a stud farm.[51,52,67,68,312] Preejaculation and postejaculation urethral swabs and semen from stallions should be cultured.[410]

Routine washing of the stallion penis with antiseptic solution before and after breeding is contraindicated because it may disturb the normal bacterial flora of the penile surface and promote growth of pathogenic bacteria such as *P. aeruginosa* and *K. pneumoniae*.[52,185,190] Washing the penis with sodium hypochlorite solution (5.25%) or dilute hydrogen chloride (HCl, 0.2%) has been suggested for the treatment of stallions with a positive culture of *P. aeruginosa* or *K. pneumoniae*.[51,197,206,340]

*References 19, 40, 87, 88, 160, 206, 265, 289, 307, 426.

Coital Exanthema

Coital exanthema is a very contagious, self-limiting venereal disease caused by equine herpesvirus type 3 (EHV-3). It is characterized by the development of painful pustular lesions on the external genitalia of stallion and mares.[151,403] The direct effect of this disease on fertility remains a subject of debate. The disease is transmitted by coitus, infected artificial insemination equipment, or gynecologic instruments.[187,274,293,294,324] In one study in Austria, 27% of Noriker stallions were seropositive.[20]

The stallion plays an important role in the epidemiology of coital exanthema. Clinical signs develop within a week of infection and consist of multiple circular red nodules on the vulva, vaginal mucosa, clitoral sinus, and perineum in mares and on the surface of the penis in the stallion. The lesions increase in size to 10- to 15-mm circular vesicles, which eventually rupture and become coalescent ulcers (Fig. 8-14). The ulcerative lesions are very painful.[350]

Prevention of coital exanthema requires examination of mares before breeding or use of artificial insemination. Clinical signs are easily recognized in both stallions and mares. Confirmation of the diagnosis is made by virus isolation from the lesions or histopathologic examination looking for characteristic inclusion bodies.[293,294] A highly sensitive and specific PCR test for the detection of virus has been recently described.[204,350]

Dourine

Dourine is defined by the Office International des Epizooties (OIE) as a "chronic or acute contagious disease of breeding solipeds that is directly transmitted from animal to animal during coitus." Dourine is probably the oldest equine venereal disease known. It is caused by the only trypanosome that is not transmitted by an invertebrate vector, *Trypanosoma equiperdum*

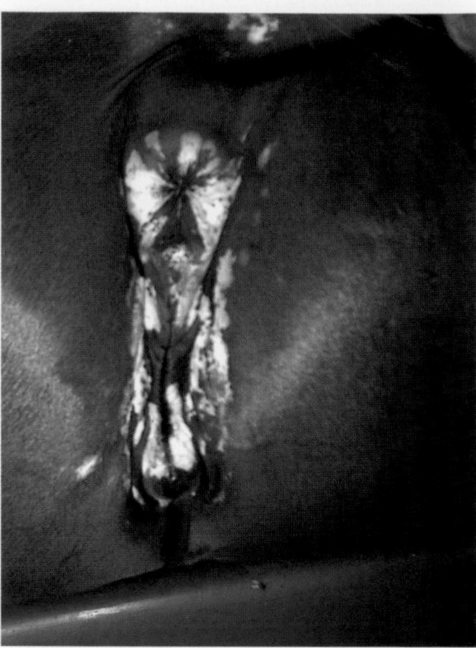

Fig. 8-14 Perineal area of mare showing old lesions of equine herpesvirus type 3 (EHV-3) infection (coital exanthema)

(see Chapter 61). It affects primarily horses and to a lesser degree donkeys.[342] Dourine had a global distribution during World War I but has been eradicated from North America and most of Europe. It is still reported in Africa (Botswana, Ethiopia, Namibia, South Africa) and Asia (Kyrgyzstan, Mongolia, Pakistan, Russia, Turkmenistan, Uzbekistan), with suspected cases reported in Germany and the Middle East.[84-86,211]

Horses with dourine typically present in one of three clinical phases. Initially, infected horses exhibit edema and fluid accumulation in the genital area starting about 2 weeks after infection. This is followed by development of the characteristic cutaneous lesions from which the disease derives its name, "dourine." The lesions are circular elevated plaques of thickened skin ranging from 1 cm to 10 cm in diameter and resembling money, or "douros." These plaques are observed mostly on the neck, hip, and ventral abdomen. Progressive nervous system compromise leads to paralysis of the hindlimbs, paraplegia, and death.

Clinical signs are highly suggestive of the disease. Dourine can be confirmed by a wide variety of laboratory tests. Complement fixation test (CFT) developed in the early twentieth century remains the internationally recommended test.[417] However, recent studies have shown that this test cannot distinguish among *T. equiperdum*, *T. evansi*, and *T. brucei*.[65,84,85,339] These cross-reactions are important from an epidemiologic point of view because some clinical signs of infection with *T. evansi* may resemble those of dourine.[84,85,150,443]

CONCLUSION: BIOSECURITY IN BREEDING OPERATIONS

Biosecurity on horse farms and in veterinary hospitals is essential to prevent introduction and spread of infectious diseases. The general approach to biosecurity and disease outbreak control is covered in depth in Chapters 66 and 67.

General principles of biosecurity for breeding farms include strict separation of transient and resident horse populations, routine quarantine of all new arrivals on the farm, and segregation of horses according to age and breeding status. Animals returning from events where commingling has occurred (e.g., breeding farms, shows) should be placed in quarantine for a minimum of 3 weeks. Prebreeding uterine culture and cytology should be required for all visiting mares, particularly those that have remained barren in the previous season. Stallions should undergo complete semen evaluation and microbiologic examination of preejaculation and postejaculation urethral swabs as well as semen. Vaccination status and previous exposure to specific disease agents should be determined.

Breeding hygiene should be strictly observed to avoid transmission of contaminants to mares. The surface of the penis can harbor several organisms that may be potentially pathogenic.[21,247,252] If artificial insemination is used, particular attention should be paid to the origin of the semen and the health certificate of stallions at collection.[68,87,231] Antibiotic-containing extenders do not eliminate risk of transmission of organisms. Quality control of semen processing, particularly shipped cooled semen, is often lacking. Health importation requirements for frozen semen should be verified for each country of origin and strictly adhered to.[266] The stallion status with regard to EVA and CEM is of particular importance. Guidelines are available for use of stallions that shed EVA virus[256] (see Chapter 14). The risk of transmission of infectious diseases by embryo transfer in horses has not been thoroughly evaluated.[264] Proper screening of the stallion, donor mares, and recipients is therefore very important. Advanced reproductive technologies, such as intracytoplasmic sperm injection (ICSI), cloning, gamete intrafallopian transfer (GIFT), and in vitro fertilization, are becoming accepted in the equine breeding industry and need to be evaluated for risk of disease transmission.

On large stud farms, foaling mares should be grouped by gestational stage. They should be monitored daily for rapid mammary development, premature lactation, or abnormal vaginal discharge. High-risk pregnancy mares should be monitored regularly by transrectal and transabdominal ultrasonography. Paddocks should be checked regularly for abortion.

A contingency plan should be elaborated for action to take in case of abortion. This plan should include proper handling (prompt submission to laboratory) of biologic tissues (placenta and abortus) and measures to isolate the aborting mare from the rest of the herd. On large farms, personnel working with pregnant and parturient mares should have no contact with other horses.

The foaling team should be educated in recognizing abnormal peripartum situations requiring urgent veterinary attention. Hygiene should be emphasized for all personnel attending or assisting in foaling.

On an individual mare level, prevention of reproductive loss from infectious diseases should focus on early diagnosis of sporadic infections that may cause permanent damage to the reproductive tract. Mares that are known to be susceptible to endometritis should be bred using minimum-contamination breeding and monitored for PMIE and treated appropriately. Corrective surgery should be performed on all mares with abnormal perineal conformation.

The potential for disease transmission by visitors should not be underestimated. Visitor contact with animals should be limited or discouraged, particularly for high-risk animals (pregnant mares and stallions). Access to a herd by the general public should be disallowed.

Prevention of introduction of diseases into the herd should also take into account other vector animals (insects, birds, and rodents) as well as proximity to other species (e.g., donkeys, wildlife). Pest control may be difficult but should not be overlooked. Regular cleaning and disinfection of the barns and common areas are critical to eliminating disease agents that contaminate housing, feeding, and equipment to minimize spread of disease by human and other fomites.

REFERENCES

See the CD-ROM for a list of references linked to the abstract in PubMed.

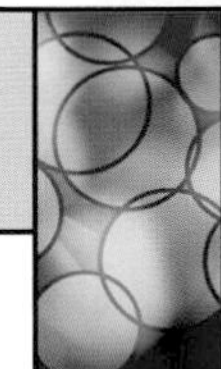

CHAPTER • 9

Urinary Tract Infections

Dana N. Zimmel

ETIOLOGY

Urinary tract infection (UTI) is caused by microbial colonization of the kidney, ureter, urine, or proximal urethra. The incidence of UTIs in the horse is low.[1-5] UTIs can be divided anatomically into *upper UTI*, involving the kidney and ureters, and *lower UTI*, involving the bladder and urethra. Ascending infections are the most common method of bacterial colonization, with the exception of septicemia-associated nephritis in neonatal foals.[6] Upper UTIs occur less frequently and can occasionally be life threatening.[4] Lower UTI is generally caused by abnormal urine flow. Urolithiasis and partial obstruction are often the cause of both upper and lower UTI in horses.

The most frequently reported bacteria in UTI include *Escherichia coli*, *Proteus*, *Klebsiella*, *Enterobacter*, and *Pseudomonas aeruginosa*.[7] Gram-positive infections in horses are less common, but *Staphylococcus* and *Corynebacterium* spp. have been isolated.[8] *Enterococcus* spp. have been identified in horses with abnormal urine flow or horses that were instrumented with a urinary catheter. Isolation of more than one organism from the urine is common. Neonatal foals receiving broad-spectrum antimicrobials can develop *Candida* infections in the lower urinary tract.[4]

The most frequent causes of UTI in the horse are bladder paralysis (Fig. 9-1), urolithiasis (Fig. 9-2), and trauma to the urethra.[4] Urethritis can result from urethral damage in geldings and stallions secondary to neoplasia, habronemiasis, or trauma to the penis or sheath.[9,10] Any alteration or obstruction to urine flow can predispose to infection. Mares are more likely to develop UTI than male horses because of their shorter urethra and the potential for fecal contamination from poor perineal conformation. In addition, mares may sustain damage to the urethra from trauma associated with foaling.

Cystitis may occur secondary to bladder paralysis, bladder neoplasia, or urolithiasis. Neurologic disease, such as equine protozoal myeloencephalitis or equine herpesvirus type 1 (EHV-1), and trauma can result in bladder paralysis. Consumption of Sudan grass and Johnson grass has resulted in ataxia and urinary incontinence in the southwestern United States from sublethal intoxication with hydrocyanic acid in the plants.[7,11,12] Conditions that inhibit bladder emptying at regular intervals encourage the growth of bacteria. Urolithiasis in the bladder can damage the mucosa lining, destroying normal defense mechanisms against microbial colonization. Obstruction of the renal pelvis, ureter, or urethra with urinary calculi may result in UTI. Unlike small animal patients, horses rarely develop UTI secondary to urinary catheterization, with the exception of sick neonatal foals.[12,13]

Pyelonephritis is rare in horses[2-4] (Fig. 9-3). The ureters attach dorsally on the bladder, providing a physical barrier to vesicoureteral reflux, which is responsible for ascending infection. Problems that disrupt this normal barrier include ectopic ureter, enlargement of the bladder from paralysis, or obstruction of urine flow from urolithiasis.[12]

PATHOGENESIS

UTIs are the result of pathogenic bacteria colonizing the urethra and then migrating to the bladder, where they multiply.[12,14] Fecal bacteria can adhere to the uroepithelial cells of the urethra when normal flora is altered by turbulent urine flow.[15]

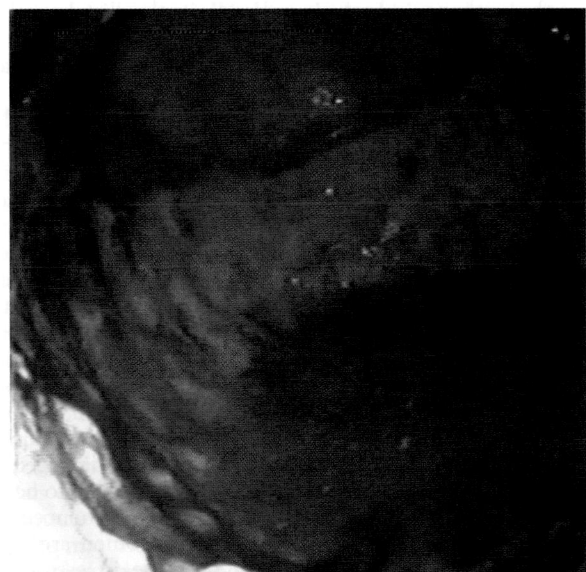

Fig. 9-1 Endoscopic image of urinary bladder of 8-year-old Quarter Horse mare with bladder paralysis and recurrent bacterial cystitis secondary to administration of alcohol tail block.

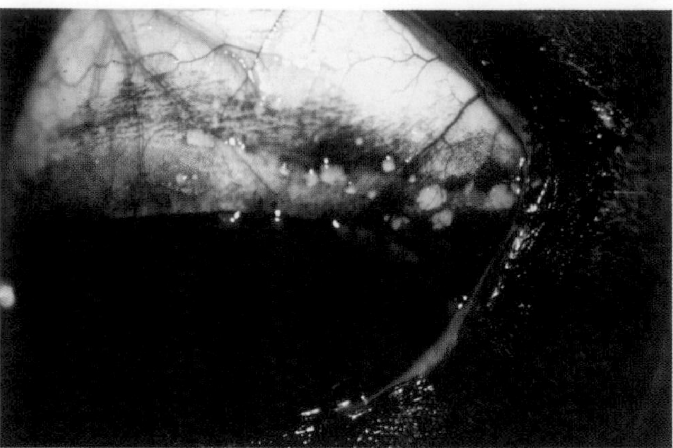

Fig. 10-3 Equine eye with numerous lymphoid follicles in perilimbal region appearing as tiny vesicles. (Courtesy Dr. Michael Davidson.)

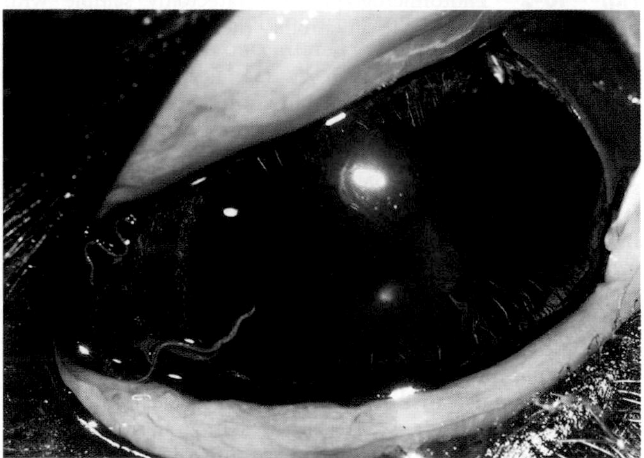

Fig. 10-4 Equine eye with two *Thelazia* larvae on corneal surface. (Courtesy Dr. Michael Davidson.)

Several bacterial species have been identified as primary etiologic agents of conjunctivitis in horses. *Streptococcus equi* subsp. *equi* is associated with regional lymphadenitis (i.e., strangles), mucopurulent nasal discharge, and conjunctivitis[32] (see Chapter 28). *Moraxella equi*[24] and *Chlamydia* and *Mycoplasma* spp.[33] have also been identified as causes of primary conjunctivitis in horses. *Histoplasma farciminosus* (epizootic lymphangitis) may result in ulcerative conjunctivitis.[26] *Aspergillus* spp. and *Rhinosporidium seeberi* can cause granulomatous conjunctivitis,[25,26] and blastomycosis has been associated with nasolacrimal disease.[26] Equine herpesvirus types 1 and 2 (EHV-1, EHV-2) can cause recurrent conjunctivitis with or without corneal ulceration[34-37] (see Chapter 13). Adenoviral infection may result in conjunctivitis with mucopurulent ocular and nasal discharge, keratouveitis, and systemic disease[26,38] (see Chapter 16). Equine viral arteritis may cause blepharedema and conjunctivitis[25,39,40] (see Chapter 14). Parasitic conjunctivitis can be caused by *Thelazia lacrimalis*, *Onchocerca* spp., *Habronema* spp., ophthalmomyiasis externa (*Oestrus ovis*), and *Trypanosoma evansi*. *Thelazia lacrimalis* can cause mild conjunctivitis and epiphora[41] (Fig. 10-4). Onchocerciasis results in depigmentation of the lateral aspect of the bulbar conjunctiva with or without uveitis[42] (Fig. 10-5). Habronemiasis results in granuloma formation with mucopurulent discharge[23,43] (Fig. 10-6). (See later discussion for more information on parasitic ocular manifestations.)

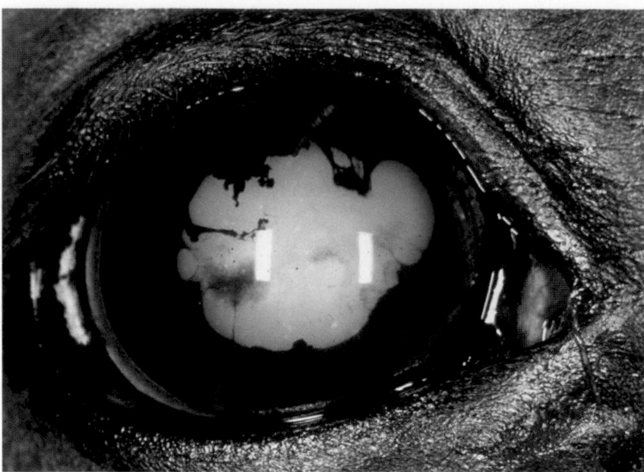

Fig. 10-5 Equine eye with chronic equine recurrent uveitis. There is conjunctival depigmentation at the temporal aspect of the globe, cataract, posterior synechia, tattered corpora nigra secondary to chronic inflammation, and a phthisical globe. Conjunctival depigmentation is a lesion typically seen with onchocerciasis infection.

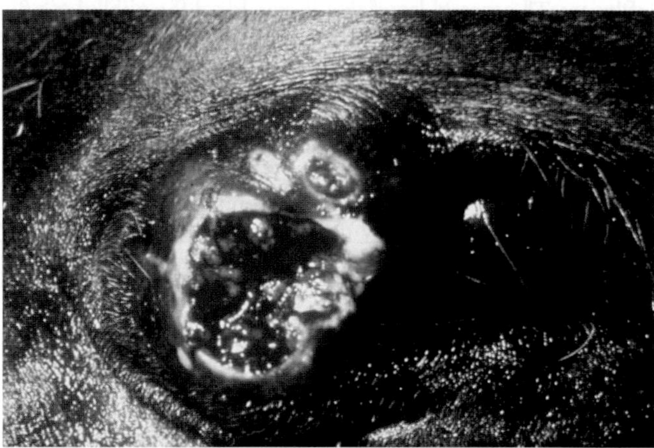

Fig. 10-6 Equine eye with granulomatous, raised, ulcerated eyelid lesion consistent with habronemiasis.

Keratitis

Infectious corneal disease in horses most often occurs secondary to corneal trauma but can also be a manifestation of primary ocular disease or systemic disease. Normal uncomplicated corneal epithelial wound healing in the horse occurs at an average rate of 0.6 mm/day.[44] Healing of corneal stromal wounds is more complicated and involves collagen remodeling and proteoglycan synthesis, eventually resulting in restoration of tensile strength.[45] The prominent anatomic location of equine eyes and the normal opportunistic bacterial and fungal periocular flora predispose equine corneas to infectious keratitis.

Infectious keratitis caused by trauma may or may not be ulcerative and may be caused by opportunistic bacterial or fungal organisms, or a combination of these. Nonspecific signs of keratitis include pain (blepharospasm, photophobia, epiphora), serous to mucopurulent ocular discharge, corneal edema, variable corneal vascularization, loss of stromal integrity (melting or keratomalacia), and secondary anterior uveitis (aqueous flare,

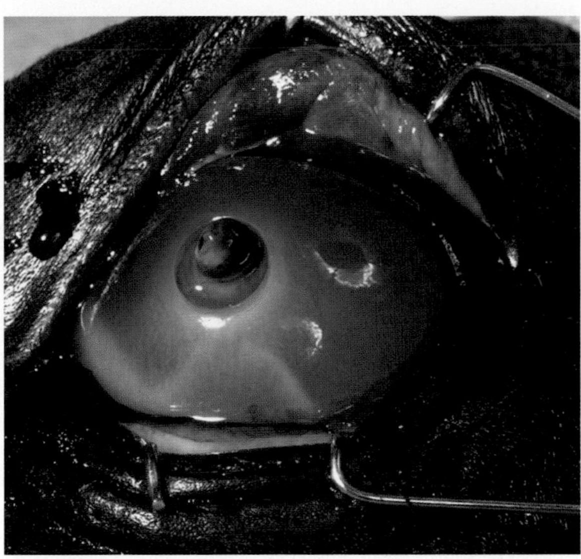

Fig. 10-7 Equine eye with axial ruptured descemetocele with iris prolapse. In addition, there is severe conjunctival hyperemia, corneal vascularization and edema, hypopyon, and fibrin in the anterior chamber.

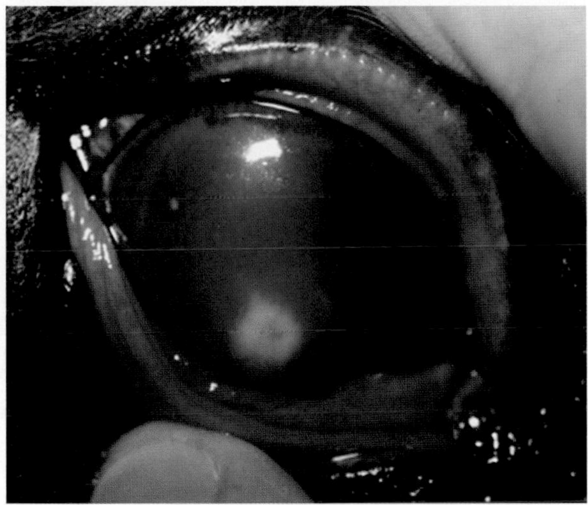

Fig. 10-8 Equine eye with creamy yellow-white, ventral paraxial, corneal stromal abscess secondary to small corneal puncture with plant material that had epithelialized, leaving fluorescein-negative lesion. There is also corneal vascularization, severe conjunctival hyperemia, and epiphora. This abscess was fungal in origin, specifically *Fusarium* spp.

hypopyon, miosis). Horses with infectious *ulcerative* keratitis will have loss of corneal epithelium and variable stromal loss. Full-thickness loss of corneal stroma that breeches Descemet's membrane will usually be plugged with fibrin and iris prolapse, with or without aqueous leakage (Fig. 10-7). This is a surgical emergency, and an ophthalmologist should be consulted. Horses with infectious *nonulcerative* keratitis will have an intact corneal epithelium, but cellular infiltration will be evident within the corneal stroma, that is, corneal abscess (Fig. 10-8). Fungal virulence factors may inhibit corneal vascularization[46,47] and reduce neutrophil infiltration and cell-mediated phagocytosis,[48]

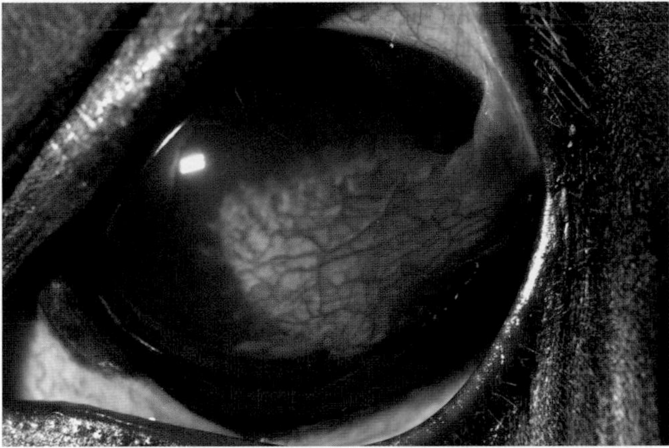

Fig. 10-9 Equine eye with conjunctival pedicle flap that has integrated well into the lesion. The eye has no residual inflammation, and the graft will usually be trimmed 6 weeks postoperatively.

impeding healing and necessitating aggressive medical and surgical intervention. In horses with progressive or perforated corneal ulceration, keratectomy with a conjunctival pedicle flap will provide diagnostic and therapeutic benefits to the patient. Stromal loss that has progressed beyond three-quarters depth may be treated with debridement, followed by synthetic or heterologous corneal grafts and a conjunctival pedicle flap (Fig. 10-9).

Primary infectious keratitis that is not associated with trauma may be caused by equine herpesvirus (EHV) and other respiratory viruses (e.g., adenovirus, influenza, Borna virus). Each of these diseases is discussed separately elsewhere in this text. EHV keratitis typically presents as superficial punctate or dendritic lesions secondary to EHV-2 infection.[34,37,46,50] Acute cases will be quite painful (blepharospasm, serous epiphora) with chemosis and conjunctival hyperemia.[46] Recurrent cases may exhibit corneal vascularization.

Diagnostic evaluation of infectious ulcerative keratitis may include evaluation of corneal cytology, culture and sensitivity, and histopathology. Nonulcerative keratitis is difficult to assess by cytology and culture and sensitivity because of the intact corneal epithelium. Definitive diagnosis of both these disorders can often be obtained at surgery by biopsy of the infected tissue. A rapid and new diagnostic test available at the author's institution is quantitative polymerase chain reaction (PCR) for fungal deoxyribonucleic acid (DNA). This assay can also be performed on formalin-fixed, paraffin-embedded tissues for retrospective analysis and may ultimately provide a more rapid and precise identification of corneal pathogens.[50a] The superficial or punctuate lesions of EHV can be identified by rose bengal stain but not always with fluorescein stain. EHV keratitis can also present as anterior stromal or epithelial punctate opacities without ulceration. This makes diagnosis difficult, and other differential diagnoses should be considered, including fungal keratitis.[46] Diagnosis of EHV keratitis is difficult, but cytology early in the course of disease may be helpful.

Infectious ulcerative keratitis that has not progressed beyond one third of the stromal depth can be treated medically. Depending on the underlying cause, topical antifungal medications (e.g., miconazole, natamycin, itraconazole with DMSO) and oral antifungal medications (e.g., fluconazole) may be necessary. All horses with corneal ulceration should be treated with topical cycloplegics (e.g., atropine, q12-24h), oral nonsteroidal antiinflammatory drugs (NSAIDs; e.g., flunixin meglumine)

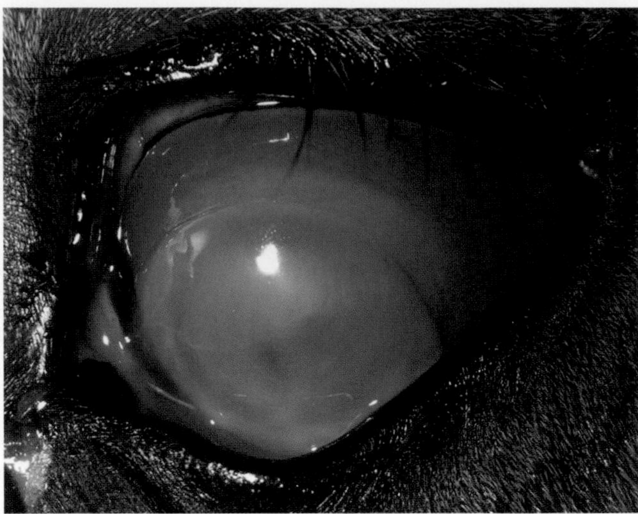

Fig. 10-10 Equine eye with large melting ulcer. The entire cornea is edematous, and there is diffuse cellular infiltrate throughout the entire cornea.

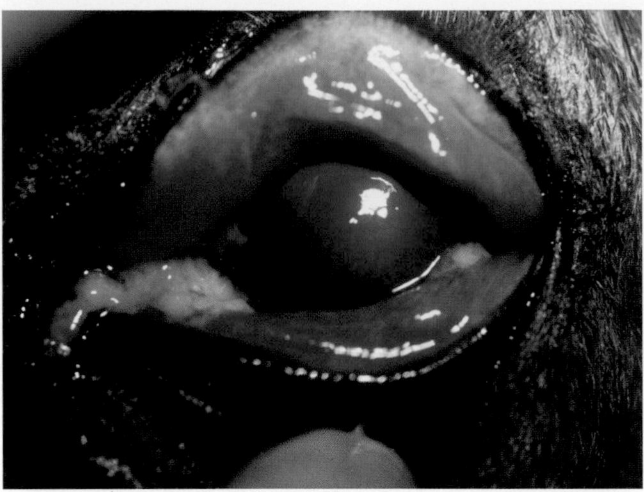

Fig. 10-11 Equine eye with acute equine recurrent uveitis (ERU). There is severe conjunctival hyperemia, mucopurulent ocular discharge, diffuse corneal edema, and enophthalmos. The intraocular structures are difficult to see because of the corneal edema.

for pain and secondary uveitis, and topical antibacterial medications (e.g., neomycin-polymyxin-bacitracin, neomycin-polymyxin-gramicidin, chloramphenicol, or ciprofloxacin, q4-6h), to prevent opportunistic bacterial growth.

Melting corneal ulcers can rapidly become surgical emergencies and should be treated aggressively (Fig. 10-10). The underlying infectious causes of melting corneal ulcers include *Pseudomonas* spp., β-hemolytic streptococci, and fungal infections. Neutrophilic infiltrates and previous corticosteroid use can predispose to melting corneal ulcers. Medical management should include compounds with antiproteolytic activity in addition to the medications just listed and appropriate antibacterial medications for the specific bacteria. Several antiproteases have been recommended for treatment of melting corneal ulcers, including 0.2% ethylenediaminetetraacetic acid (EDTA), 5% to 10% *N*-acetylcysteine, autologous serum, and topical or oral tetracycline or doxycycline. If a member of the tetracycline family is used topically, because of its bacteriostatic nature, its administration should be staggered with the bactericidal antibiotic used by at least 1 hour. Most horses with melting corneal ulcers should be examined by a veterinary ophthalmologist and will likely require surgical intervention.

Topical corticosteroids should be avoided in all horses with keratitis. Indolent or nonhealing corneal ulcers should be managed by debridement and topical antimicrobial and cycloplegic medications as well as oral NSAIDs. Grid or punctate keratotomy should be avoided because of possible underlying fungal infection.[49]

Therapy for EHV keratitis includes topical antiviral and NSAID therapies. Idoxuridine (0.1%) and trifluridine (0.3%) limit viral replication but do not kill the virus; therefore, they should be used between 4 and 12 times daily for 3 to 5 days until the condition stabilizes, then 3 to 6 times daily thereafter. Some formulations of these medications can be irritating to the eye. Topical NSAIDs include 0.03% flurbiprofen and 0.1% diclofenac and are helpful for secondary uveitis and inflammation, but they should be used with caution because they may cause recrudescence of viral keratitis in human patients. Topical corticosteroids should be avoided in horses with EHV keratitis, as well as most horses with keratitis. Oral L-lysine is useful adjunctive therapy in human and feline patients with herpetic keratitis because it limits replication of the virus as a result of its competitive antagonism with arginine.[46] There are no dose guidelines for L-lysine in horses, but empiric supplementary doses of 10 to 30 g once daily indefinitely have been suggested. Viral keratitides that are not associated with EHV are uncommon in the United States but can be treated similarly to EHV keratitis with topical antiviral and NSAID therapy.

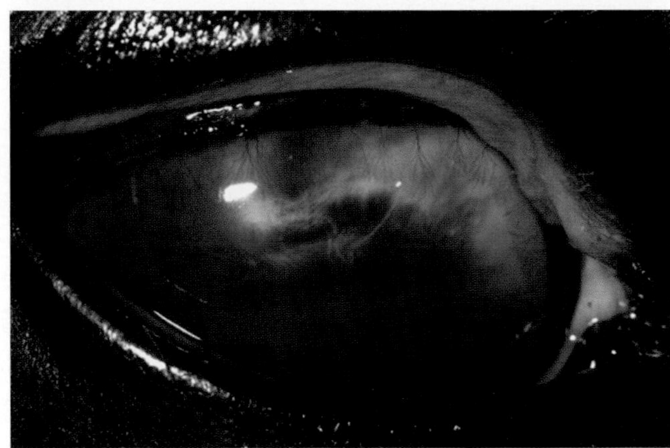

Fig. 10-12 Equine eye with ERU. There is conjunctival hyperemia, diffuse corneal edema and vascularization, a miotic pupil, and fibrin in the anterior chamber.

Uveitis

Uveitis is inflammation of the uveal tract, which includes the iris, ciliary body, and choroid. *Anterior uveitis* refers to inflammation of the iris and ciliary body, *posterior uveitis* refers to inflammation of the choroid, and *panuveitis* refers to inflammation of all components of the uvea. Clinical signs of active uveitis are nonspecific and include pain (blepharospasm, photophobia, epiphora, ocular discharge), conjunctival hyperemia, scleral injection, corneal edema, keratic precipitates, aqueous flare, hypopyon, hyphema, fibrin in the anterior chamber or vitreous, iris color change, and miosis (Figs. 10-11 and 10-12). Chronic changes include atrophy of the corpora

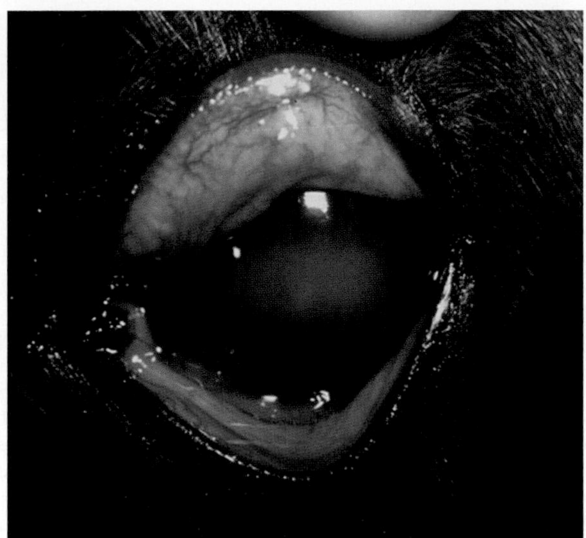

Fig. 10-13 Foal's eye with uveitis, secondary to *Rhodococcus equi* infection. There is epiphora, diffuse conjunctival hyperemia, diffuse corneal edema, and fibrin in the anterior chamber.

nigra, cataract, fibrosis of the iris, endothelial scarring, phthisis bulbi, and glaucoma. Infectious systemic causes of uveitis include viruses, bacteria, protozoa, and parasites.[51] Specific viral causes of uveitis include equine influenza virus, EHV-1, equine viral arteritis, and equine infectious anemia virus. Bacterial causes include *Leptospira* spp., *Brucella* spp., *Streptococcus* spp., *Rhodococcus equi* (Fig. 10-13), and *Escherichia coli*. *Toxoplasma gondii* may cause uveitis in horses. Parasitic etiologies include *Onchocerca* spp. and *Strongylus* spp. More detailed information regarding ocular manifestations of these organisms can be found later in this chapter.

Equine recurrent uveitis (ERU) is an immune-mediated disorder that is the leading cause of blindness in horses. Although the recurrent episodes of ERU are not directly caused by reinfection with microorganisms or parasites, numerous bacterial, viral, protozoal, and parasitic organisms have been implicated in initiating the syndrome (see Chapter 34 for discussion of the association of leptospirosis with ERU).[52]

Treatment of uveitis, regardless of cause, is aimed at decreasing inflammation in the eye, minimizing long-term damage to ocular structures, and preserving vision. Because this disease frequently has an immune-mediated basis, corticosteroids and other antiinflammatory drugs are important for treatment. Systemic and local antimicrobial therapy is also often implemented. Other therapy should be aimed at treatment of possible underlying systemic disease. Lack of response to therapy should prompt the attending clinician to consult with a veterinary ophthalmologist in a timely fashion.

SYSTEMIC DISEASES WITH OCULAR MANIFESTATIONS

Viral Diseases

Alphavirus Encephalitides

Alphaviral encephalitides (eastern, western, and Venezuelan equine encephalomyelitis) are transmitted by mosquitoes and have a typical geographic distribution[63] (see Chapter 20). When the brain stem is involved, nystagmus, strabismus, pupil dilation, and head tilt occur.[64] Systemic clinical signs include fever, conscious proprioceptive deficits, and behavioral changes. In the later stages of disease, progressive signs of cerebral or cerebrocortical and cranial nerve dysfunction may be seen and include facial, lingual, and pharyngeal paralysis; ataxia; hypermetria; circling and proprioceptive deficits or paresis of the trunk and limbs; as well as blindness.[65] Diagnosis, treatment, and prognosis for horses with alphavirus encephalitis are discussed in Chapter 20.[66,67]

Equine Viral Arteritis

Equine viral arteritis (EVA) is caused by a virus of the Arteriviridae family and is spread through inhalation of aerosolized virus or through sexual contact[68] (see Chapter 14). Horses with clinical disease may exhibit signs of upper respiratory disease, edema, fever, and abortion 3 to 8 weeks after infection.[69] Ocular signs include serous to mucoid ocular discharge, conjunctivitis, corneal opacity, photophobia, and periorbital edema. Diagnosis, treatment, and prognosis for horses with EVA are discussed in Chapter 14.[70]

Equine Infectious Anemia

Equine infectious anemia (EIA) is a chronic disease of horses caused by a virus belonging to the *Lentivirus* genus of the family *Retroviridae* (see Chapter 23). Although most infected horses show no recognizable clinical signs, other horses may present with signs that include recurrent fever, weight loss, edema, thrombocytopenia, and anemia.[71] Thrombocytopenia can result in ocular lesions, including conjunctival and intraocular hemorrhages. Choroiditis has also been described in horses with EIA.[72] Horses with subacute to chronic disease develop anemia and may experience recrudescent cycles of disease. Infected horses remain infected for life. Therefore, seropositive horses are considered infected. Diagnosis, prognosis, and prevention of EIA are discussed in Chapter 23.

Rabies

Rabies is a rapidly progressive, fatal disease caused by a neurotropic virus of the family Rhabdoviridae that may affect most warm-blooded mammals (see Chapter 19). Ocular signs rarely occur, or are not noticed, but may include prolapse of the third eyelid, blindness, nystagmus, and strabismus, most likely caused by diffuse cerebrocortical edema and hemorrhage.[72-74] Euthanasia is recommended because no treatment is available. Appropriate caution should be taken with all animals with neurologic signs, especially those not vaccinated for rabies. The most reliable diagnostic test remains the fluorescent antibody test performed on brain tissue.[73]

African Horse Sickness

African horse sickness (AHS) is a noncontagious, arthropod-borne orbivirus that affects all Equidae, although mules, donkeys, and zebras are less susceptible than horses[75] (see Chapter 15). It is endemic in sub-Saharan Africa but has not been documented in North or South America. Ocular signs may include chemosis (conjunctival edema) and bulging of the supraorbital fossae.[76] Bulging of the supraorbital fossa occurs in 10% to 20% of patients but is considered a hallmark sign of the disease; it is likely caused by retrobulbar edema and increased vascular pressure. Mortality for horses with AHS varies between 50% and 95%. Diagnosis, treatment, and prevention of AHS are discussed in Chapter 15.[77]

Equine Herpesvirus

Ocular signs have not been described in horses with EHV-1 or EHV-4 (see Chapter 13). EHV-2 is a cytomegalovirus that is not confirmed to have a primary association with systemic disease in horses but is speculated to play a role in the pathogenesis of other diseases through immunosuppression or possible transactivation of EHV-1[78-80] (see earlier discussion). Ocular signs may include serous to mucopurulent ocular discharge, conjunctival hyperemia and chemosis, superficial dendritic or punctate corneal lesions, corneal edema, and variable vascularization.[29,81] Therapy is discussed in the earlier section on keratitis.

Adenovirus

Equine adenovirus is not considered a pathogen in immunologically competent horses. The most frequent manifestation of adenovirus in the horse is lower respiratory tract disease in Arabian foals with combined immunodeficiency.[82] Bronchopneumonia is accompanied by mucopurulent ocular and nasal discharge. Conjunctival epithelial cells are histologically necrotic with intranuclear inclusions. A neutrophilic infiltrate is present in the uveal vasculature, consistent with panuveitis.[29,38]

Equine Influenza

Equine influenza is an acute respiratory tract disease caused by a virus of the family *Orthomyxoviridae*. Clinical signs of fever and serous or mucoid nasal and ocular discharge may last up to 10 days with a harsh, dry cough which persists for two to three weeks.[83,84] Fever, cough, and a serous or mucoid nasal and ocular discharge are often present along with conjunctival hyperemia.[29] Diagnosis, treatment, and prevention of equine influenza are discussed in Chapter 12.[85]

West Nile Virus

West Nile viral encephalitis is caused by a flavivirus and is considered endemic in North America, Europe, Africa, Asia, and the Middle East[86-88] (see Chapter 21). The most common ophthalmic abnormality observed in horses infected with West Nile virus is unilateral or bilateral facial nerve paralysis. Loss of menace response has also been reported, although its pathogenesis is uncertain.[89] In an outbreak of West Nile encephalitis in Italy, mild keratitis and protrusion of the third eyelid were noted in horses that recovered from the disease.[90] Some infected horses may experience blindness, presumably secondary to encephalitis (Ramiro Toribio, personal communication). In human patients, West Nile virus is reported to cause optic neuritis, uveitis, and chorioretinitis.[91,92] Diagnosis, treatment, and prevention of West Nile virus are discussed in Chapter 21.[93-96]

Bacterial Diseases

Tetanus

Tetanus occurs following infection of a wound with *Clostridium tetani*, an anaerobic, spore-forming, gram-positive bacterium found in soil worldwide (see Chapter 47). The bacteria produce three toxins responsible for clinical signs: tetanospasmin, tetanolysin, and a nonspasmogenic toxin. Tetanospasmin is responsible for the typical clinical signs associated with tetanus and inhibits the release of glycine and γ-aminobutyric acid (GABA), the main inhibitory neurotransmitters in the central nervous system (CNS).[53]

The characteristic ocular sign of tetanus in horses is rapid retraction of the globe with resulting bilateral prolapse of the third eyelid.[54] Ocular signs of advanced tetanus include ventrolateral strabismus and fixed, dilated pupils with normal vision.[55] Diagnosis, treatment, and prevention of tetanus in horses are discussed in Chapter 47.[56]

Botulism

The clinical signs of botulism are caused by a neurotoxin of the anaerobic bacterium, *Clostridium botulinum* (see Chapter 46).[57] The toxin blocks the release of acetylcholine from the presynaptic peripheral cholinergic neurons, resulting in a neuromuscular blockade and generalized muscular weakness.[58] Ocular signs associated with botulism include enophthalmos secondary to retractor bulbi spasm, upper eyelid ptosis, mydriasis, and slow pupillary light reflexes.[57,59] Sluggish pupillary light reflexes can be detected within 6 to 18 hours of toxin ingestion, ultimately leading to complete mydriasis.[57,59,60] Diagnosis, treatment, and prevention of botulism in horses are described in Chapter 46.[61,62]

Lyme Disease

Lyme disease is caused by *Borrelia burgdorferi*, a tick-borne bacterium found throughout North America, Europe, and Asia (see Chapter 35). Lyme disease (*B. burgdorferi*) causes nonspecific ocular signs that include conjunctivitis, anterior uveitis, severe panuveitis, and retinal detachment.[97,98] Ophthalmologic signs reported in human patients with Lyme disease include conjunctivitis, keratitis, uveitis, panophthalmitis, papillary edema, retinal hemorrhage, and retinal detachment.[99-101] Lyme disease–associated neurologic problems affecting the eye may include facial nerve paralysis and secondary corneal disease.[99] In areas where Lyme disease is endemic, it may account for more cases of chronic uveitis than reported. Diagnosis, treatment, and prevention of Lyme disease in horses are discussed in Chapter 35.

Equine Granulocytic Ehrlichiosis

Equine granulocytic ehrlichiosis is caused by a rickettsial organism, *Anaplasma phagocytophilum* (formerly *Ehrlichia equi*), that is also the causative agent of human granulocytic ehrlichiosis and tick-borne fever of cattle and sheep in Europe (see Chapter 42). Transmission occurs through the tick *Ixodes pacificus*. Ocular signs may include icteric sclera, conjunctival petechia, and uveitis.[102] Diagnosis, treatment, and prevention of equine granulocytic ehrlichiosis are discussed in Chapter 42.

Fungal Diseases

Cryptococcosis

Cryptococcus neoformans is a pathogenic fungus that may cause systemic infection in horses and other mammals (see Chapter 57). Ocular signs are not usually reported in horses with cryptococcosis, although there is one report of a frontal sinus granuloma with a retrobulbar mass causing exophthalmos and periorbital swelling.[139] Diagnosis is based on histopathologic evidence of fungal hyphae in tissue samples or on cytology, as well as a positive culture.

Epizootic Lymphangitis

Epizootic lymphangitis, caused by *Histoplasma farciminosum*, a fungal agent found mainly in Africa (see Chapter 57), is manifested as nodules and draining lesions of the subcutaneous lymphatic system.[140] A conjunctival form of this disease results from deposition of the organism on the ocular mucous membranes by the biting flies of the *Musca* and *Stomoxys* species. Ocular signs include serous to mucopurulent discharge, blepharedema, and conjunctival papules.[140] Disease progression leads to ulceration of the papules, which may result in obstruction and erosion of the lacrimal duct or secondary keratitis. Diagnosis is mainly by cytology and culture, although serologic assays are also available.[141] Amphotericin B is the treatment of choice, and a vaccine is available for horses in endemic areas.[140,142]

Aspergillosis

Aspergillus spp. are considered opportunistic fungi that rarely cause systemic disease in nonimmunocompromised horses (see Chapters 56 and 57). Aspergillosis is a cause of guttural pouch mycosis; ocular manifestations can include Horner's syndrome, facial nerve palsy, and blindness resulting from ischemic optic neuritis secondary to extension of disease.[143] These organisms are ubiquitous in the environment, and horses are frequently exposed. Treatment with systemic antifungal agents may be attempted; however, the prognosis is always guarded depending on the underlying disease process and the severity of the lesions.

Equine Leukoencephalomalacia

Equine leukoencephalomalacia (ELEM), also called "blind staggers" or "moldy corn disease," causes central blindness when the midbrain is affected (see Chapter 57). Severe multifocal neurologic signs, including ataxia, agitation, and seizures, may accompany the blindness associated with ELEM.[144] Chronic ingestion of moldy corn infested with *Fusarium moniliforme* and its associated mycotoxin, fumonisin B1, results in liquefactive necrosis of the white matter.[144] If one horse on the farm is affected, other horses have likely been exposed, and feed should be checked for the mold. Hepatic enzyme activities are often increased in horses exposed to the toxin and may be used as a screening test.[144] Once neurologic signs have developed, the prognosis is poor. If attempted, treatment should consist of supportive care, fluids, and administration of activated charcoal to decrease absorption of the toxin.

Parasitic Diseases

Equine Protozoal Myeloencephalitis

Sarcocystis neurona is the primary etiologic agent of equine protozoal myeloencephalitis (EPM), one of the most common neurologic disorders of horses in North America (see Chapter 59). A few reports suggest that *Neospora hughesi* may cause an identical clinical syndrome.[124] Neurologic signs of EPM vary greatly depending on the area of the CNS that is affected. If the seventh and eighth cranial nerves (CN VII, CN VIII) are affected, horses may present with signs of facial nerve paralysis or vestibular disease, respectively.[103,124,125] Ocular signs associated with facial nerve paralysis include ptosis and absence of the palpebral reflex. If the parasympathetic nucleus of CN VII is affected, neurogenic keratoconjunctivitis sicca will occur, predisposing the cornea to ulceration and secondary infectious keratitis. EPM affecting the cervical spinal cord may cause Horner's syndrome. To the authors' knowledge, there are no published reports of blindness or fundic lesions in horses with EPM. Diagnosis, treatment, and prognosis for horses with EPM are discussed in Chapter 59.

Babesiosis (Piroplasmosis)

Piroplasmosis is a hemolytic disease of horses caused by the tick-borne protozoa *Babesia caballi* and *Babesia equi* (see Chapter 60). Ophthalmic signs of babesiosis include serosanguineous ocular discharge, distention of the supraorbital fossa, blepharedema, icteric conjunctiva and sclera, and petechiae and ecchymoses of the conjunctiva.[29,130,131] Diagnosis, treatment, and prevention of piroplasmosis are discussed in Chapter 60.[132]

Toxoplasmosis

Toxoplasma gondii is a protozoa that can infect the horse, although clinical disease is rare.[133] One study examined three separate horse populations in India and found that in the few horses with ocular lesions, there was no correlation with positive titers for *T. gondii*.[134] Another serologic study of 71 horses with ocular lesions associated with ERU found no correlation with positive titers for *T. gondii*.[135] There are sporadic case reports of horses with ocular lesions associated with toxoplasmosis. *T. gondii* DNA was isolated from the retina, choroid, and sclera of both eyes of a 17-year-old pony from the United Kingdom; however, the presence or absence of ocular lesions or visual deficits was not noted.[136] There is one report of peripapillary and partial optic nerve atrophy in a horse with toxoplasmosis.[137] In a study of seven horses with chorioretinitis, five had *T. gondii* titers of 1:64.[138] One of these horses became acutely blind 4 days before presentation and had diffuse, chronic chorioretinitis in the right eye and acute chorioretinitis in the left eye. At presentation the titer was negative, although 16 days later the titer was 1:64. Postmortem histologic examination of the brain found intracytoplasmic *Toxoplasma* bodies.

Onchocerciasis

Onchocerca cervicalis is spread by *Culicoides* spp. and is a common cause of dermatitis in horses (see Chapters 58 and 62). It is thought that microfilariae migrate along vessels through subcutaneous tissue to the eyelids, then into the conjunctiva, cornea, and uvea.[145,146] Ocular microfilariae have been reported in horses, and the prevalence varies by geographic location.

The most common ocular lesion evident is depigmentation of the conjunctiva at the temporal limbal region.[42,145-147] Similar to systemic onchocerciasis, ocular disease is usually caused by an inflammatory reaction to the antigens of dead parasites releasing antigens. Other ocular manifestations include conjunctivitis, peripheral keratitis, and anterior and posterior uveitis.[145,146] Conjunctivitis and keratitis are characterized by chemosis, conjunctival follicles, corneal edema and vascularization, and subepithelial yellow-to-white corneal opacities. Keratitis is typically seen at the temporal limbus but can extend axially and may be accompanied by temporal conjunctivitis and anterior uveitis. Clinical signs of uveitis include epiphora, blepharospasm, miosis, and aqueous flare.[145,146] Signs of posterior uveitis can include peripapillary chorioretinitis and chorioretinal scarring. Although onchocerciasis is often implicated in the pathogenesis of ERU, it is difficult to ascertain the true significance of the association because of the prevalence of the parasite in the normal horse population.[148]

The goal of treatment for onchocerciasis is to reduce ocular inflammation and destroy the microfilariae.[146] Ivermectin is effective at killing microfilariae, but it will not kill the adult parasites.[146,149] Systemic therapy (e.g., flunixin meglumine or phenylbutazone) and topical antiinflammatory therapy is warranted. Topical corticosteroid and NSAID therapy should not be used if a corneal ulcer is present, except under advisement of a veterinary ophthalmologist. Treatment may initially worsen clinical signs, and the disease may recur. Lesions are nonseasonal, and older horses are more likely to be affected than younger horses.

Habronemiasis

Cutaneous habronemiasis, also known as "summer sores," is caused by aberrant intradermal migration of the larvae of *Habronema* or *Draschia* spp., which are normally found in the stomach (see Chapter 62). Lesions usually develop during the summer months in traumatized skin and are caused by a hypersensitivity reaction to dying larvae. Granulomas with necrotic centers are typically seen on the lower limbs, the urethral process, or the eye. Mineralized larvae can often be observed in the center of the lesion.

Common ocular locations for habronemiasis include the medial canthus, eyelid, conjunctiva, lacrimal caruncle, nasolacrimal duct, and third eyelid.[30,43,145,150-152] Periocular or eyelid lesions have a raised, irregular, yellow appearance often referred to as "sulfur granules." The granulomatous lesions are often covered with an exudate and are painful when touched. When the nasolacrimal system is involved, a circular lesion may develop below the medial canthus. Biopsy of the affected area should be performed to aid in diagnosis and to rule out other causes of ulcerative skin lesions. Histopathologically, central cavitations (some with nematode larvae) are surrounded by degenerate and degranulating eosinophils and granulomatous inflammation.[30]

Treatment of habronemiasis consists of an adequate deworming program that includes ivermectin, debridement of the lesions, topical and systemic antiinflammatory therapy, and adequate fly control. In severe cases, systemic corticosteroids may substantially lessen the granulomatous reaction.[30,145,153]

Thelaziasis

Ocular disease caused by *Thelazia lacrimalis* is uncommon. This filarid parasite is a commensal organism that lives in the lacrimal gland, conjunctival fornices, and nasolacrimal duct. It can cause mild blepharoconjunctivitis and dacryocystitis.[154] Diagnosis of thelaziasis is confirmed by identification of the parasite in conjunctival fluid or nasolacrimal flushes.

Setariasis

Setaria digitata and *S. equina* are nematodes normally found in the stomach. Aberrant migration of *Setaria* spp. into the eye can occur in horses, resulting in severe intraocular inflammation.[89] Clinical signs include photophobia, epiphora, corneal edema, hypopyon, aqueous flare, and miosis.[101-104] Successful surgical removal of the nematode from the anterior chamber has been reported.[102] In a pilot study, treatment with diethylcarbamazine decreased microfilaremia in horses.[105] Antiinflammatory therapy should be instituted in conjunction with antiparasitic agents.

Dirofilariasis

Intraocular migration of *Dirofilaria immitis* is less common in horses than in carnivores, although successful removal of the nematode from the anterior chamber of a horse has been reported.[145]

Echinococcosis

Echinococcus granulosus is a small tapeworm that causes hydatid disease (see Chapter 61). Dogs are the definitive hosts, and horses are considered intermediate hosts. Exophthalmos, blindness, and head shaking caused by retrobulbar cysts are the only reported ocular manifestations of hydatid cyst disease in the horse.[155,156] The only definitive treatment is surgical excision, although treatment with albendazole can decrease the size of the cyst.[155] Diagnosis is based on positive histopathologic or cytologic identification. Cysts are usually an incidental finding at necropsy, but they are of particular concern because they can cause severe disease in humans, another intermediate host.

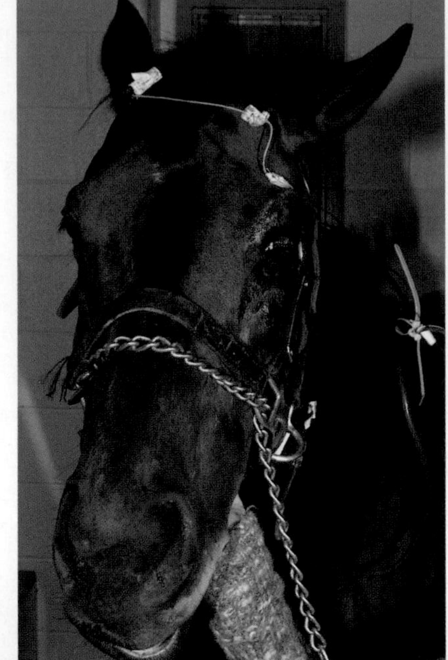

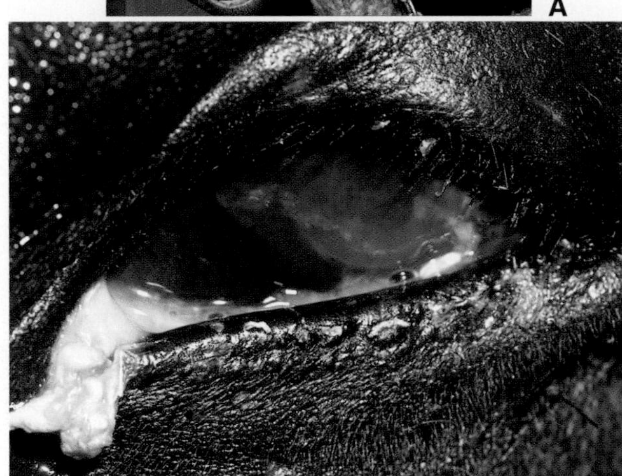

Fig. 10-14 A, Horse with facial nerve paralysis. The eye developed an infected corneal ulcer as a result of lagophthalmos. Note the dropped ear and lip. **B,** Same horse's eye. There is an infected corneal ulcer, mucopurulent ocular discharge, corneal vascularization, and enophthalmos. (A from Gilger B: *Equine ophthalmology*, Philadelphia, 2005, Saunders.)

NEURO-OPHTHALMIC INFECTIOUS DISEASES

Vestibular Disease

Vestibular signs may result from either peripheral or central nervous system diseases. Peripheral disease causes ipsilateral head tilt, horizontal or rotary nystagmus with the fast phase occurring away from the side of the lesion, falling, circling, and asymmetric ataxia without conscious proprioceptive deficits or weakness.[55,105] Common causes of peripheral vestibular dysfunction include trauma, otitis media, temporohyoid osteoarthropathy, and guttural pouch disease.[106-109] Facial nerve paralysis (Fig. 10-14) and Horner's syndrome can occur with peripheral disease because of the facial nerve and sympathetic nerve proximity to the petrous temporal bone.[105,108,109]

Central (CNS) vestibular disease presents similarly, although conscious proprioceptive deficits, generalized weakness, and involvement of multiple cranial nerves may be present.[105] Nystagmus may be rotary, horizontal, vertical, diagonal, or disconjugate (different in each eye). The direction of the nystagmus may change with head position in central vestibular disease.[55,105] Paradoxical central vestibular disease may occur with a destructive lesion near the caudal cerebellar peduncle, resulting in clinical signs contralateral to the lesion.[105] Bilateral vestibular disease is difficult to differentiate from generalized cerebellar disease; these horses do not have nystagmus or vestibular eye movements and usually exhibit a symmetric ataxia.[105] Central vestibular dysfunction is often associated with tumors or abscesses but may also be secondary to protozoal, viral, bacterial, or parasitic encephalitides.[110,111]

Diagnostic techniques for determining the underlying cause of vestibular disease in the horse should include radiographs of the skull, endoscopy of the pharyngeal region and guttural pouches, and magnetic resonance imaging (MRI) or computed tomography (CT) scan of the head. Cerebrospinal fluid (CSF) cytology and ancillary testing for viral or protozoal antibodies are indicated if CNS disease is suspected.[108,109] Caloric testing can be performed, although the test is not always reliable, and most horses will resist the procedure. In caloric testing the ear canal is irrigated with cold water, and a normal response is induction of horizontal nystagmus away from the tested side. A decreased or absent reaction indicates the side of the lesion. Brain stem auditory-evoked responses are also useful in demonstrating damage to the cochlea and CN VIII and can be used to differentiate between central and peripheral disease.[112,113] This procedure is reliable in the sedated horse. Treatment and prognosis should address the primary disease process.

Horner's Syndrome

Horner's syndrome is caused by damage or denervation along any portion of the efferent pupillomotor sympathetic nervous system. The sympathetic nervous system originates in the hypothalamus, where the central sympathetic fibers form the tectotegmentospinal tract (first-order neurons).[55] This tract descends ipsilaterally through the brain stem and lateral funiculus of the cervical spinal cord to synapse with the preganglionic cell bodies of the first to third thoracic vertebrae (T1-T3) or T4. These preganglionic sympathetic neurons (second-order neurons) leave the spinal cord through the segmental ventral roots to the paravertebral sympathetic chain, continue through the brachial plexus, and travel with the vagosympathetic trunk until they synapse in the cranial cervical ganglion caudomedial to the tympanic bulla. The postganglionic fibers (third-order neurons) join the tympanic branch of CN IX (glossopharyngeal nerve) within the middle ear and pass over the caudodorsal aspect of the guttural pouch. After the fibers exit the middle ear, they enter the cavernous sinus and join CN V (trigeminal nerve) and continue rostrally as the nasociliary nerve to innervate the orbital smooth muscles, the eyelids (including the third eyelid), and the ciliary body, iris dilator, and iris sphincter muscles.

Horner's syndrome in horses is most frequently seen secondary to guttural pouch disease.[55] Injury to the cranial thoracic spinal cord, brachial plexus avulsions, and traumatic lesions or masses involving the mediastinum, periorbital tissues, or cervical structures may also cause clinical signs of Horner's syndrome.[114-117] Iatrogenic Horner's syndrome can result from surgical ligation of the carotid artery. Other causes unique to the horse include polyneuritis equi syndrome, EPM affecting the cervical spinal cord, basisphenoid trauma, esophageal rupture, and intravenous injection with various drugs, including phenylbutazone.[118-120] Clinical signs of Horner's syndrome in horses include ptosis, relative enophthalmos, subtle miosis, regional hyperthermia, and excessive sweating on the ipsilateral side of the face.[114,121-123] Cervical sympathetic nerve damage will cause sweating of the neck, congested conjunctival and nasal mucous membranes, and inspiratory stridor.[55,122,123]

The location and cause of the lesion will determine which clinical signs are present, and the location will determine what diagnostic tests should be performed. Often, location may provide the prognosis. Phenylephrine (2% or 10%) or 1:1000 epinephrine are more readily available for the pharmacologic localization of efferent sympathetic lesions. Phenylephrine or epinephrine are direct-acting sympathomimetic drugs that will result in mydriasis within 5 to 8 minutes in postganglionic lesions caused by denervation hypersensitivity of the effector cells.[55] This test can effectively distinguish between preganglionic and postganglionic lesions during the first few weeks of clinical signs.[105] One drop of phenylephrine or epinephrine is applied to each eye (the normal eye is used for comparison), and care should be taken to use the same amount in each eye because the response is dose dependent. Mydriasis, retraction of the third eyelid, resolution of the enophthalmos, and ptosis are all positive responses to the phenylephrine test and indicate a postganglionic or third-order lesion. If a lesion localizes to the postganglionic arm of the pathway, endoscopy of the pharynx and guttural pouch should be performed. Alternatively, CT is another diagnostic option when available.

References

See the CD-ROM for a list of references linked to the abstract in PubMed.

SECTION • II
Viral Diseases

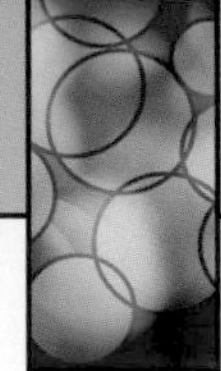

CHAPTER • 11

Laboratory Diagnosis of Viral Infections

J. Lindsay Oaks

The ability to diagnose viral infections is important for equine clinicians. Accurate and timely laboratory confirmation of a viral infection allows more effective supportive clinical management, earlier detection of complications, more accurate prognosis, more effective isolation protocols, evaluation of vaccination programs, detection of vaccination failures, and probably in the future, selection of appropriate antiviral drugs.

Unfortunately, clinically timely, sensitive, and specific laboratory assays for the diagnosis of viral infections have traditionally been challenging. Viral infections generally are detected either directly by demonstration of the virus in clinical samples or indirectly by serologic detection of antiviral antibodies in serum or other fluids. Classic methods of direct virus detection include isolation in cultures of living cells or in laboratory animals, detection of viral antigens by immunofluorescence, and electron microscopy. Although these methods form the foundations of diagnostic virology—and in some cases are still very good tests—as discussed in this chapter, their clinical utility has often been constrained by expense, long turnaround time for results, and often low sensitivity. Serologic testing has often had problems with sensitivity or specificity, as well as difficulties in distinguishing recent from past infection or between natural and vaccine titers.

Fortunately, the application of molecular biology techniques to diagnostic virology has greatly improved the clinical utility of virus testing. In particular, nucleic acid amplification tests (i.e., polymerase chain reaction, or PCR), immunohistochemistry (IHC), and enzyme-linked immunosorbent assay (ELISA)–based antigen detection tests are economical to perform, can provide results in minutes to hours, and are often very sensitive and specific. For serologic assays, newer testing formats, such as the ELISA, as well as the ability to produce highly purified and defined recombinant viral proteins or peptides for use as antigen targets, have greatly improved the sensitivity, specificity, and interpretation of antibody tests.

Despite the dramatic advances in methodology, however, many of the traditional caveats about test validation and interpretation of results remain the same. Care must still be taken not to make assumptions about the performance characteristics of any new test or testing method. Newer tests are not automatically better tests, and the sensitivity and specificity of any new test or testing method must be evaluated individually and with respect to the performance of the previous test. For example, PCR assays are often assumed to be more sensitive than virus isolation, but this is not always true. Also, regardless of the method used for detection, the significance of a virus or antibody titer identified in a clinical sample must still be interpreted in the context of the patient, the pathogenesis and epidemiology of the disease, and the host responses to that disease.

Usually the diagnostic laboratory will select the test(s) for a specific disease based on the available facilities and the current optimal test for a given virus. However, the clinician still needs to be aware of the inherent advantages and limitations of any given test and to interpret the results of the test accordingly. Moreover, understanding the various testing options may allow a clinician to select a laboratory based on the type of test offered. Appropriate sample collection and transport are also the responsibility of the clinician and critically important for good laboratory results. For a few diseases in which the assay can be performed by the clinician, such as an antigen ELISA test for influenza, the clinician will need to assume full responsibility for interpretation as well as performance of the test. Finally, good communication with the laboratory is extremely important. The ability of the laboratory to provide good service is enhanced with good clinical histories, differential diagnoses, and specific testing requests. The laboratory is also a valuable source of information about sample collection and transport, testing methodology, and interpretation of results.

The purpose of this chapter is to provide a basic description of the methods most often used in contemporary diagnostic virology laboratories, including the key advantages and disadvantages of the tests as well as concerns about interpretation, and when appropriate, to illustrate the use of a test with specific equine viral diseases. However, no attempt is made to describe comprehensively all the specific testing options or optimal sampling strategies for all the equine viral diseases. The reader is referred to the chapters on specific diseases for a more complete description of testing options.

VIRUS ISOLATION

The isolation of a virus in cell culture is the original virus detection assay.[1] The basis for this method is to inoculate a clinical specimen onto living cells in which the virus can propagate, then detect and identify any viruses that are isolated. Living cell cultures are first established in plastic wells or Petri dishes. Clinical samples are homogenized in cell culture growth media, centrifuged or filtered to remove larger debris and bacteria, treated with antibiotics to remove contaminating bacteria that may infect and destroy the cell cultures, and then inoculated onto the cells. Viral growth in the cells is detected by characteristic changes in the infected cells, called the *cytopathic effect* (CPE), caused by the virus (Fig. 11-1). When viral CPE is suspected in a cell culture, the presence of a virus as well as its identity is confirmed by additional tests, such as fluorescent-labeled antiviral antibodies, PCR for viral nucleic acids, or electron microscopy. Occasionally, clinical

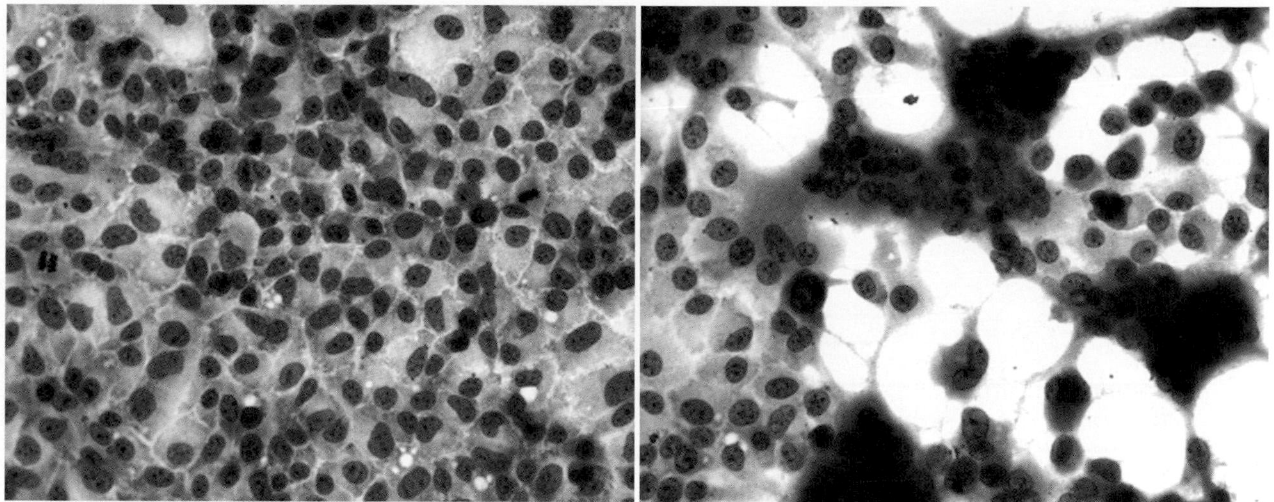

Fig. 11-1 Photomicrograph of viral cytopathic effect in cells stained with modified Wright's stain. **A,** Normal rabbit kidney cells in culture, which form an intact monolayer. **B,** Rabbit kidney cells infected with equine herpesvirus type 1, showing the resultant visible cytopathic effect. Changes include loss of cells seen as holes in the monolayer, stringing of cytoplasm between the cells, and multinucleated cells. Magnification for both panels, 400×.

samples are inoculated into laboratory animals for isolation of viruses, for example, into the brain of suckling mice for isolation of alphaviruses (e.g., eastern and western equine encephalitis viruses)[2] or into embryonated eggs for isolation of equine influenza virus.[3] Depending on the virus or virus strain and the specific cells being used for isolation, viral growth may not cause any visible changes and is called *noncytopathic.* For these virus/cell combinations, screening for the presence of virus must be done in all inoculated cell cultures by some other method, such as immunofluorescence for viral antigens or PCR for viral nucleic acids.

One of the primary advantages of virus isolation in cell culture is the potential for very good sensitivity. Because inoculated cell cultures are generally passaged serially two or three times before being called "negative," there is usually significant amplification of any virus present in the sample. However, virus isolation requires that viable virus be present in the sample, and viability may be adversely affected by sample collection and storage, timing of sample collection, postmortem interval, and sample transport. This is particularly true for fragile viruses such as herpesviruses and other enveloped viruses. Therefore, good sample collection and transport are critical for successful virus isolation. Sensitivity is also affected by the type of cells used for isolation. Different cell types vary in their ability to propagate different viruses and thus in their sensitivity of detection.[3] Therefore, most laboratories will use specific types of cultured cells or animal inoculation systems for specific viruses and thus require some guidance from the clinician about the suspected viruses.

Another advantage of cell culture is that it obtains an isolate of viable virus for evaluation of biologic properties, such as virulence, antigenic variation, and possibly, susceptibility to antiviral drugs.[1] Fortunately, with most of the common equine viral diseases, this additional information is not essential for the effective clinical management of individual cases. However, for viruses such as equine influenza or African horse sickness, the ability to type a virus or detect changes in antigenicity may explain vaccine failures or lead to changes in vaccine type.[4,5] Usually, obtaining isolates for this purpose is indicated only when there is a significant and unexplained change in the epidemiology of a particular disease. Virus isolation is also a relatively nonselective method of virus detection, which is important for the identification of new viruses. However, the search for a new virus is usually based first on unexplained viral pathology or clinical features that suggest a viral etiology. Whether the disease is caused by a change in the epidemiology of a recognized viral disease, or the appearance of a new virus, the associated investigations generally become research projects and have different goals (and sources of funding) than the routine detection of recognized equine viral pathogens.

The key disadvantages of virus isolation, in addition to the need for samples with viable virus, as previously noted, are cost and time. Maintaining cell cultures requires highly specialized facilities, equipment, reagents, and trained personnel. Virus isolation is also labor intensive. Consequently, there is considerable expense involved with this assay, and even for diagnostic laboratories that provide services at a subsidized cost, these expenses are becoming prohibitive for routine diagnostic testing. In addition, it often takes at least a week, and usually longer, to obtain results. This time frame is often not very useful for short-term clinical decision making, such as therapy, prognosis, isolation, and monitoring for complications. These limitations in particular are key reasons for replacing virus isolation with the molecular methods described next.

POLYMERASE CHAIN REACTION

Nucleic acid amplification by PCR is now one of the most common assays used to detect the presence of a virus directly in clinical samples. PCR assays have been developed for a variety of equine viral pathogens from a wide array of sample types[3,4,6-16] (Fig. 11-2).

Amplification Technique

Total deoxyribonucleic acid (DNA) or ribonucleic acid (RNA), including viral DNA or RNA if present, is extracted and purified from the sample. For RNA viruses, isolated RNA is converted to complementary DNA (cDNA) in a separate reaction by the enzyme *reverse transcriptase* (RT); therefore, PCR for RNA targets is referred to as *RT-PCR*. A heat-stable DNA polymerase is then used in a series of cyclic reactions to

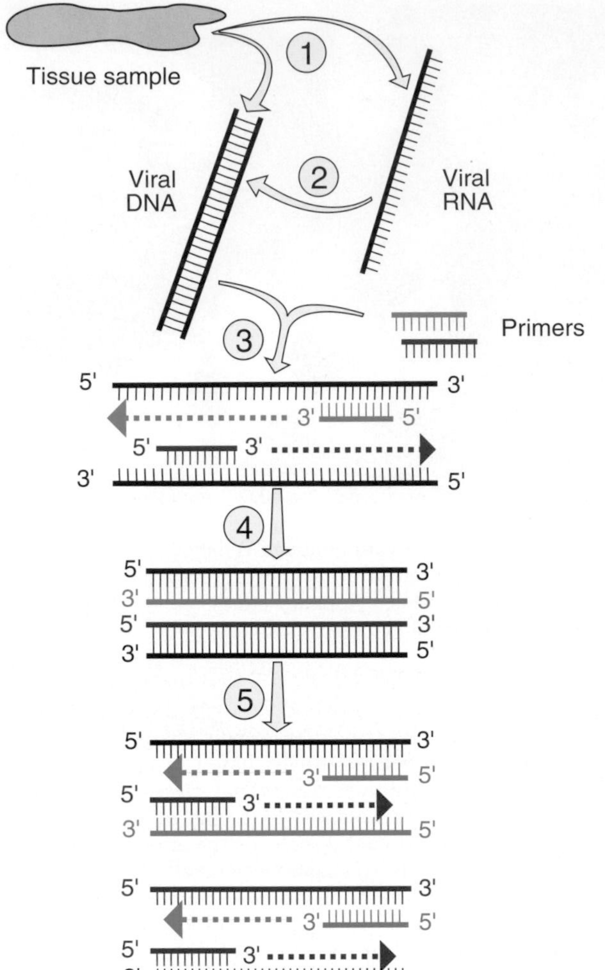

Fig. 11-2 Polymerase chain reaction (PCR) method. *1*, Viral DNA or RNA is extracted and purified from tissue or blood samples. *2*, Because the PCR method only amplifies double-stranded DNA, RNA targets are converted to DNA by the enzyme reverse transcriptase. *3*, The double-stranded DNA is denatured with heat; primers are added to the reaction along with nucleotides and with a DNA polymerase such as *Taq*. Primers bind to complementary sequences in the viral sequences, if present, and initiate copying reactions from the 3′ end of the primers. *4*, After one round of amplification, each original viral target DNA is copied, resulting in two copies of the target. *5*, The process is repeated, which results in exponential amplification of the original target sequence. *DNA*, Deoxyribonucleic acid; *RNA*, ribonucleic acid.

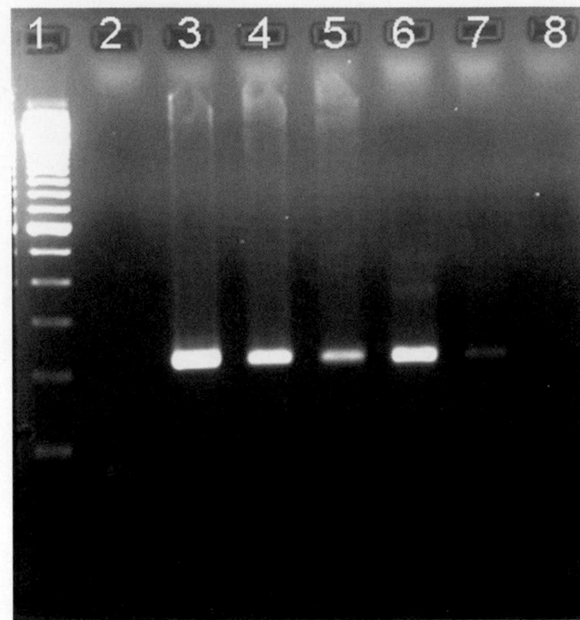

Fig. 11-3 Gel analysis of PCR reactions for equine infectious anemia virus. Following PCR, the reaction products are electrophoresed through an agarose gel and stained with ethidium bromide, which allows visualization with ultraviolet light by causing the amplified DNA to fluoresce and appear as white bands in the gel. Lane 1 is a size standard included with each gel to determine the size of the amplified DNA products. Lane 2 is a negative control. Lane 3 is a positive control. Lanes 4-8 are test samples, with positive samples in lanes 4-7 and a negative sample in lane 8.

amplify exponentially any viral DNA or cDNA sequences. The reaction is initiated and driven by two oligonucleotide primers (usually about 15-25 nucleotides in length) that are synthetically produced and complementary to a desired target sequence in the viral genome. This target sequence is selected to be unique for the virus, preventing the primers from binding to and initiating amplification of nonviral sequences in the genome of the host or other pathogens. When the primers bind to the target DNA, they allow the DNA polymerase to initiate copying of the target sequence from the 3′ end of the primer. The primers are also designed to bind to opposite strands of the double-stranded DNA target and thus initiate reactions toward each other. The heat stability of the DNA polymerase is required to prevent inactivation at the high temperatures (about 90° C) used to denature the double-stranded target for primer binding. High temperatures (usually about 55°-65° C) during the annealing part of the reaction are also used to maintain the fidelity of primer binding, because at these temperatures, binding will occur only if there is a perfect complementary match between the primer and target sequences. The other parameter important for primer selection is that they bind close enough on the target genome so that the copying reactions will efficiently copy up to the binding sites for the other primer on the opposite DNA strand. However, the *amplicons* also need to remain large enough to be detected. The optimal size for a PCR amplicon is about 150 to 800 base pairs. Because amplification is exponential, the final result of the PCR assay is a very large number of amplified DNA fragments of a specific length (i.e., the distance between the primers).

The amplicon products of PCR amplification can then be detected in several ways. The most common method is *agarose gel electrophoresis*, which separates DNA fragments based on size (Fig. 11-3). Positive reactions are identified by the detection of DNA bands of the correct size or that hybridize to sequence-specific probes.

Design Variations

Several variants of the PCR assay are designed to decrease the time necessary to perform the assay, minimize manipulations of reactions, and improve sensitivity. Decreased manipulations not only save time and labor, but more importantly, reduce the amount of amplicon contamination that inevitably occurs when opening and closing finished reactions and transferring reaction products to new tubes or analytical gels. Contaminant amplicons are notorious for their ability to get into reagents and other samples, leading to false-positive results. To avoid reaction manipulations, some assays for RNA viruses now use one-step protocols or polymerase enzymes with both RT and DNA polymerase activities, eliminating the need for separate reactions.[16-18] A common variant now is "real-time" PCR, in which amplification of either the target DNA or the cDNA is detected by the formation of a fluorescent signal in the tube, and the level of fluorescence is measured by the PCR machine during each cycle.[6,16,19] This not only eliminates the need for opening amplified reactions for gel analysis, but also allows positive and negative tests to be determined as the reaction proceeds, thus in "real time."

The sensitivity of PCR assays can be maximized by "nested" PCR.[3,7] This modification uses two sets of virus-specific primers. The first set of primers is used for an initial round of amplification as previously described. Some of this reaction product is transferred to a second PCR assay with a second set of primers that will bind to the first amplicon. Because there are two rounds of amplification, this modification allows detection of very low levels of virus. However, because of the extreme sensitivity of nested PCR, this assay is prone to false-positive results from minute levels of amplicon contamination that are very difficult to control in most laboratories. Moreover, good-quality samples from active viral infections do not usually require the sensitivity of nested PCR for detection. Thus, most laboratories avoid nested PCR assays, if possible.

Other recent variants of PCR used in human laboratories include the ligase chain reaction, strand-displacement amplification, transcription-mediated amplification, and microarray analysis.[1,19] However, these assays are not yet in widespread use for the detection of equine viruses and thus are not considered further here.

Advantages and Benefits

The key advantages of PCR assays are speed, cost, sensitivity, ability to detect nonviable virus, and in some cases, safety. Typical PCR reactions can be completed in 4 to 6 hours, allowing for results to be obtained very quickly. Although there are some initial high capital costs for equipment, most of the key steps for PCR can be performed with commercially available kits that are effective, reliable, and relatively inexpensive on a per-test basis. Thus the cost for PCR assays is usually quite reasonable compared with virus isolation. Additional setup costs for controls, gels, and size standards are required for each run, regardless of the numbers of samples tested. Consequently, unless there is a communicated need for urgency, most laboratories will accumulate some number of samples before running a test and will report results periodically.

PCR assays are generally quite sensitive because of logarithmic amplification of the target and are often comparable in sensitivity to virus isolation. However, this is not automatically true, and the performance of PCR must be assessed for each pathogen and disease. PCR is especially useful for viruses that are either slow, difficult, or unable to be propagated in cell culture, such as many of the gamma herpesviruses (e.g., equine herpesvirus types 2 and 5), papillomavirus, influenza virus, and rotavirus. PCR is also very useful to detect viruses that are fragile and prone to loss of viability during sampling or transport, such as many enveloped viruses. PCR for diagnosis of viruses that present significant hazards to laboratory personnel, such as West Nile and eastern equine encephalitis viruses, is preferable to cell culture techniques that require propagation of live virus. PCR can also be performed on DNA or RNA extracted from formalin-fixed, paraffin-embedded tissues.[14] This option provides not only good laboratory safety, but also allows a diagnosis to be made when fresh tissue samples are not available.

Disadvantages and Limitations

The main disadvantages of PCR are false-positive reactions, the lack of a viable virus isolate, detection of virus that may not be clinically relevant, and the inability to detect new or poorly characterized viruses. As noted earlier, laboratory contamination with amplicons and the resultant false-positive results are significant issues for the diagnostic laboratory. Laboratories that perform PCR routinely will have extensive and specific protocols, as well as facility design, to prevent contamination. Negative controls should be performed with each run to detect contamination if it does occur. False-positive results from nonspecific amplification may also occur if there are closely related genetic sequences either in the host genome or in other microorganisms. Good primer design, test validation, and controls usually minimize this problem. Nevertheless, the clinician should always keep in mind that a false-positive result is possible with PCR, and as with any other diagnostic test, results need to be interpreted in the context of the patient and with good clinical judgment.

PCR does not result in recovery of a viable isolate of the virus, which can be a disadvantage if biologic information about the virus is needed. However, as noted in the section on virus isolation, this information is rarely needed to manage clinical cases. Another potential problem with PCR is the detection of viruses that are not clinically relevant. This limitation is not unique to PCR, and detection of a virus in a clinical sample by any method should not automatically be assumed to be clinically relevant. For example, many adult horses may periodically shed equine herpesvirus type 1 or 4 (EHV-1 or EHV-4) subclinically in nasal secretions, and detection of these viruses by either virus isolation or PCR may or may not be important.[15,20] PCR may also detect inactive virus, such as latent herpesviral infections. This interpretive problem can be in part alleviated by sample selection based on knowledge about the pathogenesis of the disease. For example, the detection of EHV-1 or EHV-4 in nasal secretions probably indicates shedding and is much more likely to be significant than detection in neural or lymphoid tissues that may harbor latent infections.[21,22]

PCR tests can also be designed through target selection to discriminate between latent and replicating virus, for example, by detection of viral messenger RNA (mRNA) for structural genes that are only present during active virus replication. The tendency to overinterpret a positive virology result is somewhat compounded by PCR because of its ability to reliably detect viruses that in the past were difficult to detect. For example, equine herpesvirus type 2 (EHV-2), a lymphotropic gamma herpesvirus, is poorly documented as a cause of any clinical disease. However, this virus is also ubiquitous in the horse population, and testing with a highly sensitive test such as PCR is likely to give a positive result from any tissue with lymphocytic inflammation, regardless of the etiology.[11] It is important for the clinician to be aware that mammals have a normal "flora" of viruses as well as bacteria and other microbes, and the significance of virus detection must be critically evaluated, especially for viruses with a high background prevalence and that may cause subclinical infections.

Another disadvantage of PCR is that it requires existing genetic information about the virus in question to design primers. Fortunately, this is no longer a significant issue for the major equine viral pathogens, most of which have been extensively studied. However, this may cause false-negative results when there is undetected genetic variation within the primer binding sites of different strains of virus, as in equine infectious anemia (EIA) virus (JL Oaks, unpublished data). The need for prior genetic knowledge also makes PCR inherently poor for the detection of new viruses.

Viral Characterization

Ironically, however, advances in genetic sequencing that have made this technology rapid and cost-effective for routine diagnostic virology have also made PCR a powerful tool for the rapid characterization of new viruses. In this application, primers are designed to bind to highly conserved regions within a virus family or genus and amplify a portion of the genome that is variable and unique for the virus. The sequence of this unique region can then be determined and used for comparison to genetic databases, and it may either identify a well-characterized virus in an unusual disease entity or determine that the virus is a previously undescribed equine virus.

Although specific genetic information about the equine virus is not necessary, some clue as to the general identity of the virus is needed. This is most often accomplished by observing electron microscopic features, reaction with group-specific antibodies in immunofluorescence or IHC assays, or suggestive inclusion bodies within lesions. For example, this approach allowed the rapid characterization of the *Hendra virus*, a novel virus that fatally infected horses and humans in Australia in 1994,[23] and several new gamma herpesviruses associated with pneumonia in donkeys.[24]

Additional advances that combine biotechnology, molecular biology, and bioinfomatics are poised to revolutionize the detection and characterization of new viruses in both people and animals, as recently demonstrated by a sequence-independent, single-primer amplification protocol that identified two new bovine parvoviruses.[25] It should be noted that these viruses were detected as "proof of principle" rather than in the context of identifying an etiologic agent of disease. This should emphasize that with advances in our ability to detect new viruses will come a greater need to critically assess the clinical relevance of these viruses.

IN SITU METHODS: DETECTION OF VIRUS IN TISSUE SECTIONS

Histopathology

Routine histopathology on formalin-fixed, hematoxylin-eosin–stained tissue sections of biopsy or necropsy samples often provides strong supporting evidence that a lesion or disease is viral. Although rarely definitive, the distribution of lesions or necrosis and the patterns and types of inflammation are often strongly suggestive of a viral etiology. Inclusion bodies, if present, are often highly characteristic of certain viruses. For example, adenoviruses cause karyomegaly and intensely basophilic intranuclear inclusions. Most alpha herpesviruses, such as equine herpesviruses 1, 3, and 4, cause eosinophilic to basophilic intranuclear inclusions without karyomegaly. Paramyxoviruses cause both intranuclear and intracytoplasmic inclusions. Some viruses, such as lentiviruses and rotaviruses, do not typically result in inclusions in vivo. Thus, in cases where tissue samples are obtained for diagnosis, histopathology should not be overlooked for the diagnosis of viral infections. In addition, formalin-fixed, paraffin-embedded tissue samples can be used for PCR analysis, electron microscopy, and IHC.

Immunofluorescence and Immunohistochemistry

Immunofluorescence and IHC use antiviral antibodies to detect viral antigens in tissue sections. The assays technically differ only in the method used to detect bound antibody. *Immunofluorescence* uses a fluorescent label, usually fluorescein, conjugated either to the antiviral antibody itself (*direct* immunofluorescence) or to an anti-antibody (*indirect* immunofluorescence), and viewed with ultraviolet light (Fig. 11-4, *A* and *B*). Immunofluorescence is usually performed on frozen tissue sections fixed in acetone or methanol.

The antiviral antibody is referred to as the *primary antibody* and can be either immune serum from a known-infected horse or antiviral antibodies generated in laboratory animals, usually mice, rabbits, or goats. The reactivity of the antiviral antibodies is usually to (1) a single epitope for monoclonal antibodies, (2) multiple epitopes on one viral protein for monospecific antisera, or (3) multiple epitopes on multiple viral proteins for polyclonal antisera. The type of primary antibody used in a test is based on the amount of viral protein expected to be in a lesion (sensitivity) and the cross-reactivity of the antibodies with nonviral antigens in the host or in unrelated pathogens (specificity). As a general rule, *monoclonal* antibodies are highly specific, but because they only recognize one epitope, and thus fewer antibodies are able to bind to each target molecule, they may be limited in sensitivity. In contrast, *polyclonal* antisera usually provide good sensitivity because they react with multiple epitopes on multiple viral proteins, but their polyclonal composition also make them more likely to be cross-reactive and have problems with specificity. Fluorescent label directly conjugated to the antiviral antibody makes the assay quick and easy to perform, but it contributes only one label unit per antibody and tends to decrease sensitivity. Indirect procedures use an anti-antibody with a fluorescent label, referred to as the *secondary antibody*, to detect primary antibody bound to the tissue section. The use of labeled anti-antibodies usually enhances sensitivity because multiple secondary antibodies will bind to each primary antibody, effectively amplifying the signal.

An important advantage of immunofluorescence is that it can be performed rapidly. Another advantage is that it demonstrates antigen in association with lesions or affected tissues, which is supporting information that suggests the virus is relevant to the lesion. The detection of viral proteins is usually indicative of active replication, as opposed to latent infections.

The major disadvantage with immunofluorescence assays of tissues is that acetone or methanol frozen sections have poor morphology, making visualization of lesions difficult. In addition, fluorescent assays on tissues can be technically challenging to read. Finally, most immunofluorescent assays have limited sensitivity and specificity compared with contemporary immunohistochemical methods.

Immunohistochemistry is very similar to immunofluorescence but, instead of fluorescent labels, uses enzymes that are conjugated to a secondary antibody for detection of bound primary antibody. The enzyme reacts with a colorimetric substrate to cause a colored precipitate that can be viewed with standard light microscopy (Fig. 11-4, C and *D*). Immunohistochemistry is usually performed on formalin-fixed, paraffin-embedded tissue sections, which have much better tissue morphology than frozen sections, and this allows better detection of lesions and correlation of lesions with viral antigen. Formalin-fixed, paraffin-embedded tissues are also easier to process, and the chromogenic reactions are technically easier to read than immunofluorescence. More importantly, significant advances in detection systems have greatly amplified the signal generated by each bound primary antibody. For example, many standard IHC assays now use a secondary antibody conjugated to biotin, then use an avidin molecule conjugated to more biotin and the enzyme. Because each molecule of avidin can bind multiple molecules of biotin, a complex of avidin and biotin with multiple enzyme molecules is formed for each primary antibody. Haines and Chelack[26] provide a detailed overview of IHC techniques (Fig. 11-5).

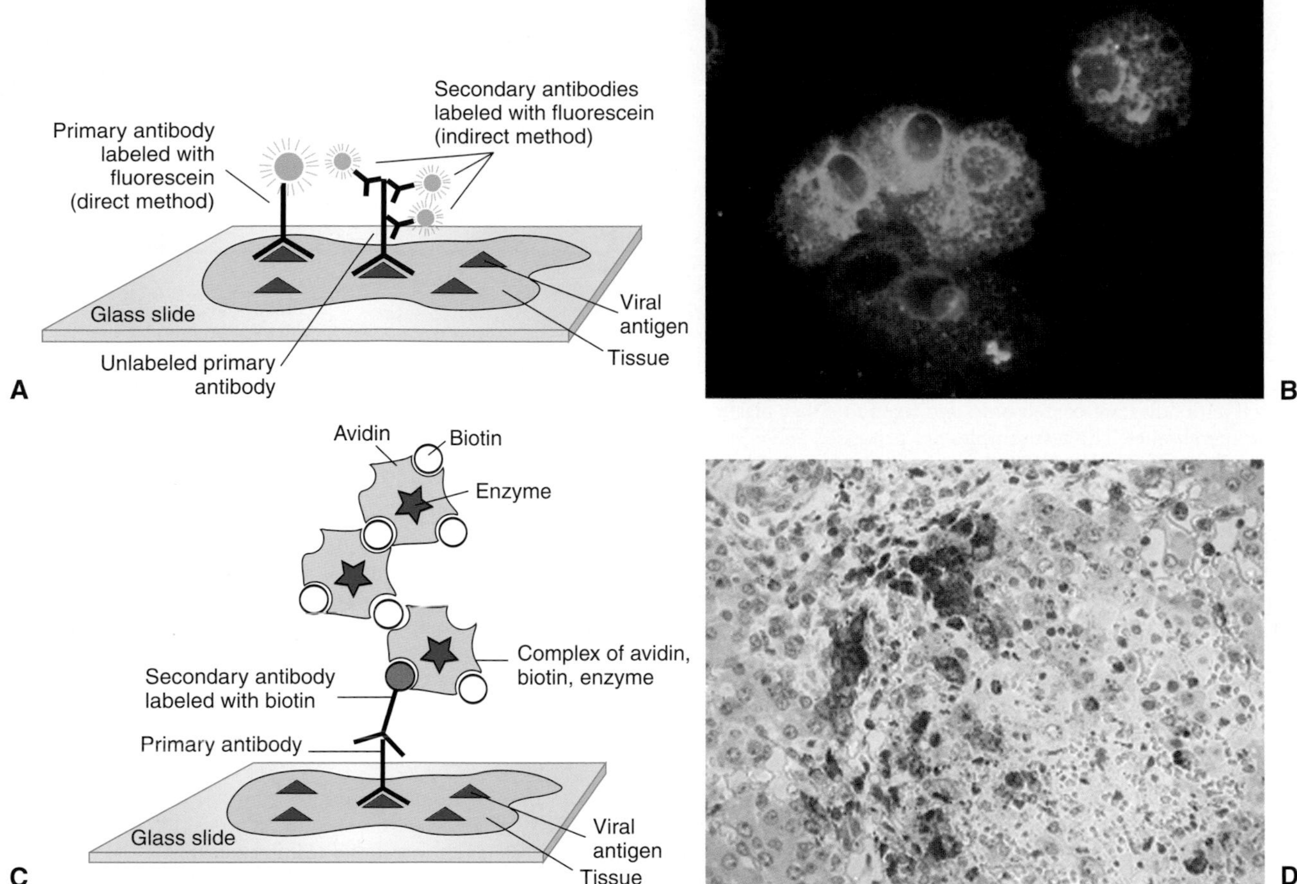

Fig. 11-4 Immunostaining methods for the detection of viral antigen in tissue samples mounted on glass slides. **A,** Immunofluorescence method, including direct and indirect protocols. **B,** Photomicrograph of equine alveolar macrophages infected with equine infectious anemia virus and detected by indirect immunofluorescence. The primary antibody is a mouse monoclonal antibody against equine infectious anemia virus; the secondary antibody is an anti-mouse IgG labeled with fluorescein. Viral antigen is indicated by the bright green fluorescence emitted from the fluorescein when the stained tissue section is observed under ultraviolet light. Magnification, 630×. **C,** Avidin-biotin immunohistochemical method. **D,** Photomicrograph of equine fetal liver from a case of equine herpesvirus type 1 abortion stained for equine herpesvirus type 1 antigen by immunohistochemistry. The primary antibody is rabbit polyclonal antisera against equine herpesvirus type 1; the secondary antibody is an anti-rabbit IgG labeled with biotin. The signal is amplified by complexes of avidin and biotin that also contain horseradish peroxidase that then reacts with a chromogen to form a red-colored precipitate. Viral antigen is indicated by the red-stained precipitate in the cytoplasm of infected cells in a necrotic focus in the liver. Magnification, 400×.

Other variations also may be used, but all are designed to amplify significantly the signal generated by each bound primary antibody.[27] The effect is to make the IHC tests very sensitive. Because of signal amplification, less primary and secondary antibodies are required for the assay, which decreases nonspecific binding and improves the test specificity. Test specificity has also been improved by recombinant protein technology, which allows greater control over the antigens used to produce the primary and secondary antibodies. Finally, in addition to being able to be performed quickly, the cost on a per-test basis is low compared to virus isolation. For these reasons, IHC is a common and effective method for the detection of a number of equine viral infections.[28-33]

In Situ Hybridization

In situ hybridization detects viral DNA or RNA in tissue sections with a labeled DNA or RNA probe that is complementary to, and thus binds to, the target viral sequence. In most other respects, in situ hybridization is very similar to IHC. In situ hybridization is typically performed on formalin-fixed, paraffin-embedded tissue sections. The DNA or RNA probes are usually labeled with a molecule such as digoxigenin, which is then detected by IHC as previously described, using a primary antibody that binds to the digoxigenin. In situ hybridization assays can be very sensitive and specific and have most of the same advantages as immunofluorescence and IHC. However, in situ hybridization is technically more

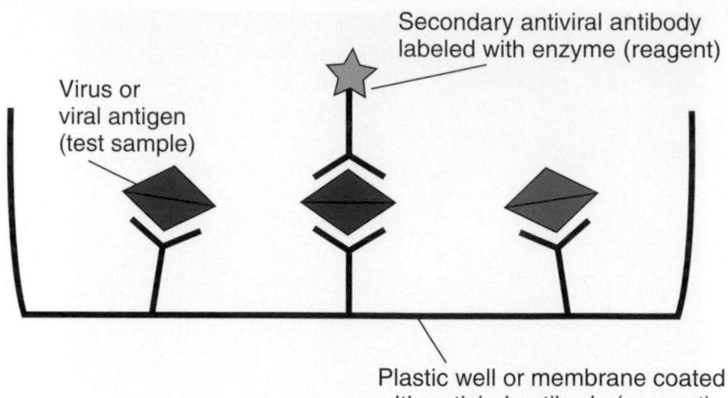

Fig. 11-5 ELISA method for the detection of antigen. Antiviral antibodies are coated onto and fixed to either plastic wells or membranes. The test samples are processed and added to the wells or membranes. If viral antigen is present, it is bound to and thus also fixed to the plastic or membrane. Following washes, another antiviral antibody labeled with an enzyme is added. This second antibody typically binds to a different viral antigen to prevent competitive inhibition of binding by the first antiviral antibody. Following washes to remove any unbound second antibody, a chromogen that reacts with the enzyme to form a color change is added. Color changes (i.e., positive reactions) can only occur if viral antigen is present in the sample.

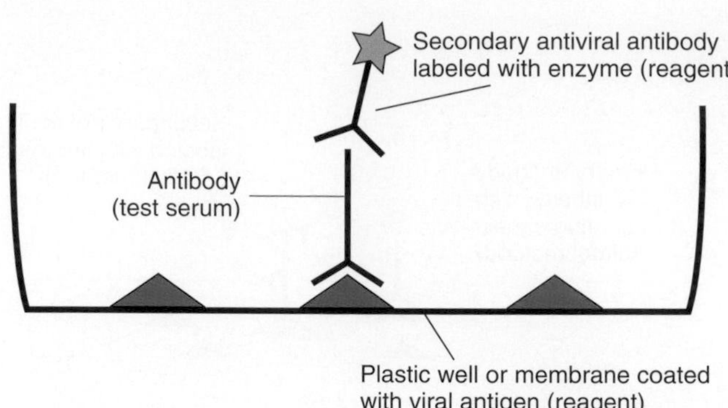

Fig. 11-6 ELISA method for the detection of antibody. Viral antigen is coated onto and fixed to either plastic wells or membranes. The test samples, generally serum, plasma, or whole blood, are added to the wells or membranes. If viral antibodies are present, they bind to and thus also become fixed to the plastic or membrane. Following washes, a secondary antibody against the isotype of the antibody being detected in the test sample (e.g., anti-equine IgG and/or IgM, and labeled with an enzyme) is added. Following washes to remove any unbound second antibody, a chromogen that reacts with the enzyme to form a color change is added. Color changes (i.e., positive reactions) can only occur if antiviral antibodies are present in the sample.

complex and relatively expensive to perform. Thus, although this method is used in research laboratories,[29,34,35] it is unlikely to be offered as a common diagnostic test.

DETECTION OF VIRUS IN CLINICAL SAMPLES

Antigen Detection by Enzyme-Linked Immunosorbent Assay

Rapid tests for viral antigen can be performed using ELISA formats that detect antigen. For this type of test, an antiviral antibody is immobilized on either a membrane or the well of a plastic plate. The test sample is then added, and if viral antigen is present, it is bound by the antibody and thus immobilized. Bound antigen is detected with a different antiviral antibody that binds to another part of the viral antigen and is visualized by generating a colorimetric reaction, as described for IHC (this antibody in effect becomes the primary antibody). The antigen ELISA method is illustrated in Figure 11-6. The most common equine viral diseases that can be diagnosed using antigen ELISA include intestinal rotavirus infection[36,37] and equine influenza.[5,38] In most cases, these tests are human kits that detect group-specific antigens that cross-react with the equine viruses. An antigen ELISA has also been described for the rapid diagnosis of African horse sickness.[39]

The key advantages of antigen ELISA tests is that they are fast, with results available in minutes. They generally are also easy to use, require minimal equipment, and are even amenable to being used stall-side. This last point is well illustrated by the widespread and successful use of human home pregnancy tests, which are antigen ELISA tests for detection of human chorionic gonadotropin in urine.

In general, although ELISA tests may have reasonable sensitivity and specificity, they are often lacking in both these parameters relative to other tests, and both false-positive and false-negative results should be expected.[5,40] Studies of the rotavirus test in cattle[40] and the influenza test in horses[5] have shown that different products may vary in sensitivity and specificity. Also, the influenza tests may detect viral antigen from horses given intranasal immunizations.[41]

To optimize the sensitivity of antigen ELISA tests, it is important to sample animals at times when viral shedding is maximal and keep in mind that this is likely to be early in the course of disease and may only be of short duration. The predictive value of tests should be maximized by careful selection of cases with appropriate supporting epidemiology, clinical signs, and laboratory evidence, and animals should not be shedding vaccine virus. Also, when the validity of the results is a concern, confirmatory tests should be considered.

Electron Microscopy

The direct visualization of viral particles in clinical specimens is another rapid test for the presumptive diagnosis of viral infection. In general, electron microscopy is of low sensitivity and requires large numbers of virions to be present for reliable detection. However, the characteristic ultrastructural appearance of different viruses gives this test good specificity for diagnosis to the level of virus family. Diagnostic electron microscopy is used routinely for diagnosis of viral enteric diseases, such as rotavirus,[36,37] in which animals with clinical disease tend to shed large amounts of virus. Electron microscopy is also used occasionally to detect unusual viral infections[42] or to support other laboratory findings.[43] Electron microscopy is also used in the laboratory as a rapid method for the presumptive identification of cell culture isolates[44,45] and can be particularly useful for selecting PCR primers that bind to family-specific or genus-specific conserved regions for genetic sequence analysis.

SEROLOGY

Testing for the presence of antiviral antibodies in serum or plasma is a classic method for the indirect detection of viral infections. Despite some limitations with interpretation, serology can still be a reliable and useful diagnostic tool. One major advantage is that collection of serum from horses is simple and relatively noninvasive, can be obtained antemortem, and lends itself to testing large numbers of animals. Serology is particularly useful for detecting infections in which virus is not easily detected by other means, as with West Nile virus (WNV),[46] EIA, and eastern equine encephalitis (EEE) virus.

Over the years, a wide variety of testing methods have been used to detect antiviral antibodies, including virus neutralization (VN), agar gel immunodiffusion (AGID) and other immunodiffusion tests, hemagglutination inhibition (HAI), indirect immunofluorescence (IFA), complement fixation (CF), Western blot (WB), radioimmunoassay (RIA), and most recently ELISA and its variants. Despite the wide array of testing formats, all these tests use some type of viral antigen as a reagent to capture antibody, if present, from a test serum sample, and then use some type of detection system to indicate that antibody has bound to the antigen. These tests can vary widely in their sensitivity, specificity, complexity, and cost. The two most common serologic test formats for equine viral diseases are the VN and ELISA tests, and only these are discussed in detail here.

Virus Neutralization

The VN test detects antibodies capable of neutralizing the infectivity of the virus. Serial dilutions of serum are mixed with a reference strain of viable virus (in this case the antigen) and incubated to allow any antibody present to bind and neutralize the virus, and then dilutions are inoculated onto cells. The presence or absence of viral growth is observed. The highest dilution (i.e., the least amount of antibody) that neutralizes infectivity is the titer. A variant of the VN test is the *plaque reduction neutralization* (PRN) test. This test is sometimes used for viruses that form distinct plaques of CPE in cell cultures, with each plaque representing a single infectious unit. The end point is defined as the dilution of serum that reduces the number of plaques by some statistically significant level (often set at >50%-90%).

Advantages of the VN or PRN tests are that they are usually highly sensitive and very specific. The key disadvantages are that these tests require living cell cultures, production and maintenance of titered virus stocks, and highly trained personnel, and they are labor intensive. Thus these tests tend to be costly and potentially cumbersome. They also require working with viable virus, which may present a laboratory hazard when testing for viruses that also infect humans.

Enzyme-Linked Immunosorbent Assay

One of the most common serologic tests currently offered is ELISA. The general principle of ELISA is that the viral antigen is bound to either a well in a plastic plate or a membrane. The test serum sample is added, and any antibody against the antigen becomes bound to the plate or membrane. After washing away unbound antibody, a secondary antibody against antibody (e.g., anti-equine IgG or IgM) conjugated to an enzyme (e.g., horseradish peroxidase) is added and will bind to any equine antibodies still present. This complex is visualized by the addition of a colorimetric substrate that reacts with the enzyme to create a visible color change. The color change is compared to controls either visually or spectrophotometrically. The antibody ELISA method is illustrated in Figure 11-6.

The primary advantages of ELISA are that it is relatively rapid and easy to perform and can be quite sensitive and specific. The sensitivity and specificity of the assay can also be manipulated by selection of antigens[48,49] and use of secondary antibodies selective for either immunoglobulin G (IgG) or immunoglobulin M (IgM).[50,51] One of the major disadvantages of ELISA is that the results are often simply reported as positive or negative, and not quantitatively to detect changes in titer. As discussed next, for diseases in which the background seroprevalence is high, fourfold or greater changes in titer are necessary to determine recent exposure. In these cases the ELISA titer must be determined for acute and convalescent sera to demonstrate recent exposure.[52-55]

Serologic Interpretation

Regardless of the test format used, there are some common themes for interpretation of serologic results. This is related in part to the biology of the disease and in part to the sensitivity and specificity of the assay. Only in selected diseases is a single positive or negative antibody result informative. A single positive or negative result is diagnostic only for persistent infections in which a positive test is synonymous with infection, such as EIA.[56] Conversely, a negative test indicates there is no infection, although the possibility remains that an animal in the early stages of infection may not yet have seroconverted. Thus, if there is a high index of suspicion that an animal is infected, a retest at a later time will be indicated. For diseases such as equine viral arteritis, in which only a proportion of animals are persistently infected (e.g., approximately 30%-60% of infected stallions), a seronegative result is good evidence for lack of infection. However, a positive test may or may not indicate persistent infection and would be an indication for additional testing, such as virus isolation.[57]

Because immunoglobulin M (IgM) is the initial antibody isotype formed transiently in a primary immune response, single antiviral IgM antibodies by ELISA may be used as a marker for acute infection and thus recent exposure,[51,52,58-60] although some individuals may have persistent IgM titers.[52] Single increased titers are also sometimes correlated to acute infection, as in EHV-1 infections. Although it is likely that either past vaccination or infection leads to more modest titers (e.g., <1:128), the natural variation in host immune responses can easily lead to overinterpretation of single titers. This type of result should at best be considered suggestive and add to the index of suspicion. Single titers may also be useful in samples from sites where no antibody should be present, except through local infection and production, such as in cerebrospinal fluid (CSF) for neurologic infections. However, the presence of serum antibody caused by leakage across the blood-brain barrier associated with inflammation or necrosis needs to be ruled out by measuring albumin quotients and IgG indices as indicators of blood contamination.[50,61]

For most viral infections, reliable detection of acute infection (i.e., recent exposure) requires demonstrating a fourfold or greater increase in titer between acute and convalescent serum samples. This applies to many of the common equine viral diseases in which there is a high background seroprevalence either from previous natural infections or from vaccination. Because most serologic tests do not distinguish vaccination and natural titers, accurate vaccination histories are also necessary to interpret serologic findings. One significant recent exception is the IgM ELISA test for WNV in which titers greater than 1:400 indicate natural infection.[59] A transient (<1 week) reaction can be seen in low numbers of horses after the first injection of WNV vaccine (Long, personal communication). Fourfold decreases may also indicate recent exposure.[52] However, decreasing titers as an indicator of recent infection are often unreliable because most viruses lead to titers that persist for months to years, and antibody decay curves are more prolonged and much less predictable than antibody production curves.

Another important concept regarding interpretation of serology is the difference in utility of screening tests versus confirmatory tests (see Chapter 65). No test is 100% sensitive and specific, and designing tests to achieve 100% sensitivity will invariably lead to loss of specificity and false-positive results; conversely, tests that have 100% specificity will lose sensitivity and are likely to have false-negative results.[62] These parameters are often set intentionally, depending on the disease in question. To test for diseases in which infected animals should not be missed, the primary serologic test will be a screening test that has very high sensitivity and that is expected to lead to false-positive results. The predictive value of a positive (or negative) test result is also a function of the prevalence of the disease in the population being tested.[62] For example, with a low-prevalence disease, there is a high statistical probability that positive results are false and that negative results are true. Therefore, positive results obtained from screening tests should be verified by a confirmatory test, which is usually a test with higher specificity and lower sensitivity. It is inappropriate to take action based on a positive test result of a screening test without confirmation, especially for a low-prevalence disease.

The sensitivity and specificity of antibody testing has been enhanced by the use of recombinant viral proteins or peptides as antigens in serologic tests. One example is testing for EIA virus, in which replacement of whole-virus antigen preparations with recombinant viral proteins has improved the sensitivity and specificity of the AGID (Coggin's) and ELISA tests.[63,64] The improvement in specificity is especially important because EIA in the United States is now a low-prevalence disease.

References

See the CD-ROM for a list of references linked to the abstract in PubMed.

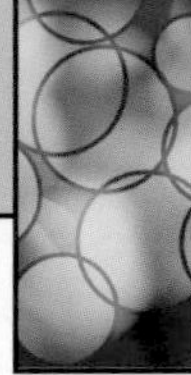

CHAPTER • 12

Equine Influenza Infection

Gabriele A. Landolt, Hugh G. G. Townsend, and D. Paul Lunn

ETIOLOGY

Influenza A viruses are members of the family *Orthomyxoviridae*, which contains enveloped viruses with segmented, single-stranded, negative-sense ribonucleic acid (RNA) genomes (Fig. 12-1). The *Orthomyxoviridae* comprise five genera: influenza A, B, and C viruses; thogotovirus; and isavirus. Influenza A viruses can be distinguished from type B and C based on the antigenic nature of their *nucleoprotein* (NP) and *matrix* (M) proteins. In contrast to influenza A viruses, which can be isolated from a wide variety of species (including horses), influenza B viruses appear to infect primarily humans. Influenza C has been isolated mostly from humans, although they have also been shown to infect pigs and dogs.[1-3] Whereas influenza A and B contain eight separate segments of single-stranded RNA, influenza C viruses possess only seven.[4]

The virions of influenza A include a host cell–derived lipid envelope, are 80 to 120 nm in diameter, and if propagated in eggs or tissue culture, have a fairly regular spherical appearance. In contrast, on initial isolation from humans or animals, influenza A viruses exhibit pleomorphism.[4] Embedded in the lipid envelope are the virus-encoded glycoproteins *hemagglutinin* (HA) and *neuraminidase* (NA), forming about 500 spikes radiating outward,[5,6] and the integral *M2 protein*, which functions as an ion channel. The HA serves as the viral receptor–binding protein and is responsible for fusion between the virion envelope and the host cell. The receptor-binding site is located on the globular head portion of the molecule and forms a pocket that is inaccessible to antibodies. Thus the amino acid residues creating the pocket (Tyr-98, Trp-153, His-183, Glu-190, Leu-194) are largely conserved among viruses.[6-9]

The HA is the major target of the host immune response, and there are five antigenic sites on the HA molecule, covering much of the surface of the globular head portion. Immune pressure is the driving force in the selection of mutants with amino acid substitutions in these antigenic sites, allowing the mutant virus to escape neutralizing antibodies *(antigenic drift)*.

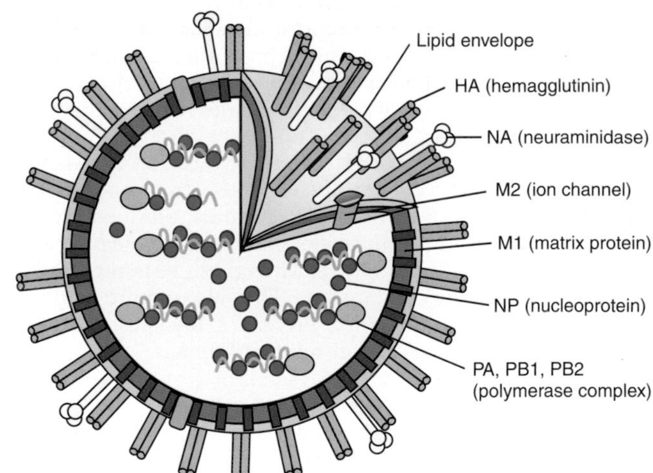

Fig. 12-1 Schematic diagram of structural components of influenza A virus. Three integral membrane proteins—hemagglutinin *(HA)*, neuraminidase *(NA)*, and the ion channel protein *(M2)*—are embedded in the lipid envelope of the virion. The matrix protein *(M1)* is thought to underlie the lipid envelope. Associated with the viral ribonucleic acid (vRNA) is the viral polymerase complex, consisting of PA, PB1, and PB2. The viral nucleoprotein *(NP)* encapsidates the vRNA segments.

The NA is the second large surface glycoprotein. It is a type II integral membrane glycoprotein[5,10] and is responsible for the cleavage of the α-ketosidic linkage between a sialic acid molecule and an adjacent sugar D-galactose or D-galactosamine.[11] Biologically, NA facilitates the mobility of the influenza virus virion by removing sialic acid residues from viral glycoproteins and infected cells, therefore assisting in the release of the budding virus particles.[12-14] In addition to its function during release of newly formed virus particles, it has long been suspected that NA also plays a role during influenza virus entry.[4,15,16] As with the HA, the NA is a major antigenic determinant and undergoes, at least partly in response to host immune pressure, substantial antigenic variation.

The most abundant virion protein is the *viral matrix protein* (M1). It is thought to underlie the envelope, serves as the major structural protein of the virion, and associates with the *ribonucleoprotein* (RNP) complexes of the virus. The eight separate RNPs of influenza A have the appearance of flexible rods[17] and are believed to consist of a segment of RNA loosely encapsidated by several NP molecules. Located at the end of each RNP are the three viral polymerase proteins PB1, PB2, and PA. The segmented nature of the viral genome is a critically important feature of the influenza A virus structure. In the event that cells are infected with two (or more) different viruses, the exchange of RNA segments between the viruses allows the generation of progeny viruses containing novel combinations of genes. This phenomenon is referred to as *genetic reassortment*[18,19] (Fig. 12-2). In theory, random incorporation of RNA segments could potentially lead to the creation of 254 new gene combinations from two parental viruses, although the recent identification of selective packaging signals within the 3′ and 5′ coding regions of the influenza virus genes suggests that the incorporation of RNA segments into the virion is only partially random.[20]

Influenza A viruses can be divided into subtypes based on antigenic properties of their HA and NA envelope glycoproteins. To date, sixteen HA subtypes and nine NA subtypes have been recognized. All the HA and NA subtypes have been recovered from aquatic birds.[2,21-24] These birds play a particularly important role in influenza epidemiology because they provide a vast global reservoir of viruses of all subtypes. Phylogenetic analyses have indicated that viruses from aquatic birds were the ancestral source of the current lineages of mammalian viruses.[21,25-27] In contrast, only a limited number of subtypes of influenza viruses have been associated with infection of mammalian species. In humans, only viruses of H1, H2, H3, N1, and N2 subtypes have circulated widely in the population[2,26,27]; only H1, H3, N1, and N2 subtypes have been consistently isolated from pigs[28-30]; and apart from occasional reports of horses infected with viruses of subtypes H1N1, H2N2, and H3N2 (usually in association with human infections),[31] equine influenza infections have been restricted to viruses of H7N7 (A/equine/1) and H3N8 (A/equine/2) subtypes.[32-35]

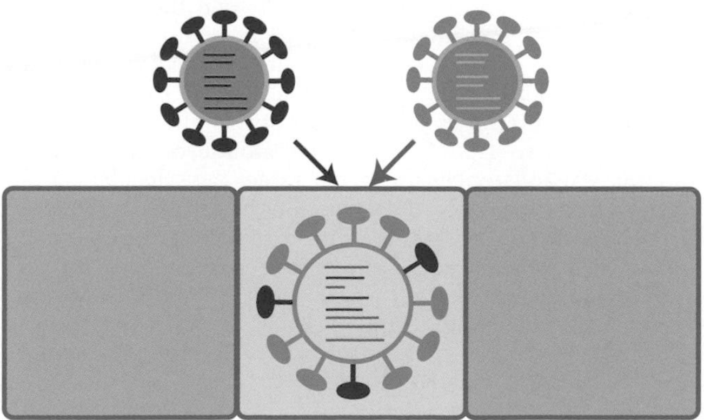

Fig. 12-2 Schematic diagram illustrating genetic reassortment. In the event that cells are infected with two (or more) different viruses, the exchange of RNA segments between the viruses allows the generation of progeny viruses containing novel combinations of genes. In theory, random incorporation of RNA segments could lead to the creation of 254 new gene combinations from two parental viruses.

Outbreaks of a disease resembling influenza have been reported as early as 1751, although the etiologic agent was not isolated until 1956.[32,33] The virus, designated A/Equine/1/Prague/56, was isolated during an outbreak of influenza in Czechoslovakia and was characterized as H7N7.[36] H7N7 influenza viruses have not been detected in the horse population since the late 1970s.[21,37,38] However, large-scale serologic surveillance demonstrated that these viruses may still be circulating at low levels in the equine population of Central Asia[27] and Eastern Europe.[32,39]

In contrast, equine-2 influenza viruses, first isolated in the United States in 1963 (A/equine/2/Miami/1/63), continue to circulate in large parts of the world, except Australia, New Zealand, and Iceland.[37,40,41] Despite intensive vaccination programs, equine H3N8 influenza infections have remained a serious health and economic problem throughout the world. In the late 1980s, severe widespread influenza outbreaks were observed in horses in South Africa,[42] in India,[43] and in the People's Republic of China,[44,45] where equine influenza viruses were not known to be circulating. The causative agent of the South African outbreak was identified as an H3N8 virus, which was most likely introduced by importation of infected horses from the United States or Europe.[37,46] The outbreaks in the People's Republic of China have been caused by both conventional strains of equine H3N8 virus and viruses that were antigenically and genetically distinguishable from other circulating equine H3N8 viruses. Phylogenetic analysis of the virus causing the 1989 epidemic showed that this virus had evolved independent of the existing equine lineage. Its genetic features were of recent avian lineage, indicating that this virus had probably spread directly to horses from the avian reservoir without genetic reassortment.[44]

Since the early to middle 1980s, the equine H3N8 influenza viruses have diverged into two distinct evolutionary lineages, European and American.* Although the circulation of both lineages initially centered largely on the geographic origin,[7] both lineages now appear to be co-circulating in Europe,[32,37,40,41,49] and to a lesser extent in the United States.[37,40,41] In the Western Hemisphere, continued genetic divergence appears to have resulted in the formation of three American-like lineages with distinct antigenic characteristics; a South American lineage, a Kentucky lineage, and a Florida lineage.[40] Although the antigenic drift of H3N8 equine influenza viruses is significant in terms of immunization, when compared to human influenza viruses, equine stains have demonstrated relatively little genetic diversion. Sequence comparisons between the prototype reference stains and more recent H3N8 influenza A virus isolates revealed 70% to 90% genetic homology.[50,51]

EPIDEMIOLOGY

Influenza is the most frequently diagnosed and economically important cause of viral respiratory disease of the horse.[52,53,54] Since first diagnosed during an epidemic of respiratory disease

*References 7, 27, 40, 41, 47, 48.

in Eastern Europe in 1956,[55] outbreaks of this disease have been observed to occur regularly throughout the world. New Zealand, Australia, and Iceland may be the only countries in the world where outbreaks of the disease have not occurred.

Experimentally, all ages and breeds of equidae may be infected with the virus.[56] Natural disease occurs in individual foals,[56-58] but only one outbreak of influenza in young foals (3-6 months of age) has been reported to date.[57] Longitudinal studies of North American racehorse populations, before the availability of highly efficacious vaccines, showed that the highest incidence of disease was observed in 2- and 3-year-old horses,[52,59] likely caused by commingling of animals that lacked previous exposure to viral antigen.[60]

In addition to age and commingling of susceptible animals, influenza-specific serum antibody concentration is a highly specific correlate of protection against infection and disease. Animals with high concentrations of homologous antibody are almost always protected against experimental challenge.[61-65] During a 3-year study of a large population of racehorses, animals with high concentrations of serum antibody had 10 to 40 times lower odds of developing disease than did horses with no detectable antibody.[59] Horses exposed to viral antigen within the past 6 to 12 months through natural infection[66] or administration of a potent killed vaccine[67] or an intranasal, temperature-sensitive, modified live vaccine[68] may show evidence of reduced clinical signs and decreased viral shedding in the presence of little or no detectable antibody.

Equine influenza has a short incubation period. Experimentally infected animals experience fever and begin to shed large quantities of virus in nasal secretions within 48 hours of infection.[68-71] Secondary bacterial infections of the respiratory tract, largely resulting from proliferation of β-hemolytic streptococci, are routinely observed[60,72-75] and are considered important in the pathogenesis of bacterial pneumonia of horses.[76-78] Influenza morbidity rates within highly susceptible groups of horses may be as high as 60% to 90%.[79-81] Mortality rates are usually less than 1%,[82] although a 1998 outbreak caused by a newly emergent strain of the virus in China was associated with a mortality rate of 20% in some herds.[83] Morbidity rates within large groups of horses with varying degrees of previous exposure to influenza antigen may range from 20% to 37%.[54,84] Outbreaks of equine influenza may occur at any time of the year, although seasonal outbreaks have been reported,[54,65] probably related to the yearly convergence of component causes (risk factors) resulting in disease at regular intervals within individual sites or geographic locations.

After natural infection, ponies were reported to be resistant to infection for 32 weeks, with partial clinical protection persisting for more than 1 year.[66] Similar data are not available for horses, although a longitudinal study of a large population of racehorses showed that horses present during an outbreak of respiratory disease in one season were significantly less likely to show clinical signs of disease during an outbreak in the following year.[59] Efficacious vaccines against equine influenza are available, and their widespread use is having a significant impact on the epidemiology of the disease. Although vaccination does not generally provide sterile immunity or full protection against clinical disease for more than a few months, the vaccination of populations of horses is reducing the frequency of disease outbreaks or the frequency and severity of clinical signs when outbreaks occur among vaccinated animals.[65,73,85-88]

Outbreaks of equine influenza occur most often when susceptible animals are congregated and kept in close contact with each other (e.g., racetracks, horse shows, sales yards, airplanes). Human studies show that spread is through direct-contact transmission with infected subjects, droplet transmission (contagious droplets greater than 10 μm and capable of being projected over moderate distances by coughing), and airborne transmission (infectious droplets less than 5 μm, capable of wide dissemination in confined environments and of reaching the lower respiratory tract of susceptible individuals).[89] No experimental studies have shown that transmission occurs through fomites, although human epidemiologic studies provide indirect evidence.[90,91] Among horses, rapid and effective spread is enhanced by a 2-day incubation period, high concentrations of virus in nasal secretions, an explosive cough, the practice of housing horses in confined spaces, and possibly, the ability of the virus to survive in wet environments (e.g., water bowls) for 72 hours and on dry surfaces (e.g., clothing, grooming equipment, vehicles, feed) for 48 hours.[91]

Anecdotal evidence suggests that disease spreads very quickly in small groups of confined animals and that all susceptible horses may become infected within 2 to 3 days. However, outbreaks occurring in large groups or populations, comprised of animals with varying histories of exposure and immunity, may last for 3 to 4 weeks,[54] thus providing at least some opportunity to institute procedures to limit the extent and severity of such outbreaks.

Recent studies show that after experimental infection, horses typically shed virus for 6 to 7 days.[68-71] Although a carrier state does not occur, subclinical infections and viral shedding are probably common, particularly after infection of partially immune animals. Partial immunity is likely in animals that have not been recently exposed or vaccinated or may be caused by mismatching of vaccine strains and circulating field virus.[73,87,92] These animals are probably important in the spread of the disease within and between groups of horses[93-95] and, along with fomites,[96-98] provide a rational explanation for disease outbreaks among horses that have not experienced direct exposure to clinically diseased animals. The international transport of subclinically affected horses has been the suspected cause of many reported outbreaks of the disease in countries or regions with large numbers of susceptible animals.[96]

PATHOGENESIS

Influenza A viruses replicate and induce pathologic changes throughout the entire respiratory tract, with the most significant pathology present in the lower respiratory tract.[2] The primary targets of influenza A viruses in mammalian species are the airway epithelial cells. After inhalation of the aerosolized virus, infection is initiated by binding of the influenza virus HA to sialic acid residues (*N*-acetylneuraminic or *N*-glycolneuraminic sialyloligosaccharides) on target cells located in the upper respiratory tract. However, for the virus to gain access to the cellular receptors, the virion first has to penetrate a mucus layer that forms a protective barrier over the cell surface. In this regard, it is thought that the viral NA promotes virus access to respiratory epithelial cells by destroying mucous glycoproteins[15] and removing decoy receptors present on mucins, cilia, and cellular glycocalix.[16]

After viral attachment, the virion is taken up into the cell through receptor-mediated endocytosis. After internalization and acidification of the endosomal compartment, the HA undergoes an irreversible conformational change,[99,100] which leads to the insertion of the hydrophobic fusion peptide into the endosomal membrane and ultimately to the fusion of the viral and cellular membranes. After membrane fusion and release of the RNPs into the cell's cytoplasm, the RNPs are actively transported into the nucleus through nuclear pores,[101] where messenger RNA (mRNA) synthesis is initiated.

During virus replication, the virus-encoded *nonstructural protein* (NS1) shuts off cellular protein synthesis by inhibiting the maturation of cellular mRNAs. NS1 is a multifunctional protein, and apart from inhibiting both polyadenylation and splicing of cellular pre-mRNAs, it also counteracts interferon (IFN)–dependent and IFN-independent antiviral responses.[102-104] This occurs by binding to the dsRNA-binding region of *protein kinase, RNA activated* (PKR), thus blocking its activation,[105] and by inhibiting the activation of IFN regulatory factor 3[106] and nuclear factor kappa B (NF-κB).[107,108]

The switch from mRNA synthesis to complementary RNA (cRNA) and viral RNA (vRNA) synthesis is believed to be triggered by an increased concentration of free NP.[109] Later in infection, the main translation products are M1, HA, and NA. These are synthesized on membrane-bound proteins and transported across the membrane of the endoplasmic reticulum (ER) by means of a *signal recognition particle* (SRP).[110,111] During transport through the ER, the proteins undergo a stepwise conformational maturation and folding, and additional processing may occur in the Golgi complex. In polarized epithelial cells, influenza viruses assemble and bud from the apical surface of the cells.[103,112,113] Interaction between the cytoplasmic tails of the HA and NA proteins and the internal proteins (most likely M1) are thought to be the main driving force behind the formation of the budding particles.[114,115] By removing carbohydrate chains from the virion and the cell surface, NA enzymatic activity is thought to be required to release the newly formed influenza virus virions completely from the cell.[12-14]

The virus spreads quickly throughout the respiratory tract, damaging the respiratory epithelial cells, particularly in the trachea and bronchial tree.[49,116] Virus replication leads to cell death, largely through virus-induced apoptosis,[117-119] and subsequent desquamation and denudation of respiratory epithelial cells. Histologic evaluation of infected respiratory epithelium reveals vacuolization and swelling of the columnar ciliated cells, accompanied by clumping and subsequent loss of cilia.[120] Consequently, tracheal mucociliary clearance is impaired, predisposing affected animals to the development of secondary bacterial infections.[34,116,121,122] Within 1 day after the onset of clinical signs, focal erosions of the respiratory cells down to the basal layer are evident. Viral antigen can be demonstrated predominantly in the respiratory epithelial cells and mononuclear cells and only rarely in the basal cell layer.[123] The disruption of the superficial cell layers allows opportunistic bacteria to invade the respiratory epithelium of both the upper and the lower respiratory tract, leading to bacterial bronchopneumonia and other complications.[2,49,123] Submucosal edema and hyperemia occur with peribronchial and peribronchiolar infiltration by neutrophils and mononuclear cells.[2,37,120] About 3 to 5 days after onset of illness, regeneration of the epithelium begins, characterized by the appearance of mitotic figures in the basal cell layer.[2] In uncomplicated cases, complete resolution of the epithelial damage takes a minimum of 3 weeks.[122,124]

Complications of equine influenza virus infections include secondary bacterial pneumonia, myositis, myocarditis, and limb edema; in rare cases, signs of encephalitis may be observed.[35,121,123] The determinants of organ tropism and virulence of influenza A viruses are polygenic, although the HA plays a pivotal role. The final processing step in HA maturation is the proteolytic cleavage of the HA precursor form (HA0) into two disulfide-linked subunits (HA1 and HA2).[125] This cleavage step is accomplished by host proteases, and because uncleaved HA cannot undergo the low-pH–induced conformational change necessary for membrane fusion, it is a prerequisite for the virus to be infectious.[126,127] The HA of most influenza A viruses (including equine influenza viruses) are usually cleaved only by a limited number of organ-specific trypsin-like proteases (e.g., tryptase Clara in the respiratory tract), so that the viruses cause only localized infections. In contrast, HAs of highly virulent influenza strains (e.g., highly pathogenic avian influenza viruses) are cleaved in a broad range of different host cells and are therefore capable of causing severe systemic infections. Thus, HA cleavability is one of the major determinants of influenza A virus tissue tropism.[128-131] In horses, however, attempts at virus recovery from the heart or brains of affected animals have been unsuccessful, and myocardial dysfunction may be caused by other mechanisms, such as an increase in the expression of inflammatory mediators (e.g., nitric oxide).[132] Alternatively, myocardial dysfunction may be caused by viral products, such as the lipid envelope.[49,121]

Finally, it has been speculated that influenza infection might predispose horses to the development of chronic obstructive pulmonary disease (COPD) and exercise-induced pulmonary hemorrhage.[35,49,121]

CLINICAL FINDINGS

Clinical signs of influenza virus infection were extensively described after its first discovery,[133] and the same clinical findings are still observed almost 40 years later. Signs of disease are typically seen 48 hours, and sometimes as early as 24 hours, after exposure to infected horses or experimental infection by intranasal instillation of virus. Pyrexia is typically present first, with temperatures sometimes exceeding 106° F (41.1° C), peaking at 48 to 96 hours after infection. A second peak of pyrexia may be observed at about the seventh day after infection. Nasal discharge follows, initially serous (Fig. 12-3), but typically becoming mucopurulent by 72 to 96 hours after infection. Coughing, sometimes paroxysmal, typically develops during this same period. Retropharyngeal lymphadenopathy is a variable but common finding, as is tachypnea. Most affected horses become anorexic at the time of the initial pyrexia, although this typically resolves in 1 to 2 days.

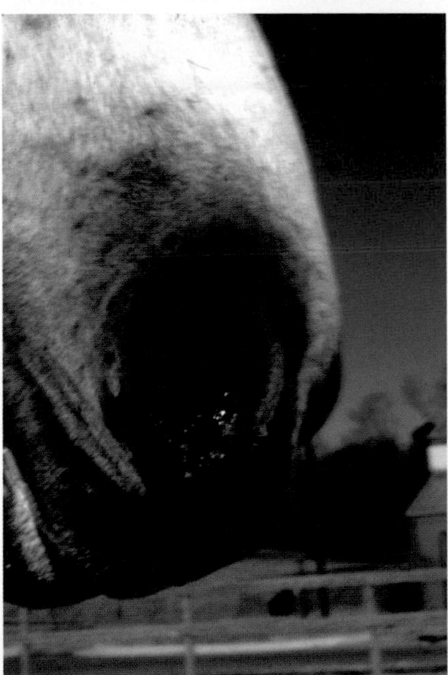

Fig. 12-3 Serous nasal discharge typical of horse with acute influenza virus infection. (Courtesy Dr. John Barneso.)

Weight loss is well documented after influenza virus infection. Clinical signs typically resolve in 7 to 14 days in uncomplicated cases, although coughing may persist for 21 days. In severe infections, lung sounds become increased in amplitude, with adventitial sounds sometimes detected. Ultrasonographic imaging of the thorax has been used to demonstrate pulmonary consolidation; pneumonia is a common sequela between 7 and 14 days after infection.[134] Persistent respiratory disease can occur beyond 14 days after infection and is thought to be the result of secondary bacterial infection.

Morbidity can approach 100% in outbreaks in susceptible populations. Mortality is typically low, although neonatal infection can be fatal,[58] resulting in severe bronchial and interstitial pneumonia. The effects of influenza virus infection in donkeys and mules is typically more severe than in horses and can result in mortality.[135] It is also important to recognize that subclinical disease with viral shedding may be common in previously vaccinated horses and represents an important source of contagion.[135] The effects of influenza virus infection can be significantly exacerbated by even moderate exercise, resulting in increased weight loss and other clinical signs.[134]

IMMUNITY

Equine influenza virus infection generates a broad range of adaptive immune responses in systemic and mucosal compartments,[71] and infection also stimulates important innate immune system responses.[136] In the horse, many investigators have demonstrated that antibody responses can be strongly associated with protection. A protective immune response, such as that following infection, is characterized by induction of influenza virus–specific immunoglobulin G isotype a and b (IgGa, IgGb) and immunoglobulin A (IgA) antibodies in both the circulation and the nasopharyngeal secretions, with the IgG isotype responses predominating in the circulation and IgA in the respiratory tract.[71,137,138]

Nasal IgA is an important mediator of protective immunity to influenza virus infection in other species,[139,140] through neutralization of viral particles at the respiratory epithelium and in the intracellular compartment.[141-143] Nasal IgA responses are a characteristic of the protective immunity that follows equine influenza infection,[137,138] and influenza virus–specific IgA-producing B lymphocytes have been detected in mucosal lamina propria and lymph nodes draining the nasopharynx of the horse.[71] Virus-specific IgG antibodies can also contribute to immune exclusion at the respiratory epithelium in a mouse model, although the lack of specialized mechanisms for transporting IgG to the respiratory surface means that its role is less important.[144] In the horse, there is evidence for local production of influenza virus–specific IgGa and IgGb at respiratory mucosal surfaces after infection,[71,145] and indirect evidence that virus-specific nasal IgGb antibody responses can contribute to a reduction in nasal shedding of influenza virus.[146] However, IgG antibody responses tend to be more short-lived in equine respiratory secretions than IgA responses.[147,148]

In the circulation, IgGa and IgGb are thought to be the principal protective IgG subisotype responses to influenza virus,[71,138] whereas IgG(T) responses are not associated with protection.[138] Circulating antibody has been measured in a number of ways in horses, including conventional hemagglutination inhibition (HI) assays, single radial hemolysis (SRH) assays, virus neutralization assays, and enzyme-linked immunosorbent assay (ELISA).[138,149] Of these techniques, SRH and ELISA may have the greatest sensitivity and utility, and it appears that SRH results correlate closely with IgGb ELISA results (Lunn and Townsend, unpublished data). Much attention has focused on the correlation between levels of circulating antibody measured by SRH tests and protection from influenza virus infection.[65] This tool has proved very useful, and SRH responses are often used to measure vaccination effect and predict protection. However, after circulating antibody responses to a prior influenza virus infection have waned, horses can remain protected against a further challenge.[66] In addition, circulating antibody responses measured by SRH to a cold-adapted, modified live influenza vaccine are almost undetectable, although this vaccine provides long-lasting protection from challenge infection.[68,150] Taken together, these observations illustrate that although circulating antibody responses are an important predictor of protection against influenza virus protection, a lack of antibody does not invariably predict susceptibility.

The role of cellular effectors in resistance to equine influenza virus infection is less well investigated. Virus-specific cytotoxic T lymphocytes (CTLs) are important for protection from influenza virus infection,[151,152] and there is a single description of the measurement of MHC-restricted CTL responses to equine influenza virus.[153] The lack of other CTL studies reflects the difficulty in detecting this equine immune response to influenza virus using available methods. Currently, influenza virus–specific lymphoproliferative responses and IFN-γ gene expression may be the best available measures of virus-specific cellular immune responses in the horse. Production of IFN-γ is an indicator of T-helper 1 (Th1) cell–mediated immunity and can contribute to immunologic protection of humans from influenza virus infection and disease.[140] Furthermore, several studies indicate an association between IFN-γ production and the concomitant generation of antigen-specific CTL responses.[154,155] A number of studies have demonstrated the development of equine IFN-γ responses to influenza virus consequent to either infection or vaccination.[71,156,157] Similarly, influenza virus–specific lymphoproliferative responses have also been associated with protective immunity.[71,145,157]

The importance of hemagglutinin (HA)–specific immune responses in protection from influenza virus infection is well known, and vaccination studies in horses using deoxyribonucleic acid (DNA) vaccination and recombinant vaccines expressing the HA gene all confirm the importance of the HA antigen for protection.[157-159] Recent studies using modified vaccinia Ankara vector vaccines have demonstrated that nucleoprotein (NP)–specific equine immune responses can also result in reduced clinical disease after challenge infection, although the degree of protection was inferior to that induced by HA vaccination.[157] Influenza virus NP is an internal viral structural protein, and therefore NP-specific antibodies are not capable of virus neutralization and do not control virus shedding in the horse[157] or other species.[160] NP typically serves as an important target antigen for cellular immune responses and can elicit cross-protective immunity to heterologous strains of influenza virus.[161] In the equine vaccination studies conducted to date, NP-specific immune responses included both lymphoproliferative and IFN-γ responses, and it is possible that NP-specific immune responses could make a significant contribution to equine immunity to influenza virus infection.

DIAGNOSIS

In a group of susceptible horses, a presumptive diagnosis of influenza virus infection can be made based on the rapid spread of an acute, febrile respiratory disease characterized by a dry, hacking cough.[49] However, laboratory diagnosis is required to confirm and differentiate influenza from equine herpesvirus types 1 and 4 (EHV-1, EHV-4), equine viral arteritis (EVA), and other respiratory pathogens. The methods presently used for diagnosis of influenza virus infections include virus isolation in embryonated chicken eggs and cell culture, antigen detection by fluorescent antibody and ELISA testing, reverse transcriptase–polymerase chain reaction (RT-PCR) assays, and serologic analyses.[49,162-165] However, many of these methods have one or more serious disadvantages, such as lack of sensitivity, long turnaround time, prohibitive costs, or the need for a high degree of technical expertise in the laboratory. Thus, to institute optimal control measures, it might be necessary to combine several of these diagnostic tools to identify the etiologic agent accurately and rapidly. The World Organization for Animal Health (OIE) publishes the *Manual of Diagnostic Tests and Vaccines for Terrestrial Animals*, currently in its fifth edition, at their website (http://www.oie.int/), which provides an extremely useful resource for current testing methodology.

Antigen Detection

Virus Isolation

Virus isolation from clinical samples is critical for epidemiologic investigation and for vaccine production and is generally carried out in embryonated chicken eggs or cell culture. In the naive horse, by the third or fourth day after infection, large amounts of virus are shed into the secretions of the respiratory tract.[34,165] Therefore the best results for virus isolation can often be achieved by collecting nasopharyngeal or nasal passage swabs within the first 24 to 48 hours after onset of clinical illness.[35] Historically, nasopharyngeal swabs obtained using a mare uterine culture swab or similar instrument have been recommended as the optimal sample type for influenza virus isolation, although a swab of the nasal mucosa provides equivalent sensitivity (Fig. 12-4). In partially immune animals the length of virus shedding is often shorter, decreasing the diagnostic sensitivity of virus isolation. Therefore it might be useful to sample more immunologically naive horses in a group to increase the likelihood of demonstrating infectious virus.[49] Nasopharyngeal or nasal passage samples are best collected using polyester-tipped swabs. Cotton swabs should be avoided because influenza viruses can adhere to the cotton fibers, decreasing the likelihood of isolating virus from the sample. The swabs should be placed in sterile viral transport medium and kept on ice until further analysis.

Traditionally, embryonated chicken eggs have been the biologic system of choice for isolating influenza viruses. At 10 to 12 days after fertilization of the egg, the sample is injected by either the amnionic or the allantoic route. After 24 to 72 hours of incubation, the allantoic or amnionic fluid is checked for hemagglutinating activity. In practice, twofold serial dilutions of the sample are prepared and mixed with a defined quantity of erythrocytes. If influenza virus is present in the sample, the HA protein binds to sialic acid–containing glycoproteins on erythrocytes. This hemagglutination activity results in the formation of a lattice.[166]

The robust yield of virus from eggs has led to their widespread use in research laboratories and for vaccine production. However, their use may be of limited value for diagnostic laboratories. Depending on the virus strain, amount of virus present in the sample, sample quality, and handling, detection of the presence of infectious virus by egg inoculation can take a minimum of 2 or 3 days. In horses with mild or subclinical infections, viral titers in nasal secretions are often low, sometimes requiring several egg passages before sufficiently high viral titers are produced to allow detection using conventional hemagglutination assays.[165] In addition, there is overwhelming evidence that the growth of influenza A viruses in eggs can lead to the selection of HA variants.[167-170] Finally, the lack of reliable high-quality chicken eggs is a serious limitation in their use.

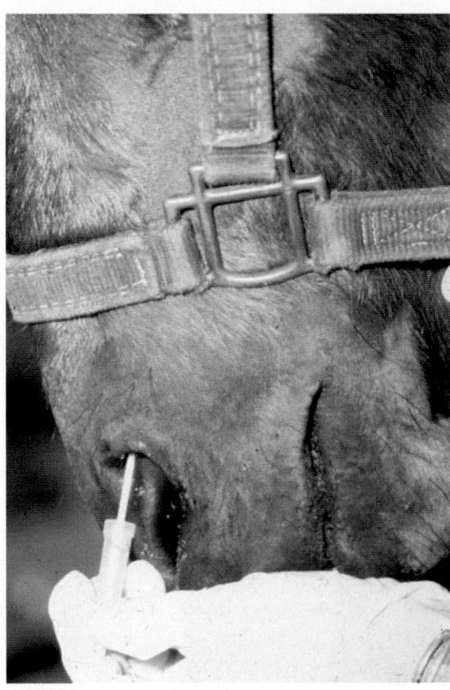

Fig. 12-4 Technique to obtain nasal mucosal swab for antigen detection or virus isolation. Short, polyester-tipped (noncotton-tipped) swab is most appropriate for sample collection. Virus isolation from a nasal mucosal swab is most sensitive for detection of equine influenza virus if obtained during the first 24 to 48 hours of fever.

Alternatively, equine influenza virus can be propagated in cell culture. Although the virus can infect a variety of primary and continuous cell lines, most cells do not support productive viral replication.[171-175] Thus the most widely used cells are Madin-Darby canine kidney (MDCK) epithelial cells. The use of cell culture for influenza virus isolation also has several limitations. For example, depending on the protocol and cell lines used, substantial differences in influenza recovery rates from clinical samples can occur.[176] In addition, MDCK cells are generally considered less permissive than embryonated chicken eggs for equine influenza viruses.[177] Finally, growth of H3 influenza viruses in MDCK cells results in the introduction of mutations in the HA.[167,178,179] A number of these amino acid substitutions were found to change the antigenicity of viruses of the H3 subtype.[178-180]

Other, less frequently used cell lines include mink lung epithelial cells (Mv1Lu) and chick embryo fibroblasts. Particularly Mv1Lu cells might provide a useful alternative system for the isolation of influenza A viruses from clinical samples. Recent studies found that Mv1Lu cells and mixtures of MDCK and Mv1Lu cells supported the replication of a wider range of influenza A virus than MDCK cells alone.[181,182]

Immunoassays

A number of ELISAs using monoclonal antibodies to detect the viral NP in nasal swab samples have been developed as a more rapid alternative to virus isolation. Although influenza A viruses can differ substantially in their HA and NA genes, the sequences of the internal genes, such as the M, NP, and the NS genes, are highly conserved among all subtypes and strains of influenza A viruses.[4] As such, a diagnostic test aimed at the detection of NP is likely to be capable of identifying a wide variety of influenza A viruses from different host species. An additional advantage of ELISA-based assays over virus isolation is that these tests are able to detect virions that have lost their infectivity during sample handling, storage, and transport to the laboratory.

Originally intended for the diagnosis of human influenza infections, an antigen-capture ELISA has been adapted for the detection of equine H3N8 viral antigen.[183,184] Briefly, to detect viral antigen, a "capture" antibody, directed against the influenza NP, is linked to a 96-well plastic plate. The clinical sample is added to the wells, and if viral antigens are present, they will be bound to the immobilized antibody. Subsequently, bound viral antigen is detected by use of a second enzyme-linked antibody. The antigen-capture ELISA was evaluated during an outbreak of equine influenza in the United Kingdom in 1989 and, when used in combination with virus isolation, was found to enhance the virus detection rate by 44%.[185] Moreover, the test was shown to be particularly useful for detection of viral antigen in samples heavily contaminated with bacteria.[49,165]

Commercial development of optical immunoassay (OIA)–based test kits, designed to detect the NP of human influenza A viruses, has facilitated the widespread use of this procedure. Two of these test kits have been evaluated for use in the diagnosis of equine influenza virus infection; the Flu OIA assay (Biostar, Boulder, Colo) and the Directigen Flu-A assay (Becton Dickinson Microbiology Systems, Cockeysville, Md). Many investigators found these commercial diagnostic kits to be useful, and frequently these assays were considerably more sensitive than traditional virus isolation. Furthermore, these OIAs proved to be highly specific and rapid, whereas virus isolation in embryonated chicken eggs required up to three passages before hemagglutination became evident.[37,186-189] Although these test kits were able to identify infected horses consistently at the peak of virus shedding, they may not be sensitive enough to detect low levels of virus shedding reliably.[7] When possible, horses with severe clinical signs during suspected influenza virus outbreaks are preferable for testing to increase the likelihood of obtaining positive results.[188]

Immunofluorescence

Employing influenza virus–specific fluorochrome-labeled antibodies, immunofluorescence (IF) is based on the immunodetection of virus-infected cells obtained from nasal scrapings or tracheal washes. Although the assay was reported to be highly sensitive and rapid,[165,190] IF requires substantial sample preparation and handling. Briefly, samples are centrifuged to separate the cells from respiratory mucous. The cells are washed, spotted onto glass slides, acetone fixed, and incubated with influenza-specific antibodies. Antigen-positive cells are detected by use of a secondary fluorochrome-labeled antibody.[49,165,190] A recent study compared the detection of influenza viruses by IF to a commercially available OIA for diagnosis of influenza virus infections in humans and found that the IF had a significantly higher sensitivity than the OIA.[190]

Reverse Transcriptase–Polymerase Chain Reaction

During the past decade, advances in polymerase chain reaction (PCR) technology and other DNA amplification techniques have resulted in these methods becoming key tools in diagnostic laboratories.[191-193] By choosing appropriate oligonucleotides, a selected region of the viral genome can be amplified. The oligonucleotides serve as primers for in vitro DNA synthesis, which is catalyzed by a special DNA polymerase isolated from a thermophilic bacterium that is stable at high temperatures. PCR is extremely sensitive and can theoretically detect a single-copy DNA in a sample. Trace amounts of RNA can be detected in the same way by first transcribing them into DNA with reverse transcriptase (RT).

RT-PCR–based assays have been used successfully for the detection of a broad range of influenza A virus subtypes from clinical samples.[164,181,190,194,195] By selecting primers specific for a region of the highly conserved M gene, such assays are capable of detecting minuscule amounts of a wide range of influenza virus strains and subtypes. In a recent study, RT-PCR was found to be a highly sensitive and specific method for the detection of influenza A viruses of human, swine, avian, and equine lineage.[164] In contrast to virus isolation, RT-PCR–based antigen detection techniques do not require the presence of viable virus,[196] and therefore the sensitivity of RT-PCR methods is often substantially higher than for virus isolation. A study comparing the results of a RT-PCR assay with virus isolation from nasopharyngeal aspirates from humans with suspected influenza virus infection found that the RT-PCR detected 83 cases of influenza A, compared with 66 cases detected by virus isolation.[190]

Although RT-PCR–based techniques have proved to be powerful tools for investigating respiratory disease caused by a variety of pathogens, the technique can also have a number of shortcomings. Because of the assay's high sensitivity, the greatest problem facing the diagnostic application of PCR is the production of false-positive results. These are often attributable to contamination by nucleic acids, particularly from previously amplified material (carryover). Any contaminant, even the smallest airborne remnant carried over from the previous PCR procedure or from a strong positive sample, may be multiplied and produce a false-positive result. In addition, a number of studies examining the sensitivity of RT-PCR–based assays on nasal or nasopharyngeal swabs have encountered false-negative results. Such false-negative results may result from the nature of the sample tested. Ribonucleases (RNases) are present in various quantities in specimens collected from the respiratory tract and may gradually digest viral RNA.[197,198] This may reduce the sensitivity of RT-PCR–based tests in clinical samples that contain large amounts of RNases and a low concentration of viral RNA. In addition, PCR assay inhibitors (e.g., lactoferrin, hemoglobin) can represent a substantial problem in diagnostic PCR-based assays.[199,200] Such PCR inhibitors were previously reported to be present in about 2% of samples from the respiratory tract.[201] Nevertheless, RT-PCR–based assays offer a more sensitive tool for the diagnosis of influenza A virus infection than conventional techniques such as culture or immunoassays.

In diagnostic laboratory settings the use of RT-PCR can be limited by cost and sometimes the availability of adequate test sample volume. To overcome these shortcomings and also to increase the diagnostic capacity of PCR, multiplex PCR assays have been developed. In *multiplex PCR,* more than one target sequence can be amplified by including more than one pair of primers in the reaction. Recently, multiplex PCR has been shown to be a valuable and cost-effective tool for monitoring the emergence of new variants and subtypes of influenza A viruses.[202,203] In addition, multiplex PCR assays have also been used successfully to screen human clinical samples simultaneously for multiple respiratory pathogens, such as influenza A and B viruses, respiratory syncytial virus, adenovirus, and parainfluenza viruses.[163,204-207] Given the advantages already demonstrated by the use of multiplex PCR assays in human and veterinary medicine, this procedure will undoubtedly prove beneficial in the diagnosis and differentiation of pathogens that commonly cause respiratory infections in horses.

Antibody Detection

In the past, serologic tests have been the key tool by which influenza infections were diagnosed. Most serologic assays are fairly easy to perform and cost-effective. In addition, a large number of samples can be collected and tested simultaneously, facilitating large-scale herd surveillance. Because many horses have been vaccinated, however, diagnosis of influenza infection can often be made only by testing paired samples (acute and convalescent titers) collected 10 to 21 days apart. Therefore, serologic testing often provides only retrospective information and subclinical infections, which may not be accompanied by seroconversion, might not be detected.[208] To diagnose influenza infection, a significant increase in titer should be demonstrated, and therefore baseline (acute) samples must be collected early in the course of infection. The tests frequently used to detect influenza-specific antibodies include hemagglutination inhibition (HI), virus neutralization (VN), complement fixation (CF), single radial hemolysis (SRH), and ELISA-based testing.

Hemagglutination Inhibition

HI tests are simple, sensitive, inexpensive, and rapid and therefore are often the method of choice for assaying antibodies to influenza A virus. The test relies on the hemagglutination activity of the influenza HA (see earlier discussion) and the ability of HA-specific antibodies to inhibit the virus from agglutinating erythrocytes (Fig. 12-5). Briefly, dilutions of serum are incubated with virus, and erythrocytes are added. After incubation, the HI titer is read as the highest dilution of serum that inhibits hemagglutination. A fourfold or greater increase in HI antibody titer is regarded as evidence of infection.[165,209] HI antibodies define subtype-specific antigens on the virus particle, thus allowing the differentiation of equine influenza H3N8 and H7N7 subtypes.[166] One of the main shortcomings of the HI test is wide interlaboratory variation, with results for the same serum sample varying as much as 100-fold.[165] A study comparing the sensitivity of HI and SRH tests on human sera found that both tests had similar sensitivity, but the interlaboratory reproducibility of HI was significantly lower.[209]

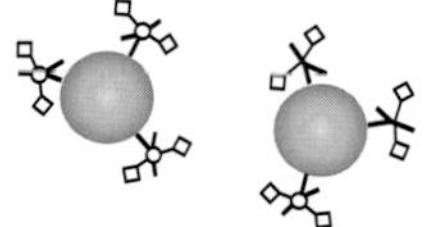

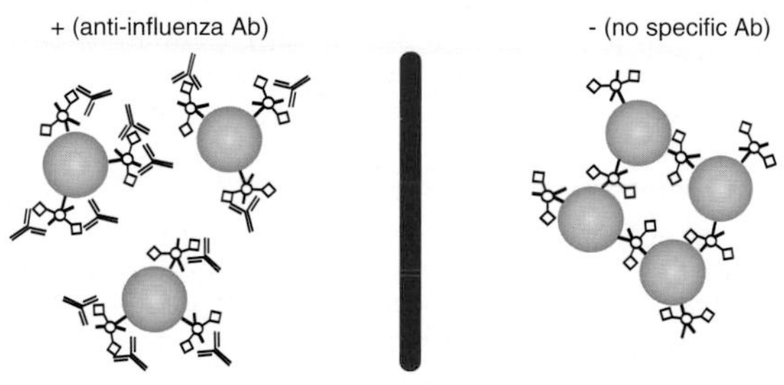

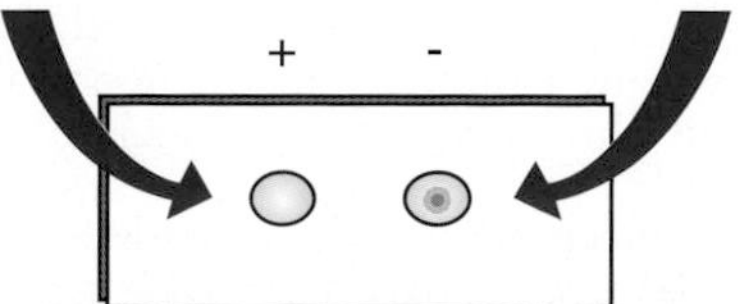

Fig. 12-5 Schematic diagram of hemagglutination inhibition (HI) assay. Chicken red blood cells *(RBCs)* agglutinate in the presence of influenza virus, but this can be inhibited by the addition of influenza virus–specific antibody *(Ab)*. HI results in cells coating the bottom of a round-bottomed test plate, whereas lack of antibody allows for clumping of cells into a pellet.

Single Radial Hemolysis

For SRH tests, sheep erythrocytes, which have previously been incubated with influenza virus, are mixed with guinea pig complement and incorporated in agarose gels (Fig. 12-6). Heat-inactivated serum samples are then added to wells cut into the gel, and the antibody titer is determined based on the zone of hemolysis induced by diffusion of the antibody-positive sample from the well.[210-212] An increase of 50% or 25 mm^2 is considered evidence of recent infection.[209] Although more labor intensive than HI assays, SRH tests have been shown to be more reproducible and more sensitive than HI.[209] Since it was found that the level of antibody measured by SRH after vaccination correlates well with the level of protection, SRH could be used to predict the level of antibody-mediated immunity and determine the need for revaccination.[165,213,214]

ELISA-Based Assays

ELISAs detecting antibodies to equine influenza HA (H3N8) have been developed as an alternative method to traditional HI tests and were found to be sensitive, rapid, and reproducible.[215] A recently developed assay employing a HA protein produced in a baculovirus expression system demonstrated broad reactivity with serum antibodies generated after infection with heterologous H3N8 influenza virus strains.[216]

Because horses are often vaccinated, and conventional serologic tests do not provide information as to whether antibodies were produced in response to infection or vaccination, an ELISA aimed at the detection of antibodies to the NS1 protein has been developed.[217] Because antibodies to NS1 could be demonstrated only in influenza virus–infected horses,[218] and NS1 is antigenically and genetically highly conserved across influenza A viruses,[219] NS1 is a good candidate for a differential diagnostic marker, capable of distinguishing infected from vaccinated horses. The assay was subsequently tested in horses that were either experimentally infected with A/equine/Kentucky/1/81 (H3N8) and A/equine/La Plata/1/93 (H3N8) or vaccinated with inactivated influenza H3N8 and H7N7 virus. The ELISA was found to be a useful tool to distinguish postvaccination antibody titers from those generated by recent infection.[217]

PATHOLOGIC FINDINGS

Given the limited mortality associated with equine influenza infection, there are few reports of gross pathologic findings, although an early publication summarizes the original studies performed when equine influenza virus infection was first recognized.[133] Subacute inflammatory disease of the nasal mucosa, pharynx, larynx, and trachea is observed. Pulmonary changes include bronchitis, peribronchitis, and perivasculitis, with subacute interstitial pneumonia, edema, and focal bronchopneumonia. Myocarditis was a variable finding. Neonatal infection with equine influenza virus can result in severe fatal bronchointerstitial pneumonia,[58] although such occurrences are rare.

Hemogram findings in equine influenza virus infection include a moderate normocytic, normochromic anemia.[133] The leukogram typically shows a leukopenia, which results from both neutropenia and lymphopenia of 3 to 5 days' duration[133,220]; neutropenia is not a consistent finding, and the neutrophil/lymphocyte ratio is often increased during

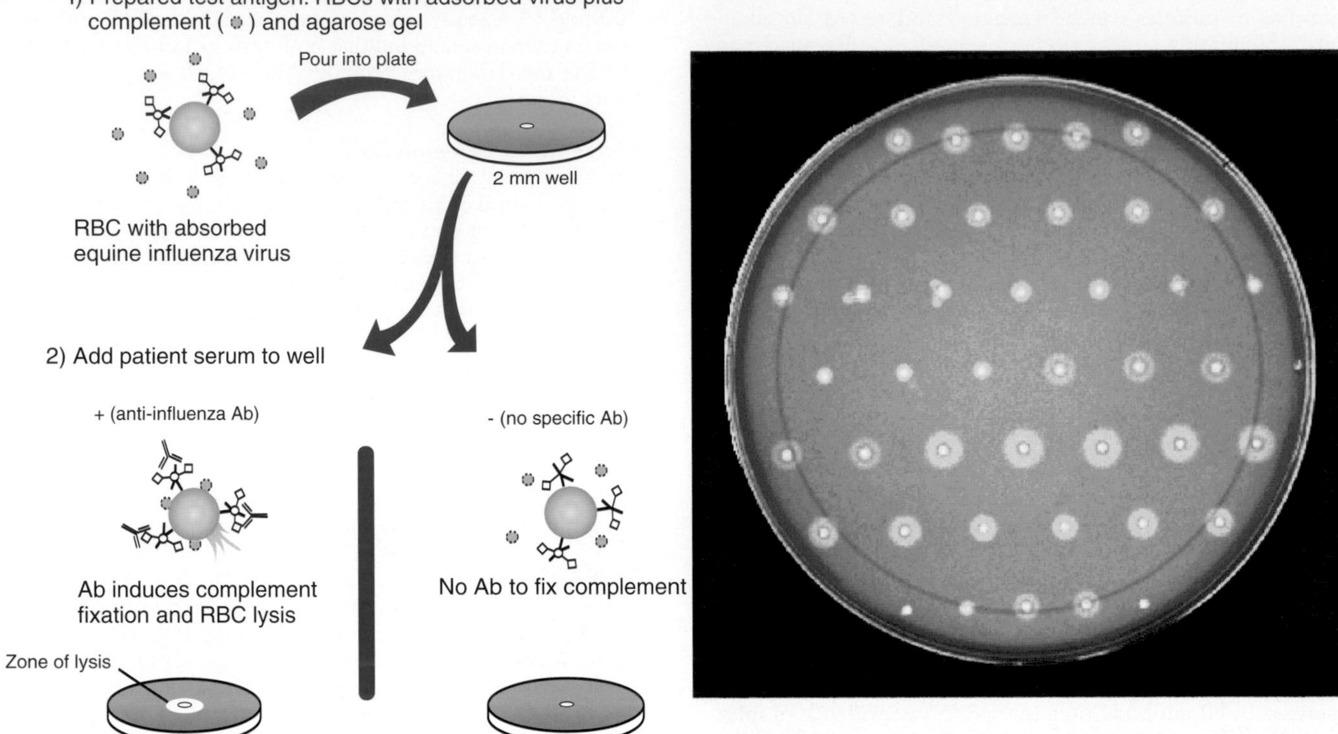

Fig. 12-6 *Left*, Schematic diagram of single radial hemolysis (SRH) assay. Sheep red blood cells *(RBCs)* coated with influenza virus and guinea pig complement are mixed with molten agar and poured in a plate. Test equine serum and control serum can be added to individual wells cut in the agar, and the zone of hemolysis corresponds to the amount of influenza virus–specific complement-fixing antibody *(Ab)* present in the test equine serum. *Right*, Typical result.

this period.[135] Monocytosis during early convalescence is a variable finding.[133]

THERAPY

Medical Therapy

Symptomatic treatment is the primary form of therapy for equine influenza virus infection and should include rest in a nonstressful environment. It is important to ensure adequate hydration, and nonsteroidal antiinflammatory drugs (NSAIDs) may reduce morbidity caused by pyrexia and myalgia. Affected animals should be monitored for development of complications such as pneumonia or myocarditis, and any horse exhibiting signs of respiratory disease beyond 10 days postinfection should be considered at high risk of secondary bacterial infection. The duration of adequate convalescence is difficult to gauge but is typically much longer than owner's expectations. Estimates for the period before horses should be returned to athletic activity vary from 50 to 100 days,[221] to a week for each day of fever.[135]

Antiviral Therapy

Vaccination of horses against influenza A viruses has been and remains the cornerstone of influenza prevention. Nevertheless, mostly because of insufficient vaccine coverage, but also a lack of protective immunogenicity in some animals, epizootics of equine influenza can cause considerable economic loss and excess morbidity and mortality. In contrast to vaccines, antivirals can be rapidly employed to combat an influenza virus outbreak. Thus, antiviral therapy could become a viable option for the protection of valuable horses in an influenza outbreak.

Two groups of influenza antiviral drugs are currently licensed for the prophylactic and therapeutic use against influenza A virus in humans: the M2 ion channel blockers and the neuraminidase inhibitors. Zanamivir and oseltamivir, the only two neuraminidase inhibitors currently licensed for use in humans,[2,222] were shown to reduce the duration of clinically significant influenza symptoms by approximately 20% in otherwise healthy adolescent and adult humans.[222-224] To date, however, their clinical effectiveness has not been tested in horses.

Amantadine (1-aminoadamantane hydrochloride) and *rimantadine* (methyl-1-adamantanemethylamine hydrochloride) target the transmembrane domain of the M2 ion channel protein. Both drugs inhibit virus replication by blocking ion channel activity of the M2 protein through allosteric inhibition. Amantadine and rimantadine have antiviral properties against all subtypes of influenza A virus.[2,225] Their primary antiviral action results from blocking the flow of H^+ ions from the acidified endosomal compartment into the interior of the virion, a process necessary for release of the viral RNPs. A second effect of both drugs is to block maturation of the HA during transport from the endoplasmic reticulum to the plasma membrane.[2,226,227]

Inhibitory concentrations of amantadine and rimantadine range from 0.03 to 1.0 μg/mL,[228] with rimantadine about fourfold to tenfold more active than amantadine.[229] In humans, amantadine and rimantadine have good oral bioavailability and very large volumes of distribution, so that local concentrations (in nasal mucus) were similar to those in plasma.[230] In horses, oral administration of amantadine was associated with substantial interanimal variation in bioavailability, ranging from very low (approximately 10%) to a maximum of 70%, and was not substantially affected by prior fasting of the horses.[231] Therefore, oral administration of amantadine in horses, although effective in some animals, might fail to produce effective plasma concentration in others. In contrast, intravenous (IV) administration of amantadine at doses ranging from 10 mg/kg every 8 hours (q8h) to 5 mg/kg q4h was suggested to be sufficient to maintain effective plasma concentrations.[231] Amantadine is excreted primarily unmetabolized in urine, and therefore the dosage must be adjusted in patients with renal insufficiency to reduce the risk of adverse effects.[222] The most common adverse effects observed as a result of amantadine therapy are central nervous system (CNS) effects.[222,232] At high doses (>15 mg/kg) the drug was reported to produce acute seizures and even death in horses.[231] In humans the concurrent use of antihistamines, anticholinergics, and psychotropic drugs is thought to enhance the neurotoxic effect of amantadine.[229]

When administered orally to healthy humans and horses, rimantadine was much less frequently associated with adverse CNS effects than amantadine.[222,233] Moreover, the bioavailability of rimantadine after oral administration in horses appeared considerably more uniform than the oral bioavailability of amantadine. The administration of 30 mg/kg of rimantadine q12h resulted in sufficiently high plasma concentrations without causing observable signs of adverse effects.[233]

Clinical trials conducted with influenza virus–infected humans and horses suggest that amantadine and rimantadine are equally effective in reducing the severity and duration of illness.[233-236] In addition, oral administration of rimantadine reduced virus load in nasal secretions, although the duration of nasal virus shedding was similar to that in the untreated controls.[233] However, the potential benefits associated with the administration of M2 ion channel blockers during an influenza virus outbreak may be limited by the rapid development of drug resistance. Amantadine-resistant and rimantadine-resistant strains of influenza A virus can be isolated in vitro and in vivo,[2] and resistant virus can develop as early as 1 day after start of treatment.[237] Such mutant viruses may then spread to susceptible contacts and cause disease, indicating that acquisition of drug resistance is not associated with attenuation of the virus.[238,239] Resistance can pose a major problem when these drugs are used therapeutically and prophylactically in close-contact environments.[240,241] In recent studies, resistance of influenza A viruses to amantadine and rimantadine was observed with a frequency of 50% or greater in children.[230,242] As discussed previously, amantadine has other limitations; the use of this drug in horses is associated with CNS adverse effects and poor oral bioavailability, making it less suited for prophylactic and therapeutic use in this species.

PREVENTION

Vaccination

Vaccination against equine influenza virus infection is a common and important practice for the control of disease, and a wide variety of vaccine formulations can be used. Inactivated vaccines remain the most common type of vaccine in use around the world, although both modified live and recombinant vaccines are commercially available. Many publications have documented the ability of inactivated equine influenza vaccines to protect against homologous viral challenge, which also demonstrates a correlation between protection and prechallenge antibody level.[63,64,243,244]

The value of inactivated equine influenza virus vaccines critically depends on the quality and quantity of viral antigen and the choice of adjuvant.[245,246] Some of the most successful inactivated vaccines have used adjuvants such as ISCOMS or carboxypolymer-based compounds (carbomer, carbopol),[64,244] and a recent North American study showed a clear advantage to carbomer-based products.[67] The use of some adjuvants, such as alum, have been associated with induction of nonprotective immune responses.[138]

Another critically important consideration is which strains of virus are used for preparation of the vaccine. Although the inclusion of the A/Equi1/H7N7 virus is no longer considered necessary for equine influenza vaccines, the evolution of two distinct lineages of the A/Equi2/H3N8 virus (European and American),[47] with consequent vaccine failure,[73] has made inclusion of examples of both lineages a desirable feature of modern vaccines.[92] However, further evolution of the American lineage H3N8 virus continues to result in failure of killed vaccines,[247] and ongoing surveillance and inclusion of viral antigens representative of contemporary circulating viruses will remain a priority.

An intranasal, cold-adapted, modified live equine influenza virus vaccine based on a Kentucky 1991 A/Equi2 virus is available in North America and provides protection for up to 12 months after a single administration, although only a 6-month claim is made on the product data sheet.[68,150] Intranasal vaccine administration is generally well tolerated in horses.[248] At the time of its introduction, this vaccine was found to protect against both European and American lineages, despite including only an example of the latter,[249] and as of this writing, it appears to have continued efficacy against contemporary circulating viruses.[67] A recombinant canary pox vector-based equine influenza vaccine (Proteq-Flu, Merial) is available in Europe and has shown excellent performance against even the most recent circulating viral lineages, including those that have overcome modern inactivated vaccines.[159] These examples illustrate the increasing role and potency of novel equine influenza vaccines not based on conventional inactivated formulations. Experimentally, there are a number of reports of alternative successful vaccination strategies, including the use of DNA vaccination,[71,145,158] and the development of a modified vaccinia Ankara (MVA) vaccine vector.[156,157] The use of the MVA vector had the particular advantage of generating nasal mucosal influenza virus–specific IgA.

Recommendations for equine vaccination are available from a variety of sources.[250,251] General recommendations are not to vaccinate in the presence of maternal immunity in foals before at least 6 months of age.[252] Vaccination of mares with inactivated vaccines that are known to generate high-titer antibody responses 2 to 6 weeks before parturition is likely to provide protection of foals through passive transfer of immunity. Initial vaccination series for inactivated vaccines should include three doses, and this approach is recommended even when data sheets only recommend two initial doses. The timing of these initial vaccinations is important. An interval of 3 to 4 weeks between the first and second dose is recommended, but a longer interval of 3 to 4 months between the second and third dose is preferred. This results in the third dose of the initial series being administered when the antibody response to the second vaccine dose has waned, and the amplitude of the antibody response to the third dose is consequently much greater.[67] This regimen of three initial doses of vaccine, with intervals of 1 month between the first and second doses and with 3 to 4 months between the second and third vaccine doses, is recommended independent of the recommendations present on data sheets. Contemporary inactivated vaccines with established protective efficacy are likely to perform well if this approach is taken, and subsequent booster vaccinations should be given at 6-month intervals in high-risk populations. The modified live cold-adapted vaccine

FluAvert I.N. (Intervet) only requires a single initial dose and is recommended for booster doses at 6-month intervals. This vaccine can protect within 7 days of administration to naive horses (Dr. Craig Barnett, Intervet, personal communication). If a known period of high risk of infection is anticipated, a booster vaccination should be given even to well-vaccinated horses 1 to 2 weeks before the risk period.

Husbandry

Control of equine influenza virus infection can be substantially addressed by adequate husbandry procedures. It is informative to review the OIE qualifications for influenza-free countries (published in the *Terrestrial Animal Health Code*, 12th edition, 2004, http://www.oie.int/). If the same criteria are met for horses entering an equine establishment, it is likely that influenza virus infection can be excluded. Specifically, horses should be isolated for 4 weeks before introduction into the horse population; horses should be fully vaccinated before admission to the isolation facility; no clinical signs of influenza should be detected during the isolation period; and no new animals should be introduced into the isolation facility during the isolation period. Some countries also perform influenza virus diagnostic testing at the beginning of the isolation period, using tests such as the Directogen ELISA (Becton Dickinson).

These criteria may be too demanding for most horse owners, but adequate vaccination and 2 weeks of full isolation on the facility could be regarded as an excellent compromise. Frequently, even this standard is difficult to achieve, and we remain heavily dependent on vaccination for protection. Nevertheless, other husbandry procedures, including segregating equine populations on horse facilities, can be valuable. This allows for potential containment of disease outbreaks, because infection moves slowly through large facilities where horse populations are segregated.[54] Shared grooming equipment and tack may increase the risk of contagion.[59]

Monitoring of vaccine response by serology has been reported to help in prevention and control of influenza virus outbreaks, and the SRH test can be used for this purpose.[65,253] Surveillance for detection of influenza virus is routinely practiced in some areas with large equine populations and offers the opportunity for early detection of outbreaks and for detection of new virus strains that may not be controlled by vaccine.[254]

PUBLIC HEALTH CONSIDERATIONS

In addition to horses, influenza A viruses infect a large variety of species, including humans, pigs, poultry, aquatic birds, sea mammals, and most recently, dogs.[255] Wild waterfowl play a particularly important role in influenza epidemiology because these birds provide a vast global reservoir of viruses of all subtypes.[22,27] Avian influenza A viruses have contributed to the generation of human pandemic viruses in 1957 and 1968. However, although influenza A viruses are occasionally directly transmitted from one host species to another (e.g., the transmission of H5N1 avian influenza A viruses to humans in Asia), biologic barriers exist that often limit such spread. This appears to be particularly true for equine-lineage influenza A viruses. Although the susceptibility of human volunteers to infection with H3 equine-lineage viruses has been demonstrated,[256] phylogenetic analyses indicate that exchange of influenza virus genes between horses and other species is limited. These findings suggest that horses may be an isolated or "dead-end" reservoir for influenza A viruses.[2,27,32]

The notable exception to this is the recent transmission of an equine-lineage H3N8 virus to dogs.[255] Transmission in this case was associated with outbreaks of respiratory disease and sudden death primarily in racing greyhounds. Viral isolation and antigen detection from clinically affected dogs with concomitant seroconversion within the same housing units support transmissibility between dogs. Although the susceptibility of dogs to influenza A viruses has been recognized,[257-260] little is known about why an equine virus was able to infect and spread among dogs with much greater efficiency than previously observed. Genetic analysis demonstrated that all the genes of this equine H3N8 were present, indicating that the rare event of passage of a whole viral genome between different host species had occurred. Analysis of virus-host interactions will be critically important to determine factors responsible for the transmission and spread of equine-lineage H3N8 influenza A virus in dogs in the United States.

REFERENCES

See the CD-ROM for a list of references linked to the abstract in PubMed.

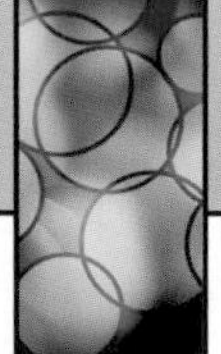

CHAPTER • 13

Equine Herpesviruses

Josh Slater

The equine herpesviruses (EHVs) are highly successful pathogens of all members of the Equidae family worldwide.[1-4] Of the nine EHVs characterized thus far, five (EHV-1 to EHV-5) infect the domestic horse, and EHV-6 to EHV-9 are associated with infections in wild equids,[5] including asses and zebra.[6-9] The EHVs are ubiquitous in both domestic and wild equid populations, and it is likely that the enduring success of the EHV as pathogens results from ancient co-evolution with the *Equidae* family and adaptation of the virus life cycle to ensure efficient spread within the equid population.

The equid herpesviruses, as with other herpesviruses that infect animals and humans, have sophisticated life cycles adapted to exploit the host animal population and ensure virus persistence. Their life cycles involve infection of multiple cell types in different tissues, with different mechanisms for evasion of the host immune response. *Latency*, in which recovered horses carry virus in a quiescent (asymptomatic) form for extended periods, is central to the success of these viruses. First, latency provides a mechanism not only for the maintenance of virus in the infected herd, but also for the introduction of virus into new herds through the movement of latently infected horses. Second, latently infected horses form a reservoir of transmissible infection through reactivation, resulting in infection of new, susceptible, in-contact horses.

In domestic horse populations the most important and most studied of the EHVs are the alpha herpesviruses EHV-1 and EHV-4. These respiratory pathogens are also responsible for abortion and neurologic disease. EHV-3 is an uncommon venereal pathogen and is not discussed in this chapter (see Chapter 8). The clinical importance of the gamma herpesviruses EHV-2 and EHV-5 is less clearly defined, although some evidence suggests that EHV -2 and EHV-5, in certain situations, may be clinically important as respiratory and ocular pathogens (see Chapter 10). There has been speculation that these viruses may act as immunosuppressive agents, predisposing to other viral infections, or may be involved in persistent, chronic fatigue syndromes.

The EHVs have a major economic and welfare impact on all sectors of the horse industry worldwide through their direct clinical effects on the horse, including respiratory disease, abortion,[10,11] and paralysis,[12] and through their effects on the horse industry, including interference with horse movement for breeding and competition. The first of the equid herpesviruses to be described were EHV-1 and EHV-4.[13-15] These viruses are closely related, but genetically and phenotypically distinct, and were originally designated as subtypes 1 and 2 of EHV-1.[16-20] These two viruses have been the subject of a major international research effort over the past five decades. This research has produced a wealth of fundamental virologic and immunologic knowledge about their pathogenesis and the interactions between these viruses and the horse.[3] This information in turn has allowed effective management control programs to be devised (embodied in the United Kingdom in the Horserace Betting Levy Board's Code of Practice; www.hblb.org.uk). From the outset, EHV research has been directed toward vaccine development; the first EHV-1 vaccines were used in 1961,[21] and there are now a variety of killed and live commercial EHV vaccines available in Europe and North America.

This chapter concentrates on equine herpesvirus type 1 (EHV-1) and type 4 (EHV-4) and reviews current understanding of their virology, epidemiology, pathogenesis, clinical disease, treatment, and prevention.

ETIOLOGY

Relevance of Virology to Clinical Practice

Advances in the understanding of the molecular biology and virology of the equid herpesviruses have greatly improved our understanding of their pathogenesis,[1,3] the immune responses required to control virus replication and spread in the host,[22] and critically the identification of key immunologic viral targets.[23,24] This information is a prerequisite for effective vaccine design.

Virology Overview

EHV-1 and EHV-4 are alpha herpesviruses (members of the *Alphaherpesvirinae* subfamily) and belong, along with bovine herpesvirus-1, suid herpesvirus-1, canine herpesvirus-1, felid herpesvirus-1, and Marek's disease virus (MDV), to the *Varicellovirus* genus, the prototypic virus of which is the human pathogen varicella-zoster virus (VZV).[25] The varicelloviruses share some similarities with the herpes simplex viruses HSV-1 and HSV-2, the cause of cold sores and genital herpes, respectively, but are genetically and phenotypically distinct. Indeed, the varicelloviruses are sufficiently different to merit care in extrapolation of data from the simplex viruses to the EHV, as with the use of the antiviral agent acyclovir to treat EHV-1 neurologic disease (see Treatment).

Each of the *Alphaherpesvirinae* has a restricted host range, typically infecting a single target species, although laboratory animal models have been employed to study many of these viruses, including EHV-1, -2, and -5, with varying success. The varicelloviruses all share common genome structure and are of broadly similar genome size.

EHV-1 and EHV-4 are closely related[26,27] but genetically and antigenically distinct with different disease profiles. EHV-1 is principally a pathogen of the domestic horse, but there is serologic evidence of occasional infection of domestic cattle and captive camelids and cervids. In contrast, EHV-4 is an exclusive pathogen of the domestic horse. In the laboratory, some aspects of EHV-1 pathogenesis can be modeled with limited success in mice[28-30] and hamsters,[31,32] but this has not proved possible for EHV-4.

Within the *Varicellovirus* genus there is a spectrum of cellular tropism from principally neurotropic viruses (e.g., VZV) to viruses that are principally lymphotropic (e.g., MDV). Equine herpesviruses types 1 and 4 lie midway along this spectrum, being both neurotropic and lymphotropic during their life cycle (see Pathogenesis). A key feature of the life cycle of EHV-1, distinguishing it from EHV-4, is that it efficiently infects a variety of cell types,[33] including respiratory epithelial cells,[34] endothelial cells,[35] neuronal cells,[36] and lymphoid cells.[37,38] EHV-4, on the other hand, has a tropism principally restricted to epithelial cells and neuronal cells and has limited potential for infection of endothelial and lymphoid cells.

The gamma herpesviruses EHV-2 and EHV-5 are principally lymphotropic, establishing functional latency in these cells.[39,40] Although viral deoxyribonucleic acid (DNA) has been detected in trigeminal ganglia,[41] reactivation from this site has not been demonstrated. EHV-2 and EHV-5 have typical *Gammaherpesvirinae* genome structures, with close similarity to saimiri and Epstein-Barr viruses.[42] They have different disease profiles from EHV-1 and EHV-4 and share no cross-protective antigens with these viruses.

Viral Genomes

In the short time since the complete genome sequences of EHV-1 and EHV-4 were determined,[43,44] partial or complete virus genomes can now be sequenced comparatively easily, and sequencing entire genomes of EHVs of interest is now a practical prospect. The availability of genome sequence, together with the molecular techniques and reagents to manipulate individual genes or groups of genes, has revolutionized understanding of EHV-1 gene function and regulation. The genomes of several EHV-1 isolates, including high-virulence and low-virulence strains, have been cloned as bacterial artificial chromosomes into *Escherichia coli*, providing a greatly improved means of studying viral gene function.[45-47] Transposon mutagenesis, a well-established technique in microbial genetics, has been successfully applied to EHV-1, providing a rapid means of screening the entire genome for virulence genes.

Virus genetics have major clinical implications for EHV-1 immunology and control programs. Identification of virulence-associated genes provides targets for live attenuated vaccines, and a complete understanding of viral gene expression and regulation provides essential insight into viral antigen targets for the immune system, a prerequisite for protein or DNA vaccination strategies.

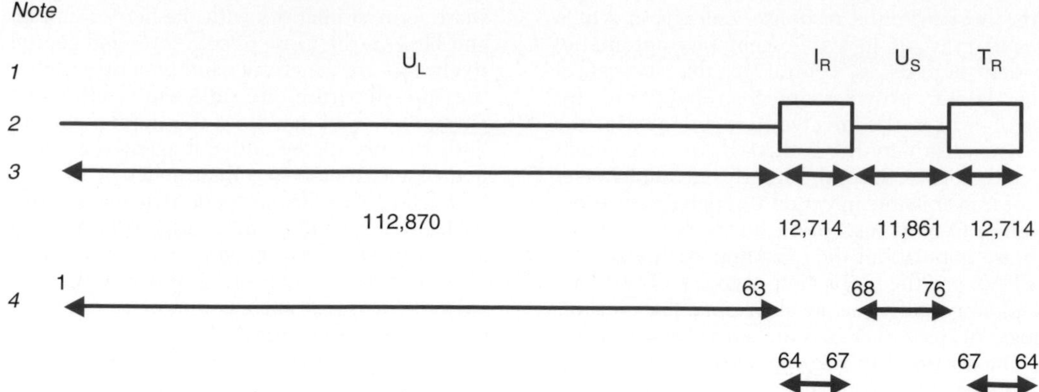

Fig. 13-1 Genome organization of equine herpesvirus type 1 (EHV-1). The genome is 150 kb in length and is predicted to encode 76 open reading frames (ORFs; genes). *Note 1*: The genome contains two unique regions; the unique long region *(U_L)* and the unique short region *(U_S)*. U_S is flanked by a repeat region creating identical, but inverted, repeats: the internal *(I_R)* repeat and terminal repeat *(T_R)* regions. *Note 2*: Schematic representation of the different genome regions. *Note 3*: Length of the different regions in base pairs. *Note 4*: Genes contained in the different regions. U_L contains genes 1 to 63; U_S contains genes 64 to 67; I_R contains genes 68 to 76; and T_R contains genes 67 to 64.

EHV-1 and EHV-4 possess linear double-stranded genomes and share the same overall genome conformation with a unique long region (U_L) joined to a unique short region (U_S) that is flanked by an identical pair of inverted repeat regions, the terminal repeat (T_R) and internal repeat (I_R) regions[43,44] (Fig. 13-1). Genes located in the repeat regions are thus represented twice in the genome. Both genomes are of similar size and share extensive sequence homology but are genetically (and phenotypically) distinct viruses. The EHV-1 genome is 150 kilobases (kb) in size and encodes 76 open reading frames (ORFs; genes), of which 63 are located in the U_L, nine in the U_S, and four in the repeat (I_R) regions (Table 13-1). The EHV-4 genome is slightly smaller (145 kb) with 76 genes, each of which has a direct positional and sequence counterpart in EHV-1. The EHV-2 genome is larger (184 kb) and contains 79 ORFs, of which 77 are predicted to code for proteins.[42]

Both EHV-1 and EHV-4 possess five unique genes (numbers 1, 2, 67, 71, and 75) that have no homologs in other sequenced herpesviruses and have been the subject of considerable research in the expectation that their products play pivotal roles in pathogenesis. Although the roles of these unique genes have not been completely elucidated, studies in vitro and in mice have failed to identify distinctive roles in pathogenesis.[48,49]

Viral Replication

The key feature of the molecular biology of EHV-1 and EHV-4 is that gene expression is tightly ordered into a highly controlled cascade.[50] The result is that the horse's immune system is

Table • 13-1

Open Reading Frames (ORFs) of Equine Herpesvirus Type 1 (EHV-1) and Predicted Functions of Their Gene Products

ORF	LOCATION	START	STOP	AMINO ACIDS	FUNCTION OF ENCODED PROTEIN
1	U_L	1298	1906	202	Unique gene with unknown function
2	U_L	2562	1945	205	Unique gene with unknown function
3	U_L	2841	3614	257	Hypothetical (unknown function)
4	U_L	4249	3647	200	Hypothetical (unknown function)
5	U_L	5874	4462	470	EICP 27; transactivator (regulatory gene)
6	U_L	7042	6011	343	Envelope glycoprotein (gK)
7	U_L	10301	7056	1081	DNA helicase-primase
8	U_L	10300	11037	245	Hypothetical (unknown function)
9	U_L	12115	11135	326	Deoxyuridine triphosphatase
10	U_L	12084	12386	100	Hypothetical (unknown function)
11	U_L	12549	13463	304	Tegument protein
12	U_L	13595	14944	449	ETIF (transactivator of IE); α-TIF homolog
13	U_L	15317	17932	871	Tegument protein
14	U_L	18083	20326	747	Tegument protein

Table • 13-1

Open Reading Frames (ORFs) of Equine Herpesvirus Type 1 (EHV-1) and Predicted Functions of Their Gene Products—cont'd

ORF	LOCATION	START	STOP	AMINO ACIDS	FUNCTION OF ENCODED PROTEIN
15	U_L	21170	20487	227	Tegument protein
16	U_L	22851	21445	468	Envelope glycoprotein (gC)
17	U_L	24234	23029	401	Hypothetical (unknown function)
18	U_L	25696	24479	405	DNA polymerase
19	U_L	26262	27755	497	Host shut-off factor
20	U_L	28859	27894	321	Ribonucleotide reductase
21	U_L	31276	28904	790	Ribonucleotide reductase
22	U_L	32916	31519	465	Capsid protein
23	U_L	33292	36354	1020	Tegument protein
24	U_L	36588	46853	3421	Tegument protein
25	U_L	47311	46952	119	Capsid protein
26	U_L	48230	47403	275	Hypothetical (unknown function)
27	U_L	48791	48369	140	DNA packaging protein
28	U_L	48763	50625	620	DNA packaging protein
29	U_L	50618	51598	326	Hypothetical (unknown function)
30	U_L	55184	51522	1220	DNA polymerase
31	U_L	55453	59082	1209	DNA-binding protein
32	U_L	59243	61570	775	DNA packaging protein
33	U_L	61432	64374	980	Envelope glycoprotein (gB)
34	U_L	64578	65060	160	Virus egress
35	U_L	67093	65153	646	Capsid protein
35.5	U_L	66142	65153	329	Capsid protein
36	U_L	68975	67212	587	DNA packaging protein
37	U_L	69897	69079	272	Hypothetical (unknown function)
38	U_L	69910	70968	352	Thymidine kinase (TK)
39	U_L	71192	73738	848	Envelope glycoprotein (gH)
40	U_L	76224	74632	530	Tegument protein
41	U_L	76793	77512	239	Hypothetical (unknown function)
42	U_L	77703	81832	1376	Capsid protein
43	U_L	82083	83027	314	Capsid protein
44	U_L	84320	83148	734	DNA packaging protein
45	U_L	84480	86600	706	Hypothetical (unknown function)
46	U_L	86620	87732	370	Tegument protein
47	U_L	88917	87886	358	Hypothetical (unknown function)
48	U_L	88947	89900	317	Hypothetical (unknown function)
49	U_L	89369	91153	594	Tegument protein
50	U_L	91135	92832	565	Deoxyribonuclease
51	U_L	92784	93008	74	Tegument protein
52	U_L	94472	93120	450	Envelope glycoprotein (gM)
53	U_L	94390	97053	887	Origin-binding protein
54	U_L	97069	99324	751	DNA helicase-primase
55	U_L	100332	99421	303	Hypothetical (unknown function)
56	U_L	102391	100130	753	Capsid protein
57	U_L	102375	105020	881	DNA helicase-primase
58	U_L	105070	105747	225	Hypothetical (unknown function)
59	U_L	106416	105877	179	Hypothetical (unknown function)
60	U_L	107116	106478	212	Hypothetical (unknown function)
61	U_L	108144	107206	312	DNA glycosylate
62	U_L	108843	108147	218	Envelope glycoprotein (gL)
63	U_L	111985	110387	532	EICP0; Early gene; transactivator (regulatory gene) (regulatory gene expression) (transactivator)
64	IR	118591	114128	1487	IE; transactivator (regulatory gene)

Continued

Table • 13-1

Open Reading Frames (ORFs) of Equine Herpesvirus Type 1 (EHV-1) and Predicted Functions of Their Gene Products—cont'd

ORF	LOCATION	START	STOP	AMINO ACIDS	FUNCTION OF ENCODED PROTEIN
65	IR	121368	122249	293	Hypothetical; possible late regulatory gene
66	IR	122862	123572	236	Late gene; homolog of HSV U_S10
67	IR	125194	124376	272	EICP22; Unique early gene; transactivator (regulatory gene)
68	U_S	126275	125019	418	Late gene; unknown function
69	U_S	126411	127559	382	Serine-threonine protein kinase
70	U_S	127681	128916	411	Envelope glycoprotein (gG)
71	U_S	129097	131490	797	Envelope glycoprotein (gp300); unique gene
72	U_S	131583	132791	402	Envelope glycoprotein (gD)
73	U_S	132899	134173	424	Envelope glycoprotein (gl)
74	U_S	134406	136058	550	Envelope glycoprotein (gEl)
75	U_S	136055	136447	130	Unique gene with unknown function
76	U_S	136783	137442	219	Tegument protein
67	TR	137966	138784	272	EICP22; unique early gene; transactivator (regulatory gene)
66	TR	140298	139588	236	Late gene; homolog of HSV U_S10
65	TR	141792	140911	293	Hypothetical (unknown function)
64	TR	144569	149032	1487	IE; transactivator (regulator of gene expression)

U_L is the unique long region of the genome; U_S is the unique short region; I_R and T_R are the internal and terminal repeat regions flanking U_S.

exposed to virus gene products in a sequential fashion, providing specific opportunities for immunologic intervention. One complete cycle of virus replication (the *lytic cycle*) takes approximately 20 hours, during which a well-ordered progression of events occurs: attachment to the host cell membrane, membrane fusion and penetration, translocation of viral DNA to the nucleus, viral DNA replication, viral protein synthesis, capsid assembly, egress from the nucleus, envelopment and egress from the cell, and death (lysis) of the cell as progeny virions are released. During these different stages of infection, viral gene transcription and regulation is sequentially regulated into three distinct phases: *immediate early* (IE), *early* (E), and *late* (L) (see Virus Proteins).[50-53] Gene products from each phase have regulatory roles that, acting in concert with host cell proteins, upregulate ("switch on") expression of other phases while downregulating ("switching off") their own phase (Fig. 13-2).

Lytic and Latent Infection Cycles

On entry to host cells, the virus enters either a lytic cycle or latent cycle of infection. These two pathways appear to be independent, to occur simultaneously, and to diverge immediately after viral entry in the cell. Virus replication is not required for the establishment of latency. The lytic cycle,

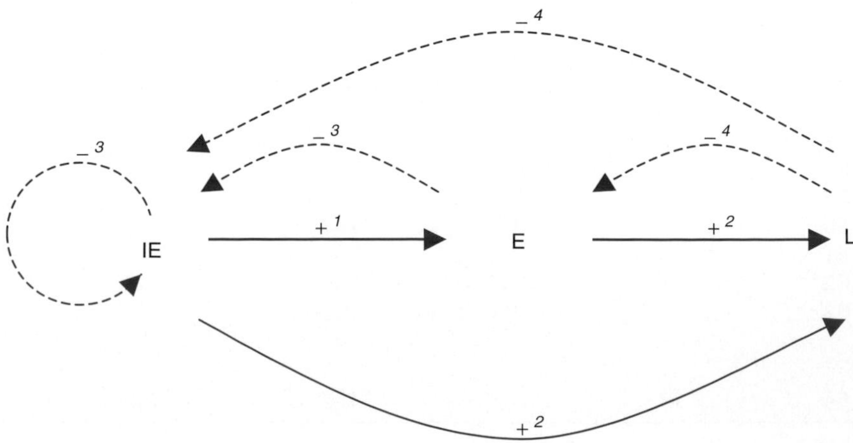

Fig. 13-2 Regulation of EHV-1 gene expression during lytic infection. Gene expression is co-ordinately regulated into three phases: immediate early *(IE)*, early *(E)*, and late *(L)*. *Note 1*: The IE protein transactivates (upregulates expression of) promoters of the E genes. *Note 2*: The IE and E proteins (EICP 22 and 27) transactivate L genes. *Note 3*: The E protein EICP 0 downregulates IE; the IE protein downregulates (autoregulates) its own promoter. *Note 4*: The L proteins downregulate expression of E genes and the IE gene.

as previously described, results in release of new virus particles from the infected cell. During the *latent cycle* of infection, viral DNA translocates to the nucleus, but the transcription and translation cascade of all gene classes is blocked, with the exception of limited transcription in the region antisense to the IE gene. This results in expression of the EHV *latency-associated transcript* (LAT).[54-56]

The mechanisms that control entry into lytic and latent infection cycles are not well understood. In the nervous and lymphoid systems, it appears that the two infection cycles occur in parallel, principally within neurons of the trigeminal ganglion and CD8+ T lymphocytes.[36,57,58] Although the genetic mechanisms responsible for suppression of gene transcription and translation in latency have not been fully elucidated, it seems unlikely to be entirely caused by antisense repression of IE gene transcription by LAT messenger ribonucleic acid (mRNA).

During latency, the genome exists in multiple copies in a continuous (circular) episomal form in the nucleus of infected cells. Latently infected cells do not express viral antigens and are thus not detectable immunologically. Latently infected cells represent a subset of neurons and CD8+ lymphocytes.[59]

The numbers of latently infected neurons within the trigeminal ganglion has not been determined; in the circulation, latently infected lymphocytes are rare and are estimated to occur at a frequency of 1 in 10^4 or 10^5. The number of latently infected lymphocytes declines over time but is increased during reactivation episodes or by exposure to new infections. The population of latently infected neurons is assumed to be stable because these are long-lived cells. It is not known whether repeated reactivations increase the number of latently infected neurons.

Periodically, the latent genome undergoes reactivation, during which a "reverse trip" occurs in which unenveloped virus capsids are assembled within latently infected cells before translocation to the respiratory epithelial surface, where they undergo envelopment and become infectious virus particles. Once delivered to the respiratory epithelial surface, virions undergo one of two fates: (1) neutralization by local mucosal immunity or (2) establishment of infection and a repeat of the events that occurred during primary infection, with shedding of infectious virus in respiratory tract secretions and possibly development of viremia[60] (Fig. 13-3). The precise details of this reverse trip from neurons of the trigeminal

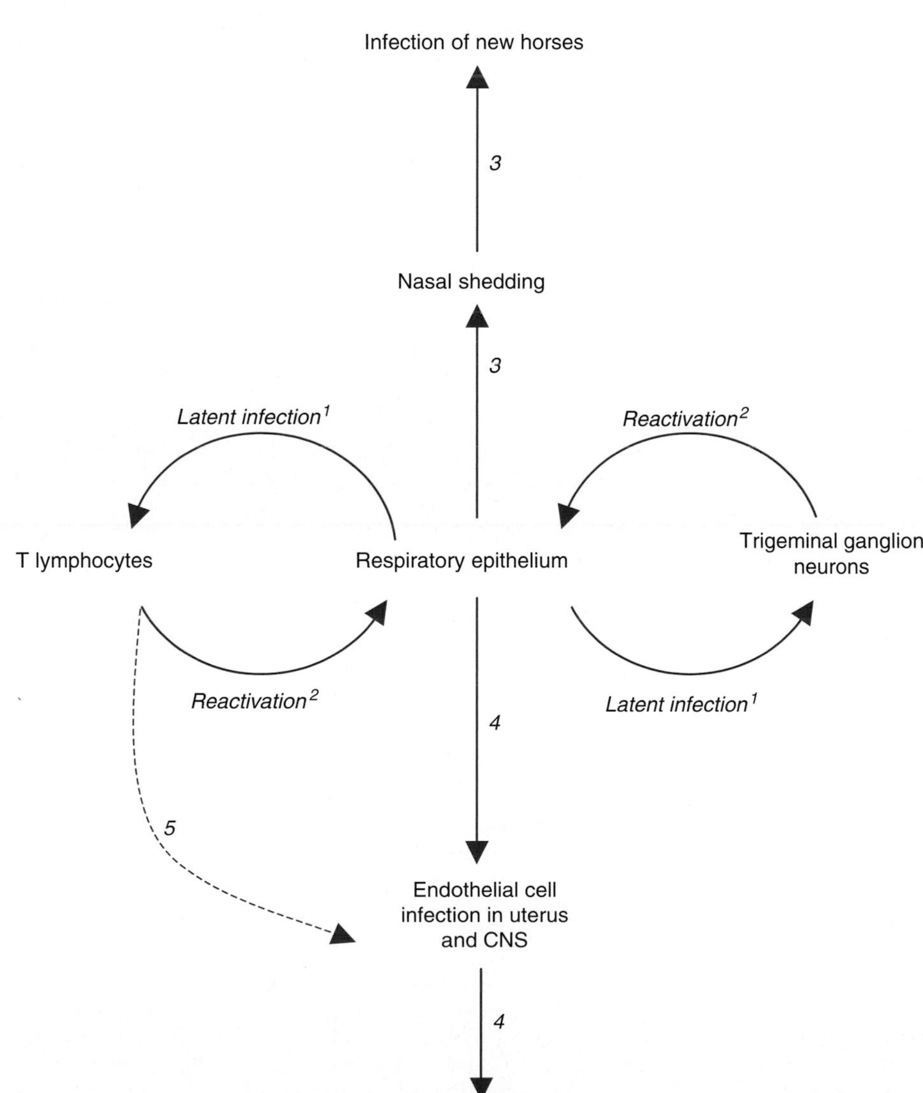

Fig. 13-3 EHV-1 latency and reactivation. *Note 1*: Latency is established in trigeminal ganglionic neurons and in T lymphocytes. *Note 2*: Reactivation from both sites delivers virus back to the respiratory epithelium. *Note 3*: Dependent on the ability of local (mucosal) immune responses to neutralize reactivated virus, reactivation may result in nasal shedding and infection of new, susceptible horses. *Note 4*: Within the reactivating horse, replication of reactivating virus in respiratory epithelium may seed a viremia (mirroring events during primary infection), with subsequent endothelial cell infection in the uterus and central nervous system *(CNS)*, resulting in abortion or equine herpesvirus myeloencephalopathy *(EHM)*. *Note 5*: It is possible that reactivation may occur locally within the uterus or CNS, with direct transfer of reactivating virus to endothelial cells in these sites.

ganglion[36] and circulating T lymphocytes[59] are not fully understood. It is assumed that the transfer of reactivating virus from lymphocytes to the respiratory epithelium involves expression of viral proteins on the surface of reactivating lymphocytes to allow cell-cell fusion and direct virus transfer. This process may also occur within the uteroplacental unit and the central nervous system (CNS), providing a mechanism for disease recurrence with reactivation.[3]

At a cellular level the molecular, cellular, or other events that control the switch from latency infection to reactivation are unknown. *Reactivation* involves a switch from latent to lytic cycle that is initiated by transcription and translation of the IE gene, inducing the lytic gene cascade as seen during primary infection. It is not known whether initiation of transcription requires a specific trigger, possibly *trans*-activation of the IE promoter by viral, cellular, or exogenous factors, or whether it occurs spontaneously. The IE promoter can be transactivated by a variety of viral and cellular proteins, including proteins encoded by EHV-2,[61] although the biologic significance in relation to reactivation is not known.

Whatever the mechanism of reactivation, it is likely that the outcome of most reactivation events, which may occur frequently at the cellular level, is neutralization of reactivating virus by mucosal immune responses, and thus prevention of virus shedding from the respiratory tract and development of viremia. Reactivation only becomes detectable at horse level, by nasal shedding or viremia, when the host immune response is compromised either by treatment with corticosteroids[60] or other immunomodulatory compounds or by a variety of management stressors,[62] including transport, illness, and hospitalization. It is not known how frequently horse-level reactivation and shedding actually occurs, but it is sufficiently frequent to maintain these viruses in the global horse population.

Viral Proteins

The virus encodes a single IE gene, 55 E genes, and 20 L genes. The 76 gene products have a variety of different functions, giving the EHV surprising complexity and comparatively sophisticated life cycles, features that greatly complicate attempts to understand pathogenesis and devise control measures. Functions have been assigned to the majority of viral proteins. At least 30 are associated with the virion, of which six form the capsid,[63] 12 are associated with the tegument[64,65] (located between the capsid and the envelope), and a further 11 are glycoproteins[66] anchored to, and projecting from, the envelope. The remaining proteins are involved with viral replication functions, including DNA replication enzymes; regulation of the viral gene cascade; and virus egress from infected cells. The regulation of the sequential cascade of viral genes into IE, E, and L phases[50] is controlled by six genes whose gene products act as transactivators and transcriptional regulators/suppressors: the IE gene (gene 64), four E genes (EICP 22, 27, 0 and TR2), and one L (ETIF) gene. Five of these genes (IE, EICP22, EICP27, TR2, and ETIF) are essential for virus replication in vitro.

The single IE protein is extremely important from an immunologic perspective because it is the first virus expressed by infected cells and, in some horses at least, contains a dominant *cytotoxic T lymphocyte* (CTL) epitope, making it a key vaccine target.[24,50,51,67-74] The 1487 amino acid IE protein is essential for virus replication and is a vital regulatory protein,[75] repressing its own promoter and transactivating expression of early and late gene promoters. It possesses different functional domains, including a DNA-binding domain responsible for binding its own promoter, a domain responsible for translocation of the IE protein to the infected cell nucleus, and a domain that binds *transcription factor IIB* (TFIIB) from the infected cell.[76-78]

Four E proteins (EICP 22, 27, 0, and TR2) have regulatory activities. EICP22 and 27 (gene 5) function synergistically with the IE protein to transactivate E and L genes, and EICP0 (gene 63) is also a powerful transactivator but is antagonistic to the IE protein and competes for the cellular transcription factor TFIIB.[47,52,77,79-85]

The late protein regulatory protein ETIF[53,86] is the product of gene 12 and is the EHV-1 equivalent of the herpes simplex virus *alpha trans-inducing factor* (α-TIF), a key transactivator that binds upstream of the IE gene and transactivates the IE promoter. ETIF is required for cell-to-cell spread; ETIF mutants produce small plaques in cell culture, and although capsids are produced, envelopment in the cytoplasm does not occur.

Glycoproteins

The 11 envelope-anchored surface glycoproteins of EHV-1 and EHV-4 play key roles in pathogenesis, including host specificity and cellular tropism.[66,87] They mediate viral attachment to and entry into cells as well as fusion of infected cells and direct cell-to-cell spread of virus. They are the principal viral immunogens, at least for humoral immunity, and are the major targets for virus-neutralizing antibody. Five glycoproteins (gB, gD, gH, gK, gL) are absolutely required for virus replication in tissue culture and are termed *essential*. The remaining six (gC, gE, gG, gI, gM, gp300) are not required for replication in vitro and are termed *nonessential*, a designation that does not translate to the in vivo situation because deletion mutants in these glycoproteins are viable but less virulent. Although convalescent horse sera recognize all 11 glycoproteins, three (gB, gC, gD) are "immunodominant," that is, are the principal viral antigens recognized by the equine host. Further features of gB, gC, and gD that have made them prime vaccine candidates are (1) they are protective in mice; (2) gB, gC, and gD deletion mutants are nonpathogenic in mice; (3) gB and gD are involved in cell-cell fusion and spread of virus; and (4) gD is involved with virus entry into cells and appears to be responsible for cellular tropism and host cell specificity.[88-99] The functions of the other glycoproteins are less well characterized; gE and gI are involved in cell-cell spread of virus, gK in cell-cell spread and virus egress, and gM in cell penetration and cell-cell spread[46,68]; gH is partially protective in mice.[100]

Taken together, it is clear that the glycoproteins are important epitopes for the humoral immune response. It is therefore likely that they will be included in future protein, subunit, recombinant, or DNA vaccines for the EHVs. Glycoproteins do not appear to be important CTL epitopes, however, and vaccines based on these glycoproteins alone are unlikely to induce efficient cellular immune responses.

EPIDEMIOLOGY

The principal reservoir of infection for EHV is latently infected horses. Environmental transmission is of most importance during outbreaks when horses are kept in close confinement and probably plays a minor role in maintenance of these viruses in the horse population. Environmental persistence of EHV is short, estimated to be less than 7 days in most conditions, with a maximum survival of 35 days.[101] The viruses are labile and easily inactivated by heat and disinfectants. Serologic surveys suggest that most adult horses have been exposed to EHV-1, -2, -4, and 5. Epidemiologic studies of stud farms suggest that infection is acquired within the first few weeks or months of life, generally before or just after weaning, from adult mares that asymptomatically shed virus[102-105] (Fig. 13-4).

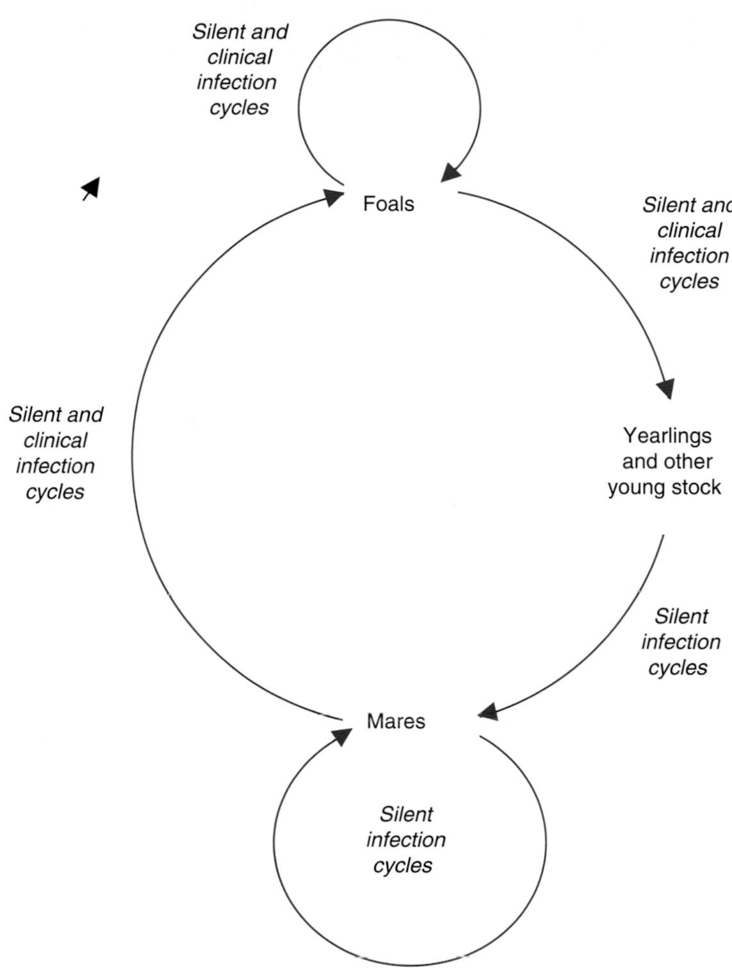

Fig. 13-4 Transmission of EHV-1. EHV-1 is transmitted through "silent" (subclinical) and "clinical" infection cycles. Adult horses (principally mares) infect foals early in life; infection is transmitted between foals and young stock. Endemic infection is maintained in mares by contact with younger stock and by subclinical transmission between mares. In all age groups, reactivation of latent virus provides the source of infectious virus to maintain endemic infection.

It is not clear whether the maintenance of endemic infection is caused by cycles of subclinical infection within the mare population or reactivation of endogenous latent infection in individual mares. The life cycles of the EHV share four main features: (1) early and widespread infection of young horses, (2) a widespread carrier (latent) state in adult horses, (3) transmission from latently infected adults to new generations of young stock, and (4) widespread "silent" adult-adult, adult-foal, and foal-foal endemic infection cycles of transmission.

Spread of Infection

Infection is spread by direct horse-to-horse contact as well as indirectly by fomites and personnel. The most common transmission route is through the respiratory tract by aerosolized droplets of respiratory tract secretions. Infection can also occur by ingestion or inhalation of droplets from surfaces. All horses with clinical disease and reactivating horses are considered to be contagious by the respiratory route, although shedding adult horses may show no overt clinical signs. Aborted foals, fetal membranes, and placental fluids contain large quantities of infectious virus and are particularly hazardous.

Latency

Latency and reactivation are key features of the epidemiology of EHV-1 and EHV-4 infections and are responsible for the ubiquitous distribution of these viruses in the horse population. The large majority of recovered horses carry latent EHV infections for extended periods, possibly for life.[57,58] Latency almost certainly also plays a key role in the biology of EHV-2 and EHV-5, since the majority of adult horses and almost all foals harbor latent infection in circulating lymphocytes. EHV-1 and EHV-4 enter into a latent state in the lymphoreticular system, in circulating and lymph node CD8+ T lymphocytes, and in neurons within the trigeminal ganglia.[36] EHV-2 and EHV-5 establish functional latency in circulating lymphocytes and trigeminal ganglia, from which virus can be reactivated in vitro.[106,107] Viral DNA can also be detected in other locations,[108] including the trigeminal ganglia,[41] but it is not clear whether virus is capable of undergoing reactivation from these other sites. These latently infected cells form, by means of periodic reactivations that result in shedding of infectious virus from the host, a transmissible reservoir of infection that maintains all the EHVs in the horse population.

Reactivation from Latency

Periodically, latently infected horses experience reactivation episodes, during which infectious virus is shed into respiratory tract secretions, with the potential for infecting other, susceptible horses. Reactivation of latent EHV-1 and EHV-4 infections from horses has been observed in field situations after transport, handling, rehousing, and weaning, and reactivation has been achieved experimentally in horses by treatment with high doses (10 times therapeutic doses) of corticosteroids.[36,109] The frequency with which reactivation occurs in response to the stresses imposed by the modern horse industry is unknown.

Reactivation is generally asymptomatic, resulting in "silent" shedding of virus, thus providing a mechanism for maintenance of endemic infection cycles and the apparently unexplained appearance of disease in closed populations of horses.

Abortion or neurologic disease may be the result of local reactivation of virus, that is, reactivation of EHV-1 within blood vessels of the uterus, placenta, or CNS, resulting in endothelial cell infection and thrombo-ischemia in those organs.[110-113] In this situation, disease occurs without prerequisite respiratory infection, nasal virus shedding, or viremia. Regardless of the sites from which reactivation occurs, it is likely that latency and reactivation are important in the epidemiology of EHV-1 abortion and neurologic disease. The majority of natural EHV-1 abortions occur singly,[114] rather than as "abortion storms,"[115] implying that abortion may have resulted from reactivation of endogenous latent virus rather than from a newly acquired respiratory infection. Such reactivations of latent EHV-1 may also explain abortions that occur many weeks or months after infection, beyond the period of viremia that follows. It is not clear whether latency is also important in the epidemiology of neurologic disease. However, it is logical to assume that endogenously reactivated virus may be responsible for isolated neurologic cases or for seeding virus into groups of horses where outbreaks of neurologic disease occur.

PATHOGENESIS AND PATHOLOGIC FINDINGS

Respiratory Tract

Following inhalation of virus or contact with infected fomites, both EHV-1 and EHV-4 replicate in upper respiratory tract epithelial cells. After experimental infection, virus can also be transiently recovered at low titer from lower respiratory tract (tracheal and bronchoalveolar) lavage samples. Virus replication causes death of epithelial cells, resulting in epithelial erosions. EHV-1 quickly spreads to cells in the underlying lamina propria, with infected (viral antigen-expressing) endothelial cells, lymphocytes, and monocytes detectable in respiratory tract–associated lymph nodes within 48 hours.[116,117] From these sites, virus-infected lymphocytes enter the circulation, resulting in a CD8+ T lymphocyte–associated viremia that disseminates virus widely, including into the uterine and CNS vascular endothelium.[118,119] In parallel, EHV-1 also rapidly gains access to neurons of the trigeminal nerve, reaching the trigeminal ganglion by 48 hours after infection, establishing latency in trigeminal ganglionic neurons.[36] Experimentally, EHV-1 shedding occurs from the respiratory tract for up to 14 days, and viremia persists for up to 21 days.[120] In the field, however, shedding and viremia may be more transient and intermittent, making detection difficult in the later stages of infection.

The detailed pathogenesis of EHV-4 infections has not been elucidated. The initial mucosal phase probably closely parallels that of EHV-1, with infection of the respiratory tract and its associated lymphoid system. EHV-4 DNA persists in the trigeminal ganglion[121] and circulating lymphocytes[58] after recovery from infection, but infectious virus has not successfully been reactivated from these sites in vitro. Most isolates of EHV-4 have low endotheliotropism, do not establish viremia, and therefore do not cause abortion or neurologic disease.[33,122] The duration of nasal shedding of EHV-4 is usually more transient than for EHV-1.

Viremia

Viremia disseminates virus to the uterus[123] and CNS and is therefore a prerequisite for these diseases. However, not all viremic pregnant mares abort, and only a very small minority of viremic horses develop neurologic disease. Local reactivation can also be responsible for these diseases without detectable viremia (see Latency and Reactivation). Viremia also delivers virus to other organs, detectable by polymerase chain reaction (PCR) assays, but does not result in clinically apparent organ dysfunction. Viremia is cell associated, primarily within CD5+/CD8+ T lymphocytes,[124,125] and free virus is rarely detected in the blood. Lymphocytes do not support lytic infection in vivo; virus can be liberated from these cells using only co-cultivation (in vitro reactivation) assays. Lymphocytes are susceptible to infection in vitro only after mitogen stimulation,[126] which also increases the efficiency of reactivation in vitro.[59] Viremia seldom occurs with EHV-4 infection, although some "high-virulence" isolates capable of inducing viremia exist, and EHV-4 DNA can be detected in circulating lymphocytes after infection.[127]

Uterus

The pathogenesis of EHV-1 abortion involves virus translocation from the circulation into the placental unit and induction of uterovascular lesions.[128] Infection of endothelial cells in the pregnant uterus causes a vasculitis that affects small arteriolar branches in the glandular layer of the endometrium at the base of the microcotyledons.[113] If these endometrial vascular lesions are widespread, the fetus may be aborted before detectable transplacental spread of virus has occurred.[129,130] Virologically negative abortions[129] in earlier EHV-1 challenges had been assumed to be caused by maternal stress or pyrexia, and the incidence of this type of abortion after spontaneous field infections is not known. However, in a survey of 241 abortions in the United Kingdom between 2001 and 2003,[130] nine were "typical" EHV-1 abortions (i.e., placenta and fetus were virus positive), whereas six were "atypical," and there was no detectable fetal infection by either PCR or immunohistochemical methods.[131] The susceptibility of uterine endothelial cells to infection with EHV-1 is low in early pregnancy compared with late pregnancy, and any potential association of EHV-1 infection with early embryonic death and resorption has not been investigated.

The pathogenesis of abortion caused by less virulent isolates of EHV-1 is not as clear,[132] because these isolates appear to have a reduced affinity for endothelial cells; however, abortion is also caused by vascular lesions and thrombo-ischemia. The rare cases of abortion that follow infection with EHV-4 are also likely to involve the capacity of certain isolates of EHV-4 for replication in uterine and fetal endothelial cells.

Central Nervous System

The pathogenesis of EHV-1 neurologic disease also involves vasculitis and thrombo-ischemia following endothelial cell infection.[133] There is little evidence for lytic virus infection of neurons or direct viral neuropathology,[134] and virus has rarely been isolated from the CNS. Affected horses demonstrate sites of vasculitis with virus antigen expression in the brain and spinal cord, with or without local hemorrhage and thrombo-ischemic necrosis.[136,137] Neurologic clinical signs therefore result from ischemic death of nervous tissue, and the virus thus causes a myelopathy, encephalopathy, or myeloencephalopathy, depending on which regions of the CNS are affected. EHV-1 neurologic syndromes are therefore generally referred to as *equine herpesvirus myeloencephalopathy* (EHM).

Virulence

There are wide variations in virulence among different isolates of EHV-1 and EHV-4. High-virulence EHV-1 strains, such as Ab4 and Army-183, are endotheliotropic, efficiently cause viremia, are abortigenic, and after experimental inoculation of horses, cause high rates of abortion and neurologic disease. Other isolates, such as V592, are less virulent, have reduced endotheliotropism, cause only "low-level" viremia, and rarely cause abortion or neurologic disease.[33,132] The availability of genome sequences for different EHV-1 strains has allowed identification of sequence variations that correlate with specific phenotypes. Small differences at genome sequence level account for marked phenotypic differences. For example, Ab4 and V592 exhibit only 0.1% difference in sequence (150 bases in 150,000). These are mostly single-base changes, causing coding changes in 31 genes. Gene 68 (U_S2) shows the highest variation rate (2%) and is now used as a phylogenetic marker for epidemiologic analysis. However, no relationship appears to exist between the phylogenetic groups generated by this method and the pathogenic potential of strains.

Dimorphism in the sequence of gene 30 (encoding DNA polymerase) does, however, provide a means of identifying paralytic strains of EHV. Two single-base changes, substituting G for A at positions 2254 and 2968, correlate with paralytic potential. The majority of nonparalytic strains possess A at position 2254, whereas the majority of paralytic viruses possess G at position 2254. It is not clear whether dimorphism in this gene is a surrogate marker for other virulence determinants because virulence may intuitively be expected to be determined multigenetically.

Immunology

Natural or experimental infection induces a solid but transient protective immune response to EHV that protects against reinfection for 3 to 6 months. During this time, there is clinical protection and sterile immunity (i.e., exposure to virus does not induce nasopharyngeal virus shedding or viremia). Exposure of mares early in gestation protects them from abortion in the later, susceptible stages of gestation. Furthermore, mares that have aborted in 1 year usually do not abort in subsequent years.[181]

The life cycle of EHV-1, and to a lesser extent EHV-4, is complex and involves infection of multiple cell types.[3] The initial mucosal colonization and replication phase of infection is rapidly followed by an *invasion phase*, during which virus enters the lamina propria and gains entry into blood vessels and lymphatics through endothelial cell infection, and a *distribution phase*, where infected lymphocytes disseminate virus throughout the horse. In parallel, latency is established. It is now clear that immune control of pathogenesis requires an integrated, multicomponent immune response, and that there are unlikely to be simple correlates of protective immunity. This is in marked contrast to "hit and run" virus pathogens with comparatively simple pathogenesis, exemplified by equine influenza viruses, for which measurement of the humoral immune response provides a simple and accurate measure of disease susceptibility and resistance.

For the EHVs, humoral immune responses alone do not provide protective immunity. An effective immune response to the EHVs requires a combination of mucosal and systemic humoral and cellular immune responses. Much of these data have come from experimental infections, and information from field infections or naturally occurring outbreaks is still scarce. The techniques and reagents required to study the cellular immune response to EHV infection have recently become available, allowing rapid progress to be made in this complex area of immunology. Although not completely elucidated, viral epitopes that drive cellular immune responses have been identified, and the relationship between MHC (ELA) haplotype and virus antigen recognition by CTL is being unraveled.

Infection induces strong systemic humoral immune responses characterized by an initial, rapid, but short-lived (<3 months) immunoglobulin M (IgM) response, followed by a slower-onset but longer-lived (>12 months) immunoglobulin G (IgG) response (see Diagnosis). The principal IgG isotypes produced are IgGa, IgGb, and IgGc. Only small quantities of immunoglobulin A (IgA) are found in the circulation in convalescent sera. In diagnostic laboratories, these responses are measured using the *complement fixation* (CF) test for the short-lived (IgM) antibody response and the *virus neutralization* (VN) test for the longer-lived (IgG) antibody response. Systemic humoral immune responses alone are not sufficient to protect horses from infection. VN antibody titers do not correlate with protection from infection. High VN titers are associated with reduced nasal virus excretion but do not influence the duration of viremia or the frequency of viremic cells in the circulation,[182] presumably because viremic cells express few, if any, virus antigens and are therefore not recognized as targets by the immune system.[183] Infection induces mucosal immune responses characterized by mucosal IgA production. In contrast to VN antibody, mucosal IgA titers do correlate with protection from infection.[184] The IgA response is short lived after a single infection but persists longer with subsequent infections. Mucosal IgA is an important first line of defense against EHV-1 infection. It is known to be neutralizing in vitro, although its function in vivo has not been fully characterized.

Infection induces both tissue (mucosal and lymphoid) and circulatory cellular immune responses mediated by CD8+ cytotoxic T lymphocytes (CTLs).[185-187] Understanding of the cellular immune response has advanced rapidly in the last 10 years, and there is abundant evidence that CTL responses are not only central to recovery from infection but also provide a correlate of protective immunity.[22,188] CTLs are the effector arm of the cellular immune response and kill infected cells that present virus antigens on their surface in the context of major histocompatibility complex (MHC) class 1 (ELA-A) molecules; that is, CTL responses are MHC-1 (ELA-A) restricted. The CTL response is directed by "professional" antigen-presenting cells (dendritic cells and macrophages). These cells are also MHC-1 restricted and work in concert with the Th1 subset of CD4+ T helper cells and an associated panel of cytokines, including interleukin-2 (IL-2), interferon-gamma (IFN-γ), and tumor necrosis factor alpha (TNF-α).[24,189] The polymorphic nature of ELA-1 molecules in the horse means that individuals vary in their CTL responses to particular virus antigens. As with other herpesviruses, MHC-1 expression is downregulated on the surface of infected cells, thus providing a means of immune evasion by the virus.

EHV-1 and EHV-4 infections cause changes in leukocyte populations in infected horses characterized by leukopenia followed by leukocytosis. The initial leukopenia consists of lymphopenia and neutropenia, with an initial depletion in CD8+ cells, and occurs between days 7 and 13 after infection. This is followed by a leukocytosis, consisting principally of a lymphocytosis, that continues to day 21 to 28 after infection. EHV-1, but usually not EHV-4, infection induces a cell-associated viremia that is associated mainly with infection of CD8+ cells, although a small proportion of monocytes and possibly CD4+ cells also become infected. In vitro, these cells are refractory to infection unless stimulated by mitogens. Both CD8+ and CD4+ cells release IFN-γ, an indirect marker of cytotoxic activity, in response to EHV-1 infection in vitro, suggesting both cell types are responsive to EHV-1.[24,189]

CTL responses to EHV were initially measured using a bulk lymphoproliferative assay.[186] Although lymphoproliferative responses increased after infection, there was no clear correlation with protection. The assay was refined by measuring the frequency of CTL precursors (CTLp) by limiting dilution analysis (LDA).[188] For the first time, this provided a correlate of protective immunity: high numbers of CTLp correlated with protection, whereas horses with low CTLp numbers were susceptible to infection. High frequencies of circulatory CTLp also correlate with protection from abortion in the face of EHV-1 challenge.[22]

The EHV-1 antigens that act as CTL targets have been mapped, providing valuable information on which virus antigens stimulate cellular immune responses. A variety of viral proteins have been mapped, including IE, several glycoproteins (e.g., gB, gC, gD), structural proteins, and proteins involved in replication. The IE protein, the first virus protein to be expressed in infected cells, is the most efficient CTL epitope. However, the ability of this protein to induce CTL responses varies with MHC haplotype; efficient responses are seen only in horses with the ELA-A3.1 haplotype.[23] A universally immunodominant CTL epitope, the functional equivalent of gB, gC, and gD for the humoral immune response, seems unlikely, but a panel of viral proteins constructed around the IE protein may fill this role.

Immune Evasion

The changes that occur in blood and pulmonary leukocyte populations after EHV-1 infection, including the lack of viral antigen expression on the surface of infected leukocytes, have led to the recognition that EHV-1, as with many of the herpesviruses, modulates the horse's immune response. Because cytotoxicity against EHV-1 proteins is MHC-1 restricted, it is not surprising that EHV-1 produces proteins that interfere with MHC-1 presentation of virus antigens as a means of evading the horse's immune response to infection.[190] Whether this *immunomodulation* represents *immunosuppression* is an area that requires further investigation. EHV-1 causes specific but incomplete downregulation of MHC-1 on the surface of infected cells that is mediated, by an unknown mechanism, by the IE, or possibly E, proteins of EHV-1.

CLINICAL FINDINGS

The clinical disease syndromes associated with EHV-1 and EHV-4 infection are well recognized. These viruses cause respiratory disease, abortion, and neurologic disease. EHV-1 is associated with all three syndromes, although the virulence of individual isolates shows considerable variation (see Virulence). EHV-4 is principally a cause of respiratory disease, although some highly virulent endotheliotropic, abortigenic isolates exist.

The role of EHV-2 and EHV-5 in clinical disease is uncertain. In most cases the virus is isolated from nasal and blood samples of apparently healthy foals and adult horses.[106,107,138] EHV-2 and EHV-5 are universally present in horse populations. The viruses can be detected (by the presence of DNA and recovery of virus from leukocytes) in 60% to 80% of adult horses and almost 100% of foals. EHV-2 is detected less frequently in nasal swabs in adult horses, but longitudinal surveys suggest the virus is frequently shed from apparently healthy foals. EHV-2 has been isolated from cases of keratoconjunctivitis in foals and weanlings[139] and is a presumed etiologic agent of some chronic superficial keratopathies in adult horses, although the evidence for this is weak (see Chapter 10). EHV-2 has been implicated in respiratory disease in foals and weanlings and isolated from the lungs of a stillborn foal. Both EHV-2 and EHV-5 have been suggested as causes of equine fatigue and poor performance syndromes, although little evidence exists to support this. Some have suggested that EHV-2 may act as an immunosuppressive agent in foals predisposing to other infections,[140] including other respiratory viruses and *Rhodococcus equi*.[141] The more detailed disease descriptions that follow relate to EHV-1 and EHV-4.

Respiratory Disease

Accumulated evidence indicates that EHV-1 is an uncommon cause of clinically apparent respiratory disease.[142-145] Several large epidemiologic surveys in Thoroughbred populations in Europe and North America have failed to associate EHV-1 with respiratory disease. EHV-4, however, is associated with respiratory disease. Both viruses generally cause self-limiting upper respiratory tract disease. In neonatal, immunocompromised, and other naive young animals, these viruses can cause severe lower respiratory tract disease (viral pneumonitis) and can lead to secondary bacterial bronchopneumonia. These foals show progressive disease with marked depression, pyrexia, tachypnea, and dyspnea. Horses experimentally infected with EHV-1 or EHV-4 show a short (1-3 days) incubation period before respiratory signs appear.[118,146] In the field, longer incubation periods of up to 10 days have been observed, presumably caused by differences in strain virulence, infective dose, and host immunity. In previously infected horses, clinical respiratory signs may be of minimal severity and of short duration,[37,116,147] or they may be completely inapparent in older horses. This applies particularly to pregnant mares and mature horses with neurologic disease; these animals usually show no respiratory clinical signs before abortion or onset of paralysis.[148] This is also the case during reactivation of latent EHV-1 or EHV-4, which usually results in asymptomatic virus shedding and viremia.

Primary infection in naive foals infected with virulent strains of EHV-1 results in clinically obvious upper respiratory tract disease.[118,120] Depression and anorexia are associated with a biphasic pyrexia of 8 to 10 days' duration, which peaks on days 1 to 2 after infection and again on days 6 to 7. Initially there is serous nasal discharge, conjunctivitis, and serous ocular discharge. The character of the nasal discharge progresses rapidly to mucoid and then mucopurulent by days 5 to 7, which is usually attributed to secondary bacterial infection (Fig. 13-5). There is progressive lymphadenopathy, principally of the mandibular lymph nodes, although occasionally the retropharyngeal lymph nodes become sufficiently enlarged to become palpable. Lymph nodes reach maximum size between 7 and 10 days after infection and can remain enlarged for many weeks. There is a biphasic change in both the circulating and the pulmonary leukocyte population consisting of an initial leukopenia caused by both lymphopenia and neutropenia, for the first 5 to 7 days after EHV-1 infection. This is followed by a leukocytosis, consisting principally of a lymphocytosis.[118,147] Coughing, in contrast to equine influenza virus infections, is not a major clinical sign in EHV infection but may be more prominent where management practices are substandard, especially with poor stable air hygiene and failure to rest the horse from training or performance activities.

On recovery from EHV-1 or EHV-4 upper respiratory tract disease, some horses may develop a "poor performance syndrome," which may be associated with nonspecific bronchial hypersensitivity and a syndrome resembling chronic obstructive pulmonary disease (COPD). Thus the economic losses associated with respiratory disease are associated not only with the costs of veterinary care and lost days training during the acute stages of infection, but also with the longer-term, detrimental effects on athletic performance.

Abortion

Pregnant mares infected with EHV-1 usually abort in the last third of pregnancy and appear refractory to abortion if virus is encountered earlier (<120 days) in gestation.[123] There are

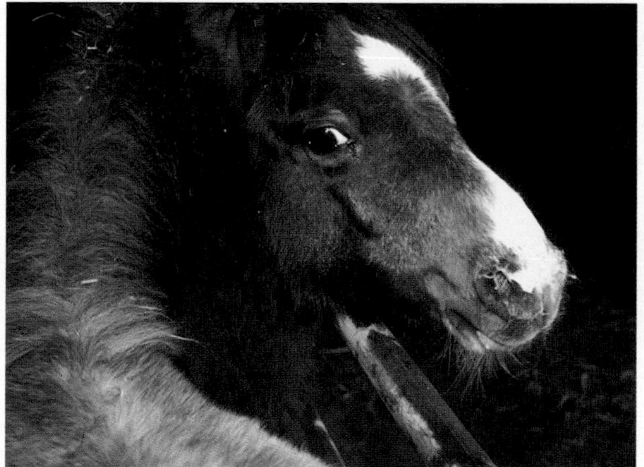

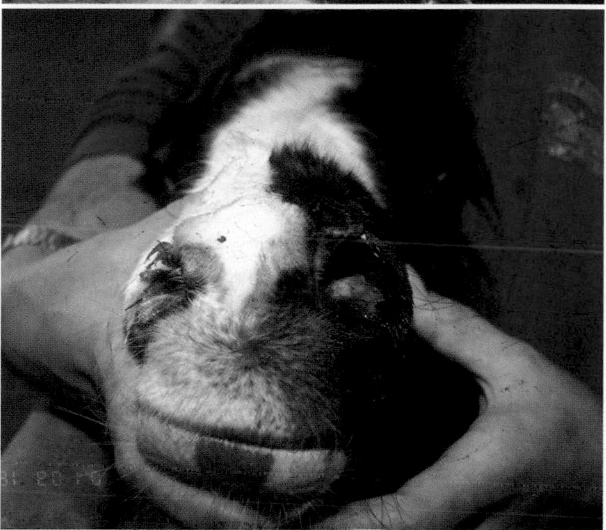

Fig. 13-5 A and B, Foals and young horses infected with EHV-1 may develop clinically apparent respiratory disease. Nasal discharge is initially serous but quickly becomes mucopurulent.

usually no warning signs, and abortion occurs precipitously.[129] Specifically, there are usually no respiratory signs before abortion occurs. Mares often abort standing up, and the foal is usually expelled within the intact amnion and may be expelled within the intact allantochorion. Occasionally a live foal is born that dies shortly after birth.[4,10] EHV-1 abortions are rare events and generally occur sporadically in individual mares.

"Abortion storms" are now extremely uncommon, presumably a reflection of the improved management measures that have been implemented as part of EHV-1 control measures on studs. However, devastating abortion storms have been recorded and remain a constant threat if scrupulous hygiene precautions are not followed.[149]

Most mares conceive successfully shortly after the abortion and foal normally the following year. Mares rarely abort from EHV-1 infection in successive years but may eventually become reinfected and abort again. Abortion is occasionally caused by "high-virulence" isolates of EHV-4,[150] with phenotypes resembling EHV-1. These isolates exhibit endotheliotropism, lymphotropism, and an ability to invade the allantochorion, causing placental and fetal ischemia.[33]

Other Reproductive Syndromes

Neonatal Foals

Neonatal EHV foal disease is rare. It is associated primarily with EHV-1 infection[12] and occasionally with EHV-4. It is not clear whether affected foals are infected in utero or whether infection is acquired, presumably from the dam, immediately after birth. Affected foals are born live but are sick at birth or become ill within 1 to 2 days. They show marked and rapidly progressive lower respiratory tract signs (dyspnea and tachypnea) caused by primary viral pneumonitis that leads to respiratory distress, hypoxia, and death. Secondary bacterial bronchopneumonia develops in foals that survive more than 2 or 3 days. These foals may survive for 10 to 14 days but eventually die from respiratory disease and a complex combination of other complications, including generalized lymphoid depletion and profound leukopenia. Occasionally, EHV-4 has been associated with neonatal foal disease and mortality.[151]

Stallions

Stallions infected with EHV-1 may develop scrotal edema, loss of libido, a reduction in sperm quality, and shedding of infectious virus (through infected leukocytes) into semen.[152,153] It is not known whether these changes affect fertility or whether venereal shedding plays a role in epidemiology, in a manner analogous to equine viral arteritis (EVA).

Neurologic Disease

Equine herpesvirus myeloencephalopathy (EHM) is sporadic and uncommon but is a potentially devastating manifestation of EHV-1 infection[154] and has been recognized clinically for many years.[155] EHV-4 neurologic disease is rare, but isolated cases have been identified. Anecdotal field evidence suggests that the neurologic disease is becoming increasingly common, leading to speculation that viruses with increased neurovirulence are circulating. However, the apparent increase in prevalence may be caused by increased awareness and improved sampling of suspected clinical cases.[156] EHM is not restricted by pregnancy, age, or gender and can occur in foals, yearlings, geldings, stallions, and both barren and pregnant mares.[157] Transmission is assumed to be through the respiratory route, although the source of infection may be endogenous reactivating virus.

Clinical signs appear during the viremic phase of infection. The interval between infection and subsequent onset of neurologic disease is usually between 6 and 10 days but may be as short as 1 day. There are invariably no premonitory clinical signs of respiratory disease, and pyrexia is likely to be the only warning clinical sign. Cases are often sporadic, but large outbreaks can occur, affecting 30% to 40% of horses on the premises.[156,158,159] Affected horses should be assumed to be contagious and precautions taken to prevent spread to other horses on the premises. It is assumed that neurologic clinical signs occur during or toward the end of the viremic phase of infection, similar to the pathogenesis of abortion.

The presentation and severity of clinical signs are highly variable and depend on the extent and location of the neurologic lesions[148,160] (Fig. 13-6). The caudal segments of the spinal cord and sacral plexus are affected most often, although outbreaks have been described in which horses develop acute-onset paralysis with cerebral signs, followed by rapid death. Clinical signs usually appear suddenly and reach their peak intensity within 2 to 3 days of onset. Neurologic dysfunction ranges from temporary ataxia and paresis to complete paralysis. The hindlimbs are usually the most severely affected, although quadriplegia has been observed. Bladder dysfunction, characterized by atony with incontinence or urinary retention,

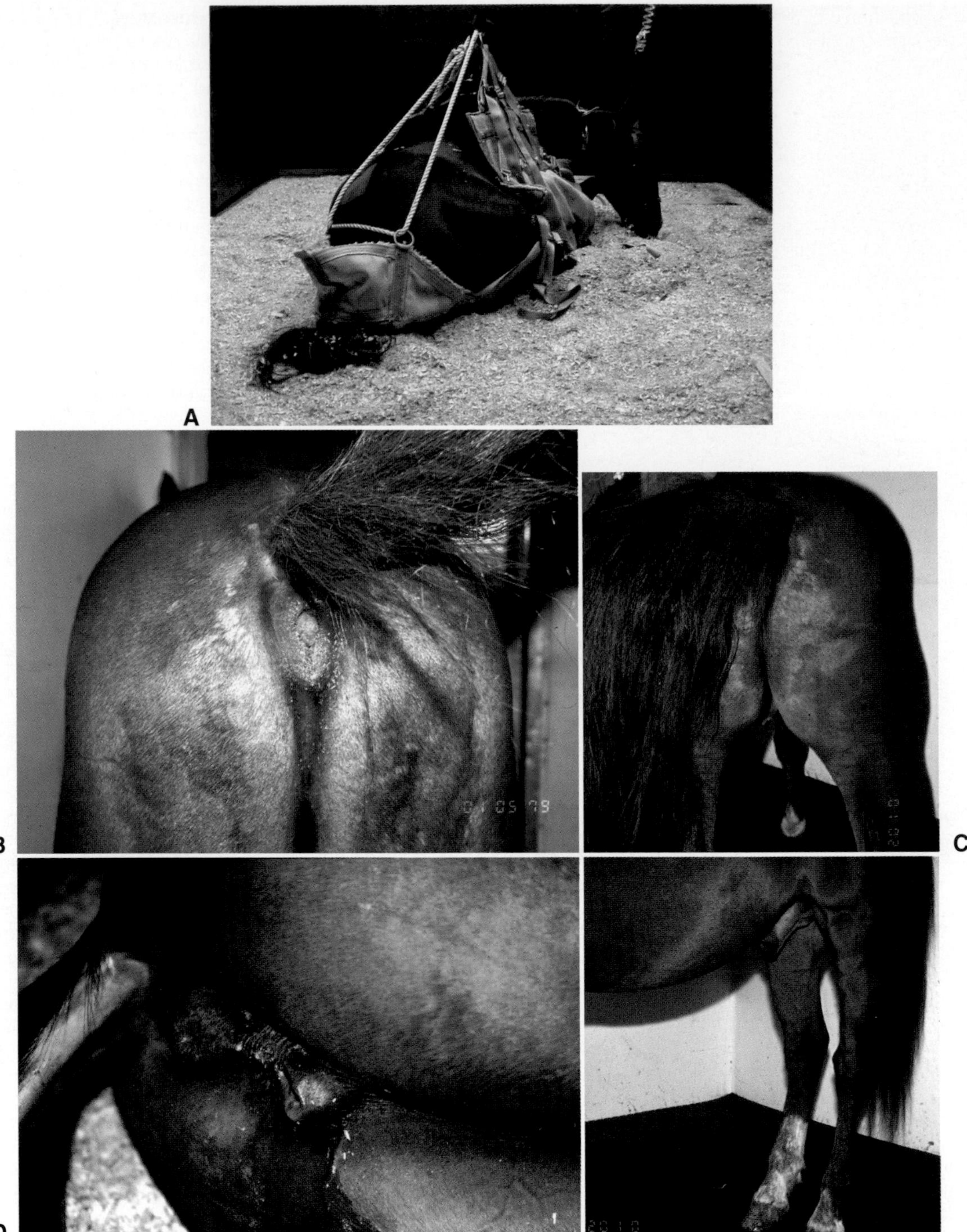

Fig. 13-6 Clinical signs in horses with equine herpesvirus myeloencephalopathy (EHM) vary in severity from mild ataxia and proprioceptive deficits to severe ataxia and recumbency requiring extensive supportive care (**A**). Other clinical signs may include loss of anal tone (**B**), flaccid paralysis of the tail (**C**), and urinary incontinence (**D**) with secondary urine scald on the hindlegs (**E**). (*A* courtesy Dr. Chris Sanchez, University of Florida.)

and cutaneous perineal and limb sensory deficits result from sacral nerve involvement. Some affected horses develop a head tilt.

The prognosis for nonrecumbent horses is favorable, but it is poor for recumbent horses, which frequently develop fatal complications (e.g., extensive myopathy, pneumonia, intussusception, bladder rupture) and require euthanasia.

DIAGNOSIS

History and Clinical Signs

Although a thorough history should be taken and a detailed clinical examination performed, it is usually not possible to diagnose any of the diseases associated with infection by EHV with certainty on clinical grounds alone. Except for infections in foals and young horses, EHV infections generally do not cause clinically apparent respiratory disease, and even then, there is little to distinguish EHV respiratory disease from that caused by other viral and bacterial pathogens. In particular, EHV-1 seldom causes obvious respiratory clinical signs in adult horses, and a common misconception is that monitoring for respiratory disease provides warning of impending abortion or EHM.

Abortion and neurologic disease (EHM) generally occur without any premonitory clinical signs apart from pyrexa, which, unless the horse is being closely monitored, is unlikely to be detected. Sudden abortion in the last third of pregnancy with the fetus still contained in the allantochorion is suggestive, but not diagnostic, of EHV-1 abortion. Abortion storms raise suspicion of EHV-1 infection in a herd, but these are rare. A presumptive diagnosis of EHM can sometimes be made with more confidence based on clinical signs, especially if more than one horse is affected, but diagnosis of individual cases on clinical grounds is difficult.

Because of these difficulties, further investigations are always required to confirm EHV disease, either by direct demonstration of virus (virus isolation, virus antigens, or nucleic acid) or indirect evidence of infection (serology). During outbreaks in particular, it is important to select rapid, sensitive, and specific diagnostic tests to enable rapid implementation of biosecurity measures and limit disease spread. In practice, the usual approach of diagnostic laboratories is to make an initial, perhaps preliminary, rapid diagnosis, followed by more time-consuming tests for confirmation (Table 13-2).

Case Selection

Correct selection of cases for sampling within an affected group is vital to gain the best-quality information from clinical pathologic investigations. Virus shedding from the respiratory tract, especially from adult horses, is generally short lived (<10 days), may be intermittent, and is most reliable soon (<5 days) after infection. All samples for direct demonstration of virus should therefore be collected from early clinical cases whenever possible. This generally means identifying in-contact horses with pyrexia but probably few or no other clinical signs because these appear later in the course of disease. Early sampling is especially important in suspected EHM cases because clinical signs appear toward the end of the viremic phase of infection, by which time virus shedding is waning or may have ceased. Diagnosis of EHV-1 abortion is perhaps the most straightforward because this is achieved using the aborted foal and placenta.

Selection of early clinical cases is also extremely important for indirect demonstration of infection using serology. Cases should be selected carefully, especially for aborting mares and EHM, because the delay between infection and appearance of obvious clinical signs may mean that the first of the paired serum samples already contains maximum titers of antibody, and a further rise on the second paired sample will therefore not occur. Although in these situations it is possible to infer evidence of infection on the basis of a *falling* titer, this can be misleading.

Direct Demonstration of Infection

Immunofluorescence

Direct immunofluorescence (IF) tests are very rapid (hours), simple tests with acceptable sensitivity and specificity that are used as the front-line diagnostic test for demonstration of virus antigens in nasal or nasopharyngeal swab samples or in frozen (cryostat) sections from aborted fetal and placental tissues. Although IF detects virus antigens expressed on the surface of infected cells and therefore does require live virus to be present in the sample, it is important to remember that its sensitivity approaches, but does not exceed, that of virus isolation.

Table • 13-2

Diagnostic Tests for Equine Herpesvirus Type 1 (EHV-1)

DIAGNOSTIC TEST	RAPID TEST?	SAMPLE REQUIRED	COMMENTS
Immunofluorescence (IF)	Yes	Airway swabs or frozen sections; fresh blood samples (for viremia)	Useful initial screening test; highly specific; false negatives occur; blood samples may be transiently IF positive
Polymerase chain reaction (PCR)	Yes	Airway swabs or lavages; blood; frozen or fixed tissue samples	Highly specific test; can differentiate between different EHVs; good sensitivity; false negatives occur
Virus isolation	No	Airway swabs and lavages; fresh blood, fetal and placental tissue samples	"Gold standard" for diagnosis; time-consuming; highly specific; false negatives occur
Histopathology	No	Fixed tissue samples	Definitive diagnosis of abortion and EHM, especially if used with ISH
Hematology	Yes	Whole blood in EDTA	May provide nonspecific evidence of virus infection
Serology	No	Serum (clotted blood samples); take two samples 10-14 days apart to demonstrate rising antibody titers	Highly specific test; provides indirect retrospective evidence of infection; early case selection important

EHM, Equine herpesvirus myeloencephalopathy; *ISH*, in situ hybridization: *EDTA*, ethylenediaminetetraacetic acid.

Polymerase Chain Reaction

Several PCR tests have been devised for the detection of nucleic acid (DNA) of the EHVs,[48,108,121,161-167] with different type-common and type-specific primers capable of distinguishing between the different EHVs.[58,168] PCR is an enyzmatic exponential DNA amplification technique that, in optimum conditions, is extremely sensitive, capable of detecting as few as 10 to 100 copies of target viral DNA.[169] However, the sensitivity of PCR tests in clinical samples is reduced, probably from the presence of inhibitors of the polymerase enzyme, other impurities within the DNA, and degradation of the viral DNA target. As for IF techniques, the sensitivity of PCR approaches that of virus isolation. PCR tests can be performed on respiratory tract swab or lavage samples, blood, or fresh, frozen, or fixed tissue samples.

The original PCR tests were nonquantitive and were incapable of estimating the amount of virus DNA present in the sample. Recently, quantitive ("real-time") PCR techniques have been devised for EHV-1 and EHV-4 that allow estimation of virus load in samples. These tests have quantified virus in respiratory tract and blood samples after experimental infection. They may have clinical application in the identification of latently infected horses, not currently possible, by measurement of virus load in leukocytes because virus copy number in latently infected leukocytes is between two and three orders of magnitude less than that in lytically infected cells.

Virus Isolation

Virus isolation remains the "gold standard" for laboratory diagnosis of EHV infections and provides unequivocal evidence of the presence of infectious virus in clinical samples (respiratory tract, blood, fetal, and placental tissue samples). The technique involves demonstration of typical *cytopathic effect* (CPE) in susceptible cell cultures inoculated with the supernatant from the sample, which can be followed by immunoassays or PCR tests to confirm the identity of the isolated virus, if required. EHV-induced CPE is normally detectable within 5 to 7 days of culture. Although false-negative results occur, because the technique requires the presence of infectious virus, virus isolation has higher sensitivity than both IF and PCR assays in clinical samples.

Histopathology

Histopathology is an essential method for confirming EHV infection in aborted fetuses and samples collected *postmortem* from horses with EHM.[170] Characteristic pathologic changes include eosinophilic inclusion bodies in airway epithelial and hepatic cells from aborted fetuses and vasculitis, often thrombosis, of CNS blood vessels. *Immunohistochemistry* (IHC) can be performed on paraffin-embedded, formalin fixed tissue sections to demonstrate virus antigen expression by infected epithelial and endothelial cells and provides valuable confirmation of the cause of vasculitis in the CNS and fetal tissues and placenta.

Viral nucleic acids (DNA) can also be detected in fixed tissue sections by *in situ hybridization* (ISH) techniques. In principle, ISH provides additional sensitivity over IHC because whereas all virus-infected cells contain viral DNA, only a proportion express viral proteins. Although DNA-DNA ISH has the potential to detect both lytically and latently infected cells, experimental evidence suggests that the technique is insufficiently sensitive to detect the low copy number of virus genomes present in latently infected cells, and that the more sensitive RNA-DNA hybridization techniques must be employed for this purpose. Practically, this means that ISH-positive cells can be taken as direct evidence for EHV infection without the need to distinguish latent, and therefore possibly irrelevant, cells from lytic infection.

Indirect Evidence of Infection

Hematology

Practitioners typically collect blood samples for hematologic analysis (total and differential white blood cell counts) from horses with suspected EHV disease. At best these samples provide nonspecific indication of a viral infection but are not diagnostic of EHV infection. Experimentally, EHV-1 and EHV-4 infections induce a biphasic change in total and differential white blood cell counts. There is an initial transient leukopenia with lymphopenia in the first 7 to 10 days after infection, which is replaced by a leukocytosis with lymphocytosis up to day 21 after infection. During the second (leukocytosis) phase, the increase in lymphocyte numbers reverses the normal ratio between neutrophils and lymphocytes (approximately 2:1) and can be regarded as a nonspecific indication of viral infection. In reality, however, the variation in hematology parameters among normal horses and the difficulties in correctly timing the collection of samples significantly limit the value of hematology, especially on single samples, to gain supportive evidence of EHV infection.

Serology

Serology can be used to gain a retrospective diagnosis of EHV-1 or EHV-4 infection and forms a valuable part of longitudinal surveillance. After infection there is an initial rapid increase in IgM antibody, detectable at 4 to 5 days, peaking at about 20 to 30 days, and decreasing to baseline values between 60 and 80 days.[171] There is a later but more sustained increase in IgG antibody, detectable 8 to 10 days after infection, peaking at 30 to 40 days, and persisting for many (>9) months. These antibodies can be measured by complement fixation (CF), measuring principally IgM antibodies;[172] virus neutralization (VN), measuring principally IgG antibodies; and enzyme-linked immunosorbent assay (ELISA). CF titers rise immediately after infection, peak rapidly, and then decay, whereas VN titers show a more gradual rise but remain elevated for extended periods. Rising CF titers on paired samples 10 to 14 days apart provide unequivocal evidence of EHV infection and can be useful during outbreaks of disease[158] when longitudinal sampling is possible. Significant increases in antibody are interpreted by most diagnostic laboratories to be a threefold to fourfold increase. A high CF titer in a single serum sample provides good preliminary evidence of infection and is a valuable initial diagnostic test in suspected EHM cases.

The longevity of VN antibodies means they are not useful for investigation of acute cases. They can be used, however, for disease prevalence surveys because they indicate historical exposure to infection. One drawback of CF and VN tests is that these antibodies are generated against epitopes common to both EHV-1 and EHV-4 and therefore do not allow differentiation between infection with the two viruses. Both type-common and type-specific ELISA tests are commercially available, although the type-specific assay, measuring antibody directed against EHV gG,[173,174] is the more useful because it differentiates between infection with EHV-1 and EHV-4.[175] As discussed earlier, appropriate case selection for serologic diagnosis is essential, and the clinician should remember that previous vaccination and maternal antibodies confound the interpretation of serologic investigations.

Cerebrospinal Fluid Analysis

Cerebrospinal fluid (CSF) from horses with EHM may have increased total protein (principally albumin) concentration without a concomitant increase in nucleated cell count.

CSF may also show xanthochromia (yellow discoloration, Fig. 13-7) caused by increased protein concentrations and red blood cell breakdown. These CSF changes, in conjunction with characteristic clinical signs, are suggestive, but not diagnostic, of EHM. Antibodies against EHV-1 in the CSF may be the result of leakage from the circulation secondary to EHV-1 endothelial cell infection and vasculitis, or other causes of vasculitis, rather than local production within the CNS and, although indicative of exposure to EHV-1, are not necessarily conclusive of EHM.

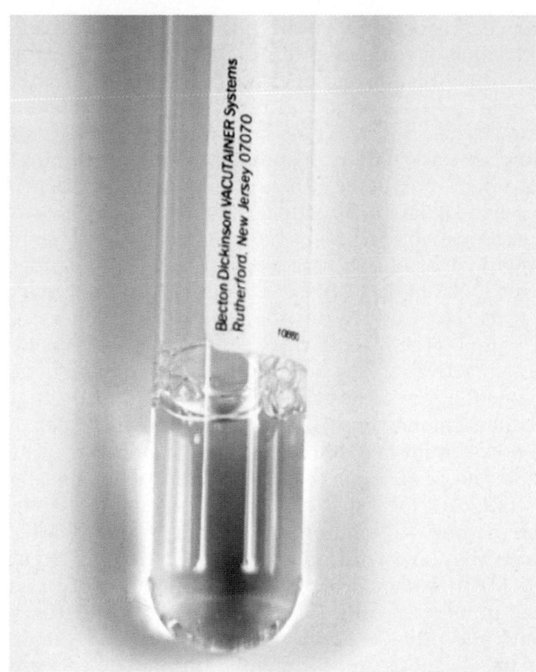

Fig. 13-7 Xanthochromic cerebrospinal fluid sample from a horse with EHM. (Courtesy Dr. Chris Sanchez, University of Florida.)

Diagnosis of Latent Infection

The ability to identify latently infected horses with accuracy would greatly assist control programs because these animals form the reservoir of transmissible EHV infection and are responsible for maintenance of infection in the horse population. Diagnosis of latent infection *antemortem* is a considerable challenge both clinically and in the laboratory. Latently infected horses cannot be identified with certainty using any of the currently available diagnostic methods (Table 13-3). There are several reasons for this: (1) latently infected horses are "silently" infected, exhibiting no clinical signs of disease; (2) latently infected cells express no virus-encoded proteins and thus escape immune detection; (3) the latent virus genome is transcriptionally silent, except for limited transcription from the region antisense to the single IE gene; (4) latently infected cells harbor a relatively small number of virus genomes; and (5) latently infected leuckocytes form only a small subset of the total leukocyte population, making them comparatively rare cells. These observations mean that the standard diagnostic tests previously described do not readily differentiate between lytic (acute) and latent infection cycles and that, with the exception of PCR and possibly VN assays, latently infected horses are generally negative using most current diagnostic tests. Leukocytes harbor detectable, latent EHV DNA for many months, possibly years, after infection and provide the only means presently available of identifying latently infected horses (the presence of VN antibodies indicates previous exposure to virus but not necessarily that latent infection has been established). Latently infected horses are more readily detectable during reactivation episodes because they shed infectious virus, often become viremic, and seroconvert.

Table • 13-3

Diagnosis of Latent and Lytic Infection Cycles Using Common Commercial Diagnostic Tests

SAMPLE SITE	DIAGNOSTIC TEST	LATENT INFECTION[1]	LYTIC INFECTION
Airway	Immunofluorescence	Negative	Positive
	Virus isolation	Negative	Positive
	PCR	Negative	Positive
Whole blood	Immunofluorescence	Negative	Positive (transiently)[2]
	Virus isolation	Negative[3]	Positive
	PCR	Positive	Positive
Serum	Serology	Positive or negative[4,5]	Positive[5]
Tissue[6]	Immunofluorescence	Negative	Positive
	Virus isolation	Negative[3]	Positive
	PCR	Positive	Positive

Note 1: Results for all assays during reactivation would be same as during lytic infection.
Note 2: There is brief expression of virus antigens during viremia.
Note 3: Direct virus isolation from fresh blood or tissue is negative during latent infection, but co-cultivation techniques are positive.
Note 4: Serum viral neutralization (VN) titers remain raised for many months, but in the absence of periodic reactivation, latent virus is likely to persist for longer than the duration of detectable VN antibody.
Note 5: During lytic infection and reactivation, complement fixation (CF) and VN antibody titers increase.
Note 6: Postmortem fresh, frozen, or fixed samples of lymph nodes and trigeminal ganglia.
PCR, Polymerase chain reaction.

Presumptive diagnosis of latent infection can be made in a horse that has (1) negative respiratory tract samples by IF, PCR, and virus isolation and negative blood samples by IF; (2) negative or positive blood samples by virus isolation (co-cultivation); (3) positive blood samples by PCR; and (4) detectable serum VN titers. It should be remembered that detection of viral DNA by PCR is not unequivocal evidence for the presence of latent infection (i.e., a functional virus genome that is capable of reactivation) because the assay detects a fragment of one virus gene, and "residual" or fragments of virus DNA in host cells will produce positive results with PCR tests. For this reason, the search for markers of "functional" latency (i.e., latent virus genome that is capable of undergoing reactivation, leading to production of infectious virus) has been a research priority. Initial optimism that latency-associated transcripts (LATs) might provide such a marker has now diminished due to technical difficulties in its detection and the realization that LATs are not universally present in cells carrying functional HSV-1 latent infection. These problems notwithstanding, the advent of quantitative PCR methods may allow differentiation of lytic and latent infection cycles in leukocytes based on estimation of virus copy number in infected cells. This would improve the utility of PCR assays and provide a comparatively rapid and simple method for the diagnosis and differentiation of acute disease and latent infection.

Diagnosis of latent infection postmortem is more straightforward. Viral DNA is detectable by PCR assays in most tissues, including respiratory tract, respiratory tract drainage lymph nodes, spleen, other lymphoreticular organs, and CNS. Co-cultivation (an in vitro test of reactivation) is the "gold standard" test for latent infection because it provides unequivocal evidence of functional (reactivatable) latent infection. Latently infected tissues do not yield infectious virus on direct culture (homogenization followed by sonication and titration of tissue supernatant on monolayers of susceptible cells) but do yield infectious virus when dispersed, viable tissue cells are cultured, perhaps for extended periods (up to three passages), with monolayers of susceptible cells. The sensitivity of this assay can be increased for latently infected leukocytes by stimulation with T-cell mitogens. Perhaps not surprisingly, only a subset of PCR-positive tissues, for both EHV-1 and EHV-4, are also positive by co-cultivation. Overall, it appears that EHV-1 establishes functional latency in the lymphoreticular system (principally CD8+ T lymphocytes) and the CNS (neurons of the trigeminal ganglion). Latent virus can be detected in fixed tissue sections using RNA-DNA ISH to detect virus genome and RNA-RNA ISH to detect EHV LATs, although these are research techniques that are not available commercially.

TREATMENT

Respiratory Disease

Horses with EHV respiratory disease are contagious and should be isolated (see Chapters 66 and 67). Exposed, in-contact horses should also be isolated. It is generally necessary to establish "clean" and "dirty" areas to separate unaffected horses from the affected horse(s) and in-contacts. Yard staff must be briefed about barrier nursing, and biosecurity precautions (which at their minimum should include the use of gloves, dedicated boots, and overalls) must be implemented. Affected horses should not be worked until at least 7 days after clinical signs have resolved and should be kept in stables with good air hygiene (dust free with low concentrations of allergens, bacteria, and irritants).

Respiratory disease is generally mild and self-limiting and does not require specific treatment. Broad-spectrum antibiotics are often administered, but seldom indicated, to prevent secondary bacterial infections. The beta-2 sympathomimetic clenbuterol stimulates mucociliary clearance and may assist in reducing airway contamination but is usually not required. Mucolytics (e.g., dembrexine) could also be considered but, again, are not usually indicated. Occasionally, horses fail to recover at the expected rate or may develop persistent post-viral syndromes, and immunomodulation therapy may be beneficial in these cases (see Chapter 72).

Abortion

Abortion occurs without warning. There is no evidence that treatment of in-contact mares with antiviral agents (e.g., acyclovir; see later discussion) assists with prevention of abortion. Once abortion has occurred, rigorous biosecurity measures should be implemented (see Control and Chapters 66 and 67). The affected mare should be examined to ensure that the entire placental unit has been expelled, which is invariably the case. In the rare cases where this does not occur, the mare should be treated for retained fetal membranes.

Ocular Disease

Cases of suspected EHV keratoconjunctivitis or chronic superficial keratitis have been treated empirically with antiviral compounds, mainly idoxuridine[39] and acyclovir[12,159] (see Chapter 10). Little pharmacologic basis exists for the use of these compounds in horses, although they have been successfully used to treat HSV keratopathies in humans. Horses with nonulcerative chronic superficial keratitis respond well to corticosteroid and cyclosporine treatment, suggesting that pathology is immune mediated, rather than directly virus induced.

Equine Herpesvirus Myeloencephalopathy

Horses with confirmed or suspected EHV-1 neurologic disease may be contagious and should therefore be subjected to the same rigorous biosecurity measures as aborting mares. Strict hygiene precautions and barrier housing are necessary because virus can be transmitted by both direct (aerosol) and indirect (fomites) means within stable yards and equine hospitals (see Chapters 66 and 67). These measures do create additional difficulties for nursing affected horses, especially those with more severe clinical signs, but are required to prevent disease spread within the hospital. Affected horses should be stabled in isolation or a geographically separate part of the yard. This may not be possible for recumbent horses, for which stables with specialized overhead equipment may be required for sling attachment. Dedicated footwear, gowns, and gloves must be worn when attending affected horses. Equipment and utensils should not be shared with other horses.

The stable should contain sufficient bedding to prevent trauma to the horse, and the environment should be quiet to prevent excitement. Recumbent horses can be successfully nursed in slings (e.g., Anderson sling), but scrupulous attention must be paid to welfare and secondary complications (e.g., skin trauma, decubital ulceration, impaction colics). An indwelling Foley catheter is required in horses with bladder paralysis, urinary retention, and overflow. Application of petroleum jelly to the perineum and an extension line to direct urine away from the perineum help to prevent urinary scalding. Urinary catheters should be maintained in a sterile fashion, but cystitis is a common complication, and prophylactic broad-spectrum antibiotics should be considered. Water intake must be carefully monitored because horses may be unable to drink the 50 to 70 mL/kg daily required to maintain hydration.

Intravenous (IV) fluid therapy is indicated for horses that are unable to drink, especially horses in slings. Attention must be paid to food intake, and a palatable high-energy, high-protein gruel should be offered. The addition of oil to the gruel can make a valuable contribution to energy intake.

Treatment of horses with neurologic disease is largely empiric because little experimental or clinical evidence exists to support many of the drugs used. No controlled studies have compared treatments in affected horses, partly because the sporadic and uncommon nature of the disease makes controlled studies in the field difficult. Based on pathologic observations that the nervous system lesion is a thrombo-ischemic injury secondary to virus infection of endothelial cells, many clinicians treat affected horses with nonsteroidal antiinflammatory drugs (NSAIDs) and antiviral drugs.[176] Dimethyl sulfoxide (DMSO, 1 g/kg diluted 1:10 in saline and given intravenously [IV] once daily for 3-5 days), corticosteroids (dexamethasone, 0.1 mg/kg IV once daily for 3 days), and NSAIDs (flunixin, 1.1 mg/kg IV twice daily for 3-5 days) are believed to aid recovery. Concern has been expressed that corticosteroid treatment may exacerbate disease by allowing continued viral replication or viral reactivation; however, this is without foundation. Although reactivation has been induced experimentally by dexamethasone treatment, this was achieved with doses tenfold higher than those used clinically. Similarly, dexamethasone treatment, even at 1 mg/kg IV, did not increase the duration or titers of virus replication during experimental challenge, whereas the T-cell immunomodulator cyclosporin-A increased both titers and duration of shedding.

The antiherpesvirus drug *acyclovir* (ACV) has been used in outbreaks of EHV-1 neurologic disease in the United States, and reports of its use have now entered the literature.[177] Although the balance of clinical opinion is that ACV treatment appears to be worthwhile, the current enthusiasm for its use should be tempered by the paucity of in vitro or in vivo experimental evidence of its efficacy against EHV-1 and also by the absence of data from controlled clinical studies in affected horses. ACV is the first-line treatment for infections with human herpesviruses HSV-1, HSV-2, and VZV and therefore seems an obvious choice for EHV-1 therapy. However, ACV is not equally active against the different herpesviruses. It has highest activity against HSV-1 and is less active against HSV-2 and VZV. Comparative in vitro inhibition studies have suggested that ACV may lack sufficient activity to be useful against the animal herpesviruses. The differential activity of ACV (and related compounds) is compounded by their low aqueous solubility and thus poor bioavailability after oral treatment: only 10% to 20% of the oral dose is absorbed. To circumvent this problem in humans, *prodrugs* (derivatives that are metabolized after oral administration to produce the active form of the drug) have been developed to increase bioavailability of ACV. Valacyclovir and famciclovir are now successfully used as oral prodrugs for ACV and the related compound *penciclovir* (PCV).

ACV is a nucleoside analog that, when activated in virus-infected cells, interferes with virus replication by preventing viral DNA synthesis. Nucleosides are the building blocks of DNA and consist of a base (adenine, guanine, thymine, cytosine, or uracil) linked to a sugar (ribose in RNA or deoxyribose in DNA) and are called adenosine, guanosine, cytidine, thymidine, or uracil, depending on which sugar they contain. Before they can be incorporated into a new strand of DNA, *nucleosides* have to be "activated" by the sequential addition of three phosphate groups to the carbon in the 5′ position of the carbon ring of the sugar to form triphosphate *nucleotides*. This process is known as *phosphorylation* and is carried out by enzymes called *kinases*. In addition to the 5′ phosphate group, the sugar ring also carries a hydroxyl group on the 3′ carbon. The new DNA strand is formed as the enzyme DNA polymerase links nucleotides together to form a polymer by sequentially adding sugars through their 5 phosphate group to the free 3′ hydroxyl group on the end of the DNA strand.

Acyclovir is acycloguanosine; it possesses the guanine base but has a linear carbon chain instead of the ribose sugar of the "normal" guanosine nucleoside; that is, ACV lacks the five-carbon sugar ring, or is *acyclic*. Critically, ACV lacks a 3 hydroxyl group and, when incorporated into the newly synthesized DNA strand, ACV therefore prevents DNA polymerase from adding further nucleotides. ACV thus blocks DNA synthesis by chain termination and competitive inhibition of the normal substrate of DNA polymerase, guanosine triphosphate. The carbon chain of ACV, in the positional equivalent of the 5′ carbon, can be phosphorylated ("activated"), but not by cellular kinases because these have low affinity for ACV. The key to the antiviral action of ACV and its selective toxicity is that only the herpesvirus enzyme *thymidine kinase* (TK), not cellular kinases, will undertake the first (of the three) phosphorylation steps required to convert acyclovir to its active form, acyclovir triphosphate. This is because herpesvirus TKs are different from cellular TKs at the amino acid level, have different substrate specificities, and possess extra enzymatic activities, making them multifunctional deoxpyrimidine kinases. In virus-infected cells only, therefore, acyclovir is converted to its active triphophosphate form by phosphorylation, initially by viral TK, which adds the first phosphate, then by cellular kinases that complete the process. In this way the active triphosphate form of acyclovir is confined to virus-infected cells and does not accumulate in uninfected cells. In infected cells the active acyclovir triphosphate is inserted into newly synthesized viral DNA by DNA polymerase in place of the "normal" nucleotide guanosine and terminates the DNA chain by preventing further addition of nucleotides to the DNA strand.

There are limited data describing either the in vitro or in vivo efficacy of ACV against any of the EHVs, including EHV-1. ACV is relatively ineffective against EHV-1 compared with the human herpesviruses[178] and is less effective against EHV-1 than the related acyclic nucleoside PCV.[179] A variety of in vitro susceptibility assays suggest that the inhibitory concentration of ACV against different EHV-1 isolates lies within the broad range of 0.44 to 7.0 μg/mL. For comparison, the estimates of inhibitory concentrations of PCV against EHV-1 range from 0.01 to 1.6 μg/mL. The accepted breakpoint for ACV resistance by HSV-1 is 2 μg/mL, which suggests that it may not be possible to achieve effective concentrations of ACV against EHV-1 in vivo, especially if oral dosing is used. There are no data for the efficacy of ACV in EHV-1 infections in horses, but in a hamster subcutaneous infection mortality model, ACV given at 100 mg/kg orally for 5 days afforded poor protection against death, with mortality rates of 70%.[180] In contrast, PCV administered at doses as low as 2 mg/kg orally provided complete protection in this model.

Clinical cases of EHV-1 neurologic disease have been treated with ACV at a dose of 10 mg/kg PO five times daily, which produced mean peak plasma concentrations of 0.287 μg/mL (range, 0.226-0.869 μg/mL),[177] a value significantly below the lowest estimate of the required inhibitory concentration for EHV-1. The five horses in this report all survived, suggesting either that the in vitro inhibitory concentration is not reflective of the in vivo situation, or that ACV treatment did not influence the outcome of infection. In contrast, an IV infusion of 10 mg/kg ACV produced peak plasma concentrations of 13.7 ± 5.9 μg/mL, suggesting that the IV route, not the oral route, is capable of achieving effective ACV concentrations in the horse.

Thus, although generic ACV is now available, making oral therapy in horses potentially affordable (estimated cost approximately $50 per day for the regime previously outlined), the limited available data raise questions about the rationale behind its use. Detailed pharmacokinetic studies in the horse coupled with rigorous in vitro inhibition testing would greatly assist clinicians in the therapeutic decision-making process. Although the oral route offers clear practical advantages over IV treatment, it seems likely that the related acyclic nucleoside PCV, or alternatively the ACV and PCV prodrugs valacyclovir and famciclovir, would be more effective for oral therapy.

VACCINATION

Effective vaccines against the EHVs must satisfy a difficult series of demands: a safe and efficient delivery route and induction of a multilayered immune response, consisting of long-lived systemic and mucosal immune responses producing serum and mucosal VN antibody, together with high frequencies of CTL precursors (CTLp) and memory B cells. This is further complicated by the influences of MHC haplotype on CTL recognition of virus antigens. Virus strain variation may have an effect, and the horse's immune status and preexisting latent infection are also likely to influence the response to vaccination. It is not surprising, therefore, that each of the currently available EHV-1 vaccines induces some, but not all, of the desired components of the immune response against EHV-1, and none produces complete protection. A general feature of all current commercial vaccines is that they induce high titers of VN antibody in adult horses, which are presumably primed by previous exposure to the EHV, but induce weaker or perhaps undetectable responses in immunologically naive animals, especially foals. There is little evidence that existing vaccines induce significant cellular immune responses.

Vaccination has been used, in combination with management measures, to control EHV-1 infection for more than 40 years.[21,191] It is difficult, however, to assess the impact of vaccination on the control of EHV disease because of a lack of randomized, controlled field studies. The first EHV-1 vaccination program was carried out in Kentucky in 1961 using a live hamster-adapted strain that protected horses for 3 months against respiratory disease. Field data also suggested a reduction in abortion frequency in vaccinated mares. A commercial vaccine (Pneumabort-K) was subsequently used extensively in Kentucky and was credited with reducing abortions; in a 3-year period, 140 of 20,223 nonvaccinated mares aborted (0.69%) compared with 14 of 6806 vaccinated mares (0.18%). An inactivated vaccine was credited with reducing abortion rates from 6.8 in 1000 to 1.6 in 1000.[192] Over a 20-year period, commercial vaccines reduced the incidence of abortion in Kentucky by almost 75%.[193] Vaccination assisted in this reduction, but the vigorous implementation of hygiene measures undoubtedly had a major impact by reducing the spread of virus, and thus the occurrence of multiple abortion storms.

More recently, a randomized control study has been carried out to assess the efficacy of a commercial inactivated combined EHV-1/EHV-4 vaccine.[194] Vaccination did not reduce respiratory clinical signs or influence viremia but did reduce nasal shedding of virus and did appear to decrease abortion. There are no data on the ability of current vaccines to prevent EHV-1 neurologic disease, and the relative rarity of this disease makes it unlikely that such data will be forthcoming. Similarly, no data are available on the use of these vaccines in an outbreak of EHV disease (respiratory, abortion, or neurologic), although from first principles it is unlikely that any of the current vaccines would induce a sufficiently rapid immune response to intervene in pathogenesis, especially for neurologic disease. There is a clinical suspicion that frequently vaccinated horses may be at increased risk of developing neurologic disease, and some veterinarians therefore believe that vaccination during an outbreak of neurologic disease is contraindicated. Vaccination of pregnant mares does not appear to be effective at blocking the cycle of silent transmission of either EHV-1 or EHV-4 on large studs.

There are currently 10 killed commercial EHV vaccines available (eight in United States and two in Europe) and two live vaccines (one in United States and one in Europe). These vaccines induce high titers of CF and VN antibody and appear to offer some protection against respiratory disease. They reduce the duration and titer of nasal virus shedding of virus but have little effect on viremia. Their effect on abortion in the field is less clear[195-198] because, again, the rarity of field abortions makes these studies difficult. These vaccines therefore *assist* with disease control and are not intended, or marketed, to provide complete protection from disease. The reasonable expectation of current vaccines should not be to produce sterile immunity but rather to reduce the severity of clinical disease and limit virus shedding from infected horses, thus reducing contagion. Vaccines should therefore be used to supplement hygiene control measures, which have a central role in reducing exposure to virus.

Extensive research continues to develop improved vaccines against EHV-1 and EHV-4. Thus far, the other EHVs have received little attention because they are less clinically and commercially important. Attention is currently focused on recombinant vaccines, using baculovirus and canary pox as vectors to deliver EHV-1 glycoproteins gB, gC, and gD, and on DNA vaccines, delivering the same glycoproteins together with candidate CTL epitopes. Efficient humoral immune responses are generated by vector vaccines or by combined approaches using DNA vaccination to prime and a protein vaccination to boost, but generation of high-frequency CTL responses remains problematic. Other research challenges are the construction of sufficiently attenuated yet immunogenic modified live-virus vaccines and the identification of appropriate adjuvants and delivery routes.

CONTROL

The control of EHV disease is by a combination of management and hygiene measures supplemented by vaccination.[158,199,200] Worldwide, EHV-1 disease control programs have three common goals: (1) prevention of disease entry onto premises; (2) limiting the extent of spread and severity of clinical disease once EHV-1 enters the premises or appears in the herd; and (3) limiting the spread of disease to adjacent premises during an outbreak. In the United Kingdom these measures are formalized into a voluntary code of practice (hblb.org.uk) that has greatly assisted in disease control.

Prevention of disease entry onto premises is not straightforward because the majority of adolescent and adult horses carry latent EHV infections. Diagnosis of latent infections is not straightforward (see Diagnosis), and in any event, exclusion of latently infected horses is impractical. To reduce the risk of disease entry into premises, new arrivals should ideally have been vaccinated before arrival and should be kept isolated from other horses until sufficient time has passed for disease to become apparent. On studs, newly arrived and "walk-in" mares should be kept strictly separate from resident in-foal mares for 56 days after covering. Mares arriving at studs to foal should be transported at least 28 days before the foaling due date. Horses that have arrived from sales or markets are at particular risk, as are any animals whose background, health, and vaccination status is uncertain. In yards with no pregnant mares, new arrivals should be kept isolated for at least 21 days and preferably 28 days after arrival because virus shedding may occur after reactivation. Minimizing management stress in resident horses, including transport, disruption of established social groups, and weaning, should assist in reducing the frequency of reactivation. If clinical respiratory or neurologic disease occurs in a new arrival, the horse should be isolated for at least 28 days from the onset of clinical signs.

Limiting the extent of spread of disease on the premises is greatly assisted by simple stock management measures (see Chapters 66 and 67). Different age groups should not be mixed, and group size should be kept as small as practicable. Pregnant mares should be isolated from other horses on the premises and should be subdivided into small groups to reduce the risk of large-scale outbreaks. Mares in the last third of pregnancy (the highest risk period for EHV-1 abortions) should ideally be housed and managed individually. Isolation areas should be rigorously maintained and located in a geographically separate area of the premises, and staff should understand and be able to apply the principles of barrier housing. As soon as disease is suspected on clinical grounds (e.g., respiratory clinical signs, abortion, stillborn foals, neonatal foal death, onset of neurologic disease), the horse should be isolated and appropriate clinical samples immediately submitted to a diagnostic laboratory (see Diagnosis). Any in-contact horses should ideally be isolated and carefully monitored for signs of disease. If the in-contact group is large, it should be subdivided. If the in-contact group cannot be isolated, it should not be moved, and horses from the group should not be mixed with horses from other groups.

Because the virus can persist in the environment, even though this is for limited periods, all discharges from the affected horse should be removed and the area disinfected using Virkon or other approved disinfectants. This is especially important after an abortion; the large volumes of infectious allantochorionic and amniotic fluids, fetal membranes, and the aborted foal present a high contagion risk. Bedding should be disinfected before disposal or destroyed by burning. Vehicles and equipment should be disinfected. If EHV-1 is confirmed, the aborted mare and exposed or in-contact horses should be kept isolated for 28 days and not mixed with pregnant mares for 56 days. Mares can be safely covered on their second estrus after abortion. Pregnant in-contact mares should not leave the premises until after foaling. Horses with neurologic disease should be kept isolated for at least 28 days. Movement of all horses on and off the premises should stop for a period of 28 days.

Limiting spread of disease to adjacent premises requires efficient and open communication among the attending veterinarian, the premises' owners, and other parties working with the affected premises. Owners of horses that have come into contact with animals on the affected premises should be informed. Care must be taken with vehicles and other fomites to avoid transmission, and these should be rigorously disinfected. Personnel should be aware that they can indirectly transmit virus. Horse movements on and off the premises should stop for at least 28 days, but pregnant mares should not leave until after they have foaled. Affected horses, especially neurologic cases, should be tested (by nasopharyngeal swabs) to make sure they are no longer contagious and are free from disease before leaving the premises.

REFERENCES

See the CD-ROM for a list of references linked to the abstract in PubMed.

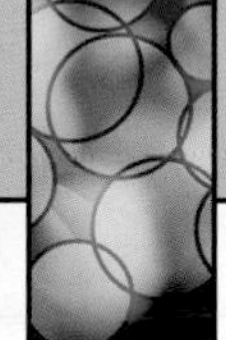

CHAPTER • 14

Equine Viral Arteritis

Udeni B. R. Balasuriya and N. James MacLachlan

Equine viral arteritis (EVA) is an infectious disease of equids that is caused by *equine arteritis virus* (EAV). EAV infection occurs throughout much of the world, although the incidence of both EAV infection and clinical EVA varies greatly between countries and among horses of different breeds. The vast majority of EAV infections are inapparent or subclinical, but occasional outbreaks of EVA are characterized by any combination of influenza-like illness in adult horses, abortion in pregnant mares, and interstitial pneumonia in very young foals.[1,2]

An extensive outbreak of EVA that occurred in Kentucky Thoroughbreds in 1984 generated widespread interest, publicity, and concern.[3-6] Since then, a number of other outbreaks have been reported from North America and Europe.[6-11] Similarly, EAV infection of horses has recently been identified in countries such as Australia, New Zealand, and South Africa that were previously thought to be largely or completely free of the virus.[12-17] This apparent global dissemination of EAV and rising incidence of EVA likely reflect the rapid national and international movement of horses for competition and breeding, as well as increased recognition of the importance of EAV infection.[3,18-22]

ETIOLOGY

EAV was first isolated from the lung of an aborted fetus after an extensive outbreak of respiratory disease and abortion on a Standardbred breeding farm near Bucyrus, Ohio, in 1953.[23,24] EVA was identified as an etiologically distinct disease after isolation of the causative virus (EAV) and description of characteristic vascular lesions.[25] EVA was distinguished from equine influenza and equine herpesviruses type 1 and type 4 (EHV-1, EHV-4), which potentially cause similar respiratory and reproductive disease syndromes in horses.[23,24] Although it was not definitively confirmed to be a new disease entity until 1953, apparent EVA was described in the late eighteenth and early nineteenth centuries as "pinkeye," "infectious or epizootic cellulitis," "influenza erysipelatosa," "Pferdestaupe," "Rotlaufseuche," and "equine influenza."[26-29]

Genome Organization and Virion Structure

EAV is the prototype virus in the family *Arteriviridae* (genus *Arterivirus*, order Nidovirales), a grouping that also includes porcine reproductive and respiratory syndrome virus, simian hemorrhagic fever virus, and lactate dehydrogenase–elevating virus of mice.[30,31] The EAV virion is an enveloped, spherical, 50- to 65-nm particle with an icosahedral core that contains a single-stranded, positive-sense ribonucleic acid (RNA) molecule of about 12.7 kilobases[31-33] (Fig. 14-1). The EAV genome includes a 5′ leader sequence and nine open reading frames (ORFs).[32,34] The two most 5′-proximal ORFs (1a and 1b) occupy approximately three fourths of the genome and encode two replicase polyproteins (pp1a and pp1ab). These two precursor proteins are extensively processed after translation into at least 12 nonstructural proteins (nsp 1-12) by three viral proteases (nsp1, nsp2, and nsp4).[31,35,36] The greatest variation in the EAV replicase gene occurs in the portion of ORF1a encoding the nsp2 protein, with considerable variation at amino acids 388 to 488.[37]

The structural proteins of the EAV virion include six envelope proteins (E, GP2b [GS], GP3, GP4, GP5 [G_L], and M) and a nucleocapsid protein (N), which, respectively, are encoded by ORFs 2a, 2b, and 3 to 7 located at the 3′ proximal quarter of the genome.[33,38-40] These structural proteins are expressed from six subgenomic viral messenger RNAs (mRNAs) that form a 3′-coterminal nested set and contain a common leader sequence of 224 nucleotides encoded by the 5′ end of the genome. Three of the minor envelope proteins (GP2b, GP3, and GP4) form a heterotrimer in the EAV particle, and the M and GP5 proteins form a disulfide-linked heterodimer.[40-42]

The greatest sequence variation in the ORFs encoding structural EAV proteins occurs in ORFs 3 and 5, which encode GP3 and GP5, respectively.[37,43-46] GP5 expresses the major neutralization determinants of EAV, and although considerable variation exists in the sequence of the GP5 protein of field strains of the virus, there is only one serotype of EAV, and all strains evaluated thus far are neutralized by polyclonal antiserum raised against the virulent Bucyrus strain.[45,47-53] However, field strains of EAV are frequently distinguished based on their neutralization phenotype with polyclonal antisera and monoclonal antibodies. Similarly, geographically and temporally distinct strains of EAV differ in the severity of the clinical disease they induce and in their abortigenic potential.[1,2,54-58] Although strains of EAV from North America and Europe share as much as 85% nucleotide identity,[37,45,57] these viruses generally segregate into clusters reflective of their geographic origins after phylogenetic analysis.[45,46]

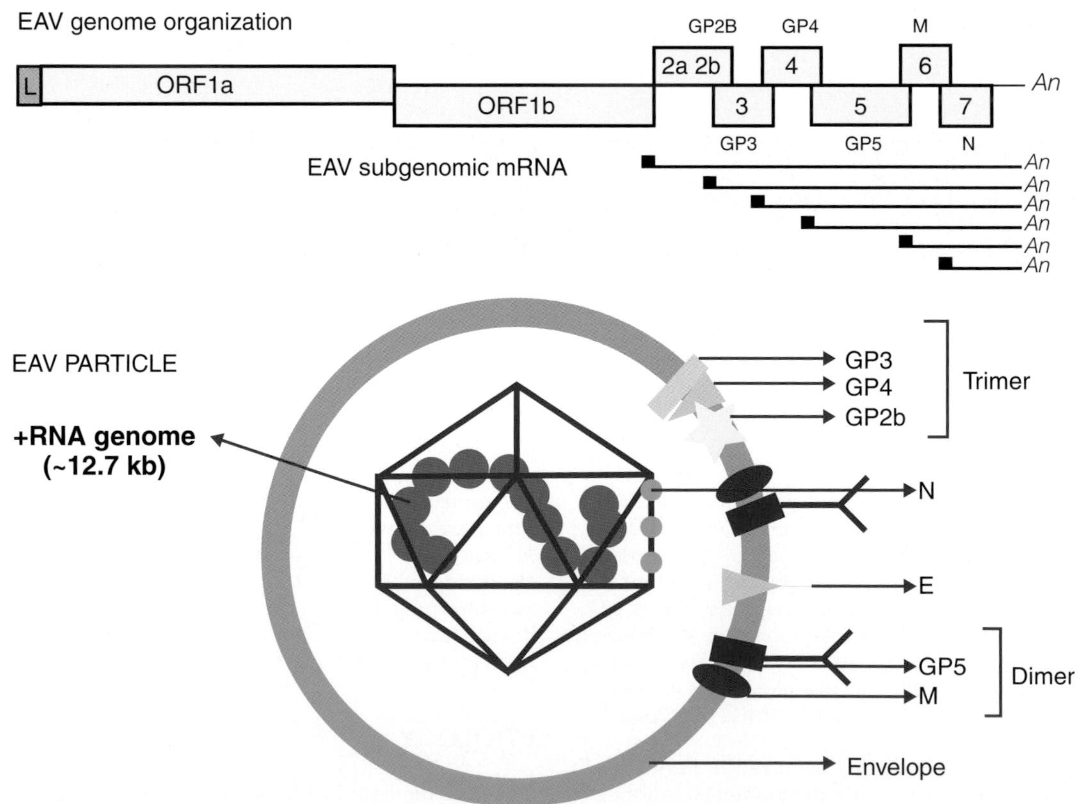

Fig. 14-1 Schematic representation of equine arteritis virus (EAV) genome organization and the virus particle.

Resistance to Physical and Chemical Agents

EAV is readily inactivated by lipid solvents (ether and chloroform) and by common disinfectants and detergents. EAV survives 75 days at 4° C, between 2 and 3 days at 37° C, and 20 to 30 minutes at 56° C. Tissue culture fluid or organ samples containing EAV can be stored at −70° C for years without significant loss of infectivity.

EPIDEMIOLOGY

Seroprevalence and Breed Predilection

EVA is a disease of the horse, but antibodies to EAV recently have been identified in donkeys in South Africa.[15,59] Serologic surveys have shown that EAV infection occurs among horses in North and South America, Europe, Australia, Africa, and Asia.[1] However, the seroprevalence of EAV infection of horses varies between countries and among equine populations within some countries. Iceland and Japan, for example, are apparently free of the virus. EAV infection is relatively common in horses in a number of European countries; studies conducted in 1973 estimated the seroprevalence of EAV infection at 11.3% of Swiss horses and 2.3% of English horses.[60,61] Similarly, approximately 14% of Dutch horses were seropositive to EAV in surveys done in 1963 and 1975.[60] In German horses, 1.8% were seropositive in a study conducted in 1987, and the seroprevalence increased to 20% in a subsequent survey in 1994.[62] In the United States (U.S.), the 1998 National Animal Health Monitoring System (NAHMS) equine survey showed that only 2.0% of unvaccinated horses in the U.S. were seropositive to EAV.[63] Similarly, resident unvaccinated California horses had a seroprevalence to EAV of only 1.9%, whereas 18.6% of horses imported into California from other countries (most often European Warmbloods) were seropositive.[64]

The seroprevalence of EAV infection varies not only between countries but also among horses of different breed and age, with marked disparity between the prevalence of infection of Standardbred and Thoroughbred horses.[65,66] EAV infection is considered endemic in Standardbred but not Thoroughbred horses in the U.S., with 77.5% to 84.3% of all Standardbreds but only up to 5.4% of Thoroughbreds being seropositive to the virus.[1,66-70] Similarly, the seroprevalence of EAV infection of Standardbred horses in California was 68.5% in 1991, versus less than 2% in all other breeds tested.[68] The seroprevalence of EAV infection of Warmblood stallions is also very high in a number of European countries; about 55 to 93% of Austrian Warmblood stallions are positive for antibodies to EAV.[71]

These profound differences in the breed-specific seroprevalence of EAV infection might reflect inherent genetic differences that confer resistance to infection. More likely, however, these differences reflect the different management practices used with individual horse breeds. Specifically, studies have not demonstrated any breed-specific variation in susceptibility to EAV infection or in establishment of the carrier state;[72] thus the number of actively shedding carrier stallions likely determines the prevalence of EAV infection in individual horse breeds. The seroprevalence of EAV infection increases with age, indicating that horses may be repeatedly exposed with increasing age.[71,73]

Outbreaks

Since the recognition of EVA in 1953, outbreaks of the disease have been reported from Switzerland,[74,75] Austria,[76,77] Poland,[78,79] Italy,[80,81] the United Kingdom,[6,8-10] Spain,[7] Netherlands,[82] Canada,[83,84] and the United States.[1,2,56,67,85-88] At least four major documented outbreaks of EVA have occurred in the U.S. since the 1953 epizootic,[54,86-88] the first at a racetrack in Kentucky in 1977.[87] Subsequent epizootics included an extensive outbreak in Thoroughbred horses in central Kentucky during the 1984 breeding season[88] and another in racing Thoroughbred horses in 1993 (>200 clinical cases) that began at the Arlington racetrack in Chicago and then spread to horses at Churchill Downs, Prairie Meadow, and Ak-Sar-Ben.[86] A well-documented outbreak of EVA occurred on a single Warmblood breeding farm in Pennsylvania in 1996, precipitated by an imported carrier stallion.[2,54] Similarly, the first recorded outbreak of EVA in the United Kingdom followed the importation of an Anglo-Arab stallion from Poland.[8,70,89]

Transmission

Transmission of EAV between horses occurs through either respiratory or venereal routes[1,24,65,90-92] (Fig. 14-2). Horizontal respiratory transmission of EAV occurs after aerosolization of infected respiratory tract secretions from acutely infected horses; high titers of EAV are present in respiratory secretions for some 7 to 14 days during acute infection.[91] However, direct and close contact is necessary for aerosol transmission of EAV between horses.[66,85] EAV also can be transmitted by aerosol from urine and other body secretions of acutely infected horses, aborted fetuses and their membranes, and the masturbates of acutely or chronically infected stallions.[16,61,71,91,93-95] Venereal transmission of EAV contained in the semen of stallions that are either acutely or chronically infected with EAV is the other important route of natural transmission of the virus.[65,92]

Persistently infected carrier stallions are the essential reservoir responsible for perpetuation and maintenance of EAV in equine populations. The persistent EAV infection that occurs in carrier stallions is highly unusual in that virus is shed only in the reproductive tract; thus, 85% to 100% of seronegative mares bred to long-term carrier stallions become infected with the virus and seroconvert within 28 days. Mares are also readily infected by artificial insemination with semen collected from shedding stallions.[56] Mares that become infected following natural or artificial breeding then can readily transmit the virus by nasal aerosol to susceptible cohorts in close proximity.[90]

Other, less common modes of transmission of EAV include congenital infection of foals after transplacental transmission of the virus in mares infected in late gestation.[96] The virus is not teratogenic, but congenitally infected foals may develop a rapidly progressive, fulminating interstitial pneumonia and fibronecrotic enteritis.[79,96-99] Lateral dissemination of EAV also can occur through fomites (e.g., personnel, clothing, vehicles, equipment),[1,61,66,85] as described during an outbreak of EVA on a Warmblood breeding farm in Pennsylvania, where virus was first indirectly spread from a carrier stallion to a susceptible horse.[54] The virus then rapidly spread by aerosol to contact horses. Similarly, EAV was spread among nonbreeding Lipizzaner stallions in South Africa by the apparent aerosolization of virus shed into bedding in the masturbates of a carrier stallion(s).[26]

Carrier State and Molecular Epidemiology

The asymptomatic carrier stallion is the essential natural reservoir of EAV, as first described more than 100 years ago when it was noted that healthy stallions could transmit so-called epizootic cellulitis-pinkeye or influenza (which likely was EVA) to mares at breeding.[28,29] The EAV carrier state was poorly defined until the 1984 epizootic in Kentucky, when studies by Timoney and McCollum unequivocally established the importance of the carrier stallion in the natural epidemiology

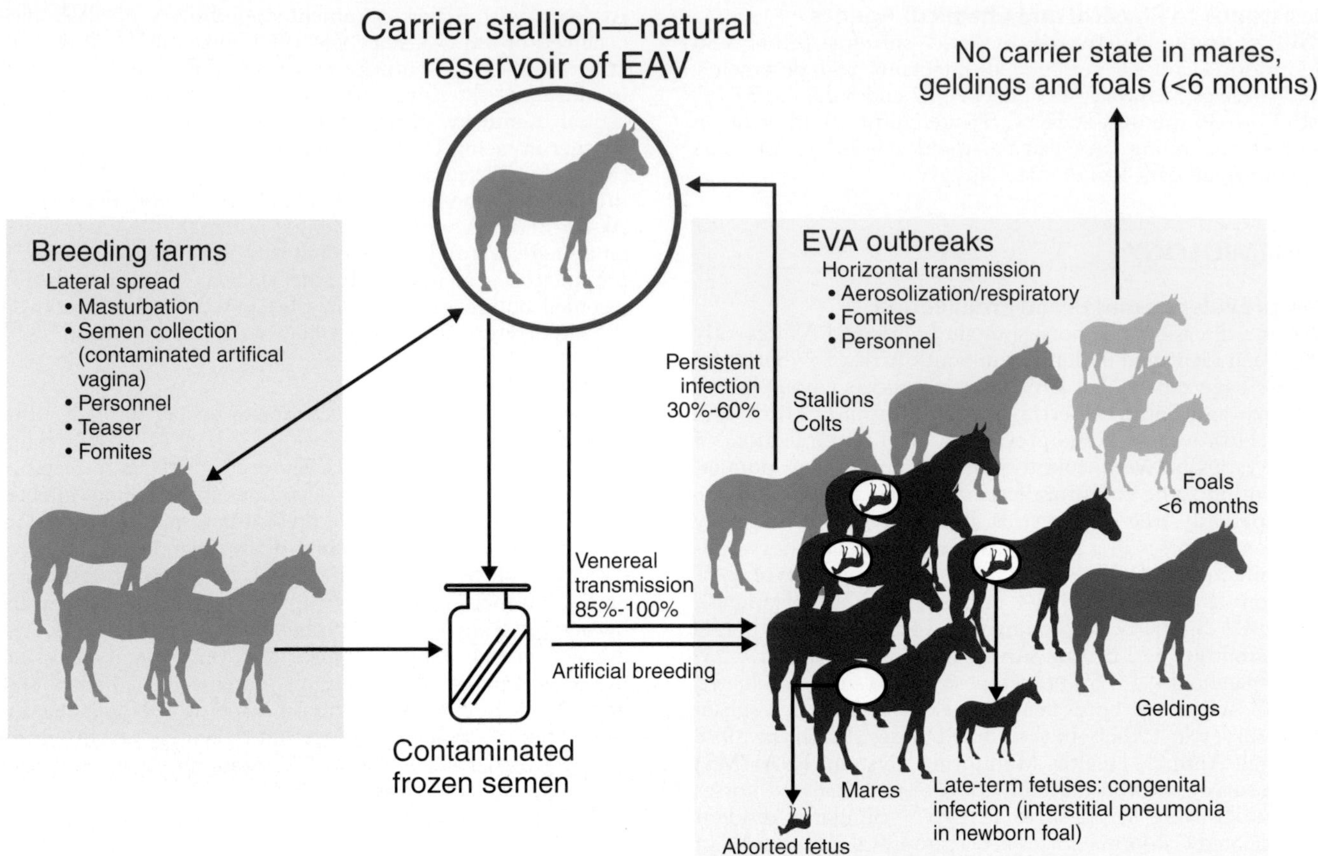

Fig. 14-2 Transmission of EAV between horses.

of EAV infection.[65,92,100,101] Specifically, Timoney et al.[92] confirmed the chronic carrier state in naturally infected Thoroughbred stallions using test matings and isolation of virus from semen and showed that 30% to 35% of stallions that were infected during the outbreak subsequently became long-term carriers.

Persistently infected stallions can be divided into three groups based on the duration of virus excretion in semen.[65,102] The *short-term*, or convalescent, carrier state lasts only a few weeks after clinical recovery, and the *intermediate* carrier state lasts for 3 to 7 months in both naturally and experimentally infected animals. The *long-term*, or chronic, carrier state can last for years and even the entire life of the infected stallion. Some persistently infected, long-term carrier stallions cease to shed virus after years of persistent infection, with no apparent later reversion to a shedding state. However, the mechanism responsible for this spontaneous clearance of EAV from persistently infected stallions is not clear. There is no convincing evidence that carrier stallions are or can become intermittent shedders of the virus or have latent infection.

Carrier stallions have moderate to high titers of serum neutralizing antibody to EAV and shed the virus constantly in their semen, but virus is not present in their blood, urine, or body secretions.[1] EAV appears to be restricted to the reproductive tract during persistent infection of carrier stallions, and highest titers of the virus consistently have been demonstrated in the ampulla of the vas deferens (>10^5 PFU/g tissue).[1,101] Virus in semen is associated with the sperm-rich fraction and not with the pre-ejaculatory fluid, and the titers of virus in sequential ejaculates vary little from the same stallion.

The mechanism of persistence of EAV in the male reproductive tract is not clear. However, studies have established that persistence of EAV in stallions is testosterone–dependent;[103,104] persistently infected stallions that were castrated and treated with testosterone continued to shed the virus in semen, whereas untreated animals ceased shedding virus. Holyoak et al.[100] studied the persistence of EAV in prepubertal and peripubertal colts and showed that EAV replicates in the male reproductive tract of a significant proportion of colts for a variable period (up to 6 months) after clinical recovery in the absence of circulating concentrations of testosterone equivalent to those found in sexually mature stallions. However, long-term persistent EAV infection does not occur in colts exposed to the virus before the onset of puberty. Similarly, persistent infection does not occur after EAV infection of mares, geldings, or fetuses.[1,104] Thus, EAV was not isolated from the reproductive tract of seropositive mares 1 month after infection,[104,105] and convalescent mares did not transmit infection to susceptible stallions during mating or to contact horses.[66,71,106]

The carrier stallion clearly is responsible for generating the genetic heterogeneity that distinguishes individual field strains of EAV. Sequence analyses of the variable ORF5 gene of strains of EAV sequentially present in the semen of carrier stallions showed that EAV behaves as a *quasispecies* (population of genetically related viral variants) during persistent infection, leading to both genetic and phenotypic divergence of the virus.[37,44,54] Outbreaks of EVA result from the emergence and spread of specific variants of EAV that are present in the quasispecies virus population in the semen of individual carrier stallions; however, the mechanisms involved in selection and emergence of virulent viral variants remain unclear. It has also been recently shown that novel variants with distinct neutralization phenotype arise during persistent infection of carrier stallions, and that the altered neutralization phenotype of these variants correlates with amino acid changes in specific regions of the GP5 envelope glycoprotein.[44,47-49,54,56] However, all the variants that arise in the course of persistent infection of carrier stallions are neutralized by high-titer polyclonal equine sera, which suggests that immune evasion is not responsible for the establishment of persistent EAV infection of carrier stallions. There also is no evidence that positive selective pressures are responsible for establishment of persistent EAV infection of stallions.[37,44]

The recent advent of molecular techniques has greatly increased our understanding of the epidemiology of EVA. For example, investigation of an extensive outbreak of EVA on a Warmblood breeding farm showed that a single virus variant present in the semen of a carrier stallion was selected and then efficiently transmitted by aerosol among other horses on the farm.[54] Thus, it appears that the considerable genetic heterogeneity afforded by the viral quasispecies likely facilitates persistence of EAV in the reproductive tract of carrier stallions. However, only some members (variants) within the quasispecies appear to be capable of efficient aerosol transmission to other horses, perhaps because of an enhanced ability to replicate within the respiratory tract. The strain of EAV that circulated during this particular outbreak was genetically stable during repeated horizontal and vertical passage in horses, unlike the diverse, quasispecies virus population in the semen of the carrier stallions on the farm.

In summary, genetic divergence of EAV occurs in the course of persistent infection of the reproductive tract of carrier stallions, leading to the emergence of novel strains of EAV, and likely compensating for the minimal virus diversity that is generated during EVA outbreaks when the virus is transmitted by aerosol. Therefore the persistently infected carrier stallion serves as the natural reservoir that harbors EAV between breeding seasons and also provides the environment in which genetic diversification of the virus occurs.

PATHOGENESIS

The pathogenesis of EVA has been studied by both the experimental inoculation (intranasal, intramuscular, intravenous) of horses with strains of EAV of different virulence and the careful evaluation of natural outbreaks of EVA.[2,58,90,91,107-113] Quantitative distribution of EAV has differed greatly between individual experiments, which likely reflects the inherent differences in the route of infection, virus dose, strain of virus, and quality of the specimens used for virus isolation.[33] Briefly, EAV is rapidly spread within the lung and bronchial lymph nodes (in 2 days) after aerosol infection, then is disseminated throughout the body through the circulation. Virus can be isolated from the nasopharynx, buffy coat, and serum for a variable time after intranasal exposure (Fig. 14-3). Virus can be isolated from the nasopharynx for 2 to 14 days after infection and from buffy coat for 2 to 19 days. Virus typically is isolated from serum or plasma for 7 to 9 days, and the disappearance of virus from serum coincides with the development of virus-specific neutralizing antibodies. Virus can be isolated from a wide variety of tissues and body fluids of infected horses beginning about 1 to 2 days after infection.[91] Apart from occasional cases where EAV has been isolated from buffy coat cells for several months after infection, and from the reproductive tract of prepubertal colts (≤6 months of age), EAV generally is not isolated beyond 28 days after infection except from the semen of carrier stallions.

The pathogenesis of EVA is not clearly defined. Many of the clinical manifestations of EVA result from vascular injury, and death in horses inoculated with the highly virulent, horse-adapted Bucyrus strain of EAV is a consequence of severe vascular damage leading to disseminated intravascular coagulation. The characteristic vascular lesions of EVA have been compared to those of Aleutian disease of mink and other immune-mediated vascular diseases.[114,115] The lesions of EVA, however, do not appear to be the result of immune-mediated injury, because they develop at only 4 to 5 days after experimental inoculation, which is not consistent with an immune-mediated process. Furthermore, arteries larger than 1 mm are affected, and neither immunoglobulin G (IgG) nor complement (C3) is present in the lesions, as would be expected if immune complexes were responsible.

Therefore, vascular injury in EVA likely results from direct virus-mediated injury to the lining (endothelium) and walls (media) of affected vessels. EAV infects and replicates in endothelial cells (ECs) and causes extensive damage to the endothelium and the subjacent internal elastic lamina, then gains access to the media of affected vessels. Increased vascular permeability and leukocyte infiltration resulting from generation of chemotactic factors lead to hemorrhage and edema around these vessels.[116,117] In addition to ECs, EAV also replicates well in macrophages in infected horses; EAV infection of cultured equine ECs and macrophages leads to their activation, with increased transcription of genes encoding proinflammatory mediators, including interleukin-1 beta (IL-1β), IL-6, IL-8, and tumor necrosis factor alpha (TNF-α).[118] Furthermore, virulent and avirulent strains of EAV induced different quantities of TNF-α and other proinflammatory cytokines from both infected ECs and macrophages. These studies strongly suggest that cytokine mediators that are produced by ECs and macrophages have a central role in the pathogenesis of EVA.

Evidence suggests that abortion after EAV infection of pregnant mares is the result of a lethal fetal infection rather than myometritis or placental damage that impairs progesterone synthesis, leading to fetal expulsion.[109] The tissues of aborted fetuses contain higher titers of virus than those of the dams from which they abort, indicating that substantial virus replication occurs in the fetus itself.[109] The stress that results from fetal infection would be expected to activate the fetal hypothalamic-pituitary axis, thus inducing abortion.

CLINICAL FINDINGS

The clinical severity of equine arteritis virus (EAV) infection of horses varies greatly.[1,58,61,96] The vast majority of EAV infections are inapparent, especially those that occur in mares bred to persistently infected stallions.[1,65,92] Outbreaks of clinical disease caused by EAV infection, equine viral arteritis (EVA), are characterized by one more of the following: abortion of pregnant mares; fulminant infection of neonates, leading to severe interstitial pneumonia or enteritis; and systemic illness in adult horses, with any combination of leukopenia and pyrexia, respiratory signs with nasal and ocular discharge, peripheral edema, hives, and persistent infection of stallions. The clinical signs observed in natural cases of EVA vary

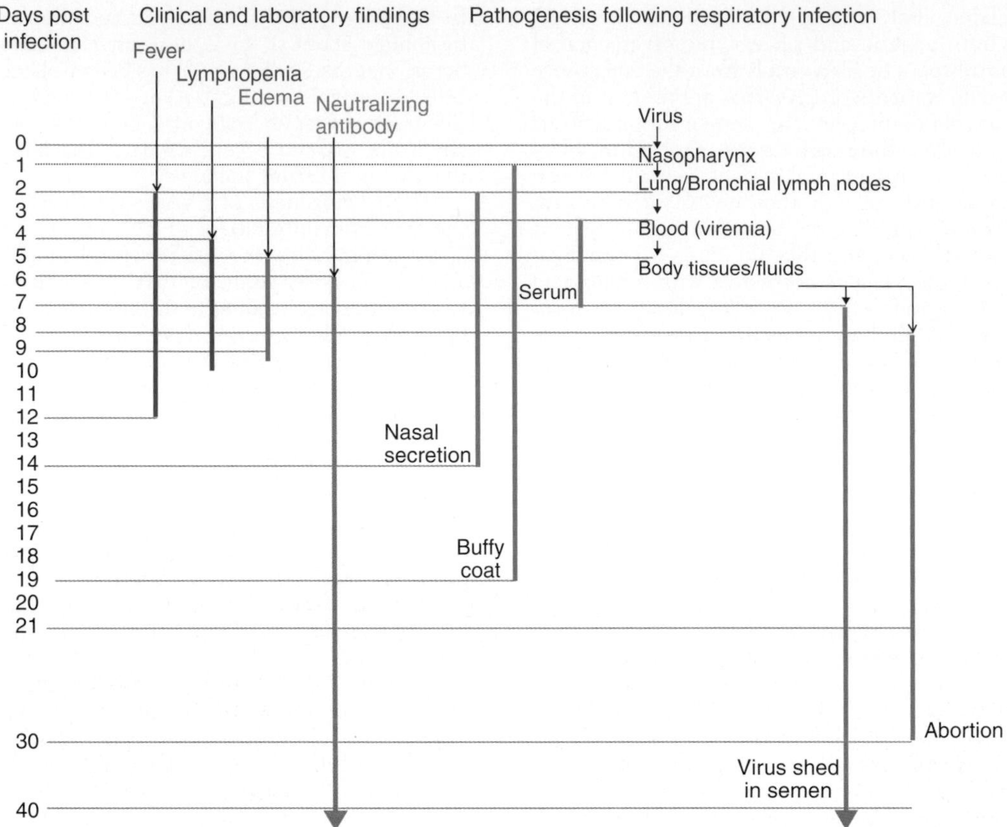

Fig. 14-3 Clinical and laboratory findings and sequential pathogenesis of equine viral arteritis (EVA) after respiratory infection. Vertical bars correspond to the chronologic occurrence of the respective clinical or laboratory findings and the distribution of virus in body tissues and secretions.

considerably among individual horses and between outbreaks and depend on factors such as the age and physical condition of the horse(s), challenge dose and route of infection, strain of virus, and environmental conditions.[1,96] Although there is only one serotype of EAV, the clinical disease produced by different virus strains ranges from severe, lethal infection caused by the horse-adapted Bucyrus strain to clinically inapparent infection.[20,66,109] Very young, old, debilitated, and immunosuppressed horses are predisposed to severe EVA.

Regardless of the infecting virus strain, the vast majority of naturally infected horses recover uneventfully from EVA. Young foals, however, can develop fatal infections that lead to severe, fulminating interstitial pneumonia,[96,98] and foals up to few months of age can develop a rapidly progressive "pneumoenteritis" syndrome. With the notable exceptions of abortion and fulminant respiratory disease in foals, mortality rarely if ever occurs in natural outbreaks of EAV. The highly virulent horse-adapted Bucyrus strain of EAV (which causes high mortality in healthy adult horses) is not representative of field strains of the virus and is best regarded as an aberration.

Clinical cases of EVA are characterized by an incubation period of 2 to 14 days (6-8 days after venereal exposure), pyrexia of up to 41° C that may persist for 2 to 9 days (Fig. 14-3), and any combination of depression and anorexia; conjunctivitis and rhinitis with nasal and ocular discharge; leukopenia; periorbital and supraorbital edema; edema of the limbs, especially of the hindlimbs; mid-ventral edema involving the scrotum and prepuce or mammary glands; urticaria that may be localized to sides of the neck or face or may be generalized over most of the body; and abortion.* Less frequently observed signs include icterus; photophobia; corneal opacity; coughing and dyspnea; abdominal pain and diarrhea; ataxia; petechiation of the nasal mucosa, conjunctiva, and oral mucous membranes; submaxillary and submandibular lymphadenopathy; and adventitious edema in the intermandibular space, beneath the sternum, or in the shoulder region† (Fig. 14-4). The most consistent clinical features of EAV infection are pyrexia and leukopenia.[112,113,122]

Abortion in pregnant mares is not preceded by premonitory signs and may occur late in the acute phase or early in the convalescent phase of the EAV infection.[1,24,83,105,122] Abortions have been documented at 3 months to over 10 months of gestation after natural or experimental infection.[1,24,90,105,116] Abortion rates in outbreaks of EVA have varied from less than 10% to between 50% and 60%.[1] Infections with the strain of EAV that caused the 1984 Kentucky outbreak resulted in an abortion rate of 71%.[90] The abortigenic potential of different strains of EAV has not been adequately compared, but it appears that strains differ in their abortigenic potential as they do in their virulence characteristics.

Stallions may undergo a period of temporary subfertility associated with decreased libido, sperm motility, concentration, and percentage of morphologically normal sperm in ejaculates during acute EAV infection. These changes can persist for up to 6 to 7 weeks after experimental EAV infection of

*References 1, 24, 55, 61, 91, 93, 95, 105, 113, 119.
†References 23, 24, 75, 83, 85, 90, 108, 120, 121.

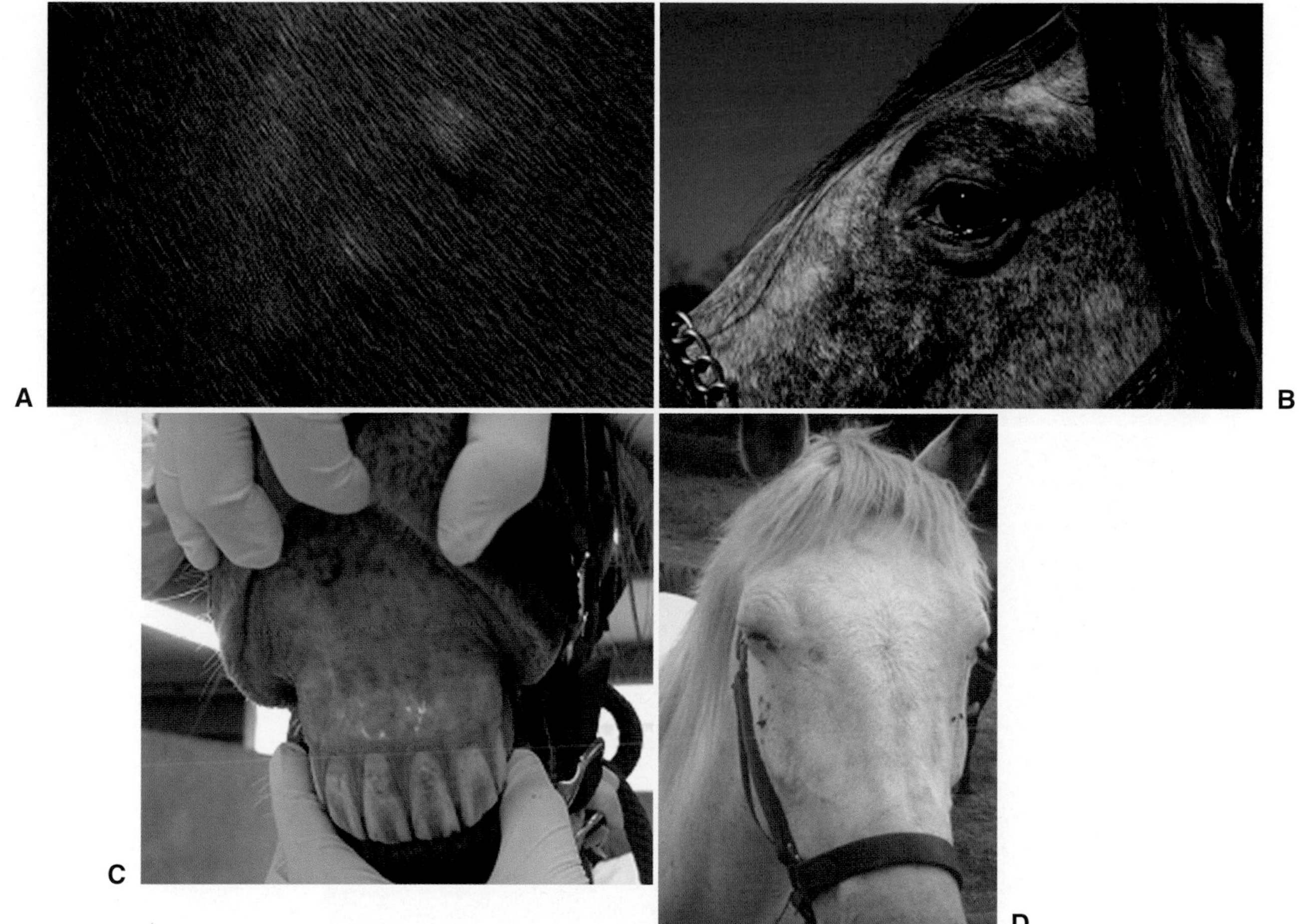

Fig. 14-4 Representative example of clinical signs of EVA after experimental inoculation of horses with virulent strains of equine arteritis virus (EAV). **A,** Urticaria; **B,** conjunctivitis and periorbital edema; **C,** mucosal petechiation; **D,** facial edema.

Continued

stallions[1,123] and are considered to result from increased testicular temperature rather than any direct virus-induced pathologic effect. Semen quality is apparently normal in persistently infected stallions, despite active shedding of the virus into the semen. Similarly, venereal infection of mares by persistently infected carrier stallions does not appear to result in subsequent fertility problems.[1]

DIAGNOSIS

Clinical EVA resembles a number of other infectious and noninfectious diseases of horses, and therefore a presumptive diagnosis based solely on the clinical signs of EVA should only be made with caution.[1,124] The differential diagnosis of EVA includes other viral respiratory tract infections of the horse (equine herpesviruses [EHV-1, EHV-4], equine influenza virus, equine rhinitis A and B viruses, equine adenovirus and Getah virus), equine infectious anemia, African horse sickness, Hendra, leptospirosis, purpura hemorrhagica, urticaria, and toxicosis caused by hoary alyssum *(Berteroa incana)*. EVA is characterized histologically by a distinctive arteritis that differentiates it from these other diseases, although vasculitis certainly is not pathognomonic of EVA. Importantly, the severity and distribution of vasculitis vary greatly between cases of EVA.

Abortion from EVA also can present a diagnostic dilemma. Differential diagnoses include EHV-1 (or rarely EHV-4), although fetuses are typically expelled without any premonitory signs in EHV abortions. EHV-infected fetuses are expelled fresh and frequently have characteristic gross lesions, whereas those infected with EAV are usually partially autolyzed and lack pathognomonic lesions.

Laboratory diagnosis of EVA is currently based on any combination of virus isolation, viral nucleic acid or antigen detection, and serology.

Virus Isolation

The most appropriate specimens for virus isolation from live horses include nasopharyngeal swabs or washings, conjunctival swabs, and citrated or ethylenediaminetetraacetic acid (EDTA) blood samples for separation of buffy coat cells. Heparinized blood is not suitable for virus isolation because of the inhibitory effect of heparin on the isolation of EAV in cell culture.[125] The sperm-rich fraction of the ejaculate is optimal for virus isolation from equine semen samples.[1] Placenta, fetal

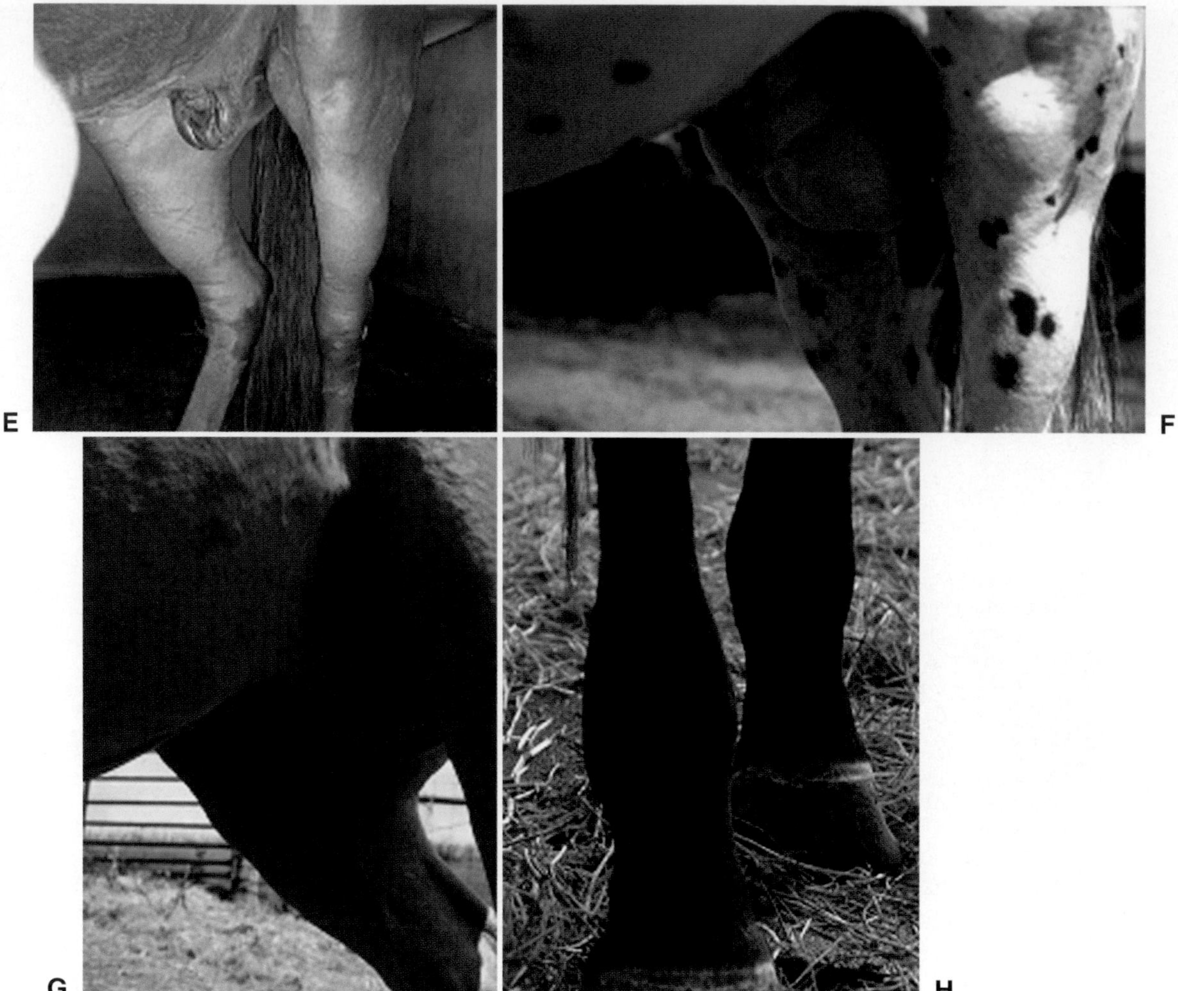

Fig. 14-4, cont'd E, preputial and hindlimb edema; F, scrotal edema; G, edema of the mammary gland; H, limb edema. (*B, D, F,* and *G* courtesy Dr. Peter J. Timoney, Gluck Equine Research Center, Lexington, Ky.)

fluids, lung, spleen, and lymphoid tissues should be collected for virus isolation to confirm cases of EAV-induced abortion. A wide variety of organs and lymph nodes associated with the alimentary and respiratory tracts should be collected for virus isolation in suspected cases of "pneumoenteric" forms of EVA in young foals.

Specimens should be collected as soon as possible after the onset of clinical signs or suspected EAV infection. Nasopharyngeal and conjunctival swabs should be immediately placed in transported medium (any cell culture medium or balanced salt solution containing 2% to 5% fetal bovine or calf serum) and either refrigerated or, preferably, frozen at −20° C or lower.[1] All other specimens for virus isolation should be packed in dry ice and dispatched by overnight delivery to an appropriate laboratory, except for blood samples, which should be refrigerated.

Cell culture isolation of EAV is usually done in the rabbit kidney-13 continuous cell line, and development of a cytopathic effect in inoculated cells indicates the presence of virus. The identity of the virus isolate should be confirmed by immunofluorescence or immunoperoxidase staining or by microneutralization assay with EAV-specific antiserum or monoclonal antibodies.

Viral Antigen Detection

Indirect immunohistochemistry is a reliable, powerful, and rapid assay to diagnose EAV infection in tissues and occasionally in skin biopsies.[126] An avidin-biotin complex (ABC) for immunoperoxidase staining using monoclonal antibodies to individual EAV proteins has been successfully used to detect viral antigens in formalin-fixed paraffin-embedded samples, as well as in frozen tissue sections.[109,127,128]

Viral Nucleic Acid Detection

Several reverse transcriptase–polymerase chain reaction (RT-PCR), nested RT-PCR (RT-nPCR), and real-time RT-PCR assays for detection of the EAV nucleic acids in cell culture supernatants and clinical specimens have been developed.[129-135] These assays target different genes (ORFs 1b, 3, 4, 5, 6, and 7), and their sensitivity and specificity vary considerably. The sensitivity of RT-PCR–based assays is significantly increased by using either RT-nPCR that incorporate two primer pairs specific for ORF 1b or real-time TaqMan RT-PCR that uses primers and a probe specific for a highly conserved region of ORF7. RT-PCR–based assays have several potential advantages over the current virus isolation procedure; however, further standardization and validation clearly will be necessary before their adoption as the standard screening assay to evaluate such clinical specimens as semen from horses scheduled for international movement.

Serologic Diagnosis

Serologic diagnosis of EVA is based on virus microneutralization and is standardized by the World Organization for Animal Health (OIE) and described in the OIE manual.[136] The assay is performed in the presence of guinea pig complement, and the CVL-Weybridge strain of EAV is used as the challenge virus in most laboratories.[137] Carrier stallions usually have very high titers of serum neutralization antibody. For serologic diagnosis of acute EAV infection, acute and convalescent sera (paired serum samples) should be collected at a 21-day to 28-day interval, and a fourfold or greater increase in serum antibody titer is indicative of seroconversion. Recent investigation demonstrates that the use of specific commercial inactivated EHV-1 and EHV-4 vaccines induce serum cytotoxicity that can interfere with accurate interpretation of the virus neutralization test, although this potential problem currently appears to affect European more than North American horses.[138] Several enzyme-linked immunosorbent assays (ELISAs) have been described that detect antibodies to EAV,[139-145] but none has yet gained widespread acceptance. The microneutralization assay remains the "gold standard" for detection of serum antibodies to EAV.

Histopathologic Examination

Tissue samples should be fixed and saved in 10% neutral buffered formalin and submitted for histopathologic examination at an appropriate laboratory.

PATHOLOGY

Descriptions of the gross and histopathologic lesions of EVA are based on examination of material derived from horses that were experimentally inoculated with the virulent Bucyrus strain of EAV or from natural outbreaks of EVA.* It is important to recognize that this highly virulent, horse-adapted strain of EAV causes a highly fulminant and often fatal infection that is not representative of the disease caused by field strains of the virus. Common gross necropsy findings in horses inoculated with the Bucyrus strain of EAV include edema, congestion, and hemorrhage in subcutaneous tissues, lymph nodes, and viscera of the thoracic and abdominal cavities, and pulmonary edema and pleural and pericardial effusion can be spectacular in fulminant cases. These gross lesions result from severe panvasculitis, with especially severe histopathologic changes in medium and small muscular arteries throughout the body, including hemorrhage, edema, and necrosis of vessel walls, with accompanying infiltration of lymphocytes and neutrophils. Similar necrosis and accumulation of inflammatory cells occurs in and around thin-walled vessels (veins and lymphatics). Vascular thrombosis and associated tissue infarction may be present in the lungs, adrenal glands, and large intestine, along with extensive lymphoid necrosis in the germinal centers of the bronchiolar and mesenteric lymph nodes. Sinuses of the bronchial lymph nodes may contain unusual, large, pleomorphic cells that resemble reactive histiocytes. Severe, diffuse interstitial lymphocytic nephritis with tubular necrosis has also been described in severe cases of EVA.[127]

*References 1, 24, 25, 91, 94, 96, 97, 105, 109, 117, 126-128, 146, 147.

The distribution of EAV antigen in infected tissues has been evaluated by both immunofluorescence and immunoperoxidase staining.[97,109,127] EAV antigen was localized to endothelium lining vessels of all calibers and types, ranging from small capillaries to the endocardium (Fig. 14-5). Macrophages in lymph nodes and many other organs also were infected. Viral antigen was demonstrated in the tunica media of infected arteries, as well as the renal tubular epithelium.[127] Immunoperoxidase staining of frozen sections of placenta and fetal tissues demonstrated that viral antigen was localized to the cytoplasm of a very limited number of cell types, including endothelial cells in arteries, veins, and lymphatics; trophoblast cells of chorioallantois; and macrophages in a variety of lymphoreticular tissues.[109,127]

Fetuses aborted after natural or experimental infections of EAV frequently do not show any obvious gross or histopathologic lesions.[23,24,108,116] Fetuses are usually partially autolyzed

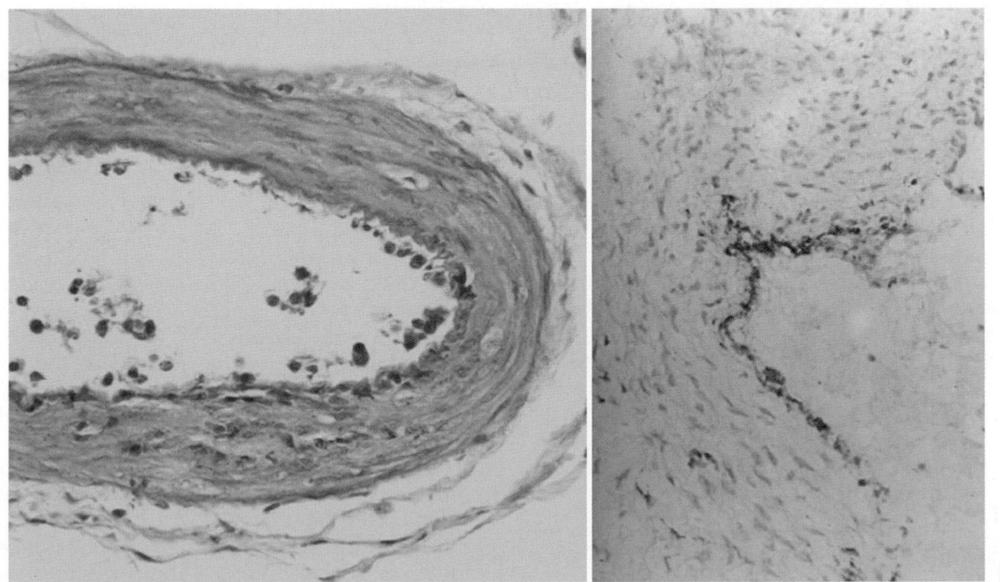

Fig. 14-5 A, Medial necrosis of muscular artery, and B, immunohistochemical staining of EAV antigen in endothelium of vessels in the placenta of EAV-infected fetus.

at expulsion and may have increased peritoneal and pleural fluid, as well as petechial hemorrhages in the mucosal linings of the respiratory and digestive tracts and on the serosal lining of peritoneal and pleural cavities. The placenta typically is grossly unremarkable and expelled with the fetus. Johnson et al.[148] described disseminated vascular lesions in the liver, adrenal gland, spleens, kidney, brain, and lymph nodes of two equine fetuses aborted during an outbreak of EVA. The placenta of one fetus had severe vasculitis with necrosis of the arterial walls. Vascular lesions also were described in several tissues of a fetus that was aborted after experimental inoculation of a pregnant mare with the virulent, horse-adapted Bucyrus strain of EAV.[109]

The gross lesions in foals with fatal EVA include diffuse severe pulmonary edema, pleural and pericardial effusion, and petechial and ecchymotic, serosal and mucosal hemorrhages in the small intestine.[96,98,99,127] Microscopic lesions include the following[127]:

- Severe interstitial pneumonia with hypertrophic type 2 pneumocytes containing intracytoplasmic EAV antigen, congestion, interlobular and intralobular edema, and extensive infiltration and accumulation of mononuclear inflammatory cells.
- Fibrinoid necrosis of the tunica media of small muscular arteries, associated with EAV antigen in the walls of affected vessels.
- Multifocal hemorrhage and lymphoid depletion in the thymus, spleen, and mesenteric lymph nodes.
- Diffuse, severe edema and multifocal hemorrhages in the intestinal submucosa and serosa.

Lesions have been described in the reproductive tract of prepubertal and peripubertal colts inoculated with EAV.[147] Acute necrotizing vasculitis involving the testis, epididymides, vas deferens, ampullae, prostate, vesicular glands, and bulbourethral glands was present during acute infection (7-14 days after infection). Multifocal accumulations of lymphocytes and plasma cells were present within the ampullae and parenchyma of the reproductive tract after 28 days.

THERAPY

As with other animal viral diseases, there is no specific antiviral treatment for horses infected with EAV. Virtually all naturally infected horses recover from EVA uneventfully, although horses with severe clinical signs should be treated symptomatically with nonsteroidal antiinflammatory drugs (NSAIDs), antipyretics to control fever, and diuretics and support wraps to reduce edema.[1,61] Breeding stallions and horses in training should be rested. There is no effective treatment for young foals with EAV-induced interstitial pneumonia or "pneumoenteritis" other than prophylactic administration of antibiotics to counter possible secondary bacterial infections. Also, no consistently effective treatment currently exists to eliminate the carrier state in stallions persistently infected with EAV other than surgical castration. However, the EAV carrier state is clearly testosterone dependent, and transient suppression of testosterone production in carrier stallions may offer therapeutic promise in the elimination of EAV infection.[1,61,103,149]

PREVENTION

Immunity

Both natural and experimental infection of horses with either virulent or avirulent strains of EAV results in long-lasting immunity against reinfection with all strains of the virus, including the most virulent strains.[23,110,120] The humoral immune response to EAV is characterized by the development of both complement-fixing and virus-specific neutralizing antibodies.[22,150] Complement-fixing antibodies develop 1 to 2 weeks after infection, peak after 2 to 3 weeks, and steadily decline to disappear by 8 months, whereas neutralizing antibodies are detected within 1 to 2 weeks after exposure, peak at 2 to 4 months, and persist for years.[1,112,113,119,150]

Minimal information is available on the cellular immune response to EAV in horses. Castillo-Olivares et al.[151] recently described EAV-specific cytotoxic T-lymphocyte (CTL) responses using peripheral blood mononuclear cells (PBMCs) from convalescent EAV-infected (experimental) ponies. The data showed that cytotoxicity induced by EAV-stimulated PBMCs was virus specific, genetically restricted, and mediated by CD8+ T cells, and that EAV-specific CTL precursors persist for at least 1 year after infection. Further studies are needed to identify the specific viral protein(s) targeted by the CTL response of EAV-infected horses.

Vaccination

A modified live-virus attenuated vaccine (ARVAC, Fort Dodge Animal Health, Iowa) is licensed for use in the United Sates and Canada for prevention of EAV infection in horses. A killed-virus vaccine (Artervac, Fort Dodge Animal Health, Iowa) is licensed for use in the United Kingdom, Ireland, France, Hungary, and Denmark.

The modified live-virus (MLV) vaccine is administered intramuscularly to horses. A small minority of horses vaccinated with this MLV vaccine develop mild febrile reactions and transient lymphopenia. Vaccine virus may be sporadically isolated from the nasopharynx and buffy coat, usually for only about 7 days but occasionally up to 32 days after vaccination.[1,94,152] Vaccinated stallions do not shed virus in either semen or urine. The MLV vaccine is not recommended for use in pregnant mares, especially during the last 2 months of gestation, or in foals less than 6 weeks of age. Apparent fetal infections with MLV after vaccination of pregnant mares have been documented, but only rarely.[153]

Maternal antibodies to EAV disappear between 2 and 6 months of age;[73,154] thus it is recommended that foals be vaccinated at 6 months of age, before the onset of puberty. Foals can be vaccinated before 6 months of age in high-risk situations, but they also should be revaccinated after 6 months of age. Vaccinated colts are resistant to development of the persistently infected carrier state after subsequent exposure to EAV. The protective immunization of prepubertal colts is therefore central to effective control of the spread of EAV infection.

Virus-neutralizing antibodies are induced within 5 to 8 days after MLV vaccination and persist for at least 2 years.[1,66] Revaccination greatly increases the serologic response of horses, providing protective immunity that persists for several breeding seasons. Although MLV vaccination provides sustained protection against clinical EVA, it does not consistently prevent infection of vaccinated horses or subsequent limited replication of field strains of the virus.[155] Vaccinated mares inseminated with semen from carrier stallions became infected, as evidenced by the transient isolation of virus from buffy coat and nasopharynx, but did not develop EVA. Furthermore, a contact seronegative mare also became infected in this same study, indicating that infectious virus was shed by the vaccinated mares. However, the MLV vaccine has been successfully used to curtail several large-scale outbreaks of EVA in the United States, including the 1984 outbreak in Thoroughbred horses in Kentucky. Since 1984, the MLV vaccine has been extensively used in control programs in several states.

The MLV vaccine is not licensed in either Europe or Japan, and an inactivated (killed) EAV vaccine containing an adjuvant (Artervac) was formulated for use in the United Kingdom after an outbreak of EVA in 1993.[156] This vaccine is also administered intramuscularly, and a booster immunization is recommended after 3 to 4 weeks and annually thereafter. Although this vaccine induces high titers of neutralizing antibodies, its ability to prevent EVA and persistent infection of stallions is less characterized than that of the MLV vaccine.

Husbandry and Control Programs

There is no established domestic EVA control program in the United States. However, the recent publication from the U.S. Department of Agriculture (USDA) Animal and Plant Health Inspection Service (APHIS), *Equine Viral Arteritis: Uniform Methods and Rules*, describes the minimum standards for detecting, controlling, and preventing EVA, as well as minimum EVA requirements for the interstate and intrastate movement of horses.[157] The EAV carrier stallion is the essential natural reservoir of the virus and has a pivotal role in the transmission and maintenance of EAV infection in horse populations.[1,65] Therefore, outbreaks of EVA can be prevented by the identification of persistently infected stallions and the institution of management practices to prevent the introduction of EAV-infected horses (Fig. 14-6).

All stallions should be tested for EAV antibodies before they are vaccinated with the MLV vaccine. A neutralization antibody dilution titer of 1:4 or greater (titer ≥4) is regarded as positive. If seronegative stallions are vaccinated, they should be vaccinated 28 days before the breeding season, or semen collection, and receive an annual booster. Vaccinated stallions should be isolated for 28 days after vaccination and receive boosters annually. Nonvaccinated seropositive stallions should be tested for virus shedding by virus isolation every 12 months or by test breeding with seronegative mares (at least two) that are monitored for seroconversion at 14 and 28 days after breeding. There is no need for vaccination of stallions that are seropositive as a result of natural infection. Young fillies and geldings benefit from vaccination before going to the track or to any environment with the potential for exposure to EAV. Vaccination of colts 6 to 12 months of age is done to prevent the future establishment of the carrier state in these animals[100,103,149] and thereby reduce the natural reservoir of EAV, which is especially important in breeds in which the infection is prevalent (e.g., Standardbreds, Warmbloods).

Stallions that are confirmed semen shedders and carriers of EAV can be used for breeding purposes provided that stringent requirements are met.[1,5,18,19,65] Carrier stallions should be kept physically isolated and bred only to mares that are seropositive from either previous natural exposure or vaccination (no less than 3 weeks previously). Mares should be kept isolated from other nonvaccinated or seronegative horses for 3 weeks after being bred to a shedding stallion or after insemination with infective semen. It is also critical that carrier stallions be isolated and collected separately to prevent contamination of collection equipment, teasers, and premises with ejaculate, because EAV can be transmitted to susceptible horses by indirect aerosol contact.

If an outbreak of EVA on a farm is suspected based on clinical signs and history, the state veterinarian should be notified,

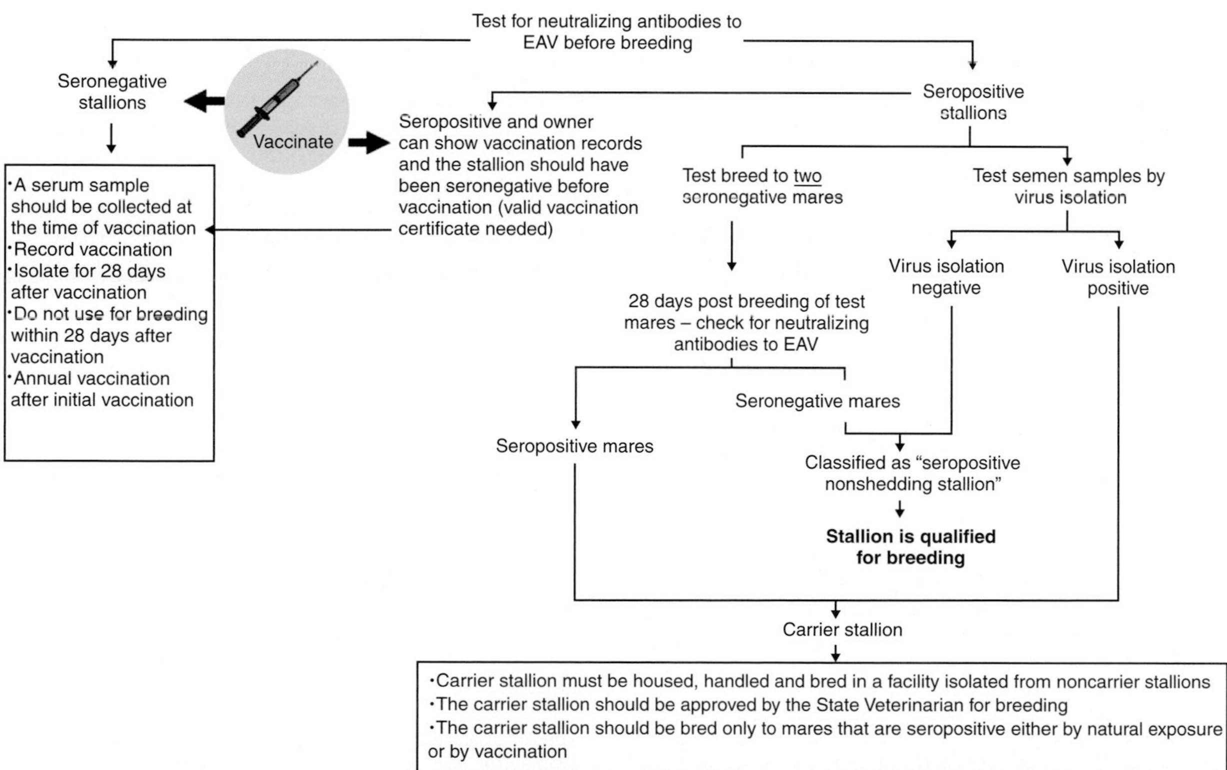

Fig. 14-6 Guidelines and minimum standards for prevention and control of EVA. (Modified from US Department of Agriculture, Animal and Plant Health Inspection Service: *Equine viral arteritis: uniform methods and rules*, Effective April 19, 2004.)

affected and in-contact horses isolated, movement of horses on and off the farm discontinued, at-risk horses vaccinated, and breeding activity stopped to prevent further spread of the virus. Diagnosis of EVA should be confirmed by laboratory testing as soon as possible. Stalls and equipment on the affected premises should be decontaminated with disinfectants. EAV is susceptible to phenolic, chlorine, iodine, and quaternary ammonium compounds. Quarantine is discontinued when no more clinical cases of EVA or serologic evidence of infection are observed for 3 consecutive weeks.

PUBLIC HEALTH CONSIDERATIONS

Equine arteritis virus (EAV) is a pathogen only of equids, and no evidence indicates that it can infect people.

ACKNOWLEDGMENTS

The authors gratefully acknowledge the advice, assistance, and intellectual input they have received over many years of productive collaborative research with Drs. William H. McCollum and Peter J. Timoney of the Gluck Equine Research Center, University of Kentucky, and specifically, for their careful and constructive review of this chapter.

REFERENCES

See the CD-ROM for a list of references linked to the abstract in PubMed.

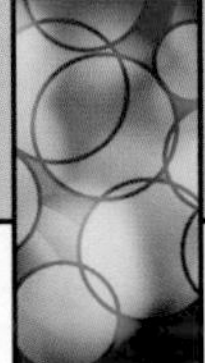

CHAPTER • 15

African Horse Sickness

Alan J. Guthrie

African horse sickness (AHS) is a noncontagious, infectious, insect-borne disease of equids caused by *African horse sickness virus* (AHSV). In horses the course of the disease is usually peracute to acute, and more than 90% of immunologically naive animals die. Clinically, AHS is characterized by pyrexia; edema of the lungs, pleura, and subcutaneous tissues; and hemorrhages on the serosal surfaces of internal organs. Mules are less susceptible than horses and donkeys, and zebras rarely show clinical signs of disease.

An Arabic document reports the first known historical reference to a disease resembling AHS occurring in Yemen in 1327.[1] Father Monclaro's report of the travels of Francisco Baro in East Africa in 1569 also reports AHS affecting horses imported from India.[1,2] Although neither horses nor donkeys were indigenous to southern Africa, they were introduced shortly after the arrival of the first settlers of the Dutch East India Company in the Cape of Good Hope in 1652.[1] Records of the Dutch East India Company make frequent reference to "perreziekte" or "pardeziekte" in the Cape of Good Hope.[2] In 1719, almost 1700 horses died from AHS in the Cape. During their exploration and expansion into the interior of southern Africa, the Voortrekkers reported severe losses among their horses.[1] Exploration of southern, central, and East Africa by Livingstone was complicated by his inability to use horses on some of his journeys.[2] Although horses die as a result of AHS every year in southern Africa, major epizootics before the 1950s occurred about every 20 to 30 years. Severe losses were reported in 1780, 1801, 1839, 1855, 1862, 1891, 1914, 1918, 1923, 1940, 1946, and 1953.[1] The 1854-55 epizootic was the most severe, with almost 70,000 horses dying, representing more than 40% of the horse population of the Cape of Good Hope.[3]

Initially, AHS was confused with anthrax and piroplasmosis. In the early 1900s, M'Fadyean,[4] Theiler, Nocard, and Sieber[1] all succeeded in transmitting the disease with a bacteria-free filtrate of blood from infected horses, confirming that the disease was caused by a virus. The pioneering research of Sir Arnold Theiler, who founded the Veterinary Research Institute at Onderstepoort in 1908, revealed the plurality of "immunologically distinct strains" of AHSV because immunity acquired against one "strain" did not always afford protection against infection by "heterologous strains."[2,5-8] Alexander[9,10] showed that viscerotropic isolates of AHSV became neurotropic but did not lose their immunogenicity after serial intracerebral passage in mice. This work led to the development of the first polyvalent vaccine against AHS in the 1930s.[11,12] Although Pitchford and Theiler[13] proposed in 1903 that AHS may be transmitted by biting insects, it was not until 1944 that Du Toit[14] confirmed that *Culicoides* species were probably vectors of both AHS and bluetongue viruses.

In endemic areas, severe losses caused by AHS have ceased since the development of polyvalent vaccine. However, the occurrence of epizootics in countries outside the endemic regions in Africa[15-17] serve as a warning that AHS may spread to areas traditionally free of the disease. AHS is one of the important diseases to consider when moving equids internationally, but movement can be accomplished safely by following appropriate quarantine and testing procedures.[18,19]

ETIOLOGY

AHSV is a member of the genus *Orbivirus* in the family *Reoviridae* and as such is morphologically similar to other orbiviruses, such as bluetongue virus (BTV) of ruminants and equine encephalosis virus (EEV; see Chapter 26).[20,21] The virion is not enveloped and is about 70 nm in diameter. It consists of a two-layered icosahedral capsid composed of 32 capsomeres.[22]

The genome comprises 10 double-stranded ribonucleic acid (RNA) segments, each of which encodes at least one polypeptide.[23] The core particle comprises two major proteins, VP3 and VP7, which are highly conserved among the nine AHSV serotypes, and three minor proteins, VP1, VP4, and VP6.[22,24] Together these proteins make up the group-specific epitopes.[25] The core particle is surrounded by the outer capsid, which is composed of two proteins, VP2 and VP5. VP2 is the protein responsible for antigenic variation.[26-28] At least three nonstructural proteins have been identified in infected cells (NS1, NS2, and NS3/3a).[29-31]

Nine antigenically distinct serotypes have been described.[32,33] Although there may be some cross-relatedness between the serotypes, there is no field evidence of any intratypic variation.[32,33] All nine serotypes have been documented in eastern[34] and southern[32,33,35] Africa, whereas serotype 9 is more widespread and appears to predominate in the northern parts of sub-Saharan Africa.[36,37]

EPIDEMIOLOGY

AHSV is biologically transmitted by *Culicoides* spp., of which *C. imicola* and *C. bolitinos* have been shown to play an important role in Africa.[38,39] The disease therefore has a seasonal occurrence, and its prevalence is influenced by climatic and other conditions that favor the breeding of *Culicoides* spp. *Culicoides variipennis*, a midge prevalent in the United States but not present in Africa, has been shown to transmit AHSV under laboratory conditions.[40] Although other insects have been suggested as possible vectors of AHSV, none has been shown to play a role under natural conditions. Biting flies may play a minor role in the mechanical transmission of AHS; however, because the viremia in horses is relatively low and AHSV is susceptible to desiccation and high temperature, this method of transmission is inefficient. AHSV can be transmitted between horses by parenteral inoculation of infective blood or organ suspensions, and it is more readily transmitted by the intravenous than by the subcutaneous route.[1]

A continuous transmission cycle of AHSV between *Culicoides* midges and zebras was shown to exist in the Kruger National Park in South Africa.[41] Under such circumstances, a sufficiently large zebra population can act as a reservoir for the virus.[42-44] Donkeys may play a similar role in parts of Africa with large donkey populations.[45] In view of the high mortality in horses, this species is regarded as an accidental or indicator host. Animals that have been infected with AHSV do not remain carriers of the virus, which explains the failure of the disease to become established outside tropical Africa, despite the occurrence of many outbreaks outside endemic areas.[1]

AHS is endemic in eastern and central Africa[2] and spreads regularly to southern Africa. In endemic areas, different serotypes of AHS may be active simultaneously, but one serotype usually dominates during a particular season. The disease is also reported from time to time in countries in North Africa, from where it has occasionally extended into the Middle East and Spain.[46,47] However, its intrusion into North Africa and countries around the Mediterranean and in Asia is impeded by the Sahara desert.[48] AHS has not been recorded in Madagascar or Mauritius.

AHS was recorded in Egypt in 1928, 1943, 1953, 1958, and 1971;[49] in Yemen in 1930; and in Palestine, Syria, Lebanon, and Jordan in 1944.[46,50-52] In 1959, AHS serotype 9 occurred in the southeastern regions of Iran. This was followed by outbreaks during 1960 in Cyprus, Iraq, Syria, Lebanon, and Jordan, as well as in Afghanistan, Pakistan, India, and Turkey. Between 1959 and 1961, this region lost more than 300,000 equids.[52,53] In 1965, AHS occurred in Libya, Tunisia, Algeria, and Morocco and subsequently spread to Spain in 1966.[54] Between 1987 and 1990, AHS serotype 4 occurred in Spain, with the source of infection being zebra *(Equus burchelli)* imported from Namibia.[16,17] AHS was also confirmed in southern Portugal in 1989 and Morocco between 1989 and 1991, with these outbreaks being extensions of the outbreak in Spain.[16,55] In 1989 an outbreak of AHS serotype 9 occurred in Saudi Arabia.[15] AHS was also reported in Saudi Arabia and Yemen in 1997 and on the Cape Verde Islands in 1999.

AHS can be distributed over great distances if equids incubating the disease are translocated by land, sea, or air.[17,56] Outbreaks have also been reported to result from wind-borne spread of infected vectors.[57]

AHS is not endemic in parts of South Africa, but each year the disease appears in the northeastern part of the country, occasionally during December but usually in January, from where it spreads southward. The extent of the southerly spread is influenced by the extent of favorable climatic conditions for the breeding of *Culicoides* midges.[48] Early and heavy rains followed by warm, dry spells favor the occurrence of epizootics. Although parts of the inland plateau of South Africa and most of the Cape Province are usually free of AHS, the disease has sometimes extended into these areas and caused serious losses. Significant losses were reported at Belfast, a town situated about 2100 meters (8000 feet) above sea level during the severe epizootic of 1923.[58] The first cases of AHS usually occur at the beginning of February, but the most serious outbreaks usually occur in March and April. Following the first frosts, which usually occur at the end of April or in May, the disease disappears abruptly. However, in the northeastern parts of South Africa, where the occurrence of frost is less common, deaths may continue to occur into May and June.[1] In recent years the southerly spread of AHS has been less extensive, probably as a result of the widespread use of a more effective vaccine, which became available in 1974.[48] Approximately 300,000 doses of polyvalent AHS vaccine are sold annually by Onderstepoort Biological Products. It is speculated that immunization of horses in these regions establishes a fairly effective "immune barrier" that seems to impede the southerly spread of the disease.[48] Outbreaks of AHS associated with the introduction of infected animals have been reported in the Cape Peninsula in 1967,[48] 1990,[59] 1999,[60] and 2004.

AHS affects primarily equine animals. Horses are most susceptible to the disease (mortality of 70%-95%), but mules are less so (mortality of 50%-70%). Most infections of donkeys and zebras are subclinical.[2,46] Generally, horses of all breeds are equally susceptible to AHS, but variation in susceptibility to the same virus in individual horses has been reported.[2] Some indigenous horses in North and West Africa, which descend from animals that have been present there since at least 2000 BC, have apparently acquired natural resistance to AHS.[61] Foals born to immune mares acquire passive immunity by the ingestion of colostrum.[62] This passive immunity progressively declines and is completely lost after about 4 to 6 months. Donkeys in the Middle East appear to be more susceptible to AHS (mortality of 3%-10%) than southern African donkeys.[46] Zebras are highly resistant to AHS and only show a mild fever after experimental infection.[63]

Dogs are the only other species that contract a highly fatal form of AHS.[64-67] All reported clinical cases in dogs have resulted from the ingestion of infected carcass material from horses that have died from AHS.[68,69] AHSV serotype 9 has been isolated from the blood of stray dogs in Egypt,[49] and antibodies to AHSV have been detected in the sera of dogs in

India[70] and South Africa.[71] However, it is doubtful that dogs play any role in the spread or maintenance of AHSV, because *Culicoides* spp. do not readily feed on them.[71] Besides zebras,[63,72-74] no other wildlife or domestic ruminants have been shown to play a significant role in the epidemiology of AHS.

PATHOGENESIS

After infection, initial multiplication of AHSV occurs in the regional lymph nodes and is followed by a primary viremia,[75] with subsequent dissemination to endothelial cells of target organs.[76] Effusions into body cavities and edematous changes of various tissues, as well as serosal and visceral hemorrhages, are consistent with endothelial cell damage. In experimental cases of AHS, high virus concentrations are found in the spleen, lungs, cecum, pharynx, choroid plexus, and most lymph nodes by the second day after inoculation. This precedes the onset of fever or detectable viremia. By the third day after inoculation, virus is present in most organs. Virus multiplication at these sites gives rise to a secondary viremia of variable duration. In horses the viremia is generally not higher than 10^5 $TCID_{50}$/mL and lasts 4 to 8 days but does not exceed 21 days. In donkeys and zebras the viremia is lower but may last as long as 4 weeks.[75] In zebras, viremia has been reported in the presence of circulating antibodies.[63]

The factors determining the course and severity of infection are not well understood. Small plaque variants produce severe clinical reactions, whereas large plaque variants of AHSV are less pathogenic.[75] Fully susceptible horses, such as foals that have lost their colostral immunity or horses that have never been exposed to the AHSV, usually develop the peracute "pulmonary" form of AHS. Exercise during the febrile stage of the disease may also precipitate this form of AHS.[50,75] During the 1959 Middle East epizootic of AHS caused by serotype 9, severe myocardial lesions with extensive areas of degeneration and necrosis of myocytes, accompanied by a marked inflammatory response, were described in fully susceptible horses, particularly those with the "cardiac" form of the disease.[77] In this form of AHS, heart failure is attributed to hydropericardium[75,78] and myocardial damage.[77] However, most natural cases of AHS are of the "mixed" form, with evidence of both pulmonary and cardiac compromise.[47,75,77]

CLINICAL FINDINGS

The clinical findings of natural and experimental cases of AHS have been described.[17,77,79-81] In experimental cases the incubation period is usually between 5 and 7 days, but possibly as short as 2 days and rarely as long as 10 days. The duration of the incubation period depends on the virulence of the virus and the dose of virus received.

"Dunkop" or "Pulmonary" Form

The "dunkop" or "pulmonary" form is the peracute form of AHS, and recovery is the exception. This form of AHS occurs when AHSV infects fully susceptible horses. In endemic areas, it is also common in foals that have lost their maternally derived passive immunity. Dunkop is also the usual form in dogs that become infected after ingestion of AHSV-infected carcass material.

The incubation period for pulmonary AHS is short, usually 3 to 4 days, and is followed by a rapid rise in temperature over 1 or 2 days, with the body temperature reaching 104° to 106° F (40°-41° C). The dunkop form is characterized by marked and rapidly progressive respiratory failure, and the respiratory rate may exceed 50 breaths per minute. The animal tends to stand with its forelegs spread apart, its head extended, and the nostrils dilated. Expiration is frequently forced, with the presence of abdominal heave lines. Profuse sweating is common, and paroxysmal coughing may be observed terminally, often with frothy, serofibrinous fluid exuding from the nostrils (Fig. 15-1). The onset of dyspnea is usually very sudden, and death occurs within 30 minutes to a few hours of its appearance. Sometimes an apparently healthy horse at work becomes listless, suddenly severely dyspneic, and dies shortly thereafter. Initially, the appetite of affected animals remains good despite the high fever and respiratory distress. The prognosis for horses with the dunkop form is extremely poor (<5% recover). If animals recover, the fever subsides gradually, but the breathing remains labored for several days.

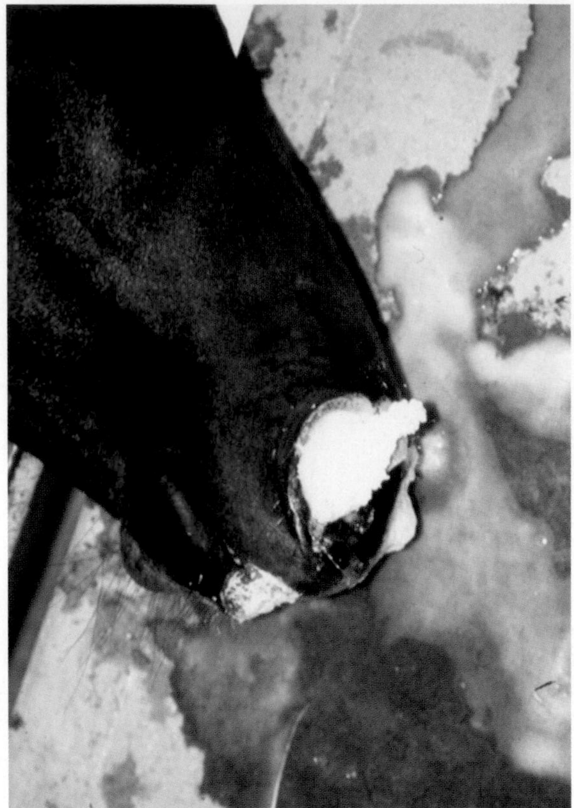

Fig. 15-1 "Pulmonary" or "dunkop" form of African horse sickness (AHS), with froth and serous fluid at nostrils caused by severe alveolar edema.

"Dikkop" or "Cardiac" Form

The incubation period in the "dikkop" or "cardiac" form of AHS is longer than the "dunkop" (pulmonary) form, usually 5 to 7 days, followed by a fever of 102° to 106° F (39°-41° C) that persists for 3 to 4 days. The more typical clinical signs do not appear until the fever has begun to decline. At first the supraorbital fossae fill as the underlying adipose tissue becomes edematous and raises the skin well above the level of the zygomatic arch (Figs. 15-2 and 15-3). The edema can later extend to the conjunctiva (Fig. 15-4), lips, cheeks, tongue, intermandibular space, and laryngeal region and may extend a variable distance down the neck toward the chest, often obliterating the jugular groove. As the swellings increase, dyspnea and cyanosis may supervene. However, ventral edema and

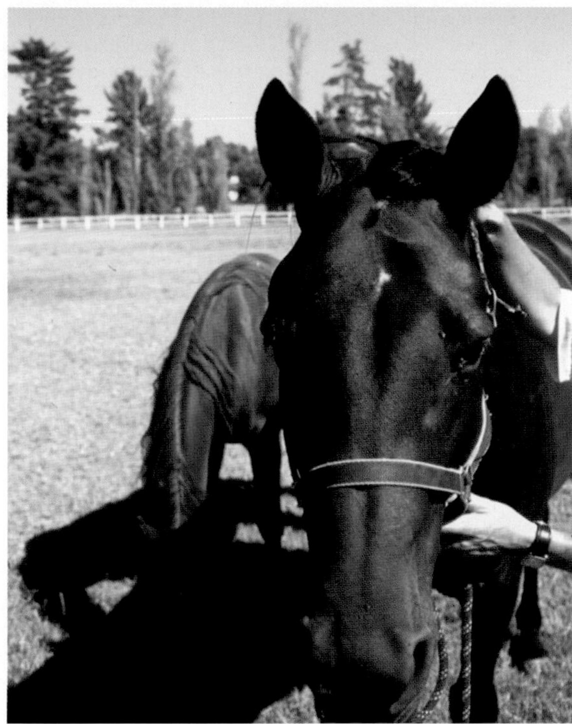

Fig. 15-2 "Cardiac" or "dikkop" form of AHS, with filling of supraorbital fossae.

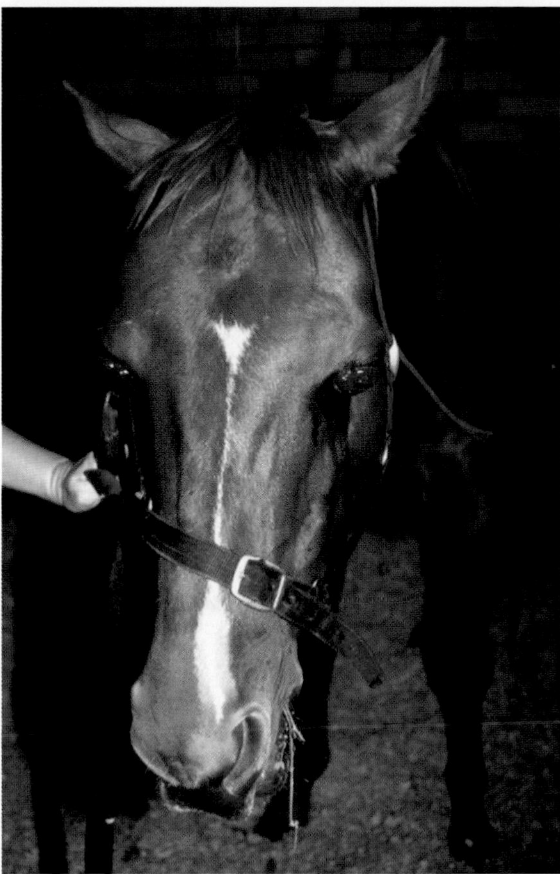

Fig. 15-4 Severe conjunctival edema and hyperemia with some hemorrhage in horse with AHS.

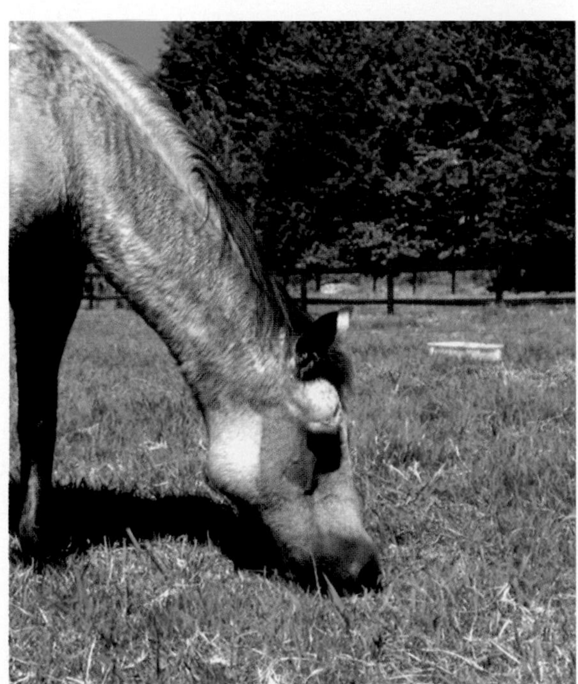

Fig. 15-3 Severe edema of head associated with cardiac form of AHS.

edema of the lower limbs are not observed. Unfavorable prognostic signs include petechial hemorrhages on the conjunctivae and on the ventral surface of the tongue; if they occur, these hemorrhages become evident shortly before death. Some animals may show signs of severe colic, repeatedly lie down, are restless when standing, and frequently paw the ground.

The course of the dikkop form of AHS is always more protracted and milder than in the dunkop form, with mortality greater than 50%. Death usually occurs within 4 to 8 days after the onset of the febrile reaction. In horses that recover, swellings gradually subside over 3 to 8 days. Paralysis of the esophagus may be a complication, particularly in patients with severe edematous swellings of the head, resulting in dysphagia.[81] In severely affected animals the esophagus becomes distended, and animals may die from foreign body pneumonia. Equine piroplasmosis is a common complication of AHS during recovery.[1,82] In such horses, icterus, anemia, and constipation are evident.

"Mixed" Form

Although the most common form of AHS, the "mixed" form, is rarely diagnosed clinically, it is seen at necropsy in the majority of fatal cases of AHS in horses and mules. Initial pulmonary signs that are mild and not progressive are followed by edematous swelling and effusions, and death results from cardiac failure. More often, the subclinical cardiac form is suddenly followed by marked dyspnea and other signs typical of the pulmonary form. Death usually occurs 3 to 6 days after the onset of the febrile reaction.

Horsesickness Fever

Horsesickness fever is the mildest form of AHS and is frequently not diagnosed clinically. The incubation period is between 5 and 9 days, after which the temperature gradually rises over 4 to 5 days to 104° F (40° C), followed by a drop in temperature to normal, then recovery. Apart from the febrile reaction, other clinical signs are rare and inconspicuous. Some animals may be depressed with partial loss of appetite, congestion of the conjunctivae, slightly labored breathing, and increased heart rate, but these signs are transient. Horsesickness fever is usually observed in donkeys and zebra or in immune horses infected with a heterologous serotype of AHSV.

DIAGNOSIS

Diagnosis of AHS is virtually impossible during the early febrile phase of the disease. Hematologic abnormalities include leukopenia, thrombocytopenia, and elevated hematocrit, erythrocyte count, and hemoglobin concentration. Hemostatic abnormalities include increased concentration of fibrin degradation products and prolonged prothrombin, activated partial thromboplastin, and thrombin clotting times.[83] A presumptive diagnosis should be possible once the characteristic clinical signs have developed. The typical macroscopic lesions of AHS on necropsy are often sufficiently specific to allow a provisional diagnosis of the disease.

The clinical signs of AHS may be confused with those of equine encephalosis (see Chapter 26). Many of the epidemiologic features of the two infections are similar. Horses with swelling of the supraorbital fossae, eyelids, or lips as a result of equine encephalosis cannot be differentiated clinically from the "cardiac" form of AHS. However, mortality from AHS is much higher than from equine encephalosis. Virus isolation and identification are essential to confirm either diagnosis.

The disseminated petechiation associated with the cardiac form of AHS may be similar to that found in animals with purpura hemorrhagica and equine viral arteritis. However, the subcutaneous edema observed in these conditions tends to be more ventral than that observed in animals with AHS. In purpura hemorrhagica the hemorrhages tend to be more severe, numerous, and widespread than in AHS. The early stages of piroplasmosis may occasionally be confused with AHS. AHS may also be complicated by piroplasmosis, and ventral edema may be severe in these horses.

AHS is foreign to almost all countries outside of sub-Saharan Africa and is an OIE-listed disease. Suspected cases of AHS must therefore be reported to the State Veterinary Authority and must always be subject to laboratory confirmation. Blood samples collected in heparin during the febrile stage of the disease or specimens of the lungs, spleen, and lymph nodes collected at necropsy and kept at 4° C (39.2° F) can be used for virus isolation.[84]

Primary virus isolation can be performed using a variety of cell cultures (BHK21, Vero, or MS cells)[49,52,85,86] or by intracerebral inoculation of suckling mice.[84] Cytopathic effects (CPEs), characterized by increased refractivity and detachment of cells, can appear 3 to 7 days after inoculation of cultures but may only become conspicuous in the second passage. After three passages, advanced CPEs develop within 2 to 4 days.[84] Serotyping of AHSV isolates is performed using virus neutralization (VN) tests employing type-specific antisera in mice,[33,87] or more often on various cell cultures.[88,89] Group-specific antibody to AHSV can be detected by using complement fixation (CF),[35,84,90] agar gel immunodiffusion (AGID),[84,90] indirect fluorescent antibody (IFA),[90,91] and enzyme-linked immunosorbent assay (ELISA) tests.[16,84,90,92,93] Serotype-specific antibody to AHSV can be detected using serum neutralizing tests.[35,84,90] CF antibody titers are of short duration,[35,50] whereas neutralizing and ELISA antibodies persist for a number of years.[94]

Several polymerase chain reaction (PCR) assays[95-98] have been described to detect AHSV and to differentiate between serotypes.[99,100] PCR-based assays are rapid, sensitive, and versatile and may supplement or replace some of the older conventional methods. Furthermore, PCR can be applied to specimens from clinical cases that do not contain live virus. Antigen-capture ELISAs that detect antigen in mammalian and insect tissue homogenates and cell culture have also been reported.[59,101,102]

PATHOLOGIC FINDINGS

Macroscopic Pathology

"Dunkop" or "Pulmonary" Form

The most striking finding in the pulmonary form of AHS is diffuse, severe, subpleural and interlobular edema of the lungs (Fig. 15-5). The lungs do not collapse on opening of the thorax and are heavier than normal. Severe hydrothorax is common, with the pleural cavity containing several liters of transparent, pale-yellow, gelatinous fluid. Subcutaneous and intermuscular edema is usually absent. Edema may also involve the mediastinum, base of the heart, and the parietal pleura.

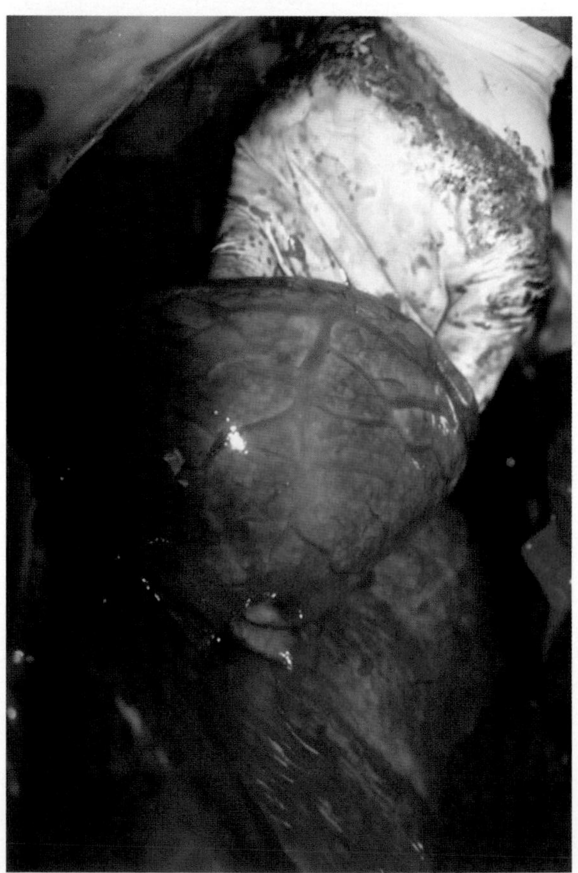

Fig. 15-5 Severe septal edema of lungs associated with "pulmonary" or "dunkop" form of AHS.

Serous fluid oozes from the cut surface of the lung. The trachea and bronchi usually contain large amounts of froth and yellow serous fluid (Fig. 15-6). Petechiae and ecchymoses are sometimes present on the mucosa of the trachea. The bronchial and mediastinal lymph nodes are severely swollen and edematous. The spleen is normal in size, with the white pulp more prominent than usual. Moderate, diffuse congestion of the mucosa of the glandular part of the stomach is a consistent finding (Fig. 15-7). Patchy congestion of the serosal surface of the small intestine and scattered petechiation on the intestinal serosa are common. There is usually some degree of ascites.

"Dikkop" or "Cardiac" Form

The most characteristic finding in the cardiac form of AHS is the presence of distinctly yellow edema of the subcutaneous and intermuscular connective tissues. The edema is particularly severe around the ligamentum nuchae. In mild cases, only the head and neck are involved, but in severe cases the edema involves the lower parts of the neck, the thorax, and shoulders. The eyelids, supraorbital fossae, and lips are often involved. The tongue may have petechiae or ecchymoses on its ventral surface and is occasionally swollen and cyanotic. Severe hydropericardium is almost invariably present. Subepicardial petechiation and subendocardial ecchymoses, particularly over the papillary muscles, are usually present (Fig. 15-8). Pale-gray areas of varying size may occur in the myocardium of horses with severe myocardial damage. The lungs are usually normal or slightly congested, and hydrothorax is rare. The lymph nodes are swollen and edematous. Mild nephrosis may be present.

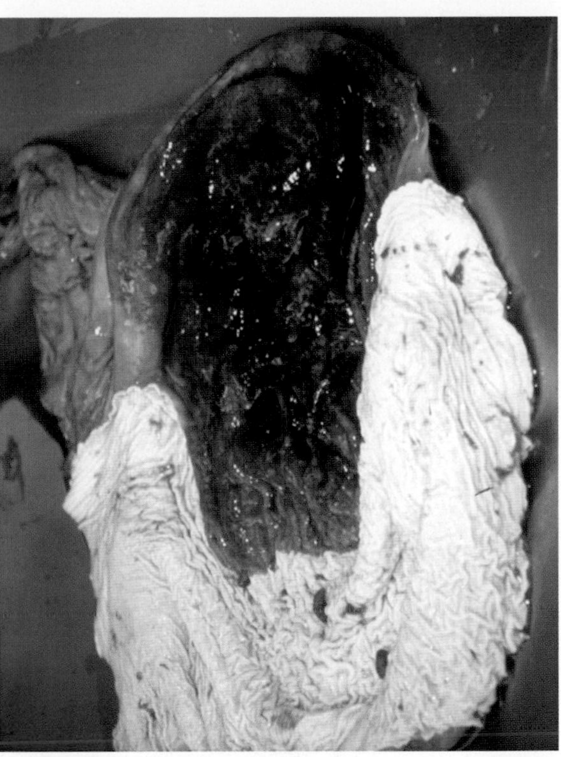

Fig. 15-7 Congestion of glandular part of stomach in horse with AHS.

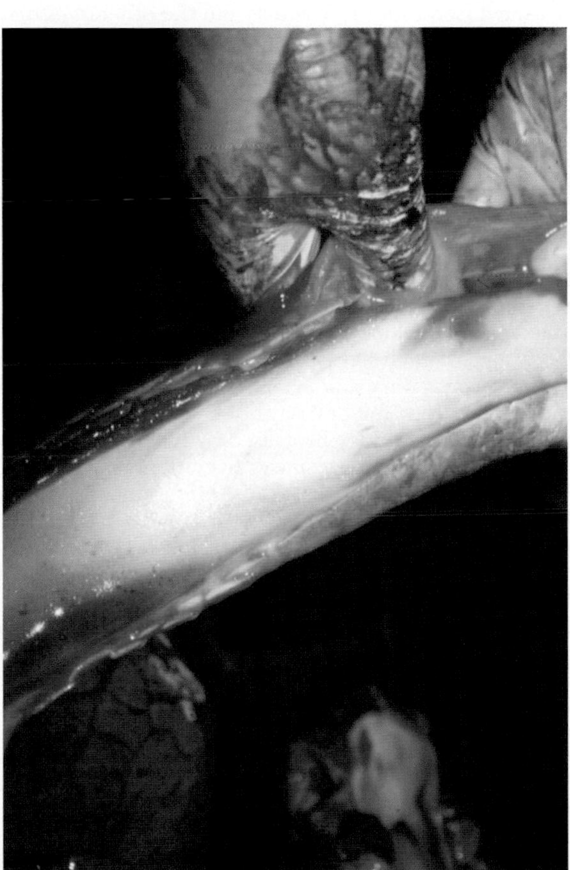

Fig. 15-6 Froth and serous fluid in trachea in horse with pulmonary form of AHS.

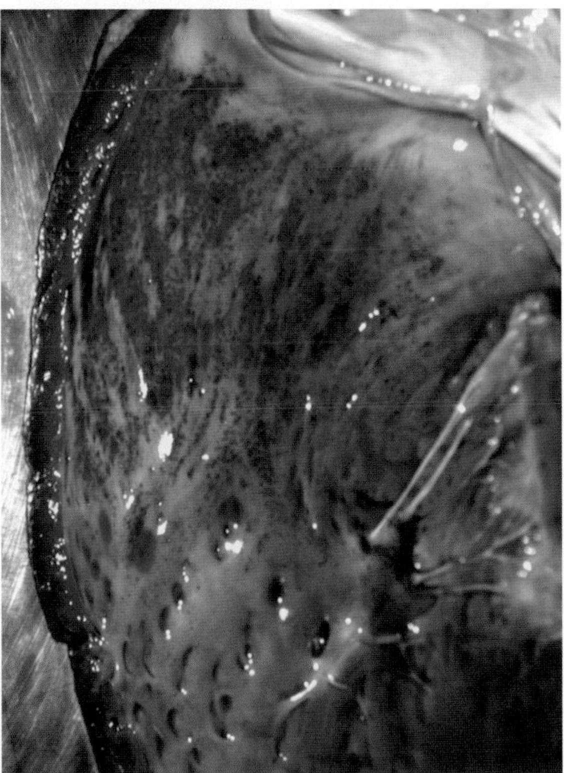

Fig. 15-8 Subendocardial hemorrhages in right ventricle of heart in horse with "dikkop" or "cardiac" form of AHS.

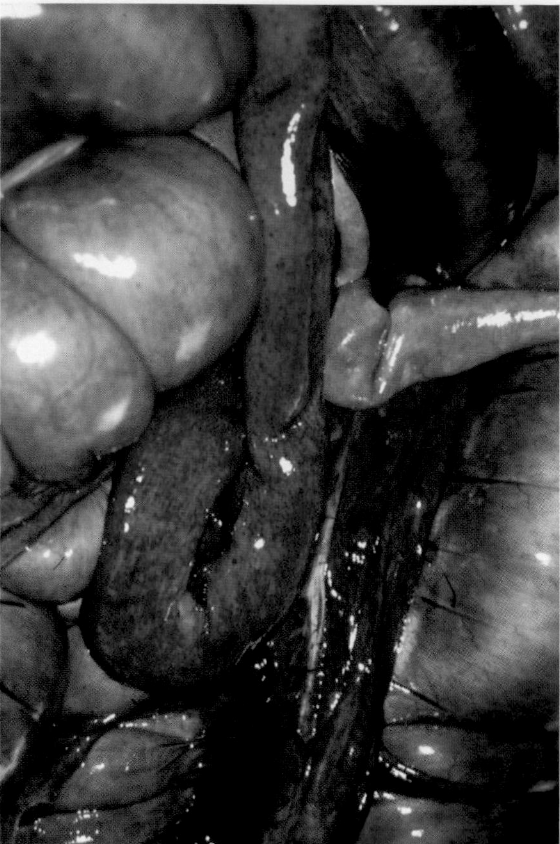

Fig. 15-9 Petechiation on surfaces of small and large intestines in horse with AHS.

Moderate to severe edema, congestion, and petechiation of the mucosa of the cecum, colon, and rectum are common (Fig. 15-9). In horses with esophageal paralysis, the esophagus is distended with a variable amount of compressed food.

"Mixed" Form

Lesions described for the pulmonary and cardiac forms of AHS and edematous infiltration are found together in animals that die of the mixed form of the disease.

Microscopic Pathology

In horses with pulmonary involvement, widening of the interlobular septa and locally extensive pockets of alveolar edema are the predominant findings.[77,80,103] Perivasculitis, characterized by edematous separation of the adventitial connective tissue of medium-sized vessels, and focal influx of mononuclear cells are evident in the lungs.[80,103] Type I pneumocytes occasionally separate from the alveolar wall.[80] The microscopic lesions in the heart vary considerably, with the myocardium appearing essentially normal in a large proportion of cases. Changes range from focal myocardial hemorrhage with no myofiber changes to acute degeneration of myocardial fibers with loss of cross-striations and occasional fragmentation of the sarcoplasm. Occasionally, this is accompanied by infiltration of inflammatory cells.[77,103] The germinal centers of most lymph nodes and the spleen show varying degrees of lymphocyte depletion and nuclear karyorrhexis.[80,103] In situ hybridization[103] and immunohistochemical staining[104] have revealed the presence of AHS viral nucleic acid or antigen in endothelial cells in the lung, heart, and spleen. Ultrastructural changes have also been demonstrated in endothelial cells in the lungs.[76]

THERAPY

There is no specific treatment for AHS. Affected animals should be provided with supportive therapy, nursed, and rested because the slightest exertion may result in death. Animals that survive should be rested for at least 4 weeks after recovery before being returned to light work. They should also be carefully monitored for complications such as piroplasmosis.

PREVENTION

Since the demonstration in the early 1930s that AHSV could be attenuated by serial intracerebral passage in mice, the immunization of horses against the disease has been greatly simplified and improved.[10,11,46,105] The first highly effective attenuated vaccine was produced in 1936.[106] Virus attenuation occurs faster during passage in cell culture than in mouse brain.[107] The size of plaques in cell culture has been found to be a marker of the virulence of AHS viruses, and therefore, large plaque variants are now selected as candidate vaccine strains.[75,84,108]

In endemic areas, annual vaccination of horses in late winter or early summer is a practical means of control. Unfortunately, prophylactic immunization against AHS cannot be relied on to protect all horses fully against infection or disease. However, horses that have received three or more courses of immunization are usually well protected against AHS. Onderstepoort Biological Products currently produces a polyvalent vaccine containing attenuated strains prepared in two components, one *trivalent* (serotypes 1, 3, and 4) and the other *quadrivalent* (serotypes 2, 6, 7, and 8).[108] Immunization consists of the administration of these component vaccines at least 3 weeks apart. Serotypes 5 and 9 are not included in the vaccines because serotypes 8 and 6, respectively, are reported to afford adequate cross-protection.

Generally, immunization has little or no side effects. A slight temperature increase may occur between 5 and 13 days after vaccination as a result of virus replication. Occasionally, individual animals vaccinated for the first time may show a severe vaccine reaction and may develop clinical signs of AHS. The simultaneous administration of several serotypes of attenuated AHS in horses usually results in the production of antibody against each serotype, although the response of individual horses may vary, and in some animals, antibody against one or more of the serotypes may not be detectable by neutralization test.[62,109] This may be caused by interference between viruses in the polyvalent vaccine or overattenuation of vaccine strains.[33,110] During the outbreak of AHS in Spain, about 10% of animals immunized for the first time with a monovalent, attenuated AHS virus serotype 4 vaccine failed to seroconvert. However, at least some of these animals are resistant to challenge.[16]

The antibody acquired from colostrum correlates well with the antibody level of the dam and determines the duration of passive immunity.[62,109] Because of possible interference of passive immunity with response to vaccination in foals born to immune mares, it is recommended that foals should not be immunized before they are 6 months of age. However, some foals acquire low levels of antibody to one or more AHS virus serotypes via the colostrum, and neutralizing antibody to individual serotypes may decline to undetectable levels shortly after birth, with a result that these foals can become susceptible to infection well before age 6 months.[109]

The risk of infection in susceptible horses can be reduced significantly by stabling them before dusk until after sunrise, because *Culicoides* spp. are nocturnal and are not inclined to enter buildings.[109] The application of insect repellents and the use of insecticides on animals also reduce the risk of infection.

After a suspected outbreak of AHS in a country previously free of the disease, attempts should be made to limit further transmission of the virus and to achieve eradication as soon as possible. It is important that control measures be instituted immediately. The control measures in epizootic situations include (1) delineation of the area of infection; (2) strict movement controls within, into, and out of the infected area; (3) stabling of all equids at least from dusk to dawn; (4) insect control measures; (5) temperatures of all equids measured for early detection of infected animals; (6) consideration of immediate vaccination of all susceptible animals with an attenuated polyvalent vaccine, pending serotyping, and subsequent use of a relevant monovalent vaccine; (7) identification of all vaccinated animals; and (8) notification of the Office Internationale des Epizooties (OIE) about the disease outbreak.[19]

The International Animal Health Code provides guidelines for the importation of domestic horses from AHS-infected countries or zones.[19] These include the housing of animals in vector-protected quarantine facilities for at least 40 days and testing for the absence of AHSV or demonstration of a stable or declining AHS antibody titer.

PUBLIC HEALTH CONSIDERATIONS

Accidental aerosol infection occurred in four workers packing mouse-brain attenuated strains of AHS vaccine at Onderstepoort Biological Products.[113] They developed nonfatal encephalitis and chorioretinitis, which resulted in partial loss of vision or blindness. These neurotrophic strains have since been removed from the AHS vaccine produced by Onderstepoort Biological Products.

REFERENCES

See the CD-ROM for a list of references linked to the abstract in PubMed.

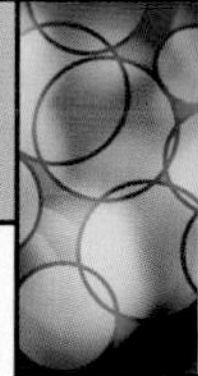

CHAPTER • 16

Miscellaneous Viral Respiratory Diseases

Michael J. Studdert

EQUINE ADENOVIRUSES

Equine adenovirus type 1 (EAdV1) causes acute upper respiratory disease, follicular conjunctivitis, bronchopneumonia, and infection of the gastrointestinal (GI) tract that is associated with production of soft feces. EAdV1 is peculiarly linked as a dominant pathogen to the uniformly fatal, inherited disorder termed *primary severe combined immunodeficiency disease* (PSCID), which affects certain Arabian foals. These foals have an inexorably progressive EAdV1 bronchopneumonia as well as EAdV1-related pathology in many other organs and tissues

Etiology

Equine adenoviruses are members of the genus *Mastadenovirus*, family *Adenoviridae*. Only a single antigenic type of equine adenovirus (EAdV1) has been isolated from horses with respiratory disease.[1,2] A second serotype, equine adenovirus type 2 (EAdV2), has been isolated from the feces of foals with diarrhea.[3] The biophysical properties of EAdV are similar to those of adenoviruses of other species. Equine adenoviruses are nonenveloped, 70 to 80 nm in diameter, and the capsid is composed of 252 capsomers; 240 hexamers occupy the faces and edges of the 20 equilateral triangular facets of an icosahedron, and 12 pentamers occupy the corners. The inner core contains the double-stranded deoxyribonucleic acid (DNA) genome, which for EAdV1 is 34.4 kilobases in length. Restriction endonuclease maps and genome orientation data were published for EAdV1,[4] and genomic sequence data for both viruses were also published.[5,6] Nucleotide sequence data for the EAdV2 genome corroborated at the molecular level that EAdV2 is distinct from EAdV1 and that the two viruses evolved separately.[5]

An adenovirus-associated virus was isolated from a foal with respiratory disease after inoculation of equine cell cultures.[7] As for adenovirus-associated viruses of other species, the equine virus is assumed to be nonpathogenic.

Epidemiology

EAdV1 occurs worldwide, and seroprevalence rates vary from less than 2% to 100%, depending on the serologic test used and the age, breed, activity, and size of the population sampled reported.[2] The prevalence of antibody to EAdV1 increases with age such that in some populations, about 70% of yearlings and 2-year-old horses have EAdV1 antibody. Serologic evidence indicates a high infection rate in the first year of life, but in some populations, 50% of horses under 1 year lack EAdV antibody and are presumably at risk for EAdV disease.[1]

All adenovirus infections appear to be followed by a latent carrier status and shedding of the virus. Studies in the Pirbright, United Kingdom, pony herd indicated that EAdV1 infections were often subclinical, and that virus may persist in the nasopharyngeal mucus for up to 68 days after primary infection.[8] EAdV1 was isolated from a foal, without clinical signs at the time of isolation, at 3 days of age.[9] It seems that foals may acquire infection from their dams or other horses in their cohort during the suckling period, even in the presence of detectable levels of maternal antibody. Thus, if there is persistent or repeated EAdV infection, the passive immunity of the foal would be converted to an active immunity, probably without significant clinical disease. Disease would develop if primary infection occurred after maternal antibody had declined, or if the foal was unable to produce an active immune response. This overview of the early natural history of EAdV1 is supported by the natural history of EAdV1 in Arabian foals with PSCID, in which the transmission pattern and consequences of infection are viewed in the absence of an active immune response.[10]

EAdV2 has been isolated in Australia and New Zealand.[3,11] Collected from widely separated geographic areas in Australia and from horses of diverse breed and age, 327 horse serums were tested for EAdV2 neutralizing antibody; 77% of these serums were positive (maximum titer, 1:640). This pattern of infection is likely to occur worldwide.

Pathogenesis

EAdV1 presumably is frequently acquired as a droplet or close-contact respiratory or ocular infection. The virus replicates in epithelial cells throughout the respiratory tract, producing lysis and sloughing of these cells and a hyperplastic response in underlying noninfected cells. Respiratory disease in foals is more severe and more likely to be associated with pneumonitis when there is total or partial failure of maternal antibody transfer (T.B. Crawford, personal communication). Recovery from disease caused by EAdV1 alone in immunologically competent horses occurs within a week to 10 days, but mixed infections with other viruses and bacteria may cause more severe and prolonged disease.[8,12] Multiple infections involving various combinations of equine herpesviruses types 1 and 4, equine rhinitis A and equine rhinitis B viruses, and equine adenoviruses were recognized in 15 of 69 outbreaks of respiratory disease of horses in the United Kingdom.[13] EAdV1 may infect cells of the GI tract and may be shed in feces, and presumably it may also be transmitted through a fecal-oral cycle. EAdV1 was isolated from neuritis of the cauda equina but was probably an incidental contaminant.[14]

Immunity

Immunocompetent foals develop EAdV1 antibody, recover spontaneously from the disease, and generally do not possess recoverable virus by day 10 after infection.[12] In experimental infections of colostrum-deprived and colostrum-fed foals, the colostrum-fed foals had less severe changes than colostrum-deprived foals.[12,17]

Reinfection by EAdV1 was found to occur frequently in a group of 16 mares and foals, and many of these infections (or reinfections) occurred in the presence of high levels of circulating antibody.[22] Immunoglobulin A (IgA) in nasal secretions is responsible for resistance to reinfection in human infections with adenovirus or rhinoviruses. A similar situation could occur in horses, when rapidly declining levels of nasal antibody after an infection could soon render the horse susceptible to reinfection, despite high serum antibody levels.

After intramuscular (IM) immunization with live EAdV1 and subsequent development of high serum antibody levels, a specific-pathogen-free (SPF) foal proved resistant to intranasal challenge with EAdV1.[17] Clinical disease did not develop and virus was not isolated, although there was a greater than twofold increase in serum-neutralizing (SN) antibody after challenge. Immunity was correlated with prior exposure to the virus and high circulating SN antibody levels.

An experimental inactivated EAdV1 vaccine elicited high antibody titers in rabbits, mice, and foals. Using nude mice as a model of T-cell immunodeficiency, it was shown that production of EAdV1 SN antibody and, to a lesser extent, hemagglutination-inhibiting (HI) antibody was T lymphocyte dependent.[23] As a measure of cell-mediated immune responses, an EAdV1-specific in vitro lymphocyte blastogenesis assay was developed and evaluated using lymphocytes from four vaccinated and two unvaccinated control horses. The four vaccinated horses showed marked increases in stimulation indices in response to EAdV1 antigen (maximum stimulation indices, 5.3-18.6).[24]

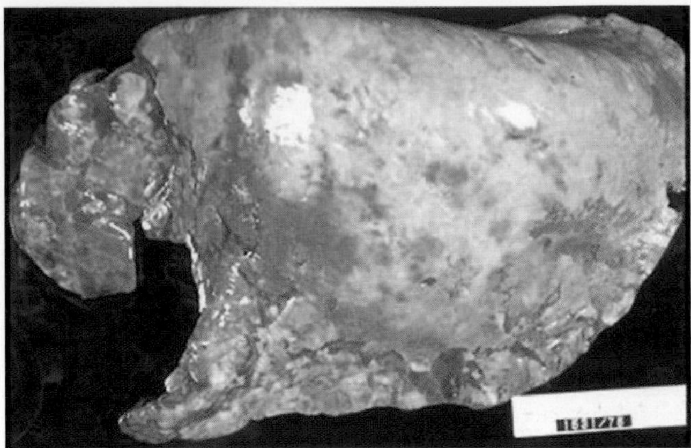

Fig. 16-1 Lung of 63-day-old, purebred Arabian foal that had primary severe combined immunodeficiency disease (PSCID). There is extensive bronchopneumonia. The lungs have failed to collapse. On the cut surface of the lung, essentially all bronchi are plugged with thick, cream-colored exudate.

As mentioned, EAdV1 is peculiarly associated as a dominant pathogen in the uniformly fatal, inherited disease syndrome, PSCID.[25,26] When first recognized in the early 1970s, PSCID was estimated to cause the death of about 3% of all purebred Arabian foals. Foals are born with a total absence of T and B lymphocytes, and PSCID is inherited as an autosomal recessive gene.[27,28] A consistent and dominant feature of PSCID is an inexorably progressive EAdV1 bronchopneumonia (Fig. 16-1); the virus also causes pathology in a wide variety of other organs and tissues in PSCID foals, including the GI tract, liver, pancreas, and bladder.

Clinical Findings

EAdV1 causes acute upper respiratory disease with nasal discharge, conjunctivitis, and bronchopneumonia and infection of the GI tract, leading to the production of soft feces. Other clinical signs include coughing after exercise and enlarged submandibular lymph nodes.[2,13] Severe or fatal bronchopneumonia has been occasionally recorded in non-immunodeficient Thoroughbred foals.[15,16]

Respiratory disease signs were described in an experimentally infected SPF foal that was cesarean delivered, colostrum deprived, and artificially reared in an EAdV-free environment.[17] The foal was healthy and 6 weeks old when infected and had been shown to be immunocompetent. After intranasal infection with EAdV1, clinical signs included mucopurulent nasal discharge, severe follicular conjunctivitis (Fig. 16-2), transient anorexia and pyrexia, and sustained tachypnea. There were no changes in blood leukocyte numbers. EAdV1 was readily isolated from nasal, conjunctival, and rectal swabs and from lung, trachea, bronchial lymph nodes, and small intestine tissue homogenates obtained after an elective postmortem at 6 days after infection.

The clinical response to experimental infection of a 4-day-old foal that received colostrum but was artificially reared from 12 hours after birth in an EAdV1-free environment, and that had a 1:320 SN antibody titer and a 1:40 HI antibody titer,

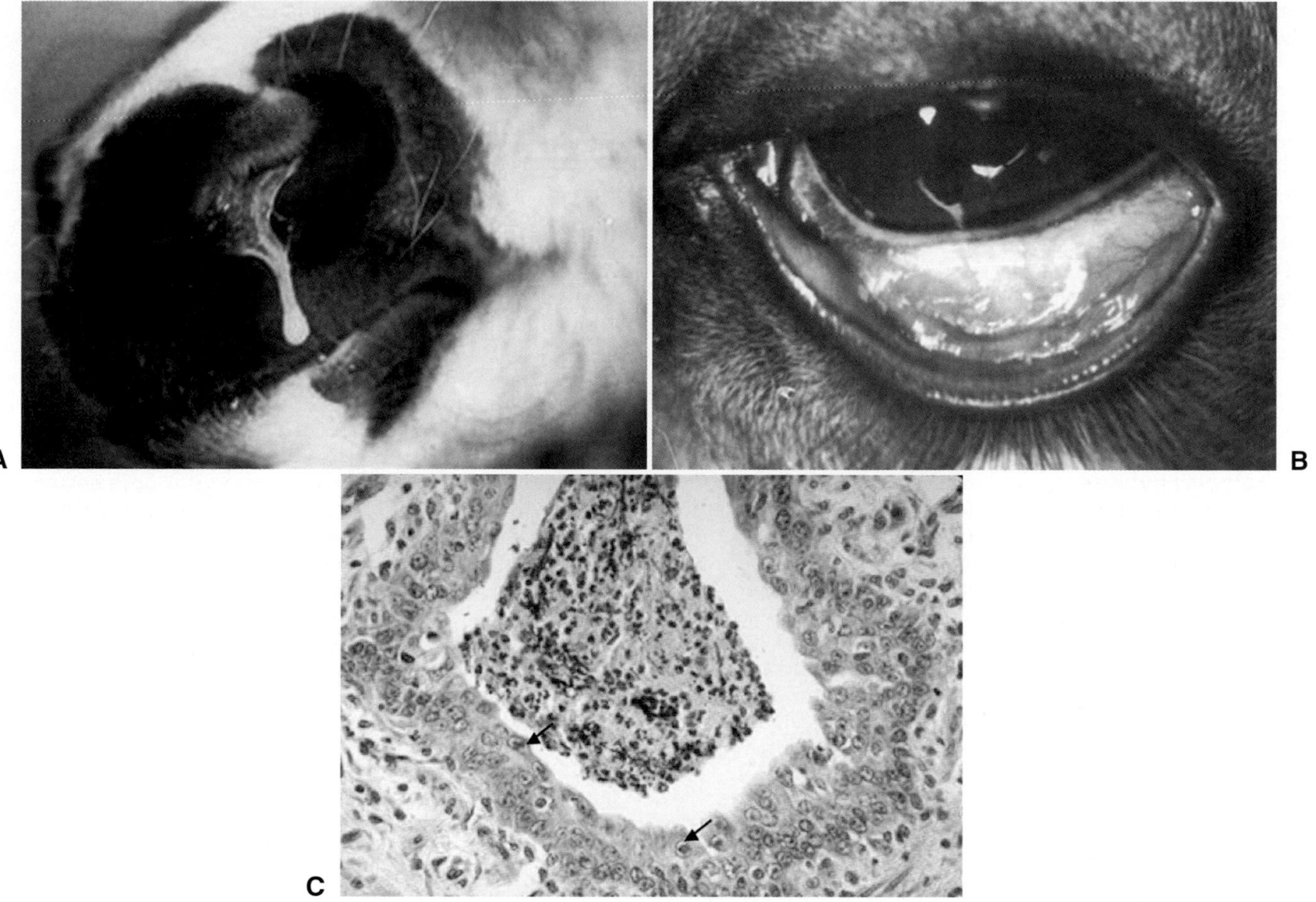

Fig. 16-2 A, Nasal discharge in 9-week-old specific-pathogen-free (SPF) foal 6 days after experimental intranasal/intraocular infection with EAdV1.[17] **B,** Conjunctivitis in the same foal 6 days after infection. **C,** Low-power image of bronchiolitis of the same foal. Note proliferation and disorientation of bronchial epithelial cells and the highly cellular bronchial exudate. Arrows indicate adenovirus inclusion bodies in nonsloughed bronchial epithelial cells.

was similar to that of the previous foal, except fever was not as marked or as sustained, the conjunctivitis was less severe, and nasal discharge was minimal.[17] EAdV1 was readily isolated from nasal and conjunctival swabs and from trachea and lung, but not from rectal swabs, small intestine, or bronchial lymph nodes, when an elective postmortem was conducted 6 days after infection.

The production of soft feces in adult horses, indicative of GI infection, has been reported as a sole manifestation of EAdV infection.[13] Replication of EAdV1 in cells of the GI tract was confirmed after experimental intranasal infection.[17]

EAdV1 was reported as a potential cause of abortion in mares, and abortion was reproduced experimentally after intrauterine inoculation of the virus.[12] However, claims for the natural occurrence of EAdV abortion are unsubstantiated.

EAdV2 was isolated from foals with severe diarrhea in which rotavirus was also present.[18] Several foals died, and at postmortem one had an intussusception. In light of experiences with a human rotavirus vaccine that was withdrawn from the market because of an increased incidence of intussusception in infants receiving the live-virus oral vaccine, it seems of interest that the 1976 case of intussusception in the foal, to our knowledge, was the first in any species associated with adenovirus/rotavirus infection.

Diagnosis

Clinical Laboratory

Virus isolation from nasopharyngeal and conjunctival swabs during the acute phase of infection is possible but not frequently reported. EAdV1 may also be isolated from rectal swabs but would need to be differentiated from EAdV2. Polymerase chain reaction (PCR) primers have been designed for the detection of both EAdV1 and EAdV2.[19] Detection of adenovirus in negatively stained preparations from fecal samples by electron microscopy (EM) is readily achieved. Immune precipitation, complement fixation, hemagglutination, HI, and SN assays have been extensively used in diagnosis and seroepidemiologic studies. EAdV1 hemagglutinates human blood group O and equine erythrocytes, but not those of sheep or chicken.[20] EAdV2 does not hemagglutinate human O, rhesus macaque, or equine erythrocytes, and accordingly, HI assays for EAdV2 have not been developed.[3]

Virus Isolation

EAdV1 and EAdV2 are highly host cell specific and have been cultivated only in cells of equine origin in which both viruses produce a cytopathic effect. On light microscopy and hematoxylin-eosin (HE) staining, intranuclear inclusion bodies are a prominent feature of the cytopathology of adenovirus-infected cells. On thin-section EM, virions assembled in the nucleus form crystalline aggregates.

Serology

Adenoviruses are typed on the basis of SN assays. Most adenoviruses hemagglutinate appropriately chosen red blood cells (RBCs), and HI assays are used for antibody detection. Hemagglutination is mediated by the knoblike tip of the penton binding to receptors on the RBC surface. Type-specific antigenic determinants defined by SN and HI assays are located on the outward-facing surface of the hexamers. EAdV1 possesses the common group-specific mastadenovirus antigen.[20] HI antibody to EAdV1, by definition, is type specific.[3,20] Extensive analysis of adenoviruses recovered from horses with respiratory disease, including PSCID Arabian foals, indicated that on SN and HI assays, all were a single antigenic type, designated EAdV1.[1,21] On SN assay, EAdV2 is unrelated to EAdV1.[3]

Pathologic Findings

As previously described, after experimental infection the colostrum-deprived SPF foal showed gross and histopathologic evidence of rhinitis, conjunctivitis, tracheitis, and pneumonia. There was both bronchopneumonia and interstitial pneumonia in affected areas of lung. Duodenal villous atrophy and idiopathic glomerular hyperplasia were also observed. EAdV antigen was detected by indirect immunofluorescence antibody staining of trachea and lung, but not in frozen sections of bronchial lymph node or small intestine. In the SPF foal that received colostrum, gross and histologic evidence of EAdV1 disease was generally similar but less severe than that observed in the SPF colostrum-deprived foal.[17]

Therapy and Prevention

There are no specific therapies for equine adenovirus infections, and vaccines have not been marketed. For both prophylaxis and therapy, as for other neonatal and perinatal infectious diseases, the provision of supplemental passive antibody either through colostrum or parenterally administered EAdV1 hyperimmune sera should be considered when there is a failure or partial failure of maternal antibody transfer.

Public Health Considerations

No human public health implications are associated with equine adenoviruses.

HENDRA VIRUS

Hendra virus, formerly known as *equine morbillivirus,* was first recognized in 1994 as the cause of an outbreak of acute respiratory disease that affected 21 Thoroughbred racehorses in Hendra, a suburb of Brisbane, Queensland, Australia. Fourteen horses died, and seven in-contact horses were euthanized. The trainer of the horses and a stable hand were infected with the virus and became seriously ill, and the trainer died.[29] A second occurrence of the disease, in Mackay, Queensland, involved two horses that died and a second human death.[30,31] Three further incidents of single, sporadic deaths in horses, as well as a suspected infection of a veterinarian who autopsied one of the horses and who recovered, all in northern Queensland, have been recorded.[32-34]

Nipah virus, which is closely related to Hendra virus, emerged as a major new disease causing respiratory disease and encephalitis in domestic pigs and humans in Malaysia in 1999. There were 265 human cases of Nipah virus infection, 106 fatal, and about 1.1 million pigs on infected premises either died or were culled.

The natural hosts of both Hendra and Nipah viruses are fruit bats (flying foxes), in which these viruses are not known to cause disease.

Etiology

Hendra and Nipah viruses are the sole members of a new genus, *Henipavirus,* in the family *Paramyxoviridae,* subfamily *Paramyxovirinae,* order Mononegavirales. Virions are enveloped with a single-stranded, negative-sense ribonucleic acid (RNA) genome that is 18,234 nucleotides in length.[35] In negatively stained electron micrographs, the virus is pleomorphic and approximately 180 nm in diameter. Unusually, the envelope is covered with two kinds of spikes that are 10 nm and 18 nm long and give the particle a "double-fringed" appearance (Fig. 16-3, *A*), which is not a feature of previously described paramyxoviruses. The nucleocapsid is 18 nm wide and has a periodicity of 5 nm[36] (Fig. 16-3, *B*). Phylogenetic analyses confirmed that Hendra virus and Nipah viruses form a distinct clade within the family *Paramyxoviridae*[37] (Fig. 16-4). Hendra virus does not agglutinate erythrocytes from a range of species, including human type O, monkey, equine, porcine, bovine, guinea pig, chicken, and goose, when tested at 4°, 22°, and 37° C, or possess detectable neuraminidase activity.

Epidemiology

Fruit bats (flying foxes) of the genus *Pteropus,* order Chiroptera, suborder Megachiroptera, are the natural hosts for Hendra virus. Antibodies were found in four Australian species of fruit bats, with up to 47% of the bats testing positive.[38,39] Of 13 wildlife animal species tested, only bats had antibodies to Hendra virus.

Transmission of Hendra virus from bats to horses seems to be a rare event. The circumstances that facilitate transmission to and among horses remain unclear, but camping under trees or housing in buildings in which bats are roosting should be avoided. Evidence suggests that urine, aborted fetuses, and reproductive fluids from infected bats may be involved in transmission.[38] After transmission to horses or humans, the virus does not appear to be highly contagious. Aerosol transmission among horses apparently is not a major mode of spread. In the original outbreak, a 5-km (3-mile) radius around the infected stables encompassed many other training stables, and the area was close to two major Thoroughbred racing and training tracks. Therefore the opportunity existed for many horses to become infected if the virus was readily transmissible. An extensive surveillance program undertaken in this area revealed no evidence of spread of infection beyond the two known, adjoining infected stables. No spread occurred to other stables contiguous with the two infected premises or to horses that shared the spelling paddock with the index case. Spread may have been inadvertently assisted by human actions. Serologic testing of more than 2500 equine sera collected from the outbreak area, a wider zone around Brisbane, and from other areas in Australia, in particular from horses with pneumonia, revealed no evidence of infection elsewhere.[29]

In the original outbreak the index case was a pregnant mare, and one of the two horses infected in the second occurrence was also a pregnant mare, suggesting that pregnancy may be a risk factor. No direct epidemiologic association was established between the Brisbane and Mackay episodes.

Pathogenesis

In horses, Hendra virus is predominantly pneumotropic but may also be neurotropic. All the equine cases and the first human case died from acute respiratory disease, whereas the second human patient died from encephalitis. Little is known about the portal of entry of the virus, the distribution and

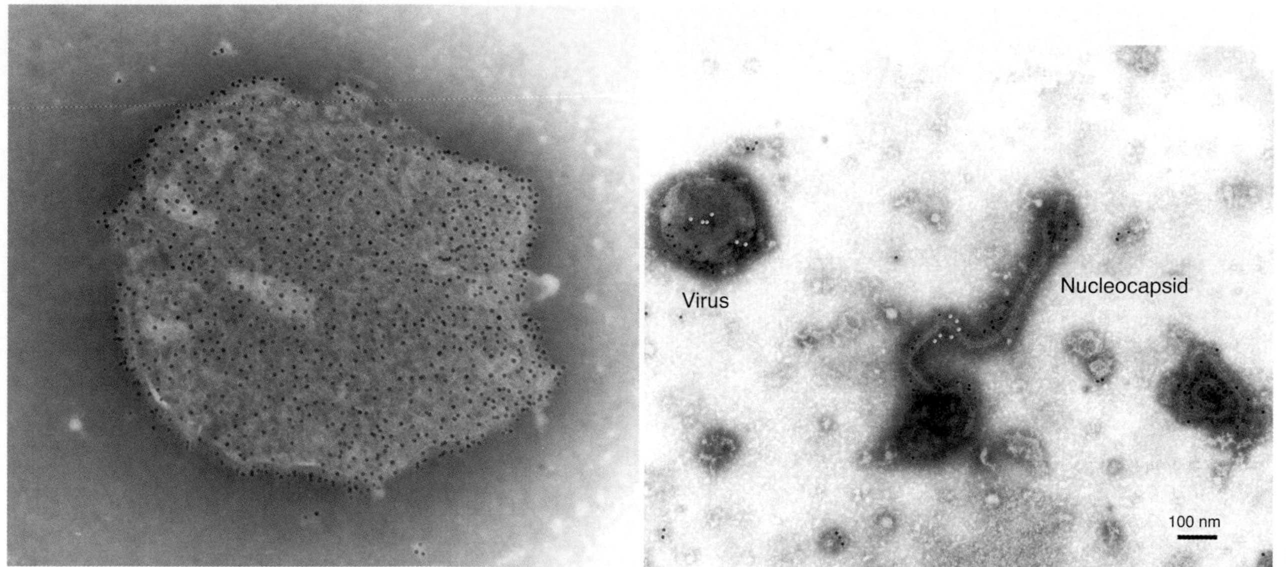

Fig. 16-3 A, Electron micrograph of negatively stained preparation of Hendra virus. Note surface projections, which are glycoprotein spikes that are of two distinct lengths. The black dots are immunogold staining of the surface glycoproteins. B, Electron micrograph of a negatively stained preparation of supernatant from Hendra virus–infected cell culture. At left is a virus particle in which the surface proteins have been immunogold labeled; some of the gold spheres are colored yellow. At right is a nucleocapsid that has been released from within a virus particle. The nucleocapsid proteins have been immunogold labeled. (Courtesy AD Hyatt, CSIRO Livestock Industries' Australian Animal Health Laboratory.)

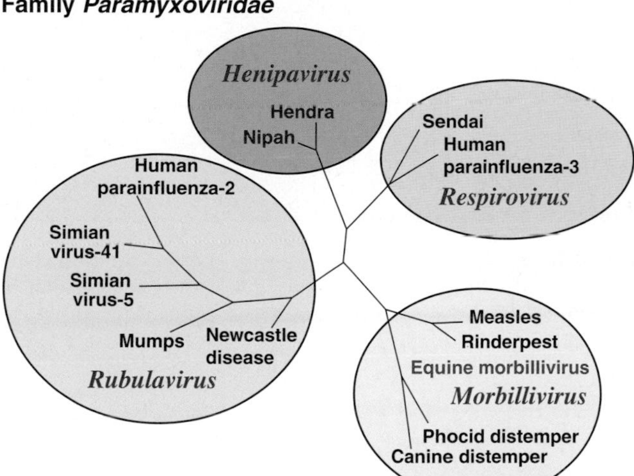

Fig. 16-4 Phylogenic relationship of Hendra virus to other members of the family *Paramyxoviridae*, based on analyses of predicted amino acid sequences of virus matrix proteins. (Courtesy Linfa Wang, CSIRO Livestock Industries' Animal Health Laboratory.)

persistence of the virus in the body, or the routes of excretion of the virus. Horses were experimentally infected subcutaneously, intraocularly, and by aerosol, and virus was detected in nasal swabs collected postmortem. Virus was isolated from the lungs, liver, kidney, lymph nodes, and heparinized blood of experimentally infected horses. The virus was isolated from the kidney of the first human case, even though specific neutralizing antibody was detected in his serum.

Hendra virus attacks vascular endothelial cells and causes pulmonary edema. The lung and brain pathologies are somewhat similar to those produced by related viruses, such as canine distemper and measles. Experimentally, cats and guinea pigs are susceptible to Hendra virus, and although some pathologic differences exist in these two species, the diseases are similar to that observed in horses.[40,41] Cats can be infected orally or parenterally and can transmit the virus to in-contact cats, although aerosol transmission of the virus was not demonstrated experimentally. There is no evidence of natural infection in cats, and serologic surveillance of cats in Brisbane yielded no evidence of feline infection. No infection or disease occurred in dogs, rats, mice, or chickens after experimental infection.[42] There was infection but no disease in fruit bats after experimental infection.

Clinical Findings

The Hendra viral disease in horses is characterized by high fever (up to 41° C [105.8° F]), anorexia, increased respiratory and heart rates, and paroxysms of coughing. This leads rapidly to severe respiratory distress, with blood-tinged, foamy nasal and oral discharge; ataxia; head pressing; tonic spasms of the neck and hindlimb muscles; and collapse. The clinical course is short, with 10 of the 13 naturally infected horses in the first outbreak dying within 36 hours of onset of clinical signs; seven of these deaths occurred within 12 hours of onset.[43] The incubation period in horses experimentally infected with tissue homogenates derived from naturally occurring cases was 6 to 10 days.[44] Two horses experimentally infected with the virus developed disease 2 and 3 days after inoculation, respectively.

Diagnosis

Clinical Laboratory

Initially, the clinical signs and postmortem findings of Hendra infection in horses were suggestive of acute African

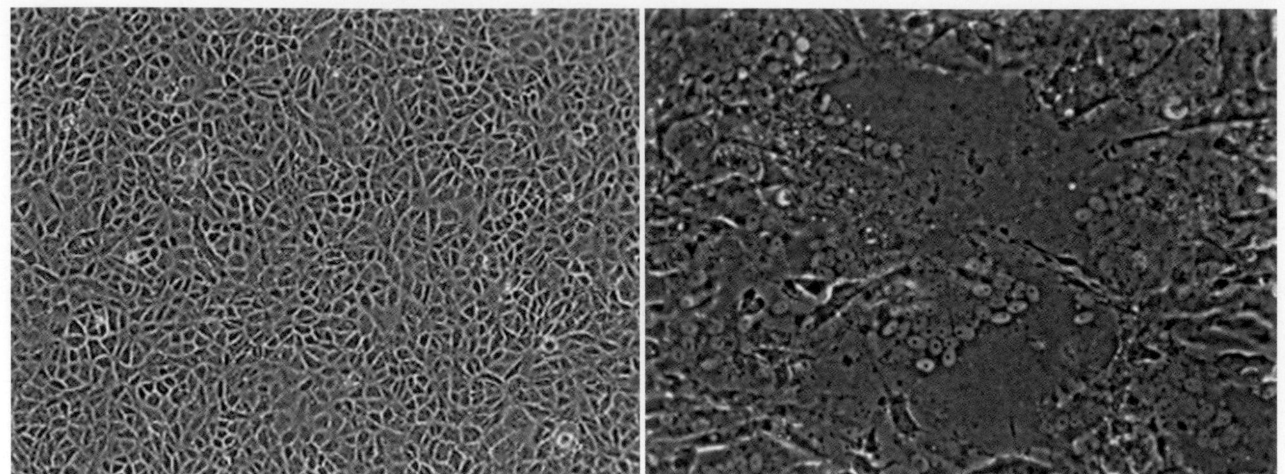

Fig. 16-5 A, Normal Vero monolayer cell culture. B, Vero monolayer cell culture 24 hours after infection with Hendra virus. Note syncytium. (Courtesy Gary Crameri, CSIRO Livestock Industries' Australian Animal Health Laboratory.)

horse sickness or virulent equine influenza. Inoculation of Hendra virus experimentally into horses reproduced the syndrome, and specific antibody was detected in all recovered horses and two infected humans in the first outbreak. The histopathology in naturally and experimentally infected horses and humans is similar, and characteristic immunofluorescence and immunoperoxidase staining of tissues can support the diagnosis.

Virus Isolation

Hendra virus may be isolated in monolayer cell cultures of Vero cells inoculated with filtered lung homogenates, although the virus can be isolated from other tissues and in cells such as primary equine fetal kidney cultured cells. Following inoculation of monolayer cell cultures a cytopathic effect was detected 3 days after inoculation (Fig. 16-5). The cytopathic effect (CPE) consisted of focal syncytium formation, which subsequently spread throughout the monolayer. Virus from a human case was isolated in LLC-MK2 and MRC5 cells, in which the CPE characterized by syncytium (multinucleate cell mass) was detected 12 days after inoculation.

Serology

Serum neutralization, enzyme-linked immunosorbent assay (ELISA), and indirect fluorescent antibody tests have been developed to detect Hendra virus.

Organism Detection

Virus isolation in cell culture, immunohistochemistry, and PCR are used for detection of Hendra virus in clinical specimens.

Pathologic Findings

The outstanding postmortem finding is pulmonary edema, which is accompanied by hemorrhage and froth in the trachea, bronchi, and bronchioles.[42,44] The lungs are congested, firm, and fluid-filled with dilated lymphatics, and fibrin tags may be seen on the pleura (Fig. 16-6). The pericardial sac may contain up to 100 mL of serous fluid. In some horses with Hendra virus infection, extensive subcutaneous hemorrhages were observed, but these may have been agonal. Histologic findings include

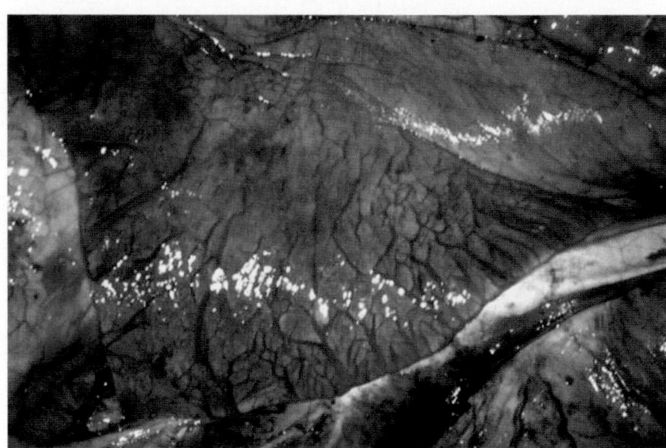

Fig. 16-6 Gross lesions in lung of horse experimentally infected with Hendra virus, showing pneumonia and dilation of lymphatics. (Courtesy CSIRO Livestock Industries' Australian Animal Health Laboratory.)

interstitial pneumonia with proteinaceous alveolar edema associated with hemorrhage, dilated lymphatics, alveolar thrombosis, and necrosis of the walls of small blood vessels. The vascular lesions are remarkable in that there are syncytia (multinucleate giant cells) in blood vessel walls, especially in the endothelium (Fig. 16-7). Nonsuppurative encephalomyelitis was present in some horses.[45,46] Intracytoplasmic inclusion bodies are present, and thin-section EM reveals characteristic nucleocapsids in the cytoplasm. Nucleocapsids were observed in negatively stained, horse lung homogenates, and these could be immunogold labeled.[36,45]

Therapy

No specific therapy exists for horses with Hendra virus infection. Because of the serious zoonotic potential of Hendra virus, therapy should not be undertaken once a diagnosis is confirmed or even suspected.

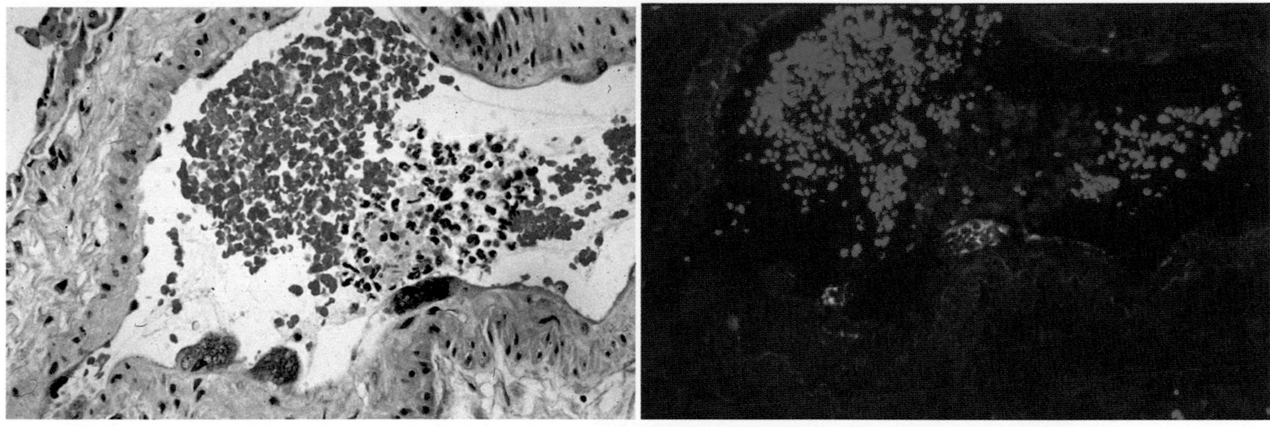

Fig. 16-7 **A,** Hematoxylin and eosin–stained section of lung of horse infected with Hendra virus (400×). Note multinucleate giant cells (syncytium) at lower left. **B,** Immunofluorescence staining of same section as in *A;* green staining indicates Hendra virus–specific antigen. (Courtesy PT Hooper, CSIRO Livestock Industries' Australian Animal Health Laboratory.)

Prevention

Vaccination

Vaccines against Hendra virus have not been developed for use in the horse. Based on the success of other paramyxovirus vaccines, such as for canine distemper and rinderpest, if developed, vaccines would undoubtedly be highly effective. Because all four incidents in horses were contained by death or euthanasia, and with no evidence of wide dissemination of the virus in horses, vaccines have not been developed.

Other Methods

Avoidance of contact with bats, particularly at critical times, can be considered. Early diagnosis and control by euthanasia are likely to remain the key preventive measures. Occurrences of the disease require immediate quarantine of the premises, controls on the movement of horses within a defined disease control zone, and serologic surveillance to determine the extent of infection. A greater understanding of the virus and the disease may allow less dramatic disease control programs to be used in the future. Information on the persistence of the virus in the environment and the possibility that recovered animals may act as carriers and potential sources of infection needs further exploration. No excretion of virus occurs from animals that recover from morbillivirus infections (e.g., rinderpest, canine distemper), and a similar situation may exist for Hendra virus.

Public Health Considerations

Although transmission to humans is a rare event, the zoonotic potential of Hendra virus must be considered when undertaking in vitro and in vivo tests and when collecting field samples from suspect equine cases. The five known occurrences of human infection involved transmission from infected horses. Surprisingly, no cases of human infection have been reported as a result of direct transmission from bats, even though many humans are bat caretakers and other humans come into close contact with bats. The testing of 150 human sera and retrospective examination of selected archived tissue specimens did not indicate any previous occurrences of human infections. Hendra virus is classified as a Biocontainment Level 4 agent, which is the highest level of security for any infectious agent. People working with the virus in the laboratory or with live animals are required to wear a biohazard suit with its own air supply and in the laboratory to work with the virus contained in an enclosed biosafety cabinet, known as a "flexible film isolator."

Case Study

The second human death from Hendra virus occurred in Mackay, 1000 km (600 miles) north of Brisbane. In August 1994 a 36-year-old sugarcane farmer assisted his wife, a veterinarian, in performing a postmortem examination on two horses that died 10 days apart on their property. Retrospective diagnosis of Hendra virus as the cause of death of the horses was made on paraffin-embedded, formalin-fixed tissue blocks.[31] Ten days after the second horse died, the farmer was admitted to the hospital with meningitis, from which he apparently recovered. Fourteen months later he was again hospitalized, and he died 25 days later after the development of seizures and paralysis of increasing severity. Postmortem examination revealed meningoencephalitis with areas of necrosis throughout the cortex. Vascular thrombosis and occasional multinucleate giant cells were present in the brain.[47] The brain tissue was positive for Hendra virus on immunofluorescence and immune EM, and thin-section EM showed viral nucleocapsids in neuronal cells.[31,36] Virus was not isolated. Both the cerebrospinal fluid and brain tissue were positive for Hendra virus on PCR, and sequencing of the PCR products showed the sequence to be identical to the Hendra virus sequence of the first isolate.[31,47] During the hospitalization period, there was a rise in Hendra virus neutralizing antibody from 1:16 at admission to 1:5792 terminally. The veterinarian who assisted with the postmortem examination did not develop clinical disease and was antibody negative.

The clinical course and pathology of this second fatal human case were very different from the first human case, in whom the predominant signs were respiratory and death occurred within 2 weeks after infection.

EQUINE RHINITIS A VIRUS AND EQUINE RHINITIS B VIRUSES

Picornaviruses are recognized causes of acute upper respiratory and systemic disease in horses. When first isolated in the 1960s, the biophysical properties of these viruses indicated

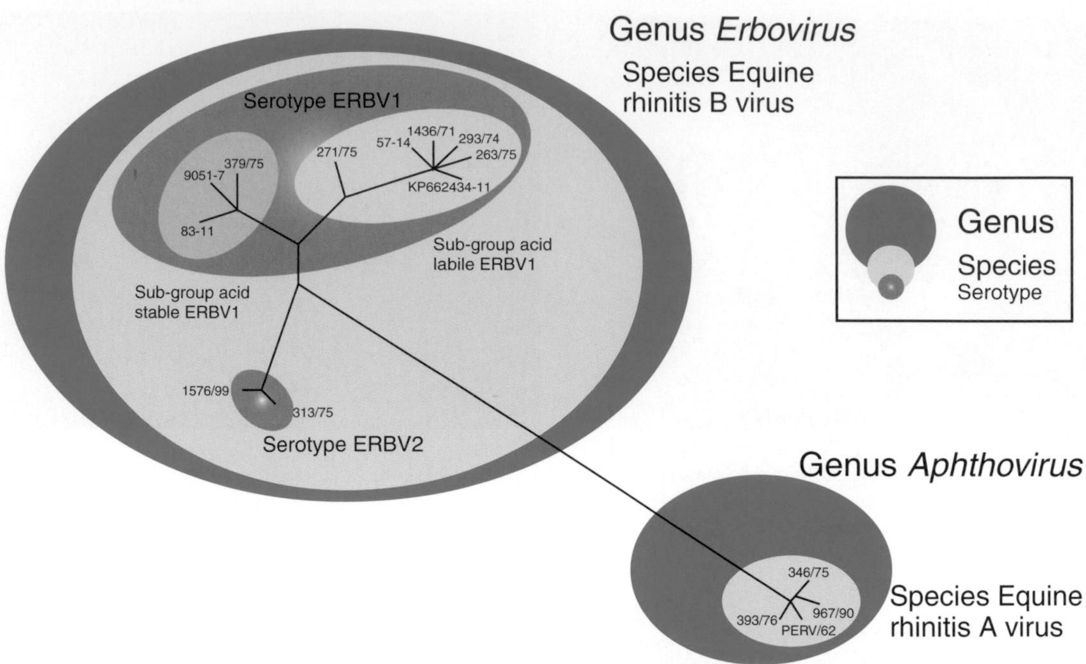

Fig. 16-8 Phylogenetic tree showing relationships among equine rhinitis viruses.

that they were members of the family *Picornaviridae*, and because the majority of the isolates were acid labile (infectivity destroyed at pH 3), they were classified in the genus *Rhinovirus*, which includes the common cold viruses of humans, and named equine rhinoviruses. Both the naming and the classification implied that the biology, including clinical diseases and pathogenesis, would parallel human common cold viruses, which are the prototypic members of the genus *Rhinovirus*.

Despite seroprevalence rates of 20% to 80% for equine rhinitis A virus (ERAV), equine rhinitis B virus type 1 (ERBV1), and equine rhinitis B virus type 2 (ERBV2), these viruses are seldom specifically diagnosed as causes of respiratory disease in horses. Their relative "neglect" may be related to the dominant position of influenza viruses and equine herpesvirus types 1 and 4 (EHV-1, EHV-4) as causes of acute upper respiratory disease in horses but is also related to a lack of sensitive, widely available and adopted diagnostic tests.

Etiology

Three acid-labile serotypes, called "equine rhinoviruses 1, 2, and 3," were originally identified. A fourth serotype, so-called "acid-stable picornavirus" (ASP), was also isolated. Sequence analysis of the genome of two strains of equine rhinovirus 1 indicated that this virus was most closely related to "foot-and-mouth disease virus" (FMDV),[48,49] and accordingly, the virus was reclassified in the genus *Aphthovirus*, although as a separate cluster (Fig. 16-8), and renamed *equine rhinitis A virus* (ERAV).[50] Until that time, FMDV had been the sole member of the genus *Aphthovirus*. Analysis of the sequence of the genome of equine rhinovirus 2 indicated that although most closely related to "encephalomyocarditis virus,"[49] a member of the *Cardiovirus* genus, it was sufficiently distinct from all other picornaviruses to be assigned as the sole member of a new genus *Erbovirus* (erb[o] for *e*quine *r*hinitis *B*) and renamed *equine rhinitis B virus* (ERBV).[50] Some ERBV1 isolates have been shown to be stable at acid pH, and these can also be distinguished from acid-labile ERBV1 by genomic sequence analysis.[51] The biologic significance to the two phylogenetically distinct clades within ERBV1 has not been established. Sequence analysis of the antigenically distinct equine rhinovirus 3 indicated that this virus was a second serotype (ERBV2) within the genus *Erbovirus*.[52] Acid-stable picornaviruses have been isolated from the respiratory tract (prototype 4442/75) and oral cavity of horses,[53,54] and it has been shown that they are a third serotype (ERBV3) within the erbovirus genus.

ERAV was first isolated and characterized in the United Kingdom by Plummer.[55-57] Subsequently, ERAV was isolated in many parts of the world.[58] Most isolations of so-called equine rhinoviruses were antigenically similar to the virus (PERV/62) originally isolated by Plummer[55] in 1962 and now designated ERAV. Hofer et al.[59] confirmed that there were at least two distinct serotypes of equine rhinovirus. The identity of a second serotype (prototype 1436/71) was confirmed by Newman et al.,[60] and after sequencing of the genome[49] and renaming,[50] this virus is now designated ERBV1. Steck et al.[61] indicated the existence of a third serotype, and genomic sequencing of the prototype strain of this virus (313/75) confirmed that it was a second member of the genus *Erbovirus*, proposed to be designated ERBV2.[53] Only one other isolation of ERBV2 from a horse with febrile respiratory disease has been reported.[79,80] The so-called acid-stable equine picornaviruses were identified as a distinct serotype[53,54] and as noted are now designated ERBV3.

Virions measure 24 to 30 nm in diameter. The genome is a single-stranded, positive-sense RNA. Virions are not inactivated by lipid solvents (ether, chloroform) or by nonionic detergents. The density of the ERAV in cesium chlorine (CsCl) is 1.455g/mL. ERBV1.1436/71 has a heterogenous buoyant density in CsCl varying from 1.40 to 1.45 g/mL.[62] ERAV is inactivated at 50° C after 1 hour and is not stabilized by 1-M magnesium chloride ($MgCl_2$), whereas ERBV1 and ASP isolates studied were stabilized by 1-M $MgCl_2$.[53,62-66] ERAV is nonhemagglutinating (human O, guinea pig, equine, and chicken RBCs).

Epidemiology

ERAV, ERBV1, and ERBV2 are spread by contact through nasal secretions and aerosol inhalation.[66,67] ERAV is also shed in urine for prolonged periods, and urine aerosol is considered an important mode of transmission.[68,69] Although labile at pH less than 6.5, ERAV may remain infectious in the environment under favorable conditions for extended periods, perhaps months.[67] Generally, ERAV is most frequently isolated, whereas ERBV1, ERBV2, and ERBV3 appear less frequently isolated. A notable exception to this view was a study of 92 horses with acute respiratory disease in Canada,[70] in which ERBV was isolated from 28 of 64 (44%) nasopharyngeal swabs from horses with acute febrile respiratory disease; of the 28 virus-positive horses, six (21%) showed a significant rise (≥fourfold) to ERBV2 antibody.

Surprisingly, ERAV is shed in urine for prolonged periods after the acute phase of infection. As a coincidental part of a study of the carrier status of equine arteritis virus in male horses, McCollum and Timoney[68] showed that 432 of 2523 (17%) postrace urine samples were positive for ERAV by virus isolation. The frequency of urine shedding was highest in 2-year-old horses (26%) and appeared to decline steadily to 5% in 8-year-old horses, although horses up to 10 years of age shed virus. There were no differences in urine shedding of ERAV between stallions and geldings. Persistent shedding in urine for up to 146 days was demonstrated in individual horses. In a study of 20 young stallions in which both nasopharyngeal and urine samples were examined for ERAV, only 1 of 11 stallions from which virus was isolated was double positive; 5 of the 20 stallions yielded virus from nasopharyngeal swabs and 7 from urine samples. A possible interpretation of these data is that virus shedding from urine is much more prolonged than shedding from the nasal cavity. Although the role of fecal and urine shedding in the transmission of ERAV has not been fully defined, from studies[68] it appears that urine is an important mode of transmission, presumably by inhalation of a urine aerosol, as also proposed by Powell.[69] McCollum and Timoney[68] did not recover ERBV1 or ERBV 2 from urine. ERAV and ERBV have been isolated from ill horses in outbreaks of respiratory disease primarily attributed to EHV-1/EHV-4 or equine arteritis virus.

ERAV, ERBV1, and ERBV2 maternal antibody was present 12 hours after suckling in foals born to antibody-positive dams. By 10 to 12 months, however, ERAV SN antibody was not detected in any of the progeny horses, whereas ERBV1 and ERBV2 SN antibodies were common (83% and 100%, respectively).[71]

In a U.S. study the overall percentage of horses less than 3 years old with SN antibodies to ERAV and ERBV was 73%, whereas 90% of horses older than 4 years were positive.[72] The prevalence of ERAV antibody in Australia indicated a maximum infection rate of 47.9% (170 of 355 serums), and accordingly at any one time, 50% of the population was susceptible.[66,71] In a study in Japan, paired serum samples were collected from 3012 racehorses that developed pyrexia at two training centers between 1980 and 1986.[73] Seroconversion to ERAV was demonstrated in 102 (3.4%), and the mean age of horses seroconverting was 2.44 years. In a study by Carman et al.,[70] 9 of 92 (10%) horses that presented with respiratory disease had a significant rise in ERAV SN antibody, suggesting that ERAV was the cause of respiratory disease in these horses; the corresponding figure as previously noted for ERBV was 6 of 28 (21%) horses.

In a more comprehensive seroprevalence study, 388 serums from 291 horses were tested for SN antibody to ERAV, ERBV1, and ERBV2.[71] The prevalence of ERAV, ERBV1, and ERBV2 SN antibodies was approximately 37%, 83%, and 66%, respectively. One part of this study included serum from 44 Thoroughbred horses obtained when they were newly introduced into a training center and their average age was 23 months, with a second sample obtained approximately 7 months later. ERAV, ERBV1, and ERBV2 SN antibody was present in 8 (18%), 34 (77%), and 39 (89%) of horses, respectively, when first bled, and in 27 (61%), 34 (77%), and 38 (86%) of horses, respectively, when tested 7 months later. Accordingly, 19 of the 44 horses (43%) seroconverted to ERAV within 7 months of entering the training stable. For ERBV1 and ERBV2, the percentage of seropositivity between the first and second samples was about the same. Notably, however, five (12%) and four (9%) of the 44 horses, respectively, seroconverted to ERBV1 and ERBV2, although this rate of seroconversion was offset by the observation that five (12%) and six (14%) of the horses, respectively, *seroreverted* (became antibody negative). Among all the horses, the average ERAV SN antibody titer was relatively high (3796), and in contrast, ERBV1 and ERBV2 titers were relatively low (average of 84 and 45, respectively) and often fell to below detectable levels (seroreverted) over time at a rate comparable to seroconversion.

In general, Thoroughbred horses 6 to 24 months of age are serologically negative to ERAV and do not seroconvert until after entering training stables. This suggests that most horses are infected with ERAV during the period of training and racing.[67,71,74]

Pathogenesis

After aerosol or indirect transmission, virus replicates in nasal epithelial cells. Viremia is a regular feature of ERAV infection. Virus disappears from the blood after onset of antibody production, although it persists in the pharynx and may be isolated from feces in small amounts (<10 $TCID_{50}$/g) for at least 1 month after infection (samples were not tested beyond this time).[57] Isolation of the virus from feces was considered curious because virus was not isolated at any time from gut, indicating that it must either infect and persist in lower gut cells or be transported from the pharynx through the bloodstream in a manner not detectable by standard virus isolation procedures. The demonstration that ERAV is shed in urine for prolonged periods, up to 146 days in one study but almost certainly longer,[68] led to a view that a persistent infection must be established in the urinary tract, possibly in the bladder.

A temporary suppression of cell-mediated immunity in Standardbred horses with decreased athletic performance, in association with symptoms such as intermittent fever and mild pharyngitis, was linked to ERAV infections.[75] In this study, lymphocyte proliferation assays to evaluate cell-mediated immunity and a bioassay for equine type 1 interferon were used as markers for detection of viral infection.

Clinical Findings

ERAV is generally considered to cause mild to severe respiratory disease,* although clinical signs may be quite variable,[59] and nasal discharge is not invariably present.[67] In many cases, infection results in subclinical disease. The incubation period is 3 to 8 days. Clinical signs in natural outbreaks of disease may include fever (41° ± 0.5° C), anorexia, and copious serous nasal discharge that becomes mucopurulent.[63] There may be coughing and severe pharyngitis. Recovery in uncomplicated cases occurs within 7 days. Lymphadenitis and abscesses of the regional lymph nodes may result from secondary bacterial infection, usually with streptococci. Where pharyngitis persists, coughing may continue for 2 to 3 weeks. Although persistent shedding of ERAV in urine and feces is presumably a consequence of prolonged infection, no disease has been linked to nonrespiratory sites of infection.[68]

*References 58, 59, 67, 70, 76, 77.

Viremia may last several days before dissipating with the appearance of circulating antibody.[56]

Plummer and Kerry[57] showed that after experimental infection of horses with ERAV, the incubation period averaged 4.25 days (range, 2-8 days). Illness was characterized by fever (up to 40.6° C), anorexia, nasal discharge, pharyngitis, and lymphadenitis involving at least the submaxillary and pharyngeal lymph nodes. Bronchitis was also recognized. Based on serologic conversions, most authors recognize that subclinical infections occur. Viremia consistently developed on average at 5.4 days (range, 3-7 days) and lasted 4.5 days (range, 4-5 days). The disappearance of virus from the blood coincided with the onset of antibody production.

ERBV infection of horses may also result in an acute febrile respiratory disease characterized by coughing and lymphadenitis and recovery, although there is persistent infection and virus shedding from the respiratory tract.[53,68,70,74,78] In contrast to ERAV viremia, urine and fecal shedding have not been recognized in association with ERBV infection.

Diagnosis

Clinical Laboratory and Virus Isolation

ERAV replicates in cultured equine cells as well as in cells from several heterologous animal species.[67] CPE was produced in primary cell cultures from horse, dog, rabbit, hamster, and monkey; in a diploid cell line of equine origin; in cell lines that included HeLa and Hep 2 from humans, rhesus monkey, and African green monkey kidney (LLC-MK2 and Vero cells); and in a rabbit kidney cell line (RK13). Of these, RK13 and Vero cell cultures were found to be efficient host systems for some ERAV strains.[56,68,79] The CPE produced occurs at 37° C (98.6° F) and resembles that produced by other picornaviruses, where infected cells round up, shrink, and show marked nuclear pyknosis, becoming refractive and eventually degenerating and detaching from the surface.[72] However, primary isolation and propagation of ERAV in cultured cells have proved difficult in some cases.[56,66] ERAV may replicate in primary equine fetal kidney (EFK), Vero, and RK13 cells without causing obvious CPE, and switching cell lines was necessary to maintain cytopathic ERAV.[81] Similarly, primary isolation of ERBV also seems to be difficult; isolation rates achieved in some studies[59,71] were not matched in other studies.[66,79,82]

These variable success rates correlating acute respiratory disease with rhinitis viruses may simply reflect the real situation at the time the samples are taken. An alternative view is that the noncultivability of the viruses from particular outbreaks may be an important factor. Variation in the susceptibility of the cell lines used for isolation or genetic variation (quasispecies) in the viruses themselves could account for higher success rates of virus isolation in some studies compared with others.

Serology

The demonstration of rising SN antibody titer in paired sera collected about 2 weeks apart will confirm a diagnosis for ERAV or ERBV infection. Other serologic tests (e.g., ELISA) generally have not been available.

Organism Detection

Reverse transcriptase–polymerase chain reaction (RT-PCR) has been developed for the detection of ERAV in nasopharyngeal swabs and other samples collected from horses with acute respiratory disease.[81,83,84] An ERBV-specific nested RT-PCR that amplified a product within the $3D^{pol}$ and 3′ nontranslated region of the viral genome was developed.[79] This RT-PCR detected all 24 available ERBV1 isolates and one available ERBV2 isolate. The limit of detection for the prototype strain ERBV1.1436/71 was 0.1 50% tissue culture infectious doses. Using this RT-PCR, DNA was amplified from 6 of 17 nasopharyngeal swab samples from horses that had clinical signs of acute febrile respiratory disease, but from which ERBV was not initially isolated in cell culture. The sequences of these six ERBV-positive samples had 93% to 96% nucleotide identity, with six other partially sequenced ERBV1 isolates and one ERBV2. ERBV was isolated from one of the six samples at fourth cell culture passage when it was shown that the addition of 20 mg/mL $MgCl_2$ to the cell culture medium enhanced the growth of the virus. The study highlights the utility of PCR for the identification of viruses in clinical samples that may initially be considered negative with conventional cell culture isolation.

Pathologic Findings

No detailed studies on the pathology of ERAV and ERBV infections have been done other than in explant organ cultures infected with ERAV.[85,86] ERAV replicated in cell and organ cultures, but was released almost exclusively from nasal turbinate epithelium. On thin-section EM, organ cultures inoculated with ERAV appeared normal, with the exception of rare, islandlike lesions in infected nasal turbinate, and virus particles were not seen.

Therapy

There is no specific antiviral therapy for rhinitis virus infection in horses. Therapy should be symptomatic and supportive. The administration of reconstituted lyophilized serum orally to protect newborn foals was proposed.[87]

Prevention

Vaccines for ERAV or ERBV have not been developed commercially. An experimental inactivated ERAV vaccine produced primary immune responses in horses, mice (including athymic *nu/nu* mice), and rabbits.[88] The problem of multiple serotypes recognized for FMDV does not occur because ERAV is antigenically and genomically remarkably stable over time and geographic location.[84] The occurrence of three serotypes of ERBV would need to be considered in any vaccine development.

Because of the inconvenience of infection in later life, planned infection programs of young horses were once advocated.[89] This suggestion, never widely adopted, would need reevaluation in light of the findings of McCollum and Timoney[68] showing that primary infection is followed by prolonged shedding of the ERAV in the urine.

Public Health Considerations

Evidence indicates that ERAV infects humans after both natural and experimental infection. A human volunteer infected with ERAV developed severe pharyngitis and swelling of the pharyngeal lymph nodes accompanied by fever, and virus was isolated from his blood.[55,56] Based on serologic data, humans may be infected with ERAV by contact with infected horses, but clinical disease or subsequent human-to-human transmission of virus was not recognized in such naturally occurring infections.[55,56,90] Kriegshauser et al.[90] tested 137 sera from veterinarians for the presence of ERAV and ERBV1 SN antibody. Four (2.7%) and five (3.6%) human sera had low levels of neutralizing "activity" to ERAV and ERBV1, respectively. The authors concluded that the risk of acquiring ERAV and ERBV1 as zoonotic infections among veterinarians appears low.

References

See the CD-ROM for a list of references linked to the abstract in PubMed.

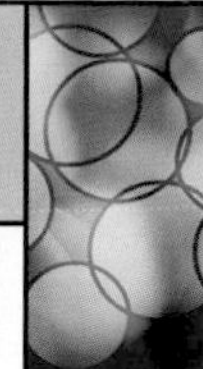

CHAPTER • 17

Equine Rotavirus

Roberta M. Dwyer

Diarrhea is one of the most common medical problems of newborn foals, and rotavirus is the most common cause of foal enteritis in the major breeding centers of Kentucky, Ireland, and England.[1,2] Both single cases of rotaviral diarrhea and severe farm outbreaks can occur. However, with the use of a commercially available vaccine, practical farm management practices, and hygiene measures, this disease can be controlled.

ETIOLOGY

The family *Reoviridae* consists of five genera: *Orthoreovirus, Orbivirus, Coltivirus, Aquareovirus*, and *Rotavirus*. These are all double-stranded, ribonucleic acid (RNA), nonenveloped viruses with a diameter of about 80 nm (Fig. 17-1). The genus *Rotavirus* is subdivided into several groups (A-G) based on differences in the group-specific inner capsid protein, VP6. Equine and other animal isolates are in group A; groups B to G cause disease in humans, swine, fowl, and other animals.[3] Further subdivision is made based on serologic assays using neutralizing antibodies to two outer capsid proteins, VP4 and VP7. Strains containing VP4 are referred to as *P* (protease-sensitive) serotype and strains containing VP7 as the G (glycoprotein) serotype.[4] Serotypes G3, G5, G8, G10, G13, and G14 and serotypes P7, P12, and P18 have been described in horses.[4-6] The G3 serotype has been identified in Kentucky and Japan and has been used in equine vaccine trials.[7-9]

Rotaviruses are stable within a pH range of 3 to 7 and are resistant to iodophor, quaternary ammonium, chlorine, and hypochlorite (bleach) disinfectants. Ethanol, phenols, and formalin can inactivate the virus.[10-12]

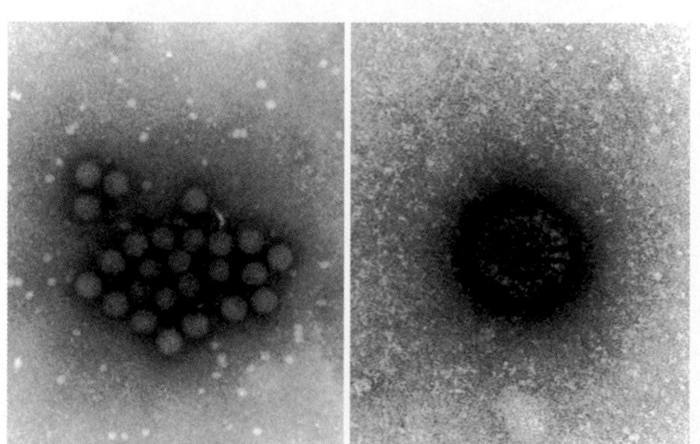

Fig. 17-1 Electron micrographs of *Rotavirus*. **A,** Particles magnified at ×135,000. **B,** Single particle magnified at ×300,000. (Courtesy Ms. Patricia Van Meter, University of Kentucky.)

EPIDEMIOLOGY

Equine rotaviruses have been detected from diarrheic foals in the United States, Argentina, Britain, Ireland, Germany, Australia, New Zealand, and Japan. Equine rotaviruses only affect foals and are considered species specific; for example, cattle rotavirus affects cattle and not horses or humans. No natural reservoir for equine rotavirus has been identified. Mares do not shed the virus,[1] except under experimental conditions.[13] However, pregnant sows can shed the virus in feces from 5 days before to 14 days after farrowing, thereby seeding the environment for piglets.[14] Considering the large concentrations of virus shed into the environment (10^{11} particles/g feces) by diarrheic animals, as well as the ability of the virus to remain viable for as long as 9 months,[15] the potential for an outbreak after the first clinical case is very real.

Rotavirus is transmitted by the fecal-oral route through contaminated feces or fomites and is highly contagious. The incubation period is 12 to 24 hours. Adult horses are not clinically affected during outbreaks of foal diarrhea, but some mares with diarrheic foals will seroconvert, indicating subclinical infection.[13] Studies of more than 400 adult horses performed in conjunction with rotavirus vaccination trials in Kentucky, Japan, and Argentina revealed a seroprevalence rate in broodmares approaching 100%.[7-9] However, these studies were conducted in concentrated horse-breeding regions, and seroprevalence in adult horses in other geographic areas may be less.

The average age of foals with rotaviral diarrhea is 75 days, with a reported range of 2 to 155 days.[1] The average duration of diarrhea in affected foals is 3 days (range, 1-9 days), with fecal shedding of rotavirus particles continuing for an average of 3 days after return of normal feces.

With appropriate supportive care, including fluid and electrolyte replacement therapy, rotaviral diarrhea has low mortality and high morbidity in foal populations. During a 3-year study of rotavirus on multiple central Kentucky horse farms, no foal had a confirmed recurrence of disease after recovery. In one study, fecal shedding of virus was demonstrated in clinically normal foals on 7 of 10 farms undergoing an outbreak of foal rotaviral diarrhea.[1,16] This shedding does not continue after resolution of disease in other foals on the farm.

PATHOGENESIS

After rotavirus enters the gastrointestinal tract, it invades and rapidly multiplies in columnar epithelial cells of the villous tips in the duodenum and jejunum.[17] This results in significant blunting of the villi and subsequent villous atrophy. The loss of these epithelial cells results in the absence of disaccharidases, especially lactase, causing a hyperosmotic solution in the intestinal lumen. This leads to malabsorption and maldigestion of nutrients and acute diarrhea. Intestinal crypt cells are not affected as they are in canine parvovirus infection. Therefore, crypt cells continue to replicate, differentiate, and eventually replace the tip cells destroyed by the virus, resulting in a self-limiting disease. Chronic diarrhea (>14 days) is not typical of rotavirus infection.

CLINICAL FINDINGS

The severity of rotavirus infection varies depending on the foal's age and immune status, the virulence of the virus, and the quantity of viral inoculum. Approximately 18 to 24 hours after ingestion of infective material, foals show signs of lethargy, decreased suckling, and diarrhea that may vary from "cow pie" to watery consistency. With watery diarrhea, the foals' tails may not be wet or stained with feces because of the projectile nature of the diarrhea. Fever may or may not be present. Younger foals are often more susceptible to severe disease because of their limited ability to self-correct fluid and electrolyte imbalances that accompany severe diarrhea (Fig. 17-2). Electrolyte imbalances may include hypochloremia, hyponatremia, hypokalemia, and acidosis. The hemogram is often normal or reveals evidence of hemoconcentration (e.g., increased packed cell volume).[18]

DIAGNOSIS

Field Testing Procedures

Commercial diagnostic assays are based on detection of VP6, the most abundant protein in viral particles.[4] Because VP6 is highly conserved across rotaviruses that affect many species, human rotavirus test kits are routinely used in equine practice and veterinary diagnostic laboratories. A fecal sample (1-3 g) or fecal swabs from affected foals should be submitted for rotavirus antigen testing by latex agglutination or other methods. Samples that can be tested within 8 hours should be held at room temperature or refrigerated. Veterinarians should contact testing laboratories for recommendations regarding storage and shipment of samples if testing cannot be performed within 8 hours of sample collection.

Results from latex agglutination rotavirus test kits are available within 10 to 15 minutes of processing the sample (Virogen Rotatest, Wampole Laboratories, Princeton, NJ) (Fig. 17-3). The Virogen Rotatest has a 100% sensitivity and 96.3% specificity compared with enzyme-linked immunosorbent assay (ELISA) for diagnosis of bovine rotavirus infection.[19] Compared with electron microscopy for identification of viral particles in pediatric stool samples, the Virogen Rotatest has a sensitivity of 86% and specificity of 95%.[20]

The ImmunoCardStat! Rotavirus is an immunogold-based, horizontal-flow membrane assay that yields results within 10 minutes. It had a sensitivity of 94% and specificity of 100% in one study of pediatric stool samples[21] and has been found useful for rapid diagnosis of bovine rotavirus infection.[22]

Other Diagnostic Options

Although electron microscopy for detection of viral particles in feces is widely considered to be the "gold standard" for

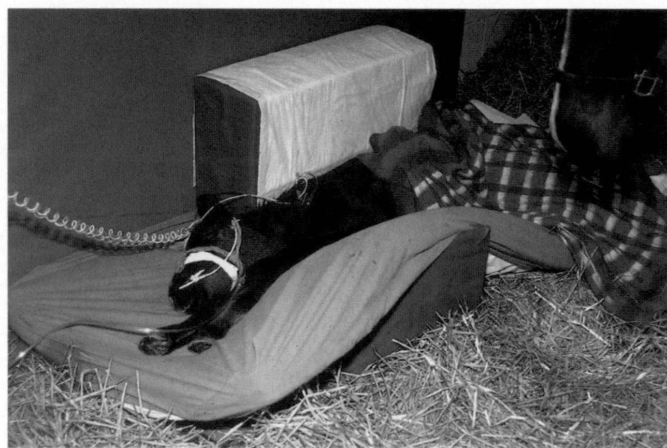

Fig. 17-2 Young foals can develop life-threatening dehydration and electrolyte imbalances from rotavirus infection, requiring intensive care.

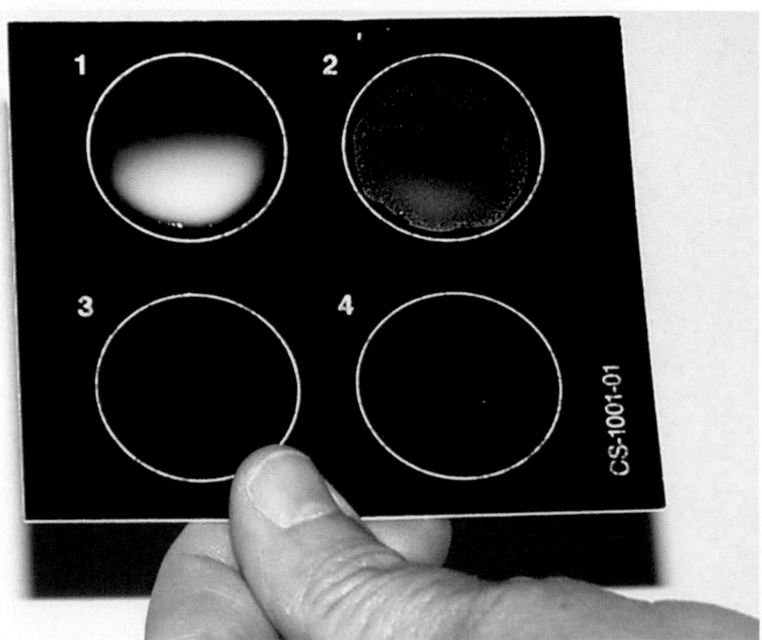

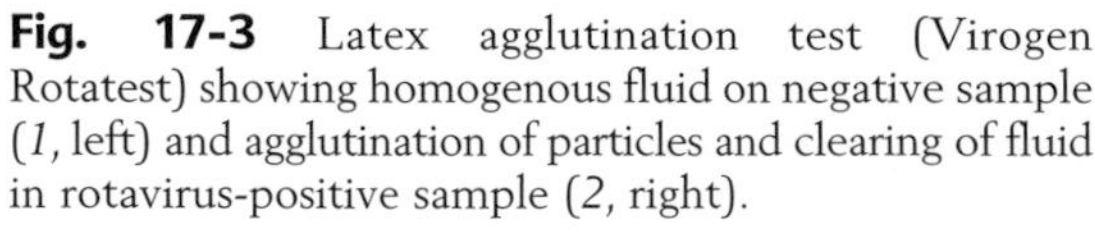

Fig. 17-3 Latex agglutination test (Virogen Rotatest) showing homogenous fluid on negative sample (*1*, left) and agglutination of particles and clearing of fluid in rotavirus-positive sample (*2*, right).

rotavirus diagnosis, this test is not routinely available and is expensive, and results may take several days. Other laboratory methods for diagnosis of rotaviral diarrhea include enzyme immunoassay,[22,23] polyacrylamide gel electrophoresis,[24] polymerase chain reaction,[25] and various molecular techniques,[25,26] all using fecal samples. Rotaviruses are extremely difficult to grow in cell culture, so virus isolation is not practical.[3] Serology for diagnostic purposes in foals is unreliable.[13]

As with testing feces for *Salmonella*, a single negative test result is not conclusive of the absence of rotavirus infection. In the author's experience, a minimum of three negative test results on samples properly obtained and stored before testing gives confidence in stating that a foal does not have rotaviral diarrhea.

A separate fecal sample should be obtained for bacterial culture to rule out other causes of foal diarrhea, including *Salmonella*, *Clostridium* spp., and parasites. Although concurrent infection with rotavirus and other pathogens is possible, several studies have concluded that most rotavirus infections in foals occur without simultaneous infection with other potential pathogens[1,2]

PATHOLOGIC FINDINGS

Mortality is low in rotavirus infections; foals less than 14 days of age are most at risk of death. In foals that die from dehydration and electrolyte imbalances, epithelial cells at the tips of intestinal villi are destroyed in the duodenum and occasionally the jejunum. The infection produces little inflammatory response in surrounding tissue.[3]

THERAPY

Isotonic fluid therapy to correct electrolyte imbalances is especially important in young foals and those that are significantly dehydrated. Adsorbents and protectants such as bismuth subsalicylate (30-60 mL PO 3-4 times/day), mineral oil, and activated charcoal may help in binding toxins and firming the feces, although owners should be aware that overuse can cause severe constipation. Feces of foals treated with bismuth subsalicylate may appear dark in color, similar to the color observed with proximal gastrointestinal tract hemorrhage. Mineral oil and activated charcoal administered by nasogastric tube may help lubricate the intestinal tract and bind toxins, respectively. In severely affected animals, parenteral nutrition may be indicated.[18,27,28] For uncomplicated rotavirus diarrhea, antibiotics are not indicated unless the animal is highly compromised or is in danger of septicemia, in which case broad-spectrum parenteral antibiotics may be used. Foals with failure of passive transfer or with hypoproteinemia secondary to diarrhea may benefit significantly from intravenous plasma transfusion.[27]

Some foals with rotavirus diarrhea may present with mild signs of colic. Pain may be controlled with appropriate doses of nonsteroidal antiinflammatory drugs such as flunixin meglumine (e.g., 1.1 mg/kg IV every 18-24 hours) or butorphanol (0.02-0.1 mg/kg IM every 4-6 hours). Frequent administration or inappropriately high doses of flunixin increase the risk for gastric ulceration in foals.[28]

Diarrhea is a significant risk factor for the development of gastric ulcers in foals. Prophylactic treatment with proton-pump blockers (e.g., omeprazole, 0.5 mg/kg IV every 24 hours followed by 1-4 mg/kg PO every 24 hours) is recommended for most affected foals. Omeprazole oral paste (GastroGard, Merial, Duluth, Ga) facilitates healing of equine gastric ulcers and is approved for treatment of foals 4 weeks of age and older. Other antiulcer medications include H_2 antagonists such as ranitidine (6.6 mg/kg PO every 8 hours) or cimetidine (12-20 mg/kg PO every 8 hours) in combination with sucralfate (1-2 g for small foals; 2-4 g for large foals). Because sucralfate may inhibit the absorption of other oral medications, it should not be administered at the same time as other drugs.[29]

Supportive care and hygiene are critically important for foals with rotaviral diarrhea to avoid pressure ulcers, scalded perianal skin, and secondary infections. Foals recumbent in filthy surroundings are predisposed to secondary problems, such as infected skin lacerations and pneumonia. Stalls should be kept as dry and clean as possible and should be heavily bedded. To prevent dermatitis between the hindlegs and in the perianal area, baby oil, zinc oxide ointment, or commercial diaper rash ointments may be applied. Should the skin become compromised, the area should be cleaned and a triple-antibiotic ointment applied.

PREVENTION

Vaccination

Since 1996, the Equine Rotavirus Vaccine (Fort Dodge Animal Health, Fort Dodge, Iowa) has had a conditional U.S. Department of Agriculture license. The vaccine contains an inactivated strain of a G3 equine rotavirus serotype (H2 strain) in a metabolizable oil-in-water adjuvant.[7] This vaccine is administered intramuscularly to pregnant mares at 8, 9, and 10 months' gestation to heighten colostral immunity. It has been safely used in thousands of mares in central Kentucky, Florida, Newmarket (UK), and other major breeding centers in the United States, United Kingdom, and Ireland. Antirotaviral antibodies are concentrated in colostrum and absorbed by suckling foals.[7,8] Ten years of clinical experience with this vaccine support its efficacy in reducing the incidence and severity of rotaviral diarrhea. The vaccine, however, is not a replacement for hygiene and meticulous husbandry practices.

Husbandry

Because rotaviruses are excreted from diarrheic foals in large quantities (10^{11} particles/g), overcrowding is a significant risk factor for outbreaks of foal diarrhea. Rotavirus can survive for months in the environment.[3] Manure and bedding from stalls of affected foals should be considered a biosecurity threat to unaffected foals. This material should not be spread on pastures, but rather composted in an area isolated from horses or disposed of according to local ordinances.

Hygiene of foaling areas is critical for disease prevention. Because rotavirus is a nonenveloped virus, it has natural resistance to disinfectants that primarily disrupt the viral lipid envelope. Prevention and control of outbreaks of rotavirus diarrhea are discussed in Chapters 66 and 67.

PUBLIC HEALTH CONSIDERATIONS

Rotavirus is not a zoonotic disease. However, universal (standard) precautions of disposable gloves and handwashing should be taken with any equine diarrheic disease.

REFERENCES

See the CD-ROM for a list of references linked to the abstract in PubMed.

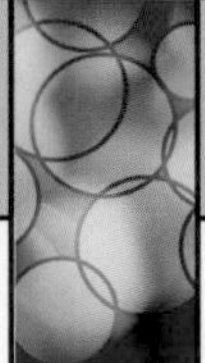

CHAPTER • 18

Coronavirus Infections

EQUINE CORONAVIRUS

Marta Gonzalez Arguedas

Coronaviruses have been identified in a wide range of animal species as causes of a variety of primarily gastrointestinal and respiratory diseases. Although coronavirus-induced enteritis has been suspected in foals with diarrhea, direct pathogenicity of equine coronavirus (ECV) in equids has not been demonstrated.[1,2]

Etiology

Coronaviruses are members of the *Coronaviridae* family, order Nidovirales, all of which are positive-sense ribonucleic acid (RNA) viruses.[3-6] The family *Coronaviridae* contains two genera, *Torovirus* and *Coronavirus*.[3,4,6-8] The coronaviruses were so named because the unusually large, club-shaped peplomers projecting from the envelope give the viral particle the appearance of a solar corona.[4,6,9] The tubular nucleocapsid is composed of a phosphorylated nucleoprotein and seems to be connected directly to a transmembrane protein, *M*, which spans the lipid bilayer three times and has only a small fraction of its mass exposed to the external environment.[4,6,8,9] Two types of prominent spikes line the outside of the virion. The long spikes, which consist of the *S* (spike) glycoprotein, are present on all coronaviruses and give them their characteristic "corona" appearance. The short spikes, which consist of the *HE* (hemagglutinin-esterase) glycoprotein, are present in only some coronaviruses.[4,6-8] Based on antigenic relationships and genetic homologies, the coronaviruses are subdivided into three antigenic groups.[1-3,7,10] ECV is a member of the group 2 mammalian coronaviruses.[7]

Toroviruses are established agents of gastroenteritis in animals, and the type species of the genus is Berne virus (BEV), a chance isolate from a diarrheic horse in 1972.[5,8,11-13] Torovirus is discussed in more detail later in this chapter.

Epidemiology and Clinical Findings

Coronaviruses are a common cause of disease in humans and domestic animals.[6] Coronaviruses have been identified in mice, rats, chickens, turkeys, swine, dogs, cats, rabbits, horses, cattle, and humans.[1,4] They cause respiratory, gastrointestinal, neurologic, and generalized infections.[8] In horses, it is believed that coronavirus infection spreads through fecal-oral transmission; however, other routes of transmission, such as respiratory and mechanical, may also be possible.[8,14] Most coronaviruses infect only the cells of their natural host species and a few closely related species.[6] In their natural host species, coronaviruses exhibit marked tissue tropism. Virus replication in vivo can be either disseminated, causing systemic infections, or restricted to a few cell types, often the epithelial cells of the respiratory or enteric tracts and macrophages, causing localized infections. Coronavirus replication takes place in the cytoplasm of infected cells.[6]

Anzai et al.[14] investigated the effect of long-distance transport of 29 racehorses (age 2 years) on serologic evidence of infection with potential respiratory pathogens, including coronavirus. Serum antibody titers to coronavirus were evaluated by serum neutralization (SN) test using bovine coronavirus (BCV), which is closely related antigenically to ECV.[7,14,15] Two horses were seropositive for BCV 1 month before transportation (dilution titers 1:10 and 1:40). These horses were transported in the same vehicle as four horses that were seronegative to coronavirus. The four seronegative horses seroconverted after transportation (titers between 1:10 and 1:20 within 1 month), but none developed clinical signs, and a direct relationship between disease and coronavirus infection could not be confirmed.[14] This study suggests that ECV may spread among horses while they are stabled together or during transport. This conclusion is consistent with serologic evidence that BCV or its related virus is widely prevalent in horses in Japan.[14,15]

Coronavirus-like particles have been observed by negative-contrast electron microscopy (EM) in fecal samples from healthy and diarrheic foals,[16-21] from one foal with combined immunodeficiency syndrome and diarrhea,[22] and from adult horses with Potomac horse fever.[23] Concurrent infections with rotavirus[18,19] and *Cryptosporidium*[22] have also been reported.

Davis et al.[2] identified a coronavirus antigenically related to BCV in a 5-day-old foal with enterocolitis. Bacterial cultures from feces were negative for enteric pathogens, and viral particles were not observed on EM. The coronavirus was identified in intestinal tissues of the foal by immunohistochemistry using BCV-specific monoclonal antibodies and in feces using an antigen-capture enzyme-linked immunosorbent assay (ELISA) designed for BCV detection.[2,7] The foal's serum antibody titer to BCV increased over an 8-day period from 1:25 to 1:100.[2]

Despite the reports of probable or possible coronavirus infection in foals, there were no definitive descriptions of ECV isolation from sick horses before 2000.[2,16,17,22,23] In 2000, Guy et al.[7] described for the first time the isolation and characterization of ECV (isolate NC99) from feces of a 2-week-old diarrheic foal. Further study of this isolate may yield important information about the role of enteric coronaviruses in equine intestinal disease.

Diagnosis

Coronavirus infection may be suspected if other etiologic agents of diarrhea in foals have been ruled out. Coronaviruses are difficult to isolate and propagate in cell culture. The diagnostic method of choice is direct demonstration of coronavirus antigens in biologic samples.[9] Negative-stain EM can be used to identify coronavirus-like particles in feces.[7,17-19,22,23] However, if viral particles are not present in sufficient numbers, EM examination may require considerable searching or may be unrewarding.[2,16]

Because of the cross-reactivity between BCV and ECV, detection of neutralizing antibody to BCV in horses provides presumptive evidence of exposure to ECV.[2,7,14,15,17] Because the presence of SN antibodies against BCV in equine sera may be a common finding, acute and convalescent samples should be examined for evidence of increasing titer.[2,14,15] Convalescent serum samples from horses with suspected ECV infection may be evaluated approximately 10 days after the onset of disease. In human patients, a fourfold increase in titer to coronavirus is indicative of recent active infection. An antemortem diagnostic panel for ECV should include assay for serum antibody titer to BCV and fecal capture ELISA evaluation for coronavirus antigen.[2]

Although coronaviruses or coronavirus-like particles have been identified in foals and adult horses with enteric disease, the pathogenicity of coronaviruses and their etiologic role in equine enteric disease remains unclear, and it is unlikely that coronavirus infection is responsible for outbreaks of diarrhea.[2,7,22,24] Additional studies are needed to determine the prevalence of ECV infection in healthy and sick horses, the occurrence of mixed infections of coronavirus and other enteric pathogens, and the relative importance of ECV as a cause of enteric disease in horses.[7]

EQUINE TOROVIRUS

Debra C. Sellon

Etiology

Equine torovirus (Berne virus) was originally isolated from a rectal swab of a horse with hepatic and gastrointestinal disease in Berne, Switzerland, in 1972.[25] It is currently classified in the *Torovirus* genus with bovine, human, and porcine toroviruses, within the family *Coronaviridae* and order Nidovirales.[26-28] The enveloped virions are pleomorphic with large protein spikes on the surface, resembling the peplomers of coronaviruses. The nucleocapsid has a tubular appearance with helical symmetry. The positive-sense RNA genome is estimated to be 20 to 25 kilobases in length with six open reading frames (ORFs). Four structural proteins have been identified: spike (S), membrane (M), hemagglutinin-esterase (HE), and nucleocapsid (N) proteins.

Epidemiology

Although originally isolated from a horse with gastrointestinal disease, a causal link between Berne virus and equine disease has not been established. Limited seroepidemiologic studies indicate that the virus is present in Europe and the United States. Neutralizing antibody is also found in the sera of other ungulates (cattle, sheep, goats, pigs), laboratory rabbits, and at least two species of wild mice (*Clethrionomys glareolus* and *Apodemus sylvaticus*).[29]

Clinical Findings

Despite widespread evidence of exposure to Berne virus, no evidence indicates that this virus is associated with clinical disease in horses or any other species. Inoculation of the virus into two foals induced neutralizing antibody without associated clinical signs.[29] Bovine torovirus has been associated with gastroenteritis in calves and possibly pneumonia in older cattle.[28,30] Human and porcine toroviruses are associated with gastroenteritis in people and pigs, respectively.[31-33]

REFERENCES

See the CD-ROM for a list of references linked to the abstract in PubMed.

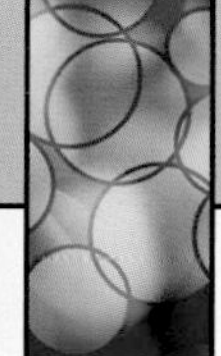

CHAPTER • 19

Rabies

Pamela A. Wilkins and Fabio Del Piero

Rabies virus (RABV) is an enveloped ribonucleic acid (RNA) rhabdovirus that induces lethal polioencephalomyelitis and ganglionitis in infected animals.[1,2] The disease is universally endemic in mammals and other warm-blooded vertebrates, except in Australia, where other types of zoonotic lyssaviruses transmitted by flying foxes (bats) are present. The disease has been excluded or eradicated from some countries, or parts of them, especially islands (e.g., Great Britain, New Zealand, Iceland).

ETIOLOGY

Viruses in the *Rhabdoviridae* family known to infect mammals belong to either the genus *Vesiculovirus* (vesicular stomatitis virus serotype New Jersey and serotype Indiana, Chandipura virus, and Piry virus) or the genus *Lyssavirus* (rabies virus and rabieslike viruses).[1,2] Lyssaviruses include six distinct genotypes that can be classified according to their degree of amino acid homology. Genotypes 2 (Lagos bat virus) and 3 (Mokola virus) are the most phylogenetically distant from the vaccinal and classic rabies viruses of genotype 1. Genotypes 4 (Duvenhage virus) and 5 (European bat lyssavirus 1 [EBL1]) are closely related to each other, with the separate genotype 6 represented by EBL2.

RABV virions are enveloped, bullet-shaped, 45 to 100 nm in diameter, and 100 to 430 nm long (Fig. 19-1). Surface projections of the envelope are distinct spikes, dispersed evenly over the whole surface (except for the quasiplanar end of bullet-shaped viruses). The uncoiled nucleocapsid is filamentous, with regular surface structure, and cross-banded. Virions contain 1% to 2% nucleic acid composed of one molecule of linear, usually negative-sense, single-stranded RNA. Nucleotide sequences of the 3′ terminus are inverted and complementary to similar regions on the 5′ end and are the same for each gene segment in species of the same genus. Virions contain 65% to 75% protein, most of which are structural. RABVs are recognized and classified through panels of monoclonal

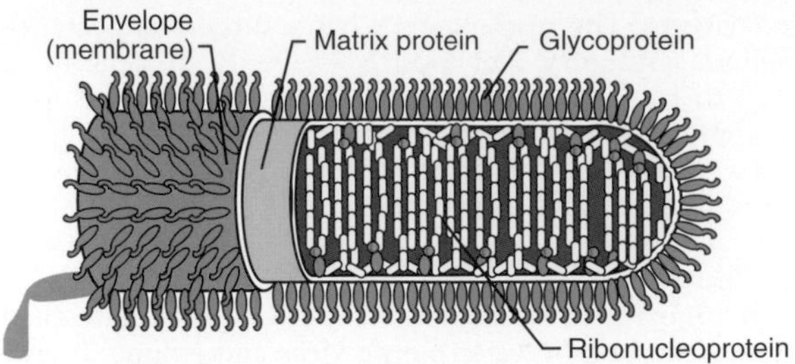

Fig. 19-1 Diagrammatic representation of rabies virus. (Courtesy Centers for Disease Control and Prevention, Atlanta.)

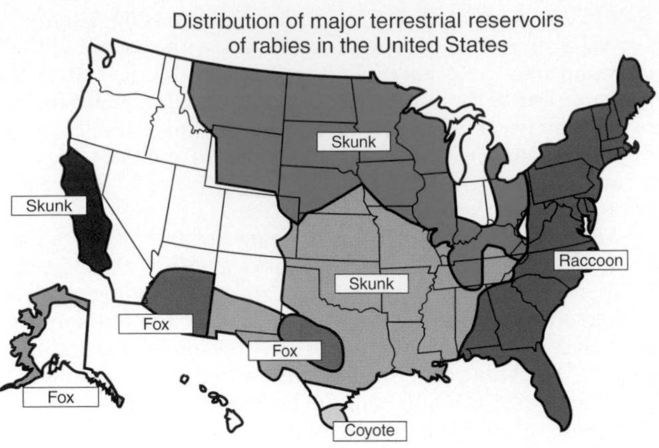

Fig. 19-2 Rabies reservoirs. Note the raccoon and skunk rabies present in the Central *(Skunk)* and Mid-Atlantic to Northeastern *(Raccoon)* distribution in the continental United States. (Courtesy Centers for Disease Control and Prevention, Atlanta.)

antibodies against nucleocapsid proteins. The pattern of antiglycoprotein reactivity of the isolates allows identification of the viral subtype.

EPIDEMIOLOGY

RABV is transmitted to warm-blooded animals by bites from infected vectors such as foxes, raccoons, skunks, bats, and vampire bats. In 2003, wild animals accounted for more than 91% of all cases of rabies reported to the Centers for Disease Control and Prevention (CDC).[3] Rabies control programs, including vaccination programs, have significantly decreased, if not eliminated, rabies in humans caused by canine variants. However, ever-increasing numbers of human cases are attributable to bat variants, a group difficult to target for rabies control by traditional methods.

In the United States, rabies infection of terrestrial mammals occurs in geographically defined regions, and transmission is usually within species, with occasional spillover to other species that rarely maintain intraspecific transmission (Fig. 19-2). Sixty-three cases of rabies were reported in horses and mules (including donkeys) in 2003, an 8.6% increase over the 58 cases reported in 2002 (Fig. 19-3). The majority of rabies in horses occurs in animals with no history of vaccination, although it may be recognized in animals not vaccinated within a year of diagnosis.[4] The increase in equine rabies in 2003 was consistent with the increase observed in raccoons, 8.9%, while the number of rabid skunks decreased by about 13%.

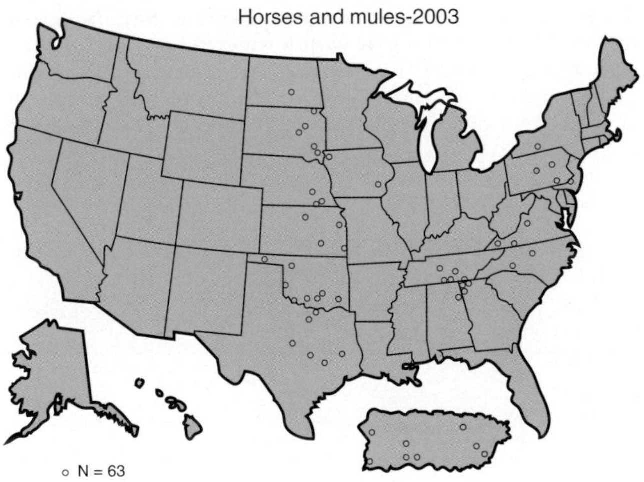

Fig. 19-3 Distribution of equine rabies cases in the United States and Puerto Rico in 2003. Note Central and Mid-Atlantic to Northeastern distribution in the continental United States. Most cases are caused by the local reservoir type, that is, Central (skunk) and Mid-Atlantic to Northeastern (raccoon). (Courtesy Centers for Disease Control and Prevention, Atlanta.)

PATHOGENESIS

The primary means of transmission of RABV is through the bite of an infected animal that inoculates saliva containing virus into tissues of a receptive animal. The virus likely replicates in muscle tissue at the site of inoculation. Rabies virus is believed to remain near the site of initial inoculation for most of the incubation period. In 1889, DiVestea and Zagari[5] showed that mortality was greatly diminished by severing the sciatic nerves of experimental animals before virus was inoculated in the footpad. This reduction in mortality is seen even when the nerves are severed several days after inoculation of virus.[6] Delayed progression of infection within muscle cells is thought to be responsible for the long incubation period of clinical rabies.[7]

Eventually, RABV binds to nicotinic acetylcholine receptors at the neuromuscular junction, the major site of entry into neurons.[8,9] The neural cell adhesion molecule, the low-affinity p75 neurotrophic receptor, and perhaps the *N*-methyl-D-aspartate NR1 receptor may also function as RABV receptors.[10-13] The virus then travels in an ascending fashion through the spinal cord to the brain or from the cranial nerves directly to the brain stem. Once transit in peripheral nerves begins, it progresses rapidly through transsynaptic neuronal spread. Virus can be observed in peripheral nerve myelin late in infection.[14] Clinical signs appear to result primarily from neuronal dysfunction secondary to drastically diminished synthesis of proteins required for maintenance of normal neuronal function.[15] After it reaches the brain, RABV is passed centrifugally to tissues and organs. It reaches the salivary glands and nasal secretions after passage down appropriate cranial nerves.[16]

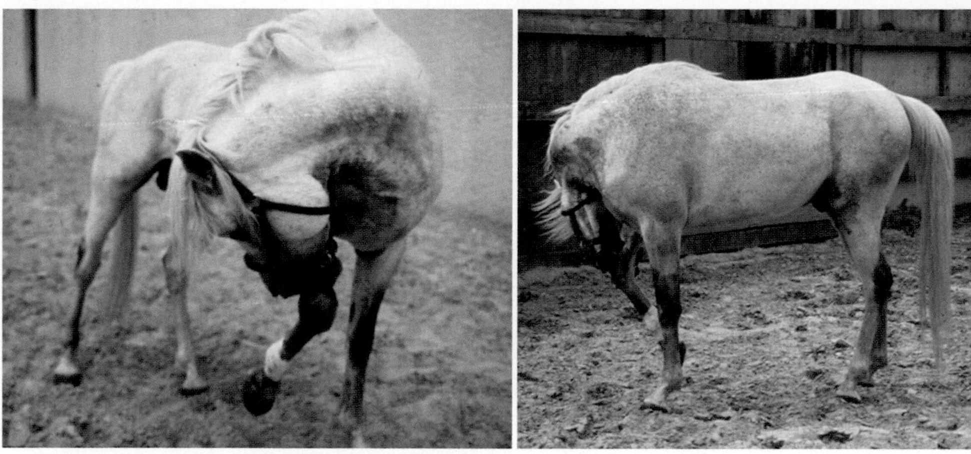

Fig. 19-4 Arabian stallion with rabies exhibiting signs of self-mutilation. Aggressive biting behavior led to human injury and rabies virus exposure, with subsequent human prophylactic treatment. (Courtesy Dr. Ian G. Mayhew.)

CLINICAL FINDINGS

Several authors have described clinical signs of rabies in horses in detail.[4,17-19] These signs range from poor racing performance to bizarre behavior and may include spinal cord, cerebral, and cranial nerve signs; apparent lameness; gastrointestinal signs; and genitourinary signs (Fig. 19-4). Clinical signs are progressive from onset until death, which usually occurs by day 10. Average survival from the onset of clinical signs is approximately 5 days. Clinical chemistry and hematology results are nonspecific and nondiagnostic. Cerebrospinal fluid (CSF) analysis reveals increased protein and lymphocytes but is not diagnostic.

Spinal cord signs are frequently observed in horses with rabies and may include subtle hindlimb lameness or shifting of weight in the hindlimbs, progressing to knuckling of one or both fetlocks. Ataxia or weakness usually follows, with paresis advancing to total pelvic limb paralysis when spinal cord signs are present. Associated signs may be constipation, tenesmus, paraphimosis in males, dribbling of urine from bladder paralysis, and flaccid tail and anus.

The classic description of encephalic signs includes evidence of progressive depression ("dumb" form) or aggression ("furious" form). Depression is often characterized by extreme obtundation, whereas aggression often includes hyperesthesia and self-mutilation. Other accentuated cerebral responses observed in rabies patients are hypersexuality with frequent mounting behavior, localized or generalized pruritus leading to self injury, tremors, seizures, alert eyes and ears despite paralysis or ataxia, blindness, head pressing, bellowing, and opisthotonos. Dysphagia, salivation, and a weak tongue may occur, often accompanied by an inability to drink, which may reflect laryngeal paralysis.

Several common diseases should be considered as differential diagnoses of rabies. In the paralytic form with spinal cord signs predominating, sacral injuries from estrous activities and spinal cord neoplasms or abscesses should be considered. In advanced rabies cases approaching coma, many encephalitides and toxic central nervous system (CNS) diseases should be considered.

DIAGNOSIS

There is no definitive antemortem test for rabies in horses. A minimum protocol for postmortem diagnosis of rabies can be found at the CDC website.*[1] Clinical signs are suggestive but nondiagnostic. CSF from rabies patients may be normal, have only increased protein values, or have both increased nucleated cells and protein. Most nucleated cells in the CSF of rabies patients are mononuclear cells. However, one report of 21 cases of rabies in horses found mononuclear pleocytosis without increases in protein concentration in five of six horses. No other antemortem tests are potentially helpful to the practicing veterinarian.

The brain from suspect animals must be submitted to a regional laboratory approved by the respective state health department for rabies testing, using CNS tissue smears and direct immunofluorescence with monoclonal antibodies. Enzyme-linked immunosorbent assay (ELISA), reverse transcriptase–polymerase chain reaction (RT-PCR) and peroxidase immunohistochemistry (IHC) are also available and reliable but are not considered official diagnostic tools.[4] These tests can be used when fresh tissue is not available or as research tools. In a simple, rapid, single-step RT-PCR test of the nucleoprotein (N) gene of RABV, a conserved set of RT-PCR primers is designed to amplify the most variable region in the N gene. The cornea impression smear test using direct fluorescent IHC is not reliable for rabies in animals. Intracerebral murine inoculation is not used as a routine diagnostic tool but can be used to propagate the virus. The fluorescent antibody virus neutralization (FAVN) test is used for the detection of antibodies against rabies virus. This test can be modified by using monoclonal antirabies antibodies and a peroxidase antimouse conjugate, instead of a fluorescent antirabies conjugate, with the results read on an automatic multichannel spectrophotometer. RABV is highly neurotropic but has been also observed in glial cells, epithelial cells of the cornea, hair follicles of carnivores, adrenal medulla, and skeletal muscle.

PATHOLOGIC FINDINGS (FIGS. 19-5 THROUGH 19-13)

Gross CNS lesions of rabies are rare in horses and may consist of focal to multifocal, mild to moderate hemorrhages. Self-trauma or aspiration pneumonia may be seen. Histologic

*http://www.cdc.gov/ncidod/dvrd/rabies/professional/publications/DFA_diagnosis/DFA_protocol-b.htm.

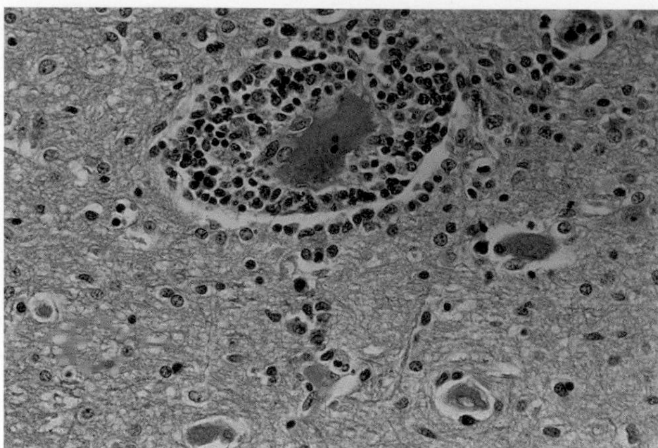

Fig. 19-5 Rabies; horse, cerebrum, neocortex. Polioencephalitis characterized by perivascular small lymphocyte cuffs, gliosis *(right)*, and neuronal satellitosis *(below)*. (Hematoxylin-eosin [HE] stain.)

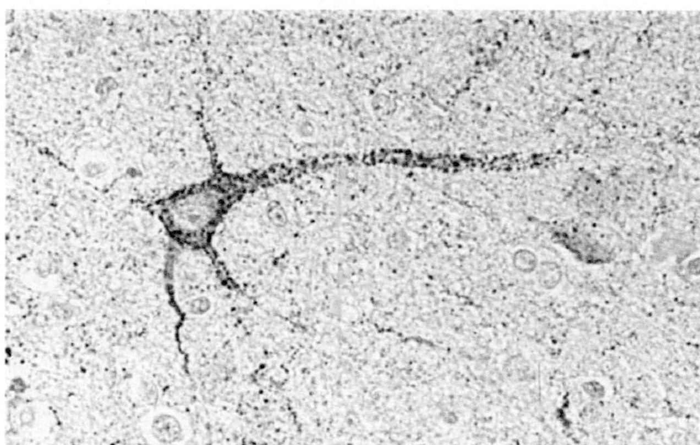

Fig. 19-6 Rabies; horse, neocortex. The cytoplasm of this cortical neuron is prominently colonized by rabies virus, which extends within the dendrites and the axon; surrounding fibers are diffusely colonized, and the astrocytes are hypertrophied. (Indirect peroxidase immunohistochemistry [IPIHC] and hematoxylin [He] stain.)

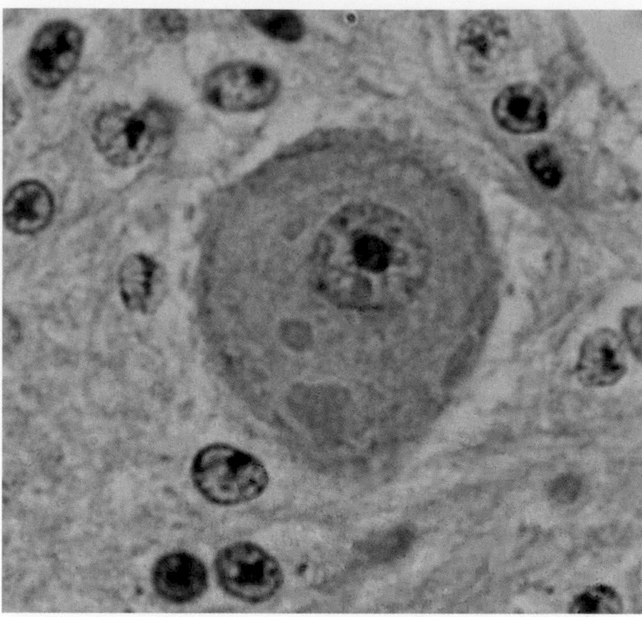

Fig. 19-7 Rabies; horse, cerebellum, Purkinje cell. Intracytoplasmic eosinophilic Negri inclusion bodies. (HE stain.)

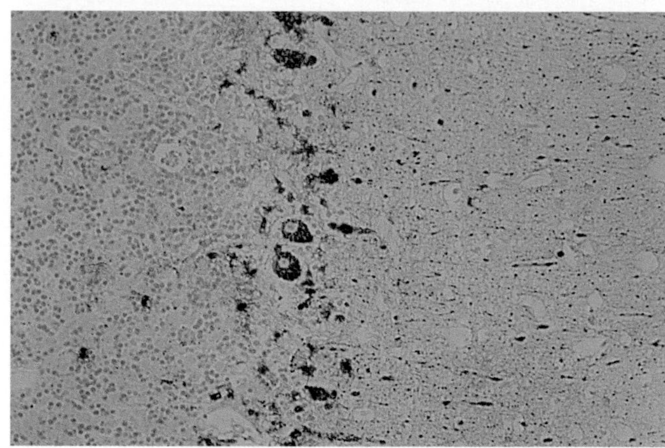

Fig. 19-8 Rabies; horse, cerebellum. Abundant intracytoplasmic rabies virus within Purkinje cells, granule cell layer *(left)*, and in particular within the molecular layers and fibers *(right)*. (IPIHC and He stain.)

lesions of rabies in horses are similar to lesions in cattle, although with more frequent neuronal vacuolization, and much less frequent Negri body formation.[4,8] There is a clear viral tropism for gray matter, neuronal cell bodies, and glial cells. Less virus antigen is found in animals euthanized early in the disease process. Histologic lesions observed in rabid animals, which died or were euthanized, consist of nonsuppurative perivascular encephalomyelitis with ganglionitis. Moderate to severe lymphocytic perivascular inflammation in gray and white matter of cerebral hemispheres with mild lymphocytic leptomeningitis is often present. In the basal nuclei, gray matter of the thalamus, and the brain stem, there is prominent inflammation with diffuse gliosis and the presence of lymphocytes in the neuropil. In these areas and in the hippocampus, neuronophagia, neuronal chromatolysis, microglial cell nodules, and proliferation of rod cells tend to be constant features. Moderate lymphocytic inflammation infiltrates the subependymal tissue of the lateral ventricles and fornix. The cerebellum contains mild perivascular lymphocytic inflammation in the molecular layer, mild lymphocytic leptomeningitis, and moderate inflammation of the white matter. Negri bodies, eosinophilic intracytoplasmic inclusions associated with accumulations of viral and cell protein (see Fig. 19-7), are observed in pyramidal cells of the hippocampus, extensively in Purkinje cells, and infrequently in the neocortex, without inflammatory changes. Mild ring hemorrhages are occasionally observed multifocally. Trigeminal ganglia are affected by severe lymphocytic inflammation with neuronal degeneration, neuronophagia, and formation of Nageotte bodies, which are aggregates of glial cells replacing a neuron (see Figs. 19-11 and 19-12).

Using indirect peroxidase IHC with monoclonal antibodies, RABV can be identified within neural cell cytoplasm and processes.[4] Often the distribution of RABV is prominent, with marked intracytoplasmic immunoreactivity of almost all neurons in every brain area and diffuse granular positivity of the neuropil of cerebral and cerebellar cortices, the thalamus, and the gray matter of the brain stem and spinal cord. RABV forms fine to large granules and 3- to 10-micron inclusion

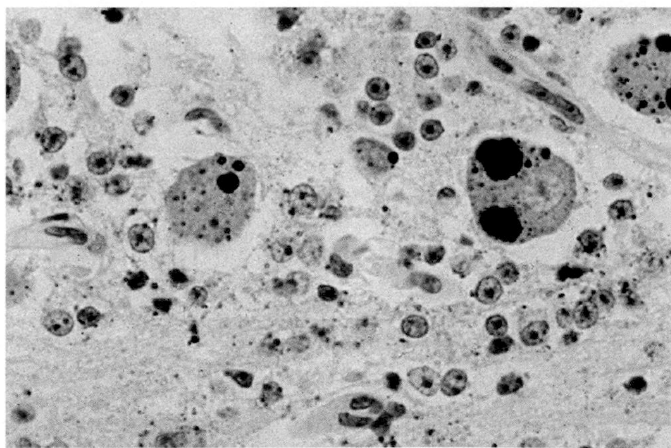

Fig. 19-9 Rabies; horse, cerebellum. Purkinje cells and granular cells contain variously sized, round to oval, often prominent, rabies virus aggregates. (IPIHC and He stain.)

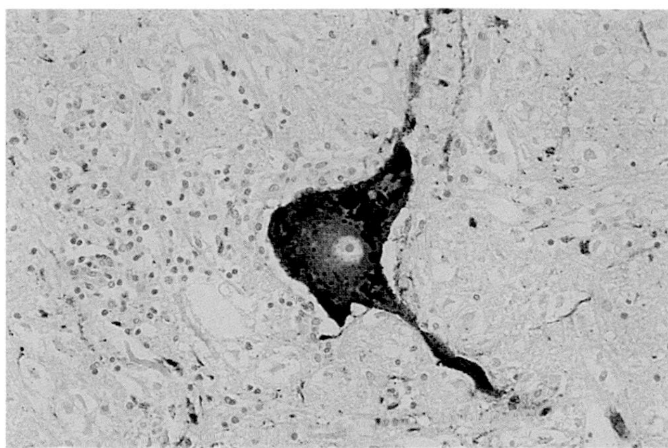

Fig. 19-10 Rabies; horse, brain stem. The cytoplasm of this nuclear neuron is heavily colonized by rabies virus, which extends within the visible dendrite and the axon; surrounding fibers also contain rabies virus, and there is moderate focal gliosis *(left)*. (IPIHC and He stain.)

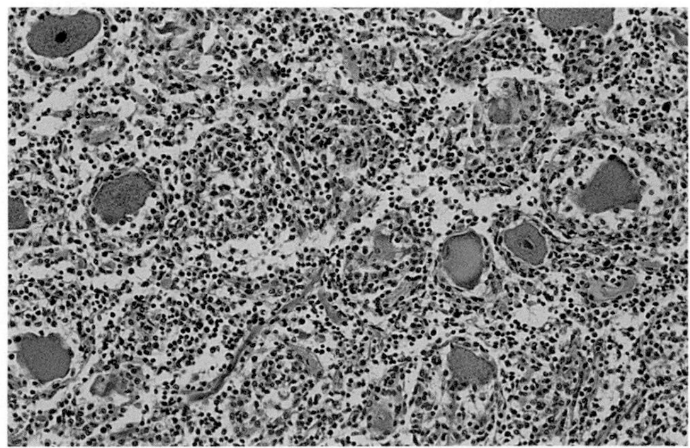

Fig. 19-11 Rabies; horse, trigeminal ganglion. Severe, diffuse lymphocytic ganglionitis. (HE stain.)

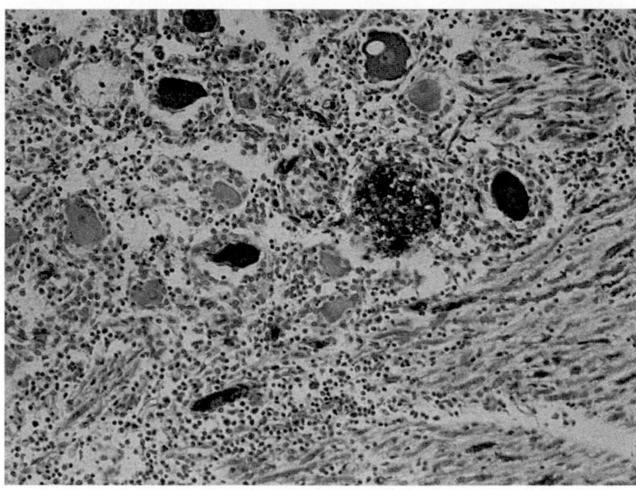

Fig. 19-12 Rabies; horse, trigeminal ganglion. Abundant intracytoplasmic rabies virus within ganglial neurons and trigeminal nerve fibers *(right)*; there is a gathering of glial cells replacing a necrotic phagocytized neuron (Nageotte body) and lymphocytic ganglionitis. (IPIHC and He stain.)

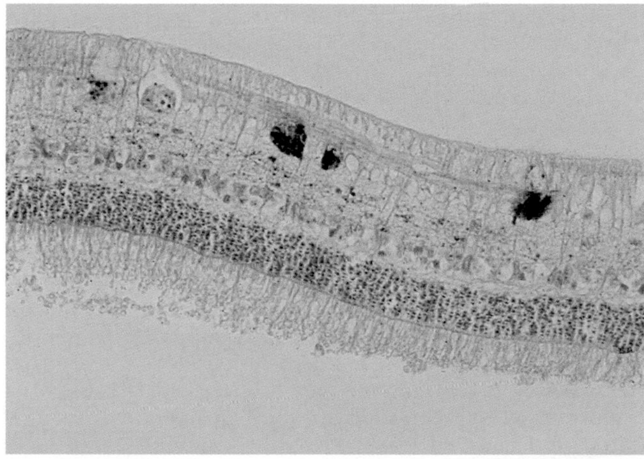

Fig. 19-13 Rabies; horse, retina. In absence of histologic lesions, the entire retinal layers contain variable quantity of granular intracytoplasmic rabies virus; particularly colonized are the ganglion cells, the inner plexiform layer, and the outer nuclear layer. (IPIHC and He stain.)

bodies that are single or multiple and distributed homogenously within the cytoplasm. RABV is predominantly observed in neuronal cell bodies, axons, and dendrites, which appear morphologically normal. There is prominent immunostaining of cortical neurons, pyramidal cells, and neurons of gyrus dentatus, as well as nuclei of the thalamus and brain stem. In the cerebellum, RABV is primarily localized within the Purkinje cells and some neurons of the granular and molecular layers. The spinal cord often contains abundant RABV in dorsal and ventral horns, with sparing of the white matter. RABV is also observed in some astrocytes and oligodendrocytes, ganglion cells of the retina and trigeminal ganglia cells, and autonomic ganglia of celiac-mesenteric ganglia. Negri bodies are reported in less than 30% of cases, and their absence should not rule out rabies as a diagnosis.

Table • 19-1

Approved Rabies Vaccines for Use in Horses (as of 2004)

PRODUCT	MANUFACTURER	DOSE	RECOMMENDED BOOSTER	ROUTE*
Monovalent (Rabies Inactivated)				
RABVAC 3	Fort Dodge Animal Health (Lic. #112)	2 mL	Annually	IM
RABVAC 3 TF	Fort Dodge Animal Health (Lic. #112)	2 mL	Annually	IM
IMRAB 3	Merial Inc. (Lic. #298)	2 mL	Annually	IM/SC
IMRAB Large animal	Merial Inc. (Lic. #298)	2 mL	Annually	IM/SC
Combination (Rabies Inactivated)				
Equine POTOMOVAC + IMRAB	Merial Inc. (Lic. #298)	1 mL	Annually	IM
MYSTIQUE II POTOMOVAC+	Intervet Inc. (Lic. #286)	1 mL	Annually	IM

**IM*, Intramuscular; *SC*, subcutaneous.

THERAPY

No known therapy is effective for treatment of unvaccinated or vaccinated horses with clinical rabies. Horses presenting with clinical signs of rabies should be isolated to prevent possible human exposure. Healthy, vaccinated horses suspected of being exposed to rabies may be quarantined for a period of observation for development of clinical signs. All species of livestock are susceptible to rabies; horses are among the most frequently infected. Horses exposed to a confirmed rabid animal and currently vaccinated with a vaccine approved by the U.S. Department of Agriculture (USDA) for that species should be revaccinated immediately and observed for 45 days (Table 19-1). Unvaccinated horses should be euthanized immediately. If the owner is unwilling to have this done, the horse should be kept under close observation for 6 months. More than one rabid horse in a herd, or herbivore-to-herbivore transmission, is uncommon. Therefore, if a single animal has been exposed to or infected by rabies, quarantine of the rest of the herd is not necessary.

Box • 19-1

*Rabies Vaccination Protocol**

Adult Horses:

Broodmares: Annually, before breeding.

Other adult horses: Annually.

Foals:

From vaccinated mares: First dose, 6 months, second dose at 7 months. Boost again at 12 months, then annually thereafter.

From unvaccinated mares: First dose, 3 to 4 months. Second dose at 12 months, annually thereafter.

*Based on vaccination guidelines of the American Association of Equine Practitioners (AAEP).

PREVENTION

The mainstays of rabies prevention are vaccination and exposure avoidance. Parenteral animal rabies vaccines should be administered only by, or under the direct supervision of, a veterinarian. Any veterinarian signing a rabies certificate should ensure that the person administering the vaccine is identified on the certificate and is appropriately trained in vaccine storage, handling, administration, and management of adverse events. This practice ensures that a qualified and responsible person can be held accountable to make certain the animal has been properly vaccinated.

A peak rabies antibody titer is reached within 28 days of primary vaccination. An animal is currently vaccinated and is considered immunized if the primary vaccination was administered at least 28 days previously and vaccinations have been administered appropriately.

Regardless of the age of the horse at initial vaccination, a booster vaccine should be administered 1 year later (Box 19-1). Because a rapid anamnestic response is expected, an animal is considered currently vaccinated immediately after a booster vaccination. Rabies is rare in vaccinated animals. If suspected, such an event should be reported to state public health officials, the vaccine manufacturer, and the USDA's Animal and Plant Health Inspection Service (APHIS), Center for Veterinary Biologics.*[2] The laboratory diagnosis should be confirmed and the virus characterized by a rabies reference laboratory. A thorough epidemiologic investigation should be conducted.

PUBLIC HEALTH CONSIDERATIONS

Rabies is considered a zoonotic disease. Although the authors were unable to find a single case of documented transmission of rabies from horse to human, the possibility is real, and all equine rabies suspects*[3] must be handled as if a significant threat to human health exists. Animals with suspected rabies should only be handled by individuals who have had appropriate rabies preexposure vaccination. A list of all "in-contact" and potential in-contact individuals, including owners and

*http://www.aphis.usda.gov/vs/cvb/ic/adverseeventreport.htm; telephone: 800-752-6255; or e-mail: CVB@usda.gov.

private parties, should be developed and kept current. It is convenient to place a clipboard near the stall housing a rabies suspect and require individuals to sign the list if they enter the stall, handle the patient, or handle biologic material from the patient. If rabies is a differential diagnosis, laboratory personnel handling body fluids obtained for diagnostic purposes should be informed of this potential. This is best accomplished by labeling all specimens obtained as "rabies suspect" on their containers and clearly stating this on any submission paperwork. Details of the CDC preexposure vaccination protocols can be found below* (at /00056176.htm).

Horses suspected of having rabies should be handled carefully, with examiners using protective gear that includes eye goggles, face shields/masks, and gloves during all examinations. Persons performing necropsy examinations on horses with suspected rabies are at increased risk of exposure to RABV, and more extensive protective measures should be considered. Individuals who move the bodies of rabies suspects should wear rubber boots, a scrub suit, double gloves (the outer glove being heavy vinyl with gauntlets), and a face shield for splash protection. Additionally, individuals who decapitate and remove brains of rabies suspects should use the protection of a Tyvek coverall (or surgical gown at a minimum) and a mist mask rated for biohazards (N95 rating or better; routine surgical masks are unacceptable for this purpose). The brain half that is submitted for rabies testing should be placed in a sealed plastic container, the external surface thoroughly cleaned with an appropriate disinfectant, and the container then placed in a second clean plastic container. Samples for rabies testing should be transported in rigid leakproof containers with the sample stabilized within the container by frozen gel packs or similar materials. The outer container should meet the federal standards for transport of diagnostic or dangerous goods.

The carcass and other specimens obtained at necropsy should not be submitted for additional studies until a negative rabies test result is obtained from the appropriate testing facility. If a positive test result is reported, all interested parties should be notified immediately, including the state veterinarian. Exposed individuals should consult their physician and local and state health authorities regarding postexposure treatment, which will vary depending on suspected level of exposure and preexposure vaccination status.

*http://www.cdc.gov/mmwr/preview/mmwrhtml/rr5309a1.htm.

ACKNOWLEDGMENTS

The authors would like to acknowledge the assistance of John Krebs, MS, from the CDC, in the preparation of the manuscript. We would also like to acknowledge the CDC for allowing free use of their images.

REFERENCES

See the CD-ROM for a list of references linked to the abstract in PubMed.

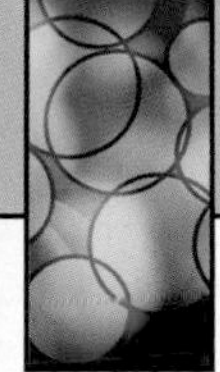

CHAPTER • 20

Equine Alphaviruses

E. Paul J. Gibbs and Maureen T. Long

The first recorded epidemic of *eastern equine encephalitis* (EEE) in horses likely occurred in Massachusetts in 1831; the first recorded human case occurred in that state in 1838.[1] In 1933, EEE virus was isolated from a horse, and it was established that epidemics of encephalitis in horses in North America were caused by two separate viruses, EEE and *western equine encephalitis* (WEE), that were segregated geographically. A related virus, *Venezuelan equine encephalitis* (VEE), causes outbreaks of encephalitis in horses in Central America, South America, Mexico, and occasionally the southern United States. Although widespread vaccination has reduced the size and number of outbreaks of EEE, WEE, and VEE in horses, the impact of these diseases is still significant because of the fulminant nature of clinical signs and high mortality rate in affected horses.

ETIOLOGY

The genus *Alphavirus* belongs to the family *Togaviridae* and includes a large number of viruses that have been isolated from horses with neurologic disease. Of these alphaviruses, eastern, western, and Venezuelan equine encephalitis viruses are the most frequently isolated from epidemics of encephalitis in horses and humans in the Western Hemisphere.[2,3] The other genus in the family *Togaviridae*, *Rubivirus*, contains no viruses of known equine significance. Togaviruses are single-stranded, linear positive-sense ribonucleic acid (RNA) viruses that are enveloped and measure 60 to 70 nm in diameter. Within the envelope there is a nucleocapsid with icosahedral symmetry composed of peplomers arranged as trimers. Each peplomer is a heterodimer composed of two glycoproteins, E1 and E2.[4]

The glycoproteins E1 and E2 are immunodominant proteins that induce neutralizing antibody.[4-6] The E2 glycoprotein induces the strongest neutralizing antibody response (both polyclonal and monoclonal) and has hemagglutinating properties, the activity of which is highly modulated by pH.[2,7,8] Both hemagglutination inhibition (HI) activity and neutralizing specificity have historically been used to differentiate viral species and their antigenic types (Table 20-1). Although these techniques are now being rapidly replaced by molecular

Table • 20-1

*Alphaviruses Reported to Cause Equine Encephalitis**

ANTIGENIC COMPLEX	ANTIGENIC SUBTYPE	ANTIGENIC VARIETY	EQUINE CLINICAL SYNDROME	DISTRIBUTION
Eastern equine encephalitis (EEE)		North American	Encephalitis	North America, Caribbean
		South American	Encephalitis	South, Central America
Venezuelan equine encephalitis (VEE)	(I) VEE	AB	Encephalitis	South, Central, North America
		C	Encephalitis	South, Central America
		E	Encephalitis	Central America
	(II) Everglades		Unknown	Florida, USA
Western equine encephalitis (WEE)	WEE	Several	Encephalitis	North, South America
	Highlands J		Rare encephalitis	Eastern North America

Modified from Weaver SC, Powers AM, Brault AC, Barrett AD: *Vet J* 157:123-138, 1999.
*Refer to text for other isolated alphaviruses that may be pathogenic for horses.

sequencing as the basis for viral classification, the common group-specific antigenic determinants are still usually defined by serologic techniques, such as fluorescent antibody (FA), complement fixation (CF), and enzyme-linked immunosorbent assay (ELISA).[7-15]

In addition to the alphaviruses that occur in the Western Hemisphere and are associated with equine encephalitis, several other alphaviruses that are potential causes of encephalitis have been isolated in the Americas and throughout the world.[16] There is only one known species of EEE virus, but it exists as separate North and South American variants with a high degree of genetic conservation between isolates.[17] North American isolates of EEE virus differ by less than 2% in their genomic nucleotide sequence analysis, even when comparing strains isolated more than half a century apart and over a 1200-mile land mass. In contrast, South American isolates can be classified as several genotypes that diverge by up to 25% in nucleotide sequence analysis.[18]

There are two antigenic subtypes of WEE virus: WEE and Highlands J viruses.[19-23] Most infections that occur east of the Mississippi River are caused by the *Highlands J* (HJ) virus.[20,24-26] Although generally considered less pathogenic for mammals than WEE virus, HJ virus has caused natural cases of encephalitis in horses and is pathogenic for domestic turkeys, pheasants, and exotic species of birds.[20,24,25] Other subtypes of WEE virus that may cause disease in North American horses include Fort Morgan and Buggy Creek viruses.[27] One WEE variant, Y62-WEE, has been identified in Russia. No equine disease has been associated with either Sindbis or Aura viruses, other members of the *Alphavirus* family.[28] Most WEE infections in the western United States are likely the result of infection with one of the several antigenic variants of the actual WEE subtype.[29] This virus is more pathogenic in horses and humans than closely related viruses, although minimal disease has been reported in humans and horses in the last decade.

Six distinct subtypes (designated by Roman numerals I through VI) and numerous varieties of viruses (designated by letter) within those subtypes are classified within the VEE virus complex.[9] The "epidemic type" of VEE viruses (types IAB, IC, and IE) are responsible for the large outbreaks of encephalitis in horses in the Western Hemisphere in the past 20 years. So-called endemic types of VEE virus are considered to be of low pathogenicity for equids under most circumstances.[29-31] These include ID and IF variants from Central America and Brazil, respectively,[9,32] type II (Everglades) virus found in Florida, three known variants of type III (Mucambo) virus, type IV (Pixuna) virus, type V (Cabassou) virus, and type VI virus. The Mucambo virus has three subtypes of potential pathogenicity for the horse.[9,33] These viruses have been isolated in Trinidad, French Guiana, western North America, and Peru. The Pixuna subtype of VEE is associated with febrile illness in horses in Brazil.[9]

EPIDEMIOLOGY

The life cycle of equine alphaviruses involves transmission between birds or rodents and mosquitoes.[34] In some cases, other domestic and wild animal species, especially species exotic to North America, such as the emu, have been affected during these outbreaks.[35] Although other RNA viruses, such as human immunodeficiency virus (HIV), have high rates of genetic evolution (up to 10^4 nucleotide changes per year), alphaviruses evolve relatively slowly, at approximately 10^2 to 10^3 substitutions per year.[22,36-39] This slow progression reflects adaptation of viruses to multiple hosts, which presumably requires more genomic conservation for maintenance in nature. There may be higher rates of viral evolution outside of North America. Despite this lower evolution rate, these viruses have the ability to adapt rapidly to new ecologic challenges. When VEE is placed in cell culture, serial passage results in stability of the substitution rate. When placed back in vivo (usually hamsters), the mutation rate of the virus increases dramatically, indicating that these viruses can rapidly change and have the potential to cause new outbreaks in new hosts and in new locales. Because alphaviruses are transmitted by arthropod vectors, clinical disease occurs during the arbovirus season of late summer and early fall in temperate zones, with year-round transmission possible in the tropics and subtropics.

Understanding the antigenic and genetic relationships among the viruses in the WEE complex has proved more challenging than for the viruses within the EEE and VEE complexes. Western equine encephalitis virus is a member of the WEE antigenic complex that includes several Old World viruses in addition to the New World viruses previously described. Phylogenetic analyses of isolates from North and South America indicate that regional WEE lineages appear to have evolved independently for several years to a few decades (e.g., genotypes in South America are apparently absent from North America).[3,25,37,40-44] However, relative homogenous genotypes of WEE are dispersed across both North and South America. This contrasts with EEE and VEE viruses, where certain virus genotypes appear to be restricted to either North or South America. WEE virus has been reported in several countries in South America (Argentina, Guyana, Ecuador, Brazil, Uruguay), but only in Argentina has it been associated with human disease and significant epidemics in horses.[23,45-47]

Eastern Equine Encephalitis

Although designated as an "eastern" virus, EEE has a wide geographic distribution. It is found as far north as eastern Canada, is dispersed throughout the Caribbean, and has been identified in Central and South America. Infection in the United States (U.S.) is primarily seen in the southeastern states but has been detected in all states east of the Mississippi River and also in a number of western states. In recent years, intense focal activity has been reported in Wisconsin, Ohio, Massachusetts, and New Hampshire.[48,49]

In the U.S., most cases of EEE in horses occur in the northern parts of Florida and the Carolinas. In total, several hundred equine cases are confirmed each year, despite the widespread availability of vaccines. In Florida, many horses that succumb to EEE are not vaccinated, are less than 3 years of age, and are stock-type horses (Long, unpublished data). There is no gender predilection. The occurrence of human disease is sporadic, with approximately 10 fatal human cases per year reported for the entire U.S.

In North America, EEE virus is perpetuated in a sylvatic cycle between avian hosts (passerine birds) and mosquitoes, primarily the ornithophilic mosquito, *Culiseta melanura*.[50-52] Indigenous passerine birds do not develop disease but develop sufficient titer viremia to allow transmission to feeding mosquitoes.[53] *Cs. melanura* is not a mammalian feeder and is not responsible for transmission between birds and mammalian hosts. However, several species of secondary or epidemic mosquitoes that feed on both birds and mammals can act as biologic vectors. These likely transmit EEE to horses, humans, and other vertebrate species. Horses and humans are clinically affected but do not develop viremia sufficiently high enough to transmit virus back to vector mosquitoes and are considered "dead-end" hosts.

Disease caused by EEE was first identified in Connecticut in 1937 in the then recently introduced exotic ring-necked pheasant. Since that time, disease in sparrows, pigeons, Pekin ducks, and Chukar partridges (all old-world species) has been reported.[54] In 1991, EEE was the cause of fatal hemorrhagic colitis in commercial flocks of emus in Louisiana. Similar outbreaks have been reported in emus and ostriches in Georgia, Florida, and other states.[55,56] Outbreaks of EEE have been recorded in intensive swine herds in southern Georgia.[57] Isolated cases of EEE in cattle, sheep, and nondomestic ungulates have also been recorded.[58-60]

The mechanism by which EEE virus overwinters (diapause) remains uncertain.[61,62] Transovarial transmission of EEE virus is not important, although it does occur in the mosquito host. In tropical and subtropical climates, the year-round mosquito/avian cycle likely obviates the need for a period of diapause in mosquito populations. In the many areas of North America with seasonal EEE activity, winters are long and severe enough such that no adult mosquito activity occurs for several months.

Culiseta melanura, a temperate breeding species of mosquito, does not readily breed in southern Florida and the Caribbean, and EEE is not an endemic disease in this relatively focal region.[63] Only sporadic reports or small epidemics of EEE disease in horses have been recorded in these areas, likely through migratory influx of viremic birds providing occasional sources of virus for secondary vectors. These secondary vectors can initiate short-term outbreaks but cannot maintain the disease endemically.

Comparatively few epidemics of EEE in horses have occurred in South America, with minimal disease reported in humans. Mosquitoes of the subgenus *Culex (Melanoconion)* in South and Central America are implicated as endemic vectors.[64] Antibody prevalence studies in birds and small rodents indicate that, in contrast with North America, small rodents are involved in the primary virus life cycle.

Western Equine Encephalitis

Since 1964, WEE has been reported in 640 people. The highest number of cases has been reported in Colorado and Texas, followed by Minnesota and California. Historically, large outbreaks of WEE have been described in horses. The virus was first identified in association with a large epizootic that occurred in the San Joaquin Valley of California in 1930. Approximately 6000 horses were affected, with a case-fatality rate of 50%.[65] This outbreak continued and spread to several western states from 1931 to 1934. Within a decade, another 300,000 equid cases were reported, with several thousand human cases. Over the last decade, reports of WEE in horses have been limited and sporadic, likely reflecting vaccination and protective immunity gained by subclinical exposure.[66,67]

Culex tarsalis is the primary vector that maintains WEE virus in an enzootic cycle with birds, especially nestling passerines,[68,69] *Cx. tarsalis* population abundance is favored by a rapid increase in temperature following a cool, wet spring, resulting in the rapid melting of snow and flooding of rivers.[70,71] This species of mosquito also has a predilection for irrigated lands as breeding sites.[72] Other ornithophilic mosquitoes become infected as the summer progresses, and the infection eventually spills over to other types of birds, mammals, and possibly reptiles and amphibians. Most, if not all, of these infections are inapparent. This in turn results in the virus becoming established in species of mosquitoes with host preferences other than birds. Transovarial transmission of WEE in North American mosquitoes, including *Cx. tarsalis*, has not been proved, and interepidemic maintenance in temperate areas by mosquitoes is therefore in doubt. Horses, even those that are obviously clinically affected, do not produce viremia high enough to infect mosquitoes.

At least two variants of WEE virus (Fort Morgan and Buggy Creek) have been isolated in western North America and are transmitted between birds by swallow nest bugs *(Oeciacus vicarius)*.[24] Neither variant is considered to be pathogenic for humans or horses. A third variant, Highlands J virus, is mainly found east of the Mississippi River and has been isolated from horses dying of encephalitis.[20,24-26,73] Information is limited on the number of horses infected with HJ virus on an annual basis.

In South America, where *Cx. tarsalis* does not occur, antibody prevalence rates in birds are lower than in North America, and the species (vertebrate and invertebrate) responsible for maintaining the virus on that continent have not been identified.[74] *Aedes albasfaciatus* has experimentally transmitted WEE virus to chickens in Argentina.[75] Other studies have demonstrated mosquitoes of the *Culex pipiens* complex are refractory to oral WEE virus inoculation. The species of mosquitoes from which WEE virus has mostly been isolated feeds principally on mammals rather than birds.

Venezuelan Equine Encephalitis

Venezuelan equine encephalitis virus is one of the most important human and veterinary pathogens in the New World.[76] The virus, both historically and very recently, has been responsible for large outbreaks of disease in both humans and horses over large geographic areas. The first recognized outbreak of VEE occurred initially in equids in Colombia and then in Venezuela in 1935 and 1936, although it is speculated to have been active in this area since 1920.[77] Documentation of human disease occurred in a Columbian outbreak in the 1960s, when an estimated 50,000 to 100,000 equids (horses, mules, donkeys) died and 250,000 humans were affected (mainly an influenza-like disease, but some cases of encephalitis and death). It is uncertain whether the 1969–1971 epidemic that was first reported in Ecuador and subsequently spread to Central America, Mexico, and Texas was directly related to this outbreak in Colombia or was caused by the use of an incorrectly inactivated subtype IAB strain vaccine.[78,79] Regardless of its cause, however, this epidemic revealed the potential for VEE to spread rapidly within an equine population, with a case-fatality rate approaching 90% in some areas.

The availability of vaccines and active surveillance throughout the Americas since the early 1970s have arguably reduced the impact of the disease in the rural regions, where VEE has traditionally been described. Nevertheless, after a long period with no evidence of clinical disease in horses, outbreaks of VEE were reported in 1993 in Chiapas, southern Mexico; in 1995 in Venezuela and Colombia; and in 1996 in Oaxaca, Mexico.[80-84] The geographically extensive outbreak in 1995 had all the initial hallmarks of the 1969–1971 epidemic. Not only did large numbers of horses, mules, and donkeys die, but there were also an estimated 75,000 to 100,000 human cases of disease. VEE viruses isolated in 1995 were genetically similar to those associated with disease in the 1960s. Although the cause of these severe cyclic disease occurrences is still a matter of intense research, it can be assumed that severe epizootic VEE may continue to occur with approximately one- to two-decade-long interepizootic periods.

Key to understanding the epidemiology of VEE is recognition of the differences in the basic biology of two transmission cycles, enzootic and epizootic, of this virus[76] (Fig. 20-1). The enzootic cycle centers around sylvatic rodents such as spiny and cotton rats, which have high natural infection rates and can develop viremia high enough to transmit VEE to mosquitoes.[85,86] Even opossums, bats, and shore birds likely are important in dispersal of enzootic virus.[87,88] The subgenus *Melanoconion (Culex cedecci)* is likely to be the most important vector of enzootic VEE.[89] This vector resides in tropical forests and swamps and feeds on small forest mammals at night. Some species of this mosquito have broader feeding patterns. Activity for this vector peaks with high ambient temperature and rainfall. Table 20-1 indicates that certain strains of virus are found only in the enzootic cycle. These viruses, subtypes I-E, II, III, and IV, tend to be of low pathogenicity for equids and do not result in high levels of viremia in horses.

Many theories exist on the origin of epizootic VEE viruses, primarily of the subtypes IAB and IC.[90,91] These viruses are associated with variable but often quite high equine mortality (20%-85%).[92] In contrast to most arboviruses in the horse, efficient amplification of the virus by equids is the hallmark of epizootic VEE. Humans usually develop a flulike illness, with only 4% to 14% exhibiting neurologic signs and symptoms.[88] Case-fatality rate for humans is approximately 1%. Several other species of mammals, including domestic rabbits, small ruminants, and dogs, develop potentially fatal clinical disease after VEE virus infection.[92] More than 100 species of

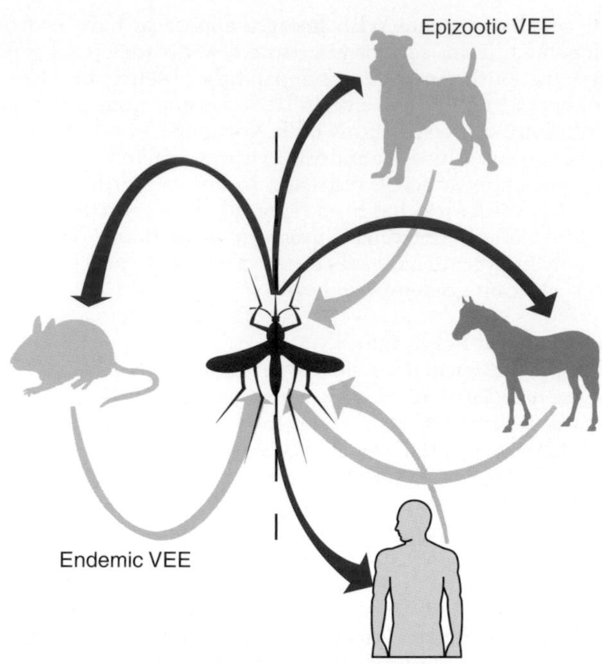

Fig. 20-1 Life cycle of Venezuelan equine encephalitis virus *(VEE)*. During the endemic cycle, VEE is maintained in a sylvatic ecosystem with a rodent reservoir (spiny rat) and mosquito vector, generally *Culex* spp. *(Melanoconion)*. On generation of an epizootic strain of VEE, multiple-vector species transmit the virus. The horse generates a sufficiently high-titer viremia to amplify the virus significantly. Several other terrestrial mammals also are susceptible to infection and develop significant viremia (including human and dog).

birds have been either virologically or serologically associated with transmission of epidemic VEE virus. Shore birds in general and herons in particular appear to be capable of serving as amplifier hosts.[93,94] Birds may develop viremia as high as 10^8 $TCID_{50}$/mL of blood.

The importance of equine infection in maintenance of epizootic VEE is evidenced by the observation that human disease has never been demonstrated in the absence of equine disease.[29] All mammalian hosts are capable of developing a high-titer viremia of approximately 10^5 to 10^7 pfu/mL for up to 5 days, but the horse is likely to be the most important mammalian host in terms of vector capacity.[76] In contrast to EEE and WEE, where horses are not considered to be a major source of virus for the vector, in VEE epidemics, horses are the most important amplifiers of virus activity.

Several species of mosquitoes from at least 11 genera have been determined to be naturally infected with epidemic strains of VEE virus.[95-102] In particular, *Psorophora confinnis*, *P. columbiae*, *Ochlerotatus sollicitans*, *O. taeniorhynchus*, and *Culex* spp. have been associated with epizootics. Virus has also been isolated from *Culicoides* spp. *(Ceratopogonidae)* and blackflies *(Simuliidae)*, but it is not known whether insects in these families are capable of biologic transmission of VEE virus.[95] During an epidemic, dogs regularly become infected and may be capable of virus amplification.[103-106] In addition, ticks, including the species *Ambylomma cajennense* and *Hyalomma truncatum*, may be capable of viral transmission.[107-111]

Several theories exist regarding the source of IAB and IC strains and how they persist in the environment between outbreaks.[112] Although molecular analyses have been used to address this, a comprehensive understanding of how epidemics in horses originate remains elusive. Isolates that are virulent for horses do not appear to be transmitted in the interepizootic period.[113,114] There is some evidence for circulation of these viruses in the interepizootic period, but no latency is associated with these infections. No evidence suggests that the epizootic strains coexist in the enzootic cycle. Mutation of enzootic strains may allow the emergence of highly pathogenic virus and initiation of epizootics.[115] This has been identified as the source of four epizootics. Some of these epizootics may have occurred secondary to the use of a modified live vaccine derived from the IAB strain.[79]

PATHOGENESIS

The alphavirus genome is 9.7 to 11.8 kilobases in length and encodes both nonstructural and structural proteins. With a 5′-methylated and a 3′-polyadenylated cap, the nonstructural proteins are encoded at the 5′ end and the structural proteins at the 3′ end of the genome.[40,116-119] Unlike flaviviruses, which translate the entire genome, only the 5′ end is translated in alphaviruses. The resultant polyprotein is subsequently cleaved by a proteinase. Viral RNA-dependent RNA polymerase is formed from two of these proteins, and complementary (negative-sense) RNA (cRNA) is transcribed.[3,120] From this template, full-length viral progeny are transcribed, and a short "subgenomic" portion is transcribed.[121-123] The latter, which has a cap at the 5′ end and a polyadenylated tail, is translated to form a polyprotein that is processed to the five viral proteins: E1, E2, E3, 6K, and C.[117,119,124-127]

Alphaviruses replicate to high titer in the cytoplasm of infected cells and exit the cell by the budding of preassembled nucleocapsids through the plasmalemma.[128,129] They cause cytopathic effects (CPEs) in a wide range of vertebrate cells in vitro, particularly embryonic avian cells.[130] Infection causes complete shutdown of host-cell protein and nucleic acid synthesis. Invertebrate cells, such as C6/36 derived from *Aedes albopictus*, are equally sensitive to infection with alphaviruses, but no CPE is apparent, and cell division is unaffected.[131]

Much of the understanding of the pathogenesis of alphaviruses comes from studies comparing the difference in pathogenicity between endemic and epidemic strains of VEE. Virulence of VEE virus correlates with viremia as opposed to specific neurovirulence per se. Low-virulence strains are more susceptible than high-virulence strains of VEE to interferons (IFN-α,β).[133,134] Comparatively, epidemic and epizootic VEE have similar ability to invade the CSF and, when inoculated intracerebrally, have similar pathogenesis even though there are differences in in vitro growth characteristics.[132] Changes in the E2 glycoprotein confer virus replication, resulting in rapid development of CPEs in vitro.[135,136] However, the relationship between pathogenesis and virus strains is more complex than just viral characteristics; while virulent strains of VEE differ in their ability to stimulate endogenous intracellular antiviral functions, ultimately mortality (in experimental models) appears to depend on genetics of the host.

Studies in mice demonstrate that neural invasion is likely to occur secondary to vascular infection or invasion through the olfactory epithelium.[137] After inoculation, there is local viral replication in fibroblasts. In young mice, there is intense replication in osteoclasts of developing bone, possibly explaining that young animals and humans are much more susceptible to severe disease.

The regional lymph node is presumed to be the site of primary viral replication after the bite of a mosquito infected with EEE, WEE, or VEE virus.[49] The reticuloendothelial system is a major target in epidemic VEE infections. The viruses cause encephalitis after hematogenous or neuronal spread. Immunity, after both inapparent infection and clinical disease as caused by EEE, WEE, and VEE, is long lasting in all species. Horses infected with EEE and WEE do not excrete infectious virus, and recovered animals are not persistently infected with virus. In humans naturally infected by mosquitoes, the common symptoms of infection with alphaviruses (fever, headache, and myalgia accompanied by leukopenia) have been attributed to circulating interferon and other soluble mediators.[12,88,138-141] The pathology in humans is similar to that in horses.

CLINICAL FINDINGS

Different strains of EEE, WEE, and VEE viruses may differ in their virulence not only for horses, but also for humans, certain domestic and wild animals, birds, and laboratory animals.[29] Clinical observations during epidemics of VEE indicate that the disease is generally less severe in donkeys (burros) and mules.[142] None of these viruses appears to cause clinical disease in their reservoir hosts indigenous to North and South America. Many human and equine infections, apart from those caused by highly virulent strains, are subclinical. When disease does occur, there are broad differences in the clinical manifestations that are produced by the three virus complexes in horses and humans.

EEE and epidemic VEE viruses are generally more neuroinvasive than WEE and endemic VEE viruses. Children and young animals of all susceptible species are more likely than adults to develop clinical CNS disease.[49,88,143-149] The incubation periods of EEE, WEE and VEE vary from 2 to 3 days to, rarely, as long as 3 weeks. Inapparent infections in horses may or may not be accompanied by fever. In clinical cases, pyrexia is the first clinical manifestation of infection.[150] Temperature has usually abated or is only moderately elevated by the time signs of encephalitis become evident. Neurologic signs are variable, but obtunded mentation, ataxia, paralysis, anorexia, and ultimately stupor occur in clinical cases (Fig. 20-2). Irregular gait, grinding of teeth, incoordination, circling, staggering, head pressing, and hyperexcitability are also observed; clinical signs are progressive in nature. Severely ataxic animals may stand by leaning against walls or other objects and sometimes stand with their hindlegs crossed. Partial or even total blindness may be evident. In severely depressed horses, the head hangs low with drooping ears, the eyelids may be slightly swollen and partly closed, the lips are flaccid, and the tongue may protrude from the mouth. The profound depression associated with these infections give rise to the common name of "sleeping sickness." Esophageal paralysis, as manifested by repeated unsuccessful attempts to drink, has also been described.

The course of disease in severely affected horses varies between 2 and 14 days. Nearly all horses with EEE die, regardless of the quality and intensity of clinical care. Horses with VEE and WEE are more likely to survive. Terminally ill horses can no longer stand, become comatose, and frequently exhibit seizure activity.

DIAGNOSIS

Clinical signs and antemortem clinical pathologic findings are not specific for alphavirus infection. Viral and other encephalitides can cause abnormal cerebrospinal fluid (CSF),

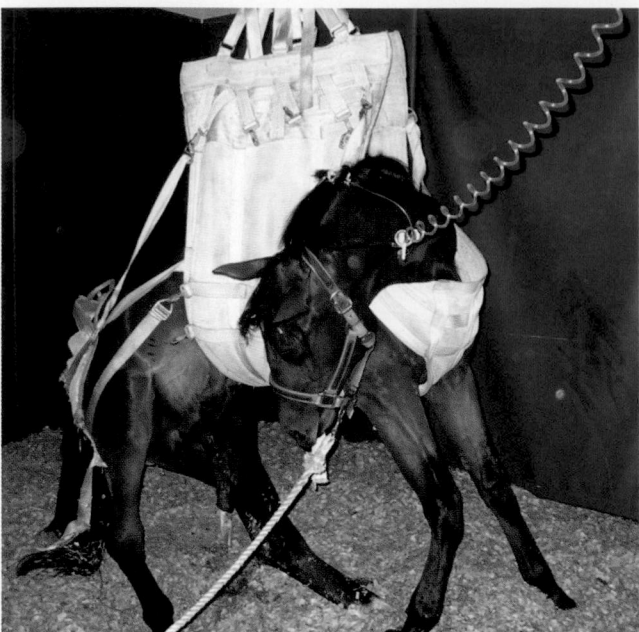

Fig. 20-2 Two-year-old Thoroughbred colt profoundly affected with EEE virus. This horse had clinical signs for approximately 36 hours. Initial signs consisted of fever and depression. The horse rapidly deteriorated and by 24 hours after onset was not arousable. This horse also had persistent priapism, a common clinical sign in male horses with encephalitis.

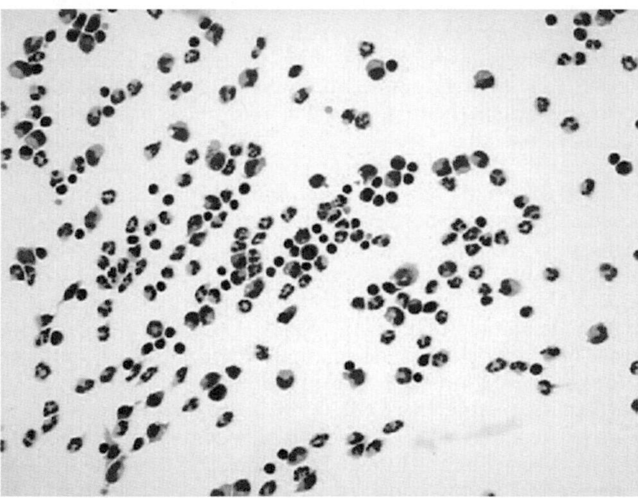

Fig. 20-3 Photomicrograph of cerebrospinal fluid (CSF) from horse with eastern equine encephalitis (EEE). This horse had exhibited clinical signs for less than 72 hours when the CSF was obtained. The CSF contains more than 50% nondegenerate neutrophils.

which usually consists, in the horse, of a moderate mononuclear pleocytosis with increased CSF protein. EEE is unique in that acute infection frequently results in a neutrophilic pleocytosis (Fig. 20-3). Because high mortality is associated with this disease, identification of a neutrophilic pleocytosis indicates probable EEE infection and offers the veterinarian a chance to prognosticate regarding the horse's survival.

It is paramount to obtain a definitive diagnosis for clinical signs of encephalitis in the horse to justify and institute effective control measures because of the risk of these viruses to the health and well-being of both humans and equine livestock. The viruses of EEE, WEE, and VEE frequently can be isolated or detected after death in brain material of diseased horses by the use of cell cultures (e.g., Vero cells), through intracerebral inoculation of suckling mice, and by detection of specific nucleotide sequences using reverse transcriptase–polymerase chain reaction (RT-PCR) technology.[11,144,151-157] Blood is an inappropriate specimen for virus recovery because usually no circulating virus is present when signs of encephalitis become apparent. In an epidemic situation, however, it may be possible to isolate the virus from nonencephalitic horses in the affected group, particularly if they have increased body temperatures. The cytopathic or lethal effects of the virus in cell cultures or experimental animals can be inhibited by the use of specific antisera, and in this way the virus involved may be specifically identified.

Currently, no reliable antemortem diagnostic tests are available to detect virus in clinically affected horses, and serology provides the mainstay of presumptive antemortem diagnosis. The demonstration of specific immunoglobulin M (IgM) antibody (dilution of 1:400) suggests recent infection.[158] The detection of IgM antibody in CSF (if available) is even more conclusive. Rising antibody titers to EEE, WEE, or VEE virus in the sera of horses that survive can be detected by testing of acute-phase and convalescent-phase sera. Even in endemic areas, it is not possible to diagnose or differentiate EEE, WEE, or VEE in the horse with any certainty based on clinical signs and epidemiologic circumstances. Rabies, hepatic encephalopathy, and equine protozoal myeloencephalitis are the major diseases that must be considered in the differential diagnosis in the Western Hemisphere. Other diseases that should be considered in the differential diagnosis are equine herpesvirus type 1 infection of the central nervous system, leukoencephalomalacia (a neuromycotoxicosis caused by the ingestion of maize infected with *Fusarium moniliforme*), and ataxia as a result of the cervical vertebral malformation.

PATHOLOGIC FINDINGS

In horses, brain lesions are thought to be the direct result of viral replication and are characterized by necrotizing encephalitis with neuronal dysfunction.[152,159-161] No consistent gross lesions are found in horses that die of EEE, WEE, or VEE. Histologically, neuronal necrosis with neurophagia, marked perivascular cuffing with both mononuclear and polymorphonuclear leukocytes, and focal and diffuse microglial proliferation are evident. The lesions are more pronounced in the gray matter than in the white matter of the brain. Lesions are most marked in the cerebral cortex, thalamus, and hypothalamus, whereas the spinal cord is mildly affected. Severe lesions usually occur more often in the cervical spinal cord than in lumbar cord segments. Organisms may be demonstrated in affected CNS tissues by immunohistochemistry.

THERAPY

No known antiviral medications demonstrate reliable activity against alphaviruses, and treatment of disease in affected horses is supportive. The survival rate for EEE infection is low compared with other infectious encephalitides. In most cases, horses die 3 to 5 days after onset of signs.

Corticosteroids should be considered as a component of therapy for horses with neurologic signs consistent with viral encephalitis and neutrophilic CSF. If administered early, corticosteroids (to reduce brain edema) and intravenous fluids may aid recovery. In human patients, treatment with methylprednisolone (1000 mg/100-kg patient) is often recommended. Administration of flunixin meglumine (1.1 mg/kg q12h IV) or other antiinflammatory medications to horses with EEE does not often result in the dramatic response frequently observed in horses with West Nile virus. Mannitol (0.25-2.0 g/kg q24h IV) may assist in the control of brain edema. Detomidine hydrochloride (0.02-0.04 mg/kg IV or IM) is effective for prolonged tranquilization.

Intravenous immunoglobin therapy has been used in humans for both its proposed neutralization of virus and immunomodulatory effects. IFN-α is a relatively common therapy; its recommendation is based on anecdotal reports in the human and veterinary literature. Limited information regarding the efficacy of IFN-α in the horse is available.

PREVENTION

The alphaviruses are not stable in the environment and are easily inactivated by common disinfectants. Both mosquito control and immunization of horses are important in control of EEE and VEE epizootics. Vector control can be achieved through reducing the breeding activities of mosquitoes by implementing appropriate water management systems, although this can be difficult in extensively rural areas.[162-165] The widespread dispersal (usually achieved by aerial spraying) of insecticides has been used successfully, although a number of critical factors need to be considered before embarking on such a step. Concern over indiscriminate spraying of insecticides can be mitigated in some circumstances if the biology of the mosquito vector is well known. For example, in northern Florida, where EEE is endemic, treating the pools of water in which *Culiseta melanura* breeds with a larvicide is often practical and economically feasible on those farms with valuable horses.[166] Swamps with soil types that support the breeding of *Cs. melanura* can often be recognized by the non-entomologist by the presence of the loblolly bay tree *(Gordonia lasianthus)*; this broadleaf evergreen tree grows to a height of about 30 feet and can easily be recognized by its white, magnolia-like flowers and serrated leaves. Risk assessment can be assisted by geographic mapping of large areas where mosquitoes breed by using thematic mappers, such as those on orbiting satellites.

Immunization of horses has proved highly effective as an adjunct to other control measures, particularly in outbreaks of VEE in which horses may serve as a source of infection for mosquitoes.[167,168] Currently, bivalent vaccines (usually consisting of formaldehyde-inactivated virus) are commercially available against EEE and WEE. These vaccines require a primary and secondary immunization schedule about a month apart, followed by biannual boosters. The vaccines are not particularly effective in protecting foals and yearling horses, for reasons that are not understood.[147] Broodmares should be vaccinated at least 4 to 6 weeks before foaling to ensure adequate colostral transfer of antibodies. Interference with production of neutralizing antibody has been demonstrated in foals that receive EEE-positive colostrum; however, immunotolerance does not occur. Vaccines should commence in foals between 4 and 6 months of age, and three injections should be given for the primary immunization series.

The 1969–1971 VEE epidemic in Central America and the southern United States was controlled partially by immunizing large numbers of horses with an attenuated VEE virus strain, TC-83.[167,168] This vaccine strain was produced by serial passage of an epidemic variant in guinea pig cell cultures. Because of concerns over the presence of low-level viremia in some horses and the possible transmission of vaccine virus between horses by mosquitoes and reversion to virulence, inactivated vaccines against VEE are now available for use in horses. These vaccines are not widely used in North America because they compromise the international movement of horses for competition and breeding.

The distinct possibility exists that VEE outbreaks could be completely prevented if sustained and widespread vaccination with live, attenuated VEE vaccines was performed in Central and South America.[76] Public health and animal industry officials should consider maintaining vast quantities of the live attenuated TC-83 vaccine. The use of the formalin inactivated vaccine (usually marketed as a multivalent antigen) is discouraged in VEE endemic areas because of the need for multiple vaccinations (and thus delayed onset of protection), short-lived immunity to VEE, lack of long-term compliance from agricultural officials and the horse-owning public in endemic locales, and concern of limited response to the live vaccine in horses immunized recently with a killed product.

Surveillance for encroachment of alphaviruses in new geographic locales is also paramount to control. Most southern U.S. states have encephalitis testing programs that offer subsidized testing for horses with suspected viral encephalitis. Enhanced passive surveillance for alphaviruses should be undertaken when environmental conditions are favorable. For example, hurricanes were implicated in the VEE outbreak in Mexico in 1995. Given that the United States has experienced intense hurricane activity in 2004 and 2005, enhanced surveillance for epizootic VEE should logically be undertaken.

PUBLIC HEALTH CONSIDERATIONS

Alphaviruses are pathogenic for people but require a vector for transmission to occur. The horse does not develop a sufficient level of viremia with EEE and WEE to act as a reservoir or an amplifying host for these viruses. In contrast, horses are considered the most important species for amplification of virus in epizootic VEE. Therefore, control measures should be implemented to limit new exposure of horses in locales that are undergoing epizootic VEE. This includes restriction of horse movement; clinically normal horses may be viremic, and the disease can be translocated. Horses should be vaccinated and sprayed frequently with permethrin-based products. Mosquito abatement efforts should be pursued. Blood and tissues from VEE horses should be handled as infectious and biohazardous materials.

REFERENCES

See the CD-ROM for a list of references linked to the abstract in PubMed.

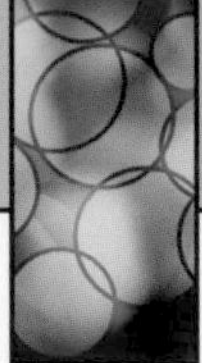

CHAPTER • 21

Flavivirus Infections

Maureen T. Long

Before the North American epizootic of *West Nile virus* (WNV), several features of flavivirus outbreaks were noted by scientists in the public health community.[1] First, outbreaks with these viruses were occurring in new locales over the previous 20 years. Second, outbreaks with apparent clinical disease were becoming more frequent. Third, enhanced pathogenicity for humans was often observed. Fourth, development of better molecular technologies demonstrated increased viral variation within this group of viruses (likely accounting for the trends just mentioned).

Emergence of new diseases or new outbreaks of previously described diseases are largely the product of globalization. This has created an interface of exotic disease and new interfacing with people, pests, and animals traveling over unprecedented distances.[1] Before 1999, the U.S. equine practitioner had little familiarity with flaviviruses. Horse owners typically did not even know these diseases existed. After WNV was first identified in the United States, the widespread outbreak in humans and horses residing in middle and northern latitudes of the North American continent was not predicted.[2-4]

Some of the most important scientific landmarks in human and veterinary health have centered on flaviviral infections. In 1900, Walter Reed and colleagues demonstrated that the causative agent of *yellow fever* (YF) was a filterable agent or virus. This was also the first agent that was determined to be transmitted by arthropods,[5] allowing the eradication of YF from coastal cities of North America and Cuba. The molecular sequencing of uncultivable *hepatitis* C *virus* (HCV) allowed development of screening tests, which has resulted in a significant decrease in transfusion-related transmission of HCV.[6,7]

ETIOLOGY

The family *Flaviviridae* consists of a pathologically active group of viruses composed of three genera that are found worldwide.[8] This group of viruses has the distinction of containing some of the most important human pathogens in the world. The genus *Flavivirus* contains many viruses (approximately 70), which are usually transmitted by ticks or mosquitoes (some are through direct contact, or the vector is unknown) and organized into groups according to cross-neutralization with polyclonal hyperimmune mouse ascites (Table 21-1). About one fourth of these viruses are of veterinary importance. The other two genera have viruses of veterinary and human importance, with the genus *Pestivirus* containing the ubiquitous *bovine diarrhea virus* (BVD), and *Hepacivirus* containing the human pathogen HCV. At least half the members of *Flaviviridae* are zoonotic.

The members of the *Japanese encephalitis* (JE) serogroup that are most likely to cause overt disease in horses are JE virus (JEV), WNV, and *Kunjin virus* (KV; an Australian flavivirus, now considered a variant of WNV).[9] Disease in horses caused by *Murray Valley fever* (MVF) is geographically restricted to the South Pacific and is sporadic in occurrence.[10-12] Several other members of this group and those belonging to the other major groups of flaviviruses have been detected serologically in horses, with limited reports of clinical disease. Published reports of experimental reproduction of disease in horses are lacking for many of these viruses (see Table 21-1). The following discussion emphasizes WNV and JEV.

As with other members of the *Flaviviridae,* WNV (and JEV) are positive–sense, single-stranded ribonucleic acid (RNA) viruses measuring approximately 50 nm.[6] The virions are spherical and enveloped with the C protein, making up a nucleocapsid of about 25 nm. Electron microscopy reveals an icosahedral symmetry of the envelope and capsid of these viruses. An approximately 11-kilobase (kb) genome contains a single open reading frame (ORF) that is translated in its entirety and cleaved into 10 viral proteins by both cell and viral proteases[13,14] (Fig. 21-1). There are three structural and seven nonstructural proteins; the structural proteins include the capsid (C), premembrane (prM) and membrane (M), and envelope (E) proteins. The nonstructural (NS) proteins, numbered 1 through 5, are cleaved after translation to form NS1, NS2A, NS2B, NS3, NS4A, NS4B, and NS5 and are required for viral replication and assembly.

The final M protein and the E protein are important in virulence for the JE group[15-20] (see Fig. 21-2). The M protein is formed from a precursor protein (prM protein), which is modified as immature virions are secreted through the Golgi network of the cell, leaving the C-terminal portion of the protein inserted in the envelope of the mature virion. The E protein is only secreted in its native conformation through association with the prM protein. The E protein is the immunodominant viral protein and exists in the virion as a β-pleated sheet arranged head to tail, with the distal ends anchored in the membrane. This protein is dimeric, held together with intermolecular disulfide bonds, and lies flat against the lipid bilayer. This large protein is important in receptor ligand binding and fusion to cells, the latter being pH dependent. There are three major domains of this protein in WNV. Domain II contains a region important to virus binding in the brain. Domain III is important for vector and host virulence.[21] In WNV, glycolysis of the E protein is strain dependent and is associated with virulence. Viral binding to glycosaminoglycan on cells changes virulence in both JEV and WNV.

The NS proteins in flaviviruses are structurally and functionally similar and are involved in synthesis of viral RNA.[22,23] The glycoprotein NS1 is essential for virus function and appears to be important for cell activation as part of viral synthesis.[24-26] NS1 is found on cell membranes of infected cells and must interact with NS4A in this process. NS2A is formed by cleavage of full-length NS2. Changes in the C-terminal of this protein results in loss of viral replicative ability.[27] In addition,

Table • **21-1**

Partial Taxonomic Structure, Host, and Primary Vector of Genus Flavivirus, *Family* Flaviviridae*

SEROLOGIC GROUP	SPECIES NAME	AMPLIFYING NONVECTOR HOSTS	PRIMARY VECTOR SPECIES	LOCATION
Tick-Borne Viruses				
Mammalian tick-borne virus group	Deer tick virus	Rodents? Bats?	*Ixodes* ticks	Australia
	Kadam virus		*Ixodes dammini*	Uganda, Saudi Arabia
	Kyasanur Forest disease virus	Monkey (?), with porcupines, rats, and mice as reservoirs	*Haemophsalis spinigera*	India
	Langat virus	Rats and other small mammals	Tick	Southeast Asia, Russia
	Omsk hemorrhagic fever virus	Rats and other small mammals	*Dermacentor*	Russia
	Powassan virus	Lagomorphs, rodents, mice, skunks, rabbit Experimental reproduction in horses	*Dermacentor andersoni*	North America, Russia
	Royal Farm virus	Small mammals, likely small ruminants	*Ixodes ricinus*	Afghanistan
	Tick-borne encephalitis virus	Dogs, sheep, goats, cattle, horses	*Ixodes ricinus*	Europe, Asian Russia, China
	Louping ill virus	Sheep and grouse	*Ixodes ricinus*	
Seabird tick-borne virus group	Refer to NCBI*	Refer to NCBI*	Refer to NCBI*	Refer to NCBI*
Mosquito-Borne Viruses				
Aroa virus group	Refer to NCBI*	Rodents	Mosquito	Venezuela
Dengue virus group	Refer to NCBI*	Human and nonhuman primates	*Aedes* spp.	Tropical/subtropical
Entebbe virus group	Refer to NCBI*	Humans, monkeys, bats	(?) Likely *Aedes*	Uganda
Japanese encephalitis virus group	Japanese encephalitis virus	Birds, pigs	*Culex* spp.	Asia, Pacific, Australia
	Cacipacore Koutango		*Culex* spp. and ticks	Senegal, Central African Republic
	Murray Valley virus	Birds: night herons and cormorants Pigs	*Culex annulirostris*	Australia, New Guinea
	St. Louis encephalitis virus	Birds	*Culex* spp.	North, Central, and South America
	West Nile virus	House sparrows (passerines), crows, birds of prey	*Culex* spp.	Africa, Middle East, Europe, North America, Central America
	Yaoundé virus	Avian	*Culex* spp.	Central African Republic
Kokobera virus group	Refer to NCBI*	Macropods, horses?†	*Culex annulirostris*	Australia New Guinea
Ntaya virus group	Refer to NCBI*	Avian Small ruminants	*Culex* spp.	Central and South Africa
Spondweni virus group	Refer to NCBI*	Unknown; sylvatic, avian	*Mansonii* spp.	Africa
Yellow fever virus group	Refer to NCBI*	Monkeys, edentates, marsupials, rodents	*Aedes* spp.	Worldwide tropical areas
No Known Vector				
Modoc virus group	Refer to NCBI*	Rodents	?	Western United States
Rio Bravo virus group	Refer to NCBI*	Bats	?	United States, Mexico

*Modified from the International Committee on Taxonomy of Viruses; http://www.ncbi.nih.gov/ICTVdb?Ictv/fs_flaiv.htm#Genus1.
†Serologic evidence only.

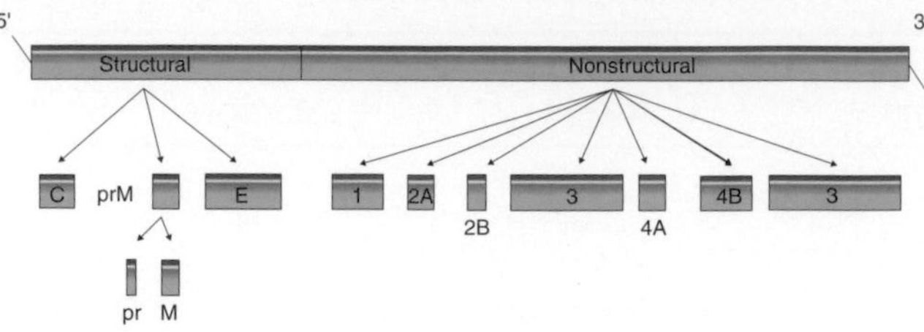

Fig. 21-1 Idealized genomic organization of members of the genus *Flavivirus*. This is a positive-sense single-stranded RNA virus consisting of two structural proteins and at least seven nonstructural proteins.

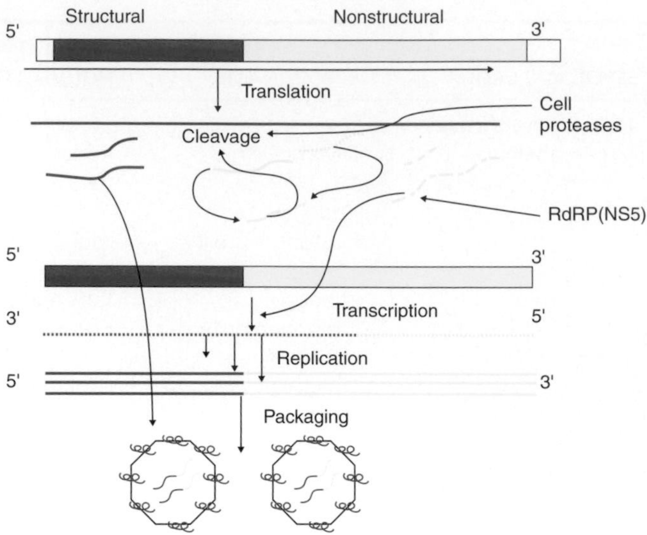

Fig. 21-2 Flavivirus replication cycle that demonstrates a first round of translation of the virus to produce proteins that are cleaved by host and viral proteases. The production of a positive-strand virus by viral proteins results in progeny that are packaged in mature virions. Rounds of translation and replication occur, and virus is released by cell lysis or, more often, budding from the infected cell.

NS2B complexes with NS3 to form a serine protease.[27-29] The NS3 protein is highly conserved between flaviviruses and, at the N-terminal, encodes a serine protease with sequences consistent with the trypsin superfamily. The C-terminal of this protein has sequences typical of RNA helicases and triphosphatases.[30] The NS4B protein appears to block antiviral cytokines.[31] The NS5 protein is essential for viral replication by forming the "cap" at the 5′ end of a genome. Viruses, as opposed to eukaryotic cells, have a type I cap at the end of the genome, which in a cytoplasmic virus such as WNV, must be formed solely by viral proteins. In addition, this is the site of the viral *RNA-dependent RNA polymerase* (RdRp), an essential protein for formation of negative-strand RNA from the genome of the positive-strand "parent" RNA virus.[31,32]

West Nile virus (and members of the JE serogroup) are thought to infect the cell through glycoprotein receptors that are likely highly conserved by hosts.[32-34] After receptor-mediated endocytosis, there is fusion of the viral membrane with membranes of the endosomal vesicle, and the nucleoprotein is released into the cytoplasm. After translation, the serine protease NS2B-NS3A, along with cell proteases, cleaves the polyprotein at multiple sites to generate viral proteins (Fig. 21-2). The RdRp copies the negative-strand RNA from the genomic RNA template. These negative-strand RNAs become templates for the synthesis of new genomic RNAs. There are likely alternating periods of replication and translation until a sufficient pool of structural proteins has accumulated. Once there is a pool of genomic RNA, virion assembly occurs in the rough endoplasmic reticulum (ER) membranes. Immature virions, still with the prM, accumulate in vesicles and are transported through the host secretory pathway, where the E and prM proteins are modified. Virions are transported to the plasma membrane in vesicles and released by exocytosis. Mammalian cells will release progeny virus within 10 to 12 hours after infection.

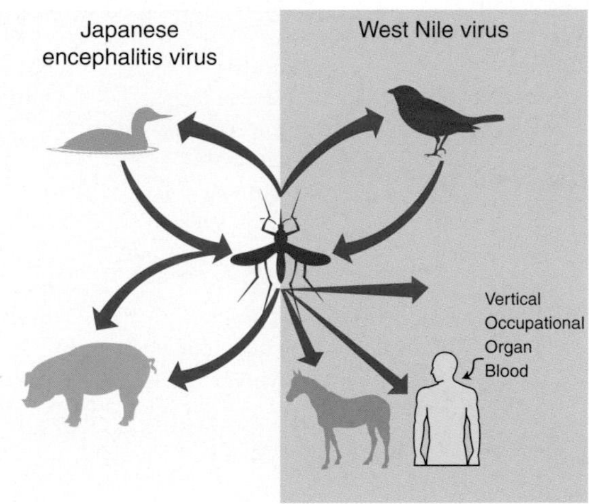

Fig. 21-3 West Nile virus (WNV) and Japanese encephalitis (JE) virus life cycle in which the primary transmission cycle is between avian or porcine reservoirs and mosquitoes. Horses and humans are aberrant hosts.

EPIDEMIOLOGY

Life Cycle

Japanese encephalitis serogroup viruses are vector-borne diseases, with transmission occurring to avian and mammalian hosts from blood meal–seeking mosquitoes[35] (Fig. 21-3). Virus is either maintained or cycled between vectors, and biologic amplification occurs within the vector species. Vertical transmission within vectors must occur for maintenance of the respective virus within a geographic area.[36] The primary nonarthropod reservoir hosts for these viruses, in which the virus is amplified and transmitted to vectors, are birds. Horses and humans are "dead-end" hosts and do not amplify the virus in quantities sufficient to infect mosquitoes. In JE, swine are considered important amplifying hosts.

Additional modes of transmission have been identified in the recent North American WNV outbreak. First, transmission through oral ingestion has been proven in both avian and mammalian hosts, and oral and cloacal shedding has been demonstrated in birds.[37-41] Second, WNV may be transmitted through contaminated blood transfusion or organ transplantation if donors are viremic.[42-46] Third, vertical transmission through placenta and milk has been demonstrated in people.[44,47,48] This last feature is important in JE and several JE serogroup virus infections.

Recent Epizootology

The largest documented outbreak of equine neurologic disease caused by a flavivirus began in 1999 with WNV encroachment into the United States (U.S.). West Nile virus was first detected in 1999 in New York City. Since that time, more than 25,000 cases of equine West Nile encephalomyelitis (WNE), with an estimated 30% to 40% case-fatality rate, have been reported in horses in the U.S. Overt clinical disease is still common in most states, with 3000 human cases and 914 equine cases reported during the 2005 arbovirus season.[49] In 2005, 119 human deaths occurred as a result of WNV infection.[50] California has reported equine mortality rates of greater than 40% for 2 years.

During 1999, WNV caused human disease in the U.S. during the weeks of July 25 to September 12, and initial surveillance identified bird mortality and equine infection as features of the disease.[51,52] Illness was detected in 60 people, with seven deaths occurring in four New York boroughs and two neighboring New York counties. During that first year, WNV was detected in four states and 12 counties by human and equine serology and testing of live and dead birds. Evidence of encroachment based on human, equine, avian, and mosquito testing was detected in 12 states and 133 individual counties in 2000, with slightly more equine cases (65) and fewer human cases (21) reported in three of those states.[53,54] For that year, 4139 dead birds representing more than 76 species were reported as WNV infected. Other seropositive mammals that year included bats, rodents, rabbits, cats, raccoons, and skunks.

The WNV outbreak reached epizootic proportions in 2001 when many equine cases and high levels of bird mortality were reported in the southeastern U.S., especially in southern Georgia and Florida.[55] WNV was reported in 27 states and 359 counties, with an expansion of the arbovirus season from June 27 to December 18 in 2001. Human illness was confirmed in 66 people, and 7333 dead birds tested positive for WNV. Corvid susceptibility became more apparent, with 5154 positive crows and 966 positive blue jays. In 2001, there were 733 confirmed cases of equine encephalomyelitis in 19 states and 127 counties.[55] In 2002, explosive WNV activity occurred in 2289 U.S. counties and 44 states, with 3389 cases of WNV disease reported in people, of which 2354 persons had neuroinvasive symptoms resulting in 201 deaths.[56] There were 4717 horses reported with confirmed WNV disease, with 30% to 35% mortality in affected horses[57] (Fig. 21-4).

By 2005, WNV had been identified in all the 48 continental U.S. states.[58] Canadian provinces reporting disease included Quebec, Ontario, Manitoba, Saskatchewan, and Alberta, with New Brunswick and Nova Scotia reporting evidence of WNV-positive birds.[59] Serologic evidence of WNV has been reported in the Latin American countries of the Dominican Republic, Mexico, Guadeloupe, El Salvatore, Puerto Rico, Cayman Islands, Jamaica, Belize, and Cuba.[41,60-65] The incidence of equine and human disease appears low for Central and South America and the Caribbean compared with the United States.[66]

Japanese encephalitis virus causes 30,000 to 50,000 human encephalitis cases annually worldwide, with endemic

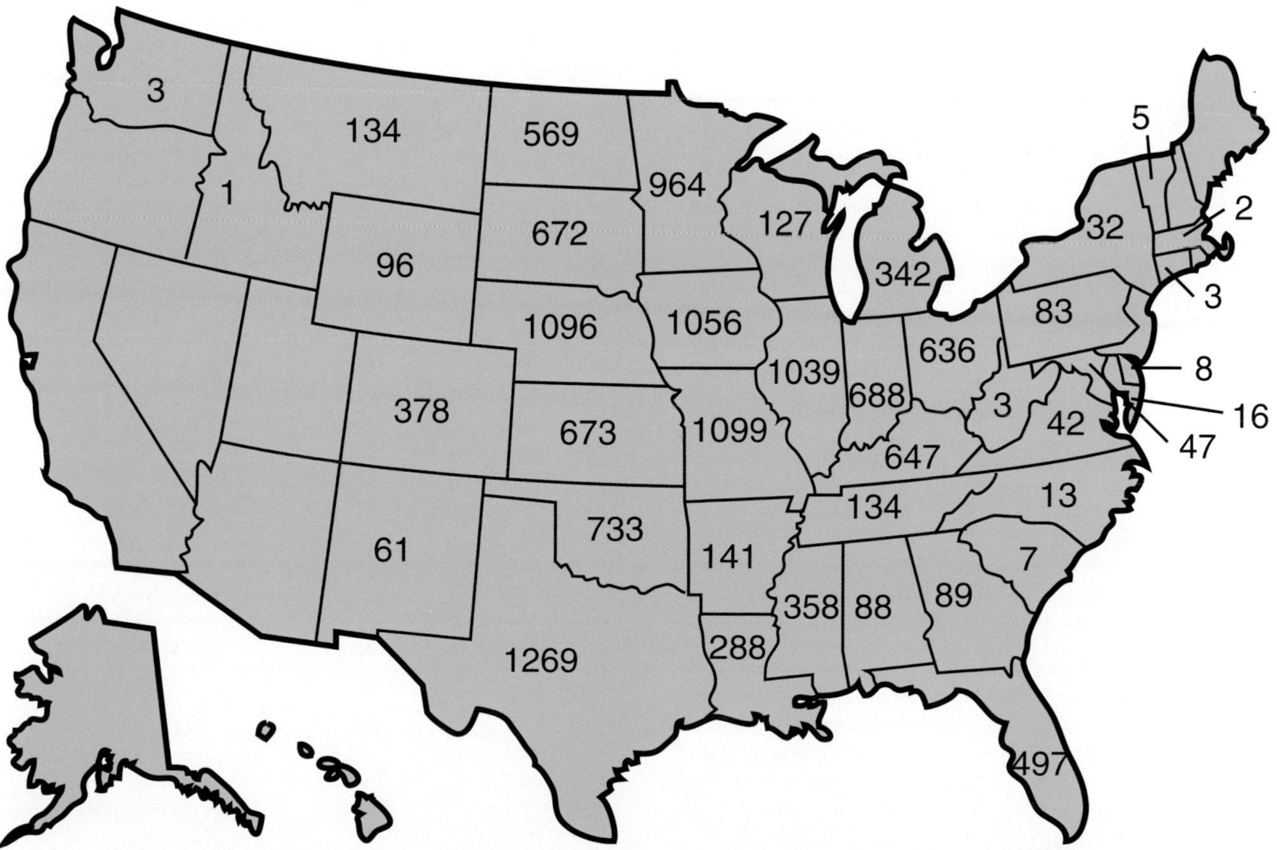

Fig. 21-4 Map of the United States depicting the numbers of reported cases of West Nile virus encephalomyelitis (WNE) in horses during 2002, the largest epizootic year since encroachment in 1999.

areas including China, the southeast region of the Russian Federation, South and Southeast Asia, and Australia. Exact numbers of horses with clinical JE are difficult to ascertain; however, there are reports of JE isolation from horses in Taiwan, China, Pakistan, and Australia in the literature since the 1980s. Outbreaks in horses have also been reported in India, Nepal, the Philippines, Sri Lanka, and Northern Thailand. Seroconversion of young horses over their first year of exposure in Hong Kong is as high as 63% in some locales.

The spread and yearly incidence of JE serogroup viruses coincides with the availability of vectors and reservoir hosts with transmission potential. Thus, outbreaks are seasonal and reflect mosquito activity. *Culex* species of mosquitoes are considered the primary mosquito vector for the JE serogroup.[41,67-70] WNV has been detected in approximately 60 species of North American mosquito, but the overall vector efficiency (moderate to high) and wide range of feeding activity of the *Culex* indicate that the North American WNV outbreak is propelled mainly by this genus.[71] Most of the data supporting this conclusion is based on vector efficiency studies under laboratory conditions, experimental feeding studies, and frequency of identification of WNV in mosquito pools.[71,72] In the northeastern U.S., more than half the WNV-positive mosquito pools are *Cx. pipiens*.[73-77] In the western U.S., populations of the highly efficient *Cx. tarsalis* constitute the majority of positive pools, with *Cx. pipiens* the next most frequently found *Culex* species.[78-80] In the southeastern U.S., *Cx. quinquefasciatus* and *Cx. nigripalpus* have the highest WNV infection rates.[81-85] In the southwestern U.S., epidemics are most often associated with positive mosquito pools of *Cx. quinquefasciatus*, *Cx. tarsalis*, and *Cx. pipiens*.[77,86-89] *Culex restuans*, frequently identified as part of the "*Cx. pipiens*" complex, is often one of the top five positive species.[71,89]

Although *Culex* is important in the epidemiology and spread of WNV, relatively little is known regarding the actual vector of transmission to the horse. Blood meal analysis suggests that *Cx. pipiens* mosquitoes are primarily avian feeders. Mammalian feeders include mainly *Anopheles quadrimaculatus*, *Coquillettidia perturbans*, and *Aedes albopictus*.[90,91] Analysis of *Cx. quinquefasciatus* has detected both human and bird blood meals, whereas *Ae. albopictus* most often contains human blood.[92] *Culex salinarius* reportedly has the most variable feeding habits, which is important for transmission between different host species. *Culex pipiens* and *Cx. salinarius* are likely the most important bridge vectors.

Experimental infection of horses through mosquito transmission studies is accomplished with *Ae. albopictus*, a common mammalian feeder and moderately efficient vector of WNV.[93,94] In studies thus far involving low numbers of horses, 9 of 10 horses became viremic, and all seroconverted to the virus. The significance of this vector under natural conditions is unknown. Members of the *Culex tritaeniorhynchus* group of mosquitoes are the most important vectors for JE, and this mosquito was used in the experimental transmission and reproduction of disease in horses.

Several species of ticks have been investigated for potential to transmit WNV. Transtadial transmission was demonstrated in one study of *Ixodes* ticks, but failed to occur in a second study with these ticks.[95,96] *Carios capensis* can transmit WNV under experimental conditions to ducklings, and *Ornithodoros moubata* can transmit WNV under experimental conditions to mice.[96,97]

A *reservoir host* is one in which a pathogen is amplified in vivo so that it can be transmitted to a vector species.[75] A blood meal taken from a mammal containing 10^5 to 10^7 plaque-forming units per milliliter (PFU/mL) of WNV results in infection of 30% to 100% of feeding mosquitoes, respectively. Humans voluntarily infected (with the Egyptian strain of WNV) developed virus titers of 10^3 to 10^5 PFU/mL. In horses the maximal titer after infection with this strain was similar.[98] Titers greater than 10^4 PFU/ml WNV in plasma are inconsistently detected in cats, and this species may be capable of short-term infectivity for mosquitoes.[99]

Viral titers capable of transmitting JEV are similar to WNV. Swine are a notable reservoir host for JE (with little indication that the same is true for WNV in the U.S.). The primary clinical manifestation of JE infection in swine is abortion. Affected litters contain weak pigs with limited survival, dead fresh term fetuses, or mummies. Semen from infected boars contains infectious virus, and the semen has decreased sperm count and motility.

To date, more than 300 species of birds have been reported as WNV positive in the U.S., with 16 new species identified during the 2005 season.[50,100] High levels of viral amplification occur in many bird species, especially Passeriformes (e.g., songbirds) and Charadriiformes (e.g., shorebirds);[40] the house sparrow is considered the most important amplifying host for WNV (Table 21-2). Although the crow is one of the most competent vectors, sparrows have a lower mortality and thus longer days of infectious virus. Strigiformes (e.g., owls) and Falconiformes (e.g., falcons) develop a viremia of shorter duration, but sufficient to infect mosquitoes. Psittaciformes

Table • **21-2**

Top U.S. Avian Hosts for West Nile Virus by Vector Competence

ORDER (FAMILY)	COMMON NAME (TOP 8 SPECIES BY LEVEL OF VIREMIA)	MORTALITY
Passeriformes *(Corvidae)*	Blue jay	High
Passeriformes *(Icteridae)*	Common grackle	High
Passeriformes *(Fringillidae)*	House finch	Moderately high
Passeriformes *(Corvidae)*	American crow	High
Passeriformes *(Passeridae)*	House sparrow	Low to moderate
Charadriiformes *(Laridae)*	Ring-billed gull	Moderate
Passeriformes *(Corvidae)*	Black-billed magpie	Moderate
Passeriformes *(Corvidae)*	Fish crow	Low to moderate

Modified from Komar N: *Adv Virus Res* 61:185-234, 2003.

(e.g., parrots) and Galliformes (e.g., game birds) develop the lowest viremias. By contrast, Anseriformes (e.g., waterfowl) are considered the most efficient avian reservoirs of JE and are essential for the spread of this virus through avian flyways.

Although corvid susceptibility has been described as unique to the North American outbreak, early studies with the Egyptian WNV strain produced high mortality in crows.[101,102] Corvids develop very high viremia with very high mortality rates from WNV, but even with their high mortality, they are likely efficient reservoirs.[37,39,40,103] Corvid susceptibility to WNV in the U.S. outbreak is an important indication of local activity and encroachment in the U.S. Dead bird counts are an important surveillance tool.

Occurrence of disease caused by JEV and WNV in horses and people reflects vector activity, seasonal in temperate regions and year-round in subtropical and tropical regions. Intense virus activity in the U.S. begins in July, with a peak incidence in September and October.[104-107] Temperature-dependent spatial modeling supports these disease dynamics, with risk increasing from 25% in late August to greater than 75% by the second week of September.[108-110] A drop in ambient temperature with soft frost usually results in a rapid decrease in reporting activity.[111,112] The appearance of disease from JE is actually highly variable depending on the locale. Seasonal occurrence of disease in specific locales should be considered to facilitate timing of equine athletic events and to tailor vaccination regimens appropriately.

Older people appear more susceptible to neuroinvasive disease from both JEV and WNV. This age bias in reporting appears true, at least for WNV, in horses.[41,50,53,113-115] Although men are more frequently affected with neuroinvasive disease, no breed or gender predilection seems to exist in horses. In one study of horses with WNV encephalomyelitis, female horses were 2.9 times more likely to die than male horses with neurologic signs.[116-118]

The remarkably explosive North American outbreak of WNV has introduced new potential hosts for the virus. Seropositive, free-ranging mammals include the big brown bat, little brown bat, eastern chipmunk, eastern gray squirrel, eastern striped skunk, white-tailed deer, and the brown bear.[41,75,100,119] Neurologic disease has been confirmed as WNV in gray squirrels and fox squirrels.[120] Alligators can have an extremely high titer of viremia and may be an important reservoir for WNV in the southeastern U.S.[119] There are reports of both farmed and free-ranging alligators with neurologic signs from which WNV has been isolated. In farm-raised alligators, cloacal shedding of virus has been demonstrated, with oral infection likely.

Serologic evidence of natural infection has been demonstrated in domestic dogs and cats.[37,38,121] Experimental infection of cats resulted in a mild transient fever in some cats and a short-term viremia high enough to possibly transmit to mosquitoes.[121] Oral transmission to cats has also been documented. New World camelids develop neurologic disease with natural exposure to WNV.[122,123]

PATHOGENESIS

Mammalian disease caused by infection with the JE serogroup viruses uniformly demonstrates predilection of these viruses for nervous tissues. Neurologic disease in the horse consists of changes in mentation, signs consistent with spinal cord abnormalities, and defects in cranial nerves of the hindbrain.[124-134] The change in behavior likely results from viral infection and pathology induced in the neurons of the thalamus, medulla, and pons, with limited viral load in the cerebrum.[126,127,135] Although the thalamus integrates all sensory input to higher centers, lesions within the midbrain and rostral pons may affect the reticular formation, which has an important role in regulation of consciousness.[134,136] The reticular formation projects to the thalamus, which in turn sends diffuse projections to the entire cortex.[134] This formation also travels directly to the base of the forebrain, which is the source of cholinergic stimulation to the entire cerebral cortex. Disturbances of the reticular formation and the midbrain may induce behavioral changes ranging from severe aggression to somnolence and even coma.

West Nile virus–induced motor deficits are multifocal, asymmetric, and primarily characterized by weakness and ataxia.[126-128,132,135,137,138] These two clinical signs are likely a reflection of brain and spinal cord disease through direct infection of the spinal cord, interruption of motor tracts in the hindbrain, and loss of fine motor control through infection of the large nuclei of the thalamus and the basal ganglia. Ataxia can be attributable to interruption of general proprioception. Although ataxia is commonly detected and could be profound, many horses have difficulty standing primarily because of profound weakness. These clinical signs are attributable to infection of the gray matter within the midbrain and hindbrain. In the spinal cord, lesions consisting of perivascular cuffing and glosis tend to increase in frequency and severity caudally, with the most severe lesions appearing in the lumbar cord compared with the cervical cord.[132] Lower motor neuron disease characterized by weakness would be a common clinical sign associated with these spinal cord lesions.

Involuntary skin and muscle fasciculations, tremors, and hyperesthesia, extremely common in WNV disease, likely result from loss of fine motor control, which is regulated mainly by the basal ganglia.[139-140] Movement disorders are detected with flavivirus infection in a long-term Parkinson-like syndrome in rats and experimental infection in monkeys.[140] Infection in the pons and medulla oblongata can explain clinical deficits of cranial nerves VII, XII, and IX.[141]

Two routes of neuroinvasion are proposed for WNV infection. In the first, WNV causes a low-level viremia, followed by replication in the lymph nodes and entry into the CNS across the blood-brain barrier.[142] The second proposes transaxonal transmission.[143] In the first theory, it is hypothesized that systemic viral infection results in local cytokine responses that increase the permeability of the blood-brain barrier to viral invasion. In particular, tumor necrosis factor alpha (TNF-α) increases vascular permeability and allows infection of peripheral nerves.[144] Evidence indicates that toll-like receptors are crucial for entry of WNV into the central nervous system (CNS), whether by neuronal or vascular route.[145,146]

Experimental rodent models demonstrate that WNV has a primary predilection for neural tissues of the vertebrate host.[142,147-149] Intraperitoneal injection of WNV (10^2 PFU) into 8- to 12-week-old mice results in dissemination into the CNS by 4 to 6 days after inoculation. The time course of infection in the hamster is similar. Experimental infection of horses results in viremia at days 3 to 5 and clinical signs in 7 to 10 days.[94,150] WNV inoculation into the CNS results in direct infection of nerve cell bodies. In rodent models, initial replication occurs in the basal ganglia, with subsequent dissemination to the cortex, cerebellum, and hippocampus.[151-155] The large neurons of the ventral or anterior horns are infected later in the course of disease.

In mammalian hosts, the actual virus load in neuronal tissues is low, indicating the possibility of another mechanism for severe neurologic clinical signs. Although cell lysis occurs with viral replication, WNV also induces apoptosis in neurons, as demonstrated in cell culture and in vivo.[151] This apoptosis can be induced by the capsid protein through the caspase-9 pathway in the mitochondria. Another mediator of neuronal injury is the host immune response. Although CD8 T cells may be important in long-term protective immune responses, lesions in brains of mice with fatal WNV are predominantly composed of $CD8^+$ T cells.[156,157]

CLINICAL FINDINGS

Japanese encephalitis and WNV produce similar clinical signs, except that fatal JEV infection in horses usually results in blindness, coma, and death, whereas these signs are relatively limited in WNE horses.[158,159] For both these infections, there is evidence of widespread subclinical infection in both people and horses. Horses develop clinical signs when infected with the neurally invasive lineage type I WNV, whereas infection with the African lineage type II viruses is universally subclinical in nature.[160,161] Kunjin virus causes milder clinical disease in horses. Infection with JEV may result in severe clinical disease in naive horses, but great variation in virulence is seen in JE viruses.

When clinically apparent disease occurs, both systemic and neurologic abnormalities are observed in horses with WNV. A mild to moderate increase in rectal temperature (38.6°-39.4° C [102°-103° F]), anorexia, and depression are the most common initial systemic signs.[124] Abdominal pain or a colic episode may be the first clinical presentation.[124,127,162,163] Gait abnormalities, including overt lameness or dragging of a limb, before development of an obvious neurologic syndrome have also been reported. Both spinal cord disease and moderate mental aberrations occur. Onset of neurologic signs is frequently sudden and progressive, and the exact course of disease in any one animal is unpredictable.

The major hallmarks of equine WNV encephalomyelitis are muscle fasciculations and changes in personality. Many horses have periods of hyperexcitability and apprehension, sometimes to the point of aggression. Frequently a quiet horse will become hyperexcitable, and an abnormally aggressive horse will become compliant. Interspersed during periods of hyperexcitability, some horses appear to have abnormalities of sudden sleeplike activity resembling narcolepsy. This can occur to the point of cataplexy, and horses may partially or completely collapse for a short period. Some horses show a persistent change of mentation, and a state of nonresponsiveness, resembling coma, results.

Fine and coarse fasciculations of the muscles of the face and neck are common. Fasciculations can be severe and can involve all four limbs and trunk, affecting normal activities such as walking, eating, and interactions with handlers and other horses. The fasciculations are most notable at the muzzle and eyelids. Eyelid activity during this period is enhanced with light, and at times horses appear photophobic.

One of the initial signs of motor abnormality is a short, slow, stilted gait, described by observers as "lameness," with laminitis being a frequent differential diagnosis at this stage. In human patients, however, bradykinesia or slow, deliberate movement is frequently described, and this may be the equine corollary.[114] Spinal abnormalities are characterized by ataxia and paresis that can be highly asymmetric or may involve only one or two of the forelimbs or hindlimbs. This state may be of short duration, or horses may become suddenly recumbent and either die or require prolonged treatment. Horses that become recumbent often need aggressive supportive care.

Cranial nerves are frequently abnormal for short periods; weakness of the tongue, muzzle deviation, and head tilt are the most common abnormalities reported. Dysphagia has been reported, with esophageal obstruction a possible sequela. A cauda equine syndrome consisting of stranguria and rectal impaction is infrequently reported.

Overall, the combination, severity, and duration of clinical signs can be highly variable. After initial clinical signs abate, about 30% of horses experience a recrudescence in signs within the first 7 to 10 days of apparent recovery. Overall, about 30% of affected horses progress to complete paralysis of one or more limbs overall. Most of these horses are euthanized for humane reasons or die spontaneously.

Many horses will improve within 3 to 7 days of displaying clinical signs. If the horse demonstrates significant improvement, full recovery within 1 to 6 months can be expected in 90% of patients. Residual weakness and ataxia appear common, with long-term loss of the use of one or more limbs infrequently described. Mild to moderate, persistent fatigue on exercise has been observed.

Experimental infection of horses with WNV and JE has been reported in the literature using mosquito and needle challenge.[94,164] In general, for every 11 or 12 WNV infections, only one horse develops clinical signs. Horses develop a low-grade viremia within 3 to 5 days after challenge. This level of virus in the horse is not high enough to transmit back to mosquitoes, confirming that the horse is a dead-end host.

DIAGNOSIS

West Nile Virus

Ancillary diagnostic testing for horses with suspected WNV infection should include complete blood count (CBC), serum biochemistry analysis, and cerebrospinal fluid (CSF) analysis.[165,166] CBC and serum biochemistry profiles of WNV-infected horses are usually normal, but basic bloodwork can rule out systemic causes of CNS abnormalities such as liver failure. WNV-infected horses may have a mild absolute lymphopenia. Horses can have elevated muscle enzymes secondary to trauma and prolonged periods of recumbency. A frequent finding is hyponatremia, which has also been described in humans with encephalitis, potentially caused by inappropriate release of antidiuretic hormone.[167,168] CSF cell counts and protein concentration may be elevated. Differential cell counts in CSF of WNV-infected horses primarily have increased mononuclear cell populations. Protein concentrations are frequently elevated (N<70 mg/dL) and the color of the fluid can be mildly xanthochromic.[166]

No pathognomonic signs distinguish WNV infection in horses from other CNS diseases, and a full diagnostic evaluation should be pursued. Infectious CNS diseases that should be considered as differential diagnoses include alphavirus encephalitis, rabies, equine protozoal myeloencephalitis (EPM), equine herpesvirus type 1 (EHV-1), botulism, and verminous meningoencephalomyelitis (e.g., *Halicephalobus gingivalis*, *Setaria*, *Strongylus vulgaris*). Noninfectious causes to consider include hypocalcemia, tremorigenic toxicities, hepatoencephalopathy, and leukoencephalomalacia. In alphavirus encephalitis and rabies, signs of cerebral involvement are characterized by behavioral alterations, depression, seizure, and coma. The appearance of seizure and coma is rare in WNV horses. Motor function is frequently abnormal in EEE and western equine encephalitis (WEE). In WNV suspects, circling and propulsive walking may occur, but head pressing is rare. Cranial nerve signs common in EEE and WEE are also common in WNV and include head tilt, pharyngeal/laryngeal dysfunction, and paresis of the tongue. Other clinical signs of alphavirus encephalitis also observed with horses with WNV infection are muscle fasciculations, hyperesthesia, excitability, blindness, somnolence, and progression to recumbency. Mortality in nonvaccinated horses with EEE is high, approximately 80% to 100% (as in rabies). The incidence of WEE in horses is fairly low in the U.S., but mortality and severity of clinical signs would be similar to WNV. Spinal disease caused by EPM is a more difficult differential diagnosis if horses with WNV are not febrile and do not exhibit excessive muscle fasciculations. Both diseases demonstrate hindbrain disease with diffuse spinal cord abnormalities.

Confirmation of WNV infection with encephalitis in horses begins with assessment of (1) whether the horse meets the case definition based on clinical signs and (2) whether the horse resides in an area in which WNV has been confirmed in the current calendar year in mosquito, bird, human, or horse.[137] Serologic testing developed by the National Veterinary Services Laboratory (NVSL) is based on detection of the immunoglobulin M (IgM) antibody response that uniformly occurs in acutely infected horses. The preferred test is an IgM-capture enzyme-linked immunosorbent assay (MAC-ELISA).[150] Horses develop a very intense IgM response on exposure to WNV that lasts approximately 6 weeks. This immunologic reaction is much more reliable than in human infection, where a more persistent IgM response is common. Most diagnostic laboratories utilize the WNV IgM-capture ELISA (MAC) for actual confirmation of disease (increases in IgM rarely occur after vaccination). The sensitivity and specificity of this test are 81% and 100%, respectively.

In the nonvaccinated horse, a fourfold change in paired neutralizing antibody titers is confirmatory of a diagnosis of WNV infection. The most common neutralizing antibody test formats are the classic plaque reduction neutralization test (PRNT) for detecting antibody response and a more recently developed microwell format.[116,125,137,150] Vaccination induces formation of neutralizing antibody, which likely confounds interpretation of the PRNT. Since the marketing of equine WNV vaccines in 2001, reliance on the PRNT for serologic confirmatory diagnosis of WNV in horses has diminished.

Other methods for confirmation of a diagnosis of WNV include postmortem detection of WNV by polymerase chain reaction (PCR), culture, and immunohistochemistry (IHC) in CNS tissues (Fig. 21-5). Several methods for detection of WNV nucleic acids in equine tissue have been described. One uses nested PCR targeting the E protein and has demonstrated sensitivity for relatively low viral loads in equine tissues.[169,170] Real-time PCR methodology has been used to detect WNV in equine tissues.[170] In the author's laboratory, the E-protein real-time primers have not detected WNV in tissues, but the NS5 target has detected WNV nucleic acids in CNS tissues, heart, and intestine of clinically affected horses.[170]

Serum titers should be evaluated for recent exposure to other encephalitides, including EEE, WEE, and EHV-1. Measurement of titers from paired sera is necessary in vaccinated horses for detecting recent exposure to these diseases. Because WNV can present with asymmetric weakness and ataxia, Western blot testing for EPM should also be performed on serum and CSF. The integrity of the blood-brain barrier during acute infection is unknown. Initial work indicates little leakage, with most WNV-specific IgM within CSF considered to be of intrathecal origin.[165]

Japanese Encephalitis

Japanese encephalitis should be suspected in horses with compatible clinical signs that reside in an area of virus activity. Diagnostic confirmatory tests include serologic assays such as neutralizing, complement fixation, hemagglutination inhibition, and ELISA tests.[171-173] All single sera testing, including IgM assays, must be interpreted with caution in horses from areas with other endemic flaviviruses. In fatal JE cases, viral isolation, PCR assays, and IHC for detection of virus in CNS tissues is confirmatory.

PATHOLOGIC FINDINGS

Flaviviruses cause polioencephalomyelitis (inflammation of the gray matter) with lesions that increase in number from the diencephalon through the hindbrain and frequently increase in severity caudally through the spinal cord.* The histologic changes within the brain, including inflammatory foci and detectable virus in the thalamus, medulla, and pons, are consistent with changes in behavior.

Gross pathologic findings are limited in WNV infection in the horse. The meninges may be congested. Small to moderately sized foci of hemorrhagic discoloration may be observed in the brain and spinal cord. These areas occur most often in

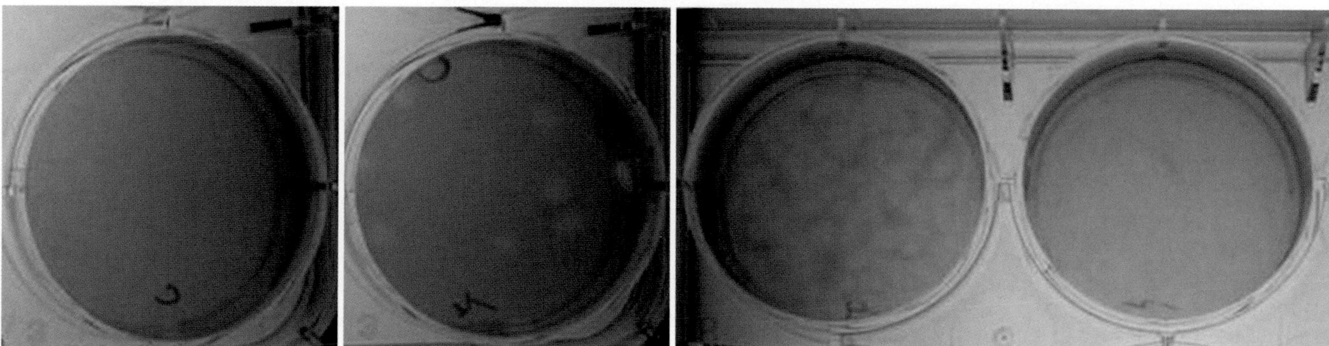

Fig. 21-5 Six-well plate exhibiting clearing of monolayer (plaques) of Vero cells as cytopathic effect of West Nile virus (WNV) infection. These plaques form the basis of the "gold standard," the plaque reduction neutralization test (PRNT), for detection of neutralizing antibody to flaviviruses.

the basal ganglia, rostral colliculus, pons, medulla, and lumbar spinal cord. Edema and softening of tissues are also common findings.

Histopathologic changes secondary to WNV infection are consistent with viral infection and neural cell death. The basal ganglia, thalamus, pons, and medulla have the highest numbers of lesions, with two to several cell layers of mononuclear perivascular cuffing. Predominantly confined to the gray matter, collections of mononuclear cells are also seen within the parenchyma (gliosis). By contrast, these lesions are limited in the cortex and cerebellum. Neuronal damage includes chromatolytic neurons and neuronophagia. Horses with long-standing disease may have areas of neuronal dropout. In the spinal cord, there is perivascular cuffing, gliosis, and damaged neurons.

THERAPY

No known antiviral medications are marketed that demonstrate reliable activity against flaviviruses, and thus treatment of disease is supportive.[124,127,177-179] In horses, the survival rate for WNV encephalitis is high compared with other infectious encephalitides. Most horses appear to begin recovery 3 to 5 days after onset of signs, which makes it difficult to assess any pharmacologic intervention accurately, when a feature of analysis is resolving clinical disease. Flunixin meglumine, 1.1 mg/kg every 12 hours (q12h) intravenously (IV), early in the course of the disease appears to decrease the severity of muscle tremors and fasciculations within a few hours of administration.

To date, much of the mortality in WNV horses results from euthanasia of recumbent horses for humane reasons. Recumbent horses are mentally alert and frequently thrash, sustaining many self-inflicted wounds and posing risk to personnel. Therapy of recumbent horses is generally more aggressive and may include dexamethasone sodium (0.05-0.1 mg/kg q24h IV) and mannitol (0.25-2.0 g/kg q24h IV). Controversy remains as to whether or not corticosteroids enhance peripheral and CNS viral load.[180-183] Detomidine hydrochloride (0.02-0.04 mg/kg IV or intramuscularly [IM]) is effective for prolonged tranquilization. Low doses of acepromazine (0.02 mg/kg IV or 0.05 mg/kg IM) provide excellent relief from anxiety in both recumbent and standing horses. Until EPM is ruled out or WNV is confirmed, prophylactic therapy with antiprotozoal medications is recommended for horses in geographic areas where *Sarcocystis neurona* infection is prevalent. Other supportive measures may include oral and intravenous (IV) fluids and antibiotics for treatment of infections that frequently occur in recumbent horses (wounds, cellulitis, and pneumonia).

A variety of treatments have been recommended for horses with WNV; however, there is limited evidence at this time to support their efficacy.[114,178,179,184-186] The recommendation for interferon alpha (IFN-α) therapy is based on anecdotal reports in the human and veterinary literature. Limited information regarding efficacy in the horse is available. In a blinded study in which children with encephalitis caused by JEV were treated with IFN-α, survival was not enhanced. In fact, length of hospitalization was increased in the IFN-α–treated group.

Therapy with WNV-specific IV immunoglobulin has also been recommended. In a blinded placebo-controlled trial with low numbers of animals, the risk for development of recumbency was less in horses receiving plasma from horses immunized against WNV (Long, unpublished data). However, plasma treatment did not change outcome and severity of WNV disease. In human patients, high-dose glutamate therapy has been suggested to prevent neuronal cell death. Another experimental therapy in mice is administration of beta-lactam inhibitors, which stimulate GLT1, a chemical that activates glutamate.

PREVENTION

Epidemiologic and anecdotal evidence exists regarding the effectiveness of vaccination against flaviviruses. Initial epidemiologic studies performed in 2000 established a point source for infection of WNV, demonstrating that outbreaks in horses may be controlled best by vaccination.[55,57,150] This finding was consistent with prior experience with JE, in which vaccines were advocated for horses before the WNV epizootic.

Presently, three vaccines are licensed for prevention of WNV viremia in the U.S. and as of 2005, at least three vaccines are available for vaccination of horses against JE.[187-191] Vaccination before the mosquito season is critical. The manufacturer's labeling instructions must be followed for induction of immunity with initial immunization. More frequent vaccination in areas with year-round mosquito seasons is highly recommended. Limited information is available regarding long-term immunity after vaccination. However, it is not expected that the initial vaccine series will provide long-term protection; antibody levels rapidly decrease after 4 to 6 months. Where these viruses are endemic, vaccination schedules should be maintained even with a decrease in the incidence of overt disease. This is evidenced by the persistence of reports of JE disease in naive horses after introduction into endemic areas. Horses that have recovered from clinical disease have long-term immunity and should not require annual boosters.

PUBLIC HEALTH CONSIDERATIONS

West Nile virus is considered a zoonotic disease. A bird reservoir maintains the virus in an endemic life cycle in the environment, allowing for transmission by mosquitoes to humans. There is little risk of disease by direct contact with an infected horse, except during postmortem examination with inappropriate handling of infected tissues. Postmortem handling of tissues should be performed with personal protection similar to that for rabies suspect cases (see Chapter 19). The ecology of horse pastures and stables with standing water, a high degree of biologic debris, and "bridge" vectors that feed on mammalian populations likely increase the risk of exposure in that environment. The same types of management tactics for prevention of disease in horses are important for people, except that there is no vaccine. Personal mosquito protection with a DEET-based product is recommended in areas with endemic disease.

The North American epidemic of WNV has demonstrated new modes of transmission, including blood-borne and occupational risks. Blood-borne transmission can occur between viremic hosts. In addition, occupational infection has occurred through necropsy of avian hosts. Veterinarians and horse owners should institute personal protection with appropriate clothing, gloves, and eye protection when coming into contact with animal tissues during the arbovirus season.

REFERENCES

See the CD-ROM for a list of references linked to the abstract in PubMed.

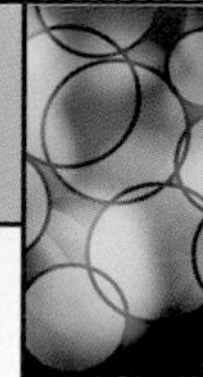

CHAPTER • 22

Borna Disease

Juergen A. Richt, Arthur Grabner, Sibylle Herzog, Wolfgang Garten, and Christiane Herden

Borna disease (BD) is a naturally occurring, infectious, usually fatal, progressive meningopolioencephalitis, predominantly affecting horses and sheep; less often other *Equidae*, cattle, goats, and rabbits; and occasionally a variety of other animal species and possibly humans.* Synonyms used in the past, such as "hot-headed disease" *(Hitzige Kopfkrankheit)*, "brain fever," "subacute meningoencephalitis," and "hypersomnia of horses," reflect the restriction of the disease to the nervous system. The current name of BD originated from a devastating epidemic among horses of a cavalry regiment between 1894 and 1896 near the town of Borna in Saxonia/Germany. More sporadic occurrence of equine BD has since been described in different areas of Germany,[52] Switzerland,[81] Liechtenstein, and Austria.[128,139] There are reports of equine BD cases in Japan,[129] but these could not be confirmed by others.[138] It is uncertain whether clinically similar cases of equine encephalitis in France, Romania, Libya, and the Near East were in fact BD. However, good reason exists to assume that BDV infections are more widely distributed because virus-specific antibodies have been demonstrated in horses from several additional countries.†

During the first decade of the twentieth century, studies of BD focused primarily on defining the etiology, pathology, and pathophysiology of the disease. Final proof for a viral etiology was presented in 1927 by Zwick et al.[147] by reproducing the disease with bacteria-free filtrates of brain homogenates from affected horses. Histopathologic studies of the brain, described in detail by Joest and Degen,[59] Seifried and Spatz,[120] and Gosztonyi and Ludwig,[33] revealed massive perivascular infiltrations, reactive astrogliosis, and intranuclear eosinophilic "Joest-Degen" inclusion bodies. The pathologic changes were preferentially localized in the limbic system, which may be connected with behavioral alterations observed in some animals.[107]

Detailed studies have been performed on the spectrum of susceptible host species and on the manifestation of the disease.[48,107,122] More recently, the causative virus, *Borna disease virus* (BDV), has been cultivated in cell cultures,[56,80] aspects of pathogenesis of the disease have been elucidated,[85,86,102-104,124] and the molecular characterization of BDV‡ and its replication strategy[21,22,115,116,130] were achieved. With the advent of a reverse-genetics system to produce infectious complementary deoxyribonucleic acid (cDNA) clones, future studies will enable detailed molecular analysis of the genome organization and gene products encoded by BDV, as well as investigation of the regulation of BDV genome expression.[88,116,118] The organization of the viral genome led to the classification of BDV in the order Mononegavirales as the new family *Bornaviridae* with the genus *Bornavirus*.

More detail on the historical background and various aspects of BD are available from Koprowski and Lipkin[68] and Richt et al.[101,102]

Mention of trade names or commercial products in this chapter is done solely to provide specific information and does not imply recommendation or endorsement by the U.S. Department of Agriculture.

*References 15, 20, 24, 48, 68, 78, 107, 108, 146.
†References 29, 39, 40, 52, 61, 144.
‡References 13, 19, 21, 22, 75, 130, 133.

ETIOLOGY

Borna disease virus is an enveloped virus with a nonsegmented, negative-sense, single-stranded (ss) ribonucleic acid (RNA) genome of 8.9 kilobases. It has the characteristic genomic organization of members of the order Mononegavirales. Some genotypic and phenotypic distinctions of BDV required the classification in the new virus family, the *Bornaviridae*. Thus, several features of BDV replication are unique compared with other members of this order, such as the nuclear site of replication and transcription, RNA splicing, and the overlap of transcription units.[21,22,115,130] In addition, there is a high degree of genetic stability and homology among wild-type and experimentally host-adapted viruses.[54,96,122] The complete sequence of the genome from several BDV isolates has been determined.[13,19,96] Phylogenetic analysis of wild-type and laboratory strains indicate distinct virus clusters corresponding to geographically endemic areas in Central Europe.[67] BDV particles are spherical, enveloped, and approximately 130 nm in diameter, with spikes 7 nm in length and a nucleocapsid 4 nm in diameter. BDV particles are released by budding on the cell surface.[66]

On the complementary positive-strand RNA (cRNA), at least six open reading frames (ORFs) can be identified. ORF I, at the 5′ end of the cRNA, encodes the 357/370–amino acid (aa) nucleoprotein, *NP* (p38/p39); ORF II encodes the 201-aa phosphoprotein, *P* (p24); ORF III encodes the 142-aa matrix protein, *M;* ORF IV encodes the 503-aa glycoprotein, *GP;* and ORF V (at 3′ end of cRNA) encodes the RNA-dependent RNA–polymerase (RdRp) of BDV, the *L* protein, which is more than 1600 aa long.[22,115,130,135] Overlapping with ORF II, the ORF x1 encodes the 87-aa BDV *p10* protein.[136] All these virus-specific proteins have been detected in BDV-infected material. Detailed studies on the function of individual BDV proteins are in progress.

Several lines of evidence, including the location on the genome, indicate that the nucleoprotein (NP) and the phosphoprotein (P), together with the L–protein, are part of the ribonucleoprotein (RNP) and therefore part of the functional BDV replication complex. BDV RNPs are infectious after transfection into susceptible cell lines.[16] BDV-p10 can also bind to the RNP complex, and it is speculated that it may act as a negative regulator of the BDV polymerase activity.[90,116,119,143] Associated with the BDV envelope are the matrix (M) and the glycoprotein (GP). The BDV-M was thought to be glycosylated, but recent studies demonstrate that it is a nonglycosylated matrix protein, similar to that found in other viruses of the order Mononegavirales.[70] Similar to the *Filoviridae* and *Rhabdoviridae*, BDV possesses a single surface glycoprotein, BDV-GP,[31,98,117] which is posttranslationally modified by *N*-glycosylation and cleavage by a subtilisin-like protease into two fragments; this is a prerequisite for the invasion of BDV into cells.[31,89,98]

RNA transcripts encoding BDV proteins are initiated at three transcriptional start sites and terminated at five transcriptional termination sites. RNA from the first transcriptional unit codes for the NP.[21,22,115,130] Alternative initiation at two in-frame AUGs results in the p38 and p39 isoforms of the NP. The RNA from the second transcription unit is bicistronic and codes for the P and p10 proteins. Similar to NP, two isoforms of P have been detected.[64] Translation of P and p10 is most likely accomplished by "leaky scanning" because no spliced products of this messenger RNA (mRNA) have been described so far.[136] RNA transcripts originating from the third transcriptional start site can be terminated at two different termination sites. In both cases, the transcripts may contain up to three introns, and depending on whether intron 1 and/or intron 2 is spliced, the respective mature mRNA can code for the M, GP, or L protein.* It can be assumed that RNA splicing may play an important role in the regulation of BDV genome expression by increasing the versatility of its primary transcripts and by providing the possibility for controlled synthesis of new BDV polypeptides.

The induction of a persistent, noncytopathic infection in cell cultures and in brain cells of a variety of animal species, the low replication rate, and therefore the difficulty in detection of virions in infected material might be the consequences of the tight control of protein expression from the third transcriptional unit. Recently, a novel strategy for viral replication-control has been postulated. BDV seems to restrict its propagation efficacy by defined 5′-terminal trimming of genomic and antigenomic RNA molecules.[105,116,118]

EPIDEMIOLOGY

To date, BD in horses has been recognized only in Germany, Switzerland, Liechtenstein, and Austria. However, the diagnosis may have been overlooked in other areas because of a lack of diagnostic effort. Seroprevalence studies demonstrate that BDV infections can occur worldwide. BDV-specific antibodies were detected in horses from many countries, including several European countries, Turkey, Israel, Japan, Iran, China, Australia, and the United States.†

Extensive studies of the seroprevalence of BDV are only reported from Germany, where BD is the most important viral CNS disease of horses. These studies demonstrate that the disease occurs predominantly in endemic regions in the central and southern parts of Germany. In contrast to the epidemic course of BD at the end of the nineteenth century, a significant reduction of BD incidence to about 0.3% was noted in an endemic region in central Germany in 1960 and from 1989 to 1996.[131] At present the incidence in endemic regions in Germany is even lower, approximately 0.02% to 0.04% in Bavaria.[36] A seasonal accumulation of cases is observed in April, May, and June, with a significant decrease in late fall and winter.‡

Most BDV infections appear to be inapparent infections, as indicated by various studies determining BDV seroprevalence. The average seroprevalence of BDV-specific antibodies in clinically healthy German horses is approximately 11.5%,[52,99] which increases significantly to 22.5% in endemic regions. In stables with diseased horses, the prevalence of BDV-specific antibodies is approximately 50%.[36] In 72% of horse stables with cases of BD, only individual animals showed clinical signs of BD. Repeated outbreaks of BD in stables are possible, although these are usually observed some time (2 months to several years) after the initial outbreak of BD.[36,99] There is no explanation for the discrepancy between the high seroprevalence and the low incidence of disease so far. The development of Borna disease after BDV infection may depend on the genetic factors, age, and immune status of the host and the genetic characteristics of the virus.

The route of transmission of BDV is uncertain. Investigations in rats showed that BDV can be shed in nasal and lacrimal secretions as well as in urine, and transmission most likely occurs through open nerve endings in the nasal and pharyngeal mucosa.[82,111] In a few cases, infectious virus could be isolated from the lacrimal and parotid glands of horses with BD (S. Herzog, unpublished results), and virus-specific RNA could be demonstrated in nasal and lacrimal secretions and saliva of such animals[73]; this was also possible in a few seropositive, inapparently infected horses.[100] However, there is no evidence of virus replication in lacrimal or parotid gland of inapparently BDV-infected horses (S. Herzog, unpublished results). This indicates that horses infected with BDV, especially with clinical signs of BD, could play a role in the transmission of BDV. To date, no evidence suggests that other animal species (e.g., rodents) play a role in the transmission of BDV.

PATHOGENESIS

Most of the currently available information regarding the pathogenesis of BDV infection is derived from studies of experimentally infected Lewis rats and recently, also from BDV-infected mice.[23,41,51,85,86] The use of genetically altered animals provides new opportunities to study the immunopathogenesis of BD in more detail. In general, it can be assumed that the virus enters the body by intranasal infection through olfactory nerve endings.[82,73,100,111] Another possible route is orally, through the trigeminal nerve.[5] After the virus enters the nervous system, it migrates along the axons of the olfactory system to the brain, where it replicates in neurons and glial cells, preferentially in the limbic system. Over time the virus disseminates throughout the central nervous system (CNS), then spreads to the peripheral nervous system and the neuronal cells of the retina.[71,72,85] Axonal transport, with consequent protection from recognition of foreign antigens by the humoral immune system, may explain the lack of neutralizing antibodies until late in infection.

In adult rats the virus demonstrates a strict neurotropism. Viral antigens and infectivity persist throughout the life of the infected animals exclusively in neural tissues; that is, the animals develop a persistent CNS infection. The occurrence of clinical signs correlates with the appearance of inflammatory lesions in the brain. In general, the inflammatory reaction consists of mononuclear cells and is centered in the limbic system, but it spreads to other areas of the brain during the course of infection. Interestingly, late after infection, the inflammation decreases despite the presence of viral antigen and infectious virus.[23,51,85,86] This might be caused by a switch from a T helper cell 1 (Th1) to a T helper cell 2 (Th2) immune response in later stages of the disease.[43] In contrast, neonatally infected rats harbor infectious virus not only in the CNS, but

*References 18, 21, 22, 115, 116, 130 135.
†References 29, 39, 40, 52, 61, 62, 107, 144.
‡References 24, 35, 36, 113, 114, 131.

also in parenchymal cells of peripheral organs.[53] Although these animals do not manifest clinical signs and inflammatory infiltrates, they shed virus in various secretions and excretions and are therefore virus carriers.[53,82]

When diseased horses and sheep were analyzed for the presence of BDV-specific RNA by the reverse transcriptase–polymerase chain reaction (RT-PCR) technique, the bulbus olfactorius, nucleus caudatus, hippocampus, and cerebral cortex of all animals were positive.[73] BDV RNA was also present in the spinal cord, eye, nasal mucosa, parotid salivary gland, lung, heart, liver, kidney, bladder, and ovaries in some animals. Presence of BDV RNA in tissues of nonneural origin could be caused by virus replication in nerve endings within these organs. In addition, BDV-specific RNA was detected in conjunctival fluid, nasal secretions, and saliva of two infected animals.[73] Interestingly, viral dissemination and persistence in the brain of BDV-infected mice is not affected by overexpression or deletion of various cytokines or chemokine receptors.[27,46,69]

Both naturally and experimentally, BDV infects a broad spectrum of warm-blooded animals, inducing persistent infection without cytolytic destruction of cells. Sequence analysis of virus isolates obtained from various animal species or tissue culture reveals a remarkable conservation of the genome. The highly conserved viral genome suggests that BDV adapts easily to various animal species without significant genetic change. The rate of production and release of infectious virus in vitro and in vivo is extremely low despite the presence of relatively high amounts of viral antigen in infected cells. This indicates an abortive cycle of viral reproduction in most cell types infected. Evidence suggests that BDV replication in brain cells and probably other cell types may be controlled by the virus through various strategies, such as direct modification of the viral genome, control of transcription, regulation of viral protein expression (e.g., ratios of BDV-N vs. BDV-P), or abrogation of BDV glycoprotein synthesis.[22,98,116,130,140] BDV can interfere with various cellular proteins or signaling cascades (e.g., neurite outgrowth factor HMG-1, neurotropin signaling, Raf/MEK/ERK pathway, activation of NF-κB) or the induction of the antiviral interferon (IFN) response.[12,32,60,93,132] This interaction with host cell function might represent additional viral strategies to spread, replicate, and persist in the CNS of its host.

Borna disease is caused by a virus-induced immunopathologic reaction.[123] This was convincingly shown in rodent systems. Infection of adult immunocompetent rats results in encephalitis and disease, whereas infection of newborn, athymic, or immunosuppressed animals leads to neither encephalitis nor disease, despite persistent high levels of virus in the CNS of these virus carriers.* Newborn infected animals appear clinically normal;[53] however, some physical, behavioral, and pathologic abnormalities are observed. Learning deficits; elevated cytokine or chemokine expression, even in the absence of inflammation; and degeneration of postnatally developing brain areas have been described.[1,95,97,110] These changes might be caused by direct effects of the virus on cell and organ functions. BDV-specific antibodies adoptively transferred into immunosuppressed, virus-infected recipients do not induce pathologic alterations or disease.[86] Neutralizing antibodies to BDV are only detectable late, if ever, after infection and might play a role in preventing generalized infection with BDV. Transfer of immune serum into immune-incompetent newborn rats could not prevent persistent CNS infection but did prevent dissemination of the virus from neural tissues to peripheral organs.[125] However, adoptive transfer of immune cells from spleen or lymph nodes of BDV-infected animals is effective in the induction of BD in immunosuppressed virus carriers.[85,86]

*References 53, 55, 85, 86, 126, 127.

Mice develop a nonpurulent meningoencephalitis with a typical neurologic disorder only when they are infected as newborns. In contrast, adult BDV-infected mice show neither obvious clinical signs nor significant inflammatory alterations in the brain.[41,109] The clinical signs of neonatal BDV-infected mice range from ataxia to paralysis of the hindlimbs. The incidence and severity of the BDV-induced clinical manifestations vary considerably between the different mouse strains used for infection. MRL/+ mice develop strong neurologic signs,[109] whereas C57BL/6 mice were clinically inconspicuous.[41] The reason for the different course of experimental BDV infection in adult versus newborn rats and mice remains unclear.

The pathogenesis of BD is somehow similar to that *observed* for lymphocytic choriomeningitis virus (LCMV) infection,[145] in which a virus-induced cell-mediated immune response causes disease. Whereas CD8+ cells are responsible for induction of LCM, CD4+ and CD8+ cells are apparently responsible for development of BD. The role of virus-specific T cells in the pathogenesis of BD was demonstrated by passive transfer of in vitro established homogenous BDV-specific CD4+ T-cell lines into immunosuppressed virus carriers. The recipients consistently developed clinical signs characteristic of acute BD.[103,104] However, evidence indicates that in addition to virus-specific CD4+ T cells, CD8+ cells are also involved in pathologic alterations.[91,95,126] These are thought to be a main effector cell in BDV-infection of mice, although there is no lysis of BDV-infected neurons observed in infected mice or rat brains. In rats as well as in mice, BDV-specific CD8+ cytotoxic T lymphocytes (CTLs) are mainly directed against the viral nucleoprotein.[45,92,112] The kinetics of CTL induction and subsequent recruitment of these cells to the brain determine the severity of BDV-induced neurologic disease. Downregulation of the functional avidity of virus-specific CD8+ T cells in experimentally infected mice seems to be involved in controlling the inflammatory reaction and facilitating viral persistence.[26] However, immune control of BDV infection could generally be achieved only by antigen-specific immune priming or adoptive transfer of BDV-specific T cells.[44,49,74,104] Taken together, these data indicate that T cells play a crucial role in the pathogenesis of BD. The severe meningoencephalitis with mononuclear infiltrates observed after BDV infection most likely represents a delayed-type hypersensitivity reaction.

As observed in the experimental rat model, brain tissues from various Equidae with natural BD have mononuclear immune cell infiltration and increased expressions of major histocompatibility complex (MHC) class I and class II antigen were described.[6,14,50] The composition of the inflammatory cell infiltrates is similar to that observed in experimentally BDV-infected rats, and therefore a similar pathogenesis of disease in naturally infected Equidae and experimentally infected rats is presumed.

CLINICAL FINDINGS

Natural BDV infection can result in peracute, acute, or subacute Borna disease with meningoencephalitis, which leads to death 1 to 4 weeks after onset of initial signs in more than 80% of animals.* In less severe cases, spontaneous recovery is occasionally observed despite a persistent CNS infection.[20,36,80,113] In up to 10% of animals with BD, a chronic, sometimes recurrent

*References 24, 35, 36, 37, 58, 99, 113, 114, 131.

course of disease is observed.[20,36,37,80,113] A bland encephalitis without obvious clinical signs is possible.[36]

The incubation period for BD after natural infection is variable, ranging from 2 weeks to several months.[113,114] In a large number of experimentally infected animals, the average incubation period was 2 to 3 months. More recently, experimental intracerebral infection of three ponies with various doses of BDV resulted in an incubation period of 15 to 26 days.[63] Two ponies were febrile for 3 to 7 days before neurologic signs occurred. The course of BD was dependent on virus dose used for infection. Whereas two ponies died after rapid onset of CNS symptoms within 28 or 30 days after infection, the third pony survived the infection without residual clinical signs. The major clinical signs were ataxia, head tilt, muscle fasciculation, hindlimb paresis, localized cutaneous hyperesthesia and hypoesthesia, and aggressive behavior, similar to signs of natural BD.[63]

Clinical manifestations of BDV infection may vary among individual animals.[37,99,131] Typical clinical signs of BD in horses are simultaneous or consecutive changes in psyche, sensorium, sensibility, and mobility and in the autonomic nervous system.* The most common clinical signs are depression with apathy, somnolence, and stupor.[5,35,36] The neurologic signs are variable and complex, depend on the course of disease, and are related to the inflammatory reaction in the areas of CNS previously mentioned.

Alterations in behavior and consciousness can be observed in early stages of BD, and these signs progressively worsen toward the final stages.[37,99] Slow-motion eating, eating arrest with chewing movements (called *Pfeifenrauchen*, "pipe smoking") (Fig. 22-1, *A*), and chewing motions without food intake, interrupted by frequent yawns or head pressing, can be present early in the course of disease and are important diagnostic clues. Recurrent fever that is resistant to antipyretic medications may occur in the initial stages of acute BD.[24,36,37,131] Prolapse of the penis without urination; rhythmic repetitive motor activities; disturbances in the mental status with lethargy, somnolence, and stupor; hyperexcitability; fearfulness; and unusual aggressiveness may be observed in variable degrees. These alterations might be caused by impairment of the limbic system, which regulates affective and compulsive behavior.[5,35,37]

Hypokinesia and abnormal postures (postural unawareness), as well as decreased skin and deep sensory reactions, are frequently observed, resulting in an impaired reaction to exogenous and nociceptive stimuli and a loss of proprioception (Fig. 22-1, *B*). Early in the course of BD, a deficit of the "cutaneus trunci reflex" and flexor reflex may be noticed.

Hyporeflexia of spinal reflexes, head tilt, and hypoesthesia with disturbances in proprioceptive sensory functions are characteristics of more advanced stages of BD. In this stage, horses may exhibit ataxia and imbalance, an abnormal reaction toward exogenous stimuli, and abnormal posture (see Fig. 22-1, *B*). Impairment of cranial nerve (CN) function as a consequence of inflammatory reactions in the respective CN nuclei, as well as direct effects on CNs, such as the trigeminal nerve (CN V), result in the development of these clinical signs: (1) dysphagia and salivation from pharyngeal paralysis (CNs IX and X), (2) decreased tongue tension and increased tongue movement (CN XII), (3) bruxism and trismus (CNs V and VII), (4) paresis of the facial nerve (CN VII), (5) nystagmus (CNs XI and VII), and (6) strabismus and miosis (CN III).[37,99]

In the final stages of BD the horse develops an increased appearance of neurogenic torticollis with torsion dystonia in the neck muscles, in some cases associated with compulsive circular walking (Fig. 22-1, *C*). A slight tremor in the head area is usually observed, followed by convulsions. Convulsions are regularly associated with head pressing, which is possibly the result of a high cerebrospinal fluid pressure caused by the inflammatory reaction in the CNS.[5,36,37,57] Loss of the pupillary reflex and strabismus are often observed at this stage,[83,113] and affected animals may lapse into a comatose condition.[5,35,36] Blindness is often observed in horses with acute BD.[5]

In more than 50% of animals with acute BD, disturbances in chewing and swallowing of food and water develop, which could limit the duration of the disease in some horses.[37,131] In the final stages of the disorder, food intake ceases, and only 20% of the affected animals are able to swallow small amounts of water. As a consequence of this lack of food intake, a fasting hyperbilirubinemia with icteric mucous membranes develops.[24,36,37]

*References 24, 37, 48, 77, 113,114, 131, 146, 147.

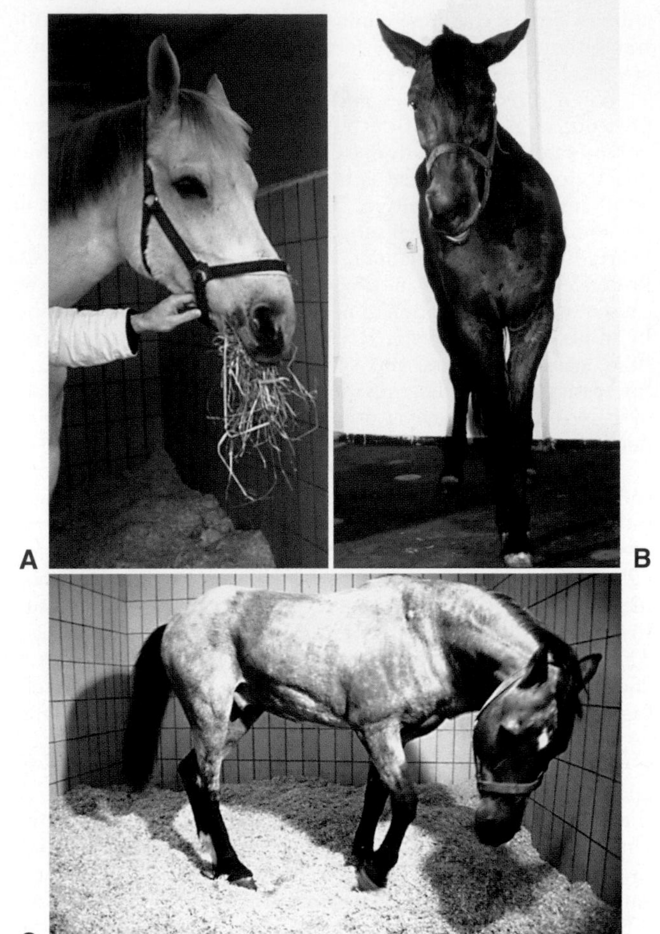

Fig. 22-1 Horses with Borna disease (BD). **A,** Seven-year-old gelding affected with somnolence and displaying characteristic arrested eating with chewing movements (called *Pfeifenrauchen*, "pipe smoking"). **B,** Two-year-old mare affected with disturbances in proprioception (abnormal posture) and paralysis of facial nerve. **C,** Seventeen-year-old Welsh Pony stallion with neurogenic torticollis and compulsive circular walking. (From Richt JA, Grabner A, Herzog S: *Vet Clin North Am Equine Pract* 16:579, 2000.)

Nonneurologic signs, such as recurrent colic, emaciation, and chronic lameness of unknown etiology, as well as behavioral abnormalities such as "head shaking," have also been described.[9] Whether these signs are directly caused by the BDV infection is not clear, but the disturbed food and water intake might be misdiagnosed as colic.[36,131]

DIAGNOSIS

Antemortem Diagnosis

Because of the multifocal appearance of brain lesions, the resulting clinical signs are not highly specific for BD. CNS infection with a variety of pathogens may result in similar signs. In countries where BD in horses is prevalent, infections with equine herpesviruses,[65,142] rabies,[38] tick-borne encephalitis,[76,134] and various bacterial diseases (e.g., botulism,[141] bacterial meningitis[28]) and parasitic diseases (e.g., verminous myeloencephalitis,[25] equine protozoal myeloencephalitis [EPM][79]) must be considered as differential diagnoses for BD. EPM often has a relatively long incubation period compared with BD.[79,137] In the Americas, besides these infections, arthropod-borne infections with alphaviruses or flaviviruses, inducing equine encephalitides, and West Nile virus (WNV) infections should be included as important differential diagnoses.

Hematologic and biochemical parameters are usually within normal limits in affected horses. Hyperbilirubinemia is frequently observed but is a nonspecific change related to decreased food intake. During the final stages of BD when convulsions occur, a high concentration of lactate may be present in the plasma.[5]

In acute disease the quantity of cerebrospinal fluid (CSF) and the concentration of CSF proteins (86.3 ± 14.8 mg/dL; 58 cases) may be increased.[26,37,131] The CSF shows a characteristic lympho-monocytic pleocytosis (56.4 ± 32.8 cells/μL) during acute and subacute BD, consistent with the presence of a nonpurulent encephalitis.[36,37,131] In chronic BD, most CSF parameters are in the normal range, except the CSF lactate concentration, which is usually increased.[36]

Because of the lack of specificity of clinical signs and laboratory abnormalities, Borna disease must be confirmed by the demonstration of BDV-specific antibodies in the serum or CSF of diseased horses,[35,37] using Western blot analysis,[52] enzyme-linked immunosorbent assay (ELISA),[18] or an indirect immunofluorescence assay (IFA)[37,56] (Fig. 22-2). IFA is acknowledged to be the most reliable method for the detection of BDV-specific antibodies. Antibody titers in sera range between 1:5 and 1:1280 and in CSF between 1:2 and 1:1280.[37,52] No correlation exists between the antibody titers and the clinical signs or the outcome of infection. Using a highly sensitive technique, the nested RT-PCR, it was possible to detect BDV RNA in cells isolated from the CSF. In acute BD, CSF pleocytosis and BDV-specific antibodies can be detected in 100% of affected horses; however, BDV-specific antibodies are often missing in peracute BD, at the beginning of acute BD, or in horses pretreated with corticosteroids.[37] BDV-specific antibodies may be found in the serum, but not in the CSF, of clinically healthy animals.[37,50]

The detection of BDV-specific RNA in peripheral blood mononuclear cells (PBMCs) has been proposed as an alternative in the antemortem diagnosis of BD.[3,84] This was not shown to be useful, however, in a study including 175 horses with or without BD.[37]

In summary, antemortem diagnosis of BD can be regarded as positive when (1) animals show neurologic signs, (2) BDV-specific antibodies are detectable in the serum, or (3) CSF and characteristic pathologic changes in the CSF are observed.

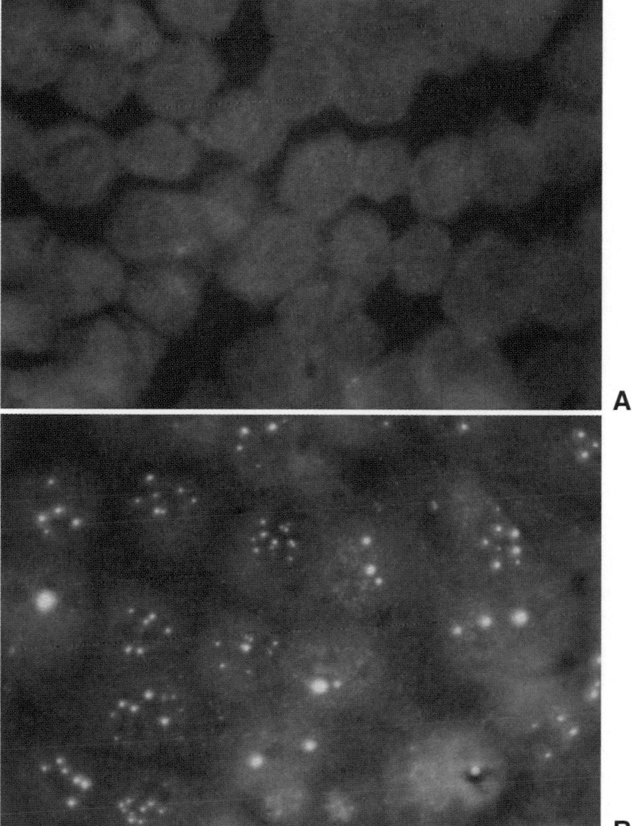

Fig. 22-2 Indirect immunofluorescence assay of horse sera with Madin-Darby canine kidney (MDCK) cells. **A,** Borna disease virus (BDV)–positive serum incubated with uninfected MDCK cells. **B,** BDV-positive serum incubated with BDV-infected MDCK cells.

Postmortem Diagnosis

The postmortem diagnosis of BD involves histopathology, immunohistochemistry (IHC), and virologic methods. Histopathologically, naturally diseased horses show a nonpurulent meningoencephalitis with more or less pronounced perivascular and parenchymal infiltrates (Fig. 22-3, *A*). Joest-Degen inclusion bodies are not always found. Details of expected histopathologic changes are described in the next section. IHC can be performed using monoclonal or polyclonal antibodies specific for various BDV proteins[5,37,50] (Fig 22-3, *B*). Monoclonal antibodies specific for the BDV nucleoprotein (p38/p39) and phosphoprotein (p24) are frequently used to detect BDV protein in the nucleus and cytoplasm of neurons, neuronal processes, and glial cells.[5,50] The same monoclonal and polyclonal antibodies can be used for the detection of BDV antigen in the CNS of infected horses by Western blot analysis.[32,33] Comparative studies indicate that all three methods, as well as nested RT-PCR, give identical diagnostic results in acute cases of BD.[37,50] The isolation of infectious BDV and the demonstration of virus-specific RNA by in situ hybridization can complete a postmortem diagnosis. These methods, however, are less suitable when the material is in a state of decomposition. In this case, IHC and Western blotting are preferred.[50]

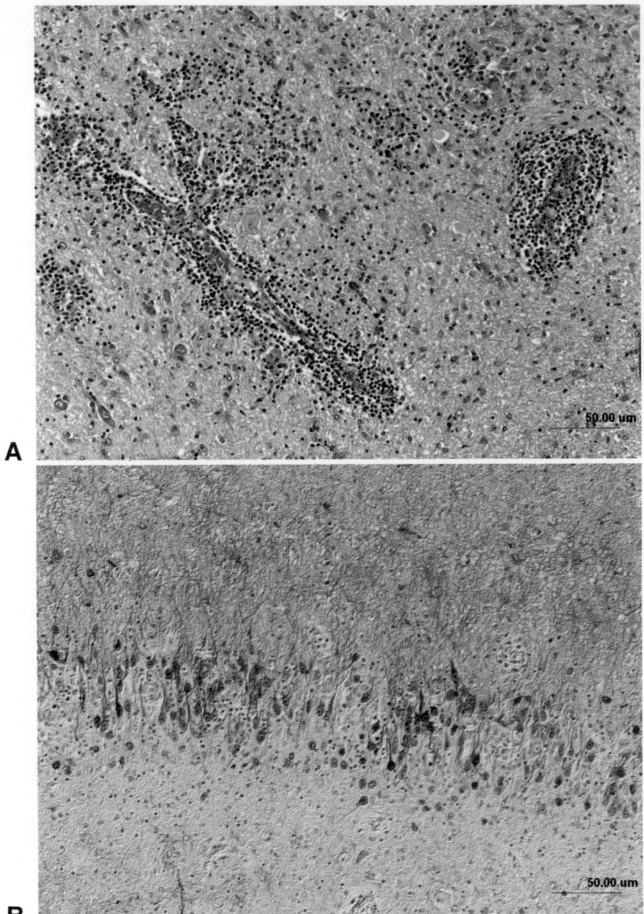

Fig. 22-3 Pathologic and immunohistochemical analysis of brain section from horse naturally infected with Borna disease virus (BDV). **A,** Photomicrograph revealing nonpurulent meningoencephalitis with mononuclear perivascular and parenchymal immune cell infiltrates. **B,** Immunohistochemical detection of the BDV nucleoprotein using the monoclonal antibody Bo 18. BDV nucleoprotein is present in the nuclei and cytoplasm of infected neurons and in neuropil.

PATHOLOGIC FINDINGS

The pathologic changes associated with BDV infection are similar in all naturally infected animals. They are restricted to the CNS (mainly in the gray matter), spinal cord, and retina. Histolopathologic examination reveals a severe, nonpurulent poliomeningoencaphalomyelitis with massive perivascular and parenchymal infiltration (see Fig. 22-3, *B*). The perivascular cuffs consist predominantly of macrophages, T lymphocytes (CD4+ and CD8+), and late after infection, some plasma cells.[6,14,23,50] Degeneration of neurons and neuronophagia are not prominent; however, a loss of pyramidal cells of the hippocampus might be observed, and a reactive astrocytosis can often be observed in all areas with inflammatory lesions. Besides the gray matter of the olfactory bulb, basal cortex, caudate nucleus, thalamus, and hippocampus, the periventricular areas, mainly in the medulla oblongata, can also be affected. No significant lesions are apparent in the cerebellum, and alterations in the spinal cord are inconsistent. In infected neurons, intranuclear eosinophilic (Joest-Degen) inclusion bodies can sometimes be observed preferentially in the hippocampus. If present, they are regarded as pathognomonic for BDV.

A peculiarity of BDV-infected rats and rabbits involves histopathologic changes in the retina, resulting in nonpurulent chorioretinitis with degeneration of rods and cones.[71,72,85,86] The loss of neurons leads to blindness. Interestingly, such alterations in the retina are not observed in horses, despite occasional observation of clinical signs of blindness. Nevertheless, viral antigen and infectious BDV can be detected in the respective neuronal cell layers in most of the affected horses.[50] An explanation for the lack of inflammation and degeneration might be that horses are euthanized before retinopathy can develop. Blindness could also be caused by the severe inflammation observed in the optic region of the thalamus.[5,50]

THERAPY AND PREVENTION

No specific therapy is available for horses with BD despite promising reports several decades ago.[58] These early studies are difficult to interpret because the diagnosis of BD was uncertain, and spontaneous recovery of horses has been observed.[36,113] A recent report recommends the use of *amantadine sulfate* (AS), a drug with antiviral activity against influenza A,[47] for treatment of BD in horses.[8] The efficacy of AS for treatment of persistently BDV-infected cell cultures and animals, however, is controversial.[8,17,42] In a small clinical study, the potential therapeutic effect of AS (2 mg/kg orally) in nine horses with acute BD was analyzed, with no effect in eight animals.[36] After 10 days of AS treatment, one horse showed a significant improvement and after 6 weeks recovered from the disease. From these preliminary data we cannot conclude whether the recovery of one horse resulted from a potential therapeutic effect of AS or from a spontaneous recovery, as observed in some horses[36] (see Fig. 22-1).

A new therapeutic strategy might be *CSF filtration* to remove cellular and soluble components.[106] CSF filtration was previously used to treat patients with Guillain-Barré syndrome[30] and also in one case of schizophrenia related to "subclinical" BDV encephalitis.[2] This approach was used to filter approximately 400 mL of CSF per day over 5 days. The method was successfully applied in two horses.[34] However, future studies are needed to evaluate its efficacy.

For the control of BD on a regional and international scale, veterinarians should constantly be reminded of the need for a careful differential diagnosis of disorders involving the CNS of horses and sheep, and data should be collected by health authorities for continuous survey.

In vaccination experiments, it was found that attenuated virus but not killed vaccines induce protection against BD.[20,87] Immunoprophylaxis with a lapinized live vaccine[148] was practiced for many years in Germany. Because the efficacy of this vaccine was questionable, it was abandoned in 1992. New data from experimental studies applying recombinant parapoxvirus constructs are promising,[49] but its use in naturally infected horses needs further investigation. Nevertheless, in view of the predominant role of cell-mediated immune responses in the development of BD, artificial stimulation of immune reactions carries a risk of exacerbation of disease.

PUBLIC HEALTH CONSIDERATIONS

Whether BDV can be described as a zoonotic pathogen is uncertain. In BDV-infected animals, CNS infection not only induces neurologic signs, but also behavioral alterations. This is obvious in animals that survive the acute phase of the disease. Such animals become somnolent, restive, and timid and show changes in social interactions. The latter effects were predominantly observed in BDV-infected tree shrews *(Tupaia glis)*, animals that are classified on the phylogenetic root of the primates.[121]

In the last decade it has become obvious that people can be infected by BDV or a BDV-like agent.* BDV-specific antibodies are present in sera of patients with various psychiatric diseases.[7,107,108] The fact that BDV-specific antibodies were also found in some clinically normal people, as was observed with horses, indicates that disease induction after BDV infection in humans and animals is only found under certain, but unknown, circumstances. Virulence of the virus and genetic predisposition of the host or other exogenous and endogenous factors might play a role in the outcome of the disease in animals and humans.

*References 4, 7, 8, 10, 11, 107, 108.

REFERENCES

See the CD-ROM for a list of references linked to the abstract in PubMed.

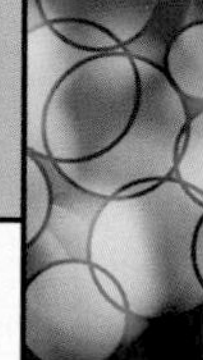

CHAPTER • 23

Equine Infectious Anemia

Robert H. Mealey

Equine infectious anemia (EIA), also known as "swamp fever," is an infectious disease of horses and other equids characterized by recurrent episodes of fever, lethargy, inappetence, thrombocytopenia, and anemia. The clinical signs of EIA were first described in horses in France in 1843,[1] and the causative agent was shown to be a filterable agent in 1904.[2] This made EIA the first animal disease for which a viral etiology was assigned. During the next 60 years, much descriptive information was obtained in the areas of EIA epidemiology, pathology, and clinical manifestation. However, little progress was made in understanding EIA pathogenesis and immunology, primarily because the virus could not be transmitted to experimental hosts other than the horse, and because the virus could not be cultivated in vitro. Not until 1967 was it demonstrated that field strains of the EIA virus could be propagated in equine leukocyte culture,[3,4] and subsequently, several EIA virus strains were adapted to more convenient equine fibroblast culture systems.[5,6] These advancements led to significant gains in the knowledge of the EIA virus, its interaction with host cells, and the immunopathogenesis of EIA.

ETIOLOGY

Equine infectious anemia virus (EIAV) is a lentivirus of the family *Retroviridae* and is closely related to other important lentiviruses, including Maedi visna virus (MVV), caprine arthritis-encephalitis virus (CAEV), bovine immunodeficiency virus (BIV), feline immunodeficiency virus (FIV), simian immunodeficiency virus (SIV), and human immunodeficiency virus (HIV). All lentiviruses cause persistent infections, and most lentiviruses cause slowly progressive disease that frequently results in death. In contrast, EIAV infection results in an acute phase, followed by recurrent clinical disease episodes that eventually subside in most horses. These horses become persistently infected, lifelong, inapparent carriers.

EIAV has a simple ribonucleic acid (RNA) genome that is only 8 kilobases in length. The genome includes three principal genes (gag, pol, env) and three regulatory genes important for viral replication and pathogenesis. The *gag* gene encodes the structural proteins needed for virus assembly and encapsidation of the genome. These proteins include the nucleocapsid (p11), capsid (p26), and matrix (p15). Gag proteins are the predominant protein components of the EIAV particle.[7] The *pol* gene encodes enzymes required for viral replication (reverse transcriptase) and integration into the host cell genome (integrase). The *env* gene encodes the virus envelope surface unit (gp90) and transmembrane (gp45) glycoproteins.

On encountering a host cell, the gp90 glycoprotein (which projects from the surface of the EIAV envelope) binds to a specific receptor on the target cell surface. Recent work indicates that EIAV binds to the newly designated *equine lentivirus receptor-1*, which is related to the family of tumor necrosis factor (TNF) receptor proteins.[8] After binding, the virus envelope fuses with the host cell membrane, and the virion is internalized. Once inside the cell, the EIAV particle uncoats, and replication begins with the production of a double-stranded deoxyribonucleic acid (DNA) copy of the RNA genome, mediated by viral reverse transcriptase. The EIAV DNA is then translocated to the nucleus, and viral integrase inserts the viral DNA into the host cell genome, where it remains as provirus. The integrated provirus utilizes host cell mechanisms for DNA replication, transcription to messenger RNA (mRNA), protein production, and assembly of virus particles. Newly assembled virions bud from the host cell, retaining a portion of the cell membrane as the envelope (Fig. 23-1). The replication cycle is repeated as the new cell-free virus particles encounter and infect new host cells.

Incorporation of the provirus into the host cell genome is a principal mechanism of EIAV persistence within the host. In addition, because reverse transcriptase lacks "proofreading" ability, mutations accumulate in the viral genome during replication.

Consequently, a tremendous number of genetic viral variants ("quasispecies") arise during the course of infection, some of which can escape established immune responses. Antigenic variation and immune escape are therefore major contributing factors to EIAV persistence.

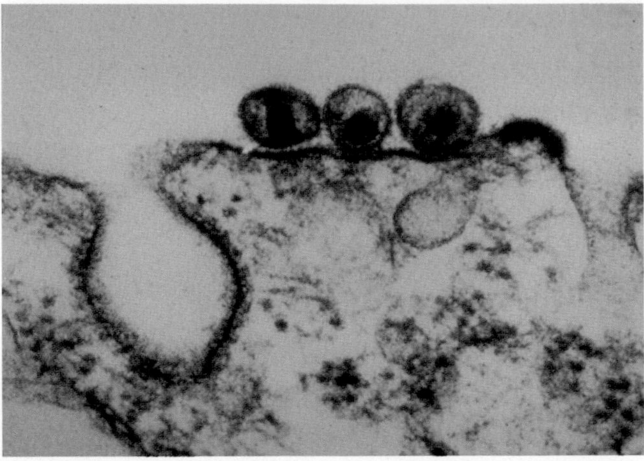

Fig. 23-1 Electron micrograph of equine infectious anemia virus (EIAV) particles budding from cell membrane of infected macrophage.

EPIDEMIOLOGY

Prevalence

Equine infectious anemia is a worldwide disease of Equidae, including horses, ponies, donkeys, mules, and zebras. Because EIAV is most often transmitted by insect vectors, the prevalence is higher in regions with warm climates. In Brazil, for example, the infection rate in certain horse herds has been as high as 50%.[7] In the United States the highest prevalence has occurred in the Gulf Coast region, which has a favorable climate for vector transmission. A reliable serologic test for EIA was developed in the early 1970s,[9,10] and this test became the basis for the EIA control program implemented by the U.S. Department of Agriculture (USDA) in 1972. As a result, the prevalence of EIA in the United States has declined from 3.09% in 1972 to 0.01% in 2003, and in the Gulf Coast region the prevalence has declined from 11.08% to 0.03% (Fig. 23-2).

However, these figures do not necessarily reflect the EIA prevalence in the general horse population because they are biased by repeated testing of high-quality horses competing in events that require negative test results. Testing is required only for horses that are entering exhibitions or competitive events, being moved interstate, changing ownership, being imported, or entering auctions or sales markets. According to the USDA National Agricultural Statistics Service, there were 5.25 million horses in the United States at the end of 1997 and 5.32 million at the end of 1998 (the most current data available at this writing).[11] According to the USDA Animal

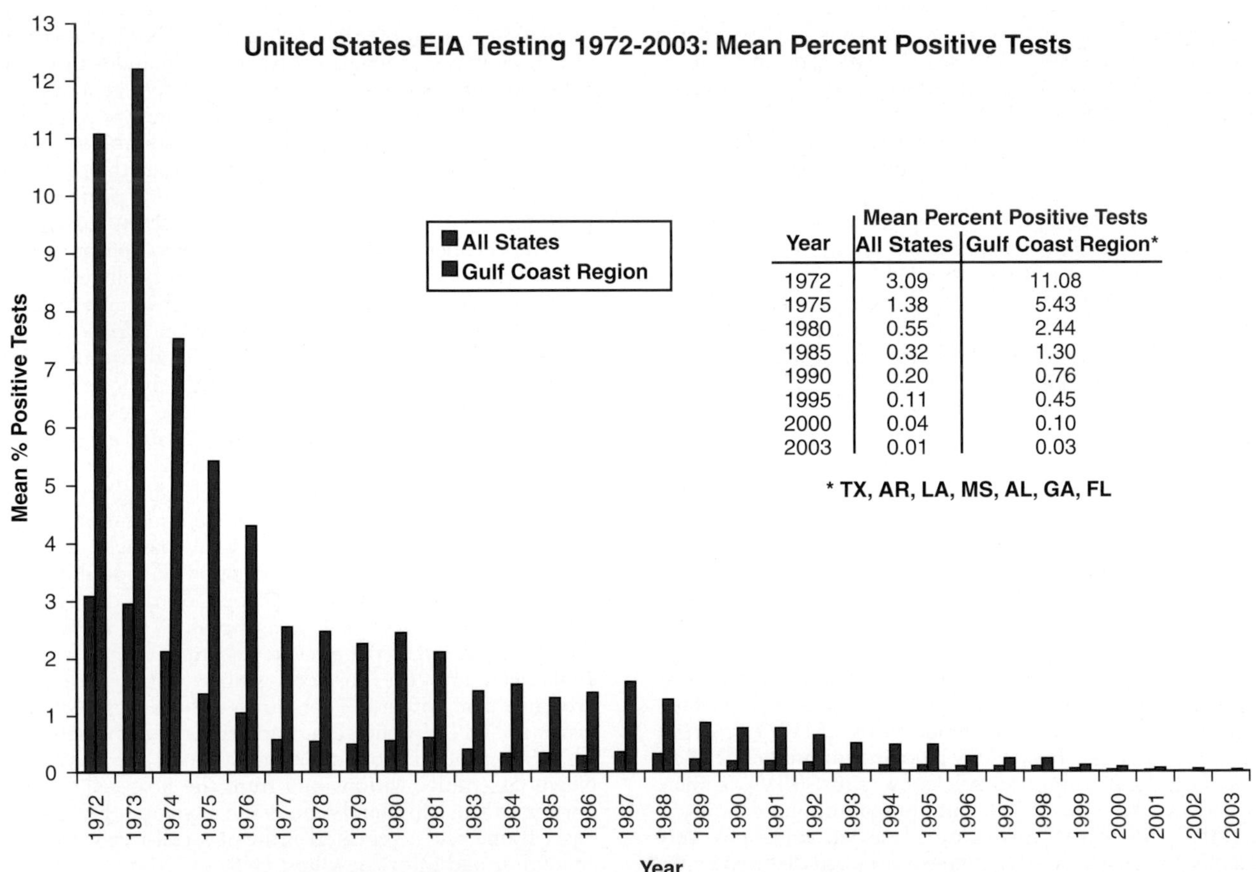

Year	Mean Percent Positive Tests: All States	Gulf Coast Region*
1972	3.09	11.08
1975	1.38	5.43
1980	0.55	2.44
1985	0.32	1.30
1990	0.20	0.76
1995	0.11	0.45
2000	0.04	0.10
2003	0.01	0.03

Fig. 23-2 Mean percent positive equine infectious anemia *(EIA)* tests for all 50 states *(red)* and for states in the Gulf Coast region *(blue)* from 1972 to 2003. (Courtesy US Department of Agriculture, Animal and Plant Health Inspection Service.)

and Plant Health Inspection Service (APHIS), 1.37 million and 1.43 million EIA tests were performed in those same years, respectively.[12] Based on these data, an average of only 26.5% of the equine population is tested annually. This figure is an overestimate because the tests performed in a given year include repetitive testing of an undisclosed number of horses.

In summary, the majority of horses in the United States are not tested, and the true EIA prevalence is not known.

Transmission

Blood from infected horses is the most important source of EIAV for transmission to susceptible horses. Transfer of blood by blood-feeding insects is the predominant means of natural transmission. Because the virus does not replicate within insect cells, insects serve only as mechanical vectors, transferring blood on their mouthparts.[13] The most important insect vectors for natural transmission are horseflies and deerflies,[7,13-16] both of which are members of the family *Tabanidae.* Stable flies *(Stomoxys calcitrans)* have also been shown to transmit the virus,[15] but they are less efficient than tabanids as natural vectors. Experimentally, a single horsefly[16] and as few as six deerflies[14] or 52 stable flies[14] can transmit the virus from acutely infected horses to susceptible horses. Studies within the past 25 years indicate that mosquitoes do not transmit EIAV.[13,17]

Several factors are critical for EIAV transmission by insect vectors. Horses with a high titer viremia and clinical disease are much more likely to transmit EIAV than are inapparent carriers with very low levels of virus in the blood. In one study, horseflies were not able to transmit virus from 10 naturally infected horses with no known history of clinical disease.[18] However, the transfer of 1 mL of whole blood from seven of these inapparent carrier horses was sufficient to cause infection in susceptible ponies, and 25 horseflies were able to transmit virus from one inapparent carrier horse that had an acute clinical disease episode 9 months previously.[18]

Vector population and feeding behavior also influence the probability of transmission. For transmission to occur, the vector must find and feed on an infected horse, be interrupted in that feeding, then find and feed on another horse within a short time. Horseflies are not able to transmit EIAV if the subsequent feeding is delayed 4 hours.[16] Tabanids inflict painful bites, contributing to their efficiency as vectors because their feeding is frequently interrupted by defensive movements made by the horse they are biting. Importantly, tabanids have large, slashing mouthparts that sever small vessels, creating a pool of blood. They imbibe blood from this extravascular pool, contaminating their mouthparts in the process (Fig. 23-3). As a result, tabanids transfer a relatively large amount of blood (up to 10 mL) when they feed on a subsequent horse.[19]

The distance separating infected and susceptible horses is another critical factor for transmission. When tabanids are interrupted in their feeding and released 1 foot (30 cm) from the initial host, 87.5% of them will return to the same horse when other horses are tethered 120 feet (36 m) away.[20] At a separation distance of 160 feet (48 m), 99% of the horseflies would be expected to return to the original horse if interrupted in their feeding. Therefore, a 200-yard (180-m) separation distance between horses adequately reduces potential EIAV transmission by tabanids. Finally, transmission is more likely when vectors are present in large numbers, explaining the higher EIAV prevalence in regions with warm climates, as well as the increased incidence during the summer months.[13]

Vertical transmission may occur in utero, at parturition, or after ingestion of infected colostrum or milk.[21-23] Transplacental transmission appears to be a rare event and is more likely when the mare develops acute clinical disease and high-titer viremia during gestation. In one study, 12 of 52 foals from

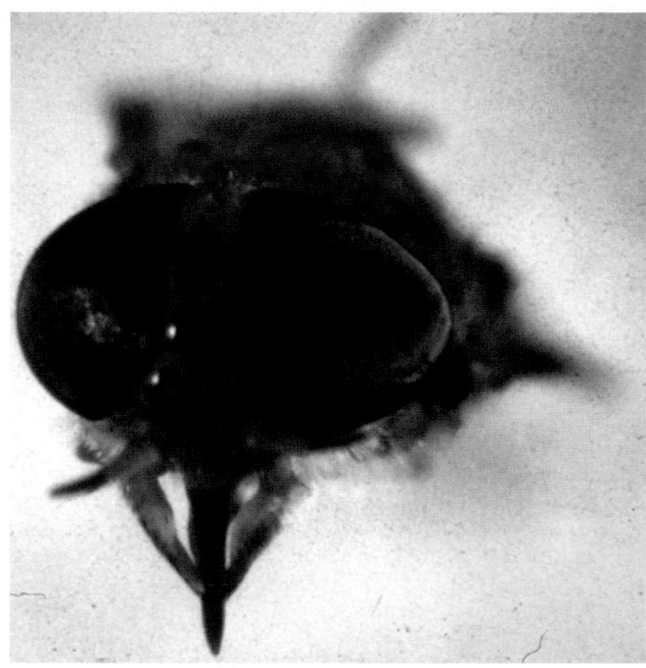

Fig. 23-3 Horsefly *(Tabanus fuscicostatus)*. Note the large mouthparts. (From Sellon DC: Equine infectious anemia. In Colahan PT, Merritt AM, Moore JN, Mayhew IG, editors: *Equine medicine and surgery*, ed 5, St Louis, 1999, Mosby, pp 2013-2019.)

EIAV-infected mares were virus positive (as determined by blood inoculation into susceptible ponies) when tested at 1 week to 6 months of age.[21] Although 7 of the 12 foals were offspring of mares that had clinical signs of EIA during gestation, transplacental transmission was confirmed in only one aborted fetus.[21] In other studies, 18 of 20 foals born to infected dams were virus negative (as determined by pony inoculation) at weaning,[24] and 29 of 31 foals from infected mares had no evidence of infection at weaning.[25] In virus-negative foals born to infected dams, EIAV-specific colostral antibody can be detected in serum for 25 to 195 days.[24,25] More recently, of 12 foals born to EIAV-infected mares in a herd of wild horses in Northeastern Utah, none was found to be virus positive by reverse transcriptase–polymerase chain reaction (RT-PCR). However, EIAV-specific colostral antibodies could be detected in the serum from these foals for up to 336 days.[26]

Venereal transmission is possible because semen from infected stallions can result in infection after subcutaneous inoculation.[22] However, breeding EIAV-infected stallions to uninfected mares did not result in transmission except for one possible case in which a mare sustained a vaginal laceration.[22] Finally, EIAV can be transmitted iatrogenically through transfusion with contaminated blood products and by the use of blood-contaminated materials, such as surgical and tattooing instruments, hypodermic needles, and dental equipment. The virus is known to survive for up to 4 days on hypodermic needles held at room temperature.[17]

PATHOGENESIS

Infection with EIAV can result in a variety of clinical, clinicopathologic, and pathologic abnormalities, including fever, lethargy, inappetence, thrombocytopenia, anemia, splenomegaly, hepatomegaly, lymphadenopathy, weight loss, dependent edema, and hemorrhage.[7,27-29] Clinical disease severity correlates with viral load, and thus depends on the level of virus replication. The virus infects macrophages, and most infected macrophages are detected in the spleen.[30] Although peripheral blood monocytes are infected, viral replication occurs primarily in mature tissue macrophages, which serve as the predominant source of the high-titer viremia during acute infection.[31] Tissue macrophages are also the primary cellular reservoir for EIAV during subclinical infection.[32] Although viral replication is restricted during periods of clinical quiescence, the virus continues to replicate at all times.[32] The spleen contains the highest level of replicating virus during acute infection, but other tissue sites of active infection include the liver, lymph nodes, bone marrow, peripheral blood mononuclear cells, lung, adrenal gland, kidney, and brain.[31-33] During inapparent infection, replicating virus can be detected in most of these same tissues, but at much lower levels.[32,33] Endothelial cell infection also occurs in EIAV-infected horses.[34]

Although the immune response to EIAV is critical for the eventual control of viral load and clinical disease, immunologic mechanisms are involved in the development of lesions and clinical disease. The infection and destruction of macrophages, as well as the observation that most of the infectious virus in the serum of infected horses occurs in the form of immune complexes,[27,28,35] are important factors in the immunopathogenesis of EIA. Infection of macrophages with virulent EIAV induces the upregulation of TNF-α, interleukin-1 (IL-1), and IL-6.[36] Elevation of the circulating levels of these proinflammatory cytokines most likely contributes to the fever, lethargy, and inappetence observed during acute disease.[36-39]

Thrombocytopenia

Thrombocytopenia is one of the earliest and most consistent detectable abnormalities in EIAV-infected horses and closely correlates with fever and viremia.[29] The pathogenesis of EIAV-induced thrombocytopenia is multifactorial. An increase in platelet-bound immunoglobulin G (IgG) and IgM during episodes of thrombocytopenia in experimentally infected horses suggests an immune-mediated mechanism.[40] However, foals with severe combined immunodeficiency (SCID) develop the same degree of thrombocytopenia as immunocompetent foals after EIAV infection.[41] Foals with SCID lack functional T and B lymphocytes and cannot mount antigen-specific cell-mediated or antibody responses.[42,43] In addition, platelet production during EIAV infection is significantly reduced in both SCID and immunocompetent foals.[41] These results indicate that suppression of platelet production is likely the predominant mechanism of EIAV-induced thrombocytopenia. Serum activities of potential negative regulators of thrombopoiesis, including TNF-α, TGF-β, and interferon-γ (IFN-γ), are increased just before, and at the onset of, thrombocytopenia in acutely infected horses.[39] Both TNF-α and TGF-β in plasma from EIAV-infected horses suppress equine megakaryocytes in vitro.[44] Additional work indicates that platelets become activated and hypofunctional in acutely infected horses, and as a result, platelet aggregates may form, which are then removed from the circulation.[45] This could represent a nonimmune mechanism of platelet destruction in EIAV-infected horses. Finally, infection of endothelial cells could promote platelet adherence and aggregation, leading to thrombocytopenia.[34]

Anemia

Anemia is a consistent clinical abnormality associated with EIAV infection, and its severity directly correlates with the frequency and duration of febrile episodes.[28] Similar to thrombocytopenia, the pathogenesis of anemia is multifactorial and includes immune-mediated erythrocyte destruction as well as decreased erythropoiesis. Early work indicated that erythrocyte life span is reduced to between 28 and 87 days (normal mean, 136 days) in EIAV-infected horses, and that both intravascular hemolysis and extravascular hemolysis occur.[46] Immune-mediated destruction is likely initiated by binding of EIAV hemagglutinin subunits to erythrocytes, which then become coated with antibody and bind the C3 component of complement.[27,28,47-49] Erythrocytes might also bind circulating virus-antibody immune complexes.[35] Intravascular hemolysis results from activation of the complement cascade through the classic pathway, whereas extravascular hemolysis occurs as a result of erythrophagocytosis by activated macrophages.[47,50,51] Complement binding requires immune responses (most likely antibody) because EIAV-infected SCID foals, which have an intact complement system, do not have C3 on their erythrocytes.[52] The fact that SCID foals become profoundly anemic indicates that suppression of erythropoiesis is an important mechanism of EIAV-induced anemia.[52] Erythroid progenitor cells are selectively suppressed by EIAV in vitro.[53] Although the exact mechanism by which erythropoiesis is suppressed is unknown, inhibitory cytokines are likely involved. In addition, iron deficiency may play a role during EIAV infection in vivo because plasma iron levels are low, as is the percentage saturation of transferrin.[54]

Immune Control

The precise immunologic mechanisms by which horses control EIAV infection are unknown. Adaptive immune responses are required to terminate plasma viremia, as evidenced by the inability of foals with SCID to eliminate the initial viremia after challenge with EIAV compared with normal foals.[52] Adoptive transfer of EIAV-specific T and B lymphocytes to a SCID foal results in functional *cytotoxic T lymphocytes* (CTLs) and neutralizing-antibody activity and is protective against EIAV challenge.[55]

Although neutralizing antibody is undoubtedly important, cellular responses are critical in the control of EIAV. Recrudescence of cell-free viremia and clinical disease occurred in persistently infected, inapparent carriers within 6 to 10 days after immunosuppression with either dexamethasone or cyclophosphamide, a time frame in which antibody titers had not changed.[56,57] One of these studies found that the induced viremia was subsequently terminated before the appearance of neutralizing antibody.[56] In addition, horses chronically infected with EIAV resisted challenge with heterologous virus, despite the lack of neutralizing antibody to the challenge strain.[58] Other researchers observed that both envelope glycoprotein subunit and inactivated whole-virus vaccines protected horses from challenge with homologous EIAV, but not heterologous virus. The observations that vaccination stimulated T-cell–mediated immunity and that protection occurred in the absence of neutralizing antibody led to the conclusion that cell-mediated mechanisms were involved.[59]

As in HIV and SIV, virus-specific CTLs are critically important in EIAV control.[60] The initial plasma viremia in acute EIAV infection is terminated before the appearance of neutralizing antibody, but concurrent with the appearance of CTLs.[60-62] The early humoral response to EIAV infection is composed primarily of nonneutralizing antibody,[63] and subsequent episodes of plasma viremia and clinical disease typically resolve before the appearance of neutralizing antibody.[63-67] CTL epitopes have been identified in several EIAV proteins, including gag, pol, env, rev, and in the protein encoded by the S2 open reading frame.[68-72] Importantly, gag p15 and gag p26 are the most frequently recognized EIAV proteins by CTL from inapparent carrier horses[69] and likely serve as important targets for protective CTL responses. Lastly, the antigenic variants that arise during recurrent viremic episodes have been assumed to be the result of selection pressure exerted by neutralizing antibody. However, recurrent episodes of viremia and clinical disease occur in the face of both neutralizing antibody and CTLs, indicating that EIAV variants arise that must escape both neutralizing antibody and CTL responses.[70] Recent work has shown conclusively that adaptive immunity drives the selection of EIAV envelope variants during acute infection.[73] Regardless, virus replication is eventually controlled in inapparent carriers, and this control is likely the result of a broad CTL and neutralizing-antibody response.

CLINICAL FINDINGS

The clinical course of EIA is variable, depending on the dose and virulence of the virus strain and the susceptibility of the horse.[74] Clinical disease may be less severe in donkeys and mules than in horses.[75] Although the distinctions are not absolute, three characteristic clinical stages of EIA have been described.[7,76]

Acute EIA occurs after initial infection with a virulent strain of EIAV. Five to 30 days after exposure, pronounced viremia can develop, resulting in fever, thrombocytopenia, lethargy, and inappetence. These signs can be mild and are often overlooked. The initial febrile episode usually subsides within a few days, although a small percentage of horses can develop a severe and fatal form of the disease characterized by persistent viremia, severe anemia, and high viral loads in most organs.[77]

After the initial disease episode, a few horses may develop an inapparent infection, but the majority of infected horses experience recurrent episodes of acute clinical disease characterized by viremia, fever, lethargy, inappetence, thrombocytopenia, and anemia. Each episode is associated with an antigenically distinct virus isolate, as defined by neutralizing antibody.[63,65-67,78-80] Clinical episodes typically last 3 to 5 days, and the interval between episodes is variable, ranging from weeks to months. Thrombocytopenia and other clinical signs resolve rapidly with the drop in viral load as each episode is terminated, and infected horses appear normal between episodes.

If clinical disease episodes become frequent and severe, the horse develops the classic signs of *chronic* EIA (a "swamper"), including anemia, thrombocytopenia, weight loss, and dependent edema (Fig. 23-4). Pale mucous membranes, petechiation, icterus, and epistaxis associated with more severe hemolytic anemia and thrombocytopenia can also be observed. Neurologic signs occasionally develop and can include ataxia and encephalitis.[81,82] However, for the majority of infected horses, episodes of clinical disease subside within a year after initial infection, and these horses become inapparent carriers of the virus. These horses are clinically normal and have very low plasma viral loads. Many infected horses never show observable signs of disease and remain inapparent carriers until infection is discovered incidentally by the detection of serum antibody during routine health evaluation. Although the risk of transmission from inapparent carriers is low, they serve as reservoirs of the virus and can transmit it under field conditions.[76,83] Transmission of infection and disease was 100% when 250 mL of whole blood was transferred from seropositive inapparent carriers to susceptible test ponies.[10] Inapparent carriers are infected for life, and treatment with immunosuppressive drugs causes recrudescence of plasma viremia and clinical disease,[56,57] indicating that environmental stress could induce a clinical episode.

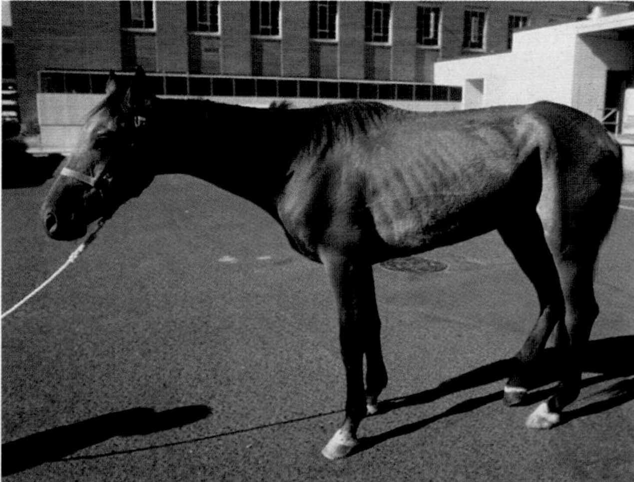

Fig. 23-4 EIAV-infected horse with clinical signs of chronic EIA (a "swamper").

DIAGNOSIS

Equine infectious anemia should be ruled out in horses showing the clinical signs of acute or chronic EIA, including recurrent fever, thrombocytopenia, anemia, petechiation, weight loss, or ventral edema. Many infected horses have no clinical signs and have no history of clinical signs. Other abnormalities in the complete blood count and serum biochemistry panel are inconsistent but can include monocytosis, leukopenia or leukocytosis, hypergammaglobulinemia, hyperbilirubinemia, hemoglobinemia, and elevation of liver enzyme levels.

Definitive diagnosis is made with serologic testing. Because EIAV is a persistent virus that is not cleared by the host, a positive serologic result indicates infection. Currently, four official serologic tests are approved by the USDA. These include the *agar gel immunodiffusion* (AGID) test, the *competitive enzyme-linked immunosorbent assay* (cELISA), the Vira-CHEK ELISA, and the synthetic antigen ELISA (SA-ELISA II). The AGID test, also known as the Coggins test, detects antibody against the EIAV gag p26 protein. The AGID test is the most widely accepted procedure for diagnosis of EIA and is highly specific; however, low levels of antibody can lead to false-negative results. The AGID test requires a minimum of 24 hours before results can be reported. The cELISA and Vira-CHEK ELISA also detect antibody against p26. They are more sensitive than the AGID, but less specific. Therefore, positive results must be confirmed with the AGID test. The cELISA and Vira-CHEK ELISA provide test results within an hour. The SA-ELISA II detects antibody to the EIAV envelope gp45 protein or the p26 protein. As with the cELISA and Vira-CHEK ELISA, the SA-ELISA II provides results within an hour, but positive results must be confirmed with the AGID test. Finally, the Western blot (immunoblot) test for antibodies against EIAV may be conducted by the National Veterinary Services Laboratory (NVSL) as a supplemental test to reach a consensus when other diagnostic tests yield contradictory results. The Western blot is not considered an official test by the USDA.

Early diagnosis may be difficult because serologic tests can be negative 10 to 14 days after infection;[10] however, most horses seroconvert by 45 days.[7,29,76] Colostral antibody usually clears by 6 months of age in noninfected foals born to seropositive mares,[76] but recent work indicates that passively acquired maternal antibody can be detected for up to 9 months with the AGID test and for up to 11 months with the cELISA.[26]

Tests that detect and quantitate EIAV in the blood are not generally used clinically, but these are routinely used in research settings. These tests are sensitive and specific and include animal inoculation, virus titration, and quantitative real-time RT-PCR. The *animal inoculation test* involves the intravenous transfer of 250 mL of whole blood from the suspect horse to a susceptible test pony, then monitoring the test pony for seroconversion and clinical signs of EIA. This test is extremely sensitive for detecting infection, including the inapparent carrier state.[10] *Virus titration* allows quantitation of infectious virus in plasma by titration in cell culture,[63] and real-time RT-PCR allows quantitation of viral RNA in plasma.[70,84] Nested RT-PCR assays (which incorporate a second round of amplification) are highly sensitive. Nested RT-PCR assays allow detection of viral RNA in plasma from inapparent carriers, as well as in plasma as early as 3 days after infection.[85] Despite their sensitivity, these RT-PCR techniques sometimes fail to detect virus in inapparent carriers with very low viral loads. All these tests that detect virus in blood are expensive and require special expertise and facilities.

PATHOLOGIC FINDINGS

In horses with acute disease, necropsy findings can include splenomegaly, hepatomegaly, generalized lymphadenopathy, ventral subcutaneous edema, vessel thrombosis, and mucosal and visceral hemorrhages[29] (Fig. 23-5). Typical tissue lesions include nonsuppurative hepatitis with infiltrates of macrophages and lymphocytes, primarily in the periportal areas[28] (Fig. 23-6). Cellular infiltrates in the kidney and other organs occur in the interstitial areas, primarily in the cortex. These cellular infiltrates are likely the result of specific immune response to viral antigens associated with infected macrophages.[28] This hypothesis is supported by the absence of typical tissue lesions in EIAV-infected SCID foals.[55,86] Glomerulonephritis is characterized by thickened basement membranes with inflammatory cell infiltrates and is associated with immune complex deposition.[87] In horses with neurologic disease, lesions include lymphohistiocytic periventricular leukoencephalitis,[82] nonsuppurative granulomatous ependymitis, meningitis, encephalitis, and plasmocytic-lymphocytic infiltration of the brain and spinal cord.[81] In inapparent carriers, necropsy results are usually normal, and tissue lesions are usually mild or absent.[7,29]

THERAPY

There is no specific therapy for EIAV infection. Equine infectious anemia is a reportable disease in the United States, and federal law prohibits interstate travel of infected animals except under special circumstances (see Prevention). If elected, supportive therapy would include isolation from other horses, minimizing stress, and providing good nursing care, nonsteroidal antiinflammatory drugs (NSAIDs), leg wraps and hydrotherapy for dependent edema, and blood transfusion for severe anemia and thrombocytopenia. Corticosteroids are contraindicated because they will exacerbate viremia and clinical disease.[56,57] Unlike other lentiviruses (e.g., HIV, SIV, FIV), EIAV does not cause profound immunodeficiency. However, high levels of viremia can induce transient immunosuppression.[88,89] Therefore, antimicrobial drugs may be indicated during febrile episodes to help prevent secondary bacterial infections.

PREVENTION

Equine infectious anemia is a reportable disease in the United States. Although developing a protective vaccine is of considerable interest and is the focus of federally funded research, no approved vaccine exists for EIA. Therefore the USDA control program is designed to maintain a low prevalence by detecting EIAV-infected horses and removing them from the population, decreasing the likelihood of transmission. Although specific procedures and requirements may vary between individual states, the following categories of horses must be tested for EIA using an official test performed by an approved laboratory: (1) horses being imported, (2) horses being entered into exhibitions or competitive events, (3) horses being moved interstate, (4) horses changing ownership, and (5) horses entering auctions or sales markets. When a positive test is obtained, the horse is placed under quarantine and retested for confirmation. Horses that are confirmed EIA positive are called "reactors." All horses that were within 200 yards (180 m) of the reactor are considered exposed and are also held under quarantine.

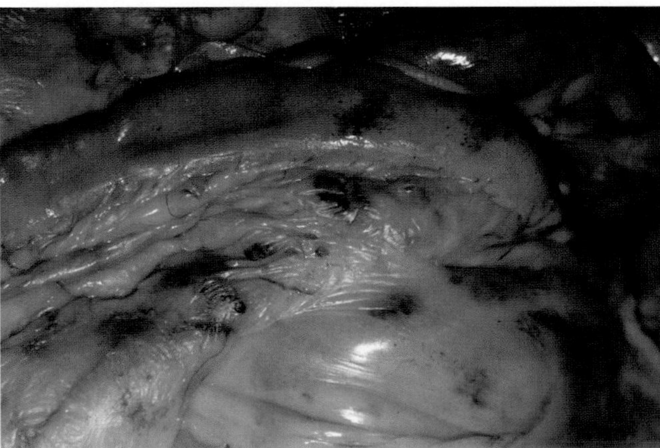

Fig. 23-5 Necropsy of EIAV-infected horse with acute EIA. Note the icteric mesentery and the numerous serosal and mesenteric hemorrhages.

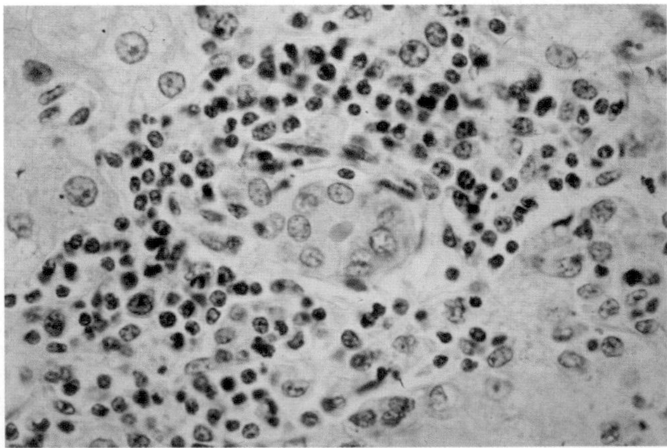

Fig. 23-6 Liver section from EIAV-infected horse (hematoxylin-eosin stain). Note the periportal accumulation of lymphocytes and macrophages.

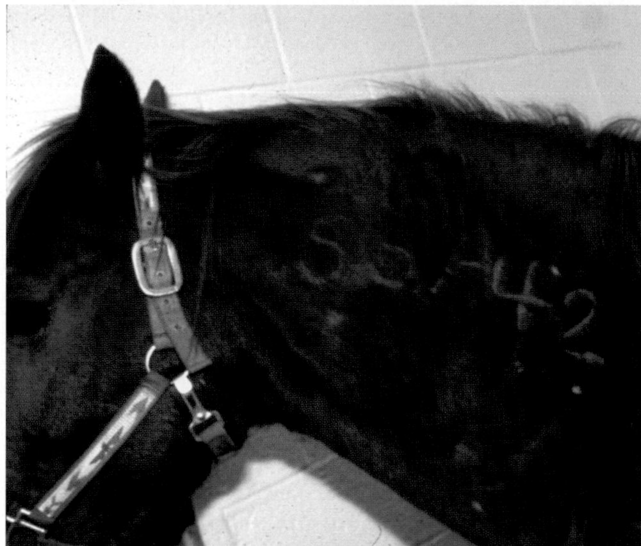

Fig. 23-7 Branded EIA "reactor." The number "55" is the individual horse identification number, the letter "A" designates the horse as an EIAV reactor, and the number "42" designates the state in which the horse was identified. (From Sellon DC: Equine infectious anemia. In Colahan PT, Merritt AM, Moore JN, Mayhew IG, editors: *Equine medicine and surgery*, ed 5, St Louis, 1999, Mosby, pp 2013-2019.)

These horses are tested at 30- to 60-day intervals, and any additional reactors are removed. The quarantine is lifted if all exposed horses are negative at least 60 days after the last reactor was removed.

There are several approved methods for removing an EIAV-infected horse from the general population. Humane euthanasia is most common. The horse could also be moved directly to an approved slaughter facility in a truck or trailer that has been officially sealed. Horses that are not immediately euthanized or shipped to slaughter must be permanently identified with a brand (Fig. 23-7) or lip tattoo. After permanent identification, a positive horse may be quarantined on the premises with a 200-yard (180-m) separation distance from all other equids. The quarantine area and the quarantined horse must be periodically monitored by regulatory personnel to ensure that the provisions of the quarantine are not violated. Alternatively, the horse may be moved under permit to a federally inspected slaughter facility or a federally approved diagnostic or research facility.

There are several recommended procedures for minimizing the risk of EIAV transmission. First, all horses should be tested annually as part of a routine equine health program. This is especially important in areas with increased prevalence, such as the Gulf Coast states. New horses added to a herd should always be tested, and an EIA test should be part of every prepurchase evaluation. Blood and plasma donors should always be screened for EIAV infection. Needles and syringes should never be used to inject more than one horse, and dental equipment, surgical instruments, stomach tubes, and any other multiple-use equipment should be free of blood contamination and adequately sterilized between procedures. Finally, rigorous environmental and on-animal vector control, especially for horseflies, deerflies, and stable flies, will minimize natural transmission of EIAV.

PUBLIC HEALTH CONSIDERATIONS

Equine infectious anemia virus only infects *Equidae,* and therefore EIA poses no public health risk.

REFERENCES

See the CD-ROM for a list of references linked to the abstract in PubMed.

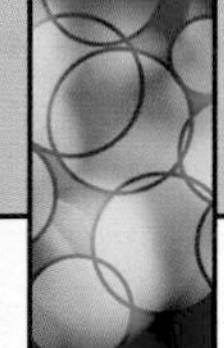

CHAPTER • 24

Vesicular Stomatitis

Brian J. McCluskey

ETIOLOGY

Vesicular stomatitis viruses (VSVs) are members of the family *Rhabdoviridae,* which includes viruses that infect vertebrates, invertebrates, and many plant species.[1] The viruses of this family that are known to infect mammals are in two genera, *Lyssavirus* and *Vesiculovirus*. Rabies is the most well characterized and most devastating virus of the *Lyssavirus* genus; VSVs are the prototype viruses of the *Vesiculovirus* genus. VSVs are bullet shaped and generally 180 nm long and 75 nm wide.[2] The nucleocapsid, or ribonucleoprotein (RNP) core, and lipoprotein envelope surrounding the RNP core are the two major structural components of VSVs. Extending from the outer surface of the envelope are spikelike projections.[1] The genome of VSVs consists of a single strand of negative-sense ribonucleic acid (RNA) and is composed of five genes, N, P, M, G, and L, representing the nucleocapsid protein, phosphoprotein (a component of the viral RNA polymerase), matrix protein, glycoprotein, and the large protein (a component of the viral RNA polymerase), respectively.[1]

Although there are many members of the *Vesiculovirus* genus, two are of particular interest in the United States, *vesicular stomatitis virus–New Jersey* (VSV-NJ) and *vesicular stomatitis virus–Indiana* (VSV-IN). These two viruses are similar in size and morphology but generate distinct neutralizing antibodies in infected animals. Thus, although considered distinct viruses, they are often distinguished only by terming one serotype "New Jersey" and the other serotype "Indiana."[3] Other members of the *Vesiculovirus* genus include Cocal, Jurona, Carajas, Maraba, Piry, Calchaqui, Yug Bogdanovac, Isfahan, Chandipura, Perinet, and Porton-S.[1] Cocal and Alagoas are subtypes of VSV-IN and have been associated with disease in animals in South America. Piry, Chandipura, and Isfahan produced only mild lesions in experimentally infected animals.[4] The remaining vesiculoviruses have been isolated from arthropods, mammals, or both but are not associated with disease.[1]

EPIDEMIOLOGY

Disease in United States

The first report of vesicular stomatitis (VS) in the United States was in 1916. However, anecdotal reports from the Civil War period leave little doubt that VS was occurring in horses during that time.[5] In 1926 an extensive outbreak of VS occurred in New Jersey in which approximately 750 cattle on 33 farms were affected. The disease appeared in very few horses. The agent was isolated and determined to be distinct from the Indiana strain isolated in the previous year. This new strain of VS was termed "vesicular stomatitis New Jersey strain."[6] Over the next six decades, VS occurred sporadically throughout the United States. Only states in New England appear to have been spared incursions of VS.

In the 1990s, three outbreaks of VS occurred in the southwestern United States. On May 9, 1995, the first case of VS was confirmed in Las Cruces, New Mexico. A "case" was defined as an animal with positive virus isolation or serologic test results, in combination with clinical signs consistent with VS. Bridges et al.[7] have provided an extensive review of this outbreak. Briefly, 1162 investigations were conducted in 42 states during the outbreak. VS was confirmed in six states, including Colorado (165 premises), New Mexico (186 premises), Utah (6 premises), Texas (1 premises), Arizona (1 premises), and Wyoming (8 premises). Overall, 78% of the positive premises housed horses that were positive for VS, 22% of positive premises housed cattle that were positive for VS, and there was one VS-positive llama. All cases where virus isolation was successful were caused by the VSV-NJ serotype.

McCluskey et al.[8] have provided a detailed review of the 1997 outbreak. The index case for this outbreak in the United States was identified on May 27 in Yavapai County, Arizona, after a report of suspicious vesicular lesions in a horse by a private practitioner. During the 1997 outbreak, 689 investigations for suspect VS occurred in 40 states. There were 380 (55%) premises identified as housing animals positive for VS in four states: Arizona, Colorado, New Mexico, and Utah. Similar to the 1995 outbreak, clusters of cases occurred in the Albuquerque, New Mexico, and Grand Junction, Colorado, areas. However, unlike the 1995 outbreak, a large number of cases were identified in the counties east of the Continental Divide in Colorado, extending from Pueblo as far east as Brush, Colorado. Nationwide, horses comprised 704 of 802 (88%) of the examinations conducted for suspect VS, and 362 of 374 (97%) positive premises had horses positive for VS. Cattle comprised 78 of 802 (10%) of the examinations conducted, and 12 of 374 (3%) positive premises had positive cattle. No premises had both positive cattle and positive horses. Both VSV-NJ and VSV-IN were isolated from clinical cases.

In 1998 the index case of VS occurred in a horse in Tularosa, New Mexico; virus isolation was confirmed as VSV-IN on May 18. Overall, 130 of 232 (6%) investigations nationwide were positive for VS. A total of four states were affected, including Texas (1 positive premises), Colorado (102 positive premises), New Mexico (12 positive premises), and Arizona (15 positive premises). Premises where an equid was positive for VS represented 99% of all positive premises. Only 1 premises housed cattle positive for VS, and this occurred in only one cow.

In 2004 a total of 294 positive premises were identified in three states (Colorado, New Mexico, and Texas) and in 2005, 445 positive premises were identified in nine states (Arizona, Colorado, Idaho, Montana, Nebraska, New Mexico, Texas, Utah, and Wyoming). In both the 2004 and 2005 outbreaks the virus isolated was VSV-NJ. The outbreak in 2005 occurred over the widest geographic area since the 1980s.

VS is endemic on Ossabaw Island, Georgia, where cattle, raccoons, white-tailed deer, horses, and feral swine are seropositive to VSV-NJ.[9,10] Serologic data indicate that transmission occurs annually, is seasonal, and is associated with maritime forest habitat.[11] Clinical disease is rare and is only observed in feral swine.

VS is a disease of the Western Hemisphere. Although only one endemic focus of disease occurs in the United States, areas throughout South America, Central America, and Mexico are considered endemic for VS. There are reports of endemic VSV and other vesiculoviruses in Brazil,[12,13] Argentina,[14] Columbia,[15] and other South American countries.[12] Extensive research in Costa Rica has demonstrated the endemic nature of the virus and the disease.[16-19] Work conducted by the author in El Salvador also indicated that the virus and disease are endemic in that country. A review of VS in Mexico revealed that cases occurred in every year between 1981 and 1995, with both serotypes identified in most years. VS has a national distribution in Mexico, although most cases occur in the southern states of Chiapas, Veracruz, and Tabasco. Disease is considered endemic in the central area of Mexico, but at a lower level than in southern states; viral activity in the northern area of Mexico is sporadic.

Transmission

Vesicular stomatitis viruses are considered arboviruses because they use insect vectors as their primary means of transmission. Although experimental and epidemiologic evidence for the role of arthropods as biologic vectors in the transmission of VSV is convincing, the mechanisms of virus acquisition by arthropod hosts and potential amplification of disease and the identity of reservoir hosts remain an enigma. Propagation of VSV outbreaks may be enhanced by movement of infected horses and spread by direct contact between infected and uninfected mammalian hosts.

Arthropod Vector Transmission

Outbreaks of VS in the southwestern United States typically begin in late spring or early summer and continue through late fall, with northward progression of disease over this period. Index cases for outbreaks in the United States are usually identified in southern New Mexico or Arizona. Both the temporal and the spatial characteristics of VS outbreaks suggest an association with arthropod abundance. New cases occur as warmer weather induces insect hatches and cease when cold weather predominates, inhibiting vector hatches.

The evidence for arthropod transmission of VSV is most compelling for sandflies *(Luzyomia shannoni)* and black flies (Diptera: *Simulidae*). Other species of insects may also be

Table • 24-1

Insect Genera from which Vesicular Stomatitis Viruses Have Been Isolated

GENUS	COMMON NAME	TRANSMISSION
Tabanus	Horsefly	Yes
Chrysops	Deerfly	Yes
Aedes	Mosquito	Yes
Culex	Mosquito	Yes
Culicoides	Biting midge	Yes
Musca	Housefly	No
Hippelates	Eye gnats	No
Simulium	Black fly	Yes
Lutzyomia	Sandfly	Yes
Stomoxys	Stable fly	Yes

competent biologic or mechanical vectors of VSV. Table 24-1 contains species of arthropods from which VSV have been isolated.

On Ossabaw Island, VSV-NJ has been isolated from sandflies, and virus activity, as measured by seroconversion in feral swine populations, corresponds to the seasonal appearance of sandflies.[20,21] Sandflies feed on feral swine, white-tailed deer, and to a lesser extent, horses and raccoons in that environment,[22] but neither swine nor white-tailed deer are competent amplifying hosts of VSV-NJ for sandflies.[23,24]

Black flies are competent experimental vectors for VSV-NJ, and this virus has been isolated from *Simulidae* trapped in the wild during outbreaks of VS.[25,26] *Simulium vittatum* (black fly) females intrathoracically infected with virus transmit infectious virus in their saliva after 10 days.[25] Efficient transmission of VSV-NJ occurs between infected and noninfected black flies co-feeding on nonviremic deer mice, suggesting that black flies could act as a transfer vector between nonviremic vertebrate hosts and domestic livestock.[27,28] Clinical disease was detected in two of three horses when VSV-NJ–infected black flies fed on their lips and muzzle.[29] Subclinical infection, as indicated by seroconversion, occurred in one horse when feeding was restricted to the thorax.

The flight range of potential VSV insect vectors vary, but none would be adequate to explain the often large distances observed between either individual or clusters of infected premises. Analysis of backward wind trajectories during the VS outbreaks in 1982 and 1985 suggest the feasibility of infected insects being transported for long distances on wind currents and subsequently landing on noninfected premises many miles away.[30]

Transport of Infected Animals

During the VS outbreak in 1983, disease entered California through transport of infected cattle purchased in Idaho.[31] The only case of VSV infection identified in Texas during the 1995 outbreak was caused by movement of a horse from an area in New Mexico that was experiencing increased VSV activity into Texas. This horse apparently had become infected in New Mexico and subsequently exhibited clinical signs of VSV infection after being moved to Texas.

Direct-Contact Transmission

Transmission of VSV by direct contact with an infected animal was observed when pigs were experimentally inoculated with VSV-NJ.[32] Seronegative pigs in contact with experimentally infected pigs were monitored daily for clinical disease, evidence of virus shedding, and seroconversion. Transmission occurred only when infected pigs had visible lesions. Resultant infections ranged from subclinical to clinical, with development of vesicular lesions. Seronegative pigs shed virus as early as 1 day after contact with infected pigs.

Reservoirs

Arboviruses generally use vertebrate hosts as reservoirs for transmission by arthropods. A vertebrate reservoir is normally infective for hematophagous insects when viremic. However, viremia has not been detected in livestock species that exhibit clinical signs of VS. Many vertebrate species have serologic evidence of exposure to VSV and may serve as reservoirs of infection. Table 24-2 lists select species from which antibodies to one or both VSV serotypes have been detected.

Bats *(Myotis lucifugus lucifugus)* subcutaneously inoculated with Cocal VSV were viremic for 10 days when housed at 22° C (71.6° F) and for 16 days when maintained in hibernation conditions.[33] These periods of viremia may be caused by active virus replication within the bats or may merely represent persistence of the original experimental inoculum. Virus is recoverable from spleen, liver, and brain homogenates for up to 8 months after experimental infection of immunocompetent Syrian hamsters with VSV-IN.[34] In deer mice *(Peromyscus maniculatus)*, a potential reservoir species in the southwestern United States, VSV-NJ can be demonstrated by

Table • 24-2

Wild Vertebrates Identified to Have Antibodies to Vesicular Stomatitis Viruses

SPECIES	COMMON NAME
Alouatta villosa	Howler monkey
Antilocapra americana	Pronghorn antelope
Antilope cervicapra	Blackbuck
Aotus trivirgatus	Night monkey
Artibus spp.	Fruit bat
Baiomys taylori	Pygmy mouse
Bassaricyon gabii	Olingo
Bradypus infuscatus	Sloth
Canis latrans	Coyote
Cervus elaphus	Elk
Coendu rothschildi	Porcupine
Dasypus novemcinctus	Armadillo
Didelphis virgianus	Opossum
Felis rufus	Bobcat
Lepus californicus	Jackrabbit
Lynx rufus	Lynx
Meleagris gallopavo	Wild turkey
Mus musculus	House mouse
Mephitis mephitis	Skunk
Myocastor coypu	Nutria
Neotoma mexicana	Wood rat
Odocoileus virginianus	White-tailed deer
Odocoileus hemionus	Mule deer
Ovis canadensis	Bighorn sheep
Peromyscus maniculatus	Deer mouse
Procyon lotor	Raccoon
Saguinus geoffroyi	Marmoset

immunohistochemistry in central nervous system tissues and the heart for up to 5 days after inoculation.[35]

Risk Factors

A case-control study of horses, cattle, and sheep on 395 premises in Colorado, New Mexico, Utah, and Arizona identified management factors affecting the risk of animals developing VS in the southwestern United States.[36] Animals with access to a shelter or barn have a reduced risk of developing VS. This effect is more pronounced for equine premises. Risk of developing disease is increased where animals have access to pasture. On all premises where owners report increased insect populations and where animals are housed less than 1/4 mile (0.4 km) from a source of running water, chances of developing VS are increased.

A retrospective case-control study of 52 premises with VS-positive animals, 33 with no VS-positive animals, and eight nearby premises determined potential risk factors for VS in Colorado in 1995.[37] Premises-level and animal-level data, including management practices and ecologic variables, were collected. Premises with at least one seropositive animal in 1996 were significantly more likely to be case premises in 1995 than were control premises. For case premises, there was an association between serologic status of the animals in 1996 and clinical disease status in 1995. No significant premises-level or animal-level risk factors were identified in this study.

PATHOGENESIS

The molecular basis of VSV pathogenesis is typical of viral infections, with a series of events terminating in the release of progeny virions and cell death. Virus attaches to cell surface receptors through the G-protein spike. Penetration and uncoating of viral particles occur, and transcription and replication commence. Ultimately, new viral particles are assembled at the cellular plasma membrane. The matrix (M) protein plays a specific role in the attachment of condensed nucleocapsids to the plasma membrane and to subsequent budding of the new virions.[38] Inhibition of cellular RNA, DNA, and protein synthesis occurs before cellular rounding that results from M-protein–induced disruption in the cytoskeleton.[39]

Infection of epithelium with VSV induces intercellular edema in the malphigian layer, and the epithelial cells become separated by vacuolar cavities.[40,41] Cellular necrosis occurs concomitant with edema; cells shrink in size but do not undergo lysis. The infiltration of inflammatory cells, including granulocytes and monocytes, eventually results in cellular lysis. Vesicles develop when the necrotic, edematous mucosa breaks free from underlying tissue, forming a cavity filled with cellular exudates. Separation occurs at the basal layer (stratum basale) of the epithelium. Intercellular fluid accumulation, cellular necrosis, and inflammatory cell infiltration result in vesicle formation within 48 hours of experimental inoculation. Vesicles rapidly disappear resulting from seepage of edema fluid.

CLINICAL FINDINGS

The clinical signs of VSV infection occur in cattle, horses, swine, and rarely in llamas (Figs. 24-1 through 24-4). Signs follow a typical viral incubation period of 3 to 7 days. An initial febrile period is followed by ptyalism in cattle and horses.[42-44] Lesions of the oral mucosa present as raised, blanched, and rarely, fluid-filled vesicles. The dorsolingual surface is often affected, but the gingival surfaces, palate, and mucocutaneous junctions may also exhibit lesions.[43] Vesicles are very short lived and rupture, leaving ulcerations and erosions. Lesions often coalesce to form large, denuded areas of oral mucosa with epithelial tags. Vesicular and ulcerative lesions outside the oral mucosa occur on the snout of pigs, teats of cattle, and coronary bands of pigs, cattle, and horses. Teat lesions are not as common as oral lesions but may be associated with severe secondary cases of mastitis. Lesions of the feet typically manifest as coronitis, with edema and inflammation extending from the coronary band proximally up the lower leg. Foot lesions are much less common than oral lesions in outbreaks in the southwestern United States.

Crusting or scabbing lesions of the muzzle, ventral abdominal wall, prepuce, and udder may appear in affected horses. These lesions typically start as discrete, small (approximately 1-cm) erosions that quickly coalesce so that large, crusted or scabbed areas are observed. These lesions are often located in areas of the body favored by hematophagous arthropods. Vesicular stomatitis viruses have been isolated from these crusting or scabbing lesions.

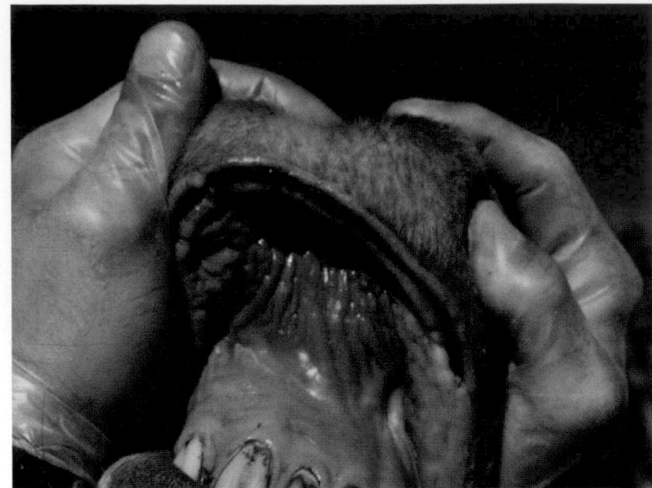

Fig. 24-1 Ulceration of oral mucosa at mucocutaneous junction in horse caused by vesicular stomatitis virus (VSV) infection.

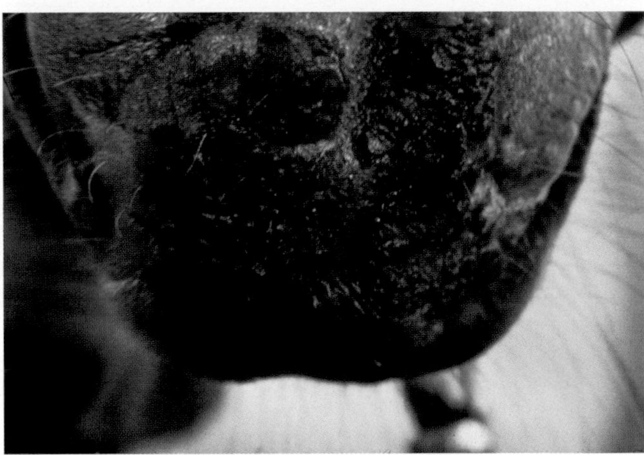

Fig. 24-2 Crusting lesion of horse's muzzle caused by infection with vesicular stomatitis virus serotype New Jersey (VSV-NJ).

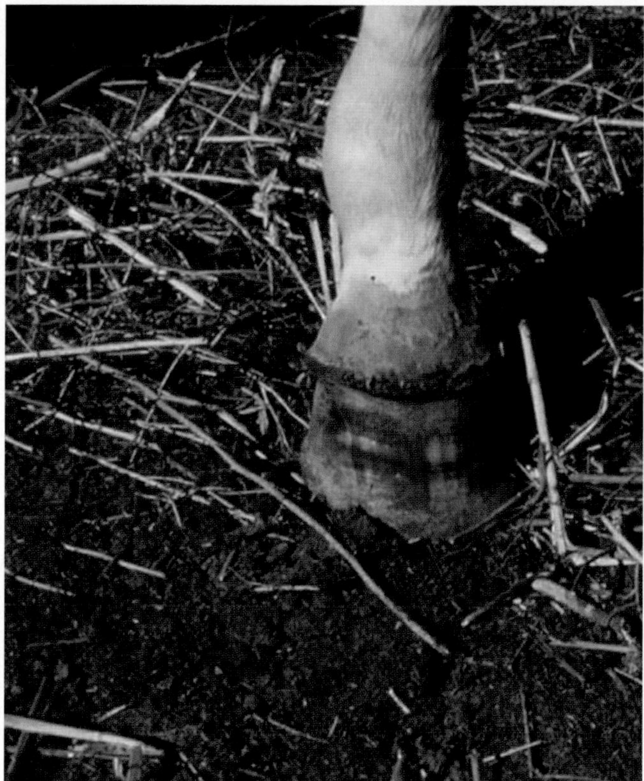

Fig. 24-3 Coronitis caused by VSV-NJ infection.

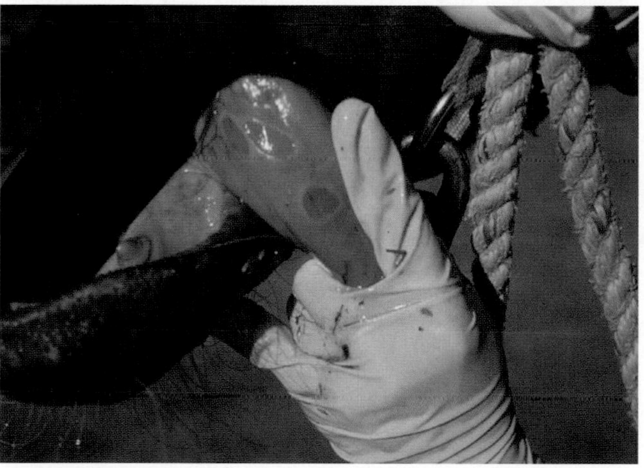

Fig. 24-4 Lingual vesiculation and ulceration in horse caused by VSV infection.

Stomatitis and other ulcerative, erosive, or vesicular diseases not caused by VS also occur in horses. McCluskey and Mumford[45] provide an extensive review of the differential diagnosis of VS in horses. Trauma of the oral and nasal cavities and coronary bands from any cause is the primary differential diagnosis for VS in horses. Sunburn is also often confused with VS. Very few infectious agents, other than VSV and other vesiculoviruses, have been definitively associated with vesicle formation in horses. In some cases, infections with equine arteritis virus, Jamestown Canyon virus, caliciviruses, and equine herpesviruses may result in oral ulcers and erosions. Wood shavings of the *Simaroubaceae* family (containing the compounds quassin or neoquassin) used as bedding material can cause apparent "outbreaks" of ulcerative stomatitis in groups of horses, as can physical trauma induced by coarse forage or plant awns, including triticale hay.

Cantharidin is the toxin contained in blister beetles (*Epicauta* spp.), which may be present in baled alfalfa hay. Ingestion of the beetles can cause vesicular or ulcerative lesions as well as severe systemic signs. Adverse reactions to the administration of pharmaceuticals or over-the-counter medications, including nonsteroidal antiinflammatory drugs (NSAIDs), may cause ulceration or erosion of the oral mucosa, generally in combination with systemic manifestations.

Pemphigus foliaceus, equine exfoliative eosinophilic dermatitis and stomatitis, squamous cell carcinoma, and melanoma can mimic the clinical picture of vesicular stomatitis. Recently, several apparent outbreaks of ulcerative stomatitis were reported in horses in the United States and New Zealand. Extensive investigations failed to determine any infectious or other cause for these outbreaks. The most significant differential diagnosis for VS in nonequine species is foot-and-mouth disease, which does not occur in horses.

Subclinical infections are common in livestock during outbreaks of VS. One study reported disease prevalence of 44.7% in horses on 17 premises, with a seroprevalence of 61.0%. Only 4.5% of cattle on the 17 premises investigated showed clinical signs, whereas 67.6% were seropositive to VSV-NJ.[46] Another study, also conducted during the 1982 outbreak in the southwestern United States, indicated disease prevalence ranging from 0% to 30%, with the seropositivity ranging from 14% to 100%.[47] Extensive herd testing conducted on an equine operation in 1995 confirmed the extensive nature of subclinical infections. Ranch census indicated the presence of 98 horses at the time VS was first diagnosed on August 22. Blood sampling and oral examination were performed on all horses at 30 days, and horses without clinical signs were rebled at 60 days. Overall, 25 of 98 (26%) horses examined were considered clinically affected with VS at the 30-day examination. Affected horses had active and healing ulcers on the oral mucosa; one horse had flulike signs consistent with the initial stages of VS. Of the 98 horses tested, 64 (67%) were positive by the *competitive enzyme-linked immunosorbent assay* (cELISA), and 73 (77%) were positive by the *virus neutralization test* (VNT). Horses negative on the first test were rebled 34 days later (60 days), and of the horses retested because of a negative first test, 3 of 25 were positive (12%) by the VNT. The retested animals, combined with the original horses tested, provided an overall seroprevalence of 81% by the VNT.

DIAGNOSIS

Three approaches to diagnosis of VSV infection are available: (1) antibody detection through a variety of serologic tests, (2) virus detection through isolation methods, and (3) detection of viral genetic material by molecular techniques.

Detection of antibodies to VSV is accomplished by VNT, *complement fixation test* (CFT), or ELISA. The VNT is considered the standard serologic test for VSV antibodies. The World Animal Health Organization (OIE) recognizes the VNT as a prescribed test for international trade.[48] Samples with detectable antibody at greater than a 1:40 dilution are considered positive for international trade purposes. The CFT is also recognized as a prescribed test for international trade purposes, and samples with titers greater than 1:5 dilution are considered positive.[48]

Numerous ELISAs have been developed for detection and quantitation of VS antibodies,[49-51] but most recently the cELISA has become the serologic test of choice for screening purposes during outbreaks of VS in the United States. The cELISA is considered a prescribed test for international trade by the OIE. A sample is considered positive if the absorbance is greater than or equal to 50% of the absorbance of the diluent control.

An ELISA capable of detecting the immunoglobulin M (IgM) class of antibody to VSV (mcELISA) was developed after the 1982 outbreak of VS in the southwestern United States.[52] It facilitates detection of recent exposure to VSV. This assay is not a prescribed test for international trade as determined by the OIE.

A comparison of the most common diagnostic tests for VSV (VNT, CFT, cELISA, mcELISA) by examination of experimentally inoculated animals indicates that the cELISA performs comparably to the VNT. The relative sensitivity and specificity of the cELISA compared with the VNT is 88% and 99%, respectively.[53] Positive mcELISA and cELISA responses consistently appear 1 to 2 days before CFT seroconversion, but all animals revert to mcELISA-negative status by 49 days after exposure. In a recent report, comparison of the VNT and cELISA on 1106 samples collected from cattle on sentinel farms in Costa Rica indicates very good agreement between the two tests.[54] The current serologic diagnostic testing scheme employed during outbreaks of VS in the United States is to screen samples with the cELISA for both serotypes of virus. Positive tests are confirmed by the VNT and CFT.

For virus isolation, vesicle fluid, epithelial tags, or swabs from fresh lesions are the ideal diagnostic sample. Vesicular stomatitis viruses are easily propagated in cell culture and induce cytopathic effects (CPEs) on an assortment of cell types, including Vero, BHK-1, and IB-RS-2 cells.[48] Fluorescent antibody (FA) staining using conjugates specific for VSV-NJ and VSV-IN may be employed for serotype differentiation.[55]

The detection of genomic sequences of VSV may be used to identify the presence of virus in tissue or swab samples. A *polymerase chain reaction* (PCR) assay to detect the phosphoprotein gene of VSV-NJ (but not VSV-IN) is more sensitive in detecting positive samples than is virus isolation from tissue.[56] A heminested PCR using the genomic sequence of the L protein as the primer detects the presence of VSV-NJ and VSV-IN even when viable virus is not present.[57] A reverse transcriptase–PCR (RT-PCR) for simultaneous detection of foot-and-mouth disease, swine vesicular disease, and vesicular stomatitis virus is able to differentiate between VSV-NJ and VSV-IN.[58] A single-tube multiplex PCR for detection of VSV-NJ and VSV-IN in insect pools can detect either Indiana or New Jersey or both serotypes with as little as 20 femtograms of total RNA. Viral RNA can be detected in macerates containing two infected mosquitoes in pools of 10 to 30 noninfected mosquitoes.[59]

The report of a potential *foreign animal disease* (FAD) by a practitioner initiates standardized investigation procedures by animal health officials (see Chapter 68). The private veterinary practitioner is of paramount importance in this diagnostic scheme, and practitioners trigger the process by calling an animal health official. One of three different officials may be contacted: the nearest foreign animal disease diagnostician (FADD), a specially trained animal health official, if the practitioner knows these officials; the state veterinarian's office; or the Animal and Plant Health Inspection Service, Veterinary Science (APHIS-VS), area veterinarian in charge (AVIC) office.

The decision on whether to initiate this process is often difficult for a practitioner, and individuals have varying thresholds of when to report. Practitioners' concerns about what they should report and when are justified. Although the investigation and laboratory support of the investigation are provided at no charge, the effects of quarantines or hold orders imposed on a premises can have an adverse financial impact on horse owners and potentially strain relationships between practitioners and their clients. A practitioner's first call to the local FADD or AVIC may be merely to discuss their observations before formally reporting suspicious lesions or signs. The AVIC ultimately determines if an FAD investigation will be initiated. Early and frequent discussions between practitioners and animal health officials are encouraged as a way to eliminate crisis responses. Animal health officials depend on practitioners to report suspicious findings, and in most states, practitioners are obligated to do so. Animal health officials expect practitioners to report suspect FAD as soon as possible. Delays in reporting may have catastrophic effects on disease control, so "erring on the side of caution" is a reasonable response and will be supported by animal health officials.

Reasonable approaches to quarantine are generally the rule during the initial phases of an investigation. Quarantines and hold orders are issued judiciously by the state veterinarian's office (federal quarantines are issued only when national emergencies are declared) and in many situations apply only to the affected animal(s) (placed under movement restrictions). Owners are obligated to follow the restrictions inherent in the quarantine; practitioners are not expected to assist in ensuring that these restrictions are followed. The continued medical care of the affected animal remains the responsibility of the practitioner and owner, and the practitioner should employ biosecurity and biocontainment measures to prevent the spread of disease.

All investigative procedures conducted by the FADD are done at no charge to the owner or practitioner. Blood, tissue, and other samples are collected by the FADD and submitted to laboratories specializing in the diagnosis of FADs, either the National Veterinary Services Laboratory (NVSL) in Ames, Iowa, or the Plum Island Animal Disease Center in New York. State and university diagnostic laboratories are not routinely used for diagnostic testing. Samples collected by practitioners may be submitted by the FADD, but in most situations, new samples are collected. In rare instances, private practitioners submit biologic samples directly to the laboratories.

The FADD, with input from the AVIC, determines the priority to assign to sample processing. *Priority 1* samples may actually be hand-carried to the laboratory by the FADD. These samples have diagnostic studies begun as soon as they arrive at the laboratory. *Priority 2* samples are sent by next-day air and are processed the same day they are received if the shipment reaches the laboratory before 4 PM; otherwise, tests are begun the following day. *Priority 3* samples are also sent by next-day air and processed according to accession order. Samples are generally tested only for suspected FAD, with diagnostic tests for non-FADs on a differential list conducted only in rare circumstances on a case-by-case basis.

Results for all sample priority levels are sent by telephone, fax, or e-mail to the AVIC and then forwarded to the FADD. It is generally the responsibility of the FADD to provide results to the owner and referring veterinarian immediately after receiving results. If test results are negative for an FAD, quarantines and hold orders are released, and further diagnostic procedures and testing are the responsibility of the owner and veterinary practitioner.

THERAPY

Vesicular stomatitis is typically short lived and self-limiting. No specific treatment is indicated, and most horses recover in 7 to 14 days. Even in severe cases, supportive care is adequate. Strict biosecurity practices, including wearing disposable protective gloves and washing hands frequently, should be instituted to prevent the spread of disease among horses and to human handlers (see Chapters 66 and 67).

Frequent rinsing of lesions with mild antiseptic solutions or application of topical antibiotics may help prevent secondary bacterial infections. Softening of grain or pellets with water may ease mastication when oral lesions are present and help prevent weight loss. Dehydration of sufficient severity to require intravenous fluid support is rare.

PREVENTION

The concept of using a virulent live VSV as a vaccine was first proposed in the 1920s.[60] Cattle inoculated intramuscularly with VSV did not develop lesions and when challenged with virus locally were resistant.

A special license was obtained from the U.S. Department of Agriculture (USDA) in 1967 to produce and sell a live VSV-NJ lyophilized vaccine. Sale of this vaccine in the United States was discontinued in 1972.[61] The same vaccine was used in Guatemala for many years with reported success.

A commercially available, killed–VSV-NJ vaccine was used in Colorado during the 1985 outbreak, but serologic data regarding its immunogenicity and efficacy are not available. A field trial to examine the humoral response to this vaccine was conducted in a 350-cow dairy.[62] Two doses of this formalin-killed cell culture–derived vaccine were administered intramuscularly 30 days apart to lactating and nonlactating adult cattle. Geometric mean titers peaked 21 days after the second vaccination at 1:530 and declined to a geometric mean titer of 1:65 by 175 days after vaccination. The lack of detectable antibody in the control group of cattle indicates that exposure to wild-type virus did not occur, and therefore the efficacy of the vaccine could not be ascertained.

A similar study was conducted during the 1995 VSV outbreak. Three commercial dairies approved to use a killed autogenous vaccine produced from a 1995 isolate of virus were enlisted in a field trial.[63] Serum samples were collected from all cattle in the study before vaccination, and all were determined to be free of antibodies to both VSV-NJ or VSV-IN. Two doses of vaccine were administered 14 days apart. All vaccinated cattle generated serum neutralizing antibodies to VSV-NJ, but immunity waned quickly to low levels by 250 days after vaccination. There was no indication that wild-type virus infected livestock on these operations or on nearby operations, so vaccine efficacy could not be determined.

A DNA vaccine that expresses the glycoprotein gene of VSV-NJ elicits neutralizing antibody responses in mice, calves, and horses.[64] Manipulation of the VSV genome may ultimately lead to novel attenuated live-VSV vaccines that are safe and efficacious. One such strategy currently under investigation is the translocation of the N gene, which reduces mortality in mice without reduction in the ability to generate a protective immune response.[65]

PUBLIC HEALTH CONSIDERATIONS

Three laboratory workers infected with VSV through exposure to experimentally infected animals[66] complained of fever, general malaise, and muscle pain. Two of the individuals handled experimentally infected cattle, and the third was splashed with virus-containing material while harvesting infected allantoic fluids. Mild stomatitis was observed in two of the three individuals. Recovery was complete and rapid without specific therapy. Although no virus was isolated from any of these individuals, high neutralizing antibody titers to VSV-NJ were detected.

In the 1950s, laboratory workers at the Agricultural Research Laboratory in Beltsville, Maryland, were routinely tested for VSV complement-fixing antibodies.[67] A summary of this work indicated that VS in humans appears as an acute, self-limiting infection with signs similar to influenza. Overall, 96% of laboratory workers and animal handlers had positive titers to VSV, although only 57% of those with positive titers could recall having clinical signs.

An investigation of owners and handlers of infected cattle was conducted during an outbreak of VS in 1965.[68] Forty-one persons were interviewed, and specimens were collected for virus isolation and serologic testing. Eight persons who lived or worked on ranches where cattle were confirmed to have been infected with VSV-IN had serologic evidence of exposure to VSV. Fever, general malaise, myalgia, nausea, and pharyngitis were observed. Vesicular lesions of the gums occurred in two people.

A study of veterinarians, research workers, and regulatory personnel exposed to VSV during an outbreak in Colorado in 1982 revealed that the prevalence of neutralizing antibody was higher in exposed persons with clinical signs than in those without a history of clinical illness.[69] Higher risk of seropositivity was observed for individuals who examined the oral cavity of infected animals, who had open wounds on hands or arms, and who examined horses rather than cattle. Overall, infection rates among exposed humans were low.

REFERENCES

See the CD-ROM for a list of references linked to the abstract in PubMed.

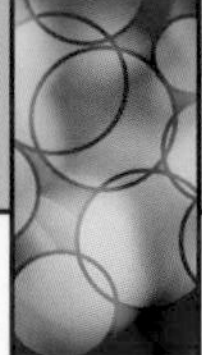

CHAPTER • 25

Papillomavirus Infections

Debra C. Sellon

Equine papillomavirus types 1 and 2 have been isolated from acquired *papillomas* (warts) and *aural plaques* in young horses. A large number of studies have implicated bovine papillomavirus types 1 and 2 in the pathogenesis of equine *sarcoid*, a form of nonmetastatic cutaneous fibrosarcoma, but a causal link has not been confirmed by fulfilling Koch's postulates. Each of these disorders is discussed separately in this chapter.

EQUINE WARTS

Etiology

Cutaneous papillomas (warts) are proliferative skin lesions caused by infection with *Equus caballus* papillomavirus type 1 (EcPV-1). Lesions are most often observed on the muzzle and lips of young horses (Fig. 25-1) but may also appear on ears, eyelids, genitalia, or distal limbs.[1] Papillomaviruses are small, nonenveloped, double-stranded deoxyribonucleic acid (DNA) viruses that are associated with epithelial proliferations in many vertebrate species.[2] EcPV-1 has been isolated, characterized, and cloned from equine warts.[3] A second mucosotropic equine papillomavirus, designated EcPV-2, has been isolated from papillomas affecting the genital area of horses. EcPV-2 differs from EcPV-1 in restriction endonuclease digestion pattern.[3,4]

Congenital equine papillomatosis is much less common than acquired disease.[5-11] Congenital lesions do not spontaneously regress, but surgery is usually curative.[11] Although in utero infection by a latent papillomavirus in the dam has been suggested as an etiology of these lesions, there has been no genetic or antigenic evidence to support this.[8,12]

Epidemiology

Most horses with cutaneous papillomatosis (warts) are less than 3 years of age. There are no breed or gender predilections. Disease can be spread by fomites or by close contact with affected horses. Spread is common when young horses are brought together in large groups for show, sale, or breeding.[1]

Pathogenesis

In 1951, Cook et al.[13] demonstrated that intradermal or subcutaneous injection of filtrates of equine papillomas results in growth of typical papilloma lesions within 60 to 70 days. Inoculation by skin scarification produces similar results. Lesions regressed spontaneously within 50 to 100 days. Similar injections into calves, lambs, dogs, rabbits, and guinea pigs did not result in lesions.[13] Natural infections are thought to require contact of virus with damaged skin (environmental trauma, ectoparasites, ultraviolet light damage).[11] The incubation period is estimated at approximately 60 days and may be influenced by the dose of virus, route of exposure, and immunity of the host.[11,14]

Histopathologic studies of naturally occurring equine warts suggest that lesions are initiated by basal cell hyperplasia without viral antigen production. As lesions develop, there is prominent acanthosis with cellular swelling and fusion, as well as marked hyperkeratosis and parakeratosis.[15] Hypomelanosis of lesions may be related to a disturbance in melanin synthesis.[16] Regression of papillomas is associated with an increase in the number of hyperfunctional Langerhans' cells at the dermal-epidermal junction and infiltration of T lymphocytes.[17] Natural immunity is strong, and warts disappear spontaneously 1 to 6 months after they initially appear.[11]

Clinical Findings

Horses with equine cutaneous papillomatosis usually have multiple lesions, most frequently on the muzzle and lips but occasionally occurring on the distal limbs, genitalia, ears (Fig. 25-2), and eyelids.[1,11] Equine warts vary in size from 0.1 to 2 cm in diameter. When they first appear, warts are often slightly raised, flat, smooth, and flesh colored. As they proliferate in number and size, they become verrucous, gray, and hyperkeratotic with development of fronds, resulting in a cauliflower-like appearance.[1] Single or multiple lesions may be oval or irregular in outline, dry, gray or red in color, and with rough, wrinkled, or smooth surfaces. Depigmentation may occur as warts slough.

Diagnosis

A diagnosis of equine warts is usually obvious based on history, clinical signs, and age of the affected horse. Additional diagnostic testing is rarely performed. If needed, cutaneous biopsy would provide a definitive diagnosis. Verrucous sarcoids resemble warts in their gross appearance and predilection for the face. Proliferative lesions in older horses should be considered sarcoids until proved otherwise.

Pathologic Findings

Biopsy of papilloma lesions reveals epidermal hyperplasia and papillomatosis without connective tissue proliferation. Ballooning degeneration of epidermal cells, clumping of keratohyaline granules in the cytoplasm, and basophilic intranuclear inclusion bodies may be observed.[1,11,15]

Therapy

A variety of therapies have been proposed for equine warts. However, most lesions resolve spontaneously within a few months of appearance, making it difficult to ascertain the true efficacy of any therapeutic intervention. If lesions persist beyond 6 to 9 months, an underlying immune deficiency should be suspected.

Most horses with warts do not require treatment. If removal is necessary for immediate esthetic enhancement, cryosurgery with a two-cycle, freeze-thaw-freeze technique is a valid treatment. Chemical cautery with *trifluoroacetic acid* is also considered safe and effective. A solution of 25 g anhydrous trifluoroacetic acid, 3 g water, and 20 g glacial acetic acid is applied to affected tissues only. Adjacent tissues should be protected with petroleum jelly. Applications are repeated on the fourth and seventh days after initial treatment.[1] Topical treatment with *podophyllin* (50% podophyllin; 20% podophyllin in 95% ethyl alcohol; 2% podophyllin in 25% salicylic acid) and undiluted medical-grade *dimethyl sulfoxide* (DMSO) may be used once daily until remission occurs. There is no scientific evidence to support the theory that surgical excision of some lesions enhances or hastens regression of remaining lesions. Recurrence after surgical excision has been reported.[1,11] A variety of immunomodulatory drugs, including mycobacterial cell wall extracts and *Propionibacterium* extracts, have also been recommended for treatment of equine warts.

Autogenous vaccines for treatment of equine warts are controversial, and to the author's knowledge, there are no scientific reports documenting their efficacy. Bovine wart vaccines are not efficacious in horses.

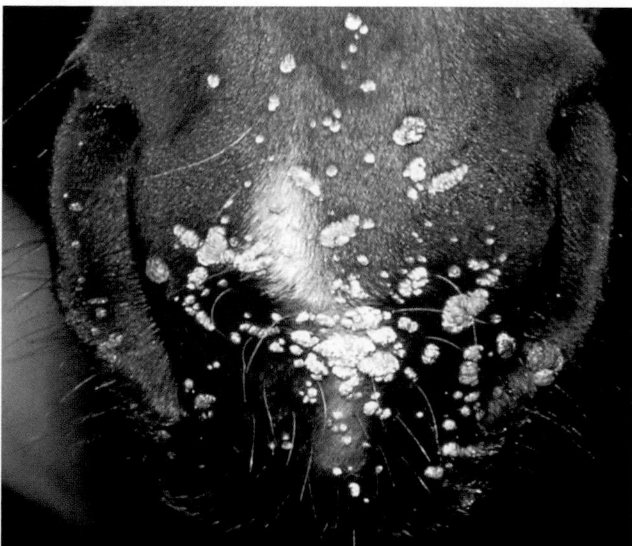

Fig. 25-1 Typical appearance of warts on muzzle and lips of young horse. (Courtesy Dr. Melissa Hines.)

Prevention

Affected horses should be isolated from uninfected animals. Skin trauma from the environment or ectoparasites should be minimized. Disinfection of premises and equipment with formaldehyde or lye is recommended after exposure to a horse with warts.[1,11]

Public Health Considerations

There are no reports of human disease secondary to equine papillomavirus infection.

AURAL PLAQUES

Etiology and Pathogenesis

Aural plaques (papillary acanthoma, hyperplastic dermatitis of the ear) are raised, depigmented lesions on the inner surface of the pinnae of the ear.[11,18-20] Papillomavirus has been demonstrated in these lesions by electron microscopy (EM) and immunohistochemistry (IHC).[21] The pathogenesis of aural plaques in horses is unclear. Lesions often appear worse in the summer and fall, possibly because of fly irritation.

Clinical Findings

There are no age, breed, or gender predilections for occurrence of aural plaques in horses.[11] Lesions are often bilateral and progress from small, smooth, depigmented papules and plaques to larger, often coalescent, hyperkeratotic plaques (Fig. 25-3). Aural plaques do not spontaneously regress, and they may be more active in the summer, possibly in association

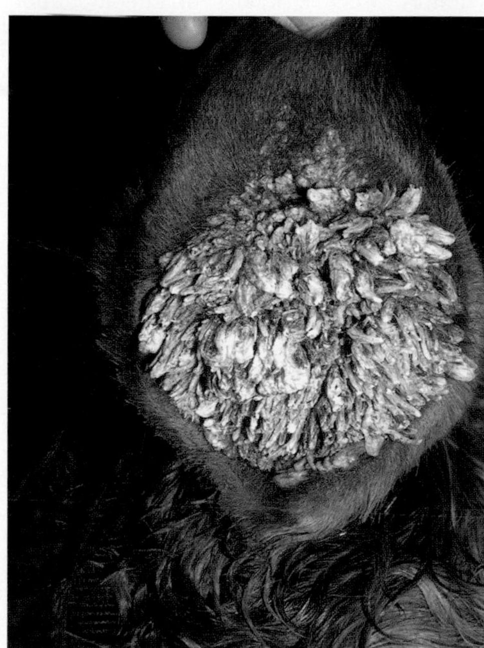

Fig. 25-2 Severe, frondlike warts in ear of yearling Quarter Horse.

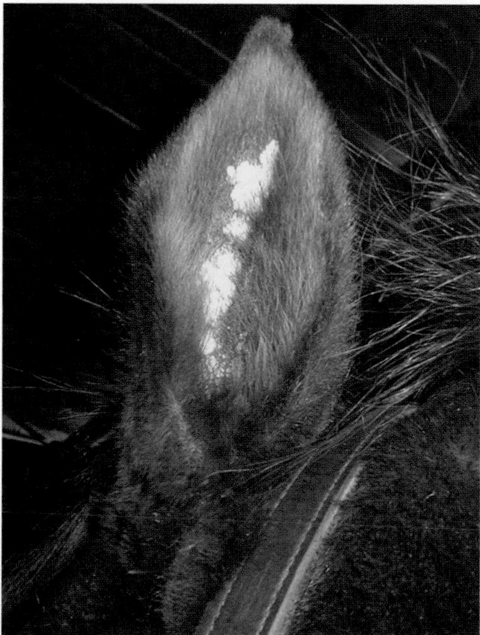

Fig. 25-3 Aural plaques in ear of horse. (Courtesy Dr. Erin Groover.)

with black fly bites. Plaques are not sensitive, pruritic, or painful but may be considered esthetically displeasing by owners. Similar lesions may occur around the anus and vulva.[11,22]

Diagnosis

The diagnosis of aural plaques is usually made on the basis of clinical signs. Biopsy is usually not indicated, but if performed, lesions appear histologically identical to verruca plana, a wart-like disease of humans, with epithelial proliferation and epidermal hypomelanosis.[22]

Treatment and Prevention

To the author's knowledge, there are no reports of successful treatment of equine aural plaques.[11] These lesions do not spontaneously regress. Use of fly repellents is recommended to minimize secondary irritation or infection of lesions.[22]

SARCOIDS

Sarcoids are locally aggressive but nonmetastatic, fibroblastic skin tumors of equids. They are the most common neoplasm of horses, donkeys, and mules. They may occur on any part of the body but have a predilection for the head, ventral abdomen, and legs. These tumors are seldom life threatening but may cause esthetic and performance-limiting problems, depending on their location, size, and rate of growth. A variety of therapies have been proposed, with minimal to moderate success. Recurrence of tumor after treatment is a significant problem regardless of the type of treatment attempted.

Etiology

A viral etiology for equine sarcoids was postulated as early as 1936 by Jackson.[23] In 1948, Olson demonstrated that intradermal inoculation of horses with cell-free extracts from bovine skin tumors containing *bovine papillomavirus* (BPV) caused lesions resembling equine sarcoids.[24,25] Ragland et al.[26] described an epizootic of equine sarcoid in 1966 and confirmed the ability to induce sarcoidlike lesions in horses by inoculation with BPV in 1969.[27,28] Lesions regressed spontaneously, and inoculated horses developed a humoral immune response to BPV. Subsequent studies by a variety of investigators have demonstrated the presence of DNA and ribonucleic acid (RNA) from BPV types 1 and 2, or closely related viruses, and expression of the BPV types 1 and 2 major transforming protein, E5, in equine sarcoids.[29-46] BPV DNA can be detected from normal skin of horses affected with equine sarcoid and, to a lesser extent, on the skin of unaffected horses, suggesting the possibility of viral latency.[32,34,41,47]

Papillomaviruses are small, nonenveloped viruses with icosahedral symmetry, 72 capsomers, and a double-stranded, circular DNA genome. They are classified on the basis of their species of origin and the degree of homology with other papillomaviruses isolated from the same species.[48] Most papillomaviruses infect epithelial cells, causing proliferative lesions described as warts, papillomas, or condylomas; however, some types infect fibroblasts with resultant fibroepithelial tumors. Lesions induced by papillomaviruses are usually benign and self-limiting. Some papillomaviruses are oncogenic; in particular, *human papillomavirus* (HPV) types 16 and 18 are associated with cervical carcinoma.[36] All the open reading frames (potential coding regions) of the viral genome are located on a single strand of viral DNA. The early region of the genome encodes proteins necessary for cell transformation (E5, E6, and E7) and replication and transcription regulatory proteins E1 and E2. The late region codes for structural capsid proteins (L1 and L2). The early and late gene regions are separated by a regulatory region containing the origin of replication and many of the control elements for viral transcription and replication.[48]

Bovine papillomaviruses are the causative agents of bovine warts. At least six distinct bovine viruses are associated with either fibropapillomas or papillomas. The group of viruses associated with bovine fibropapillomas (BPV types 1, 2, and 5) are most often identified in association with equine sarcoids.[49,50] Sequence analysis of BPV DNA from equine sarcoids suggests the possibility of equine sarcoid-specific variants of BPV.[44,45]

Despite the strength of evidence linking BPV with equine sarcoid lesions, there is no evidence of a productive infection with release of infectious progeny virions in horses. Viral DNA exists episomally in equine cells and does not integrate in the host cell genome.[39,51] This conclusion is supported by the lack of detectable antibodies to BPV in naturally affected horses, the inability to transmit sarcoids experimentally using equine tissue extracts, and the inability to identify viral particles in sarcoid lesions using EM or immunoperoxidase staining.[30,52]

Bovine papillomavirus is very resistant to physical and chemical inactivation.[32] It remains viable after 30 minutes at 67° C (152.5° F), is stable at a pH between 4 and 8, is stable in ether, and survives in 50% glycerol when frozen or lyophilized.[53] These properties suggest that BPV may be able to survive for a long time in the environment.[32]

Suggestions that other viruses may be causally related to equine sarcoid are unsubstantiated. A retrovirus identified in a cell line originating from an equine sarcoid was determined to be an endogenous virus that was unrelated to the sarcoid.[54,55] Equine cutaneous papillomaviruses, the etiologic agent of equine warts, are not causally related to equine sarcoids.[3]

Epidemiology

Equine sarcoids are the most common dermatologic neoplasm in horses, donkeys, and mules worldwide, accounting for an estimated 20% of all equine tumors[56] and as many as 90% of all skin tumors.[57] The incidence of sarcoid tumors in the general population of horses is not known. Sarcoids accounted for 0.7% of all equine cases presented to the Cornell University Veterinary Hospital between 1975 and 1987 and to the Ohio State University between 1976 and 1985.[58]

Sarcoid tumors most frequently develop when horses are 3 to 6 years of age, but lesions may occasionally be observed in yearlings.[58] Equine sarcoids appear less likely to develop in horses after 7 years of age.[59-62] Young male equids are at increased risk of disease.[45,61,63,64]

No evidence indicates that castration increases the risk of paragenital sarcoids in donkeys.[63] In cool northern climates, sarcoids are most often observed on the head and abdomen of horses; in warmer climates the limbs are more frequently affected.[58] It remains uncertain whether contact with cattle is a risk factor for equine sarcoids.[23,64] However, a donkey living in close contact with affected donkeys is more likely to develop sarcoid tumors than the average donkey.[65]

Evidence for genetic predisposition for development of sarcoid tumors includes varying disease prevalence in specific breeds,[64,66,67] increased incidence of lesions in some equine families,[26,68,69] and an association between sarcoid susceptibility and the major histocompatibility complex (MHC)–encoded class II allele ELA W13.[67,70-72] Sarcoids may occur in any breed of horse, but they are seen more frequently in Quarter Horses and less frequently in Standardbred horses than in the general equine population.[64,66,67] Several studies have shown that the frequency of the ELA W13 allele in horses with sarcoids is high regardless of breed. However, the majority of horses with the W13 allele never develop a sarcoid tumor, suggesting that environmental factors (most likely BPV) and other genetic factors are also important for disease development.

Pathogenesis

The manner by which BPV induces equine sarcoid lesions is uncertain. Hypotheses include transmission of virus by direct or indirect contact with infected horses and cattle and transmission by insects.[36,65,73] Although the physical properties of BPV suggest that it might be capable of surviving for a long time in the environment, extensive environmental surveys have not been performed. One study was unable to identify BPV DNA in the environment of affected and healthy horses, except for the environment of one horse living in contact with a cow with warts.[32] Genetic sequences specific for BPV have been identified from skin of normal horses with no sarcoid lesions and from normal skin of horses with sarcoid tumors, suggesting the possibility of viral latency.[32,34,41,47] Nucleic acid from BPV cannot be demonstrated in lymphocytes, liver, spleen, or lymph nodes of affected horses.[44,74,75]

Regardless of the manner of initial contact with BPV, it is clear that BPV alone is insufficient to induce sarcoid lesions in horses. The immunologic status of the horse, genetic background, and skin trauma may play a role in initiation of disease.[32]

Sarcoid lesions may arise spontaneously or may occur at the site of a prior wound. Rubbing or biting at truncal or limb lesions may precede appearance of lesions on lips and eyelids. Indirect transmission by tack is also possible. Metastasis to internal organs has not been reported. Recurrence after surgical resection, cryotherapy, immunotherapy, or chemotherapy is common.

Clinical Findings

Although sarcoid tumors may occur on any part of the body either singly or in clusters, the most common sites are the head, ventral abdomen, groin, axillae, and limbs.[57,59,76] Approximately 30% to 50% of affected horses have multiple lesions.[11] Lesions are usually firm on palpation because of fibroblastic proliferation. The overlying epidermis may be thick, rough, and hyperkeratotic or ulcerated. Sarcoid tumors may occur in the subcutaneous tissues as firm, movable masses with an intact covering of grossly normal skin.[59,77] Nodular, subcutaneous sarcoids are most likely to occur in the groin, sheath, or eyelid region (Fig. 25-4). These lesions may progress to typical ulcerated fibroblastic sarcoids with time or traumatic insult.

The gross appearance of sarcoids may vary, but lesions are generally classified as one of four types: verrucous, fibroblastic, mixed verrucous and fibroblastic, or occult.[78] Lesions may be pedunculated or sessile.

Verrucous sarcoids resemble equine warts, with a dry, horny, cauliflower-like surface that is partially or totally hairless[79] (Fig. 25-5). These sarcoids are usually small to medium in size, measuring less than 6 cm in diameter. They can remain static in size and shape for years but may undergo transformation and become fibroblastic if traumatized.[79] Verrucous sarcoids appear more frequently around the face, body, groin, and sheath areas.[59]

Fibroblastic sarcoids are firm, fibrous nodules within the dermis that often become ulcerated and may become quite large (>20 cm diameter) (Fig. 25-6). Differential diagnoses include granulation tissue, squamous cell carcinoma, cutaneous habronemiasis, and pythiosis. *Mixed verrucous and fibroblastic sarcoids* have characteristics of both types of tumors.

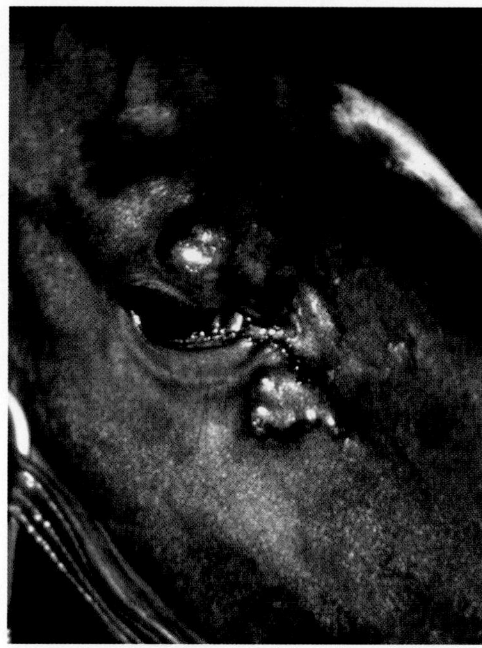

Fig. 25-4 Nodular, subcutaneous sarcoid of eyelid of horse. (Courtesy Dr. Melissa Hines.)

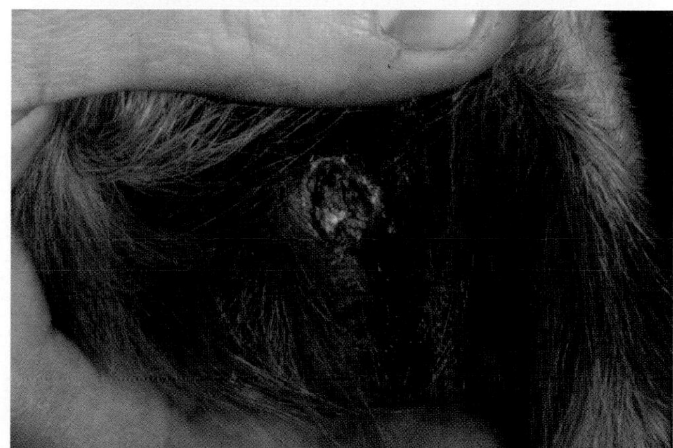

Fig. 25-5 Verrucous sarcoid on ear of horse. (Courtesy Dr. Wendy Duckett.)

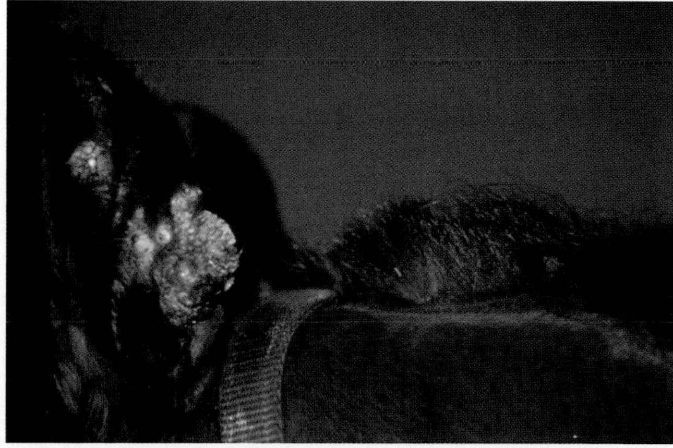

Fig. 25-6 Fibroblastic sarcoid on ear of horse.

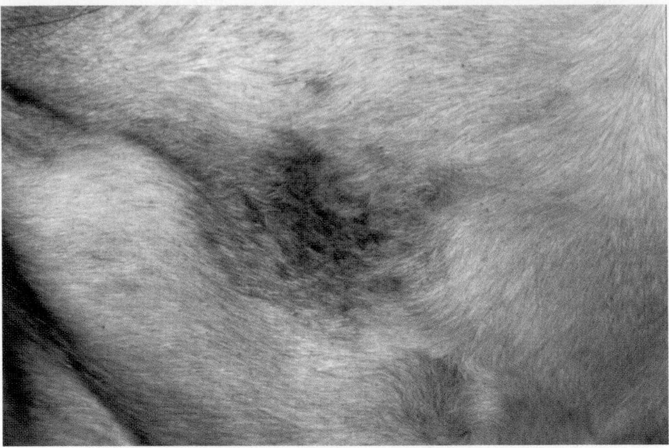

Fig. 25-7 Occult sarcoid on shoulder of horse. (Courtesy Dr. Wendy Duckett.)

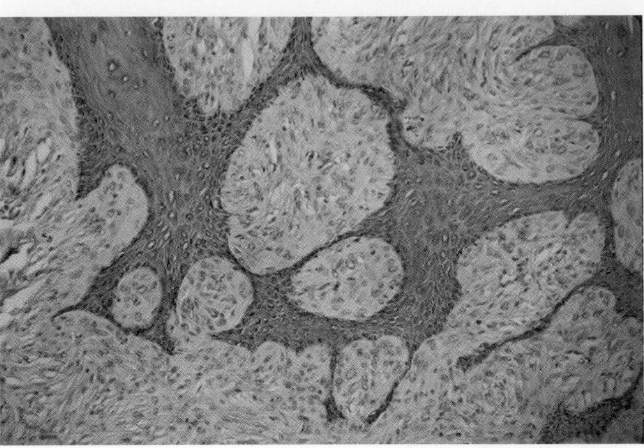

Fig. 25-8 Photomicrograph of equine sarcoid, with characteristic spindloid cells and elongate rete pegs of adjacent epidermis.

Occult sarcoids are slow-growing tumors that are flat with slightly thickened skin and a mildly roughened surface[79] (Fig. 25-7). This presentation is partially or totally devoid of hair and seems to favor areas of the body with sparse hair growth, including the skin around the mouth, eyes, neck, and medial aspects of the forearm and thigh. Trauma to occult sarcoids, surgical or otherwise, can stimulate fibroblastic proliferation of the tumor and should be avoided if possible. Differential diagnoses for occult sarcoids include dermatophytosis, dermatophilosis, demodicosis, staphylococcal folliculitis, onchocerciasis, and alopecia areata.[55,57]

Diagnosis

Diagnosis of sarcoid tumors in horses is usually suspected on the basis of characteristic clinical signs. Because lesions may grossly resemble papillomas, granulation tissue, fungal or bacterial granuloma, habronemiasis, solar keratosis, squamous cell carcinoma, neurofibroma, melanoma, and fibrosarcoma, histologic examination of biopsy specimens is required for a definitive diagnosis. Biopsy of static verrucous and occult sarcoids is usually not indicated because intervention may prompt transformation into an aggressive, fibroblastic type of lesion.[80] Partial removal of a sarcoid tumor may stimulate aggressive regrowth of tissue. If possible, wide excision of the entire mass should be performed at biopsy to decrease the likelihood of recurrence. Because autotransplantation of an equine sarcoid tumor may occur, surgical instruments that contact the tumor should not be used on healthy adjacent skin.[79]

Samples should be submitted to an appropriate diagnostic laboratory in 10% neutral buffered formalin. Small tumors may be submitted intact; representative samples should be cut from the excised tumor and submitted if lesions are large. Biopsy samples should be examined by an experienced veterinary pathologist to facilitate an accurate diagnosis. The most common incorrect diagnoses usually are fibroma, fibrosarcoma, neurofibroma, and granulation tissue, the subsequent treatment of which may lead to inappropriate therapy.[57]

Pathologic Findings

Histologically, equine sarcoids are characterized by fibroblastic and epidermal proliferation with associated epidermal hyperplasia and dermoepidermal activity.[11,26,68] The dermis contains collagen fibers and fibroblasts in a classic whorled, tangled, or herringbone pattern, and mitotic figures may be numerous (Fig. 25-8). Tumor cells are spindle or fusiform to stellate shaped. Fibroblasts at the dermoepidermal junction frequently orient perpendicularly to the basement membrane in a picket-fence pattern.[11] If present, the overlying epidermis is hyperplastic and hyperkeratotic. Occult sarcoids may exhibit only focal epidermal hyperplasia and hyperkeratosis, with underlying junctional fibroblastic proliferation.[11] The junction between tumor and normal tissue is not always clear, making it difficult to assess surgical margins histopathologically.[79]

Therapy

A wide variety of therapeutic strategies have been proposed for treatment of equine sarcoid tumors. The specific treatment selected should be determined after consideration of the tumor site, size, type, and aggressiveness; clinical experience of the attending veterinarian; and the availability of services, equipment, and facilities.[59,81] Static verrucous and occult sarcoids are usually not treated because intervention may prompt transformation to an aggressive, fibroblastic type of sarcoid.

Determining the comparative efficacy of treatment for equine sarcoid tumors is difficult because of the large variation in tumor size, location, and treatment methods. Almost all reports of treatment efficacy originate from large veterinary referral hospitals, where horses treated for sarcoid tumors are likely to have large, multiple, recurrent, and highly aggressive tumors. Success rates for therapy in this population may be expected to be less than success rates in private practice, where horses tend to have solitary, less aggressive lesions.

Surgical Resection

Surgical resection, even with wide margins of normal tissue, is not generally recommended as a sole therapy for equine sarcoids because of a recurrence rate estimated at 50% to 64%, usually within 6 months.[82] Instead, surgical resection (including normal tissue margins of 0.5-1.0 cm) is best used to debulk tumors and improve the effectiveness of adjunctive therapies (e.g., cryotherapy, laser surgical excision, hyperthermia, irradiation, photodynamic therapy, immunotherapy, chemotherapy). Split-thickness skin grafts may facilitate epithelial covering of the wound with faster healing, less granulation tissue, and a better cosmetic result.[59,81,82]

Cryotherapy

Cryotherapy with liquid nitrogen is a common adjunctive therapy for equine sarcoids after surgical debulking of lesions. One-year cure rates for cryotherapy are estimated at 70%

to 100%.[57,83-91] Horses are sedated or anesthetized to facilitate restraint during the procedure. Lesions are frozen two or three times to –20° to –30° C, with complete thawing to room temperature between each freeze. Monitoring tissue temperature with cryoprobes diminishes the likelihood of inadvertent freezing of sensitive normal tissues in the area and ensures complete freezing of the tumor. Thermocouple needles are placed in the subcutaneous tissues beneath the tumor and along the periphery of the lesion. Treated tissues undergo necrosis, with local swelling and inflammation. Healing occurs by secondary intention or delayed closure, which may result in scarring or regrowth of white hair from damage to hair follicles.[82] The average time to complete healing is 2.4 months (range, 1.0-3.5 months).[92]

Adverse consequences of cryotherapy are usually related to damage to adjacent normal tissues and facial nerve paralysis; septic arthritis, loss of the upper eyelid, and evisceration of the globe have been described.[86,90] There are limited reports of spontaneous regression of multiple sarcoids after cryotherapy of one or two lesions, suggesting that cryotherapy may enhance the immune response of the horse.[90] Because spontaneous regression occurs, however, no scientific data support intervention solely to induce remission.

Carbon Dioxide Laser Therapy

Recently, carbon dioxide (CO_2) laser therapy has been advocated for treatment of equine sarcoid tumors, with a success rate (no recurrence at the same site for 6 or 12 months) of 62% to 81%.[93,94] Animals presenting with multiple sarcoids were more likely to experience tumor recurrence, which was significantly lower in donkeys than in horses.[94] Approximately 58% of equids in one study developed new sarcoid lesions elsewhere on the body after laser therapy.[94] Swelling is minimal after laser resection, and the horse exhibits minimal pain to palpation of the surgical wound. If sufficient normal skin is available, primary closure of the surgical site can be performed.[57] Treatment with CO_2 laser requires specialized equipment and training, limiting its use to universities and a few private veterinary specialty hospitals.

Hyperthermia

Radio-frequency current–induced hyperthermia resulted in sarcoid tumor regression, with no recurrence at 7 to 12 months in three horses.[95] There have been no additional reports of its use since 1983, however, making it difficult to assess the efficacy of this modality for sarcoid therapy.

Irradiation

Brachytherapy of sarcoid tumors provides continuous delivery of a high radiation dose directly to the tumor while sparing adjacent healthy tissue. Isotopes used for interstitial brachytherapy of equine sarcoids include permanently implantable seeds of radon-222 or gold-198; removable needles of radium-226, cobalt-60, or iridium-192; and iridium-192 seeds. Response rates range from 50% to 100%.[57] Brachytherapy has been particularly useful for treatment of small periorbital sarcoids, with success rates of up to 95%.[57,96,97] In a study of 155 horses treated with iridium-192 interstitial brachytherapy for periocular tumors, adverse effects included palpebral fibrosis (10.4%), cataract (7.8%), keratitis and corneal ulceration (6.9%), permanent hair loss (21.7%), and hair dyspigmentation (78.3%).[97]

The use of brachytherapy is severely limited by the need to maintain a horse in a radiation safety–approved area and the need to comply with all state and federal radiation safety laws. Hyperthermia may be combined with brachytherapy for synergistic tumor killing.[98]

Photodynamic Therapy

Photodynamic therapy involves the administration of a photosensitizer to a patient. The drug accumulates in tumor tissue and is activated by visible light to a higher energy state from which free radicals and reactive oxygen are formed. Intratumoral injections of the photodynamic agent hypericin into three sarcoid tumors on a donkey resulted in an 81% reduction in tumor volume at the end of therapy (25 days) and a 90% reduction after 2 months.[99] Further evaluation of this type of therapy is needed before it can be recommended for general use.

Immunotherapy

Immunotherapy with an attenuated strain of *Mycobacterium bovis* (bacille Calmette-Guérin [BCG]), mycobacterial cell wall preparations in oil, and mycobacterial cell wall skeleton–trehalose dimycolate combinations have been widely used for treatment of equine sarcoids, especially periocular lesions.[11,57,100,101] Treatments are administered by intralesional injection every 2 to 3 weeks for an average of four treatments.[11] Debulking before initiating intralesional therapy is recommended. Inflammatory reactions with ulceration and necrosis are common within minutes to days of injection. Some patients experience fever, increased white blood cell count, and general malaise.[102] Occasional reports of anaphylactic reactions after repeated use of BCG have led to recommendations that horses be medicated with flunixin meglumine and corticosteroids before BCG injection.[11,103] Intralesional BCG injections have also been associated with lymphangitis[102] and septic arthritis.[104] Reported response rates for treatment of periorbital sarcoids with BCG range from 69% to 100%, with best results for treatment of fibroblastic and nodular lesions.[92,101,104] Remission rate with BCG therapy of sarcoid lesions elsewhere on the body is approximately 48%, with the poorest response reported for lesions on the legs and in the axillary region.[92] Complete resolution of lesions may require 6 weeks to 1 year or more.[92,102,103,105]

Controlled studies of immunotherapy for equine sarcoids using agents other than BCG are lacking. Systemic immunomodulator therapy with nonviable *Propionibacterium acnes* (EqStim, Neogen Corporation, Lansing, Mich) has been advocated for treatment of equine sarcoid.[59] Protocols include intralesional or intravenous injections once weekly for 6 to 8 weeks, with eventual necrosis and sloughing of the lesion.

Autogenous vaccines have been proposed as immunotherapeutic agents for equine sarcoid tumors.[62,106-108] In 1999, Kinnunen et al.[106] reported the use of an autogenous vaccine in 21 horses. All horses had surgical debulking of tumor, and resected tissue was used to prepare vaccine. Only 1 of 12 horses with a primary tumor had a recurrence of tumor after therapy. In contrast, four of nine horses with recurrent tumors before this study had recurrences after treatment with autogenous vaccine. However, disease-free intervals for both groups of horses were significantly longer than for horses treated with conventional surgery alone.[106] Sarcoid regression has been reported in several horses with refractory sarcoid after transplantation of tissue from one horse into another horse.[59] However, the transfer of tumor tissue and tumor extracts carries a risk of tumor production rather than tumor regression, as well as risk of transmission of other infectious diseases. Because other types of therapy work well for many horses without these risks, this type of therapy is not recommended.[59]

Chemotherapy

A variety of topical and intralesional chemotherapy protocols have been described for treatment of horses with sarcoids. These therapies are usually applied after surgical debulking of a lesion but may be efficacious as a sole therapy for small tumors. Administration of chemotherapeutic agents should be undertaken with caution to avoid human contact with potentially toxic agents. Gloves and appropriate protective eyewear should be worn for topical application and intralesional injection of most agents.

Daily topical application of *5-fluorouracil*, a fluorinated pyrimidine antimetabolite that interferes with DNA biosynthesis, or *podophyllin*, an irritant cathartic, has been used successfully to treat some sarcoid lesions.[59,77,82] Treatment may be continued for up to 90 days. Topical 5-fluorouracil cream applied daily to occult and verrucose periorbital lesions (not directly on margin of eyelid) was successful in eliminating lesions in six of nine horses.[101] The other three horses improved, but lesions recurred in a fibroblastic form over the next 3 to 36 months.

A bloodroot extract containing *Sanguinaria canadensis*, puccoon, gromwell, distilled water, and trace minerals (Animex, NIES, Las Vegas, Nev) has been used to treat a variety of skin lesions, including equine sarcoids.[59] It preferentially kills tumor cells and the lesion sloughs in 7 to 10 days. Another bloodroot plant extract product (XXTERRA, Larson Laboratories, Fort Collins, Colo) is marketed for treatment of equine sarcoids, with claims of changing the antigenicity of the sarcoid cells so that the immune system recognizes them as foreign with resultant tissue rejection.[59,77,82] Product literature instructs that the paste be applied topically to the lesion and covered with a bandage for 4 to 5 days. Application of the product with bandaging should be repeated until the lesion sloughs. Controlled studies demonstrating efficacy of these chemotherapeutic agents are not available.

An experimental topical ointment containing a variety of heavy metals and the antimitotic compounds 5-fluorouracil and thiouracil (AW-3-LUDES) was described by Knottenbelt and Kelly[101] but is not widely available. The ointment is applied daily or every other day for three to five treatments. A response is anticipated in 5 to 10 weeks with necrosis and sloughing of sarcoid tissue. Caution must be exercised if this compound or other chemotherapeutic agents are used for treatment of periorbital sarcoid. Inadvertent contact between these agents and sensitive ocular tissues can result in serious adverse consequences.

Intralesional injections or implants of chemotherapeutic agents result in a high local drug concentration for extended periods. Implants may consist of a high-molecular-weight collagen matrix that contains a chemotherapeutic agent (cisplatin or 5-fluorouracil) and a vasoactive modifier such as epinephrine.[59,82] Alternatively, sterilized sesame oil may be used to slow drug release and increase tumor/plasma drug concentration ratio. Intratumoral treatment of 19 horses with cisplatin (Platinol, Bristol Myers Squibb, Princeton, NJ) resulted in a 1-year disease-free period for 87% of horses.[109] Theon et al.[110] also reported a 92% and 77% relapse-free survival rate at 1 and 4 years, respectively, after surgical debulking combined with perisurgical wound injection of cisplatin and sesame oil injections.

Perioperative cisplatin in sesame oil injections are recommended when surgical debulking results in a site that cannot be surgically closed and an open wound that is less than 5 cm in largest diameter. The first treatment is administered at surgery. Instructions for preparation of the drug from powder are available.[111] Tumor dosage is planned as 1 mg of cisplatin per cubic centimeter of tissue to be injected. All visible tumor and a margin of normal tissue of 1 to 2 cm should be injected. The target volume is injected through multiple sites using a parallel-row or field-block technique. Rows of injections should be 0.6 to 0.8 cm apart. Number and frequency of treatments vary with differing protocols. A standard therapy may include four intratumoral treatment sessions at 2-week intervals.[111] All treatment effects from intralesional cisplatin in sesame oil are local. Acute inflammatory reactions may occur but usually resolve quickly. Phenylbutazone or flunixin meglumine may be administered if necessary to minimize discomfort.

Cisplatin is mutagenic and carcinogenic, and the reader is referred to other sources for a detailed discussion of appropriate chemotherapy precautions to protect the health of the owner and the veterinarian.[111]

Prevention

To the author's knowledge, there are no management strategies or treatment techniques to prevent development of sarcoid tumors in horses.

Public Health Considerations

There is no evidence that BPV is infectious for humans, and sarcoid tumors of horses are not considered a zoonotic disease.

References

See the CD-ROM for a list of references linked to the abstract in PubMed.

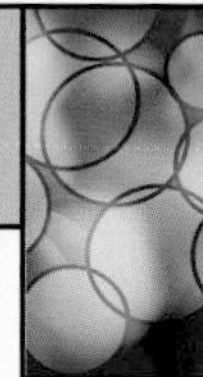

CHAPTER • 26

Miscellaneous Viral Diseases

Kenneth W. Hinchcliff

EQUINE ENCEPHALOSIS

Etiology and Epidemiology

The *equine encephalosis virus* (EEV) is an insect-borne orbivirus that is transmitted by a variety of *Culicoides* spp.[1] and is closely related to bluetongue and epizootic hemorrhagic disease viruses.[2] EEV has characteristics in cell culture similar to African horse sickness virus[3] (see Chapter 15). Seven serotypes[3-8] of EEV infect equids of southern Africa, including Kenya, Botswana, and South Africa.[4]

The virus replicates to varying degrees in midges depending on species of midge and strain of the virus. The genetic and phenotypic stability of EEV strains is unknown, and the potential exists for emergence of new strains or recognition of currently undetected strains. Variations in pathogenicity are not recognized but might exist. The observation of increased rates of seasonal seroconversion to a specific serotype, with ongoing low level of infection by other serotypes, suggests independent persistence of EEV serotypes in a maintenance cycle.[4]

Horses, donkeys, and zebra in southern Africa frequently have antibodies to a group epitope of EEV, indicating widespread infection of these equids. In South Africa, 77% of 1144 horses, 57% of 518 horses, 49% of 4875 donkeys, and up to 88% of zebra have antibody to EEV.[1,4-6] Elephant seldom have antibodies to EEV.[6] Zebra foals develop antibodies to the virus within months of losing their maternally acquired passive immunity.[8]

Clinical Findings

The equine encephalosis virus acquired its name after original isolation from a horse with clinical signs of neurologic disease. The clinical importance of EEV is uncertain but appears to be limited. Seroconversion in closely managed horses without evidence of clinical disease suggests that infection by the virus is asymptomatic in most cases. However, the disease associated with infection by EEV is poorly documented, and given the high prevalence of infection, EEV might be falsely incriminated as the cause of disease in some situations. Most infections are subclinical based on the high seroprevalence rate and lack of reports of disease outbreaks.

Clinical signs typically attributed to EEV infection include fever, lassitude, edema of the lips, acute neurologic disease, and enteritis. Abortion has anecdotally been associated with infection by EEV. Disease associated with EEV has not been recorded in donkeys or zebra.[1]

Diagnosis

Characteristic abnormalities in serum biochemistry or hematology are not reported. Antibodies to the virus are detected by serum neutralization assays (which are serotype specific) and enzyme-linked immunosorbent assay (ELISA), which is not serotype specific. A group-specific, indirect sandwich ELISA detects EEV antigen and does not cross react with African horse sickness virus, bluetongue virus, or epizootic hemorrhagic disease virus.[7]

Pathologic Findings

Necropsy examination of affected horses reveals cerebral edema, localized enteritis, degeneration of cardiac myofibers, and myocardial fibrosis, but whether these abnormalities are attributable to EEV is unclear.[3] Definitive diagnosis is difficult, if not impossible, at present because of the high prevalence of seropositive animals and the poorly defined clinical and necropsy characteristics of the disease.

Treatment and Prevention

No recognized measures exist for treatment, control, or prevention of EEV infection, and there is no vaccine.

Public Health Considerations

The equine encephalosis virus does not appear to cause disease in humans.

GETAH AND ROSS RIVER VIRUSES

Etiology

Getah virus and Ross River virus are classified in the *Alphavirus* genus within the Semliki Forest complex of the *Togaviridae* family. These are small, enveloped viruses with a single-stranded, positive-sense ribonucleic acid (RNA) genome. These viruses are discussed under the same heading because of the similarities in their cladistic classification, ecology, and clinical signs in horses. *Getah virus* causes disease in horses and pigs, whereas *Ross River virus* causes disease in humans and, arguably, horses.

Epidemiology

The geographic range of Getah and Ross River viruses is distinctive; Getah virus is reported from Japan, Hong Kong, Southeast Asia, Korea, and India, and Ross River virus is found in most areas of continental Australia, Tasmania, West Papua and Papua New Guinea, New Caledonia, Fiji, Samoa, and the Cook Islands.[9] Reports from the 1960s document antibodies to Getah virus in animals in Australia, but the presence of this virus in Australia has not been confirmed using modern techniques that can differentiate antibodies to Getah virus from those of the related Ross River virus and other viruses in this complex. There are no reports of disease caused by Getah virus in Australia. Considerable sequence homology exists between Getah and Ross River virus genomes.[10] There is geographic genetic variability among isolates of Ross River virus and temporal, but not geographic, variability among isolates of Getah virus from Southeast Asia and Japan.[11,12]

Both viruses are arthropod borne, and infection is through the bite of an infected mosquito. The virus is maintained in the mosquito-vertebrate-mosquito host cycle typical of arboviruses. The definitive, amplifying vertebrate host for Getah virus is unknown, although a number of vertebrates, including horses, cattle, and pigs, can be infected by the virus. Horses and pigs become viremic and presumably can infect mosquitoes, although this does not appear to have been confirmed experimentally. The life cycle of Getah virus has not been explicated. The virus is assumed to be maintained in a mosquito-pig-mosquito cycle in those areas with year-round mosquito activity.[13] Persistence of the virus in areas where mosquito activity is seasonal has not been explained, and whether transovarial or transtadial transmission occurs within the mosquito population is not reported. The vertebrate hosts of Ross River virus include a large number of eutherian, marsupial, and monotreme mammals and birds.[9] Macropod species, including kangaroos and wallabies, are assumed to be the most important amplifying hosts, although this is debated.

During outbreaks of disease it is suspected that Getah virus is spread by horse-to-horse contact, based on the rapidity of spread among horses, the short duration of the outbreak, and the lack of mosquito activity at the time some horses developed the disease.[14,15] However, experimental evidence suggests that this route of spread is likely of limited importance in propagation of epidemics because of the low concentration of virus in nasal and oral secretions of infected horses and the large inoculum required to cause disease in horses by the intranasal route.[16]

The prevalence of serologic evidence of infection of horses by Getah virus in Japan ranges from 8% to 93%, depending on the region of the country in which the samples were collected and the disease history of the band or stable of horses.[14,17] Seroprevalence was 17% in India and 25% in Hong Kong.[16,18] These results confirm the widespread incidence of subclinical infection of horses by Getah virus in endemic areas.

There is a similarly high incidence of Ross River virus infection of horses in endemic regions of Australia. Prevalence of seropositive horses in Queensland, an area with likely year-round mosquito activity, was approximately 80%, whereas that of horses around the Gippsland lakes in southern Australia, a region with seasonal mosquito activity, was 50%.[19] These high rates of infection, in the absence of similarly high rates of clinical disease, suggest that Ross River virus is minimally pathogenic in horses. This also increases the likelihood that seroconversion or virus isolation from horses with clinical abnormalities is a chance event and not causally related.

Clinical Findings

The disease syndrome caused by infection by Getah virus is better defined than that of Ross River virus, but infection by either virus appears to cause disease in horses with several clinical features in common.[14,15,19,20] Disease associated with *Getah virus* infection is characterized by pyrexia, edema of the limbs, and an abnormal gait, often described as "stiffness."[14,15] Eruptions of the skin, urticaria, and submandibular lymphadenopathy are reported in some horses with the disease in Japan, but not in India. The clinical disease persists for 7 to 10 days. Abortion is not a feature of the disease, and foals born of mares that have had the disease during gestation are normal.[14] Subclinical infection is very common.

The disease associated with *Ross River virus* infection of horses is typified by pyrexia, lameness (including "stiffness"), swollen joints, inappetence, reluctance to move, and mild colic.[19,20] The duration of disease caused by Ross River virus in horses is uncertain, and some veterinarians believe the disease can persist for weeks to months or recur in horses. Some are skeptical regarding the pathogenicity of Ross River virus in horses because the disease syndrome is not well characterized. Descriptions of the disease are based on a small number of horses that demonstrated viremia concurrent with development of clinical signs of disease or on larger number of horses with serum antibodies to the virus. Horses infected experimentally with Ross River virus have minimal clinical signs of disease.[21] Reports of disease are insufficient to determine if characteristic or diagnostic abnormalities in serum biochemistry or hematology occur in affected horses.

Diagnosis

Hematologic abnormalities induced by *Getah virus* infection in horses include lymphopenia. Increases in serum activity of muscle-derived enzymes, such as creatine kinase, are not characteristic of the disease. Affected horses can have mild to moderate hyperbilirubinemia secondary to inappetence.[14]

Diagnosis of disease caused by Getah virus is achieved by detection of clinical signs consistent with the disease, isolation of the virus from blood of affected horses, and seroconversion to the virus.[12] Interpretation of serologic data from horses in Japan is hindered by the widespread use of a vaccine against Getah disease that induces detectable antibodies to Getah virus in serum.[17,22]

Diagnosis of infection by *Ross River virus* is achieved by virus isolation from serum or heparinized blood samples collected during the acute phase of the disease or by detection of serum antibodies to the virus.[20] Detection of immunoglobulin M (IgM) antibodies to Ross River virus is indicative of recent infection, whereas detection of immunoglobulin G (IgG) antibodies is indicative of more distant infection. Seroconversion confirms exposure, and presumably infection, by the virus. Isolation of Ross River virus has been achieved from horses with IgM antibody to the virus, but not with IgG antibody, likely because of the temporal pattern of antibody appearance in blood of infected horses.[20] In addition to culture of the virus in mice or tissue culture, Ross River virus can be detected in blood and synovial fluid using a reverse transcriptase–polymerase chain reaction (RT-PCR).[21]

It is important to remember that subclinical Ross River virus infection of horses in endemic regions is very common, and that this high rate of subclinical infection increases the risk of incorrect attribution of clinical abnormalities to infection by the virus. Clinical abnormalities in a horse with Ross River viremia or serum antibodies to the virus may not be attributable to infection by Ross River virus.

Pathologic Findings

Reports of postmortem examination of horses with disease caused by Getah virus are limited to experimental studies because the disease is typically not fatal. Horses with disease induced by inoculation with pathogenic Getah virus typically have mild changes, including atrophy of splenic and lymphoid tissue, with destruction of lymphocytes, and perivascular and diffuse infiltration of focal skin lesions by lymphocytes, histiocytes, and eosinophils. Lesions in the central nervous system are equivocal and limited to mild perivascular cuffing in the cerebrum and small hemorrhagic foci in the spinal cord.[23]

There are no reports of postmortem examination of horses with confirmed disease caused by Ross River virus.

Treatment and Prevention

Treatment of horses with Getah or Ross River virus is supportive. Affected horses might benefit from administration of analgesics and antipyretics such as phenylbutazone. Administration of antimicrobials is not indicated in uncomplicated cases.

An inactivated virus vaccine is available in Japan for immunization of horses against disease caused by Getah virus.[17] The vaccine, which is combined with that for Japanese encephalitis, is considered effective. For both Getah virus and Ross River virus, minimizing the exposure of horses to infected mosquitoes is prudent, although the efficacy of this technique in preventing infection is unknown. During outbreaks of disease caused by Getah virus, it is prudent to isolate affected horses, given the potential for horse-to-horse spread of the virus.

There is no vaccine to prevent infection or disease of horses by Ross River Virus.

Public Health Considerations

Disease of humans caused by Getah virus has not been documented. Disease associated with Ross River virus infection is common in humans in Australia, with an estimated 4800 cases per year, and much larger numbers during epidemics of the disease.[24] The horse is believed to be an amplifying host of the virus because experimentally infected horses can infect mosquitoes.[25] The disease in humans is characterized by mild pyrexia and constitutional signs initially, with subsequent development of a rash on the skin and oral lesions. Arthritis or arthralgia is common and affects primarily the wrists, knees, ankles, and small joints of the extremities. These signs and symptoms can persist for 2 to 3 months, and the disease can relapse.[26]

BUNYAVIRIDAE

A number of viruses in the *Bunyaviridae* family cause disease in horses in the Western Hemisphere.[27] The viruses are maintained in a mosquito-vertebrate host-mosquito or a midge-vertebrate host-midge cycle, with horses occasionally being infected and developing signs of neurologic disease.

The *California serogroup* of viruses are mosquito-transmitted viruses of the family *Bunyaviridae* that can cause acute encephalitis in horses.[28,29] There are 12 serotypes isolated in Africa, Europe, Asia, North America, and South America.

Snowshoe hare and Jamestown Canyon viruses have been isolated in Canada and California and have the potential to cause disease in people. The *snowshoe hare virus* is the most widely occurring arbovirus in Canada and is maintained in an amplification cycle involving small mammals (e.g., snowshoe hares) and mosquitoes, primarily of the *Aedes* genus.[29] One horse with clinical signs of acute encephalitis recovered completely in 1 week, with seroconversion to the snowshoe hare serotype of the California serogroup of viruses.[30] Approximately 15% of horses in southern California have antibodies to *Jamestown Canyon virus*.[31] The virus has been isolated from vesicular lesions in a horse.[32]

The *Cache Valley virus* has been isolated from a clinically normal horse, and the high seroprevalence of specific antibody suggests enzootic transmission.[33]

The *Main Drain virus* has been isolated from a horse with severe encephalitis in California.[28] Clinical findings included incoordination, ataxia, stiffness of the neck, head pressing, inability to swallow, fever, and tachycardia. The virus is transmitted by rabbits and rodents and by its natural vector, *Culicoides varipennis*.

OTHER VIRUSES AFFECTING HORSES

The *Powassan virus*, a member of the *Flaviviridae* family, occurs in Ontario and the eastern United States and produces a nonsuppurative, focal necrotizing meningoencephalitis in horses.[34] Approximately 13% of horses sampled in Ontario in 1983 were serologically positive for the virus. Experimental intracerebral inoculation of the Powassan virus into horses resulted in a neurologic syndrome within 8 days.[35] Clinical findings include a "tucked-up" abdomen, tremors of the head and neck, slobbering and chewing movements resulting in foamy saliva, stiff gait, staggering, and recumbency. Pathologically, a nonsuppurative encephalomyelitis, neuronal necrosis, and focal parenchymal necrosis are seen. The Powassan virus has not been isolated from the brain.

Nigerian equine encephalitis, a disease with low morbidity but high mortality, is characterized by fever, generalized muscle spasms, ataxia, and lateral recumbency of 3 to 5 days' duration. The virus has not been identified.[36]

Nipah virus is a cause of encephalitis in humans and pigs in Southeast Asia.[37] The virus is a member of the *Henipavirus* genus (which includes Hendra virus; see Chapter 16) that is transmitted from frugivorous bats (*Pteropus* spp.) to pigs, among which it spreads horizontally to other pigs and humans. Horses can be exposed and develop antibodies to the virus, and there is one anecdotal report of dilated meningeal vessels in a horse from which Nipah virus was isolated.[38]

Salem virus has been isolated from horses but does not appear to cause disease in this species.[39]

REFERENCES

See the CD-ROM for a list of references linked to the abstract in PubMed.

SECTION • III

Bacterial and Rickettsial Diseases

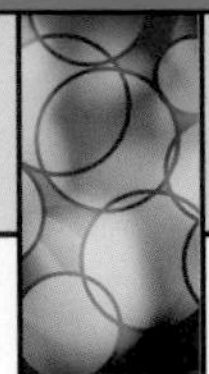

CHAPTER • 27

Laboratory Diagnosis of Bacterial Infections

Barbara A. Byrne

This chapter is designed to aid the veterinary clinician in collecting samples for bacterial culture, understanding the methods used to detect bacteria, interpreting results, and ensuring that optimal results are received from the microbiology laboratory.

DIRECT MICROSCOPIC EXAMINATION

The direct microscopic examination of samples taken from sites of suspected bacterial infection is an essential component for detection and interpretation of microbial isolation and identification results. A variety of staining methodologies can be used to examine clinical specimens. The most common methods include the Gram stain and Wright's (or Diff-Quik) stain. Less frequently used stains include acid-fast and silver stains.

Samples should be examined for the presence and type of inflammation. Wright's or Giemsa stain is preferred for this evaluation because most cells are poorly recognized with Gram stain. The smear should be evaluated for inflammatory cells such as neutrophils and macrophages and the morphologic condition of the cells. Degenerate cells, characterized by swollen nuclei, loss of cytoplasmic detail, and nuclear destruction, are highly suggestive of a septic process and indicate that a culture should be performed on the sample. Wright's stain will also detect bacteria, although the Gram-staining characteristics will not be apparent. The presence of both intracellular and extracellular bacteria is consistent with an infection rather than mere contamination. Bacteria are frequently observed when samples are obtained from normally colonized sites such as mucous membranes; however, they should not be accompanied by inflammation if only normal flora is present.

If fixed tissue sections are the only sample available for evaluation, several staining techniques can be used. With the standard hematoxylin and eosin (H&E) stain, bacteria will appear blue in color. Several silver-based staining methods are available to better visualize bacteria. These stains may be particularly helpful to observe leptospiral organisms in tissues. Available tissue Gram-staining techniques include the Brown and Brenn method, which can be used to identify the Gram reaction of organisms in fixed tissues.

Every sample submitted for bacterial culture should receive a *Gram stain* to facilitate detection of bacteria. This methodology is rapid, is simple to perform, and can give vital information regarding the potential pathogens present. Examination of the Gram-stained specimen can indicate the relative number of bacteria present. The Gram reaction, either gram positive or gram negative, and bacterial morphology can be used to develop a list of possible etiologies that can be used for empiric antimicrobial drug selection (Table 27-1). The observation of bacteria with specific morphologic and staining characteristics is consistent with the presence of anaerobic bacteria and indicates that the sample should also be incubated anaerobically (Fig. 27-1). For example, observation of large, gram-positive rods or long, tapered gram-negative rods suggests *Clostridium* spp. or *Fusobacterium* spp. infection, respectively. Failure to observe bacteria on a Gram stain does not rule out an infection because bacteria need to be present in fairly high numbers, 10^4 to 10^6/mL, to be detected.

Some artifacts appear similar to bacteria in a Gram stain. As noted, the Gram stain is not particularly useful for identifying inflammatory cells because they usually stain gram negative with poor detail. Portions of cells, particularly the nucleus, can stain gram positive and may even look similar to dense clumps of gram-positive cocci in thick preparations. Therefore, it is best to look for bacteria in areas of the smear that are less dense. Equine respiratory secretions contain abundant mucus that stains gram negative. Occasionally, these strands can appear as long, gram-negative rods. They can be differentiated from true bacteria by their variation in size and length and irregular thickness.

Acid-fast (Ziehl-Neelsen) or *modified acid-fast* (Kinyoun) *stains* can be used to help identify members of the nocardioform-actinomycete group of bacteria, including *Mycobacterium* spp. (acid fast), *Rhodococcus equi* (weakly acid fast), and *Nocardia* spp. (weakly acid fast). Bacteria that are acid fast retain the stain carbolfuchsin and appear bright pink because of the waxy outer membrane containing mycolic acid (Fig. 27-2).

Direct detection of bacterial antigen in a sample can be accomplished using immunologic techniques such as direct immunofluorescence or immunohistochemistry. These techniques utilize antibody specific for the target organism and bind bacteria within the specimen. Bound antibody is subsequently visualized using fluorescent or light microscopy, respectively. Diseases for which these techniques are used include detection of *Leptospira* in urine and *Clostridium* in tissues such as liver or muscle. Fluorescent antibody testing can be a rapid means for diagnosis of specific infections, but it requires antibody specific for the organism and fresh or frozen specimens or tissues.

SAMPLING FOR BACTERIAL CULTURE

Indications

Clinical signs suggestive of, but not pathognomonic for, bacterial infections include fever, pain, and swelling. Clinicopathologic findings consistent with a bacterial infection include increased white blood cell (WBC) count with a neutrophilia and possibly a left shift, increased plasma fibrinogen and other acute-phase protein concentrations, and hyperglobulinemia. All these findings are unlikely to be present, and their absence does not rule out the possibility of infectious disease. Cytologic examination of fluid or cells collected from the site of a suspected infection generally reveals neutrophilic inflammation and in some cases a granulomatous or pyogranulomatous response. Degenerate neutrophils are a strong indication that a septic process is present, and bacterial culture should always be performed.

Table • **27-1**

Gram Stain Reaction and Morphology of Common Bacterial Pathogens of Horses

PATHOGEN	MORPHOLOGY
Gram-Positive Organisms	
Streptococcus equi subsp. *equi*	Cocci, often in long chains
Streptococcus equi subsp. *zooepidemicus*	Cocci, often in short chains
Rhodococcus equi	Pleomorphic coccobacilli
Corynebacterium pseudotuberculosis	Pleomorphic coccobacilli, diphtheroid
Dermatophilus congolensis	Cocci, "railroad track"
Actinomyces spp.	Rods, coccobacilli to filamentous and branching
Staphylococcus aureus	Cocci
Clostridium difficile	Rods
Gram-Negative Organisms	
Escherichia coli	Rod
Klebsiella spp.	Rod
Actinobacillus spp.	Rod
Pasteurella spp.	Rod
Salmonella spp.	Rod
Pseudomonas spp.	Rod
Leptospira spp.	Curved rods
Bacteroides spp.	Rod
Fusobacterium necrophorum	Rods, tapered ends

Samples Most Appropriate for Culture

Ideally, specimens from sites that are normally sterile, such as joint fluid, peritoneal fluid, and blood, are the best samples to collect for culture because any bacteria isolated are likely causative. Culture of clinical samples obtained from sites that are colonized with bacterial flora, such as nasal or oral mucous membranes, will usually yield normal bacterial flora of that region (Box 27-1). This may result in spending the client's money and expending the laboratory's efforts needlessly to identify many nonpathogenic bacteria. Because many of these bacteria can also be opportunistic pathogens, it is difficult to determine if they are causing the clinical condition. For example, collection of purulent discharge from the nasal passage of a horse will certainly yield bacteria that are potentially pathogenic, such as *Streptococcus equi* subsp. *zooepidemicus*, but their detection does not mean this bacterium is the cause of the discharge. It is preferable to identify the specific site of infection, such as sinus, guttural pouch, or lung, and collect the sample for culture from that location.

Several exceptions to this rule can be made. In general, if the clinician is trying to detect a pathogen not present in colonized sites in clinically normal animals, the laboratory can specifically target identification efforts toward that organism or use selective media to enhance pathogen detection. Detection of *Streptococcus equi* subsp. *equi* from a nasal or pharyngeal swab would be appropriate because the microbiology laboratory can focus on β-hemolytic streptococcal isolates for definitive identification. Box 27-2 provides a list of specimens to be collected for bacterial culture of different body systems.

Methods for Collection

Tissue (collected as an aspirate or biopsy) and fluids are the best samples to collect for bacterial isolation. In general, larger samples increase the likelihood that a causative pathogen will be isolated because the sample can be centrifuged to concentrate any bacteria. Samples should be collected as aseptically as possible and placed in a sterile container. Submission of samples in a syringe is acceptable, but the needle should be removed

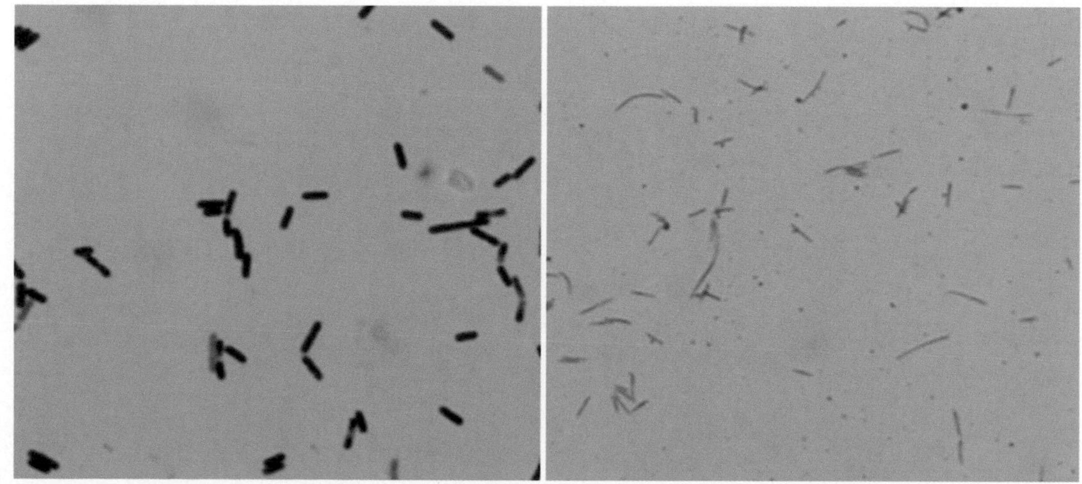

Fig. 27-1 Gram stain of two anaerobic rods demonstrating characteristic morphology. **A,** *Clostridium perfringens*. **B,** *Fusobacterium necrophorum*.

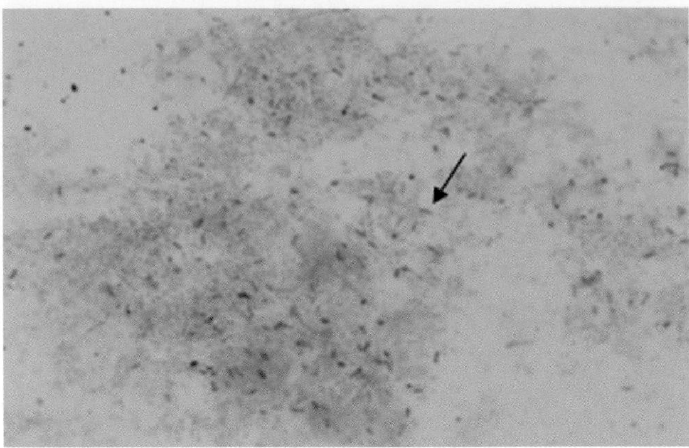

Fig. 27-2 Kinyoun acid-fast stain of *Nocardia* spp. Acid-fast bacteria *(arrow)* appear bright pink or fuscia colored.

Box • 27-1

Common Normal Bacterial Flora of Horses for Selected Sites

Oral and Nasal Cavities and Pharynx

- *Streptococcus equi* subsp. *zooepidemicus*
- *Streptococcus* spp. (nonhemolytic or α-hemolytic)
- *Pasteurella*
- *Escherichia coli*
- *Actinomyces* spp.
- *Enterobacter* spp.
- *Actinobacillus* spp.
- Anaerobes, including *Peptostreptococcus anaerobius, Bacteroides fragilis, Bacteroides* spp., *Fusobacterium* spp.

Skin

- *Streptococcus*
- *Staphylococcus aureus*
- Coagulase-negative staphylococci
- *Micrococcus*
- *Corynebacterium* spp.

Lower Genitourinary Tract

- *Streptococcus* spp.
- *E. coli*
- *Enterobacter* spp.
- *Bacillus* spp.
- *Staphylococcus* spp.

Ocular Conjunctiva

- *Streptomyces* spp.
- *Staphylococcus* spp.
- *Bacillus* spp.
- *Streptococcus* spp. (α-hemolytic, β-hemolytic)
- *E. coli*
- *Moraxella* spp.
- *Acinetobacter* spp.

and the syringe capped to avoid inadvertent injury and introduction of bacteria to personnel. Swabs are not the best choice for sampling because they hold only a small amount of material, and some swabs are made of substances that inhibit bacterial growth. Occasionally, however, a swab will be the only choice for sampling. Swabs are often not appropriate for fecal or intestinal cultures because of their inadequate sample volume. It is best to submit multiple samples in individual containers to eliminate the possibility of cross-contamination.

Suspected Anaerobic Infection

The clinician should decide before submission whether anaerobic culture is necessary so that the sample can be handled appropriately (see Chapters 44, 45, and 48). For example, when emphysema is detected within a tissue, such as in necrotizing myositis, anaerobic culture would be indicated. Likewise, anaerobic infections are common in abscesses, pneumonia, and pleuritis of horses. Anaerobic culture of tissues from an animal that has been dead for many hours may not be worthwhile because anaerobes will proliferate and disperse throughout the carcass. For example, observation of gram-positive rods typical of *Clostridium* spp. in muscle in a 24-hour-old carcass would not be indicative of clostridial myonecrosis.

Many anaerobes are highly sensitive to oxygen and will die during transport if not protected appropriately. Therefore, they should be stored and transported in an environment that minimizes their exposure to the atmosphere. Tissues or a generous volume of fluid (several milliliters) are the best samples for anaerobic culture. If a swab must be used for an anaerobic culture, it should be placed in a semisolid transport medium, such as anaerobic transport media or Port-a-Cul (BD Diagnostic Systems), to minimize air exposure. Tissues should be at least 1 × 1 cm. If very small tissue or fluid samples are available for sampling, they should be placed in transport

Box • 27-2

Samples and Tissues to Select for Common Conditions and Diseases of Major Organ Systems

- *Septicemia:* Blood culture.
- *Pneumonia:* Tracheal secretions, best collected by transtracheal aspiration.
- *Enteritis* or *colitis:* Feces more appropriate than swab of rectal contents to collect sufficient volume for enrichment to detect pathogens. At necropsy, select from the site closest to the lesion.
- *Genitourinary system* (including abortion): Multiple samples needed, and submission of entire selection for culture and microscopic examination is best to optimize identification of the etiology (abortion): fetal stomach contents, liver, lung, heart, fetal heart blood, spleen, placenta, dam serum (for serology). A guarded swab is optimal for culture of the uterus.
- *Nervous system:* Cerebrospinal fluid, or brain/spinal cord at necropsy.
- *Integumentary system:* Skin biopsy or aspiration of unruptured pustule/vesicle.
- *Musculoskeletal system:* Joint fluid, bone, affected muscle (e.g., necrotizing myositis).

media as well. Aerobic swabs are unacceptable for anaerobic culture and will not be set. Even anaerobic swabs poorly support anaerobic organisms and should only be used for short-term (a few hours) transport to the laboratory. Similarly, liquid should be placed on top of the transport media and pushed down into the gel to preserve the anaerobic environment.

Blood Culture

Neonatal foals are the equine patients at greatest risk for septicemia or bacteremia (see Chapter 6). However, blood culture may also be considered in older foals and adults when bacteremia or septicemia is suspected. Many systems are available for culturing blood, including conventional broth-based, biphasic broth-based, and lysis-concentration/filtration methodologies.

The conventional *broth-based method* uses bottled liquid-broth medium into which the patient's blood is inoculated. The amount of blood necessary varies with the volume of broth. Generally, a 1:10 blood/broth ratio is used. Most broth culture systems contain sodium polyanetholesulfonate (SPS) to inactivate bactericidal components of the blood inoculum and act as an anticoagulant. Inoculated broth is incubated at 37° C for 24 hours, then sampled for direct examination, Gram stain, and subculture onto solid media to isolate colonies. If no growth is detected, the broth is sampled again at 48 hours and 1 week after inoculation or when macroscopic changes such as turbidity or gas bubbles are observed. The broth method will require a minimum of 48 hours before colonies can be detected. The broth culture medium allows proliferation of bacteria before subculture and will help to detect bacteria present in low numbers. However, this can also be a disadvantage because contaminating bacteria will proliferate and could easily outnumber the "true" pathogen, resulting in misidentification of the causative bacterium. The *biphasic broth-based method* uses a broth medium for culture enrichment and a solid-agar medium that can be inoculated directly from the broth, decreasing the likelihood of inadvertent contamination of the broth.

Lysis systems lyse phagocytes, and the sample is either centrifuged or filtered to concentrate the bacteria. The resulting pellet is plated to solid culture media. The *lysis-centrifugation system* allows detection of bacteria within 24 hours of collection, and the number of bacteria can be enumerated. It is more sensitive than conventional broth methods.[1] Additionally, this system has advantages for isolation of fungi and *Mycobacterium* spp.[1,2]

Although rare, anaerobic infections can be identified with either a broth or lysis method if a pre-reduced solid medium (e.g., *Brucella* blood agar) and incubation under anaerobic conditions are used for culture. However, in the author's experience, the broth method will more reliably detect anaerobic bacteria, probably because the large volume of liquid preserves the anaerobic environment and allows proliferation of anaerobes that could be present in very low numbers.

It is best to collect at least one culture before administration of antibiotics, but the horse owner or farm manager may have already given antimicrobial drugs before the veterinarian's arrival. If the animal has been treated before blood collection, testing is still possible because both methods (broth, lysis) will dilute the drug to subtherapeutic levels, and SPS will inactivate some aminoglycosides. Additionally, broth blood culture media can be obtained that contains a resin that will absorb antibiotic drugs. A recent study performed in vitro demonstrated that when blood containing therapeutic levels of an aminoglycoside was inoculated with *Escherichia coli* and subsequently inoculated into broth blood culture medium, bacteria could be recovered more readily from the resin-containing blood culture broth than media without the resin (N. Pusterla, personal communication). However, these resins may not completely inactivate newer antimicrobial drugs, such as ticarcillin, imipenem, and aztreonam.

Because bacteria may only be present in the blood intermittently, several samples should be obtained. Even in foals with septicemia, the number of organisms in each milliliter of blood may be quite low; therefore a larger volume of blood for culture, such as 10 mL, is preferred to a smaller volume, such as 1 to 2 mL.

Many protocols can be followed for appropriate sampling for bacteremia; one is presented here. Up to four blood samples may be submitted in a 24-hour period. After clipping and shaving the site for venipuncture, the area is thoroughly disinfected by repeated application of 10% povidone-iodine or other suitable skin antiseptic and allowed to dry. Although not ideal, an intravascular catheter can be used for collection of one sample, but the access port must also be thoroughly disinfected. The stopper on the blood culture bottle or lysis-centrifugation tube should be cleaned with alcohol and allowed to dry. Two samples should be taken from two different sites approximately 10 minutes apart. Antibiotic administration can then be started. The final two cultures can be taken any time within the next 24 hours. These last two samples should be collected immediately before the next antimicrobial drug administration, when the drug concentration is likely to be at its nadir. This timing will increase the likelihood of detecting bacteremia; sampling from different sites will help to distinguish contaminating bacteria from pathogenic bacteria. The causative organism should be cultured from more than one sample and is almost always present in a pure culture. The presence of multiple colony or bacterial types suggests contamination.

Joint Culture

Isolation of bacteria from joints can be difficult. Bacterial numbers are very low in adults compared to neonatal foals with septic arthritis. Joint fluid is a sample that is relatively easy to collect, but false-negative culture results are common.[3] A biopsy of synovial membrane might enhance bacterial isolation, but this recommendation is controversial, and the sample is difficult to obtain, often requiring general anesthesia and arthroscopy. Joint fluid can be inoculated into blood culture broth to allow proliferation of bacteria in very low numbers, increasing the likelihood for detection of the causative bacterium. However, contaminating bacteria will also amplify in the broth culture and can confound interpretation of the results. Alternatively, joint fluid can be concentrated using a lysis-centrifugation blood-culture system. In humans, use of a lysis-centrifugation method is superior to broth inoculation.[4]

Wounds

Sampling a fresh wound at the time of first treatment can be of doubtful utility because the results will demonstrate contaminating organisms that may or may not lead to infection. Culture of an established wound with signs of infection (e.g., heat, swelling, discharge) is clearly indicated. The superficial areas of the wound should be thoroughly cleaned and debrided before obtaining a sample; otherwise, superficial bacteria will be isolated. Culture of deep regions, including a biopsy of affected tissues, is most likely to lead to identification of the causative bacterium. Aspiration of fluid from deep tissues is an additional method that is useful for sample collection.

Sampling for Enteric Infections

The major bacterial pathogens cultured from horses with enteritis include *Salmonella* spp., *Clostridium perfringens*, and *Clostridium difficile* (see Chapters 38 and 44). Samples for culture of intestinal contents should be collected, whenever possible, from the site of the lesion rather than merely collecting fecal material. This is especially important for suspected clostridial enteritis. Intestinal, fecal, and mesenteric lymph node samples are generally enriched to detect *Salmonella* spp. When submitting samples, be sure to indicate the likely pathogen(s) causing the clinical signs, and include the age of the horse.

Clostridial Enteritis

Anaerobic cultures from fecal material of horses are not routinely done at all microbiology laboratories. Therefore, clinicians submitting samples from horses with suspected *C. perfringens* enteritis should specifically request culture for *Clostridium*. In cases of *C. perfringens* enteritis or enterotoxemia, intestine from the affected region is preferred over feces at necropsy. The intestine should be collected within 1 to 2 hours of death because clostridial organisms will rapidly proliferate throughout the intestine immediately after death, increasing the chance of isolation. Thus, in cases with a long postmortem interval, isolation of *Clostridium* is of doubtful significance. Positive isolation should be correlated with the presence of appropriate histologic lesions. Currently, only a few diagnostic laboratories offer detection of *C. perfringens* toxins alpha, beta, iota, or epsilon for typing (other than the enterotoxin), making confirmation of a causative role of *C. perfringens* in enteritis difficult. An enzyme-linked immunosorbent assay (ELISA) is available to detect *C. perfringens* alpha, beta, and epsilon toxins in intestinal samples, but this test alone is insufficient for definitive diagnosis of *C. perfringens* enterotoxemia.[5] Many laboratories can perform genetic testing on isolates to identify toxin genes.

If *Clostridium difficile* enteritis is suspected, be sure to include this request on the history form because broth enrichment, specialized media, and toxin testing are required for this organism. Several commercial kits may be used to identify *C. perfringens* enterotoxin (of unknown or doubtful significance in horses), *C. difficile* toxin A, and *C. difficile* antigen (Triage *C. difficile* panel, Biosite Diagnostics) or *C. difficile* toxins A and B (TOX A/B QUIK CHEK, Techlab). These tests can provide a means for rapid diagnosis of *C. difficile* enteritis. (For further discussion of diagnosis of clostridial enteritis in horses, see Chapter 44.)

Ocular Infections

The most common indication for culture of ocular tissues is the presence of a corneal ulcer, particularly those that are healing poorly or melting (see Chapter 10). A culturette may be used to sample the cornea, but gentle scraping to collect a small amount of tissue will more likely yield a causative organism. Although most bacteria typically associated with ocular infections are readily cultured in the laboratory, some infections are caused by streptococci that require additional nutrient supplementation (e.g., chocolate agar, *Staphylococcus* feeder streak) to be isolated successfully.[6]

Botulism and Tetanus

Not all laboratories have the capability to detect botulinum toxin or *Clostridium botulinum* (see Chapter 46). The best way to diagnose botulism is detection of toxin in blood or intestinal contents of the animal; however, many tests have low sensitivity. Sampling the suspected origin of the toxin (feed, water) for presence of toxin or *C. botulinum* culture is the best approach. These samples can be sent to the microbiology laboratory, then forwarded or submitted directly to the laboratory equipped to perform the assays to speed analysis.

Clostridium tetani is difficult to grow and frequently is not isolated from affected animals (see Chapter 47). However, the laboratory can perform smears to identify typical gram-positive bacilli that could be causative. In most cases, however, tetanus is a clinical diagnosis.

SAMPLE TRANSPORT

Samples should be kept cool and shipped to the appropriate laboratory as soon as possible after collection. Samples are best shipped on ice or frozen gel pack by overnight delivery to prevent leakage. Some bacteria might survive freezing, but their fewer numbers in the tissue will decrease the likelihood of isolation. In hot weather, samples will warm up quickly, so additional cold packs may be needed. If possible, avoid shipping over the weekend, when samples may sit in warm locations before delivery to the laboratory on Monday. All samples should be contained within a sealed container (e.g., bag, tube, swab), and a second sealed container should surround the specimen in case the primary container breaks or leaks. Absorbent material should also be placed in the package in case of leakage.

SUBMISSION

To familiarize the clinician with isolation procedures in the bacteriology laboratory, it is important to explain how samples are set for bacterial isolation. Not all samples are inoculated on all types of media to isolate every possible bacterial species, particularly from colonized sites such as the gastrointestinal tract. Some sites should be normally sterile, in which case all organisms present should be identified. Organisms that require special culture characteristics (e.g., anaerobes), fastidious growth, or enrichment procedures are handled in special ways to enhance or select for their isolation (Box 27-3). The type of media and conditions used to isolate and identify bacteria in the laboratory are determined by the horse's signalment, history, and clinical findings specified by the clinician, as well as the source of the sample. Thus, it is important that the clinician provide a limited history, if possible, and any lesions or clinical signs detected. Likewise, if a particular bacterial species is suspected, it should be included so that the appropriate culture conditions are applied. The laboratory can then use this information to establish any specialized culture conditions needed to detect suspected agents.

Notify the laboratory if your list of differential diagnoses includes a disease highly infectious for humans, such as anthrax, coccidioidomycosis, histoplasmosis, blastomycosis, and mycobacterial infections. Even if the infection is not contagious to

Box • 27-3

Examples of Fastidious Organisms or Those Requiring Specialized Media or Culture Conditions

- *Mycobacterium* spp.: other than atypical mycobacteria
- *Mycoplasma*
- Anaerobes
- *Clostridium:* different media used for various species
- *Leptospira*
- *Listeria:* cold enrichment for neural tissues
- *Salmonella:* selection and enrichment
- Nutritionally variant *Streptococcus*

humans directly from the animal, some pathogens, such as the dimorphic systemic fungal infections, are highly infectious to laboratory workers when grown in culture. Warning the laboratory that these pathogens might be present will allow appropriate protective precautions to be implemented.

INTERPRETATION OF ISOLATION AND IDENTIFICATION RESULTS

Most laboratories will provide the clinician with results that include the Gram stain findings from the sample submitted, bacterial species identified, and their relative quantity. Results obtained from culture and isolation should be interpreted in the context of the organism(s) identified, Gram stain and cytology results, source of the sample, whether a mixed bacterial population was identified, quantity of bacteria, and clinical presentation.

Any bacterium isolated from a normally sterile site should be considered significant if the microscopic examination is consistent with a septic process and the organism matches the Gram stain. Isolation of some bacterial species will lead the clinician to suspect contamination, such as *Bacillus* spp., α-hemolytic *Streptococcus*, and coagulase-negative *Staphylococcus*. These organisms, when found as part of a mixed bacterial population in the sample in low quantity, can be contaminants. Although any of these bacteria can cause infection given appropriate circumstances, the clinician should carefully evaluate all findings before concluding they are the primary cause of a disease process.

If the culture is collected from a site normally colonized with bacterial flora, it is expected that a variety of bacteria will be identified. If a bacterial species identified is not part of the normal flora for the site, it could be related to the disease condition. Bacteria present in very high numbers relative to other species could be directly related to the clinical signs; however, their proliferation could be in response to a condition, not the cause.

Results from urine cultures should always include quantification of bacterial numbers in colony-forming units per milliliter (CFU/mL). Because the lower genitourinary tract is colonized with bacteria, urine samples, whether collected by catheterization or free catch, will almost always have some contamination. Bacteria in concentrations greater than 40,000 CFU/mL from a midstream free catch or 1000 CFU/mL in a catheterization sample are considered significant; 20,000 to 40,000 CFU/mL by midstream catch and 500 to 1000 CFU/mL by catheterization are considered suspicious for infection.[7] Urinalysis and cytology results should also reflect an active sediment consistent with infection.

MOLECULAR METHODS FOR DETECTING BACTERIAL PATHOGENS

Advances in genetic techniques have allowed development of several methods to detect and identify bacterial pathogens. Most use the basic concept that complementary single strands of deoxyribonucleic acid (DNA) hybridize to one another. DNA polymerases, DNA restriction enzymes, hybridization, and gel electrophoresis are all tools utilized in these techniques.

Polymerase Chain Reaction

The most common technique is the polymerase chain reaction (PCR). This method amplifies target DNA in vitro using a thermostable DNA polymerase. In short, the PCR reaction uses DNA oligonucleotides specific for the target that prime the polymerase reaction after binding; a DNA polymerase and nucleotides are used to synthesize a copy of the target DNA. Multiple cycles in which the DNA is melted to make single strands, annealing where the temperature is lowered to allow primer binding, and extension for DNA copying lead to many copies of the target DNA, which can then be more easily detected. The DNA product is visualized using agarose gel electrophoresis. Theoretically, 10^9 or more copies can be made from a single target DNA molecule; but in practical use, most assays require the presence of 10 to 1000 targets (bacteria).

A more recent variation of the PCR reaction is *quantitative* or *real-time* PCR. This technique uses the general PCR reaction, but as the DNA copies are synthesized, a fluorescent reaction is generated. A fluorescent molecule is intercalated in the target DNA and released as a copy is made, or a fluorescent-labeled probe specific for the target sequence is displaced by the growing DNA chain (TaqMan, Applied Biosystems) (Fig. 27-3). An advantage of the quantitative PCR is that the reaction and detection can take place simultaneously, reducing the time for testing and results. Also, the test has increased sensitivity, and the probe displacement allows additional specificity.

PCR is best used to detect bacteria that cannot be cultured in vitro, are difficult to cultivate, take a prolonged time for isolation and identification, or are present in such low numbers that culture is inadequately sensitive. The technique is rapid and extremely sensitive. Bacteria for which PCR has been used to enhance detection include *Lawsonia intracellularis*, *Streptococcus equi* subsp. *equi*, *Anaplasma phagocytophilum*, and *Neorickettsia risticii*.[8-12]

Another application of PCR is for detection of bacteria within the joint, where cultures are frequently negative in adults despite a high suspicion of bacterial infection based on cytology. Bacteria are broadly targeted by using primers that recognize all eubacterial 16S ribosome genes (rDNA). One study demonstrated that PCR followed by reverse line blot hybridization (a method to determine species of bacteria amplified) was more sensitive for detecting joint sepsis (89%) than culture and isolation alone (38%) or culture following incubation in blood culture broth (78%).[13,14] One further advantage of PCR is that it can be performed on archival frozen or formalin-fixed tissues when the organism is no longer viable. Detection of bacterial messenger ribonucleic acid (mRNA) by PCR can also be conducted to verify that the organism was viable in the tissue.

PCR detection of pathogens has several disadvantages. The technique is expensive and requires some specialized equipment, depending on the methodology used. There must be adequate sample to allow extraction of DNA for the PCR reaction, and some samples will contain substances that interfere with the reaction, leading to false-negative results. Something must be known about the target organism so that appropriate oligonucleotide primers can be used. Even if broadly recognizing 16S rDNA primers are used, additional sequencing must be performed to identify the pathogen present. Thus, it is difficult or impossible to identify novel agents. Furthermore, PCR does not yield a bacterial isolate to use for antimicrobial sensitivity testing. Because no isolate is obtained, it also is difficult to compare isolates between patients to understand the molecular epidemiology and ecology of the infection. Although the sensitivity of PCR is very useful, contamination of the PCR reaction or sample can easily occur, leading to false-positive results. It is essential that the laboratory performing these tests have adequate positive and negative controls to interpret results.

Use of DNA probes is an older technique in which DNA isolated from a sample is hybridized with a labeled DNA

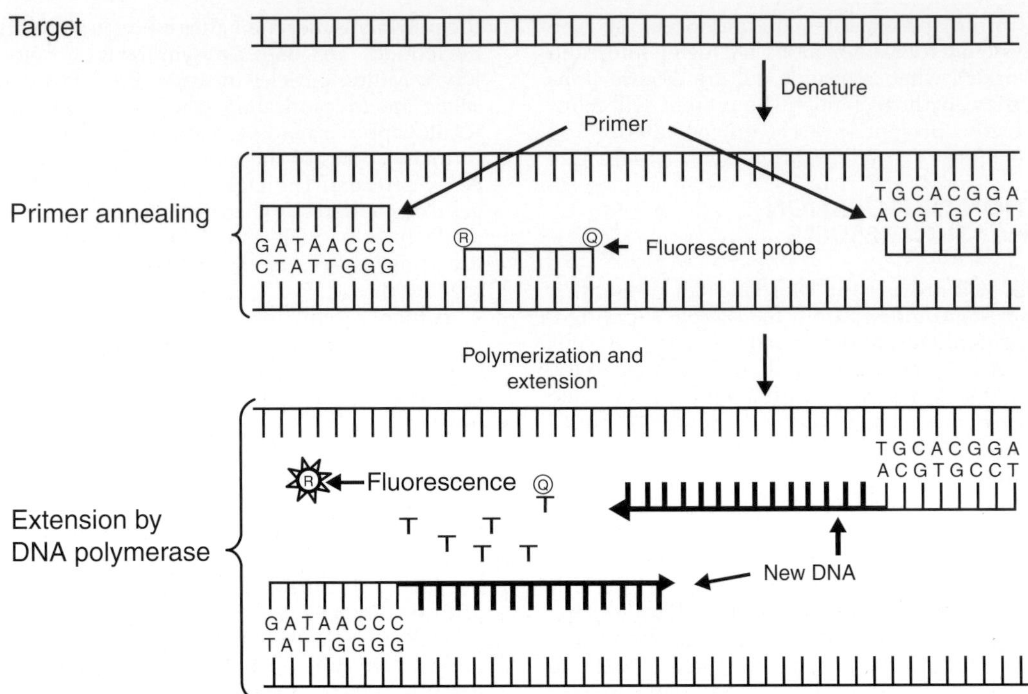

Fig. 27-3 Quantitative polymerase chain reaction (PCR) using the TaqMan technology. PCR reaction amplifies target DNA with multiple cycles of denaturation, annealing, and elongation of new DNA strands. A probe complementary to the target sequence is labeled at the 5′ end with a fluorescent reporter molecule, *R*, and at the 3′ end with a quencher, Q, that dampens fluorescence. As DNA polymerization occurs, the Taq polymerase digests the probe, releasing the fluorescent molecule. The resulting fluorescence can be measured as repeated cycles release additional reporter fluorescence.

probe specific for a particular pathogen. The probe technique is less sensitive than PCR because there is no amplification step and about 10^4 DNA copies/mL are required for most detection methods.[15] This technique has largely been replaced by more sensitive PCR assays; however, DNA probes can be useful to identify bacterial species in amplified DNA products or on bacterial isolates.

Toxin Gene Detection

Molecular methods may also be used to further characterize isolated bacteria. PCR and *multiplex* PCR, where multiple oligonucleotide primers are used in a single reaction, have been developed to detect toxin genes in *Clostridium perfringens* and *Escherichia coli*.[16] PCR methods are currently being developed and used by research and human bacteriology laboratories to detect antimicrobial resistance genes.[17] The use of microarrays to detect bacterial pathogens and antimicrobial resistance genes, although a research tool at this time, may eventually be important for resistant-gene characterization.[18-20]

Molecular Epidemiology

Identification of related isolates can be very useful for investigation of outbreaks and nosocomial infections. A variety of techniques, including *pulsed-field gel electrophoresis* (PFGE), may be used to genotype isolates in order to determine the relatedness between isolates of the same species. This technique can be used to explore whether bacteria have a similar source in a disease outbreak and to evaluate clonal spread of highly virulent bacteria.[21,22] In PFGE genotyping, genomic DNA is isolated from the bacterium and digested with an endonuclease that cuts infrequently, resulting in extremely large DNA fragments. These fragments are separated by PFGE, and a banding pattern results. The banding pattern can be compared for similarity between isolates. Bacteria with the same PFGE profile, or "fingerprint," are considered related.[23,24]

ANTIMICROBIAL SUSCEPTIBILITY TESTING

Indications

Antimicrobial sensitivity testing should be considered whenever a bacterial pathogen is isolated. Some bacteria will have a predictable sensitivity pattern, so most laboratories elect not to perform sensitivity testing. These organisms include *Streptococcus*, *Corynebacterium*, and *Actinomyces* species. Often, sensitivity of a particular organism to antimicrobial drugs can be inferred from observations of results from the practice population. Sensitivity testing is always indicated for a number of pathogens, however, because their susceptibility to different drugs can vary and resistance can be acquired rapidly. These pathogens include *Pseudomonas* spp., *Staphylococcus* spp., and all enteric organisms, such as *E. coli* and *Klebsiella* spp. Failure to respond to appropriate antimicrobial therapy is another strong indication for sensitivity testing.

Methods

The two major methods for testing antimicrobial drug sensitivity are *agar diffusion*, most frequently using the Kirby-Bauer method, and *broth dilution*, where microdilution techniques are most common. All testing and interpretation should be performed in accordance with recommendations of the Clinical and Laboratory Standards Institute (CLSI, formerly the National

Committee for Clinical Laboratory Standards [NCCLS]) so that results are highly repeatable and able to be compared between laboratories (http://www.nccls.org). In the agar diffusion method, bacteria, at a single concentration, are spread over Mueller-Hinton agar, and disks impregnated with the drugs to be tested are placed on the lawn. The plates are incubated 18 to 24 hours, and the diameter of the *zone of inhibition*, or the area where bacteria do not grow, is measured. Zone size correlates with sensitivity (Fig. 27-4). The advantages of the Kirby-Bauer method are ease, little need for specialized equipment, and the different drugs to be tested can be changed readily. Disadvantages are that some bacteria grow poorly or not at all on the media, and *minimum inhibitory concentration* (MIC) cannot be determined.

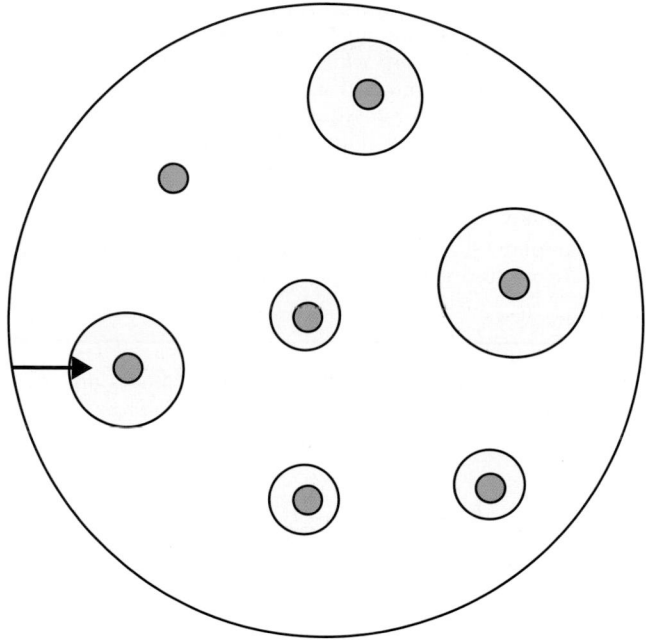

Fig. 27-4 Diagram illustrating Kirby-Bauer disk dilution antimicrobial sensitivity testing. Arrow indicates zone of inhibition.

When broth microdilution methodology is used, a set concentration of bacteria is inoculated into each well of a 96-well plate containing an antimicrobial drug. A number of drugs can be tested on each plate at the discretion of the laboratory. Each drug is tested at several different concentrations; twofold dilutions are centered around the plasma levels expected in the patient when the drug is administered at recommended dosages. The plate is incubated 18 to 24 hours and each well examined for growth. Growth in a well indicates that the bacterium is not sensitive to the drug at that concentration. The lowest drug concentration at which there is no growth is considered the MIC (Fig. 27-5).

Interpretation

CLSI establishes interpretation of antimicrobial sensitivity testing as sensitive, intermediate, or resistant, based on either the diameter of the zone of inhibition or the MIC. In the broth microdilution method, a "breakpoint" is used, or the highest concentration of drug at which the bacterium would be considered sensitive. The interpretations have been established using in vitro testing and in vivo clinical responses to the antimicrobial drug at corresponding concentrations. When an MIC is determined, a drug with an MIC greater than the breakpoint concentration is considered resistant and indicates that the MIC is above drug concentrations obtained in vivo at label or recommended dosages. The "sensitive" interpretation indicates that the drug is expected to be effective against the tested bacterium at label or recommended dosages. A "resistant" interpretation means that the drug is unlikely to be effective against the bacterium tested. An "intermediate" interpretation suggests that for drugs that have flexibility in the dosage range, the drug could be effective at the higher recommended dosages. The standards do not indicate the ability to penetrate to the

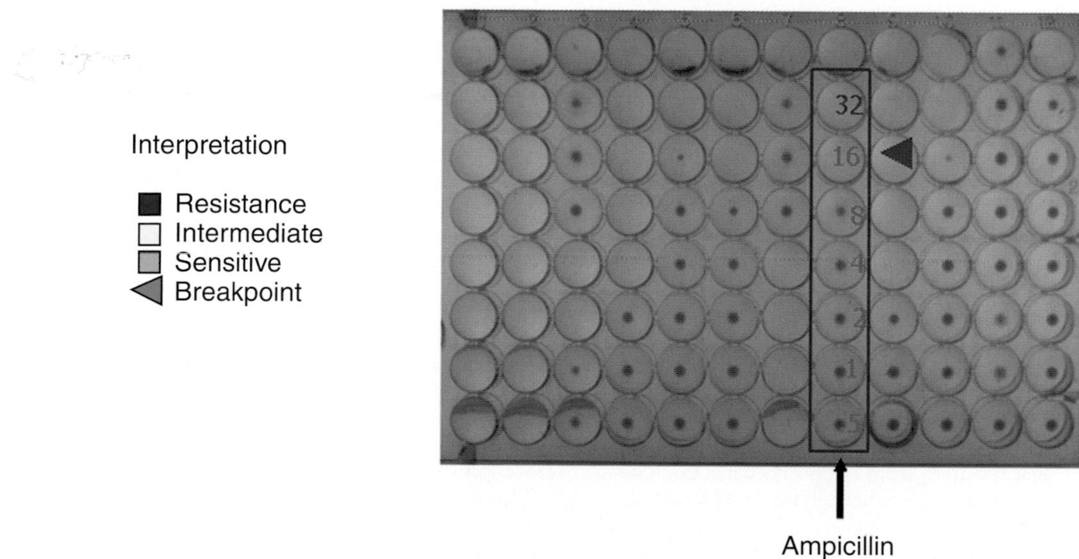

Fig. 27-5 Broth microdilution antimicrobial sensitivity testing. Drug concentrations of ampicillin are indicated in micrograms per milliliter (μg/mL). Arrowhead indicates the "breakpoint," or the highest concentration at which the bacterial minimum inhibitory concentration (MIC) is interpreted as sensitive. Growth in wells is seen as a dark pellet. Growth above the breakpoint would indicate resistance to the drug. MIC for ampicillin for this bacterium would be 16 μg/mL and interpreted as "sensitive."

site of infection or conditions found at the site. In several cases the predicted sensitivity in vitro does not correspond to clinical efficacy, particularly when the organism is intracellular or within a body compartment that is difficult to penetrate, such as the central nervous system.

SEROLOGIC DIAGNOSIS OF BACTERIAL DISEASES

Several bacterial infections can be diagnosed serologically by detection of antibody specific to the pathogen. The presence of antibody indicates exposure to the bacterium. Infection may have occurred in the past and been cleared or may be ongoing, depending on the organism and the test used. Serology results must be interpreted in light of the clinical presentation, the prevalence of the organism in the region, and the equine population at risk. Ideally, the serologic test will have little or no cross-reactivity with other bacteria, will be sensitive enough to detect low levels of antibody, and will be highly repeatable. The organism should not be part of the normal flora or one to which horses are regularly exposed; a positive result could merely indicate exposure, and many horses would have a positive result. Quantitative serologic tests (e.g., ELISA) can be helpful to follow the course of infection where rising antibody levels indicate recent exposure or infection.

Serologic testing is most useful to diagnose disease caused by bacteria that are difficult or impossible to isolate, such as *Leptospira* spp. (Chapter 34), *Lawsonia intracellularis* (Chapter 36), *Anaplasma phagocytophilum* (Chapter 42), *Neorickettsia risticii* (Chapter 43), and *Borrelia burgdorferi* (Chapter 35). Additional conditions that indicate use of serology include infections for which it is difficult or impossible to obtain a sample, as in horses with a suspected abdominal abscess.

Interpretation of a positive serologic test can be difficult because a positive test could mean that the horse was only exposed to the pathogen and does not have an active infection. Detection of IgM specific for the targeted organism aids interpretation, since IgM is an immunoglobulin that is synthesized in the acute active stages of disease. A commercially available diagnostic ELISA detects immunoglobulin G (IgG) to the M protein of *Streptococcus. equi* subsp. *equi* infection (see Chapter 28).

Blood should be collected in a serum (red-top) tube and allowed to clot fully. Subsequently, the sample should be centrifuged shortly after collection and the serum removed and transferred to a new sterile tube to avoid contamination with bacteria. Blood stored on the clot for prolonged periods may hemolyze, which can interfere with some serologic tests. If the sample will not be used within a few days, it should be stored frozen to preserve antibody integrity.

REFERENCES

See the CD-ROM for a complete list of references linked to the abstract in PubMed.

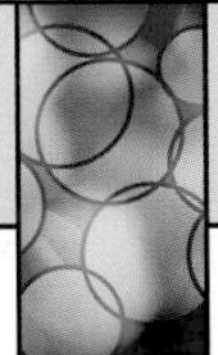

CHAPTER • 28

Streptococcal Infections

OVERVIEW

Debra C. Sellon

The streptococci are gram-positive, catalase-negative, facultative anaerobic, coccoid or ovoid bacteria. The numerous species of streptococci may be described on the basis of the nature and extent of their hemolytic activity as *alpha-hemolytic* (α-hemolytic), *beta-hemolytic* (β-hemolytic), and *nonhemolytic* species (Fig. 28-1). The most significant streptococcal pathogens in human and veterinary medicine are β-hemolytic, producing complete clearing of blood agar medium because of lysis of erythrocytes in the media. In α-hemolytic reactions, erythrocytes are not completely lysed, and growth is surrounded by greenish color of the agar resulting from streptococcal action on hemoglobin (see Chapter 27). Nonhemolytic streptococcal species have no effect on blood agar.[1]

In 1928 an American bacteriologist, Rebecca Lancefield, published a study of the chemical composition and antigenicity of hemolytic streptococci. In 1933 she described a classification of streptococci into groups according to their ability to induce production of antibodies that cause precipitation of streptococci from solution. These groups are now known as the Lancefield groups. The Lancefield group A streptococci, most notably *Streptococcus pyogenes*, are the most important streptococci in human medicine; in contrast, the group C streptococci *S. equi* subsp. *zooepidemicus* and *S. equi* subsp. *equi* assume greater importance in equine medicine. Although the Lancefield groupings remain phenotypically useful, it is now known that unrelated species of β-hemolytic streptococci may produce identical Lancefield antigens and that strains that are genetically related at the species level may have heterogenous Lancefield antigens.[1] Molecular analysis of streptococcal organisms have revealed that the bacteria formerly classified as group D streptococci, or enterococci, are better classified in the separate genus *Enterococcus* (see Chapter 30) and the group N streptococci, or lactococci, should be classified in the genus *Lactococcus*.

This chapter discusses individually the major streptococcal pathogens of horses, including *S. equi* subsp. *equi*, *S. equi* subsp. *zooepidemicus*, and *S. pneumoniae*. A variety of other streptococcal infections have been described in horses as nonspecific commensal organisms or sporadic etiologic agents of disease. Notable among these reports for the severity of associated disease, streptococcal toxic shock was reported in a horse in which *Streptococcus mitis* was cultured from the blood.[2]

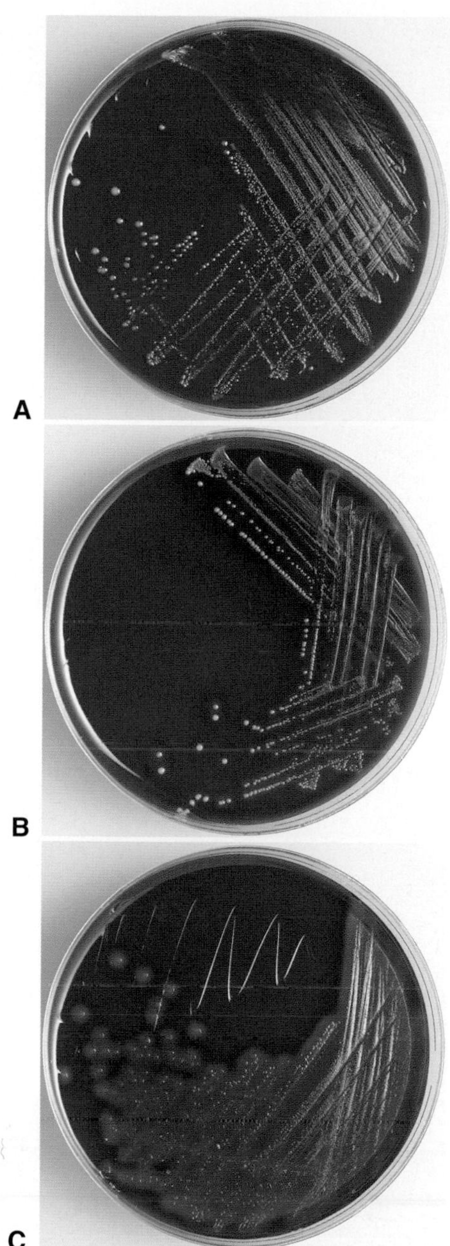

Fig. 28-1 Cultures of streptococci on blood agar. **A,** Nonhemolytic streptococci; note the absence of a zone of hemolysis around the colonies. **B,** Alpha-hemolytic streptococci; note the greenish discoloration because of partial hemolysis. **C,** Beta-hemolytic streptococci; note the complete zone of hemolysis and clearing of agar around the bacterial colonies.

STREPTOCOCCUS EQUI SUBSP. *EQUI*

Corinne R. Sweeney, Peter J. Timoney, J. Richard Newton, and Melissa T. Hines*

Disease caused by *S. equi* subsp. *equi* infection in horses, commonly referred to as "strangles," was described in early veterinary science literature and first reported by Jordanus Ruffus in 1251. Although its official name is *S. equi* subsp *equi*, there is compelling evidence that it is derived from an ancestral *S. zooepidemicus* as a "genovar" or "biovar" of the latter. The descriptive term *S. equi* is still appropriate based on its widespread usage in the scientific literature over the past century and is used in this discussion.

*Modified from Sweeney CR, Timoney JF, Newton R, Hines MT: *Streptococcus equi* infections in horses: guidelines for treatment, control and prevention of strangles, *J Vet Intern Med* 19:123-124, 2005.

Etiology

Streptococcus equi is a gram-positive coccoid bacterium that typically appears in pairs or chains. Colonies on blood agar plates are mucoid, honey colored, and surrounded by a wide zone of beta hemolysis. Its colony morphology is identical to that of *S. equi* subsp. *zooepidemicus* (see later discussion), and it must be differentiated by its inability to ferment lactose and sorbitol. There is only one known antigenic type of *S. equi*, which may be a clone or biovar of the closely related *S. equi* subsp. *zooepidemicus*.[3-5]

Virulence factors for *S. equi* include a nonantigenic hyaluronic acid capsule, hyaluronidase, streptolysin S, streptokinase, immunoglobulin G (IgG) Fc-receptor proteins, pyrogenic exotoxins (e.g., SePE-I, SePE-H), peptidoglycan, and the antiphagocytic M protein (SeM).[5] Evidence also exists for a leukocidal toxin.[6] Virulent isolates of *S. equi* are almost always highly encapsulated, producing mucoid colonies, whereas avirulent isolates lack a capsule.[7,8] The capsule appears to inhibit significantly the ability of neutrophils to bind, ingest, and kill the organism. It also facilitates the function of proteases and toxins within the organism and is required for the function of SeM.[5] The oxygen-stable enzyme streptokinase S is responsible for the β-hemolysis observed with *S. equi*. Binding to erythrocytes results in formation of a transmembrane pore and irreversible osmotic lysis of the cell.[9] At least four pyrogenic mitogens, SePE-H, SePE-I, SePE-K, and SePE-L, are expressed by *S. equi*.[5] These molecules stimulate T cells nonspecifically to proliferate and release proinflammatory cytokines, resulting in an acute-phase response with high fever, neutrophilia, and hyperfibrinogenemia. These clinical responses may be neutralized by antibody generated during convalescence or by active immunization with each mitogen.[10]

The M proteins of streptococci are antiphagocytic, acid-resistant fibrillar molecules that project from the cell wall surface in an arrangement whereby two identical molecules are coiled around each other.[5] The M protein of *S. equi* (SeM) is approximately 58 kilodaltons. Its antiphagocytic action is a result of binding of fibrinogen to the N-terminal half of the molecule and IgG to the central region.[11-13] This interaction masks C3b-binding sites on the surface of the bacteria and inhibits the alternative C3 and classic C5 convertases.[14] The M protein of *S. equi* is highly conserved with little variation in size or antigenicity between isolates, except for some isolates from long-term guttural pouch carriers that have in-frame deletions representing about 20% of the SeM gene.[15,16] Loss of SeM expression by *S. equi* results in loss of virulence, but not infectivity, for ponies.[17]

Epidemiology

Transmission

Purulent discharges from horses with active and recovering strangles are an important and easily recognizable source of new *S. equi* infections among susceptible horses (Fig. 28-2). Transmission of infection occurs when there is either direct or indirect transfer of *S. equi* within these purulent discharges between affected and susceptible horses. *Direct transmission* refers to horse-to-horse contacts, particularly through normal equine social behavior involving mutual head contact. *Indirect transmission* occurs through the sharing of contaminated housing, water sources, feed or feeding utensils, twitches, tack, and other less obvious fomites, such as the clothing and equipment of handlers, caretakers, farriers, and veterinarians, unless appropriate barrier precautions are in place to prevent spread of *S. equi*.

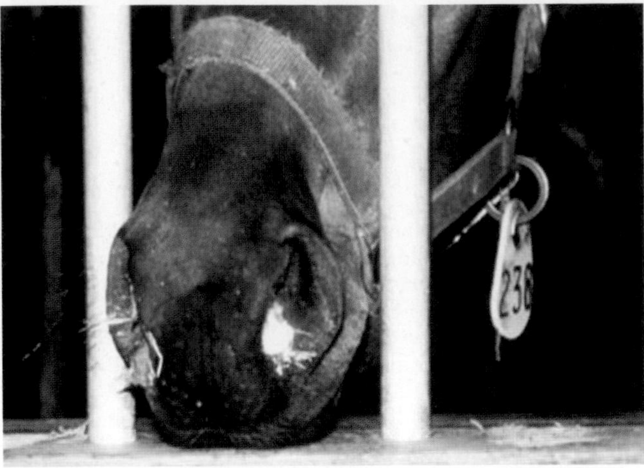

Fig. 28-2 Purulent nasal discharge in horse with strangles.

Inapparent Carrier Horses. Transmission of *S. equi* that originates from outwardly healthy animals incubating the disease or that are inapparent carriers of the organism in their upper respiratory tract has been the focus of recent investigation.[18-22] Normal nasal secretions are assumed to be the source of infection in these animals. Evidence indicates that a moderate proportion of horses continue to harbor *S. equi* for several weeks after clinical signs have disappeared, even though the organism is no longer detectable in most affected horses by 4 to 6 weeks after total recovery. In this situation the source of infection may not be readily apparent, and clinical signs may appear unexpectedly in animals with close contact to these carriers.

Horses that are fully recovered from the disease but continue to be infectious for prolonged periods through periodic shedding of *S. equi* are referred to as *long-term, subclinical carriers* and can be a source of infection for susceptible animals.[18-22] Introductions of these animals to herds may be a source of new outbreaks, even in well-managed groups of horses. Adequate control for strangles cannot be achieved without recognition of this category of animal and implementation of appropriate methods for detection and treatment.

The best recognized site of carriage of *S. equi* among subclinically infected horses is the guttural pouch. This structure becomes infected in the early stages of disease, following rupture of the adjacent retropharyngeal lymph nodes through the floor of the pouch (Fig. 28-3). It is likely that short-lived guttural pouch empyema is the most frequent outcome of uncomplicated drainage of retropharyngeal lymph node abscessation. The carrier state develops in approximately 10% of affected animals, resulting in chronic empyema of the pouches. Should the purulent material persist in the guttural pouch, inspissation occurs with formation of discrete masses known as *chondroids*. Chondroids may occur singly or multiply, sometimes in very large numbers (Fig. 28-4). Chondroids formed after strangles can harbor *S. equi*, based on culture and by histologic demonstration of the organism on the surface of and lining the fissures within these structures (J.R. Newton, unpublished data). In some animals, guttural pouch empyema with *S. equi* infection may persist without clinical signs for many months or even years. Approximately 50% of horses with guttural pouch empyema cough sporadically, and some may have an intermittent unilateral nasal discharge.

Environmental Persistence of *S. equi*. Currently, there is a lack of field-based proof for prolonged environmental persistence of *S. equi*. A suspension of bacteria survived for 63 days on wood at 2° C and for 48 days on glass or wood at 20° C. The absence of co-infection with normal environmental flora in this study might have prolonged the survival because *S. equi* is sensitive to bacteriocins produced by environmental bacteria.[23] Its survival time is decreased in the presence of other soil-borne flora.[24]

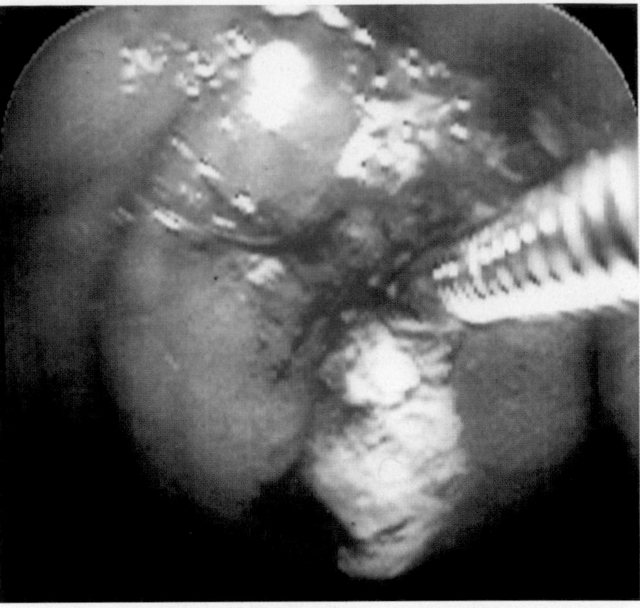

Fig. 28-3 Endoscopic examination of horse with strangles. Abscessed retropharyngeal node has ruptured into the guttural pouch after being touched by the endoscopic biopsy instrument.

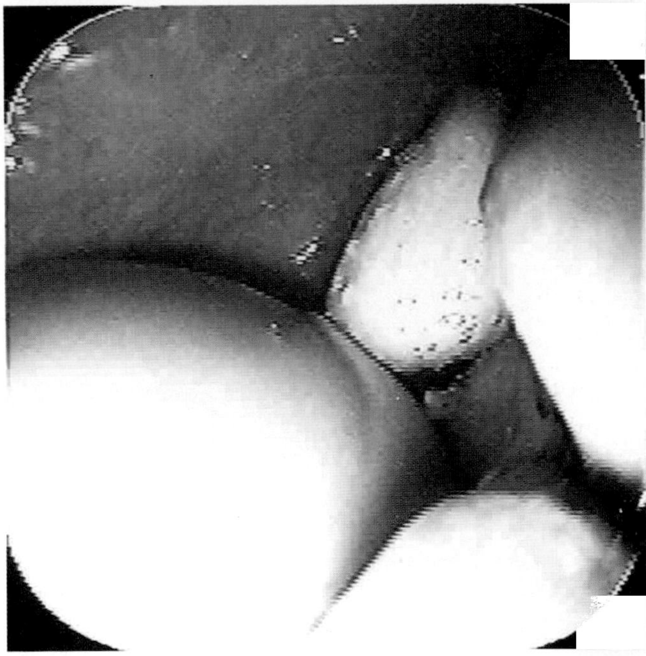

Fig. 28-4 Endoscopic examination of guttural pouch of horse with chondroids.

Pathogenesis

S. equi enters through the mouth or nose and attaches to cells in the crypt of the lingual and palatine tonsils, as well as to the follicular-associated epithelium of the pharyngeal and tubal tonsils. A few hours after infection, the organism is difficult to detect on the mucosal surface but is visible within cells of the epithelium and subepithelial follicles. Translocation occurs in a few hours to the mandibular and suprapharyngeal lymph nodes that drain the pharyngeal and tonsil region. Failure of neutrophils to phagocytose and kill the streptococci appears to be caused by a combination of the hyaluronic acid capsule, antiphagocytic SeM protein, Mac protein, and other undetermined antiphagocytic factors released by the organism.[5,24] This culminates in accumulation of many extracellular streptococci in the form of long chains surrounded by large numbers of degenerating neutrophils. Bacterial enzymes such as streptolysin and streptokinase may contribute to abscess formation by damaging cell membranes and activating plasminogen.

Although strangles predominantly involves the upper airways, including the guttural pouches and associated lymph nodes, metastasis to other locations occasionally occurs. Spread may be hematogenous or through lymphatic channels, which results in abscesses in lymph nodes and other organs of the thorax and abdomen. This form of the disease has been known as "bastard strangles." Bacteremia occurs on days 6 to 12 in horses inoculated intranasally with virulent *S. equi*.[25]

The first clinical sign of infection is a rapid increase in rectal temperature to 103° F (39.4° C) or higher between 3 and 14 days after exposure. This is associated with release of the pyrogenic mitogens. In addition, blood fibrinogen concentrations and white blood cell and neutrophil counts increase. Abscess development is rapid and is often accompanied by lymph accumulation in afferent lymphatics.

Nasal shedding of *S. equi* usually begins after a latent period of 4 to 14 days and ceases between 3 and 7 weeks after resolution of the acute phase of disease.[5,24] In some horses, shedding persists beyond this period; these animals may continue to harbor *S. equi* in their guttural pouches or other areas of the upper respiratory tract for months or years.[18,20]

Approximately 75% of horses develop solid immunity to *S. equi* after recovery from infection.[8] The other 25% of infected horses are susceptible to reinfection within months, probably because of a failure to produce or maintain adequate concentrations of appropriate mucosal and systemic antibodies.[5] Strong SeM-specific mucosal immunoglobulin A (IgA) and IgGb responses occur after infection in most horses. The development of mucosal and serum antibody responses are independent; local responses require local antigenic stimulation.[8] Local anamnestic responses contribute to protection if the horse is reexposed. Older horses with residual immunity have limited susceptibility to *S. equi* and often develop a mild form of strangles termed "catarrhal strangles."[24] Despite the lack of classic clinical signs of strangles, these horses will shed virulent *S. equi* in nasal secretions in sufficient numbers to be a serious threat of transmission of disease to younger, more susceptible horses.

Colostrum from mares that have recovered from strangles contains IgGb and IgA with specificities similar to those found in the nasopharyngeal mucus of convalescent horses.[26] These antibodies recirculate to the nasopharyngeal mucosa after a foal ingests colostrum and provide resistance to infection until approximately the time of weaning.

Although it is widely believed that the SeM protein is a major protective antigen, it is clear that other antigens are also important. An SeM-negative mutant of *S. equi* used as an intranasal vaccine protected horses against subsequent experimental challenge with virulent bacteria.[17]

Several aspects of *S. equi* pathogenesis are important to consider in the design and implementation of strangles control programs (Box 28-1).

Clinical Findings

Strangles is characterized by abrupt onset of fever followed by upper respiratory tract catarrh, as evidenced by mucopurulent nasal discharge (see Fig. 28-2) and acute swelling, with subsequent abscess formation in submandibular and retropharyngeal lymph nodes (Fig. 28-5). The term *strangles* was coined because affected horses sometimes were suffocated by enlarged lymph nodes that obstructed the airway. Severity of disease varies greatly depending on the immune status of the animal. Older horses often exhibit a milder form of the disease characterized by nasal discharge, small abscesses, and rapid resolution of disease, whereas younger horses are more likely to develop severe lymph node abscesses that subsequently open and drain (Fig. 28-6).

Fever is the first clinical sign and persists as lymphadenopathy develops and abscesses mature. Pharyngitis causes dysphagia, and affected animals may become anorexic or reluctant to eat and often stand with the neck extended. Attempts to swallow food and water may be followed by reflux of these substances from the nares. Depression and listlessness are common signs. Pharyngitis, laryngitis, and rhinitis may occur and contribute to bilateral nasal discharge, which is serous initially and rapidly becomes mucopurulent and then purulent, profuse, and tenacious. Accumulation of purulent exudates may cause a snuffling or rattling upper respiratory sound. Nasal and ocular mucosae may become hyperemic, and there may be purulent ocular discharge from which *S. equi* might be isolated.

Lymphadenopathy is a major clinical sign (see Figs. 28-5 and 28-6). The submandibular and retropharyngeal lymph nodes are involved with about equal frequency in *S. equi* infections and become swollen and painful about 1 week after infection. The first sign of lymphadenopathy is often hot, diffuse, painful edema. Serum may then ooze from the overlying skin for several days, as the lymph node abscesses mature before rupturing to drain tenacious creamy pus, which does not have a foul odor. Other lymph nodes of the rostral neck (parotid, cranial cervical, and retropharyngeal) are also frequently involved and may abscess. Retropharyngeal lymph nodes may drain into and cause empyema of the guttural pouch. Natural drainage of these deeper abscesses to the skin may take several days or weeks, and the swelling can exert pressure on the pharynx, larynx, trachea, and esophagus, causing severe dyspnea, stridor, and dysphagia. Retropharyngeal lymph node abscessation is not always associated with swelling that can be appreciated externally. Periorbital abscesses can cause marked swelling of the eyelids. Abscesses of the lymph nodes at the thoracic inlet can cause severe tracheal compression, asphyxia, and death. Coughing is not a significant feature in most cases, although some horses develop a soft, moist

Box • 28-1

Aspects of Pathogenesis Important in Control and Prevention of Strangles

- Shedding does not begin until 1 or 2 days after onset of pyrexia. New cases can therefore be isolated before they transmit infection.
- Nasal shedding persists for 2 to 3 weeks in most animals. Persistent guttural pouch infection may result in intermittent shedding for years.
- Field and experimental data support the conclusion that disease severity depends on challenge load and duration.

cough that becomes more productive and increasingly severe as the disease progresses. Squeezing the larynx will often cause marked pain, stridor, and gagging, followed by a retching cough and extended neck position when the neck is released. Expulsion of large quantities of pus from the nose or mouth with coughing usually indicates empyema of the guttural pouch.

Manifestations Associated with Severe Lymph Node Enlargement

Abscessation, particularly of the retropharyngeal lymph nodes, may result in obstruction of the upper respiratory tract. The enlarged lymph nodes may compress the pharynx, larynx, or trachea, necessitating a tracheostomy in severe cases (Fig. 28-7). Temporary laryngeal hemiplegia, resulting from damage to the recurrent laryngeal nerve from enlargement of either the retropharyngeal or the anterior cervical lymph nodes, may also contribute to dyspnea. Four of 15 horses with complicated strangles had upper respiratory tract obstruction requiring tracheostomy, and death was attributed to the obstruction in two of these horses.[27] Dysphagia may also occur as a result of lymph node enlargement or guttural pouch empyema.

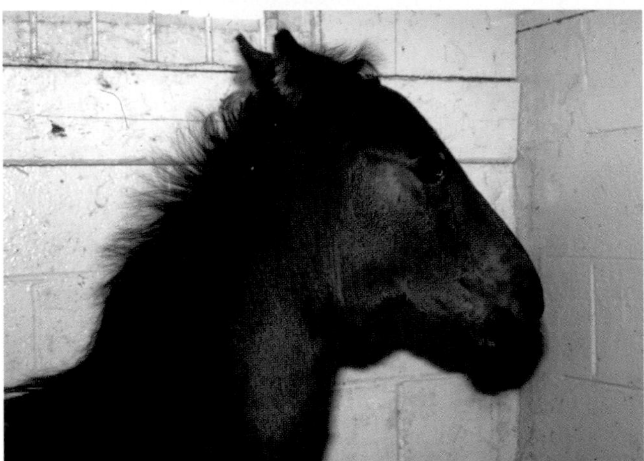

Fig. 28-5 Enlarged, abscessed submandibular lymph node in foal with strangles.

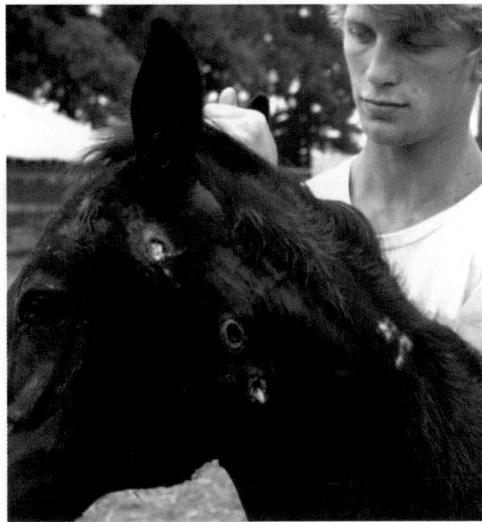

Fig. 28-6 Multiple rupture sites of abscessed retropharyngeal and submandibular lymph nodes in foal with strangles.

Complications Associated with Metastatic Spread of Infection

Internal Infection. Approximately 20% of horses with strangles experience some type of complication, and the presence of complications greatly increases the case-fatality rate.[27,28] Of 74 horses with strangles on a 235 horse farm, 15 (20.3%) had complications; case-fatality rate in horses with complications was 40% compared with an overall case-fatality rate of 8.1%.[27] Complications with strangles include spread of infection to parts of the body other than the head and neck, immune-mediated processes, and agalactia in mares.[24]

S. equi may potentially infect any anatomic site. The term *bastard strangles* is often used to describe metastatic abscessation. The organism may spread hematogenously, through lymphatic migration or close association with a septic focus, as when connecting structures (e.g., cranial nerves) allow transport of the organism or when there is direct aspiration of purulent material.

Common sites of infection include the lung, mesentery, liver, spleen, kidneys, and brain. Respiratory distress may be caused by tracheal compression resulting from enlargement of the cranial mediastinal lymph nodes. Suppurative bronchopneumonia is an important sequela of strangles. Of 15 horses with complications associated with strangles, five had pneumonia or pleuropneumonia, and three of five deaths were attributed to pneumonia, making this the most common complication resulting in death.[27,29] In a previous study, 22 of 35 animals with complications (62%) died of pneumonia secondary to strangles.[28]

Another important complication of strangles is extension of infection to the sinuses or guttural pouches.[27] In a general study of guttural pouch empyema, *S. equi* was isolated in

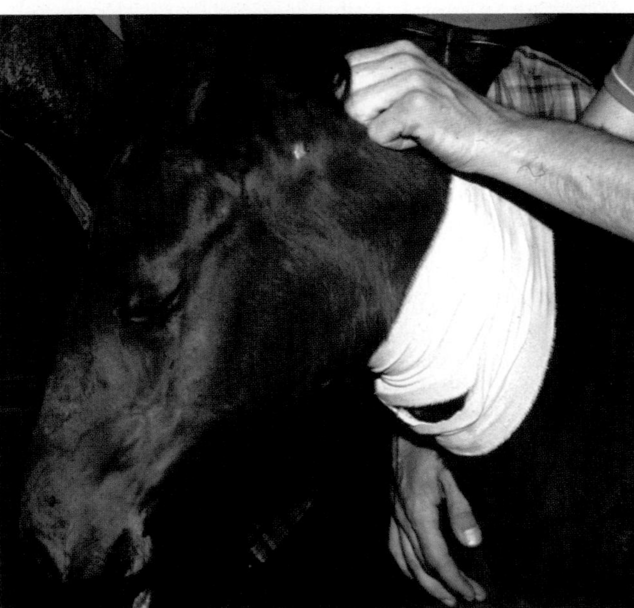

Fig. 28-7 Temporary tracheostomy in midcervical region of foal with strangles. The tracheostomy alleviated the severe dyspnea associated with strangles in this foal. The tracheostomy tube and the site of insertion must be cleaned twice daily to keep the airway free of purulent debris.

ichthammol or a hot pack may be applied to promote maturation of the lymph node abscess, although objective controlled data supporting the use of these techniques are lacking. Surgical drainage of lymphadenopathies is sometimes indicated if abscesses do not rupture spontaneously; however, it is critical to wait until the abscess has matured and thinned out ventrally. Earlier surgical intervention may only result in minimal exudate drainage and continued lymph node swelling, because the abscess has enough internal structure (honeycomb loculations) to block drainage through a single surgical incision. Daily flushing of the open abscess with a 3% to 5% povidone-iodine solution should be continued until the discharge ceases.

The use of NSAIDs such as phenylbutazone or flunixin meglumine may improve the horse's demeanor by reducing fever, pain, and inflammatory swelling at the site of the abscesses. This in turn may encourage eating and drinking. Consideration must be given to the complications seen after NSAID use in dehydrated and anorectic horses.

Even in the face of detectable lymphadenopathy, if the horse is febrile, depressed, anorexic, and especially, manifesting dyspnea as result of partial upper airway obstruction, antibiotic therapy is indicated to decrease abscess size and prevent complete airway obstruction. Rarely, affected horses may require intensive supportive therapy, including IV fluids, feeding by nasogastric tube, and tracheostomy (see Fig. 28-7). An animal requiring a tracheostomy should be given systemic antimicrobial drugs to prevent secondary bacterial infections of the lower respiratory tract.

Some clinicians believe that antibiotic therapy after abscesses have ruptured is indicated because it may hasten recovery, improve appetite, and reduce loss of body condition.

Horses with Complications

Horses that develop complications from strangles should receive appropriate symptomatic and supportive therapy, as previously discussed with the clinical findings associated with each type of complication.

Drugs of Choice for Therapy

Penicillin is generally considered the drug of choice for the treatment of nonpneumococcal streptococcal disease, with alternative drugs used depending on ease of administration or the site of infection. Other agents for therapy include cephalosporins and macrolides. Based on in vitro antimicrobial susceptibility testing, in which testing methods follow Clinical and Laboratory Standards Institute (CLSI) guidelines, the majority of *S. equi* isolates are susceptible to trimethoprim-sulfadiazine (TMS). However, this may or may not translate to in vivo efficacy. Many veterinarians have anecdotally indicated that horses with strangles have improved with TMS treatment. Although evidence suggests that TMS did not eliminate *S. equi* subsp. *zooepidemicus* infection in tissue chambers implanted subcutaneously in ponies, the study did not determine its effectiveness against *S. equi*.[42]

S. equi is consistently sensitive to penicillin, which is thus considered the antibiotic of choice. Laboratories handling hundreds of *S. equi* strains have noted no emerging antibiotic resistance to penicillin by *S. equi* or *S. equi* subsp. *zooepidemicus* (J.F. Timoney and J.R. Newton, personal communications). The incidence of resistance to most other drugs is low, with the exception of aminoglycoside resistance, including gentamicin, which is consistently observed.

Prevention

Vaccination

Most horses develop a solid immunity during recovery from strangles, which persists in more than 75% of animals for 5 years or longer.[43,44] This indicates that stimulation of a high level of immunity is biologically feasible given appropriate presentation of protective immunogen(s). The basis of acquired resistance to strangles is not completely understood but is believed to reside in part in antibodies to SeM and other immunogens unique to *S. equi*. There is evidence that immunity in horses resistant to reinfection is mediated at the mucosal level and functions to block entry of *S. equi*. However, systemic immunity after parenteral inoculation of avirulent, live *S. equi* is also protective. Together, these findings indicate that optimum immunity may require both systemic and mucosal responses.

Earlier bacterin-type vaccines have been superseded (North America and Australia) by adjuvant extracts of *S. equi* prepared by hot acid or by mutanolysin plus detergent extraction. Hot acid cleaves and removes acid-resistant proteins, and carbohydrate mutanolysin (muramidase) hydrolyzes the bacterial cell wall, releasing intact surface proteins in the presence of detergent. Both types of vaccine are potent and contain the immunogenic SeM. However, the efficacy of extract vaccines has been disappointing, with little published data to support significant protection. One study suggested a reduction in the clinical attack rate of 50% in vaccinates a few weeks after the final booster.[45] Adverse reactions include soreness or abscesses at injection sites and occasional cases of purpura hemorrhagica.

An attenuated, nonencapsulated strain of *S. equi* with defects in carbohydrate utilization and designed to mimic the immunity provided through natural infection stimulated a high level of immunity against experimental challenge.[38] Safety issues include residual virulence with formation of slowly developing mandibular abscesses in a small percentage of vaccinates, nasal discharge, and occasional cases of immune-mediated vasculitis (purpura). Because the vaccine contains live *S. equi*, accidental contamination of remote injection sites will result in abscess formation at these locations. Therefore, ideally, no other vaccinations are given concurrently or given before administration of the intranasal vaccine.

Extract vaccines are administered intramuscularly or subcutaneously and elicit serum antibody responses 7 to 10 days later. Naive horses and foals require a schedule of two or three doses at an interval of 2 weeks. Booster doses are given once annually. Pregnant mares may receive a booster a month before the expected date of foaling. Horses known to have had strangles in the previous year should not be vaccinated. Horses with signs of strangles also should not be vaccinated. During an outbreak, only horses that have no known direct contact with strangles cases or the exudates from these cases should be promptly vaccinated. No published data show that vaccination with the avirulent, nonencapsulated strain Pinnacle I.N. (Fort Dodge Animal Health, Fort Dodge, Iowa) in the presence of exposure is detrimental. However, development of immunity after vaccination takes approximately 2 weeks. Additionally, there is a real risk of transmitting the virulent, wild *S. equi* to other horses as they are vaccinated.

Live vaccine should be administered only to healthy, nonfebrile animals free of nasal discharge. Vaccine is given in a schedule of two doses at 2- to 3-week intervals. Annual booster doses are recommended. Live vaccine should not be used during an outbreak except in horses that have no known contact with infected or exposed animals.

Transfer of passive immunity to the foal mainly involves antibodies of the IgGb isotype, which are distributed to the serum and nasal secretions. Prepartum vaccination of the mare significantly increases colostral levels of these antibodies. Foals from vaccinated mares have significantly higher titers of SeM-specific IgGb, but not IgA, in mucosal washes during the first 2 months of life, although colostral levels of SeM-specific

IgA are significantly increased by vaccination. Resistance of the foal to strangles during the first months of life appears to be mediated by IgGb in mucosal secretions and milk, and not by IgA. No data are available about colostral antibody levels after administration of the intranasal vaccine administered to broodmares.

Quarantine and Bacteriologic Screening

Prevention of strangles through quarantining and screening is difficult to achieve, especially without specific measures to reduce the risk of inadvertent introduction of *S. equi* infection through subclinical carriers. The owner, farm manager, or trainer should always be questioned as to the possible exposure of the animal to strangles.

Prevention through quarantining and screening is particularly difficult where frequent moving and mixing of horses occur during the breeding season and at racetracks, and where strangles outbreaks have not been appropriately investigated and controlled.

Wherever possible, animals being introduced to a new population of horses should be isolated for 3 weeks and screened for *S. equi* by repeated nasopharyngeal swabs or lavages. This should be done in accordance with the protocol outlined for controlling outbreaks (i.e., three samples taken at weekly intervals), with samples tested for *S. equi* by culture and PCR and animals testing positive kept in isolation for further investigation and treatment.

High standards of hygiene should also always be maintained to avoid indirect transmission between quarantined and resident horses.

Control of Outbreaks

Outbreak Investigations. Investigation of strangles outbreaks should begin with an interview of horse owners to obtain a detailed history and to evaluate the potential extent of the disease problem. The review should identify affected groups of horses and allow the geography of the premises and the management practices to be assessed for further risks and future opportunities for disease control.

A practical disease control strategy should then be agreed on and implemented (Table 28-2). This strategy may need to be adapted to the individual circumstances of specific premises and outbreaks and can be summarized as follows:

- All movements of horses on and off the affected premises should be stopped and segregation and hygiene measures implemented immediately.
- Cases of strangles and their contacts should be maintained in well-demarcated "dirty" (i.e., *S. equi*–positive) quarantine areas.
- Rectal temperatures should be taken at least once daily during an outbreak to detect, promptly segregate, and possibly treat new cases.
- The aim of the control strategy, after bacteriologic screening, is to move horses from the "dirty" to "clean" areas where nonaffected and noninfectious horses are kept.
- Every precaution should be taken to ensure high hygiene standards throughout the premises for the duration of the outbreak.
- Screening of all convalescing cases after clinical recovery and their healthy contacts should be conducted using swab or lavage of the nasopharynx, with special care taken to maintain good hygiene and avoid inadvertent transmission between horses during sampling.
- Swabs or lavage fluid should be collected at weekly intervals after recovery over several weeks and tested for *S. equi* by conventional culture and PCR.
- Because PCR can detect dead as well as living bacteria, positive PCR results are regarded as provisional, subject to further investigation.
- Because the vast majority of cases of subclinical long-term carriage of *S. equi* appear to occur in the guttural pouches of recovered horses, endoscopy of the upper respiratory tract and guttural pouches should be performed in all outwardly healthy horses in which *S. equi* is detected, either by culture or PCR.
- Lavage samples from guttural pouches should then be tested for *S. equi* by culture and PCR.
- Sites such as the cranial nasal sinuses or tonsils should be considered in horses that continue to harbor *S. equi* in the absence of pathology or *S. equi* infection of the guttural pouches.

Carriers with *S. equi* Infection of Guttural Pouches

Detection. Diagnosis of *S. equi* infection associated with guttural pouch empyema with or without chondroids following strangles is best achieved by direct visual assessment of both pouches using endoscopy. Cytologic assessment and culture and PCR for detection of *S. equi* in lavage samples collected by a sterile disposable catheter passed through the biopsy channel of the endoscope are recommended to accompany visual examination, because infection and inflammation may be present in the absence of obvious and visible pathology. Diagnosis of guttural pouch empyema with or without chondroids may also be made by radiography of the guttural pouch area, although changes may not be visible in all cases.

S. equi may be cultured from lavages collected by direct percutaneous sampling of the pouch, although this is not recommended because of the high risk of injury to important anatomic structures in the region.

Treatment. Appropriate methods of treatment of guttural pouch empyema in individual horses depend on the consistency and volume of the material within the pouches. Repeated lavages of pus-filled pouches by rigid or indwelling catheters using isotonic saline or polyionic fluid, with subsequent lowering of the head to allow drainage or use of a suction pump attached to the endoscope, assist in the elimination of empyema. Sedation aids in implementation of the endoscopy and facilitates drainage of flush material from the guttural pouches by lowering the horse's head.

Administration of both topical and systemic benzylpenicillin appears to improve treatment success rate. Verheyen et al.[30] have reported on the method of delivering a gelatin-penicillin mix (Box 28-3). The gelatin-penicillin mix is more effective at remaining in the pouches than a straight aqueous solution and is a useful way of delivering a large dose of penicillin where it is needed. Instillation is easiest through a catheter inserted up the nose and endoscopically guided into the pouch opening. The catheter works best with the last 1 inch bent at an angle to aid entry under the pouch flap. Recommendations include elevating the horse's head after infusion.

Topical instillation of 20% (w/v) acetylcysteine solution has also been used to aid the treatment of empyema. Acetylcysteine has a denaturing and solubilizing activity by disrupting disulfide bonds in mucoprotein molecules, thus reducing mucus viscosity and theoretically facilitating natural drainage. Erythema of the mucus membranes lining the guttural pouch has been observed after instillation of 20% (w/v) acetylcysteine solution. More long-standing cases, in which there is inspissation of the purulent material that does not readily drain into the pharynx, are more difficult to treat topically because they can be refractory to large-volume irrigation. Use of a memory-helical polyp retrieval basket

Table • **28-2**

Goals and Associated Measures Used to Control Transmission of S. equi *on Affected Premises*

GOAL	MEASURES
1. To prevent the spread of *S. equi* infection to horses on other premises and to new arrivals on the affected premises.	Stop all movement of horses on and off the affected premises immediately and until further notice. Horses with strangles and their contacts should be maintained in well-demarcated "dirty" (i.e. *S. equi*– positive) quarantine areas. Clustering of cases in groups should allow parts of the premises to be easily allocated as "dirty" and "clean" areas.
2. To establish whether convalescing horses are infectious *after* clinical recovery.	At least three nasopharyngeal swabs or lavages are taken at approximately weekly intervals from all recovered cases and their contacts and tested for *S. equi* by culture and polymerase chain reaction (PCR). Horses that are consistently negative are returned to the "clean" area.
3. Investigate all outwardly healthy horses in which *S. equi* is detected either by culture or PCR.	Endoscopy of the upper respiratory tract and guttural pouches.
4. To eliminate *S. equi* infection from the guttural pouches.	Healing of lesions through a combination of flushing and aspiration with saline and removal of chondroids using endoscopically guided instruments. Topical and systemic administration of antimicrobials to eliminate *S. equi* infection.
5. To prevent indirect cross-infection by *S. equi* from horses in the "dirty" area to those in the "clean" area of the premises.	Personnel should use dedicated protective clothing when dealing with infectious animals and should not deal simultaneously with susceptible animals. If this is unavoidable, infectious horses should be dealt with *after* susceptible animals. Strict hygiene measures are introduced, including provision of dedicated clothing and equipment for each area, disinfection facilities for personnel, and thorough stable cleaning and disinfection methods. When cost is not a factor, consideration should be given to destruction of this equipment after eradication of the infection. After removal of organic material from stables, all surfaces should be thoroughly soaked in an appropriate liquid disinfectant or steam-treated and allowed to dry. This should be repeated if possible. Manure and waste feed from infectious animals should be composted (inactivation of bacteria by heat) in an isolated location. Pastures used to hold infectious animals should be rested for 4 weeks. Care should be taken to disinfect water troughs at least once daily during an outbreak. Horse vans should be hosed clean and disinfected after each use.

Box • **28-3**

Gelatin-Penicillin to Treat S. equi *Infection of Guttural Pouches*

To make 50 mL of gelatin-penicillin solution:

1. Weigh out 2 g of gelatin (Sigma G-6650 or household grade), and add 40 mL of sterile water.
2. Heat or microwave to dissolve the gelatin.
3. Cool gelatin to 45° to 50° C.
4. Add 10 mL of sterile water to 10 million units (10 megaunits) of sodium benzylpenicillin G.
5. Mix penicillin solution with the cooled gelatin to make a total volume of 50 mL.
6. Dispense into syringes, and leave overnight at 4° C to set.

through the biopsy channel of the endoscope allows nonsurgical removal of chondroids, even when present in large numbers and in conjunction with empyema (J.R. Newton, unpublished data). When combined with topical and systemic antimicrobial treatment, this is usually sufficient to cure severe guttural pouch lesions. Surgical hyovertebrotomy and ventral drainage through Viborg's triangle carry inherent risks of general anesthesia and surgical dissection around major blood vessels and nerves, as well as *S. equi* contamination of the hospital environment (see Chapter 1). Scarring of the pharyngeal openings of the guttural pouch may preclude both natural drainage of purulent material and endoscopic access to the guttural pouches. Such animals may require conventional surgical or endoscopically guided laser treatments to break down scar tissue and allow access to the pouches.

Hygiene Measures. Particular care should be taken with hygiene measures during strangles outbreaks to prevent indirect transfer of *S. equi* from infectious horses (including potential subclinical carriers) to susceptible animals (see Chapter 66 and 67). Personnel should use dedicated protective clothing when dealing with infectious animals and should not deal simultaneously with susceptible animals. If this is unavoidable, infectious horses should be dealt with after susceptible animals. Only dedicated equipment should be used for infectious horses and thoroughly disinfected between animals. When cost is not a factor, destruction of equipment should be considered after eradication of the infection. In disinfecting stables used by infectious horses, care should be taken to ensure thorough cleaning to remove all organic material. Particular care must be taken with feed and water troughs, as well as wooden fencing or other wooden surfaces. Manure and waste feed from infectious animals should be composted in an isolated location. Personnel dealing with susceptible animals should avoid contact with waste from infectious horses.

After removal of organic material from stables, all surfaces should be thoroughly soaked in an appropriate liquid disinfectant or steam-treated and allowed to dry; this should be repeated if possible. After thorough cleaning and soaking in liquid disinfectant, wooden surfaces should be treated with a suitable preservative or sealed with epoxy paint. Pastures used to hold infectious animals should be rested for 4 weeks; no evidence exists for prolonged survival of *S. equi* on pastures. Care should be taken to disinfect water troughs at least once daily during an outbreak. Horse vans should be hosed clean and disinfected after each use.

S. equi does not present any additional problems with disinfection of equipment than do any other bacterial species. Normal commonsense approaches should be adopted at all times, such as ensuring physical removal of visible organic material and using an appropriate disinfectant with proven action against *S. equi* and following the manufacturer's guidelines on dilution.

The Horserace Betting Levy Board in the United Kingdom has established guidelines on strangles in its Codes of Practice, which can be viewed at the following Web address:

http://www.hblb.org.uk/hblbweb.nsf/Codes%20of%20Practice%202004.pdf

Public Health Considerations

Cases of *S. equi* infection in debilitated humans have been reported.[46-49] Animal handlers, caretakers, veterinary practitioners, pathologists, and equine postmortem attendants should take particular care to avoid unnecessary contamination from infectious horses, especially avoiding respiratory and oral contamination by purulent material. *S. equi* is highly host adapted, however, and infections of humans have rarely been confirmed.

STREPTOCOCCUS EQUI SUBSP. *ZOOEPIDEMICUS*

Debra C. Sellon

Etiology, Epidemiology, and Pathogenesis

Streptococcus equi subsp. *zooepidemicus* is a Lancefield group C β-hemolytic streptococcus that is considered a part-mucosal commensal of the oral cavity, pharynx, and respiratory tract of horses. It causes disease as an opportunistic pathogen of the respiratory tract (rhinitis, bronchitis, pneumonia) and reproductive tract (endometritis) of horses after virus infection, heat stress, or tissue injury.[5,6,50-55] This organism is the most frequently isolated pathogen from equine joints, lymph nodes, nasal cavities, and lungs.[5]

S. equi subsp. *zooepidemicus* shares 98% DNA homology with *S. equi* subsp. *equi* but can be differentiated microbiologically by its ability to ferment lactose and sorbitol, but not trehalose. *S. equi* subsp. *zooepidemicus* lacks an antiphagocytic M protein (SeM) and the pyrogenic exotoxins SePE-I and SePE-H as well as homologs of a small number of other surface exposed or secreted proteins.[5] Isolates from the tonsils and pharynx of horses are almost always nonencapsulated. Although hyaluronidase is produced by some strains, it is not generally regarded as a virulence factor.[5] *S. equi* subsp. *zooepidemicus* possesses an M-like surface protein (SzP) that is the basis for strain typing and varies at the N-terminal and central regions.[56] Most horses harbor many antigenic types of *S. equi* subsp. *zooepidemicus* in their tonsils, a possible source of opportunistic infection of the respiratory tract.[55,57] Serotype and type of SzP appear to be unrelated to clinical source of isolates from the lungs, joints, uterus, fetus, or other sites in the horse.[58] However, isolates from the lungs of horses with streptococcal pneumonia are clonal, indicating infection with a single antigenic strain of the bacteria.[55]

Serum antibodies to the SzP proteins of *S. equi* subsp. *zooepidemicus* are opsonic and protective in mice and may contribute to protection in horses.[59] Specific IgA and IgG antibodies in nasopharyngeal secretions may play a role in protection.[5] However, the prolonged and frequent upper airway infections of young foals suggest that effective immunity is not acquired until later in life.[19,60]

Clinical Findings

S. equi subsp. *zooepidemicus* is associated with several clinical syndromes in horses. It causes endometritis in "susceptible mares" (see Chapter 8) and is one of the most frequent causes of infectious abortion and placentitis,[61,62] resulting in significant annual losses to the industry. *S. equi* subsp. *zooepidemicus* is the most common bacterial isolate from horses with pneumonia[63,64] and shipping fever (see Chapter 1).[6] There is growing evidence of close involvement with repeated respiratory tract infections in young animals up to 3 or 4 years old.[19,60,65,66] It has also been associated with lower airway inflammation in foals and Thoroughbred horses in training.[50,65,67-69] A longitudinal study of the microorganisms associated with lower airway disease in training Thoroughbreds revealed that most horses experienced at least one episode of disease annually (mean duration, 9.4 weeks). Seroconversion to known respiratory viruses occurred in only 7.5% of cases.[60]

Therapy

Most β-hemolytic streptococci from horses are susceptible to β-lactam antibiotics, including penicillin, ampicillin, and ceftiofur. Many isolates are also susceptible to trimethoprim-sulfonamide combinations and oxytetracycline. Specific therapy will depend on the site and severity of disease. (See Chapters 1 and 8 for treatment of respiratory tract and reproductive tract infections, respectively.)

Prevention

Prevention of equine disease caused by *S. equi* subsp. *zooepidemicus* is difficult because of the opportunistic nature of the infection. Control is best achieved by decreasing stress and treating predisposing medical conditions or stressors (e.g., viral infection, transport, uterine fluid accumulation) appropriately and promptly. Immunization of mares with bacterial extracts provides some resistance to endometritis caused by this organism.[70] However, development of vaccines for prevention of infection is unlikely to be practical because of the widespread strain variations, opportunistic nature of infection, and the concern of glomerulonephritis associated with immune complex formation.[36,71,72]

Public Health Considerations

There are numerous reports of *S. equi* subsp. *zooepidemicus* infection of people.[73-76] Outbreaks of glomerulonephritis have been linked to consumption of unpasteurized milk and cheese products contaminated with *S. equi* subsp. *zooepidemicus*.[71,72,77-80] Also, the many reports of *S. equi* subsp. *zooepidemicus* bacteremia,[81-89] meningitis,[74,81,82,90,91] and arthritis[92,93] in people have frequently been traced to animal contact.[74,86,94,95] A fatal case of toxic shock–like syndrome, with evidence of superantigen production, was attributed to infection with this streptococcal organism.[96]

Despite these reports of human disease caused by *S. equi* subsp. *zooepidemicus* infection, this is considered a rare zoonosis, especially when the frequency of human exposure to the organism is considered.

STREPTOCOCCUS PNEUMONIAE

Debra C. Sellon

Etiology

Streptococcus pneumoniae is a non–β-hemolytic streptococcus occasionally isolated from healthy horses and those with respiratory tract disease.[60,97-101] It is a facultative anaerobe, and its growth in culture can be enhanced by a carbon dioxide–enriched environment.[97] *S. pneumoniae* is an important cause of community-acquired pneumonia (pneumococcal pneumonia), meningitis, and septicemia in people, although oropharyngeal carriage in healthy people is common.[1] This organism may also cause pneumonia in calves,[102,103] goats,[104] and guinea pigs.[105] It has caused pneumonia experimentally in dogs[106] and rabbits.[107]

Pathogenesis

Only *S. pneumoniae* capsule type 3 has been isolated from horses.[19,97,101] Although more than 80 different capsule types have been isolated from people, capsule type 3 is recognized as a particularly pathogenic strain and is associated with a higher mortality than other types of pneumococci.[108] The capsule of *S. pneumoniae* is a T-cell–independent immunogen that is protective in human adults but not immunogenic in young children.[19] The purified type 3 capsule is immunogenic in ponies less than 9 months of age,[19] consistent with the theory that the immune system of the neonatal foal is more mature than that of the human infant.[109]

Clinical Findings and Therapy

S. pneumoniae has been isolated from the respiratory tract of healthy horses and on several occasions from the lungs of pneumonic foals.[97,98] As in people, the incidence of inapparent carrier status seems to be higher in young horses.[97] *S. pneumoniae* is associated with lower airway disease in training Thoroughbreds, although with a lower prevalence than *S. equi* subsp. *zooepidemicus*.[99,110] Experimental infection of ponies produced lobar pneumonia, with inflammation in the trachea typical of the disease seen in training horses.[100]

Horses with *S. pneumoniae* respiratory tract disease should be treated with appropriate antimicrobial therapy based on antimicrobial sensitivity testing. Most isolates are expected to be susceptible to β-lactam antibiotics. Additional symptomatic and supportive care should be provided if indicated.

Public Health Considerations

The isolation of *S. pneumoniae* from the respiratory tract of horses suggests the possibility of zoonotic infection; however, this has not been demonstrated to date. Transmission of *S. pneumoniae* between calves and their handlers was described by Romer,[103] who suggested that infection was transmitted from handlers to animals.

REFERENCES

See the CD-ROM for a list of references linked to the abstract in PubMed.

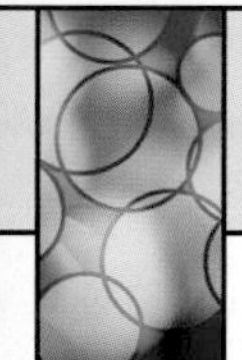

CHAPTER • 29

Staphylococcal Infections

J. Scott Weese

ETIOLOGY

The genus *Staphylococcus* consists of a group of approximately 50 different species and subspecies of gram-positive cocci, many of which are opportunistic pathogens in horses. Staphylococcal species are typically divided based on the ability to produce coagulase (Box 29-1). They are also often divided into major and minor pathogenic species based on the incidence and nature of disease. Most major pathogenic species are coagulase positive, and the two most important staphylococci in equine medicine are the coagulase-positive species *Staphylococcus aureus* and *S. intermedius*.[1] Coagulase-negative staphylococci (CoNS) can be pathogenic, but infection with these species is most common in hospitalized or otherwise compromised hosts.

Many species are part of the normal microflora, particularly of the nasal passages and skin. In humans, *S. aureus* is most often found in the anterior nares, and studies have reported colonization rates of 29% to 38% in healthy individuals.[2,3] The majority of people intermittently carry *S. aureus* in their nasal passages, whereas some may never be colonized and others are persistently colonized. *Staphylococcus epidermidis* is the predominant staphylococcal species on skin surfaces, and other CoNS can be found on a variety of body surfaces. *Staphylococcus intermedius* is uncommon in humans.

Box • 29-1

Examples of* Staphylococcus *Species Based on Coagulase Production

Coagulase positive	*Coagulase negative*
S. aureus	*S. epidermidis*
S. intermedius	*S. xylosus*
S. delphini	*S. equorum*
S. schleiferi subsp. *coagulans*	*S. schleiferi* subsp. *schleiferi*
*S. hyicus**	*S. lentus*
	S. sciuri
	S. capitis
	S. haemolyticus

*Variable coagulase reaction.

Fig. 29-1 Pulsed-field gel electrophoresis (PFGE) of methicillin-resistant *S. aureus* (MRSA) isolates obtained from horses during an outbreak. All isolates are indistinguishable and are consistent with CMRSA-5 (USA500), the clone that accounts for the vast majority of MRSA infections in horses in North America.

Body site colonization has not been evaluated as extensively in horses. Nagase et al.[4] reported isolation of staphylococci from the skin of 89.5% of horses. *Staphylococcus sciuri* was the predominant species, with lesser numbers of *S. xylosus, S. saprophyticus, S. hominis, S. epidermidis*, and *S. capitis*. *Staphylococcus sciuri* and *S. xylosus* predominated in another study of normal skin.[1] Other studies have reported the predominance of CoNS or nonhemolytic staphylococci on the skin over joints.[5,6] Fewer studies have evaluated staphylococcal colonization of other body sites. Yasuda et al.[7] reported isolation of *S. sciuri* or *S. lentus* from the nares and pasterns of 13 of 100 mares in Japan. Staphylococci, predominantly *S. aureus* and CoNS, may be found as part of the conjunctival microflora of normal horses.[8,9]

The emergence and dissemination of antimicrobial resistance in pathogenic staphylococci are of tremendous concern in human medicine and an increasing problem in equine medicine. Certain patterns of antimicrobial resistance among staphylococci have been recognized for years and are not unexpected. In particular, resistance to penicillin is widespread. Other patterns of resistance are more recent and continue to evolve.

The most significant multidrug-resistant *Staphylococcus* species in human medicine is methicillin-resistant *S. aureus* (MRSA). MRSA is one of the most important nosocomial pathogens and is associated with increased morbidity, mortality, duration of hospitalization, and treatment costs.[10,11] Mortality rates of 50% for bloodstream infections and 33% for MRSA pneumonia have been reported, and outbreaks in medical facilities are a concern.[12] Methicillin resistance in MRSA is mediated by production of an altered penicillin-binding protein (PBP) that possesses low affinity for beta (β)-lactam antimicrobials. Clinically, MRSA isolates are resistant to all β-lactam antimicrobials and are frequently resistant to a variety of other antimicrobial classes, and few treatment options may be available.

Recently, it has become evident that MRSA is an emerging pathogen in horses (Fig. 29-1). Hartmann et al.[13] reported postoperative MRSA infection in a horse, and Seguin et al.[14] reported nosocomial MRSA wound infections in 11 horses over a 13-month period at a teaching hospital. Indistinguishable MRSA isolates were also taken from three hospital personnel in the latter study, and it was speculated that hospital personnel were the source of equine infection. Weese et al.[15] reported MRSA colonization or infection in 79 horses in a teaching hospital and on horse farms. A later study identified MRSA colonization in 46 of 972 (4.7%) horses on farms in Ontario and New York.[16] As part of an equine MRSA screening program, community-associated MRSA colonization was identified in approximately 2.5% of horses admitted to a teaching hospital, and colonization at the time of admission was a risk factor for development of MRSA infection during hospitalization.[17]

Methicillin resistance is common among coagulase-negative *Staphylococcus* spp., including commensal species, although methicillin-resistant CoNS are not considered to be as important clinically as methicillin-resistant coagulase-positive staphylococci. Methicillin-resistant CoNS were isolated from the nares or skin of 29.5% of healthy horses in one study, with *S. epidermidis* being the most common species.[18]

PATHOGENESIS

Staphylococci can possess an impressive array of virulence factors that enable them to colonize and cause disease. Most virulence factors have been identified in *S. aureus*, but some may also be found in other staphylococci. Exozymes, including coagulase, protease, hemolysins, hyaluronidase, collagenase, lipase, and nuclease, facilitate colonization and growth in vivo and are possessed by virtually all *S. aureus* isolates and variably by other species.[19] Additional virulence factors may be possessed, particularly by *S. aureus*. Staphylococcal enterotoxins (SEs), also classified as "pyrogenic staphylococcal superantigens," are produced by various coagulase-positive staphylococci and are primarily associated with food poisoning in humans.[19,20] These toxins are typically associated with *S. aureus;* however, SE genes have also been found in *S. intermedius*. SEs have been identified in *S. aureus* and *S. intermedius* of equine origin,[21-23] but the role of SE in equine disease is unclear.

Toxic shock syndrome toxin (TSST-1) is another pyrogenic staphylococcal superantigen and is associated with staphylococcal toxic shock syndrome in humans.[19] TSST-1 is unique in its ability to cross intact mucosal surfaces, and systemic disease can result from localized infections. Toxic shock syndrome associated with TSST-1 has been reported in a horse.[24] Exfoliative toxin (sET) is responsible for skin exfoliation in staphylococcal scalded-skin syndrome in humans[25] and has been associated with skin infection in a horse.[26] The *Panton-Valentine leukocidin* (PVL) is associated with tissue necrosis and is emerging as an important virulence factor, particularly in community-associated MRSA infection.[27-29] This toxin has not yet been identified in any tested equine isolates.[15]

The mere presence of staphylococci in or on a host does not mean that disease is occurring or will occur. Staphylococci are opportunists, and one or more risk factors typically must be present before disease can occur. Risk factors for development of clinical infection in humans include surgery, trauma, concurrent infection, skin lesions, and immunocompromise.[27,30,31] Other risk factors presumably exist and may not be obvious. This is highlighted by the increasing incidence of community-associated MRSA infection in people without traditionally accepted risk factors.[32-34] Risk factors for development of staphylococcal disease in horses have not been adequately evaluated but are likely similar to those reported in humans.

The source of staphylococci in equine infection is often not identified. Potentially pathogenic staphylococci may originate from the endogenous microflora of the infected horse, in-contact horses, or in-contact humans. The relative importance of these potential sources is unclear. Endogenous MRSA is a source of infection in some horses,[17] but whether this is true for other staphylococci is unclear. Transmission of staphylococci between horses is probably common based on the behavior of the species, which involves frequent contact with the nares of other horses and exploratory behavior that results in contact with feces or items (e.g., buckets) that have been in recent contact with other horses. The clinical significance of this is unclear, although transmission of MRSA between horses with subsequent development of disease has been identified.[15]

Human handlers and veterinary personnel could be a source of equine infection or colonization because of the prevalence of staphylococcal colonization on human skin and the frequency of contamination of hands from contact with the nares. Normal human-horse interaction involves frequent human hand–to–horse nose contact, creating an opportunity for transmission of staphylococci in either direction. Humans are also directly involved in procedures that compromise the body's protective mechanisms, such as surgery, intraarticular injection, and intravenous (IV) catheter placement, and in the care of wounds and other compromised sites. Handling of neonatal foals, particularly contact with the umbilicus, is also an opportunity for staphylococcal transfer.

CLINICAL FINDINGS

The clinical presentation of staphylococcal infection can be quite variable and depends on the location of infection, virulence of the involved strain, and host factors. Severity of disease can range from mild local infection to septicemia and toxemia. Many studies have reported only a general classification of "staphylococci," hampering the ability to identify the relative importance of varying species. In general, most staphylococcal infections are characteristic opportunistic infections, particularly involving wounds and surgical sites, although primary infections of a variety of body sites have been reported. Staphylococci are important causes of septic arthritis after intraarticular injection, with one study isolating staphylococci from 86% of cases.[35] It is unclear whether origin of these infections is inadequately prepared skin or the hands of veterinary personnel.

Coagulase-Positive Staphylococci

Staphylococcus aureus is believed to be the most important *Staphylococcus* species in equine medicine, and most information regarding equine staphylococcal infections involves this organism. Infections of wounds and incisions, subcutaneous tissues (cellulitis), bones and joints, and skin are most frequently reported.[1,36,37] There are also numerous reports of *S. aureus* septic arthritis and tenosynovitis,[38,39] and *S. aureus* is the most common cause of postarticular injection septic arthritis.[35] A variety of other infections have been reported, including pyelonephritis, tracheitis, metritis, lymphangitis, fistulous withers, pleuritis, meningitis, and sinusitis.[1,15,40]

Infections by *Staphylococcus intermedius* are less common but tend to be similar to those caused by *S. aureus*.[1] In a study by Biberstein et al.,[36] skin infections accounted for the majority of *S. intermedius* infections, although the sample size was only nine cases. *S. intermedius* arthritis, tenosynovitis, and osteomyelitis have been identified[41] (J.S. Weese, unpublished data), as have lymphangitis and sinusitis.[1,40]

Staphylococcus hyicus has also been implicated as a cause of pastern dermatitis ("greasy heel"), postarticular injection septic arthritis, and fistulous withers.[1,35,42]

Coagulase-Negative Staphylococci

Coagulase-negative staphylococci, particularly *Staphylococcus epidermidis*, have also been identified in septic arthritis, tenosynovitis, osteomyelitis, and other musculoskeletal infections.[35,38,43-45] More often, CoNS are associated with nosocomial infections. IV catheters are particularly prone to development of complications in hospitalized horses, and CoNS are the main bacteria isolated from catheters at the time of removal.[46] Bacteremia, septic arthritis, and wound or incision infections may also occur, particularly in neonates (J.S. Weese, unpublished data). Postoperative methicillin-resistant *S. epidermidis* infection has been reported.[47] There is a report of isolation of *S. epidermidis* from cerebrospinal fluid (CSF), although the clinical significance was not clear.[48] Metritis *(S. xylosus)* and otitis *(S. warneri)* have been reported.[1,40]

Multidrug-Resistant Staphylococci

Multidrug-resistant staphylococci do not tend to cause different types of infections compared with susceptible species, but the outcome may be worse. Wounds and postoperative infections predominate in reports of MRSA infections,[13,14] although catheter site infections, pneumonia, osteomyelitis, septic arthritis, and bacteremia have also been identified.[15]

DIAGNOSIS

Most staphylococci, particularly the clinically relevant species, are easy to isolate using standard culture methods (Fig. 29-2). Therefore, diagnosis can be achieved in most cases through submission of an appropriately collected sample for bacterial culture. Joints are an exception; it is often difficult to isolate infectious agents from septic joints.[39]

Typically, laboratories will report coagulase-positive staphylococci to the species level, but occasionally they report isolates as only coagulase-positive or coagulase-negative staphylococci. This may not be adequate, particularly in terms of multidrug-resistant coagulase-positive staphylococci, which could be MRSA and for which additional infection control measures may be indicated. Identification of coagulase-positive isolates to the species level should be requested (Fig. 29-3). Speciation of CoNS is less important.

All *S. aureus* isolates should be tested for methicillin resistance, which may not be performed by all diagnostic laboratories

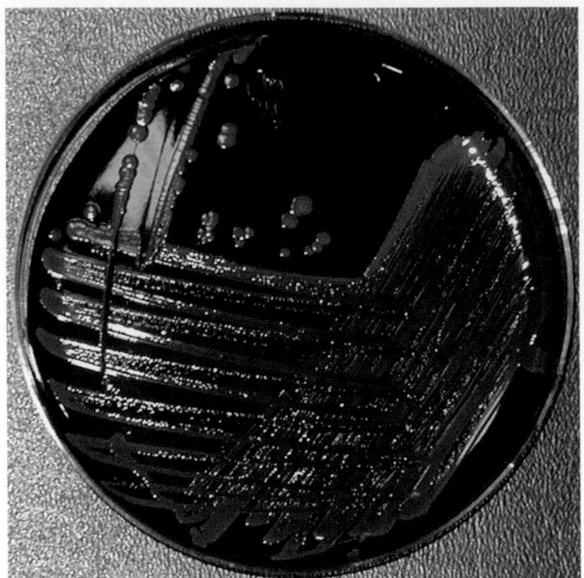

Fig. 29-2 Colony morphology of *Staphylococcus aureus*. Note the large, robust colonies and beta hemolysis that is characteristic of *S. aureus*.

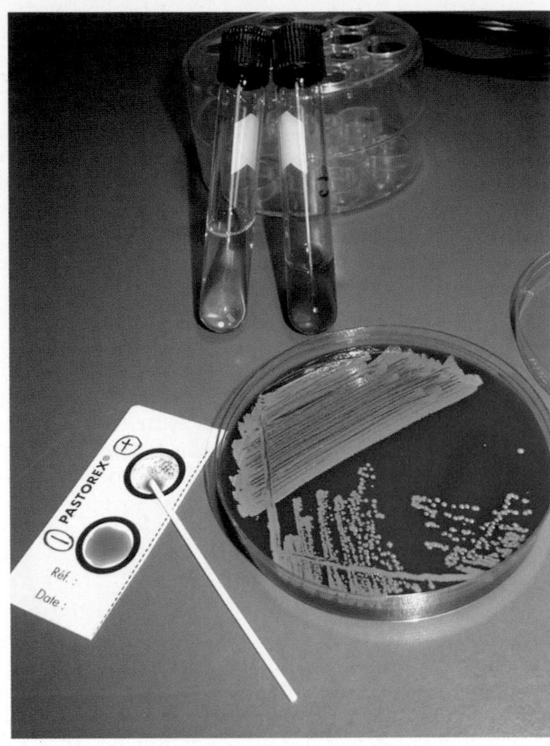

Fig. 29-3 It is important that staphylococci are identified to the species level. Some of the tests used for this purpose are depicted here: *clockwise from top*, carbohydrate fermentation, colony morphology, and *S. aureus* latex agglutination test.

at this time. Even though methicillin is not used clinically, it is important to know whether an *S. aureus* is an MRSA because of the inherent resistance to all β-lactam antimicrobials and the potential for transmission to other horses and people. Methicillin resistance is evaluated using oxacillin because it is more stable than methicillin in vitro; oxacillin-resistant staphylococci are methicillin resistant.

Although identification of *S. aureus* is usually straightforward, problems have recently been reported with the predominant MRSA clone in horses.[15] This clone can be very weakly coagulase positive or can appear coagulase negative, which may result in misclassification as "coagulase negative *Staphylococcus*." An *S. aureus* latex agglutination test should be performed on all equine staphylococcal isolates to ensure that clinically relevant *S. aureus* organisms are identified. Further, delayed oxacillin resistance may be encountered in vitro. Testing methodologies that use short incubation times (i.e., 18 hours) may not detect methicillin resistance. Confirmation of methicillin resistance can be performed with PBP2a latex agglutination test or PCR for detection of the *mecA* gene.[49]

It is important to consider the ecology of *Staphylococcus* spp. when interpreting culture results. Because staphylococci may be found on many body sites in normal animals, isolation does not necessarily indicate disease. In particular, isolation of *Staphylococcus* spp. from the oral cavity, nasal cavity, pharynx, vagina, or skin may simply be identification of the normal microflora. Coagulase-negative staphylococci have been identified in the lower airways of normal horses after exercise,[50] presumably a transient situation arising from movement of commensal flora from the upper airways; therefore, identification of CoNS in tracheal aspirate or bronchoalveolar lavage (BAL) samples in recently exercised horses must be interpreted with caution. Staphylococci can also be isolated from free-flow and catheterized urine samples from healthy horses, although at lower numbers (<20,000 CFU/mL and ≤500 CFU/mL, respectively) than would be expected with an infectious process.[51]

The technique used for sample collection should be considered when determining the relevance of culture results. For example, a deep culture of a postoperative infection from an area that had been externally cleaned is likely more relevant than a quick, superficial swab of an infected site or body surface. The high prevalence of staphylococcal colonization of humans can further complicate interpretation of results, because contamination of the diagnostic sample by hand contact could result in a false-positive result.

The clinical significance of isolation of CoNS from infected sites is sometimes debated because CoNS are often considered to be minimally pathogenic. CoNS may colonize sites with infections caused by other agents or may be present as a co-infection, but the potential for CoNS infection should not be dismissed, particularly in hospitalized animals.

Screening for horses that are colonized with MRSA may be indicated after identification of a colonized or infected horse. Nasal swabs appear to be most sensitive for MRSA screening in horses. Standard cotton-tipped culture swabs are inserted approximately 10 cm (4 inches) into the nasal passage and withdrawn while dragging against the nasal mucosa. Enrichment culture of nasal swabs increases the sensitivity of testing.[16]

TREATMENT

Treatment of staphylococcal infections will depend on the location and severity of infection and the antimicrobial sensitivity of the isolate. Culture and sensitivity (C&S) testing is essential to guide treatment. In certain situations, staphylococcal infection should be considered likely and initial treatment prescribed accordingly. In particular, it has been suggested that iatrogenic septic arthritis should be treated as penicillinase-producing staphylococcal infection until proved otherwise.[35,38]

Table • 29-1

Antimicrobial Susceptibility (% Susceptible) of Coagulase-Negative Staphylococci from Clinical Infections in Horses

		ANTIMICROBIAL										
SOURCE	***n***	**Ami**	**Pen**	**Rif**	**Amp**	**Ceft**	**Enro**	**Gent**	**Tet**	**TMS**	**Chlor**	**OXA**
Clinical infections*	18	89	50	72	50	78	94	83	78	67	92	14
Musculoskeletal infections†	14	80	29	NT	36	NT	NT	79	75	58	93	33

Ami, Amikacin; *Pen*, penicillin; *Rif*, rifampin; *Amp*, ampicillin; *Ceft*, ceftiofur; *Enro*, enrofloxacin; *Gent*, gentamicin; *Tet*, tetracycline; *TMS*, trimethoprim-sulfonamide; *Chlor*, chloramphenicol; *Oxa*, oxacillin (methicillin); *NT*, not tested.
*Unpublished data from JS Weese. Clinical isolates from the Ontario Veterinary College.
†Data from Moore RM, Schneider RK, Kowalski J, et al: *Equine Vet J* 24:450-456, 1992.

Table • 29-2

Antimicrobial Susceptibility (% Susceptible) of Coagulase-Positive Staphylococci from Clinical Infection in Horses

		ANTIMICROBIAL										
SOURCE	***n***	**Ami**	**Pen**	**Rif**	**Amp**	**Ceph**	**Enro**	**Gent**	**Tet**	**TMS**	**Chlor**	**Oxa**
Musculoskeletal infections*	48†	100	29	NT	27	100	NT	71	74	79	96	90
Various infections‡	50	92	24	94	54	86	98	78	80	80	94	92

Ami, Amikacin; *Pen*, penicillin; *Rif*, rifampin; *Amp*, ampicillin; *Ceph*, cephalosporin; *Enro*, enrofloxacin; *Gent*, gentamicin; *Tet*, tetracycline; *TMS*, trimethoprim-sulfonamide; *Chlor*, chloramphenicol; *Oxa*, oxacillin (methicillin); *NT*, not tested.
*Data from Moore RM, Schneider RK, Kowalski J, et al: *Equine Vet J* 24:450-456, 1992.
†Not all antimicrobials were tested with all isolates.
‡Unpublished data from JS Weese. Clinical isolates from the Ontario Veterinary College.

Topical therapy may be effective in uncomplicated superficial (e.g., wound, incision) infections. Silver sulfadiazine; a combination of 1% silver sulfadiazine and 0.2% chlorhexidine digluconate; fusidic acid; mupirocin; or vancomycin may be useful.[52-55] Allicin (garlic extract) and tea tree oil have in vitro antistaphylococcal activity; however, efficacy in treating clinical infections is unclear.[56-58] If topical therapy alone is chosen, patients should be monitored closely for progression of local disease or development of bacteremia and systemic disease.

Local or regional antimicrobial perfusion may also be useful in some cases (see Chapter 5). A limited study of regional limb perfusion with gentamicin (1 g) was successful in the treatment of experimentally induced *S. aureus* septic arthritis.[59] Intraosseus infusion of gentamicin with the horse standing might also be useful for treatment of orthopedic infections.[60]

In most situations, systemic antimicrobial therapy is required for treatment of staphylococcal infections. Drug choices should be based on in vitro antimicrobial susceptibility in combination with other patient and drug factors (e.g., penetration, concentration, activity at site of infection, drug interactions). "Antibiogram" information is very important because of the variability in antimicrobial susceptibility and the paucity of published data regarding susceptibility patterns. Tables 29-1 and 29-2 summarize antibiogram data from a few limited studies. The usefulness of older studies is questionable because of the continuing emergence of antimicrobial resistance among staphylococci.

Most staphylococci, including up to 90% of *S. aureus* isolates from humans and animals, are resistant to penicillin.[61,62] If there is a reasonable suspicion of staphylococcal infection, penicillin should not be used initially. This is particularly true in infections such as postinjection septic arthritis, in which staphylococci are highly likely to be involved. Resistance to other antimicrobials is variable. In general, staphylococci are susceptible to β-lactamase–resistant penicillins, cephalosporins, trimethoprim-sulfonamide combinations and fluoroquinolones. Judicious-use principles should be considered when choosing the appropriate antimicrobial.[63]

Multidrug-resistant (MDR) staphylococci may be seen, and initial treatment may need to be changed after C&S testing. The potential for resistance and initial treatment failure highlights the need for submission of appropriate culture species. The concern regarding MDR staphylococci appears to be highest in veterinary hospitals and large breeding farms.[16]

If MRSA infection is suspected, such as a characteristic secondary infection developing on a farm with endemic

Table • 29-3

Antimicrobial Susceptibility (% Susceptible) of Equine Methicillin-Resistant **Staphylococcus aureus** ***(MSRA) Isolates from Horses***

NO. OF ISOLATES	Oxa	TMS	Ami	Rif	Gen	Chl	Enro	Tet	Imi	Ery	Doxy	Van	Fus	Mup
44*	0	0	95	70	14	95	36	0	100	75	NT	100	NT	NT
67†	0	21	100	18	2	100	NT	4	100	14	22	100	100	100

*Data from Weese JS, Rousseau J, Traub-Dargatz JL, et al: *J Am Vet Med Assoc* 226:580-583, 2005.
†Data from Weese JS, Archambault M, Willey BM, et al: *Emerg Infect Dis* 11:430-435, 2005.
Oxa, Oxacillin; *TMS*, trimethoprim-sulfonamide; *Ami*, amikacin; *Rif*, rifampin; *Gen*, gentamicin; *Chl*, chloramphenicol; *Enro*, enrofloxacin; *Tet*, tetracycline; *Imi*, imipenem; *Ery*, erythromycin; *Doxy*, doxycycline; *Van*, vancomycin; *Fus*, fusidic acid; *Mup*, mupirocin; *NT*, not tested.

MRSA or in a horse that is colonized with MRSA, β-lactam antimicrobials should not be used pending C&S testing results in potentially serious infections. Initial therapy should ideally be commenced based on an understanding of the antibiogram of previous MRSA isolates from the farm or hospital, while trying to avoid the use of important broad-spectrum antimicrobials.

Although β-lactam antimicrobials will be ineffective, it is important to remember that not all MRSA isolates are highly drug resistant (Table 29-3). Some community-associated MRSA strains may be resistant only to β-lactam antimicrobials. Common antimicrobials can be highly effective if the isolate is sensitive in vitro, provided the chosen drug is able to achieve therapeutic levels at the site of infection. Therefore, identification of an MRSA infection does not mean that "big-gun" antimicrobials are required, particularly in non–life-threatening infections. However, high-level resistance to multiple antimicrobial classes does occur,[64,65] and many MRSA isolates will be resistant to all antimicrobials present on typical veterinary antimicrobial panels. Any good diagnostic laboratory should offer an expanded antimicrobial panel when MDR pathogens are isolated, either routinely or on request. An expanded panel should be requested for all MRSA isolates.

Veterinary use of drugs that are important for treatment of critically ill patients in human medicine is controversial. Emergence of MDR pathogens such as MRSA increases the pressure to use these drugs, which could be accompanied by further development of resistance and increased scrutiny of antimicrobial-use practices in veterinary medicine. In situations where MDR pathogens are more likely to be encountered (e.g., tertiary care referral centers), development of antimicrobial-use guidelines is wise to dictate if and when certain antimicrobials may be used.

PREVENTION

Because horses may harbor a variety of staphylococci as commensal organisms, methods of decreasing the development of disease are more important than decreasing exposure (except for MDR strains). Good general management, prompt treatment of illnesses, proper wound care, judicious antimicrobial therapy, judicious use of invasive devices, proper disinfection of surgical equipment, and the use of appropriate aseptic practices for surgery and intraarticular injection may all play a role in prevention of staphylococcal disease.

Horses that are infected or colonized with MRSA should be considered infectious. They should be isolated and handled with barrier precautions, including gloves, gowns (or dedicated coveralls or laboratory coats), and overboots (or dedicated boots). The entire stall environment can be contaminated, as can medical or handling items,[66] so barrier precautions should be used whenever the stall is entered or potentially contaminated items are handled. Any items that have been in contact with the horse or the environment should be disinfected or discarded after use. Staphylococci are susceptible to all common disinfectants, provided that concentration and contact time are adequate and organic debris does not inhibit disinfection.

Isolation of horses may be more difficult on farms than in equine hospitals. On a farm, prevention of nose-to-nose contact between horses is essential. Colonized horses should be housed such that they cannot come into direct contact with other horses. One problem that may be encountered, particularly in public stables, is the potential for transmission of MRSA to people or transmission between horses by people. The horse's nose is often touched during normal horse-human interaction, creating a risk of contamination of the person's hands. The risk of MRSA transmission should be adequately explained and displayed if a colonized or infected horse is in a public area.

At the Ontario Veterinary College, an MRSA control program was created after recognition of community-associated and nosocomial MRSA infection and colonization, with transmission of MRSA to hospital personnel. Nasal swabs for MRSA enrichment culture are collected from all horses on admission, weekly during hospitalization, and at discharge. Glove use is mandatory for contact with any horse. Hand hygiene has been emphasized, and alcohol-based hand-sanitizer dispensers have been placed throughout the hospital. Horses from farms with known endemic MRSA are isolated on arrival until a negative nasal swab is obtained. Dedicated medical and handling equipment is used for each horse.

PUBLIC HEALTH CONSIDERATIONS

The main public health concerns associated with equine staphylococcal infection involve MRSA. Transmission of MRSA between horses and humans is being increasingly recognized and is of concern for the horse industry and the veterinary profession. One study reported a prevalence of MRSA colonization of 13% in horse personnel on farms in Ontario and New York, with all colonized humans carrying the characteristic "equine" strain.[16] Acquisition of MRSA by veterinarians and subsequent transmission to household contacts and other patients have been documented.[15] Although the risk of clinical disease in otherwise healthy humans is unclear and likely low,

MRSA skin infections have been reported in people working with colonized horses[15] (J.S. Weese, unpublished data). The risk of zoonotic transmission is probably highest on breeding farms and in equine hospitals because of the frequency and nature of contact.

Preventing the acquisition of MRSA by veterinary personnel is important for two main reasons: to prevent disease in personnel and to prevent colonization and subsequent transmission of MRSA to other equine patients.

One area that requires closer scrutiny is therapeutic riding programs. An unknown percentage of individuals participating in these programs are presumably at higher risk for development of disease, based on underlying disease and immunosuppressive treatments. If these individuals were exposed to MRSA through a therapeutic riding program, they could be at greater risk of developing disease. Although these risks have not been adequately evaluated, veterinarians working with therapeutic riding programs should be prepared to discuss disease risks (not limited to MRSA) with program coordinators. Screening of horses in these programs for MRSA colonization should be considered.

The risk of transmission of other staphylococci, particularly other MDR strains, is unclear. Presumably, other staphylococci can be transmitted between horses and humans, although the clinical significance of non–methicillin-resistant strains is likely of lesser importance on an individual and population basis.

REFERENCES

See the CD-ROM for a list of references linked to the abstract in PubMed.

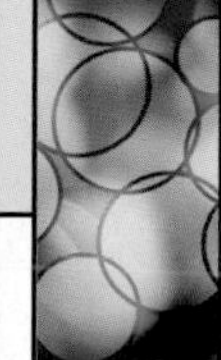

CHAPTER • 30

Miscellaneous Gram-Positive Bacterial Infections

CORYNEBACTERIUM PSEUDOTUBERCULOSIS

Sharon J. Spier and Mary Beth Whitcomb

Etiology

Corynebacterium pseudotuberculosis is a gram-positive, pleomorphic, rod-shaped, intracellular, facultative anaerobe with worldwide distribution. It is the etiologic agent of ulcerative lymphangitis, external subcutaneous abscesses, and internal infection in horses. In North America, disease is most prevalent in the southwestern United States, but cases of *C. pseudotuberculosis* infection have been reported throughout the United States. Infection has been reported in sheep, goats, cattle, buffalo, camelids, equids, and humans.

Corynebacterium pseudotuberculosis grows well at 36° C (96.8° F) on blood agar in 24 to 48 hours, and it forms small, pinpoint-diameter, whitish, opaque colonies surrounded by a weak zone of hemolysis. Because of the high content of lipids in the bacterial cell wall, particularly corynomycolic acid, the colonies spatter in a flame and can be pushed across the agar surface.[1] The high content of lipids may facilitate survival of the organism in macrophages.[2]

Two species-specific biotypes of *C. pseudotuberculosis* have been identified based on differences in nitrate reduction,[3] and deoxyribonucleic acid (DNA) fingerprinting techniques have revealed multiple strains.[4-7] Biotypes isolated from small ruminants are nitrate negative, whereas those from horses are nitrate positive. From the result of DNA studies, the terms "biovar equi" for nitrate-positive and "biovar ovis" for nitrate-negative strains were proposed.[3] Natural cross-species transmission does not seem to occur between sheep and horses; however, cattle can have infection from either biotype.[3]

Epidemiology

Three forms of *C. pseudotuberculosis* infection have been described in horses: ulcerative lymphangitis or limb infection, external abscesses (Fig. 30-1), and internal infection. *Ulcerative lymphangitis* presents as severe cellulitis, with involvement of lymphatic vessels in one or more limbs and multiple draining ulcerative lesions. In a retrospective study of *C. pseudotuberculosis* infection in horses from California, horses with ulcerative lymphangitis comprised only 1% of the cases, whereas external abscesses occurred in 91%, and internal abscesses in 8% of the cases.[11] Horses of all breeds and gender may develop any of the three forms of disease, although mares may be overrepresented and Thoroughbreds underrepresented in studies by Doherr.[16] In one recent study of internal infection, mares seemed to be overrepresented.[20]

The portal of entry of this soil-borne organism is thought to be through abrasions or wounds in the skin or mucous membranes. Many insects have been incriminated as vectors for the transmission of the disease to horses, and recent studies have shown that *Haematobia irritans*, *Musca domestica*, and *Stomoxys calcitrans* can act as vectors for this disease[12] (Figs. 30-2 and 30-3). The regional location of abscesses suggests that ventral midline dermatitis predisposes to infection. Because of the variable incubation period, ventral midline dermatitis may not be present during maturation of the abscesses.

Temporal and spatial analysis suggests that the disease can be transmitted through horse-to-horse contact or from infected to susceptible horses by insects, other vectors, or contaminated soil; the incubation period is 3 to 4 weeks.[13] The organism survives for up to 2 months in hay and shavings and more than 8 months in soil samples at environmental temperatures.[14,15]

The incidence of disease fluctuates considerably from year to year, presumably because of herd immunity and environmental factors such as rainfall and temperature. To date, the

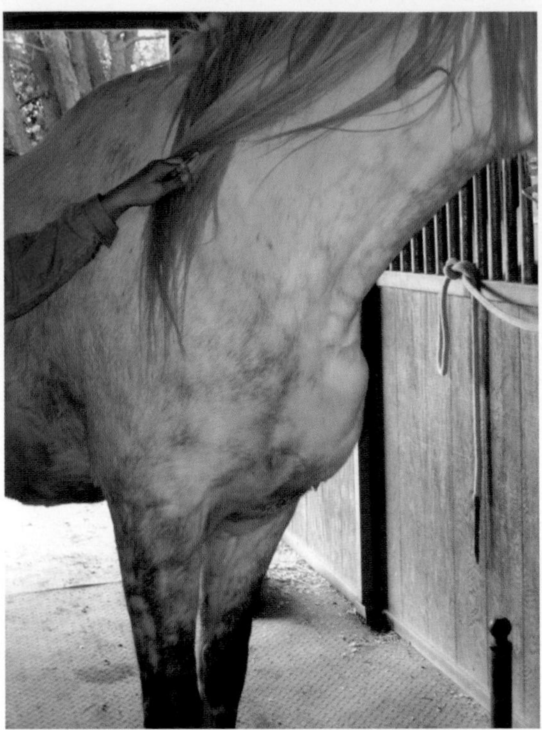

Fig. 30-1 Typical pectoral abscess caused by *Corynebacterium pseudotuberculosis*.

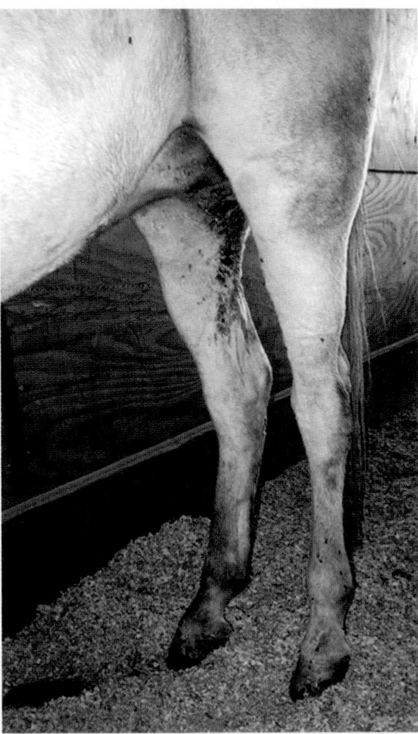

Fig. 30-2 Houseflies *(Musca domestica)* feeding on exudate draining from abscess. Flies are vectors for *C. pseudotuberculosis* infection in horses.

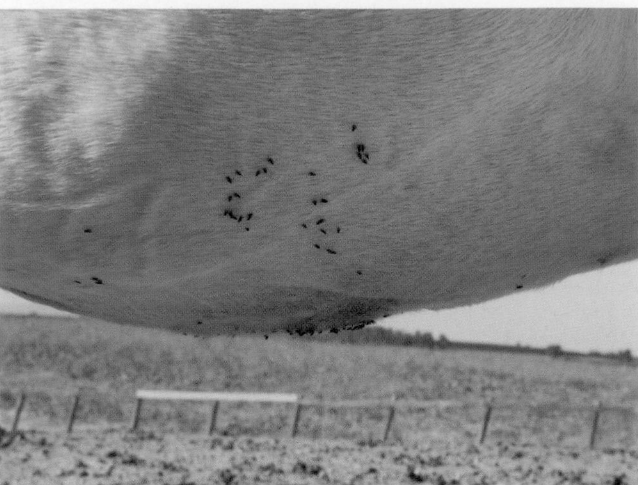

Fig. 30-3 Horn flies *(Haematobia irritans)* feeding on the ventral midline of horse. Ventral midline dermatitis is a predisposing factor for *C. pseudotuberculosis* disease in horses, and the bacteria can be found in this species of fly.

definitive environmental factors supporting the spread of infection have not been determined.[16] Disease incidence is seasonal, with highest number of cases occurring during the dry months of the year, which is late summer and fall in the southwestern United States, although cases may be seen all year. Horses with internal infection are more frequently seen 1 to 2 months after the peak number of cases with external abscesses.[17]

Horses of all ages may be affected, although the low incidence of disease in foals less than 6 months of age suggests that passive transfer of immunoglobulins offers protection in foals born in endemic areas. A case-control study in an endemic area revealed young adults (<5 years) and horses in contact with other horses on summer pasture had increased risk of infection. Horses housed outside or with access to an outside paddock appeared to be at higher risk than stabled horses.[18]

Pathogenesis

The pathogenesis of *C. pseudotuberculosis* infection in horses is poorly understood. The incubation period appears variable; temporal and spatial clustering studies by Doherr et al.[13] revealed an incubation period of 7 to 28 days. Bacteria are phagocytosed after entry into the host but continue to replicate. Intracellular survival of *C. pseudotuberculosis* has a key role in the formation of abscesses and is possibly mediated by two virulence factors: bacterial cell wall lipids and *phospholipase D* (PLD) protein exotoxin. The bacterial cell wall lipids may facilitate survival in macrophages, whereas the PLD exotoxin has profound effects on survival and multiplication within the host. The PLD toxin may directly affect phagocytic cells or inactivate complement and reduce opsonization of the bacteria. The exotoxin also increases vascular permeability, enhancing the spread of infection both locally and through the lymphatics. The subsequent vascular changes permit bacterial spread to additional locations, including regional lymph nodes. Humoral and cell-mediated immune responses ultimately develop, clearing the bacterial infection.[19]

Recovery generally is complete within 2 to 4 weeks, although rarely horses develop persistent or recurrent infections lasting for more than 1 year. In one study, 91% horses had complete recovery with no recurrence of infection in subsequent years, implying a long-lasting immunity.[11] In 9% of affected horses, however, infections persisted more than 1 year or recurred as external or internal abscesses.[11] In sheep and goats, studies have shown that acquired humoral and cellular immune responses develop after infection and that macrophages acquire the ability to kill the organism.[19] Similar studies have not been performed in horses.

Corynebacterium pseudotuberculosis produces various exotoxins, which play a role in virulence; the most studied is PLD. Phospholipases are a heterogenous group of enzymes that share the ability to hydrolyze one or more ester linkages in glycerophospholipids. Although all phospholipases target phospholipids as substrates, each enzyme has the ability to cleave a specific ester bond. Thus, qualifying letters (e.g., A, B, C, D) are used to differentiate among phospholipases and to indicate the specific bond targeted in the phospholipid molecule. PLD is important in the pathogenesis of the disease by its action on cell membranes, causing hydrolysis and degradation of sphingomyelin in endothelial cells and increasing vascular permeability.[8] The bacterial PLD is similar to the PLD of the brown recluse spider, which explains the presence of pain and edema at the site of infection. Targeted mutagenesis of PLD in *C. pseudotuberculosis* reduced the ability of this bacterium to establish a primary infection or cause chronic abscess formation in regional lymph nodes. These results indicate that PLD is a virulence determinant of *C. pseudotuberculosis*, increasing the persistence and spread of the bacteria within the host.[9] The synergistic activity of *C. pseudotuberculosis* exotoxins with the exotoxins of *Rhodococcus equi* in lysing red blood cells in agar forms the basis for the synergistic hemolysis inhibition test.[10]

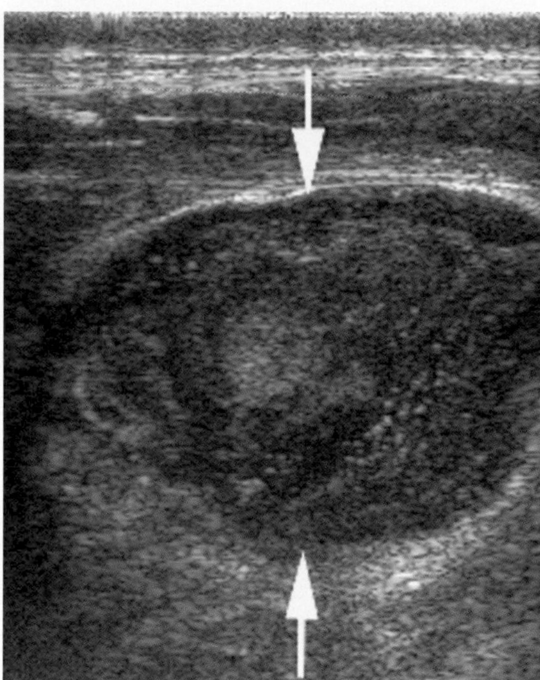

Fig. 30-4 Ultrasound image of pectoral abscess demonstrating exudate with mixed echogenicity surrounded by thin hyperechoic capsule *(arrows)*. The abscess is approximately 3 to 4 cm in diameter.

Clinical Findings

External Abscesses

External abscesses may occur anywhere on the body but most frequently develop in the pectoral region and along the ventral midline of the abdomen (see Fig. 30-1). This form of infection is commonly known as "pigeon fever," because of the large size of the pectoral abscesses with the appearance of a pigeon's breast, or "dryland distemper," because of its prevalence in arid geographic regions. Abscesses contain tan, odor-free, purulent exudate and are usually well encapsulated. Additional sites with a predilection for abscess formation include the prepuce, mammary gland, axilla, triceps, limbs, and head. Other less common areas are the thorax, neck, parotid gland, guttural pouches, larynx, flanks, umbilicus, tail, and rectum. Septic joints and osteomyelitis have been reported.[11] Horses may have an abscess involving a single site or involving multiple regions of the body. It is common to observe multiple subcutaneous abscesses coursing along a suspected lymphatic.

Clinical signs most frequently associated with external abscesses are edema, fever, and nonhealing wounds. Other clinical signs include lameness, ventral dermatitis, weight loss, depression, anorexia, and mammary gland or preputial swelling. Generally, horses with external abscesses do not develop signs of systemic illness, although one-quarter will develop fever.[11] If signs of systemic illness are present, further diagnostic testing to rule out internal infection is warranted. In cases of external abscessation, a large area of edema is often observed in the area of abscess formation. As the abscess matures, this area becomes hard and painful. Some abscesses become quite large, particularly in the pectoral region. Abscesses typically have a thick capsule and can cause severe lameness if located in the axillary, triceps, or inguinal region.[11] Maturation can be slow and drainage difficult to establish if the abscess lies deep to muscle.

After drainage is established, either by spontaneous rupture or lancing, most horses recover within 10 to 14 days without complications. The abscesses may contain from 5 to 400 mL of thick, tan, purulent exudate. Ultrasonography may aid in determining the best location for drainage of external abscesses (Fig. 30-4). The case fatality for horses with external abscesses is very low (0.8%).[11]

Clinical pathologic abnormalities that may be observed include anemia of chronic disease, leukocytosis with neutrophilia, hyperfibrinogenemia, and hyperproteinemia. These hematologic parameters can occur with either internal or external abscesses but are more consistently observed with internal abscesses.

Internal Infection

Approximately 8% of affected horses develop internal infection, which is associated with a case-fatality rate of 30% to 40%.[11] In a retrospective study, infection was localized to a specific organ(s) in 90% (27/30) of horses. Involvement of multiple internal organs was identified in 37% (10/27) of horses. The organs most often involved were liver and lungs, with kidney and spleen being affected less often. Abdominal ultrasonography was a useful diagnostic tool to identify affected abdominal organs specifically[17,20] (Figs. 30-5 to 30-8).

A diagnosis of internal infection is based on clinical signs, clinicopathologic data, serology, diagnostic imaging, and bacterial culture. The most common clinical signs are concurrent external abscesses, decreased appetite, fever, lethargy, weight loss, and signs of respiratory disease or abdominal pain. Other signs observed in horses with internal abscesses include ventral edema, ventral dermatitis, ataxia, hematuria (caused by renal abscesses), and infrequently, abortion. The median age in two studies was 7 and 8 years, with a range of 1 to 23 years.[11,20]

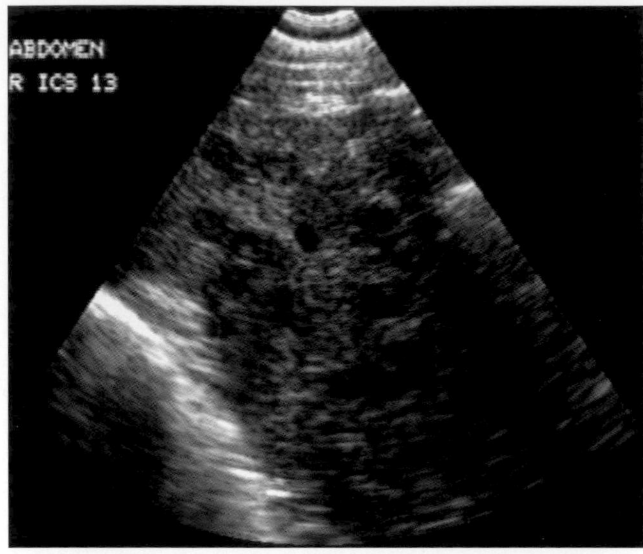

Fig. 30-5 Abnormal right liver lobe showing multiple hypoechoic abscesses producing mottled appearance to liver. The liver lobes were enlarged with rounded margins. Ultrasound image was obtained from the right 13th intercostal space with a 3.5-MHz sector transducer at a scanning depth of 14 cm.

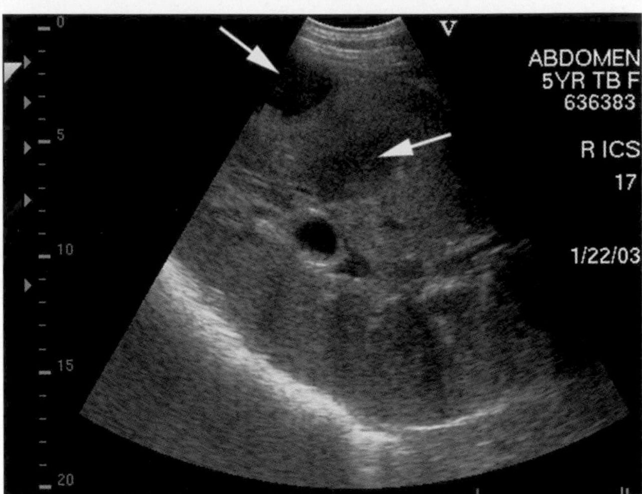

Fig. 30-7 Abnormal right kidney with two small hypoechoic abscesses, one involving the cortex and one involving the renal medulla *(arrows)*. Urine was culture-positive for *C. pseudotuberculosis*. This mare was pregnant at the time of the examination and aborted her fetus within 48 hours. The renal abscesses resolved with antimicrobial therapy. Ultrasound image was obtained from the right 17th intercostal space with a 3.5-MHz curvilinear transducer at a scanning depth of 20 cm.

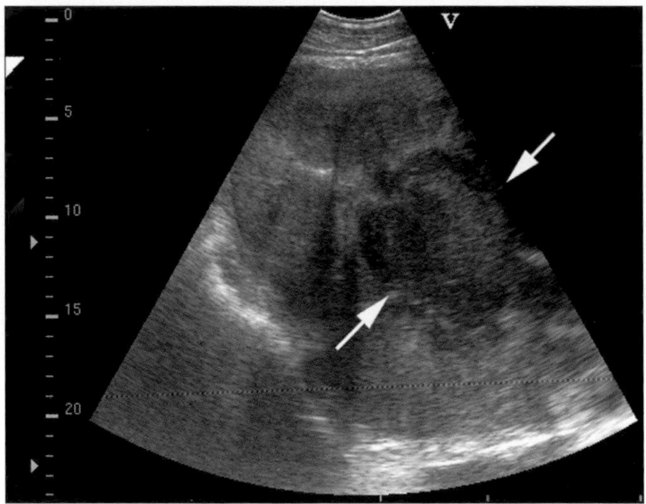

Fig. 30-6 Solitary right renal abscess *(arrows)* in mare with history of weight loss. Aspiration of this abscess yielded a large quantity of purulent material. The size of this abscess did not change with antimicrobial therapy. Ultrasound image was obtained from the right 16th intercostal space with a 3.5-MHz curvilinear transducer at a scanning depth of 25 cm.

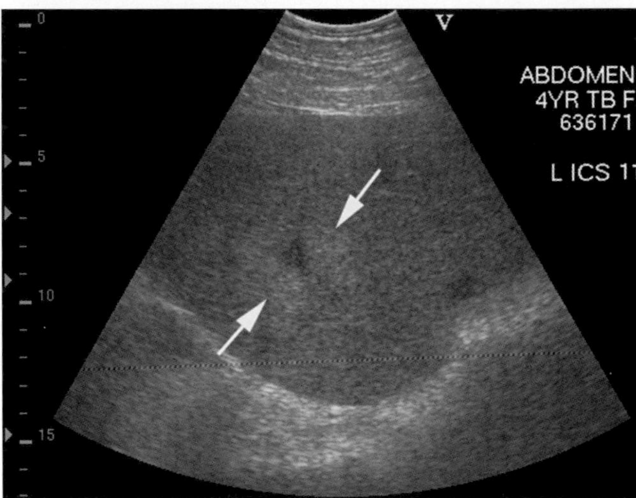

Fig. 30-8 Abnormal spleen with area of increased echogenicity surrounding small hypoechoic area, consistent with splenic abscessation *(arrows)*. Clinical signs resolved after a long course of antimicrobial therapy. Ultrasound image was obtained from the left 11th intercostal space with a 3.5-MHz curvilinear transducer at a scanning depth of 17 cm.

Anemia of chronic disease, leukocytosis with neutrophilia, and elevated fibrinogen are common features of infection, particularly in horses with internal abscesses[11] (Table 30-1). Leukocytosis with neutrophilia was seen in 36% and 76% of horses with external and internal abscesses, respectively. Hyperproteinemia, caused by increased serum globulin concentrations, was observed in 38% and 59% of horses with external and internal abscesses, respectively.[11]

Peritoneal fluid is frequently abnormal in horses with abdominal abscesses. However, peritoneal fluid analysis may be normal if abscesses are located retroperitoneal in the kidneys without involvement of other abdominal structures. *C. pseudotuberculosis* was isolated from 32% of samples of peritoneal fluid from affected horses.[11] Failure to isolate the organism from peritoneal fluid does not rule out the disease. The organisms could be located retroperitoneal, sequestered

Table • 30-1

Values of Key Clinicopathologic Data in 30 Horses with Internal* Corynebacterium pseudotuberculosis *Infection

CLINICOPATHOLOGIC DATA	MEAN ± SD	RANGE
Hematocrit (%)	33.9 ± 7.2	23.4-50.0
Total white blood cell (WBC) count (cells/μL)	19,297 ± 9485	6400-53,420
Neutrophil count (cells/μL)	16,080 ± 9109	2944-49,627
Platelet count (cells/μL)	228,967 ± 86,280	15,000-449,000
Fibrinogen (mg/dL)	670.0 ± 306.4	100-1600
Total protein concentration (g/dL)	8.7 ± 1.5	6.3-12.1
Globulin concentration (g/dL)	6.7 ± 1.8	3.5-10.5
Synergistic hemolysis inhibition (SHI) titer	2611	64-20,480

Data from Pratt SM, Spier SJ, Vaughan B, et al: *J Am Vet Med Assoc* 227:441-448, 2005.

within a thick capsule, or suppressed by local factors or nucleated cells.

Ulcerative Lymphangitis

Ulcerative lymphangitis is the least common form of *C. pseudotuberculosis* seen in horses in North America, although this form of disease has been reported worldwide. Limb swelling, cellulitis, and draining tracts following lymphatic vessels are seen. Horses often develop severe lameness, fever, lethargy, and anorexia. Aggressive medical therapy is necessary, or the disease may become chronic, resulting in limb edema, lameness, weakness, and weight loss.[1]

Diagnosis

Culture

The typical clinical presentation of single or multiple, maturing pectoral abscesses, with or without ventral midline abscesses, is highly suspicious of *C. pseudotuberculosis* infection. Culture of the characteristic tan or blood-tinged, odorless exudate is diagnostic. Bacteriologic culture of aspirates or draining abscesses readily yields growth of moderate to large numbers of organisms on blood agar in 24 to 48 hours. The colonies appear small, white, and opaque. Gram stain reveals gram-positive pleomorphic rods. Equine isolates reduce nitrate (unlike strains from small ruminants). In horses with internal infection, samples obtained by ultrasound-guided aspiration from affected organs can also yield a positive culture.[17-20]

Serology

Without a positive bacterial culture, the practitioner must rely on hematology, clinical chemistry, and serologic testing to support a diagnosis. Hematologic changes are nonspecific and indicative of a chronic inflammatory response. Serologic testing using the *synergistic hemolysis inhibition* (SHI) test can be a useful aid in the diagnosis of internal abscesses.[10,11] The SHI test measures immunoglobulin G (IgG) to the exotoxin of *C. pseudotuberculosis* and is available through the California Animal Health and Food Safety Laboratory System in Davis, California. Serology is generally not helpful for diagnosis of external abscesses and may be negative early in the course of disease and even at the time of abscess drainage. Positive SHI titers must be interpreted carefully, after appropriate consideration of clinical signs, to distinguish active infection from exposure or convalescence. Both published and unpublished data from the University of California suggest that a reciprocal titer of 256 or greater is indicative of active infection. Horses with internal abscesses generally have SHI titers of 512 or higher. In one study of internal infection, SHI titers ranged from 512 to 20,480.[20] Titers of 16 or lower are considered negative, whereas titers between 16 and 128 are considered suspicious or indicative of exposure.[21] These are only general guidelines, however, because there is considerable overlap in results from horses with active disease, exposure, and recovery from infection. Experimental inoculation of horses with a bacterin-toxoid developed from *C. pseudotuberculosis* produced increased SHI titers equivalent to those seen with active infection; the protection offered from this bacterin has not been proved to date.

Ultrasonography

Ultrasonography is extremely useful for diagnosis of internal infections in horses, not only for identifying affected organs, but also for defining the nature and extent of involvement of abdominal viscera. Abdominal ultrasound permits documentation of involvement of specific organs in the absence of clinicopathologic evidence of disease involving these organs. Abdominal ultrasound may be used for collection of transcutaneous liver and kidney biopsies and aspirates of abscesses for a definitive diagnosis (see Fig. 30-8). Thoracic ultrasound should be performed in affected horses to determine the severity of pulmonary disease (Fig. 30-9). Serial examinations can be used to evaluate response to treatment. Examinations should be performed using low-frequency (2.5-3.5 MHz) and medium-frequency (5 MHz) ultrasound transducers. Complete examination of the abdomen consists of both right and left paralumbar fossa regions, all intercostal spaces from the ventral lung margins to the costochondral junctions, and the ventral abdomen from the sternum to the inguinal region. Presence of peritoneal fluid and abnormalities of the liver, spleen, kidneys, stomach, duodenum, small intestine, cecum, and large colon can be observed.

Hepatic abnormalities associated with *C. pseudotuberculosis* infection in horses include hepatomegaly, multiple small hypoechoic areas resulting in a "moth-eaten" appearance, and discrete, circular, anechoic to hypoechoic areas (see Fig. 30-5). Renal abscessation may appear as a single large (10-15 cm in diameter) area or multiple anechoic to hypoechoic areas involving either the cortex or the medulla[17] (see Figs. 30-6 and 30-7). Splenic abnormalities may also be observed and include small, irregularly shaped, hypoechoic areas without obvious encapsulation (see Fig. 30-8). In horses with pulmonary involvement, examination of the thorax may reveal presence of pleural defects ("comet tails"), consolidation, pleural effusion, or pericardial effusion (see Fig. 30-9).[20]

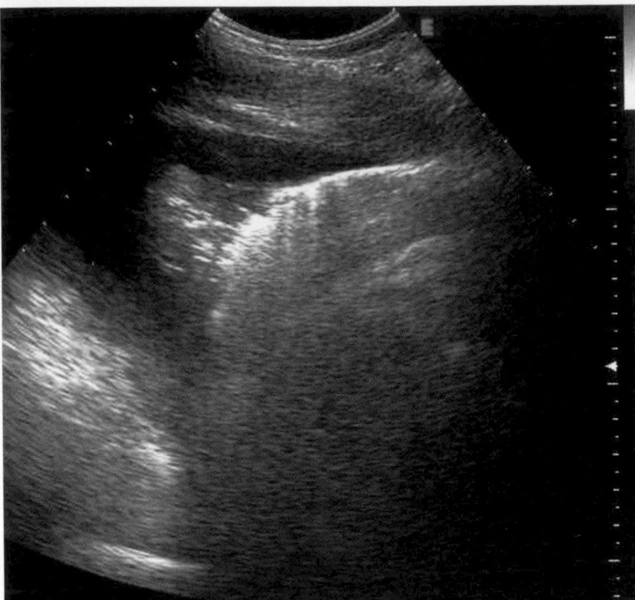

Fig. 30-9 Cranioventral consolidation with moderate pleural effusion in mare with pneumonia secondary to *C. pseudotuberculosis*. The small hyperechoic areas within the consolidated lung represent air trapped within the small airways. The image was obtained from the right sixth intercostal space with a 3.5-MHz curvilinear transducer at a scanning depth of 16 cm.

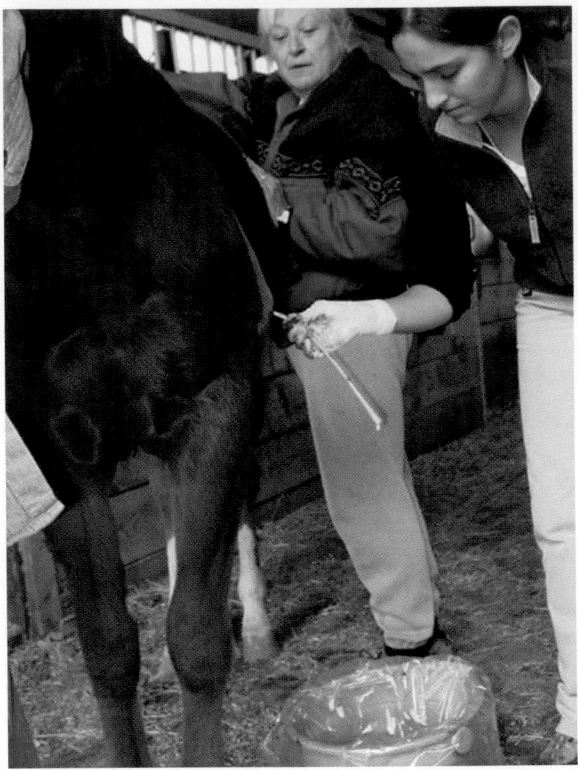

Fig. 30-10 Deep abscess in left triceps muscle was causing severe lameness in this yearling gelding. The lameness was relieved after insertion of a polyvinyl chest tube to drain the abscess.

Early diagnosis of internal infection caused by *C. pseudotuberculosis* is important for a successful outcome but is often difficult because of the insidious onset and nonspecific nature of clinical signs, which may include anorexia, fever, lethargy, and weight loss. In endemic areas, horses that have had an external abscess in the previous 6 months and then develop signs of systemic illness should be suspected of having internal *C. pseudotuberculosis* infection, as should horses with compatible signs residing on a property where other horses have had external abscesses. For horses with this history, ultrasonography and serologic testing are recommended as an aid for diagnosis of internal infections.

Therapy

External Abscesses

The treatment regimen must be individualized for each horse depending on the severity of disease, including the presence of systemic illness (e.g., fever, anorexia), the extent of soft tissue inflammation, the maturity of the abscess, and the ability to establish drainage of pus. Establishing drainage is the most important treatment and ultimately leads to faster resolution and return to athletic performance. The proximity of the fibrous abscess capsule to the skin varies, often being less than 1 cm deep for ventral midline abscesses, to greater than 10 cm for deep pectoral, axillary, triceps, or inguinal abscesses (Fig. 30-10). Aspiration and drainage of superficial abscesses are easily performed; the use of diagnostic ultrasound is helpful for localization of deeper abscesses and to judge maturity of the abscess and proximity to the skin. If the abscess is immature or cannot be safely incised, subsequent ultrasound examinations may be necessary to establish the ideal time to lance into the abscess. The abscess contents and lavage solutions (e.g., saline with or without antiseptic) should be retrieved and disposed of to prevent further contamination of the immediate environment.

Antimicrobial therapy is indicated for treatment of horses with ulcerative lymphangitis or internal abscesses. The use of antimicrobials for external abscesses is not necessary in most horses and may prolong the time to resolution.[11] Antimicrobial therapy may be justified when signs of systemic illness (e.g., fever, depression, anorexia) or extensive cellulitis are present. Horses with deep intramuscular abscesses that are lanced and draining through healthy tissue may also benefit from antimicrobial therapy.

Corynebacterium pseudotuberculosis is susceptible in vitro to many antimicrobials typically used in horses, including penicillin G, macrolides, tetracyclines, cephalosporins, chloramphenicol, fluoroquinolones, and rifampin, but some isolates may be resistant to aminoglycosides.[7,22,23] Several factors should be considered when choosing an antimicrobial: the intracellular location of the organism, the presence of exudate and a thick abscess capsule, anticipated duration of therapy, cost of the drug, and convenience of administration. Despite in vitro susceptibility, the nature of the bacteria and the copious exudate render certain antimicrobials ineffective for some cases. Trimethoprim-sulfa (5 mg/kg based on the trimethoprim fraction, twice daily orally) and procaine penicillin (20,000 U/kg twice daily intramuscularly) are highly effective for treatment of external abscesses, especially on the ventral midline. Rifampin (2.5-5 mg/kg twice daily orally) in combination with ceftiofur (2.5-5 mg/kg twice daily intravenously or intramuscularly) appears highly effective for treatment of internal abscesses. Internal abscesses have reportedly responded to procaine penicillin (dose as above), trimethoprim-sulfa (dose as above), potassium penicillin (20,000-40,000 U/kg four times daily intravenously), as well as erythromycin estolate (15-25 mg/kg twice daily orally).

Internal Infection

Antimicrobial therapy is indicated for the treatment of horses with systemic infection caused by *C. pseudotuberculosis*.[11] The median duration of antimicrobial therapy in a recent study was 36 days and ranged from 7 to 97 days. A variety of antimicrobials to which *C. pseudotuberculosis* is susceptible were used to treat these internal infections (Table 30-2). Rifampin was used in combination with another antimicrobial in the majority of horses. Rifampin alone was used for continued treatment in horses after initial treatment with a combination of rifampin and another antimicrobial.[18] Thoracic and abdominal ultrasound are useful to monitor response to therapy. Ultrasound findings, in addition to clinicopathologic data, aid in the decision-making process for continued antimicrobial therapy in these cases.

The overall mortality associated with internal infections is reported to be 30% to 40%,[11,20] but horses that did not receive antimicrobial therapy had a 100% fatality rate.[11] Antimicrobial therapy for treatment of internal abscesses and ulcerative lymphangitis must be continued for 1 to 6 months. Resolution of infection is determined based on clinical signs, normal clinical pathologic values, and decline in immunoglobulin concentrations. Some horses with very high SHI titers remain seropositive for up to 1 year because of the lengthy half-life of IgG (21 days) and for other reasons that are unknown. Under such situations the clinician should monitor a steady decline in serum SHI titers to *C. pseudotuberculosis*. Purpura hemorrhagica or vasculitis has been reported in horses with systemic infection requiring concurrent therapy with antimicrobials and corticosteroids.[11]

Ulcerative Lymphangitis

Horses with ulcerative lymphangitis or cellulitis should be treated early and aggressively with antimicrobials, or residual lameness or limb swelling may occur. Typically, intravenous (IV) antimicrobials (ceftiofur or penicillin G) alone or in combination with rifampin (orally) are used until lameness and swelling improves, and then therapy with oral antimicrobials such as trimethoprim-sulfamethoxazole or rifampin is continued to prevent relapse. The time to resolution in one study was approximately 35 days.[11] Physical therapy, including hydrotherapy, hand walking, and leg wraps, as well as administration of nonsteroidal antiinflammatory drugs (NSAIDs), are also recommended.

Table • **30-2**

Antimicrobial Drugs Used to Treat 30 Horses with Internal* C. pseudotuberculosis *Infection

ANTIMICROBIAL	NO. OF HORSES	NO. ALSO WITH RIFAMPIN
Rifampin	19	—
Trimethoprim-sulfa	11	3
Gentamicin	10	—
Ampicillin	9	4
Ceftiofur	9	7
Penicillin G	5	3
Cefazolin	2	—
Enrofloxacin	2	2
Erythromycin	2	—

Data from Pratt SM, Spier SJ, Vaughan B, et al: *J Am Vet Med Assoc* 227:441-448, 2005.

Prevention

Until a protective bacterin or toxoid is developed for horses, horse owners in endemic areas must rely solely on good sanitation and fly control and avoid unnecessary environmental contamination from diseased horses to prevent *C. pseudotuberculosis* infection in their horses. Presently, there is no evidence that diseased horses within a stable should be quarantined, but strict insect control should be implemented. Proper sanitation, disposal of contaminated bedding, and disinfection may reduce the incidence of new cases. Proper wound care is also important to prevent infection from a contaminated environment.

A commercial bacterin-toxoid is available for use in small ruminants (Caseous D-T, Colorado Serum Co., Denver; Glanvac 6 TM, Pfizer Animal Health, Australia).[24] The safety and effectiveness of this product has not been tested in horses. The inability experimentally to reproduce the disease as seen in horses in endemic areas and the sporadic nature of disease complicate research efforts.

NOCARDIOSIS

Marta Gonzalez Arguedas

Nocardiosis is a localized or disseminated bacterial disease of a large variety of animals and of humans caused by *Nocardia* spp.,[25-28] which are soil saprophytes that act as opportunistic pathogens.[25,29] In humans and domestic animals, *Nocardia* causes suppurative to granulomatous tissue reactions, which are most severe in immunosuppressed individuals.[30] *Nocardia* infections in horses are rare. When they do occur, they are usually associated with significant derangements in the host immune system.[30-32] The most common manifestations of disease are pulmonary and pleural disease or nodulo-ulcerative cutaneous lesions.

Etiology

Members of the *Nocardia* species are gram-positive, aerobic, saprophytic, nonmotile, non–spore-forming actinomycetes.[25,27,28,33,34] Nocardiae appear as long, slender, branching filaments with a tendency to fragment into rods and cocci.[34] When cultured, these organisms produce aerial filaments.[27,34] Components of the cell wall, especially mycolic acid, render *Nocardia* species partially acid-fast.[24,27,28,34]

Although most nocardial infections in horses are caused by *Nocardia asteroides*,[27,29,30,34] Deem and Harrington[26] reported a case of fatal pleuropneumonia in a 15-month-old Quarter Horse colt with histologic lesions characteristic of pulmonary nocardiosis in which *Nocardia brasiliensis* was isolated from the lung and bronchial lymph node.

Pathogenic nocardiae are obligate aerobes growing over a wide temperature range (10°–50° C [50°–122° F]).[24] *Nocardia* spp. will grow on most nonselective media used routinely for culture of bacteria, fungi, and mycobacteria.[28,33,37] However, in specimens containing mixed flora (e.g., respiratory secretions), nocardial colonies are easily obscured by those of more rapidly growing bacteria. Nocardiae normally appear within 2 to 7 days on most routine bacteriologic media.[37,38] Their relatively slow growth often results in the cultures being discarded before the nocardiae can be visualized.[27,37] The colony surface, waxy to powdery to velvety depending on the abundance of aerial growth, becomes wrinkled with age.[25,33,37,43] Although the colonies are usually white when first visible, most *Nocardia* spp. produce carotenoid-like pigments that result in colonies with various shades of yellow, orange, pink, or red.[25,27,43]

With the widespread use of molecular methods of identification, the number of recognized *Nocardia* spp. is increasing, and members of the genus *Nocardia* are becoming increasingly difficult to identify using phenotypic criteria.[35] Currently, more than 30 species are included in the genus.[25,36]

Molecular analysis demonstrates that *N. asteroides* includes several species with similar biochemistry, structure, and antimicrobial resistance: *N. asteroides, N. abscessus, N. cyriacigeorgica, N. farcinica, N. nova*, and *N. transvalensis*.[25,28,36-38] These species together are referred to as the *N. asteroides* complex.[25,36-38] It is important to note that all the literature about nocardiosis in horses was published before these species were recognized, and therefore it is impossible to determine the clinical relevance of each individual species in horses. For purposes of simplicity, the discussion that follows will use the former name of *N. asteroides*.

Epidemiology

Nocardiae are present in most environments and found extensively worldwide. They are saprophytic, making up an important component of the normal soil microflora, and are often associated with water.[25,33,38] Nocardial infections may be acquired through inhalation[27,33,34,38] or by traumatic percutaneous introduction of organisms.[33,38] Dust, soil, and plant material serve as vehicles.[25,27] In humans, intestinal nocardiosis may result from ingestion of the organism;[27,34] however, this form of infection has not been reported in horses. Infection is not considered contagious.[33] Transmission between or among animals and persons has not been demonstrated to occur.[26,37,38] Nocardiosis is not considered a zoonotic disease.[33]

In the horse, pulmonary and generalized infection appears to require profound constitutional and immune disturbances and should be considered an opportunistic infection.[25,31,34] In a review of 16 horses with nocardiosis admitted to the Veterinary Teaching Hospital, University of California, Davis, over an 18-year period, almost 90% had an underlying immunosuppressive problem.[31] The two horses that survived had local infections associated with trauma. The remaining 14 cases were associated with concurrent serious systemic illnesses and compromised immune systems that would have led to the death of the horses in the absence of nocardiosis. From the same study, the prevalence of nocardiosis in equine patients from 1965 to 1983 was 16 of 180,000 (0.009%). Two entities emerged as predominant conditions linked with systemic or pulmonary nocardiosis in horses: severe combined immunodeficiency of Arabian foals and pituitary pars intermedia dysfunction.[31] It appears that the circumstances favoring nocardiosis infection in horses closely parallel those recognized in human medicine, where the majority of patients with clinically recognized *Nocardia asteroides* infection have underlying debilitating and/or immunodepressant conditions.[25,26,31,38-40]

Pathogenesis

The outcome of infection with *N. asteroides* is largely determined by the ability of a given strain to resist the initial neutrophil leukocyte response and subsequent attack by activated macrophages and cell-mediated immunity.[27,37] Macrophages and neutrophils by themselves are insufficient to control infection by virulent strains of *N. asteroides*.[27] In vitro, virulent *N. asteroides* can grow within and destroy macrophages.[33] The resistance of this species to oxidative killing by neutrophils and monocytes has been attributed to nocardial catalase and superoxide dismutase.[25,27,33,37,41] In contrast, less virulent strains of *N. asteroides* are capable of surviving within macrophages in an altered cellular state called an "L-form."[27] L-forms are microbial variants that lack a structurally intact cell wall; some may revert to the parental form when the inducing condition is removed. L-forms of *Nocardia* spp. can be recovered from clinical material obtained from patients and may explain the occasional late relapse of nocardial infections.[27,37] The cell wall of nocardiae possesses mycolic acids that contribute to virulence by resisting killing by macrophages.[33] Several bacterial toxins, including hemolysins, have been identified in association with *N. asteroides* but are not thought to be widespread or important virulence factors.[27,37]

Nocardia spp. do not elicit an effective humoral immune response, and B lymphocytes are considered unimportant in the protective response. Protective immune responses are T-cell mediated.[27,37,41,42]

Clinical Findings

Nocardiosis can be a localized or disseminated infection.[39,43] A chronic course is usual, but in immunologically incompetent patients, disease may be acute in onset and rapid in progression.[43] Nocardiosis is infrequent in the horse; however, the following clinical forms have been recognized: pulmonary nocardiosis, disseminated nocardiosis, cutaneous and mycetomatous lesions, and rarely, abortion.[27,30,33,39]

Pulmonary Nocardiosis

Clinical signs are related to severe pulmonary infection and may include increased respiratory rate and effort, cough, and nasal discharge.[37] No specific clinical signs are diagnostic for pulmonary nocardiosis, and the clinical presentation of disease may run the full spectrum of either acute or chronic pulmonary infection. There may be pneumonia, abscess formation, or pleural involvement[27] (Fig. 30-11).

Disseminated Nocardiosis

Disseminated or systemic nocardiosis is characterized by widespread abscess formation in two or more organs of the body.

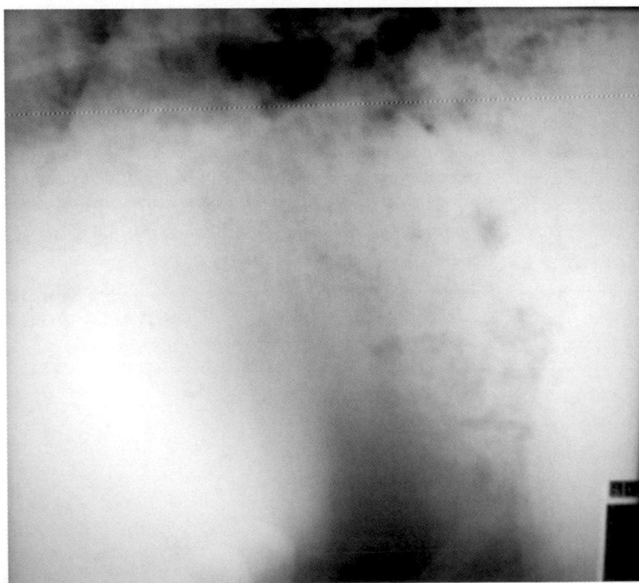

Fig. 30-11 Lateral radiographic view of thorax of 21-year-old Arabian gelding with disseminated nocardiosis secondary to pars intermedia pituitary dysfunction. (Courtesy Dr. Robert Mealey.)

After establishment of primary pulmonary nocardial infection, the organism may be disseminated hematogenously, leading to extrapulmonary disease.[27,28,37] Any anatomic location can be involved.[27] In people, the most frequently affected sites include the central nervous system and eyes (especially the retina), skin and subcutaneous tissues (Fig. 30-12), kidneys, joints, bone, and heart.[28,37]

Localized Cutaneous and Subcutaneous Nocardiosis

Rarely, *Nocardia asteroides* has been reported to cause dermatitis without systemic lesions in horses.[44] This form of disease usually occurs after traumatic introduction of *Nocardia* spp. into the skin. After the organism breaches the integrity of the skin, localized bacterial growth may progress sufficiently to induce an inflammatory response with accumulation of polymorphonuclear leukocytes (PMNs), leading to cellulitis or pyoderma. Often the infection becomes circumscribed to form an abscess.[27] Skin lesions appear as firm, painless, slow-growing subcutaneous nodules, which can occur anywhere on the body. The lesions may ulcerate and discharge a thick, odorless, grayish white or yellowish material.[44] Because the initial response to *Nocardia* is pyogenic, self-limited cutaneous lesions have the same appearance as diseases caused by other pyogenic bacteria, such as *Staphylococcus* and *Streptococcus* spp.,[27] and they may be disregarded or treated as staphylococcal in origin.[27,37]

Nocardia-Induced Mycetomas

Mycetomas are chronically progressive, destructive subcutaneous infections. Mycetomas caused by fungi are called *eumycetomas*, whereas those caused by the actinomycetes are *actinomycetomas*. The most common bacteria isolated from equine actinomycetomas are *Actinobacillus* spp., *Nocardia* spp., and *Actinomyces* spp. Regardless of causative agent, the organism usually gains entrance to the body through traumatic inoculation. The mycetoma most often starts as a painless nodule developing at the site of the injury, days to months after the injury. This nodule increases in size and may eventually become purulent and necrotic. Pus may discharge through sinus tracts. Chronic granulomatous inflammation with concomitant swelling and enlargement of the surrounding areas occurs, with the formation of multiple secondary nodules and draining sinus tracts. The exudate from these nocardial mycetomas may contain "grains" (sandlike particles) similar to those seen in actinomycosis. The granules represent small colonies of the infecting agent surrounded by masses of inflammatory cells.[27,37,44-47]

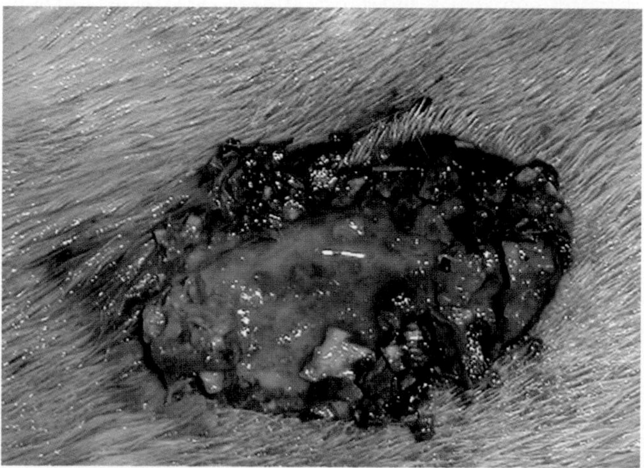

Fig. 30-12 Ulcerative skin lesion on ventral abdomen of the horse described in Figure 30-11. (Courtesy Dr. Robert Mealey.)

Abortion

Nocardia spp. have been recorded among the genital flora of clinically healthy mares.[48] *Nocardia* spp. have been associated with sporadic abortions in cattle and swine but rarely are associated with abortion in horses.[30] Bolon et al.[29] reported two cases of abortion in an Arabian and a Thoroughbred mare during the sixth gestational month. Both mares had a history of repeated failure to carry foals to term and were apparently healthy. Fetal necropsies revealed lesions in lung, liver, and placenta. The chorion was mottled, white and red, opaque, and in the Arabian fetus, avillar. Filamentous bacilli within the lungs of both fetuses, the liver of the Arabian, and the chorion of the Thoroughbred were gram positive, silver positive, and acid-fast positive. *Nocardia asteroides* was cultured from the uterus of the Arabian mare.[30]

Nocardioform placentitis is the term used to describe a distinct type of placentitis of horses that was first diagnosed in 1986 at the University of Kentucky, Livestock Disease Diagnostic Center[47] (see Chapter 8). Although similar to members of the genus *Nocardia* in morphology, the cause of this condition is the gram-positive, branching, filamentous bacterium *Crossiella equi*, a microorganism unrelated to *Nocardia*.[25,54] Recently, another filamentous actinomycete, *Cellulosimicrobium (Cellumonas) cellulans* (formerly *Oerskovia xanthineolytica*), has also been associated with nocardioform placentitis.[50]

Pathologic Findings

Nocardiosis is a predominantly suppurative process, but granulomatous or mixed responses may occur. Tissue destruction with the formation of abscesses is characteristic of all clinical forms of nocardial disease.[27,37,38,43] Exudates are sanguinopurulent and sometimes may contain small (<1 mm in diameter), soft granules consisting of bacteria, neutrophils, and debris.[25] *Nocardia asteroides* is isolated most often from the lungs (Fig. 30-13). Other tissues from which *N. asteroides* has been isolated or identified are tracheal fluid, cornea, skin lesions, brain, spleen, peritoneal fluid, pleural fluid, lymph nodes, pericardial abscess, uterus, incision from repaired rectal tear, liver, and kidney.[30,31,51] Pulmonary lesions grossly resemble those described for nocardial infections in humans and other primates.[51] There may be necrotizing abscesses that are not encapsulated or sharply circumscribed, solitary masses, reticulonodular infiltrates, large irregular nodules (frequently with cavitation), interstitial infiltrate, and pleural effusion.[27] The most frequently observed change is fibrinohemorrhagic pleuritis.[51] Other gross and histopathologic findings may include necrosuppurative lymphadenitis, necrosuppurative nephritis and ulcerative suppurative dermatitis.[33]

Diagnosis

Confirmation of a diagnosis of nocardiosis depends on the cytologic and bacteriologic evaluation of appropriate specimens[38] (Fig. 30-14). Clinical laboratory findings are not specific and may include evidence of an inflammatory or infectious process as well as evidence of immunosuppression. Thus, lymphopenia, left shift, toxic neutrophils, neutrophilia, hyperfibrinogenemia, and hyperglobulinemia or hypoglobulinemia are possible.[26,51]

Direct Examination

Gram-stained smears of *Nocardia*-infected samples reveal rod-shaped to coccoid forms and gram-positive branching filaments. Most strains are partially acid-fast.[25,33,41] Gram staining is the most sensitive method by which to visualize and recognize nocardiae in clinical specimens.[38] Modified acid-fast

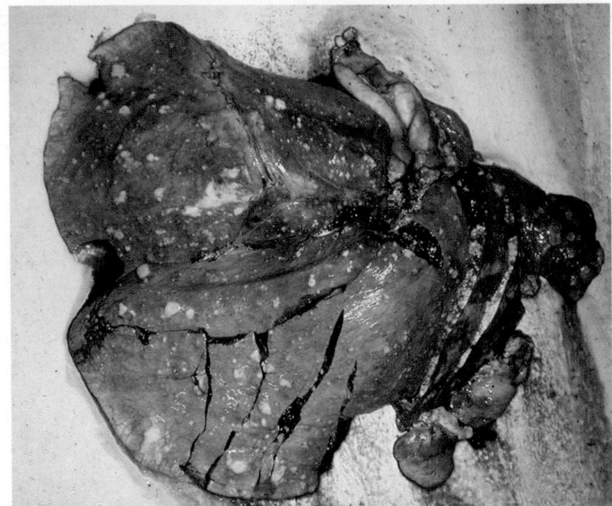

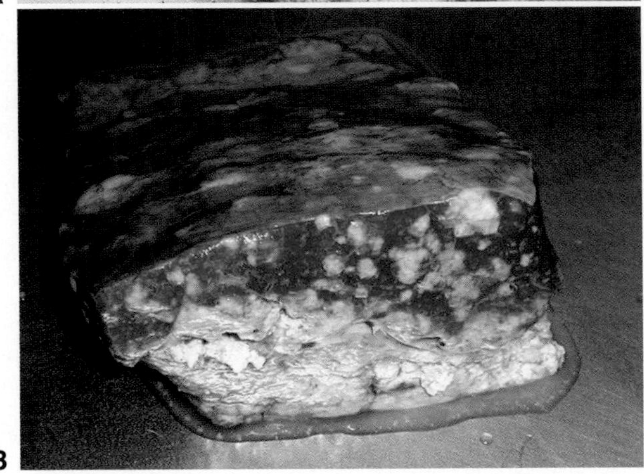

Fig. 30-13 A, Gross appearance of lungs of the horse described in Figure 30-11. Note the numerous areas of abscessation. B, Cut section through an affected area of lung. (Courtesy Dr. Robert Mealey.)

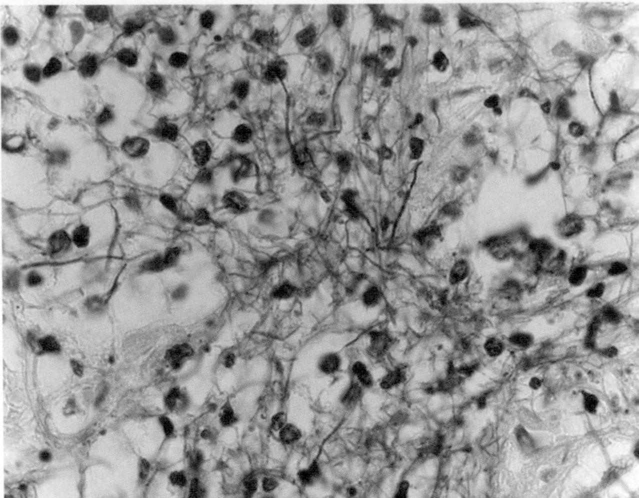

Fig. 30-14 Photomicrograph of lungs of the horse described in Figure 30-11. Note the numerous long, rod-shaped to filamentous bacteria typical of *Nocardia*. (Courtesy Dr. Robert Mealey.)

staining is not reliable (may vary with the strain and culture media used) and should be used only to confirm the acid fastness of organisms detected by Gram staining.[37,38]

Isolation and Identification

Standard collection and transport procedures suitable for bacterial and fungal cultures are adequate for isolation of *Nocardia* (see Chapters 27 and 49), but refrigeration of specimens should be avoided because some *Nocardia* strains lose viability at low temperatures.[25,37]

Serologic Testing

Major problems arise with developing serodiagnostic methods because the host infected with nocardiae usually develops a minimal, nonspecific antibody response.[27] Serologic tests (immunodiffusion, complement fixation, enzyme-linked immunosorbent assays) and cutaneous hypersensitivity tests using extracellular antigen to detect nocardial infection in cattle and dogs are of uncertain sensitivity and are not generally available.[25,38] Currently, no serodiagnostic test is routinely used to confirm nocardial infection in human patients.[27,37]

Molecular Identification

Conventional methods for identification of *Nocardia* spp. (growth characteristics, colony and microscopic morphology, biochemical and antimicrobial susceptibility testing) are insufficient to distinguish among some members of the *N. asteroides* complex.[25,27,33,36-38] At present, molecular methods used to identify the nocardiae to the species level include restriction endonuclease analysis of an amplified portion of the 16S ribosomal ribonucleic acid (rRNA) gene, polymerase chain reaction (PCR)–restriction endonuclease analysis of the amplified 65 *hsp* gene, and sequencing methodologies (e.g., of 16S rRNA or DNA).[25,38,52] An experimental study demonstrated that the diagnosis of nocardiosis by seminested PCR in mice is a rapid and more sensitive test than culture for detection of *Nocardia* in blood and different visceral organs. This method has the additional advantage over culture techniques of being able to detect L-forms of *Nocardia* in clinical specimens, which otherwise fail to grow on routine isolation medium.[53]

Therapy

Clinical experience has shown that successful therapy of nocardiosis requires the use of antimicrobial drug(s) in combination with appropriate surgical drainage.[37,39] When possible, abscesses, empyemas, and serosal effusions are treated by surgical debridement, drainage, and lavage. Granulomatous proliferations require excision.[25,26,33,37] Initial selection of a therapeutic regimen should take into account the site and severity of infection, host immune status, potential drug interactions or toxicity, and the species of *Nocardia*. Antimicrobial susceptibility testing is recommended as a guide to therapy, but such testing may be misleading, and discrepancies between in vitro data and clinical outcome are well documented.[33,37,38]

In horses the selection of antibiotic and duration of therapy are based on human medicine. In people, sulfa-containing antimicrobials are the treatment of choice for nocardiosis caused by *N. brasiliensis* and *N. asteroides* complex and have resulted in substantial improvement in outcome.[28,33,37-39] In human patients with primary cutaneous infection, trimethoprim-sulfa is sufficient in combination with appropriate surgical debridement. In severely ill or immunosuppressed patients, two or more drugs, which usually include a sulfa-containing agent, are frequently prescribed despite a lack of clinical data supporting the efficacy of combination therapy.[37,38] Amikacin has been used successfully, usually in combination with other agents, including sulfonamides, in patients with nocardiosis involving several different body sites and in immunocompromised patients. Synergy between trimethoprim-sulfa and amikacin has been demonstrated in vitro.[37] Other potentially efficacious choices include amoxicillin-clavulanate, third-generation cephalosporins, newer macrolides, imipenem, and other aminoglycosides.[37-39]

Clinical improvement is generally evident within 5 to 10 days after initiation of therapy.[37] In human medicine, recommendations on the duration of therapy are empiric and based on reports of relapse after sulfonamide therapy of different duration. Long-term antimicrobial treatment (6-12 months) may be necessary to avoid relapses.[26,33,37,38,43] The clinical outcome depends on the site and extent of disease and underlying host factors.[28] For horses with pulmonary and disseminated nocardiosis, the prognosis is poor because most of these patients are severely immunocompromised or debilitated. Prognosis is usually good in patients with only skin involvement.[31]

Public Health Considerations

As noted earlier, intestinal nocardiosis in humans may result from ingestion of the organism.[27,34] Transmission between or among animals and persons has not been demonstrated.[26,37,38] Nocardiosis is not considered a zoonotic disease.[33]

ANTHRAX

Maureen T. Long

Bacillus anthracis has a special place in world history and microbiology because anthrax was the first disease for which a causal relationship to a bacterium was demonstrated.[54-56] In 1877, Robert Koch injected a pure culture of sporulated organisms into animals and caused lethal anthrax. In 1881, Pasteur successfully demonstrated the ability of attenuated organisms to protect sheep from clinical anthrax. Before the widespread availability of a vaccine in the 1930s, anthrax was one of the most important causes of mortality in herbivores worldwide.

Etiology

Bacillus anthracis is a large, gram-positive rod (3-5 μm long) that forms spores and is cultivated both aerobically and anaerobically. This organism is often confused with *Bacillus cereus* and must be differentiated by morphologic and biochemical characteristics.[54] Specifically, *B. anthracis* is nonhemolytic, has a capsule, and is nonmotile.[54,57] Gamma phage will lyse the organism, and *B. anthracis* is positive on a "string of pearls" test.[54,58]

Epidemiology

Bacillus anthracis has a vegetative and a spore state.[54,60] Classic theory maintains that sporulation provides a state of low nutrient requirement for the organism, allowing maintenance in the environment, usually soil, for decades.[60-62] In general, spores can survive temperature extremes and favor alkaline conditions. They also survive tanning and processing of hides.[60]

The most common route of natural infection for animals is thought to be ingestion, but inhalation and skin penetration may also occur.[62] There may be concomitant damage to mucous membranes. Mechanical infection by biting flies has been demonstrated experimentally; this transmission likely occurs seasonally in areas with high incidence and has been particularly associated with outbreaks of anthrax in wildlife in Russia and Australia.[60,63-66] Climatic stressors allow reliable prediction of anthrax outbreaks.[60,63,65,67-69]

With climatic change, outbreaks of anthrax occur in infection cycles. A harbinger of infection occurs with the sudden death of one or two animals that have been recently introduced into an area.[54,62] These infected carcasses contaminate the soil with *B. anthracis*.[59,61,63,66,68-72] The next or secondary infection cycle involves multiple animals who develop anthrax after exposure to contaminated soil (or carcasses).

Anthrax is a reportable disease in the United States; suspected or confirmed cases must be reported to the state veterinarian. In addition, *B. anthracis* is listed as a Category A bioterrorism agent. Although the fall of 2001 focused attention on human anthrax and this organism as a terror threat, animal anthrax has always been present in the United States.[60,68,69,73] In fact, 2000 and 2001 were banner years for anthrax in animals (www.aphis.usda.gov). In 2000 the North Dakota Red River Valley (80 horses and cows), South Dakota (9), Nevada (32 cows), and Minnesota (10 cows) had animal losses to anthrax. In Nebraska, several cattle deaths were suspected to result from anthrax. In June through October 2001 and 2002, deaths were reported in cattle, deer, bison, water buffalo, and elk in Texas, South Dakota, Minnesota, North Dakota, and California. Texas reported 1638 animal cases of anthrax in 2001. In 2005, 109 cases of animal anthrax cases were confirmed in 16 North Dakota counties.* The Ames strain isolated from human outbreaks originates from a trail that crosses West Texas to Mexico in which the soil is heavily laden with *B. anthracis*.

Animal and human anthrax has a worldwide occurrence, and only notable recent reports are reviewed here. A large seasonal outbreak occurred in western Alberta, Canada, in 1999.[63,67] The outbreak was widespread, affecting seven cattle farms. One horse also died due to anthrax. This outbreak resulted in movement restrictions and vaccination of 650 livestock on the identified farms and 25,000 animals in the surrounding vicinity. More than 1585 bison carcasses were disposed of during 11 outbreaks that occurred in Alberta and adjacent territories.[63]

Since 1950 the U.S. Centers for Disease Control and Prevention (CDC) has been involved in the investigation of numerous anthrax outbreaks involving animals in Texas, North Dakota, Iowa, Pennsylvania, Louisiana, Wyoming, California, Connecticut, North Dakota, Missouri, New Jersey, Oklahoma, and Ohio.[60] Infection has likely occurred in many other states with animal infection only reported locally.

Risk factors associated with recent outbreaks have been identified.† In the Alberta outbreak, old anthrax graves and weather patterns were highly associated with occurrence. There was a long, dry spring followed by heavy rainfall. In this and other studies, farms with poor drainage and soil with a high degree of organic content were involved, rather than arid soil with minimal vegetative support.[68,69,76,77] During an outbreak, *B. anthracis* is found throughout the epizootic environment. Besides soil, positive samples have included hay, biting flies, and feed (from contaminated bone meal). *B. anthracis* may undergo rounds of germination and sporulation depending on soil conditions. An outbreak of anthrax in the Yamal peninsula identified blood-sucking insects and organic substances in the soil as risk factors for recurring outbreaks. Only vaccination in this region actually breaks the cycle of high numbers of wild ungulates and livestock developing disease.

Pathogenesis

The mammalian incubation period is 1 to 7 days for respiratory and gastrointestinal (GI) anthrax.[54,62,78,79] Susceptibility to disease is greatest for cattle, followed by sheep, then horses and goats.[62] These differences in susceptibility may result from

*www.agdepartment.com/Progarms/lavistock/BOAH/2005 Anthrax.pdf.

†References 56, 59, 60, 63, 65-69, 71, 72, 74, 75.

differences in oral and GI physiology and frequency of transmission. Pigs frequently develop clinical anthrax after exposure to *B. anthracis* but are the only species that may spontaneously recover (many still die).[75,80]

Ingestion is likely the primary route of inoculation for most animals; a break in the mucous membranes is considered important for development of disease.[56,81] There is an initial round of primary replication in the regional lymph nodes.[62] The organism enters the bloodstream through lymphatic drainage, with resultant bacteremia, septicemia, toxemia, and dissemination to all major organs. Proliferation of lethal toxin is considered the primary cause of death.

Classically, three clinical forms of anthrax are described in animals and people. *Cutaneous* disease is most often observed in people working with animal hides and hair contaminated with *B. anthracis* spores.[60,81,82] This form results in gelatinous edema, which leads to a "malignant pustule." After a necrotic ulcer forms, the organism can disseminate to give rise to classic septicemia, which is usually fatal. *Pulmonary* anthracic disease is common in people or animals that inhale spores.[78,79,83-85] An acute hemorrhagic mediastinitis occurs that is rapidly fatal. Cattle and other animals may inhale spores in dusty environments, leading to a vegetative state and localized pulmonary infection that eventually disseminates. *Gastrointestinal* disease occurs from oral ingestion. In people, confinement of infection to the GI tract is rare.[62] A process similar to cutaneous infection occurs, except that the mucosa is the site for invasion, pustule formation, and ulceration. This infection has an extremely high mortality rate.

The ability of *B. anthracis* to evade the immune system, undergo rapid vegetative proliferation, and elaborate toxin are critical steps in the pathogenesis of anthrax.[86,87] The bacterium has a poly-D-glutamyl capsule that protects against complement and phagocytosis.[57,88] Anthrax toxin has three components: *protective antigen* (PA), *lethal factor* (LF), and *edema factor* (EF).[86,87,89] The toxin uses the PA molecule to bind to the cell surface; because PA is important in binding, antibodies that recognize this protein usually neutralize the activity of toxins.[80,89,90] LF is required to mediate the fatal effect of *B. anthracis*. EF is required for extravasation of intercellular fluids into subcutaneous and peritoneal compartments and interstitial spaces on infection with *B. anthracis*. This toxin is an adenylate cyclase protein. Different combinations of these toxins lead to specific manifestations of pathology.[86,87] The combination of PA and LF must be present for lethality. If EF and PA are complexed, these proteins produce edema. When all three toxin components are present, the organism causes necrosis of cells with edema and is lethal.

Clinical Findings

Most of the clinical signs of anthrax, other than sudden death, have been described in cattle, the species in which anthrax is most frequently reported.* Most natural cases of anthrax in horses are associated with disease in cattle. A peracute form of anthrax is most often observed early in an outbreak. Cattle are either found dead or with premonitory signs of fever (lasting 1-2 hours), muscle tremors, dyspnea, and congestion of the mucous membranes, followed by collapse and death with discharge of bloody fluid from nostrils, mouth, anus, and vulva. Animals with acute disease have a high fever lasting approximately 48 hours, increased heart rate, anorexia, and ruminal stasis. Animals are severely depressed with congested mucous membranes. Abortions can occur, or if lactating, blood-stained milk may be observed. In cattle, bloody diarrhea is common. Edema of the head, limbs, and perineum occurs. Terminally, affected animals collapse and die.

Although not as frequently diagnosed with *B. anthracis* infection as cattle, horses do develop disease and die from anthrax.* After an incubation period of about 3 to 7 days (can be as short as 1 day or as long as 7 days), horses usually develop the acute form of anthrax, although sudden death may occur. Initial clinical signs frequently include colic, with presenting signs that may resemble those of acute enteritis. These horses progress to high fever with dyspnea. Subcutaneous edema of the ventral neck, thorax, and abdomen may be seen, especially with mediastinal involvement. Ventral edema involving the prepuce and mammary gland is postulated to be secondary to local transmission from insects.

Pigs frequently acquire infection as a result of being fed infected carcasses.[54,75,92] Although they can demonstrate the same clinical signs as cattle with anthrax, pigs usually have a characteristic edema of the throat and head, often severe enough to obstruct the airway and throat. A blood-stained, frothy discharge occurs from the nose or mouth. There are petechial hemorrhages of the skin.

Diagnosis

Clinical Pathology

Because sudden death or a short course of fatal disease is the hallmark of anthrax, blood testing from affected horses or any other livestock species is extremely uncommon.[54,92,93] Should one have the unfortunate experience of examining a blood smear, an extremely high level of bacteremia is the most notable observation. Aspirated edema fluid also contains organisms. A new methylene blue stain performed on blood or edema fluid demonstrates chains of vegetative cells that are large, square, gram-positive rods. The nonstaining internal spores are centrally located with an ellipsoid shape.

Diagnostic Testing

If a sample for culture is obtained, initial identification of *B. anthracis* is through the basic microbiologic features discussed earlier. Much safer for laboratory personnel is the inoculation of guinea pigs for lethality or fluorescent antibody testing of smears of froth, blood, or splenic aspirate.[94] Serologic and molecular-based techniques are important for identification of the specific strain of *B. anthracis*.[92,94-96] Strain typing to determine the origin of exposure in people is a priority when bioterrorism is suspected. Molecular-based techniques have been developed for environmental monitoring and likely pose an alternative to inadvertent culture of body fluids.

Treatment

Usually, anthrax is rapidly fatal in horses, and it is unlikely that there would be an opportunity for therapy of an animal showing clinical signs at diagnosis. Careful examination of other exposed animals for disease should be performed. Close monitoring of any exposed horses may result in timely administration of antimicrobial agents. Antimicrobials recommended for prevention and treatment of anthrax include penicillin, tetracyclines, and fluoroquinolones.[54,60,97,98] Recent outbreaks in people support the use of fluoroquinolones as a first-line antimicrobial in suspected *B. anthracis* infection.[98,99] Intravenous administration is highly recommended. Single or short-duration administration of prophylactic antibiotics is recommended for exposed people and is an option for horses.[99] Supportive care is essential and consists of cardiovascular support in the form of fluid and oncotic therapy. Intranasal oxygen may alleviate signs of dyspnea.

*References 61, 62, 65, 68, 69, 71, 73, 91.

*References 61, 62, 68, 69, 71, 73, 91.

Pathologic Findings

If an animal dies of disease consistent with anthrax in an endemic area, it is best not to open the carcass.* Not only is this important for human safety, but it is also exceptionally important for long-term control by minimizing environmental contamination. Collection of blood in a closed system or a splenic aspirate obtained percutaneously is recommended to facilitate confirmation of the diagnosis. Blood clots poorly in affected animals, and thus a sample may be obtained for an extended time after death.

The pathologic hallmark of anthrax is the absence of rigor mortis, with passage of blood from body orifices.[62,79,83,84,101] Blood from these sites and blood drawn at the time of death fails to clot. Petechiae and ecchymoses are widespread, with large quantities of blood-stained serous fluid within body cavities. Severe mediastinal edema, enteritis, and splenomegaly are common. In particular, the spleen has a "blackberry jam" appearance.

Prevention

Although not routinely available in the United States, vaccines are available for prevention of anthrax in cattle in other countries.[91,99,102-105] Use of cattle vaccines in horses is controversial and is not recommended in the guidelines of the American Association of Equine Practitioners. Injection site reactions and severe edema after vaccination have been described. However, immunoprophylaxis has been demonstrated as useful in cattle and experimental models of disease.† If disease and subsequent exposure to *B. anthracis* are identified or suspected in horses, methods should be implemented to prevent additional disease in horses and to minimize risk of human disease. Animals should have all external debris removed by thorough bathing with soap and water. If there is gross contamination of an animal, a 0.5% hypochlorite solution can be used. The efficacy of a chlorhexidine scrub for decontamination of animal hair is unknown. Animals should be moved immediately away from sites that have been exposed to anthrax-laden carcasses.

Maintenance of the vegetative state is essential for carcass disposal.[63,70,100,108] In its vegetative form, *B. anthracis* is quite labile;[54] the putrefactive process actually destroys most bacteria within the carcass. Site contamination comes from body fluids that, on exposure to air, allow sporulation of bacteria in these samples.

Some controversy surrounds the optimal methods of disposal of anthrax-suspect carcasses. The World Health Organization (WHO) recommends incineration of closed carcasses as the best method. The alternative to this is heat treatment or rendering of closed carcasses. Burial is considered the final choice in disposition and should occur quickly with minimal damage to the carcass. Veterinarians and public health professionals are key personnel in determining whether or not a specific method is appropriate in a given situation.

Several factors should be considered if carcasses are to be incinerated. The most important aspect is ensuring complete incineration, including the ventral parts of the carcass.[70] The soil from the site can be burned separately from the carcass or actually torched. Controversy exists as to whether or not there are bacteria in the "updrafts" of the burned carcasses; however, most microbiologists and public health agencies discount this as a true risk for human disease or bacterial dissemination. *B. anthracis* has been isolated from the ashes of incinerators, but bacterial counts are very low and associated with poor incinerator hygiene.

Rendering, done properly, is analogous to autoclaving. In the nonsporulated state, this organism is susceptible. However, the processing step could result in exposure of the carcass to air. The carcass must be "broken" down in a closed system for best practices. All wastewater must be autoclaved.

Burial must be deep so that scavengers do not disturb the bodies before putrefaction has occurred. If spores are buried, climatic, geologic, animal, and human upheavals can result in exposure years later if a burial site is disturbed.

Public Health Considerations

The zoonotic risk of *B. anthracis* cannot be minimized, and the occupational risk of exposure in veterinarians is very high compared with the risk of intentional human-to-human transmission.[56,59,60,81] Personal protection when handling anthrax-suspect animals should be complete, including gloves, boots, protective suits, and respiratory and eye protection. This protection must be maintained throughout all environmental and equipment decontamination processes. Complete bathing is recommended after handling any tissues or animals. In some situations, prophylactic antibiotic therapy is recommended if exposure is thought to be high or inadvertent through improper attention to personal protection. Animal hide, hair, and wool can contain spores, and people at occupational risk should seek immediate medical attention if skin or respiratory signs occur. Considerations of *B. anthracis* as a bioterrorist agent are discussed elsewhere.[92,95,103]

ENTEROCOCCAL INFECTIONS

Debra C. Sellon and J. Lindsay Oaks

Enterococci are gram-positive bacteria that occur singly, in clusters, or in chains. In 1984 the new genus *Enterococcus* was proposed to include the genera *Streptococcus faecalis* and *S. faecium*.[109] There are now at least 23 species classified in the genus *Enterococcus*. Enterococci are more hardy and environmentally resistant than the streptococci, growing at temperatures ranging from 10° to 45° C (50°–113° F) and surviving for as long as 30 minutes at 60° C (140° F). They can grow in solutions up to 6.5% NaCl and at a pH of 9.6.[110]

Enterococci are normal commensal flora of the GI tract of humans and many animal species. Although present at comparatively low numbers (<1% of total adult human intestinal microflora), they are important medically because of their growing significance as nosocomial pathogens.[111-113] They are the third most common isolate from human blood infections,[114] the most frequent isolate from surgical site infections in intensive care units,[115] and the second most common nosocomial pathogen in the United States.[116]

Enterococci have been identified as the cause of numerous types of opportunistic infections in horses and other domestic animals. However, at least at this time, equine enterococcal infections are typically sporadic. Most enterococcal strains encountered in veterinary medicine are not especially virulent, are associated with low morbidity and mortality, do not exhibit high-level resistance to antimicrobials, and are not related to outbreaks of nosocomial strains. Often, their isolation from culture of clinical samples is clinically irrelevant because the organism is merely present as an environmental contaminant rather than as a causal pathogen for infection.

At least five factors might contribute to the establishment of *Enterococcus* as a nosocomial pathogen in a patient: (1) the ability to acquire or develop resistance to many common antimicrobial drugs; (2) the ability to transfer this resistance to other, more pathogenic organisms; (3) the presence of a variety of virulence factors; (4) access to an extraintestinal site; and (5) the transmission of enterococci by the hands of health care workers or through other fomites. Growing evidence indicates that a subset of enterococcal strains may be particularly

*References 59, 60, 64-66, 68-70, 73, 100.
†References 80, 91, 99, 102, 103, 105-107.

virulent and have the propensity to cause outbreaks of nosocomial disease within health care facilities. Surface virulence factors, such as aggregation substance, Ace (adhesin of collagen of *E. faecalis*), *E. faecalis* adhesion molecule, and enterococcal surface protein, may facilitate the binding of enterococci to epithelial surfaces, and the formation of vegetative lesions and may contribute to pathogenicity.[111,113] Putative secreted virulence factors include cytolysin/hemolysin and gelatinase.[113] At this time the significance of these virulence factors in vivo is uncertain because their presence does not seem to correlate with isolates from patients who have died because of enterococcal infections.[112,117,118] Antimicrobial resistance and the ability to survive in a variety of environments make enterococcal organisms particularly suited to establishment of nosocomial infections.[111]

As a group, the enterococci are intrinsically resistant to many antimicrobial agents typically used in veterinary medicine, including penicillins, cephalosporins, and low concentrations of aminoglycosides. The low level of intrinsic resistance to aminoglycosides is the result of an inability of the drug to cross the enterococcal cell membrane.[111] As a result, combination therapy with a β-lactam and an aminoglycoside is synergistic and frequently efficacious clinically. Currently, in routine antimicrobial susceptibility testing, most equine isolates are susceptible to ampicillin and resistant to aminoglycosides (because of low-level intrinsic resistance). Based on the recommendations for treatment of enterococcal infections in humans,[119] for ampicillin-susceptible enterococcal isolates, monotherapy with ampicillin is likely to be effective for superficial infections (e.g., urinary tract, soft tissue) in immunocompetent patients. However, for more serious infections (e.g., endocarditis, osteomyelitis) improved clinical responses are seen when the cell wall–active agents are combined with aminoglycosides. The β-lactam drug damages the bacterial cell membrane, facilitating uptake and microbicidal activity of the aminoglycoside.

In addition to their intrinsic antimicrobial resistance, enterococci are able to acquire genetic elements that confer high-level resistance to β-lactams, aminoglycosides, and glycopeptides (e.g., vancomycin). Vancomycin resistance was first reported in 1986 and has spread rapidly since that time.[120] In strains that exhibit high-level resistance to aminoglycosides, combination therapy with a β-lactam will not result in synergy, and there is no benefit from addition of aminoglycosides. Although no consensus exists on the optimal therapy of these resistant strains, high doses and continuous infusions of ampicillin or vancomycin are usually recommended. Therapy with cephalosporins and trimethoprim-sulfa combinations is generally ineffective against enterococci regardless of their in vitro susceptibility profiles. Acquired resistance to chloramphenicol, fluoroquinolones, rifampin, and tetracyclines is common, and these drugs appear to be only bacteriostatic and result in poor clinical responses when used to treat serious enterococcal infections.[119]

LISTERIOSIS

Melissa T. Hines

Listeria monocytogenes is a bacterial pathogen of worldwide distribution that causes disease in humans and a variety of animal species. In veterinary species, listeriosis is of most importance in ruminants. Clinical disease is uncommon in horses, but sporadic cases of septicemia, encephalitis, abortion, and ocular disease have been reported. Because of the small number of equine cases, specific information on equine listeriosis is limited.

Listeria bacteria are gram-positive rods that are facultative anaerobes.[121] There are several species within the genus, and although *Listeria ivanovii* has occasionally been associated with abortion in ruminants, *L. monocytogenes* is considered the only species of major clinical significance. Based on somatic and flagellar antigens, 16 serotypes of *L. monocytogenes* have been identified, with almost all cases of animal and human infection being caused by serotypes 1/2a, 1/2b, 4a, and 4b.[121,122]

Listeria monocytogenes is ubiquitous in the environment and has been found in a variety of samples, such as soil, water, vegetation, and silage.[121,122] The organism is frequently shed in the feces of carrier animals, and although information in horses is limited, in one study in Germany, approximately 5% of horses shed *L. monocytogenes*.[123] Fecal contamination is generally thought to be the most common source of the organism, but *L. monocytogenes* can also be found in urine, uterine discharge, aborted fetal tissues, and milk. In the environment the organism can survive for long periods, multiplying in a wide range of environmental conditions, including temperatures of 4° to 45° C (39°–113° F).[121,122] The organism can grow over a pH range of 5 to 9, often reaching high numbers in poorly preserved silage or decaying vegetation when the pH rises above 5.4. The association between clinical listeriosis and silage in ruminants has resulted in the disease sometimes being referred to as "silage disease." Similarly, in Iceland, an association is believed to exist between listeriosis in horses and feeding silage.[124] In three foals with listeriosis, however, none of the foals or their dams had been fed silage, and the source of infection was undetermined.[125]

The most common route of infection in listeriosis is ingestion, although infection may also occur through the nasal mucosa, conjunctiva, or wound contamination.[121,122] Some proposed routes of infection in neonatal foals include ingestion from the environment or infected mare's milk, inhalation, through the umbilical remnant, and transplacental infection.[125-128] *L. monocytogenes* is an opportunistic pathogen, and clinical disease is thought to occur when the host's resistance is decreased as a result of stress factors such as concurrent disease, climate, pregnancy, a large infective dose, or immunodeficiency. Although no specific risk factors have been identified in most equine cases, meningoencephalitis and septicemia caused by *L. monocytogenes* were reported in an Arabian foal with combined immunodeficiency, and *Listeria* keratitis was reported in a horse previously treated with topical corticosteroids.[129,130]

Listeria monocytogenes is a facultative intracellular organism that invades both phagocytic and nonphagocytic cells. The organism can be found in multiple tissues but has a predilection for the intestinal tract wall, reproductive tissues, and medulla oblongata. A number of virulence factors are involved in the pathogenesis of listerial infection, including listeriolysin O, a hemolysin that allows the internalized listeriae to escape from the phagosome. Once within the cytoplasm, the listeriae proliferate and induce polymerization of host cell actin, which ultimately serves to move the bacilli toward the cell's periphery, where projections of the infected cell's cytoplasmic membrane invaginate into adjacent cells, allowing the listeriae to enter that cell directly. As with many intracellular organisms, immunity to *L. monocytogenes* is thought to be primarily mediated by cellular responses.[121,122]

Listeria monocytogenes has been reported as an uncommon cause of septicemia and systemic disease in foals from birth to 5 months of age and in adult horses.[124-129,131,132] Clinical signs include depression, anorexia, fever, diarrhea, and abdominal pain. Weakness, seizures, ataxia, jaundice, and respiratory distress have been reported as well. Abortion resulting from *L. monocytogenes* has also been reported in mares.[133,134] Bacterial ulcerative keratitis has been described in two equine cases;[130,135] these horses showed no evidence of concurrent systemic listerial infection. In most other species, ocular listerial infection is usually associated with other forms of infection, such as meningoencephalitis, but primary corneal infection has been reported.[135-137]

Diagnosis of listeriosis is generally established by microbiologic culture.[121] PCR has also been described but has not been used in horses.[138,139] Cytologic examination of a direct smear from infected tissue, such as corneal scrapings or aborted tissue, may reveal gram-positive rods consistent with *Listeria*.[121,130] At necropsy, histopathology, culture, and immunohistochemistry can be helpful in establishing a diagnosis.[121,126] It may be difficult to culture organisms from the brain in neural listeriosis, presumably because the organisms are intracellular and present in low numbers. In general, serology had not been useful in the diagnosis of listeriosis because of both the prevalence of positive titers in healthy animals and the cross-reactions with other organisms.[121,140,141]

Listeria monocytogenes is typically susceptible to many antibiotics. However, isolates from a corneal scraping and from blood cultures from three foals were all resistant to ceftiofur.[125,130] The isolates from the foals were susceptible to several antibiotics, including amikacin, gentamicin, ampicillin, penicillin, cephalothin, chloramphenicol, amoxicillin with clavulanate, doxycycline, erythromycin, rifampin, and trimethoprim-sulfamethoxazole.[125] Because of the limited number of cases, it is difficult to give an accurate prognosis, but some foals and adults with clinical listeriosis have responded to systemic antibiotic therapy.[124-129,131,132] Listerial keratitis has resolved after topical antibiotic therapy.[130,135]

Listeria monocytogenes is considered a zoonotic agent.[121,122] Clinical listeriosis in people occurs most often in pregnant women and immunocompromised patients. Possible sources for human infections include exposure to contaminated soil and food or to human and animal carriers. Most human epidemics have been traced to food sources of animal origin. In a study in Brazil, 9 of 121 samples (7.4%) of horsemeat for human consumption were positive for *L. monocytogenes*.[142] Direct transmission from animals to people is uncommon.

REFERENCES

See the CD-ROM for a list of references linked to the abstract in PubMed.

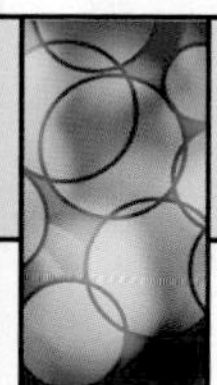

CHAPTER • 31

Dermatophilosis

Rosanna Marsella

Dermatophilosis is a common pustular and crusting skin disease of horses caused by *Dermatophilus congolensis*.[1] Various names have been used to describe this disease in horses, including streptothricosis, cutaneous actinomycosis, rain rot, mud fever, and dew poisoning.

ETIOLOGY AND EPIDEMIOLOGY

Dermatophilus is a gram-positive, non–acid-fast, facultative anaerobic, branching actinomyces.[2] Genotypic and phenotypic variation between isolates has been demonstrated.[3-5] *Dermatophilus* has a distinct life cycle and exists in two morphologic forms, hyphae and zoospores.[6,7] *Hyphae* are composed of filaments that break into coccoid cells. These cells mature into flagellated *zoospores*, which represent the infective stage.[8]

The natural habitat of *Dermatophilus* is unknown.[1,9] Many attempts to isolate the organism from the soil have failed,[10] even when soil samples were collected from the immediate environment of diseased animals.[11] In one study, however, *Dermatophilus* was isolated from the soil, and its survival appeared to depend on the type of soil and the water content.[12] Organic matter has a protective effect on the microorganism. Because the pathogenicity of *Dermatophilus congolensis* was preserved in soil, it is hypothesized that soil could act as a temporary reservoir for the organism. *Dermatophilus* can also survive in the skin of animals that are clinically normal, potentially acting as source of infection once favorable conditions are present.[13,14] Crusts from affected animals represent an important source of contagion for spreading lesions on the same animal and possibly the infection of other animals in the same herd.[15]

PATHOGENESIS

Establishment of infection with *D. congolensis* appears to depend on a variety of factors, including the virulence of the strain, the general health of the animal, skin trauma, and moisture.[16] Zoospores germinate, producing hyphae under favorable conditions. Hyphae penetrate the epidermis and spread from the initial area, triggering an inflammatory response.[17,18] Coccal cells are released from crusts to establish new sites of infection.

Virulence of the Strain

Strain differences in virulence affect the ability of *D. congolensis* to establish infection in the host.[19-22] Isolates from the same animal species or from the same geographic location are not always closely related genetically.[23] More specifically, variability may be observed in hemolytic activity on blood agar,[24] phospholipases,[25] proteases and lipases,[4,26] mucoid nature of colonies, motility, flagella density and polarity, capsule width, restriction enzyme profiles of bacterial deoxyribonucleic acid (DNA), protein electropherotype, and carbohydrate content. Hemolytic activity and enzyme activity of proteins and lipids appear to be important determinants of infectivity.[5] *Dermatophilus* also produces ceramidases,[27] which are thought to play a role in the pathogenesis of the disease through their protective and cell regulatory functions in the epidermis.

The extracellular products of *Dermatophilus* have proteolytic activities,[28] including the ability to digest keratin, which could play an important role in the establishment of the infection.[29,30] Zoospores are the most likely source of extracellular proteases, and their ability to function at a wide pH range enables the bacterium to adjust to the pH variations of inflamed skin.[30] Because the stratum corneum is filled with lipids and proteins,[31] it is reasonable to speculate that *D. congolensis* may use lipases and proteases to penetrate this barrier. Proteases may have a role in acquisition of nutrients and may initiate or inactivate host inflammatory protease cascades or cytokines.

Skin Trauma and Insects

Dermatophilus is unable to infect intact skin but can readily infect traumatized skin.[32] Various insects and ticks play a role as vectors for the transmission of *Dermatophilus* and as causes of trauma, which makes the skin more susceptible to the infection.[33,34] The inflammatory response triggered by biting flies provides a suitable growth medium for *Dermatophilus*.

Climatic Conditions and Host Factors

Moisture causes the release of infective zoospores of *D. congolensis*,[1] with resultant increased incidence of this disease during wet seasons and heavy rainfall.[9,32,35,36] Rainfall contributes to the infection in several ways, such as increasing the population of hematophagous flies, which cause skin damage and initiate inflammation at feeding sites, and contributing to maceration, which decreases the barrier function of skin. Increased temperature and humidity have been hypothesized to play a role as well. Zoospores are attracted by low concentrations of carbon dioxide and repelled by high concentrations.[37]

Host factors that influence susceptibility to infection include poor body condition, malnutrition,[38-40] stressful conditions, and glucocorticoids.[41] Resistance in some animals may have a genetic component and appears to be associated with major histocompatibility complex (MHC) haplotypes and variation in serine composition.[37,42]

Immune Responses to *Dermatophilus*

Both humoral and cell-mediated responses are triggered by infection with *D. congolensis*.[43-47] Resistance to infection may be related to antibody production,[48] T-cell activation,[49] and nonspecific immune mechanisms, such as epidermal hyperproliferation and neutrophil chemotaxis.[50-52] Several reports, however, indicate that no correlation exists between serum antibodies and resistance[53,54] Therefore, it is likely that location of antibodies may be more important than serum titers.

As the hyphae of *D. congolensis* spread in the epidermis, antigens are released that are captured by Langerhans' cells and presented to T cells at the site of infection. Dense accumulations of mononuclear cells are found in infected skin. Chronic lesions contain both CD4+ and CD8+ T lymphocytes in equal proportions, whereas acute lesions on their way to resolution contain primarily CD4+ T cells.[55] Cytokines secreted by T cells may be responsible for epidermal proliferation.

CLINICAL FINDINGS

The clinical features of dermatophilosis are fairly characteristic.[56] The primary lesions are papules, which mature into pustules. Because pustules are transient, only epidermal collarettes and areas of focal alopecia are often seen (Fig. 31-1). Lesions easily become exudative, and hairs are matted together to form thick crusts in which the hairs are embedded[57] (Fig. 31-2). When crusts are removed, the underlying skin is often eroded, painful, and prone to bleeding (Fig. 31-3). Purulent exudate may be observed in active lesions, whereas chronic lesions tend to have dry crusts with more diffuse scaling and alopecia (Figs. 31-4 and 31-5).

The distribution of lesions is also characteristic of *Dermatophilus*.[58] The rump, dorsal thorax, and face are usually affected when lesions are triggered by heavy rainfall (Figs. 31-6 and 31-7). The saddle area may be most affected in

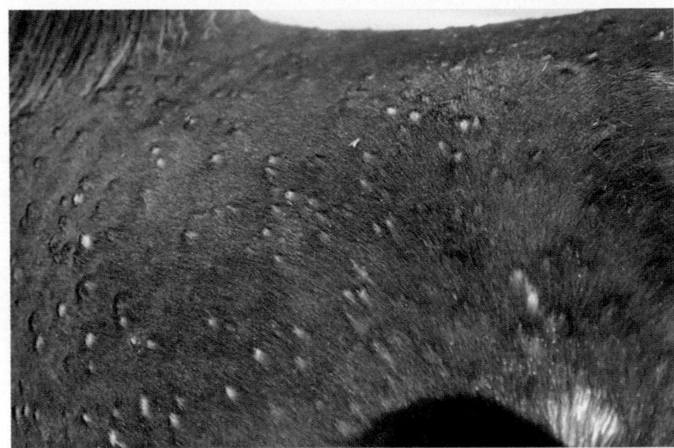

Fig. 31-1 Focal areas of alopecia on dorsal area of horse with dermatophilosis.

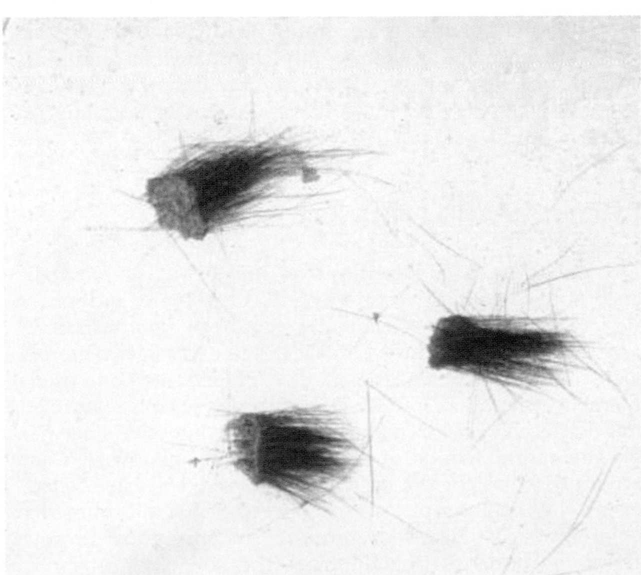

Fig. 31-2 Typical "paintbrush" appearance of crusts observed with dermatophilosis. The hairs are matted and become embedded in the crust.

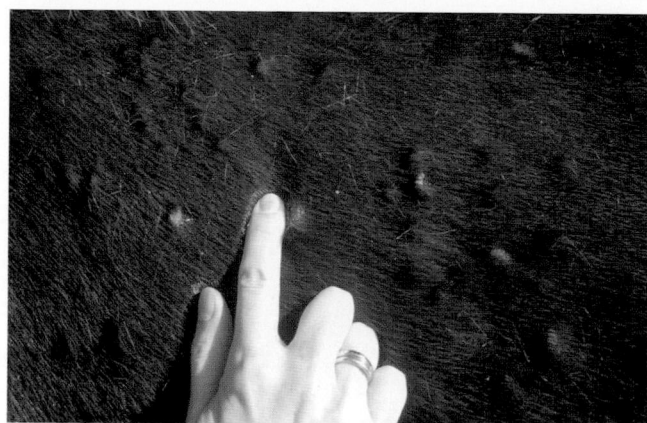

Fig. 31-3 Area underneath the crusts is often eroded and sensitive to the touch.

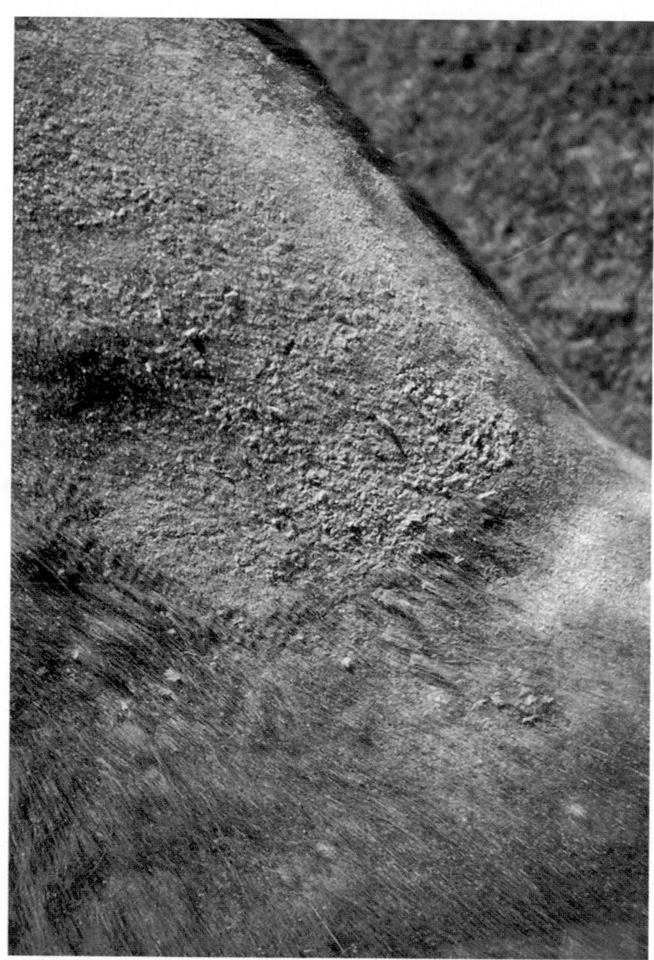

Fig. 31-4 Chronic dermatophilosis is characterized by dry skin and diffuse scaling.

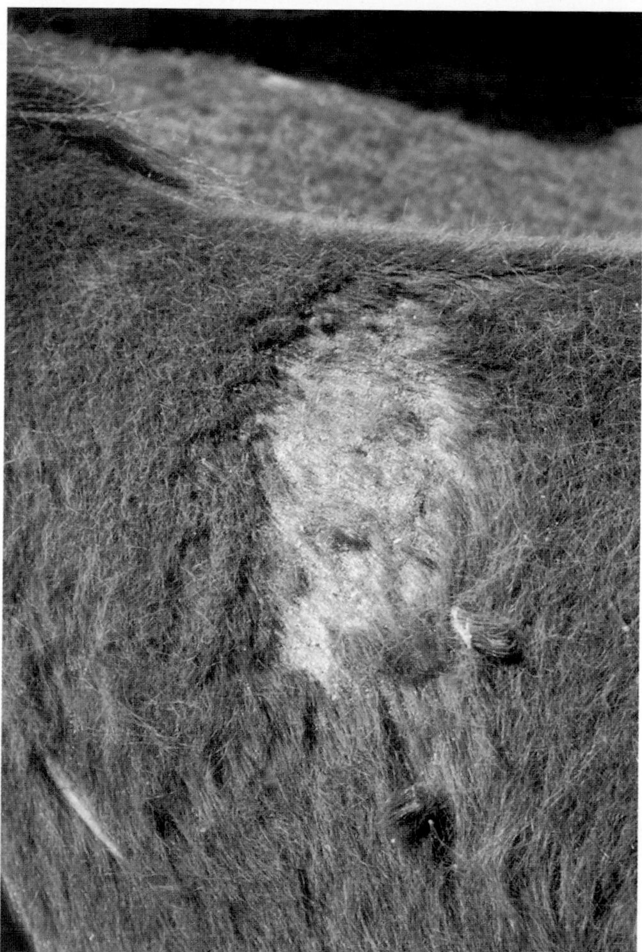

Fig. 31-5 Focal areas of alopecia coalesce to form more extensive alopecia and scaling in a horse with dermatophilosis.

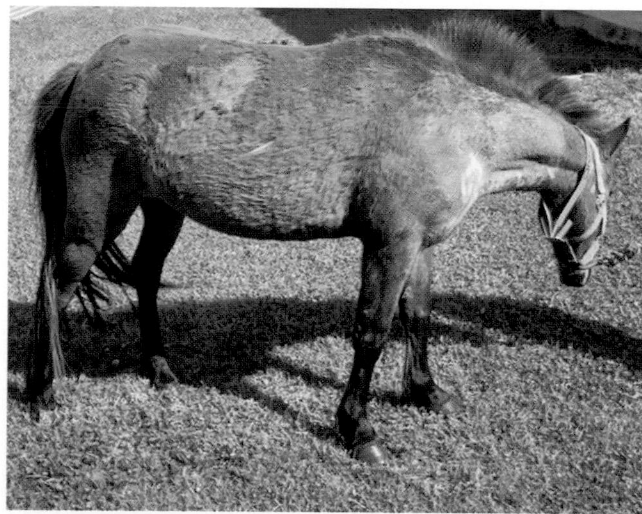

Fig. 31-6 The dorsum is often affected in horses that develop dermatophilosis after heavy rainfall.

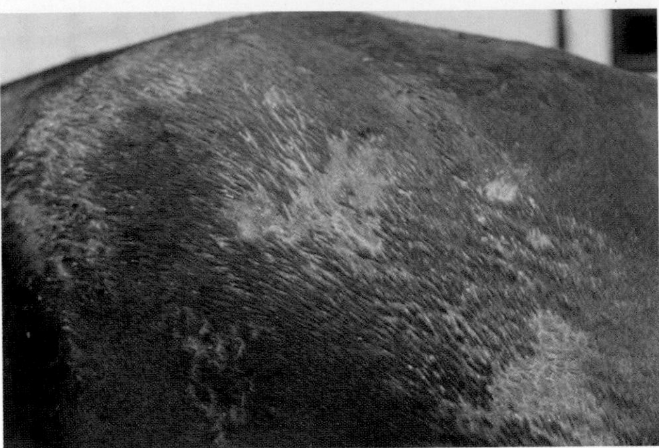

Fig. 31-7 The rump area may be affected by scaling and alopecia in a chronic case of dermatophilosis caused by excessive exposure to rain.

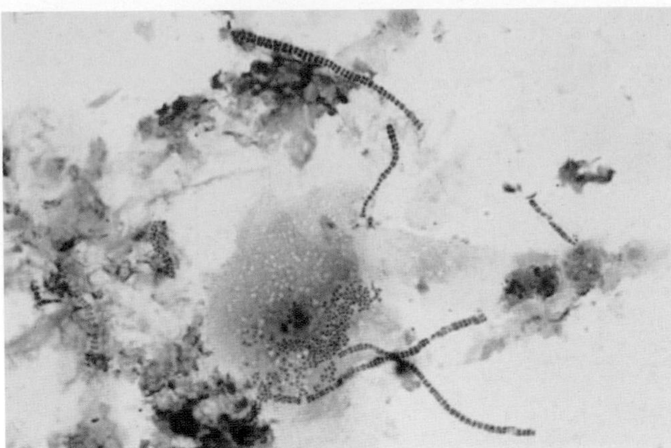

Fig. 31-8 *Dermatophilus congolensis* in cytologic preparation stained with Diff-Quik. Note the typical "railroad tracks" appearance of this bacterium.

horses, where trauma and moisture result from riding. In some horses, lesions are primarily found on the distal limbs (e.g., pasterns, coronets, heels). In these horses, lameness and edema may be present. Horses with white areas may develop severe erythema at these sites; photosensitization has been hypothesized to be involved in the pathogenesis of these lesions.

DIAGNOSIS

Diagnosis of dermatophilosis is based on suggestive history, typical clinical signs, and supportive cytology and histopathology, if necessary.[59] In horses with generalized distribution, bacterial folliculitis caused by *Staphylococcus*, dermatophytosis, demodicosis, pemphigus foliaceus, and generalized granulomatous disease should be considered as differential diagnoses.[60] Dermatophilosis involving distal limbs must be differentiated from contact dermatitis, contact photosensitization, atypical dermatophytosis, pastern folliculitis, and pastern leukocytoclastic vasculitis.

Cytology

For a definitive diagnosis, a portion of a crust should be minced and mixed with a few drops of water on a glass slide, air-dried, heat-fixed, Gram-stained, and examined microscopically. Touch preparations of the soaked undersurface of a new crust may also be useful to identify the organism. Diff-Quik can be used as a rapid staining technique to identify the organism. When present, *D. congolensis* is observed under oil immersion as branching organisms. The filaments can usually be seen dividing both transversely and longitudinally into thick bundles of coccoid forms (Fig. 31-8). In chronic cases, cytology may be negative, and it may be necessary to culture the organism.

Histology

Crusted lesions should be selected for biopsies, and care should be taken that crusts are sectioned and embedded, even when they lift off the biopsy, because the most characteristic microscopic feature is a stratified or layered crust. Crusts are made of alternating layers of parakeratotic and orthokeratotic keratin and accumulations of degenerating neutrophils.[61] Large numbers of organisms are usually present within the crust in acute cases. Severe epidermal hyperplasia, suppurative luminal folliculitis, intracellular edema, and perivascular infiltration of the dermis with neutrophils (especially in acute lesions), mononuclear cells, and plasma cells (especially in chronic lesions) are also often observed. Organisms are best visualized using Giemsa or Brown and Brenn stains.

Culture

Dermatophilus congolensis grows easily on blood agar when incubated at 37° C (98.6° F) with increased carbon dioxide. If severe secondary infection is present, other organisms may overgrow the plate, and special isolation techniques may be necessary.

THERAPY

One of the most important components of clinical management for horses with dermatophilosis is to keep animals dry. Most horses recover spontaneously within a month of being moved to a dry environment. Topical therapy is also important. Various products have been used for treatment of equine dermatophilosis. Benzoyl peroxide shampoos are antibacterial[62] and keratolytic, helping with the removal of crusts. Topical therapy should be applied at least once weekly. Shampoo should be allowed to contact the skin for 10 to 15 minutes. Excessive scrubbing should be discouraged because it leads to trauma in the hair follicles and increases the risk of furunculosis. It is important not to share grooming tools between affected and nonaffected horses to minimize spread of the organism. For localized lesions, topical mupirocin (Bactoderm), a drug with excellent antibacterial properties and skin penetration, may be used.[63,64]

Systemic antimicrobial therapy may be necessary for treatment of horses with severe or generalized dermatophilosis. *Dermatophilus congolensis* is usually sensitive to a variety of antibiotics,[65] including erythromycin, penicillin, sulfonamides, and gentamicin. Most often, penicillin (22,000 IU/kg) is used for short-term treatment, and trimethoprim-potentiated sulfonamides (15-20 mg/kg twice daily) are used for longer treatment periods (minimum treatment period of 3 weeks). Treatment should be extended 7 to 10 days past the clinical resolution of lesions to minimize the likelihood of a relapse. Horses should be monitored for development of colitis and bone marrow suppression. Unfortunately, previously infected animals may not develop immunity and may relapse when favorable conditions are present.

PREVENTION

The most effective method for prevention of equine dermatophilosis is to minimize exposure to excessive moisture and insects. Insect repellents (e.g., 2% permethrin, FlyPel) should be applied at least once daily in tropical climates where high humidity and rainfall are present. Topical antibacterial therapy with antibacterial shampoos (e.g., benzoyl peroxide) is also helpful to decrease the bacterial load on the skin.

PUBLIC HEALTH CONSIDERATIONS

Dermatophilosis is a rare zoonosis. In people it can cause pitted keratolysis, painful or pruritic folliculitis, or subcutaneous nodules.[66-68] Immunosuppressed individuals may be more susceptible to disease.[69]

REFERENCES

See the CD-ROM for a list of references linked to the abstract in PubMed.

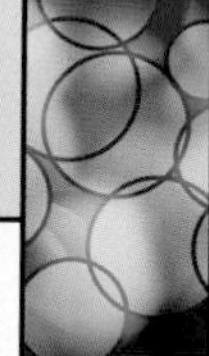

CHAPTER • 32

Rhodococcus equi

Melissa T. Hines

Rhodococcus equi infection was first described in horses in 1923.[1] It is now recognized worldwide as a major cause of disease in foals 3 weeks to 6 months of age. The most common clinical manifestation is *pyogranulomatous pneumonia*, although a variety of other clinical problems may be identified. The disease has the potential to cause significant losses, especially on farms where it is enzootic. Infrequently, *R. equi* causes infection in adult horses, generally thought to be associated with immunosuppression. *R. equi* has been isolated from a wide variety of species, including cats, dogs, goats, cattle, camelids, pigs, crocodiles, and other indigenous animals. Clinical disease is uncommon in these species, and infection is often localized. *R. equi* is now considered an important pathogen in immunocompromised human patients, particularly those infected with human immunodeficiency virus (HIV).

ETIOLOGY

Rhodococcus equi, previously known as *Corynebacterium equi* and *Mycobacterium equi*, is a facultative intracellular bacterium that resides within macrophages.[2,3] Rhodococci belong to the family *Nocardiaceae*, order Actinomycetales. *R. equi* is a pleomorphic, gram-positive organism with a rod-coccus life cycle.[2,4] Depending on growth conditions and the phase of the life cycle, it may appear either coccoid or as long rods or short filaments with rudimentary branching. The organism is aerobic, nonmotile, asporogenous, and partially acid-fast. In vitro, optimal growth occurs at 30° C (86° F) and at a pH between 7.0 and 7.5.[3,5]

Rhodococcus equi is a member of a unique phylogenetic group within the Actinomycetales, known as the *mycolata*.[2,6] This group contains a number of pathogenic genera in addition to *Rhodococcus*, including *Mycobacterium*, *Corynebacterium*, and *Nocardia*. The distinguishing feature of the mycolata is their distinct, lipid-rich cell envelope that contains mycolic acids, a large proportion of which are linked to the peptidoglycan-arabinogalactan cell wall polysaccharide and (glyco)lipids. This characteristic cell envelope forms a permeability barrier to hydrophilic compounds, which makes some type of permeability pathway necessary for the bacteria. Two channel-forming proteins, or *porins*, have been identified in *R. equi*.[7] The unique mycolic acid–containing cell envelope of *R. equi* is of clinical significance because it is thought to play a role in survival of the bacteria under harsh conditions, such as those within macrophages, and may also influence antibiotic susceptibility patterns.[6-8]

The numerous different strains of *R. equi* include both virulent and avirulent variants. Strains may be identified by a variety of characteristics, including the degree of virulence, serotyping, and restriction endonuclease (RE) digestion of genomic and plasmid deoxyribonucleic acid (DNA).[9-16] In one study, 44 strains were identified among 209 isolates, with five strains accounting for more than half the isolates.[17] It was determined that a small number of strains account for clinical disease, and that in some cases, disease may be caused by simultaneous infection with multiple strains.

Virulent strains of *R. equi* are characterized by their ability to survive and replicate within macrophages (Fig. 32-1). This ability is associated with the presence of a large virulence plasmid of approximately 80 to 90 kilobases (kb), which was initially identified in isolates from diseased foals.[12-14,18] A number of different strains carry the virulence plasmid, and these strains appear to be geographically widespread.[17] The DNA from the virulence plasmids of various isolates have been analyzed by RE digestion, and based on the digestion patterns, at least 10 distinct but closely related plasmids have been identified.[19-26]

The virulence plasmid has been sequenced and contains 69 open reading frames in three functional regions.[27] Two of these regions contain genes that are similar to those encoding proteins involved in conjugation and in plasmid replication, stability, and segregation. The presence of genes resembling

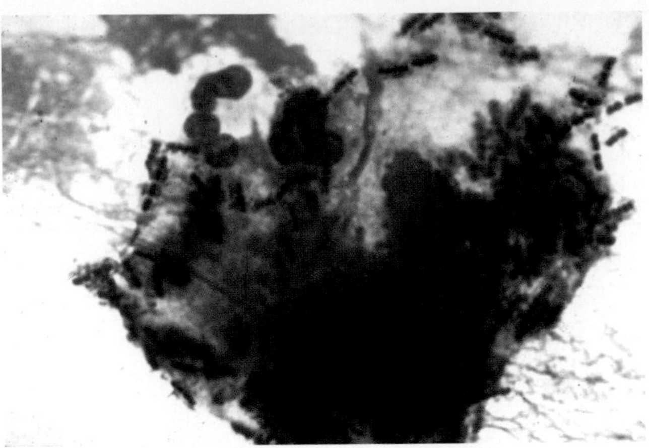

Fig. 32-1 *Rhodococcus equi* in equine macrophage. Virulence is associated with the ability of *R. equi* to survive and replicate within macrophages.

those required for conjugation suggests that the virulence plasmid may be transferred from virulent to avirulent strains, although this has not been demonstrated. The third region of the virulence plasmid is a 27.5-kb pathogenicity island that encodes seven related *virulence-associated proteins* (Vaps A, C, D, E, F, G, and H) and four additional extracellular proteins. The first Vap to be identified was *VapA*, a highly immunogenic surface lipoprotein of 15 to 17 kilodaltons (kDa).[12,13,18,28] Of the VapA homologs, all are expressed except for VapF. Vaps C, D, and E are secreted, but unlike VapA, are not anchored to the cell wall.[29] The genes of the virulence plasmid show little homology with known genes in other species, making predictions of function difficult and suggesting that *R. equi* employs novel virulence mechanisms. Two of the proteins that have homologs in other bacteria are transcriptional regulators. Although the precise functions of the Vaps are unknown, it is known that the virulence plasmid expressing VapA is required for pathogenicity in foals.[6,14,15] Also, VapA is necessary for the replication of *R. equi* within macrophages and increases the cytotoxicity of *R. equi* for murine macrophages.[14,30-32]

Gene expression by bacteria is often regulated by complex networks that respond to environmental signals. In *R. equi*, expression of VapA is influenced by environmental conditions, with maximal expression occurring at high temperature (37° C [98.6° F]) and low pH (6.5).[33,34] At least five environmental signals, including temperature, pH, oxidative stress, magnesium and iron, contribute to the regulation of gene expression within the pathogenicity island.[6,29,35-37] Because the conditions that upregulate expression generally tend to be present when there is bacterial interaction with the host, the pattern of gene expression is consistent with the role of these genes in virulence.

Virtually all clinical isolates of *R. equi* from horses contain the virulence plasmid and express VapA, but this is not true of isolates from other species.[6,15,24,38-41] A second plasmid, 79 to 100 kb in size, has been identified that expresses VapB but not VapA.[6,15,42,43] Although this plasmid has not been associated with naturally occurring disease in foals, it can cause disease after experimental inoculation and appears to be of intermediate virulence.[44] In isolates from swine, 60% are positive for VapB, whereas other isolates lack a plasmid.[45] In human patients affected with *R. equi*, strains may contain VapA or VapB or may lack a virulence plasmid.[42,46] It is unclear if the severely immunocompromised status of the majority of human patients with *R. equi* allows relatively avirulent organisms to produce disease or if there are distinct, species-specific virulence determinants.

EPIDEMIOLOGY

Rhodococcus equi is widespread in soil samples and in the feces of herbivores, especially horses.[47-57] Because *R. equi* is present on virtually all horse farms, exposure of horses is common worldwide, and the majority of horses have antibodies to *R. equi*. In soil samples the greatest numbers of organisms are found in surface soil, with almost no bacteria found at a depth of 30 cm (1 foot) or more.[56] *Rhodococcus equi* can be isolated from the feces of adult horses, reaching numbers of 10^2 to 10^3/g of feces.[50,54-56] This generally represents acquisition from contaminated soil and passive intestinal carriage in adult horses, rather than actual colonization of the intestine.

In foals, *R. equi* can be first isolated from the feces at about 1 to 2 weeks of age, with most foals becoming positive by 4 weeks of age.[54,58] Up to the age of about 3 months, *R. equi* can actively multiply in the intestine of foals, reaching concentrations of 10^4 to 10^5/g of feces or higher and then declining to adult concentrations. Foals with rhodococcal pneumonia often swallow sputum infected with large numbers of virulent organisms, which may then multiply in the intestine, resulting in high numbers in the feces and significant environmental contamination.

Under suitable conditions, *R. equi* can multiply further in the environment. *Rhodococcus equi* grows substantially better in soil enriched with feces than in soil alone, and it is hypothesized that the organic acids in manure, such as acetate and propionate, support growth.[5] The organism tends to replicate better at a relatively warm temperature and in a neutral soil (pH 7.3) compared with an acidic soil (pH <5.5).[5] In addition, decreased soil moisture and decreased pasture cover have been associated with high numbers of environmental *R. equi*.[59] In some cases, a single gram of soil may contain millions of virulent *R. equi*.[50,54-56,60]

Inhalation of dust particles containing virulent *R. equi* is the major route of infection in foals. Experimentally, aerosolized bacteria and intratracheal and intrabronchial inoculation of bacteria in foals can produce pulmonary lesions similar to those of natural infection.[61-63] In one study, *R. equi* was isolated from the air in stalls, with the number of organisms in the air increasing on dry, windy days.[55] A study of six farms found poor correlation between the numbers of virulent *R. equi* in air samples and soil samples on a given farm.[59] Although ingestion is a common route of exposure, in most cases it does not result in clinical disease.[50,54,64,65] Rarely, *R. equi* infection is acquired through contamination of a wound.[66,67] Once infection is established, *R. equi* may disseminate to distant sites by hematogenous spread.

Foals are generally exposed to *R. equi* early in life, but the time when foals actually become infected has not been well established. It has long been thought that the age of onset of clinical disease is associated with the period of waning maternal antibody.[50,54,68] However, one study concluded that foals are infected much earlier, during the first several days of life.[69] This study was based on a retrospective analysis of the age at onset of clinical signs and the age at death caused by *R. equi* pneumonia using Sartwell's model to determine if there was a logarithmic normal distribution consistent with a point source of infection. The interpretation of these data has been controversial, and although it is accepted that foals developing *R. equi* pneumonia can be infected in the first week of life, it has been proposed that infection is not limited to this period.[70] Experimental studies show that foals remain susceptible over a wider age range.[44,61-63,70] Currently, no experimental data support the long incubation period (30–90 days) that would be necessary in some cases if all foals that develop rhodococcal pneumonia after natural exposure were infected in the first few days of life.[44,61-63,70]

Exposure of foals to *R. equi* is common because the organism is present on most horse farms, but the prevalence of clinical disease is highly variable. On many farms the disease is unrecognized, whereas on others it is either sporadic or enzootic. The prevalence varies widely between farms and years, with rates ranging from 0% to 100%.[50,71-76] Many enzootic farms have prevalence rates of 13% to 25%. The mortality rate is also highly variable, with death or euthanasia occurring in 0% to approximately 30% of cases.[71,73,76-78]

A number of theories have been proposed to explain the difference in prevalence between farms. Although it was initially proposed that the prevalence of rhodococcal pneumonia correlated with the number of *R. equi* bacteria in soil, this was not supported by soil cultures.[49,79-82] Subsequently, it was hypothesized that farms with enzootic disease were more heavily infected with virulent strains of *R. equi* than those farms where the disease was not present. Although initially supported by Takai et al.,[57] other studies have not supported this theory.[23,83] Martens et al.[83] compared 33 farms with *R. equi* and 33 farms without a history of *R. equi* and found no significant associations between disease status and isolation of *R. equi* from soil or detection of VapA in soil isolates. These findings suggest that it cannot be determined whether foals on a given farm are at increased risk of developing rhodococcal disease based on soil culture and VapA results.

Several epidemiologic studies have assessed *risk factors* for the development of rhodococcal disease, evaluating variables such as soil geochemistry, breeding-farm characteristics, management and preventive health practices, and foal-related factors.[72,84-87] Although study results have varied somewhat, some general risk factors have been identified. Farms with large acreage, large numbers of mares and foals, and a population of transient mares and foals are at high risk for foals developing rhodococcal pneumonia.[85,86] High foal density is associated with an increased risk of farms being affected by *R. equi* in one study, but a subsequent study found no association.[85,86] There has been no evidence that poor farm management or lack of attention to preventive health practices contributes to the probability of rhodococcal pneumonia.[85,87] The role of housing has been evaluated, but the significance of the findings is unclear. In one study, having concrete floors in the foaling stalls was associated with an increased risk of developing disease, whereas in a second study, housing foals in stalls with dirt floors appeared to increase risk.[85,87] The investigators recommend that these results be interpreted with caution until more data are available. One study evaluated soil samples from affected and unaffected farms for multiple factors, including pH, salinity, and nitrate, and found no association between any soil factor and the *R. equi* disease status of the farms.[72] In another study, rhodococcal pneumonia was associated with an environment that participating veterinarians subjectively determined to be moderately to severely dusty.[85] One theory currently under investigation is that foals developing rhodococcal pneumonia are born to mares that shed high numbers of organisms in their feces, but as yet, no data support this hypothesis.

Limited studies have attempted to identify *host factors* of foals that influence the outcome of exposure to *R. equi*. To identify differences between foals that become affected and those that remain healthy on enzootic farms, Chaffin et al.[88] evaluated hematologic and immunophenotypic parameters in foals at 2 and 4 weeks of age before the onset of clinical disease.[88] Foals with a CD4/CD8 ratio of less than 3.0 appeared to have a higher risk of developing rhodococcal pneumonia. In addition, the number of segmented neutrophils was lower in foals that subsequently became affected compared with foals that remained healthy. However, the significance of these findings is unclear because the data were confounded by farm-related differences, and there was considerable overlap between values for affected and unaffected foals. Flaminio et al.[89] found that absolute and proportional B-cell concentrations were greater in foals with active *R. equi* pneumonia than in healthy foals of the same age. It has also been suggested that genetic factors may play a role in susceptibility to *R. equi*, because limited data suggest an association between foal death caused by *R. equi* and the type of transferrin, an iron-binding protein with differing genotypes and variable bacteriostatic properties.[90] Another hypothesis is that infection of foals with equine herpesvirus type 2 (EHV-2) is a predisposing factor for invasion of the respiratory tract by *R. equi*.[91,92] At this time, host factors that influence susceptibility to *R. equi* in foals are poorly understood.

PATHOGENESIS

Mechanisms of Disease

The infectivity of *R. equi* is limited to cells of the monocyte/macrophage lineage, and the basis of this organism's pathogenicity is its ability to replicate in and eventually destroy macrophages.[6,15,32] *R. equi* strains cured of the virulence plasmid are unable to survive and replicate in macrophages and are avirulent for foals and mice.[12,13,15,63] Specifically, it has been demonstrated by targeted "knockout" mutants that VapA is necessary for full virulence in mice, as well as for multiplication in ex vivo murine macrophages.[30] Thus, although the function of the virulence plasmid is not fully understood, it appears to be essential for full virulence. Defining the precise mechanisms by which rhodococci survive and replicate within macrophages, as well as the role of the virulence plasmid, is key to understanding the pathogenesis of the disease.

The means by which *R. equi* enters the macrophage may influence survival within the cell. Bacteria interact with a surface receptor on the macrophage and are internalized by phagocytosis, becoming enclosed in a portion of the macrophage plasma membrane, forming a phagosome. The specific phagocytic receptor involved mediates differences in internalization mechanisms and macrophage activation. *R. equi* appears to bind primarily to macrophages through fixation of complement after activation of the alternative complement pathway, then binding to the macrophage complement receptor type 3 (CR3), also known as Mac-1 (CD11b/CD18).[93,94] In general, complement receptor–mediated phagocytosis is not associated with a high level of production of reactive oxygen intermediates and proinflammatory mediators, possibly allowing the organism to avoid antibody-associated macrophage-killing pathways.[95] Brumbaugh et al.[96] reported that phagocytosis of *R. equi* by equine macrophages was not associated with a functional respiratory burst. In contrast to complement receptor–mediated phagocytosis, entry into the cell through the Fc receptor after opsonization with specific antibody is associated with significantly enhanced killing of *R. equi* by equine macrophages.[6,97,98] The presence of the virulence plasmid does not appear to influence the uptake of *R. equi* by macrophages because both virulent and avirulent strains are phagocytosed to a similar extent.[31,99]

Once within the macrophage, virulent strains of *R. equi* continue to multiply within the membrane-enclosed vacuoles, whereas avirulent strains multiply at low levels initially and cease to grow after approximately 6 hours.[8,32] The means by which virulent *R. equi* avoids the killing mechanisms of macrophages are not fully understood. Initially, a lack of phagosome-lysosome fusion was reported.[97,98] It now appears that there is a complex alteration of the normal phagocyte maturation process, which is at least in part regulated by the virulence plasmid. Based on studies with murine macrophages, Toyooka et al.[99] reported that phagosome-lysosome fusion occurred with both virulent and avirulent *R. equi*, but that the phagolysosomes containing virulent organisms were not as acidic as those containing avirulent organisms. Also in murine macrophages, Fernandez-Mora et al.[100] demonstrated that *R. equi*–containing vacuoles progressed normally through the early stages of phagosome maturation, but that maturation was ultimately blocked. This block in maturation was regulated by the presence of the virulence plasmid. Strains with the virulence plasmid maintained a nonacidified compartment for 48 hours, whereas strains lacking the plasmid acidified progressively.

Ultimately, the replication of *R. equi* within macrophages results in the death of the host cell. In vitro, macrophage degeneration is apparent by approximately 8 hours after infection and is marked by 24 hours.[97,98] The cytotoxicity is linked to virulence, although the exact mechanisms are unclear. Virulent *R. equi* bacteria are cytotoxic for murine macrophages, and the cytotoxicity is strongly upregulated by the presence of VapA-expressing plasmids.[31] Isolates with a VapB-expressing plasmid are less virulent and have a lower cytotoxic potential, whereas isogenic strains without a plasmid are avirulent with a very low cyotoxic potential. The cytotoxicity requires viable bacteria. Cell death occurs by necrosis rather than apoptosis.

A number of additional factors may play a role in the pathogenesis of *R. equi*. The polysaccharide capsule, the presence of lipoglycans, mechanisms of iron acquisition, and the enzyme cholesterol oxidase, termed "equi factor," may all contribute to virulence.[8,15,101] Some evidence suggests that the length of the mycolic acid carbon chain in the cell envelope influences virulence, because strains of *R. equi* with longer mycolic acid carbon chains are more lethal in mice and cause greater granuloma formation than those with shorter mycolic acid carbon chains.[8,102] The modulation of cytokine production by virulent strains may contribute to pathogenicity.[103] Virulence is linked to resistance to β-lactam antibiotics in a study of non–plasmid-containing *R. equi* strains isolated from humans.[104,105] However, a study of *R. equi* isolated from infected foals and soil from affected and control farms found no significant correlation between β-lactam resistance and either the presence of VapA or the disease status.[83]

Large numbers of cells migrate to the site in response to infection with *R. equi*, ultimately resulting in granuloma formation. There is an influx of neutrophils, and one early hypothesis stated that a defect in neutrophil function contributed to disease; however, neutrophils from foals are fully bactericidal.[94,97,106-108] The precise signals that influence granuloma formation are largely unknown, but it is clear that a complex network of cytokines and chemokines is involved. Granulomas may help contain and control infection but may also contribute to the pathology of disease; they are associated with the secretion of several inflammatory mediators and may allow proliferation of organisms and cause the loss of pulmonary function.[109]

Immunity to *Rhodococcus equi*

The mechanism of protective immunity to *R. equi* has important implications for the control of disease. Although the outcome of exposure to *R. equi* is clearly affected by the dose and virulence of the organism, the host immune response is also important. Virtually all foals are exposed to *R. equi* early in life, but most do not develop disease. Adult horses are essentially resistant to infection because of the acquisition of protective immunity. Thus, it appears that most foals are capable of developing effective immune responses, which subsequently protect them for life. The mechanisms of this protective immunity are not fully understood. Because *R. equi* is a facultative intracellular pathogen, much emphasis has been placed on the role of cellular immunity. However, it appears that *all* aspects of the immune system are involved in protection from *R. equi*.

Role of Innate Immunity

The replication of *R. equi* in nonactivated resident macrophages is critical to the pathogenesis of disease, but at the same time the killing of *R. equi* by activated macrophages can be important in the control of infection. Mice with macrophages that are deficient in either of two radical-generating pathways have an increased susceptibility to infection with *R. equi*.[110] Macrophage activation by *R. equi* in mice involves toll-like receptor 2 (TLR-2).[111] This may be significant because human neonates have diminished TLR-induced responses compared with adults, and it has been hypothesized that inefficient TLR-2 signaling may contribute to the enhanced susceptibility of neonatal foals to *R. equi*.

Neutrophils may also be important in controlling *R. equi* early in the course of infection. The induction of a neutrophil deficiency in mice during the first week after experimental rhodococcal infection resulted in more severe disease and in significantly increased tissue concentrations of *R. equi*.[112]

Role of Antibody

As noted earlier, the unique age-related susceptibility of foals to *R. equi* has long been thought to be associated with the waning of maternal antibody. Although the explanation is probably more complex, antibody does appear to play a role in immunity to *R. equi*. Some mechanisms by which antibody may contribute to immunity include blocking the initial stages of cellular infection, altering the route by which bacteria enter the macrophage, and decreasing the bacteria's ability to arrest maturation of the phagosome.

Several lines of evidence support a role for antibody in protection against *R. equi*, in addition to the observation that the age of onset of disease in foals typically coincides with the waning of maternal antibody. Antibodies to *R. equi*, including antibodies to the 15- to 17-kDa antigen of virulent *R. equi*, are widespread in horses and are found in the majority of foals within the first 3 months of age.[13,113-116] An inverse correlation may exist between antibody concentrations and disease severity and prevalence.[98,114,115,117] After challenge of immune adult horses with virulent *R. equi*, an antibody response is characterized predominantly by increases in concentrations of immunoglobulin G subtypes IgGa and IgGb, which are important antibody isotypes in opsonization and complement fixation.[118] During in vitro experiments by Hietala and Ardans,[97] opsonization with *R. equi*–specific antibody increased phagosome-lysosome fusion and significantly enhanced the killing of *R. equi* by alveolar macrophages from foals.

Additional evidence supporting a role for humoral immunity in protection against *R. equi* comes from studies of passive immunization through the administration of *hyperimmune plasma* (Box 32-1). Several studies investigating the protective effect of hyperimmune plasma have been performed in both mice and foals. The results in mice have been variable, with some studies indicating that hyperimmune serum was not

Box • 32-1

Commercial Sources of* R. equi *Hyperimmune Plasma

Lake Immunogenics, Inc.
348 Berg Road
Ontario, NY 14519
585-265-1973 or 800-648-9990
lakeimmunogenics.com
Plasvacc USA, Inc.
1535 Templeton Road
Templeton, CA 93465
805-434-0321 or 800-654-9743
plasvaccusa.com
Veterinary Immunogenics, Ltd.
Carleton Hill
Penrith
Cumbria
CA11 8TZ
United Kingdom
+44 (0) 1768 863881
veterinaryimmunogenics.com
PRO-SER S.A.
Av. N. Alem 1698
(2752) Capitan Sarmiento
Buenos Aires, Argentina
(054-11) 15-4420-1757
labproser.com.ar

protective against experimental challenge and others indicating a protective effect.[28,119,120] Similarly, studies in foals have had varied results. The administration of hyperimmune plasma does not always have a significant protective effect, but it does prevent or reduce the severity of pneumonia in foals that are either experimentally or naturally *R. equi* infected.[73-75,121-125] Hyperimmune plasma does not alleviate clinical signs or alter the course of the disease when administered to foals 7 days after experimental challenge with *R. equi;* thus it appears that the protective components in immune plasma are primarily effective in the prevention of infection.[122]

It is uncertain which specific components of hyperimmune plasma are responsible for enhancing protection against *R. equi*. In addition to immunoglobulin, hyperimmune plasma contains a number of substances, including fibronectin, interferon, complement factors, and cytokines. In a study by Hooper-McGrevy et al.,[126] the same degree of protection was provided by purified immunoglobulin specific for VapA and VapC as by hyperimmune plasma, suggesting that immunoglobulin was the primary component of hyperimmune plasma that conferred protection, and that specific antibodies against VapA and VapC were protective. In contrast, Perkins et al.[123] found no difference in the incidence and severity of disease after experimental challenge with *R. equi* in colostrum-deprived foals given either normal equine plasma or hyperimmune plasma. Because the survival rate for foals in both groups was approximately 70% without antibiotic therapy, both normal and hyperimmune plasma were thought to provide some protective effect, although there was no untreated control group. The researchers therefore concluded that either only a small amount of antibody was sufficient to enhance protection, or that factors in the plasma other than immunoglobulin were responsible for the protective effect.

Several studies have evaluated the protection provided by the ingestion of colostrum from mares immunized against rhodococcus. Martens et al.[127] found that the passive immunization of foals by ingestion of colostrum from mares immunized with live *R. equi* did not provide protection against experimental challenge. Similarly, in field studies by Madigan et al.,[74] in which pregnant mares were immunized with an *R. equi* bacterin, and by Prescott et al.,[124] in which pregnant mares were immunized with a VapA extract, foals were not protected from natural infection with *R. equi*. In contrast, in a field study by Cauchard et al.,[128] in which pregnant mares were immunized with either VapA protein antigen or whole killed *R. equi*, vaccination did appear to provide protection. In general, the protection provided by colostrum has not been as consistent as that with hyperimmune plasma. One possible explanation for this difference is that factors in plasma other than antibody significantly contribute to protection. An alternative explanation is that the isotypes of antibody necessary for protection may not be present in high concentrations in colostrum. Furthermore, the specific immunogens or immunization protocols employed may not induce sufficient concentrations of antibody or antibody with the appropriate antigen specificity.

Although antibody contributes to protective immunity, by itself it does not afford complete protection. The humoral response appears to be most important in the initial stages of infection. The immune response to *R. equi* is complex, and ultimately, optimal control of the disease involves cell-mediated immunity, as would be expected for an intracellular pathogen.

Role of Cellular Immunity

Considerable evidence supports the importance of cell-mediated immunity in the control of *R. equi* infection. Much of this evidence comes from a mouse model of rhodococcal disease, although there are some data in horses. In mice, both CD4+ and CD8+ T lymphocytes contribute to immune clearance of *R. equi* from the lung.[129-131] Mice that lack CD8+ but not CD4+ T lymphocytes are able to clear infection completely in the period studied, whereas mice lacking CD4+ but not CD8+ T lymphocytes are able to decrease bacterial numbers significantly in the lung.

Studies have emphasized the role of CD4+ T lymphocytes because these cells appear to be both necessary and sufficient for clearance of *R. equi*.[129-131] CD4+ T lymphocytes are further characterized as T helper 1 (Th1) or T helper 2 (Th2) cells, depending on their cytokine secretion patterns.[132] These CD4+ subtypes have been best defined in mice. CD4+ Th1 cells secrete primarily interferon gamma (IFN-γ), a potent activator of macrophage microbicidal activity. In comparison, CD4+ Th2 lymphocytes secrete predominantly the interleukins IL-4, IL-5, and IL-13, which potentiate the humoral immune response. In mice, secretion of IFN-γ by CD4+ Th1 lymphocytes appears to be absolutely required for clearance of *R. equi*.[130] Adoptive transfer of a *R. equi*–specific CD4+ Th1 cell line mediates clearance in immunodeficient nude mice that normally are unable to control pulmonary bacteria.[131] In contrast, nude mice that receive an *R. equi*–specific CD4+ Th2 cell line are unable to clear bacteria and develop prototypic pulmonary lesions.

CD4+ T lymphocytes are critical in the control of rhodococcal infection, but CD8+ T lymphocytes contribute as well. These CD8+ cells probably act through multiple mechanisms to decrease bacterial numbers. One of their effector functions is the ability to produce IFN-γ. Another possible important function is the recognition and lysis of *R. equi*–infected cells, as demonstrated for the related pathogen, *Mycobacterium tuberculosis*.[133,134]

Limited data in horses support the observations in mice that protective immunity to *R. equi* involves both CD4+ and CD8+ T lymphocytes. Adult horses challenged intrabronchially with virulent *R. equi* do not develop clinical disease and effectively clear bacteria from the lung in association with increased numbers of CD4+ and CD8+ lymphocytes at the site of infection.[135] T lymphocytes from bronchoalveolar lavage (BAL) fluid of challenged horses proliferate when stimulated with *R. equi* antigen, and both CD4+ and CD8+ T lymphocytes from the site express IFN-γ. In addition, T lymphocytes from the blood and BAL fluid of adult immune horses have *R. equi*–specific cytolytic activity.[136] These cytotoxic T lymphocytes (CTLs) appear to be primarily CD8+ and have the ability to kill in a major histocompatibility complex (MHC) class I, unrestricted fashion.

CLINICAL FINDINGS

Clinical disease caused by *R. equi* is most common in foals 3 weeks to 6 months of age, with signs most often developing before age 4 months.[73,76,77,79,137] Respiratory tract disease occurs most often, although other systems may be affected as well, either independently or in conjunction with lung involvement. In a retrospective study of 61 foals seen at a referral center for rhodococcal pneumonia, the prevalence of extrapulmonary disorders was 66%, although this percentage is higher than what some clinicians recognize.[138] General clinical signs often associated with rhodococcal disease, regardless of the site of infection, include fever, lethargy, and decreased appetite.

Rhodococcal infection may remain subclinical in some cases. When clinical disease does develop, it is often insidious in nature. Because of the foal's ability to compensate and the slow spread of infection, early clinical signs are often subtle, making the disease difficult to detect. Although infection is generally chronic, clinical signs often appear acutely when the disease becomes severe, leading to the description of an "acute on chronic" disease. A small percentage of foals exhibit a subacute form of the disease, in which they may be found dead or in acute, severe respiratory distress with high fever. These foals often have a poor prognosis.[91]

Pulmonary Disease

The most common manifestation of *R. equi* infection in foals is chronic pyogranulomatous bronchopneumonia with abscessation and associated suppurative lymphadenitis.[76,79,80,137] Zink et al.[137] confirmed the presence of suppurative pneumonia in 115 of 131 cases of *R. equi* infection. In a review of 40 cases of equine lung abscesses, 32 cases were identified in foals 6 months of age or younger, with *R. equi* cultured from 13 of 34 cases and *Streptococcus zooepidemicus* cultured from 20 of 34.[139] Occasionally, *R. equi* is cultured with other pathogens, including *Pneumocystis carinii*.[140] *Rhodococcus equi* has rarely been cultured from foals with the syndrome of bronchointerstitial pneumonia and respiratory distress, but it is not believed to be the primary cause of this condition.[141]

It is important to minimize stress during the physical examination of foals with suspected rhodococcal pneumonia so as not to exacerbate respiratory distress. The most prominent clinical signs include tachypnea and increased respiratory effort, characterized by abdominal effort and nostril flaring. Tachycardia is often present. In severe cases, mucous membranes may be cyanotic. The presence of a cough and mucoid to mucopurulent nasal discharge is variable. Generally, affected foals are in good body condition, although weight loss may be present in some chronic cases.

Findings on auscultation of the lung are variable and often do not correlate well with the severity of pneumonia. The sensitivity of auscultation may be enhanced by inducing the foal to breathe deeply using a rebreathing bag or cupping a hand over the nostrils for a few seconds if the foal is stable enough to tolerate this procedure. Inspiratory and expiratory crackles and wheezes may be audible and are often most prominent cranioventrally. In some cases, only large airway sounds are present, suggesting consolidation. With severe consolidation or extensive peripheral abscess formation, lung sounds may be decreased. This may also indicate pleural effusion, although effusion is seen only occasionally in association with rhodococcal pneumonia.[142] In one case, respiratory distress was identified in association with a focal mediastinal abscess without concurrent pulmonary involvement.[143] Thoracic percussion, as well as ancillary diagnostic aids such as radiography and ultrasonography, may help detect areas of consolidation, abscessation, or pleural fluid.

Abdominal Disease

Enterocolitis, typhlitis, abdominal abscesses, peritonitis, and adhesions have been reported in association with *R. equi*.* In the review of 131 cases by Zink et al.,[137] approximately 50% of foals with *R. equi* that had bronchopneumonia on necropsy also had intestinal lesions, and an additional 4% of foals had intestinal lesions without pneumonia. However, of the foals with intestinal lesions, only 38% had any history or clinical signs related to intestinal disease.

The predominant signs in those foals with intestinal involvement that do manifest clinical signs are colic and diarrhea. In chronic or severe cases, there may be a loss of body condition. Some foals develop significant ascites, resulting in a marked "pot-bellied" appearance. These foals generally have extensive granulomatous inflammation of the colonic mucosa and submucosa with involvement of the mesenteric lymph nodes, causing lymphatic obstruction with an increased concentration of protein in the abdominal fluid and circulating hypoproteinemia. Chances for survival decrease with extensive abdominal disease.

Nonseptic Polysynovitis

An immune-mediated polysynovitis has been documented in approximately one third of *R. equi* cases[77,138] (Fig. 32-2). Although all joints may be affected, this condition appears to be most common in the tibiotarsal and stifle joints.[77] Degree of joint effusion is variable, but unlike cases of septic arthritis, there is no or minimal lameness. Evaluation of synovial fluid reveals a nonseptic mononuclear pleocytosis with no bacterial growth.[77,146,147] Histologic examination of the synovium reveals a lymphoplasmacytic synovitis.[146,147] In horses with nonseptic arthritis, the effusion generally resolves as the rhodococcal infection clears.

It is hypothesized that the presence of immune complexes in the joint leads to an acute reactive arthritis.[146] Immunoglobulin was demonstrated within the synovial membrane using fluorescein-labeled antiequine IgG in three affected foals.[147] Additionally, rheumatoid factor activity, which results from antibodies directed against the Fc portion of autologous or heterologous immunoglobulin, was identified in the synovial fluid of a foal with *R. equi* pneumonia and reactive arthritis.[146]

*References 76, 137, 138, 142, 144, 145.

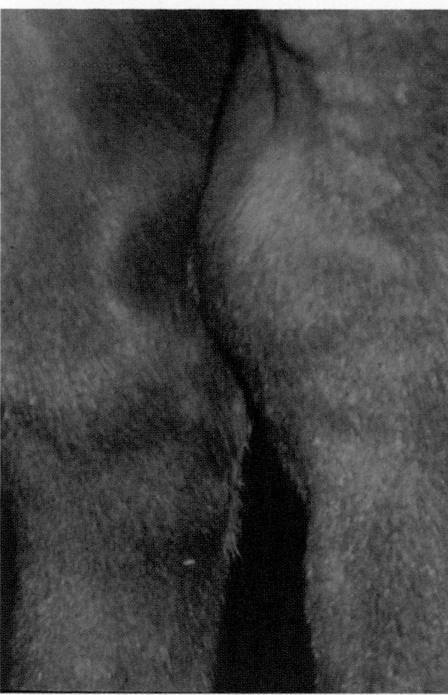

Fig. 32-2 An immune-mediated polysynovitis may be recognized in association with *R. equi* infection. Although any joint may be affected, the tibiotarsal and stifle joints appear to be most often involved. Typically, joint effusion occurs, with minimal or no lameness.

Bone and Joint Disease

Septic arthritis and osteomyelitis may be observed either alone or with other signs of rhodococcal disease.[76,137,148-151] These conditions can be distinguished from immune-mediated polysynovitis by the degree of lameness along with cytologic evaluation and culture of joint fluid or aspirates. Some foals have an associated cellulitis. Treatment includes aggressive local therapy in addition to systemic antibiotics.

Several cases of *R. equi* vertebral osteomyelitis have been reported, and the question has arisen whether this condition is becoming more common.[152-157] In general, early signs of vertebral osteomyelitis may include a stiff gait, reluctance to move, and pain on palpation. However, the diagnosis is usually not made until the infection extends to the epidural space, causing signs of spinal cord or nerve root compression, such as paresis, ataxia, paralysis, or cauda equina syndrome. The specific signs will vary depending on the severity and site of the lesion. Although radiography may be useful in the diagnosis, in four of six cases, radiographs were normal despite the presence of extensive lesions on necropsy.[154,155,157] Therefore, nuclear scintigraphy, computed tomography, or magnetic resonance imaging may be indicated.

Diseases of Other Body Systems

A variety of other conditions have been sporadically recognized in association with *R. equi*.[66,67,76,138] These include ulcerative lymphangitis, cellulitis, subcutaneous abscesses, abscesses of the submandibular lymph nodes, nephritis, renal abscesses, and hypopyon (Fig. 32-3). Some cases of cellulitis without any internal involvement may be secondary to wounds or damage to the skin by the larvae of *Strongyloides westeri*.[158] Hepatitis, cholangitis, and hepatoencephalopathy as well as uveitis and panophthalmitis have also been reported.[76,137,138,159,160]

R. equi has rarely been isolated from aborted equine fetuses and infertile mares.[137,161-165] The significance of isolating the organism has been unclear in some cases, but *R. equi* has been confirmed as a cause of placentitis and abortion with fetal pneumonia.[164,165] However, despite the frequent occurrence of *R. equi* in equine feces and soil samples, it is rarely recognized as a cause of equine abortion.[166,167]

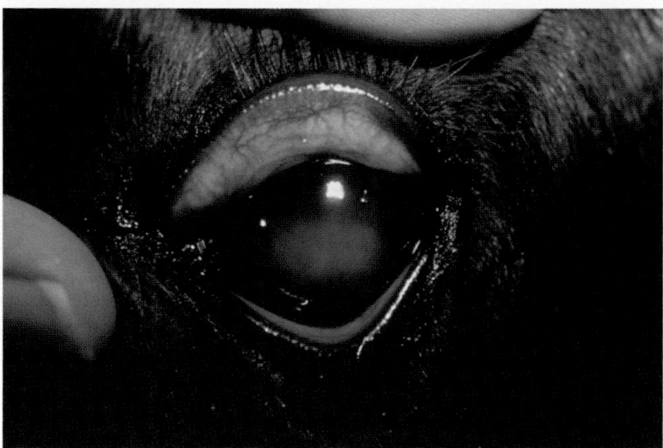

Fig. 32-3 Hypopyon associated with *R. equi* in a foal.

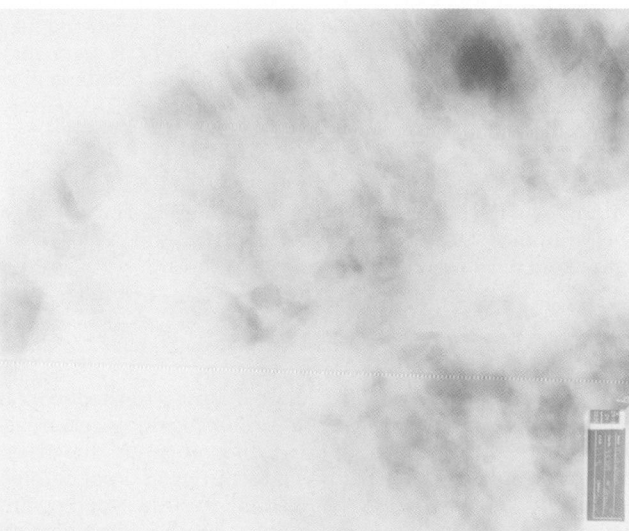

Fig. 32-4 Thoracic radiograph from adult horse with *R. equi* pneumonia. There is a severe, multifocal, coalescing alveolar pattern. Rhodococcal disease is uncommon in adult horses and is generally thought to be associated with immunosuppression. Clinically, the most common manifestation in adults has been suppurative bronchopneumonia, similar to that recognized in foals.

Infection in Adult Horses

Rhodococcal disease is uncommon in adult horses because most adults are immune to infection. However, sporadic cases have been reported.[137,168-173] As in foals, the most common clinical signs are related to suppurative bronchopneumonia (Fig. 32-4). Occasionally, pleuritis may be recognized. Other reported signs include intestinal disease, lymphadenitis, wound infections, and osteomyelitis. In both cases in which the organism isolated from adult horses was assessed, the virulence plasmid was present.[170,171] It is thought that adult horses

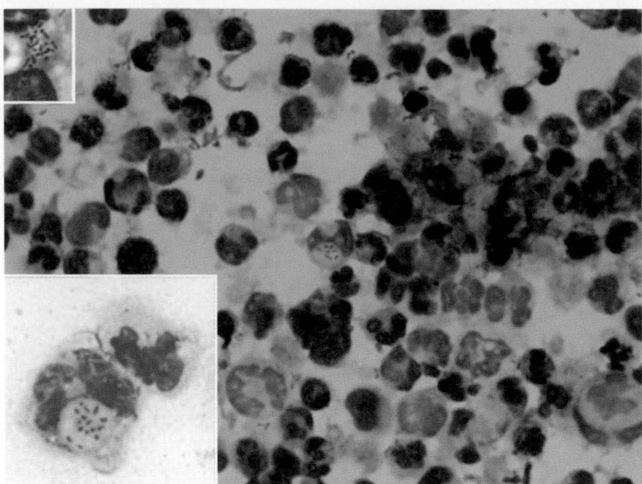

Fig. 32-5 Cytology of tracheobronchial fluid from foal with rhodococcal pneumonia. There is increased cellularity, characterized primarily by macrophages and neutrophils. Intracellular organisms are often identified in macrophages *(top inset)* and may also be found within neutrophils *(bottom inset)*. *R. equi* may appear coccoid or as rods or short filaments with rudimentary branching. It is often described as "coccobacillary." (Courtesy Dr. Andrea Bohn.)

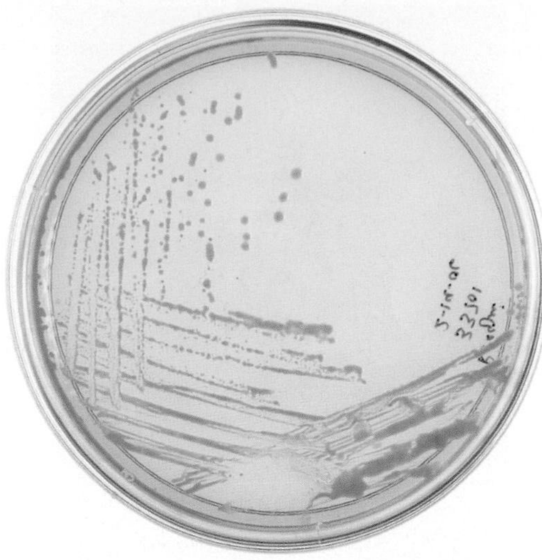

Fig. 32-6 *Rhodococcus equi* in culture. Colonies are typically irregularly round, smooth, semitransparent, and mucoid. After several days in culture, colonies often develop a characteristic salmon-pink color.

with *R. equi* infection are immunocompromised, and although the immune status has not been assessed in every case, immunodeficiency was reported in two cases.[169,173]

DIAGNOSIS

The ability to make a rapid, accurate diagnosis of rhodococcal pneumonia is important because early recognition and treatment of the disease can improve the prognosis. Based on clinical signs alone, it is difficult to distinguish pneumonia caused by *R. equi* from that caused by other pathogens. The isolation of *R. equi* by culture or the identification of *R. equi*–specific DNA by polymerase chain reaction (PCR) provides definitive diagnosis. However, a variety of additional tests can be supportive.

Cytology

The presence of intracellular gram-positive pleomorphic rods on cytologic evaluation of fluid specimens supports a diagnosis of rhodococcal infection (Fig. 32-5). However, the organisms may be present in low numbers and may be difficult to detect. Sweeney et al.[77] reported that organisms were seen on cytology of tracheobronchial fluid in 61% of 48 culture-positive foals, whereas in 22% of these foals, no bacteria were seen, and in 17%, only bacteria other than *R. equi* were identified. An indirect fluorescent antibody (IFA) technique has been described for acetone-fixed specimens; 33 of 53 (62.3%) tracheal aspirates from foals with experimentally induced rhodococcal pneumonia had a positive IFA result.[174]

Culture

Culture and subsequent phenotypic analysis of the isolate by classic morphologic and biochemical tests has been the "gold standard" for the diagnosis of *R. equi*. Typically, the organism is cultured from a tracheobronchial aspirate, which may be obtained by a variety of techniques.[174,175] When collecting the sample, the clinician must consider stress to the patient because some foals are in severe respiratory distress. Other samples, such as joint fluid or peritoneal fluid, can be cultured as appropriate based on the case.

Colonies of *R. equi* will usually appear on solid media within 48 hours of aerobic culture, although in some cases, longer incubation is necessary, especially for samples collected from foals that have been treated with antibiotics.[3,76,174,176] Occasionally, the organism may be isolated only under anaerobic conditions after antimicrobial therapy.[176] Colonies of *R. equi* generally appear irregularly round, smooth, semitransparent, and mucoid (Fig. 32-6). They typically have a characteristic salmon-pink color, which may not develop until 4 to 7 days in culture. Other pathogens may be isolated concurrently with *R. equi*.[77,177]

It is generally assumed without further testing that the isolates of *R. equi* from clinically ill foals are virulent strains. However, isolates can be analyzed for the presence of virulence plasmids and virulence-associated antigens.[38,175,178,179]

The reliability of culture of tracheobronchial aspirates in the diagnosis of rhodococcal pneumonia has varied among studies.* In some studies, essentially all foals in which *R. equi* was isolated from the lung parenchyma at necropsy had positive antemortem cultures from tracheobronchial fluid, but in other studies the results have not been as consistent. Combining the results of three studies, Giguere et al.[182] reported that 86% of foals with positive *R. equi* cultures at necropsy had positive antemortem cultures of tracheobronchial fluid. Sellon et al.[181] compared PCR, serology, and culture for the diagnosis of *R. equi* pneumonia in 56 foals with respiratory tract disease. Using the final clinical diagnosis of the attending clinician as the reference standard for diagnosis of *R. equi*, microbiologic culture was found to have a sensitivity of 57.1% and a specificity of 93.8%, making it less sensitive than PCR. In a study of experimentally induced rhodococcal pneumonia in foals, *R. equi* was consistently isolated by culture of tracheal aspirations, and culture was found to be more sensitive than either PCR targeting VapA or IFA staining of tracheobronchial aspirate cells using a monoclonal antibody against VapA.[174]

*References 64, 76, 78, 139, 180, 181.

R. equi may occasionally be isolated from the trachea as a contaminant. In one study on a farm with enzootic rhodococcal pneumonia, 77 of 216 foals with no signs of respiratory disease had positive cultures of tracheobronchial fluid.[183] These data raise the possibility that PCR tests may also be positive in cases where *R. equi* is not causing clinical disease. Therefore, it is important to interpret culture and PCR results in the context of the entire case, including the physical examination findings, laboratory evaluation, and diagnostic imaging.

Samples in addition to the tracheobronchial aspirate may be positive for *R. equi* in some cases of rhodococcal pneumonia. Although blood cultures are not routinely performed in foals with suspected *R. equi* infection, cultures have occasionally been positive in horses with natural or experimental infection.[76,181,184] In contrast, blood culture appears to be a sensitive means of diagnosis in human patients with *R. equi*.[185] Positive cultures of nasal swabs or feces cannot be taken as evidence of rhodococcal disease. The inhalation of dust from the environment may result in contamination of the upper airways and positive nasal swabs. *R. equi* can be cultured from the feces of many normal horses.[48,58,186,187] Negative fecal cultures are not helpful in ruling out infection. Despite that infected foals often swallow contaminated sputum, in one study only 5 of 30 foals (17%) with confirmed *R. equi* pneumonia had positive fecal cultures.[183] Based on another study, weekly quantitative fecal cultures have been advocated as an aid in the early diagnosis of *R. equi* enteritis because the bacterial count per gram of feces increased at the onset of clinical signs.[187]

Nucleic Acid Amplification and Polymerase Chain Reaction

A number of PCR techniques have been developed to amplify either chromosomal or plasmid DNA of *R. equi* in a variety of samples.[188-195] Using primers for VapA, virulent strains of *R. equi* can be rapidly identified. It is also useful to identify chromosomal DNA because the virulence plasmid is not present in many strains isolated from environmental samples or from species other than horses, particularly human patients. Although PCR can be a valuable diagnostic test, it should be used in conjunction with standard microbial culture because multiple bacterial pathogens may be present.

The PCR has generally been shown to be rapid and reliable, although the results of individual studies assessing its accuracy have varied. With as few as 10 to 100 organisms, *R. equi* can be identified and virulent strains differentiated from avirulent strains within 12 to 24 hours.[188,189] In the study of 56 foals with respiratory tract disease by Sellon et al.,[181] in which the reference standard was the final clinical diagnosis of the attending clinician, the PCR of tracheal wash fluid using primers that recognized the VapA virulence plasmid had a diagnostic sensitivity of 100% and a specificity of 90.6%, making it a more sensitive diagnostic test than culture or serology. Analysis of serum samples had a sensitivity of only 12.5% and a specificity of 88.9%, whereas analysis of nasal swabs had a sensitivity of 50% and a specificity of 88.9%. In the study of experimentally induced rhodococcal pneumonia by Anzai et al.,[174] PCR of tracheal aspirates, although more rapid than culture, was less sensitive in the diagnosis of *R. equi*. Recently, Harrington et al.[195] evaluated a real-time quantitative PCR for detection and quantitation of virulent *R. equi* in experimental studies and found it to be highly specific and more sensitive than standard PCR for the detection of *R. equi* in tracheobronchial fluid. The increased sensitivity of this method could facilitate the rapid and accurate diagnosis of *R. equi* pneumonia in foals, and evaluation in clinical cases is warranted.

Serologic Tests

Serologic assays developed to detect *R. equi*–specific antibodies include several enzyme-linked immunosorbent assays (ELISAs), an agar-gel immunodiffusion (AGID) test, and synergistic hemolysis inhibition (SHI) assays.[114,174,196-207] Variations among the assays are primarily based on differences in the test antigen preparation. These assays have been used in various studies to assess the humoral immune response to *R. equi*. It has also been proposed that serologic testing could be used in the diagnosis of rhodococcal infection.

Sellon et al.[181] and Giguere et al.[182] assessed an AGID test in the diagnosis of *R. equi;* both studies found the sensitivity to be 62.5%, and the specificity was 75.9% and 53.8%, respectively. Two studies critically evaluated the performance of several serologic assays for the diagnosis of *R. equi* in foals; the first evaluated three ELISAs, an AGID, and SHI assay, and the second evaluated four ELISAs and the AGID assay.[207,208] None of the serologic assays in either study differentiated between diseased and clinically normal foals. One study evaluated the testing of paired sera, but this failed to improve the diagnostic accuracy.[207] In both studies, antibodies, including those specific for VapA, were found in many foals regardless of their disease status. Some antibody could be maternally derived, but because titers increased significantly over time in all assays, this suggests that foals are routinely exposed to *R. equi*, including virulent strains. It has been suggested that serologic tests may be of more value as a diagnostic test if used on nonenzootic farms, but this has not been assessed.[206,207]

Ancillary Diagnostic Tests

Clinical Pathology

A complete blood count (CBC), fibrinogen, and serum biochemistry profile can provide useful information in the evaluation of patients with suspected rhodococcal infection.[76] However, the abnormalities generally are nonspecific, reflecting the presence of inflammation. *Hyperfibrinogenemia* is the most consistent laboratory finding, although rare cases may have normal fibrinogen concentrations. Neutrophilic leukocytosis with or without monocytosis is also common. Most studies show significant variation in fibrinogen concentrations and white blood cell (WBC) counts both within foals known to be infected with *R. equi* and compared to foals infected with another pathogen, limiting the value of these tests as specific diagnostic tests or prognostic indicators.[77,139,177,182] Thrombocytosis, which is often associated with acute or chronic inflammation, has also been reported in conjunction with *R. equi* infection, but this finding is variable.[76,184] Hyperglobulinemia may be seen in some foals. The CBC and serum chemistry profile also allow for evaluation of the patient's hydration status.

Serum amyloid A (SAA) is an acute-phase protein that has been proposed as a useful inflammatory marker in infectious disease. In one limited study, foals with *R. equi* had increased concentrations of SAA.[209] Concentrations of SAA decreased in recovered foals before fibrinogen concentration and neutrophil count decreased, suggesting that SAA concentrations could be useful in monitoring treatment response. A study that evaluated SAA concentrations in foals before and during clinical signs of rhodococcal pneumonia found that concentrations of SAA were variable among foals with *R. equi* pneumonia and could not be used reliably either as an ancillary diagnostic tool or as a screen for early detection of disease during the first month postpartum.[210]

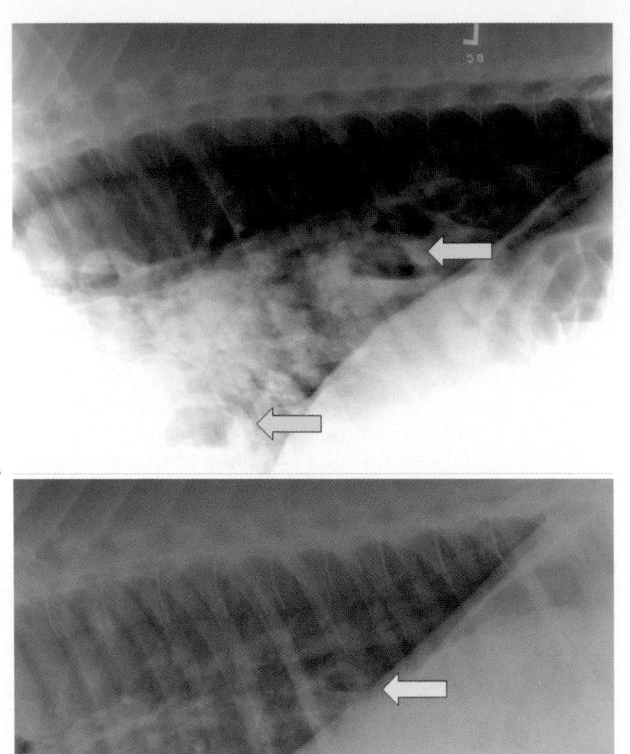

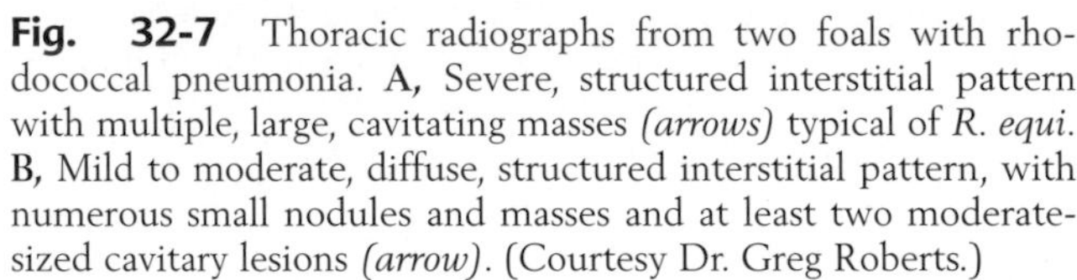

Fig. 32-7 Thoracic radiographs from two foals with rhodococcal pneumonia. **A,** Severe, structured interstitial pattern with multiple, large, cavitating masses *(arrows)* typical of *R. equi*. **B,** Mild to moderate, diffuse, structured interstitial pattern, with numerous small nodules and masses and at least two moderate-sized cavitary lesions *(arrow)*. (Courtesy Dr. Greg Roberts.)

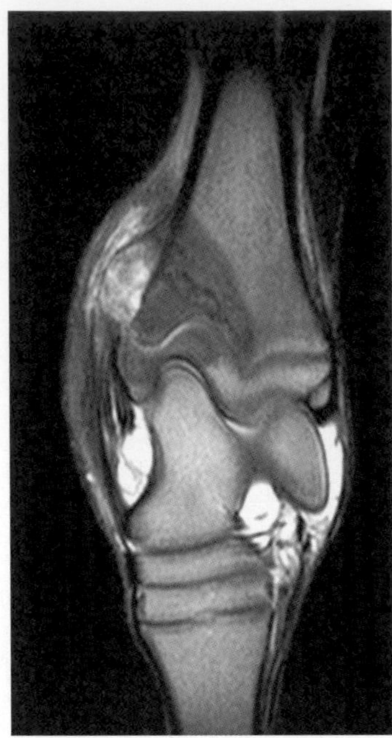

Fig. 32-8 Magnetic resonance imaging (MRI) of left tarsus of foal with septic physitis, metaphysitis, and epiphysitis caused by *R. equi* (coronal proton-density image). There is a decrease in signal from the medial aspect of the tarsus and extending beyond the midline. Fluid in the soft tissue on the medial aspect most likely represents purulent material. The lesion in the tarsus demonstrated by MRI was much more extensive than that visualized radiographically. (Courtesy Drs. Kelly Farnsworth and Pat Gavin.)

Diagnostic Imaging

Thoracic radiography is frequently used to evaluate foals with suspected *R. equi* pneumonia.[76,77,174,177,211] Typically, there is a prominent alveolar pattern with regional consolidation. Often, discrete nodular and cavitary lesions compatible with pulmonary abscessation are seen, and in some cases, gas is detectable within the abscesses (Fig. 32-7). Evidence of tracheobronchial lymphadenopathy may be present, characterized by nodular densities displacing the trachea dorsally. Although the results of studies correlating the severity of radiographic lesions and prognosis have varied, radiographic findings generally should not be used as a primary prognostic indicator because many surviving foals have had severe lesions.[76,77,177]

Radiographic evidence of pulmonary abscessation in foals strongly suggests *R. equi* infection. However, other pathogens, such as *Streptococcus zooepidemicus*, can also cause abscessation and should be considered, especially in foals over 3 months of age.[139] In addition, radiographic evidence of abscessation may be absent in some cases of rhodococcal pneumonia, and only a mild to severe bronchointerstitial pattern may be recognized. In foals with severe respiratory distress and a marked bronchointerstitial pattern, the syndrome of sporadic bronchointerstitial pneumonia should be considered. The cause of this syndrome is not known, and although occasional cases have cultured *R. equi*, its role in the pathogenesis is unclear.[141] A miliary pattern characterized by distinct reticulonodular lesions was described in three of five foals concurrently infected with *R. equi* and *Pneumocystis carinii*.[140]

Thoracic ultrasonography (US) is a practical means of assessing the thorax and can yield valuable information in the evaluation of *R. equi* pneumonia.[76,212,213] Because US does not image lesions with overlying aerated lung, the technique is primarily useful in identifying peripheral lung involvement and may not evaluate the full extent of the lesions as accurately as radiography. In most affected foals, however, peripheral lesions are present.[212,213] When thoracic US was compared with radiography in 17 foals with confirmed *R. equi* pneumonia, the findings were essentially in agreement in 15 of 17 foals.[212] Lesions were identified by US in the remaining two foals, but were less severe than those identified by radiography. It was concluded that US may be an accurate imaging modality for detection of pulmonary pathology caused by *R. equi*.[212]

Advanced imaging techniques, such as computed tomography (CT), magnetic resonance imaging (MRI), and scintigraphic imaging, may be indicated in some foals with *R. equi* infection, especially when there is extrapulmonary involvement. High-resolution CT has been used to define lesions in human patients with *R. equi* pneumonia.[214] CT was used to diagnose a mediastinal abscess causing severe respiratory distress in a 4-month-old foal with an atypical clinical presentation of *R. equi*.[143] MRI and CT have been used to diagnose septic physitis in foals (Fig. 32-8). Scintigraphic perfusion imaging was used to demonstrate pulmonary perfusion defects in affected areas of the lung in four foals with experimental rhodococcal pneumonia.[121] The findings correlated well with radiographic and necropsy lesions.

PATHOLOGIC FINDINGS

The gross lesions characteristic of *R. equi* pneumonia are multiple firm nodules separated by congested and partly atelectatic lung (Fig. 32-9).[61,62,64,137,183] The nodules vary in size, with some foci coalescing to form large lesions. Occasionally, multiple miliary pyogranulomatous foci are present. Although the distribution of lesions may be variable, lesions are bilateral in most cases and are most severe in the cranioventral regions, as is typical of bronchopneumonia. In some cases, however, lesions are distributed widely throughout the lung, especially in rapidly progressive cases. The lesions are often described as abscesses when circumscribed and as suppurative bronchopneumonia when less well defined. They consist of areas of caseous necrosis, and in most cases there is no distinct fibrous capsule around the necrotic tissue. The presence of pleural fluid is uncommon. Grossly, the bronchial lymph nodes are often swollen and edematous, and caseonecrotic foci may be present.

Histologically, the lesions are predominantly pyogranulomatous. Early lung lesions are characterized by a cellular influx into the alveolar spaces, consisting largely of macrophages and multinucleate giant cells with fewer neutrophils. Intact bacteria are typically observed within macrophages and giant cells. Lymphocytes and plasma cells are present in moderate numbers, primarily in the alveolar septa and other interstitial zones. As the disease progresses, necrosis involves the alveolar septa and spreads to affect large areas of the pulmonary parenchyma, producing the caseous necrotic foci observed macroscopically. Numerous degenerate bacteria-laden macrophages are present. Frequently, a pyogranulomatous lymphadenitis is also present histologically.

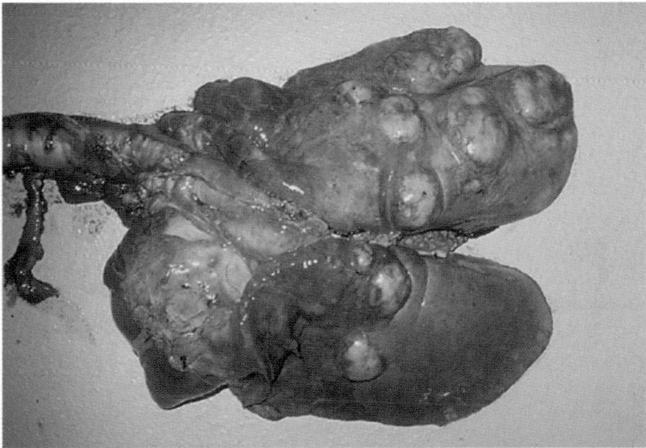

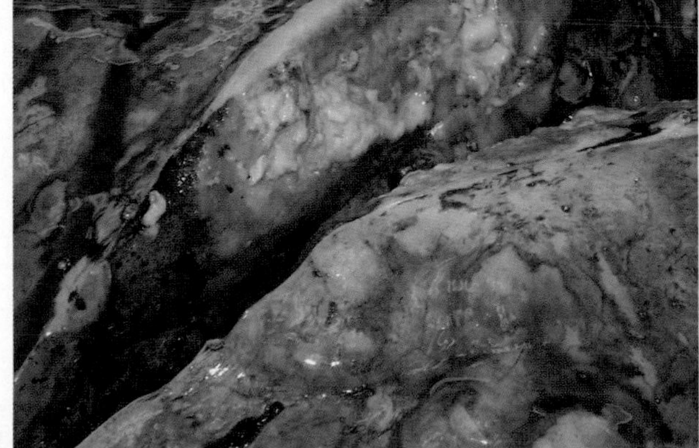

Fig. 32-9 **A,** Multiple pulmonary abscesses characteristic of *R. equi* pneumonia. **B,** Caseous exudates on cut section of rhodococcal abscess. (Courtesy Dr. Seth Harris.)

The most common sites involved in *R. equi* infection other than the lung are the intestinal tract and mesenteric lymph nodes. There is a multifocal enterocolitis and typhlitis, associated primarily with Peyer's patches in the ileum and areas of lymphoid tissue in the cecum and colon. Similar to the bronchial lymph nodes, mesenteric and colonic lymph nodes may be enlarged and have caseonecrotic foci. Occasionally a large abdominal abscess will form, most often in a mesenteric node. Peritonitis and adhesions may be present. Histologically, the intestinal lesions consist of pyogranulomatous inflammation of lymphoid tissue with fibrinonecrotic ulceration of the overlying epithelium.

The lesions of *R. equi* infection may be more widespread, suggesting hematogenous dissemination of the organism. Some of the lesions identified include septic arthritis, vertebral osteomyelitis, hypopyon (see Fig. 32-3), and ulcerative lymphangitis. Abscesses may develop at almost any site, and dermal, hepatic, renal, and splenic abscesses have been described, among others. Lesions of placentitis and fetal pneumonia in an aborted fetus have been reported in association with *R. equi* infection.[171]

R. equi can be isolated from tissues at necropsy in most cases. When only formalin-fixed tissue specimens are available for diagnostic evaluation, immunohistochemistry can be used as a diagnostic aid.[216-219] An immunohistochemical method is useful in the rapid detection of *R. equi* in impression smears obtained postmortem from tissues at necropsy.[219] This method is as sensitive as bacterial culture. To identify virulent *R. equi* specifically in tissues, monoclonal antibodies directed against the 15- to 17-kDa antigens associated with virulence have been used.[217,218]

THERAPY

Antimicrobial Therapy

Rhodococcus equi is sensitive to a wide variety of antimicrobial agents in vitro, but in vitro susceptibility does not always correlate with efficacy in vivo.[76,77,220,221] For example, aminoglycosides appear to be highly active against *R. equi* in vitro. However, in one case series, none of the 17 foals treated with gentamicin and penicillin survived despite all isolates being susceptible to gentamicin in vitro, whereas 13 foals treated with erythromycin and rifampin survived.[77] Because R. *equi* is a facultative intracellular pathogen that causes pyogranulomatous inflammation, effective antimicrobials must have good tissue and macrophage penetration and function in a relatively acid environment.

Treatment of foals with the macrolide antibiotic *erythromycin* in combination with *rifampin* began in the late 1980s (Table 32-1). The use of this combination significantly improved the success of treatment from a survival rate of approximately 20% to 30% to 60% to 90%.[76-78,222-224] Rifampin and to a lesser extent erythromycin are lipid-soluble antibiotics capable of intracellular penetration. Both erythromycin and rifampin are concentrated in granulocytes and macrophages by an active mechanism. The drugs are usually bacteriostatic but may be bactericidal at high concentrations. Use of erythromycin and rifampin in combination is recommended because they are synergistic in vitro and in vivo and because the development

Table • **32-1**

Antibiotics Frequently Used to Treat* Rhodococcus equi *in Horses

DRUG	DOSAGE
Erythromycin (estolate, stearate, phosphate ethylsuccinate, lactobionate)	25 mg/kg orally (PO) every 6 to 8 hours (q6-8h) or 37.5 mg/kg PO q12h
Azithromycin	10 mg/kg PO q24h
Clarithromycin	7.5 mg/kg PO q12h
Rifampin	5-10 mg/kg PO q12h or 10 mg/kg q24h

In most cases, erythromycin, azithromycin, or clarithromycin is given in combination with rifampin. In one study, clarithromycin-rifampin was found to be the most effective therapy.[71]

of resistance to either drug is decreased when used in combination.[76,220,225]

Two drugs closely related to erythromycin, *azithromycin*, an azalide, and *clarithromycin*, a semisynthetic macrolide, have been investigated as alternatives to erythromycin for the treatment of *R. equi* infections in foals. Compared with erythromycin, these drugs are more chemically stable, have a greater bioavailability after oral administration, and achieve higher concentrations in tissues and phagocytic cells. Studies of the pharmacokinetics and in vitro susceptibility of *R. equi* have been performed with both antimicrobials.[221,226-228]

The efficacy of azithromycin, clarithromycin, and erythromycin were compared in a retrospective study of foals admitted to a referral hospital.[71] Foals were treated with erythromycin stearate ($n = 24$; 25 mg/kg every 6 hours [q6h], 25 mg/kg q8h, or 37.5 mg/kg q12h), azithromycin ($n = 20$; 10 mg/kg q24h), or clarithromycin ($n = 18$; 7.5 mg/kg q12h). All foals except one in the azithromycin group were treated concurrently with rifampin (5 mg/kg q12h, 10 mg/kg q12h, or 10 mg/kg q24h). The results indicated that clarithromycin-rifampin was superior to erythromycin-rifampin or azithromycin-rifampin. There was no advantage of azithromycin-rifampin over traditional therapy with erythromycin-rifampin except for the convenience of once-daily dosing. These results may not necessarily apply to a situation where foals are screened and treatment is started early before establishment of severe lung lesions. Differences in the duration of therapy among treatment groups were not evaluated in this study, but many horses with rhodococcal infection require prolonged antibiotic therapy regardless of the treatment protocol. Treatment is frequently continued for 4 to 8 weeks, although a shorter duration of therapy may be sufficient if the disease is recognized early.[76,77,229] In some affected foals, such as those with well-established abscesses or osteomyelitis, a longer treatment period may be indicated. Criteria often used for the cessation of therapy include resolution of clinical signs, normalization of plasma fibrinogen concentrations, and radiographic or ultrasonographic resolution of lung lesions.

The use of erythromycin in foals is associated with a number of adverse effects, including diarrhea, hyperthermia, and respiratory distress.[230-232] In a study of 143 pneumonic foals, the risk of adverse effects was greater in foals treated with erythromycin than in foals treated with trimethoprim-sulfamethoxazole or penicillin.[230] Of the 73 foals treated with erythromycin, either alone or in combination with rifampin or gentamicin, 26 (36%) developed diarrhea, 18 (25%) develop hyperthermia, and 11 (15%) developed respiratory distress. Colitis has been observed in mares of foals being treated orally with erythromycin-rifampin, and in one study, *Clostridium difficile* was cultured from 5 of 11 (45%) of such mares with diarrhea.[233,234] Although many cases of antibiotic-associated colitis are self-limiting in both foals and mares, occasional cases are severe and fatal. In the study comparing erythromycin, azithromycin, and clarithromycin, diarrhea was observed in 17% of foals treated with erythromycin, 5% of foals treated with azithromycin, and 28% of foals treated with clarithromycin.[71] No difference was found between the groups in the proportion of foals that developed severe diarrhea requiring fluid therapy. The incidence of hyperthermia and respiratory distress resulting from antimicrobial therapy was not critically evaluated because both are common clinical signs in foals affected with *R. equi*.

The majority of *R. equi* isolates are sensitive to erythromycin, clarithromycin, azithromycin, and rifampin, but resistant strains have been encountered.[146,220,221,235-240] Resistance to erythromycin and especially rifampin can develop rapidly, particularly when these drugs are used as monotherapy. There is significant cross-resistance between the macrolides.[241] *R. equi* isolates from foals have been documented to develop resistance to rifampin after monotherapy with rifampin and to both erythromycin and rifampin during therapy.[146,237] Anecdotally, the development of resistance to clarithromycin and azithromycin in treated foals has also been observed.

It is occasionally necessary to consider alternative antimicrobials to the macrolide/rifampin therapy because of diarrhea, resistance, or financial concerns. In some horses, especially those with mild *R. equi* pneumonia, a trimethoprim-sulfonamide combination (15-30 mg/kg q8-12h) has been effective.[242] A combination of trimethoprim-sulfonamide and rifampin has been suggested, but pharmacokinetic and efficacy data are not available. Enrofloxacin (5 mg/kg orally q24h) alone or in combination with other antibiotics (ceftiofur or rifampin) has been used successfully to treat a limited number of foals with culture-confirmed *R. equi* pneumonia.[76] However, administration of enrofloxacin to foals may result in lameness, joint effusion, and cartilage lesions.[76,243-245] In foals in which significant diarrhea develops, intravenous erythromycin lactobionate (5 mg/kg diluted in saline and administered as a slow infusion q6h) has been recommended.[76] The use of an aminoglycoside in combination with either erythromycin or rifampin is controversial; it was demonstrated in vitro that activity against *R. equi* was diminished when these drugs were used in combination.[76,220,225] In a clinical study of 72 foals, however, the survival rate and ability to race as 3-year-olds were similar for foals treated with gentamicin and rifampin as for those treated with erythromycin and rifampin.[246]

Many antimicrobial agents have been used in the treatment of human patients with rhodococcal infections.[46,247] Protocols for immunocompromised human patients with serious infections often include two or three drug regimens. Antimicrobials typically used include vancomycin, imipenem, aminoglycosides, ciprofloxacin, rifampin, and erythromycin.

Additional Therapy

Additional therapy may be required depending on the specifics of the case. If a pathogen is isolated in addition to *R. equi*, a third antimicrobial may be indicated depending on the susceptibility of the organism. Supportive care is important, including maintaining adequate nutrition and hydration, as well as maintaining foals in a cool, well-ventilated environment. Arterial blood gas (ABG) assessment will help determine if oxygen therapy is indicated. Bronchodilators, such as aminophylline, theophylline, clenbuterol, and albuterol, are rarely helpful clinically.[76] In addition, concurrent administration of erythromycin and to a lesser extent clarithromycin, with either aminophylline or theophylline, may result in increased plasma concentrations of these bronchodilators, potentiating their toxicity. Nonsteroidal antiinflammatory drugs should be used judiciously to reduce fever and improve attitude and appetite. Although data are limited, based on an experimental model of *R. equi* pneumonia in foals, specific hyperimmune plasma was ineffective in treating disease once infection was established.[122] In cases with infection at a site other than the lungs, such as septic arthritis or osteomyelitis, local therapy may be indicated.

Prognosis

The survival rate for foals with *R. equi* pneumonia varies from 60% to 90% with current antimicrobial therapies.[71,73,77,78,222] Clinical and hematologic variables associated with survival from rhodococcal pneumonia have varied widely between studies. In a retrospective study of 115 cases from six veterinary medical teaching hospitals, the overall survival rate was 72%.[223] Foals that did not survive were more likely to have extreme tachycardia (heart rate >100), to be in respiratory distress, and to have severe thoracic radiographic abnormalities than were foals that survived. Clinicopathologic abnormalities were not associated with survival. The proportion of foals that survived was significantly higher in Standardbreds (80%) than in Thoroughbreds (61%). In a study of 81 foals, overall survival was 69%.[71] Radiographic scores, heart rate, and fibrinogen concentrations were significantly higher in nonsurvivors, whereas arterial oxygen and platelet counts were significantly higher in survivors. Only fibrinogen concentration was retained in the logistic regression model. There was no significant difference in survival among breeds. In another study of 39 foals, respiratory rate, temperature, WBC count, and fibrinogen concentration were higher in nonsurvivors.[177]

The prognosis has generally been poor in cases of rhodococcal osteomyelitis. However, some horses respond to aggressive treatment. A 4-month-old colt that presented for urinary incontinence associated with a *R. equi* diskospondylitis of S2-S4 responded to treatment with erythromycin, rifampin, bethanechol, and curettage of the lesion.[157] Similarly, in adult horses the prognosis has generally been poor, possibly because of delayed identification of the problem and underlying immunosuppression. A 2-year-old Quarter Horse with osteomyelitis of the pelvis did respond to treatment with erythromycin and rifampin.[172]

Several studies have attempted to evaluate the long-term effects of *R. equi* pneumonia on pulmonary function and athletic performance. In a study by Ainsworth et al.,[248] five horses recovered from rhodococcal pneumonia, and five healthy controls were evaluated by endoscopy, radiography, hematologic and BAL analyses, and pulmonary function testing. There were no significant differences in these parameters between groups, suggesting that horses that recover from *R. equi* pneumonia do not have detectable evidence of residual lung damage. The pulmonary function of seven Standardbreds that had recovered from *R. equi* pneumonia was evaluated during intense treadmill exercise, and gas exchange was not compromised compared with reference values for normal Standardbreds.[249]

A number of studies have evaluated racing performance. In one study of 11 horses previously affected with *R. equi* pneumonia, seven of them eventually raced, and four of the seven won races.[250] In a subsequent study by Ainsworth et al.,[223] 54% of foals (45/83) surviving *R. equi* infection eventually raced at least once, compared with 65% of foals in the general population. No physical examination, laboratory, or radiographic findings were identified that were predictive of whether foals went on to race. The racing performance of foals that went on to race was not significantly different from that of the general U.S. population of racing horses. Thus, although *R. equi* infection was associated with a decreased chance of racing as an adult, the performance of those foals that did go on to race was not impaired. Similarly, in a study by Bernard et al.,[251] *R. equi* in foals did not have a negative influence on racing performance, as evaluated by 2- and 3-year-old race earnings.

PREVENTION

Decreasing the Size of Infective Challenge

The outcome of exposure to *Rhodococcus equi* is partially determined by the size of the infective challenge, as with most infectious diseases. Therefore, practices targeted at decreasing the number of organisms in the environment could affect the incidence of disease. Although a number of management practices have been recommended theoretically to decrease exposure to *R. equi*, data supporting their efficacy are limited. In addition, studies aimed at identifying practices that influence the risk of disease have often had conflicting results, making it difficult to make specific management recommendations.

Farms affected with *R. equi* pneumonia tend to have large numbers of mares and foals.[76,85,86] One explanation for this is that because *R. equi* is frequently present in horse manure and may reach high numbers in the feces of foals, where it can replicate in the intestinal tract, a larger number of mares and foals may result in greater environmental contamination with *R. equi*. Alternatively, a larger number of mares and foals may simply increase the probability that a farm has a foal that develops *R. equi* pneumonia. Studies evaluating whether an association exists between high foal density and disease, as well as between mare and foal numbers and disease, have had varying results.[85,86] However, it has been suggested that both decreasing the number of mares and foals on a farm and decreasing the density could minimize *R. equi* infection.

Horse manure is believed to contribute to environmental contamination not only because it often contains bacteria, but because it contains volatile fatty acids that enhance the growth of *R. equi* once in the environment.[5,54] Therefore, it has been recommended to remove horse manure frequently from stalls, paddocks, and pastures and either not to spread manure on pastures as fertilizer or to compost the manure before spreading.[60,76,252] In epidemiologic studies, however, manure removal programs did not significantly alter the risk for development of *R. equi* pneumonia.[85,87] There were no significant differences between control farms and affected farms in whether horse manure was spread on pastures or composted before spreading.[87] The highest concentrations of bacteria in manure are generally found in the feces of infected foals, because these foals swallow sputum with large numbers of virulent organisms, which may then multiply within the intestine. Thus, although *R. equi* is not thought to be highly contagious between horses, preventive recommendations include isolating infected foals and removing their manure promptly to decrease environmental contamination.[60,76,252]

R. equi infection has anecdotally been linked to raising foals in a dusty environment, but it has been difficult to document this objectively. Cohen et al.[85] demonstrated an association between *R. equi* pneumonia and the veterinarians' report of a dusty environment, whereas Chaffin et al.[87] failed to show such an association. However, it has been theorized that efforts to reduce dust in the environment, such as reseeding and irrigating to promote growth of grass, as well as using water sprinklers in paddocks, may reduce aerosolization of dust particles that might be laden with *R. equi* and may help decrease the incidence of rhodococcal infection.

One study demonstrated that foals from farms with enzootic *R. equi* were significantly less likely to have foaled in a pasture than in a stall or small paddock.[85] Stall confinement may expose foals to high concentrations of microorganisms and poor ventilation, contributing to the development of disease. Further investigation is needed to evaluate the effects of environmental management procedures on the prevalence of *R. equi* infection.

Early Detection of Disease

The early recognition of *R. equi* pneumonia may reduce losses and limit the duration, and thus the costs, of therapy. Because obvious clinical signs are often not apparent until the disease is advanced, a number of approaches have been recommended for early diagnosis. Higuchi et al.[204] suggested that physical examination of foals at 30 and 45 days of age was useful for early diagnosis of *R. equi* infection on enzootic farms. Similarly, Prescott et al.[253] found that twice-weekly complete physical examinations with careful auscultation of the thorax was successful in the early diagnosis of infection and in preventing mortality. Serologic surveillance has also been recommended, but it is unreliable.[76,207,208]

Other strategies for early detection of *R. equi* pneumonia include serial monitoring of WBC count and fibrinogen concentration and thoracic US. A prospective study of 162 foals from a farm with enzootic *R. equi* infection evaluated the efficacy of WBC count, fibrinogen concentration, and the AGID test for early identification of *R. equi*–infected foals.[182] Although both WBC count and fibrinogen concentration were useful in detecting early *R. equi* infection, the WBC count was more sensitive and specific. It was recommended that WBC counts of foals should be evaluated monthly on farms with enzootic *R. equi* infection. Foals with WBC concentrations of 13,000 cells/μL or greater should receive a careful physical examination, and foals with WBC concentrations of 14,000/μL or higher should be considered candidates for additional diagnostic testing, such as thoracic radiography or US. Serologic testing using the AGID was not accurate in predicting disease. Thoracic US of foals starting at 30 days of age and repeated at 2-week intervals until 16 to 20 weeks of age may be effective in reducing subclinical and clinical disease associated with *R. equi*.[213]

Prophylactic antibiotic use has been anecdotally recommended to reduce disease caused by exposure to *R. equi*. This practice is controversial in part because of concerns about the selection of antibiotic-resistant bacteria. The efficacy of this recommendation in preventing disease is currently under investigation, but no data are yet available.

Passive Immunization

Hyperimmune plasma is often administered intravenously to foals in an effort to prevent *R. equi* pneumonia. In some studies, this practice has been effective in significantly reducing the incidence of rhodococcal pneumonia after experimental or natural challenge.[74,75,121,124] However, other studies have failed to document a statistically significant protective effect.[73,123,125] For example, in a randomized clinical trial of 165 Thoroughbred foals on a farm with enzootic pneumonia, 19.1% of foals receiving plasma developed *R. equi* pneumonia compared with 30% of nontreated foals.[73] This difference was not statistically significant. Despite the somewhat varying results, the generally beneficial effects and relative safety of administering hyperimmune plasma have made its use relatively common. In a study of 65 enzootic farms, 36 (56%) administered hyperimmune plasma.[85]

The optimal protocol for the administration of hyperimmune plasma has not been determined, and differences in the timing of administration may account for some of the variability between studies. Optimally, plasma should be given before exposure to *R. equi*, based on studies that demonstrated no benefit when hyperimmune plasma was administered after experimental challenge.[122] The exact time of exposure of most foals is unclear but likely occurs early in life, especially on enzootic farms.[69,70] Administration of hyperimmune plasma too early may result in a waning of passively transferred antibodies to nonprotective concentrations when some foals are still susceptible. Most studies have administered approximately 1 liter of plasma between 1and 60 days of age.[73-75,125] In the study of 165 foals on an enzootic farm, 950 mL of plasma was administered at 1 to 10 days of age and again at 30 to 50 days of age.[73] Because the majority of treated foals that developed pneumonia did so before the administration of the second liter, it was postulated that administration of the second dose at an earlier age may have been more beneficial. The ideal time for hyperimmune plasma administration may vary from farm to farm.

Active Immunization

The development of an effective vaccine for *R. equi* would clearly be beneficial to the equine population and has been an area of active research. Most foals exposed to virulent *R. equi* mount a protective immune response and remain immune as adults, which suggests that the induction of protective immunity by active immunization should be possible. However, the development of an efficacious vaccine has proved difficult despite the use of multiple strategies for active immunization of mares and foals.

One major challenge in developing an effective vaccine is the ability to stimulate the correct type of immune response (i.e., the protective phenotype) in a neonatal foal. Because of immunologic naivete, foals may have a diminished ability to mount a protective immune response of the required magnitude rapidly enough to prevent infection. Although specific information related to neonatal immunity in foals is limited, the immune responses of neonates appear to differ both quantitatively and qualitatively from those of adults.[254-258] The differences in the immune system during the first few weeks of life have been variously described as a state of immunologic immaturity, a relative immunodeficiency, or immunodeviance. With respect to cellular immunity, neonates are thought to have a Th2 bias and a diminished ability to generate the type 1 responses necessary for clearance of intracellular pathogens. Another possible challenge to immunization of neonatal foals is overcoming potential interference by maternal antibody. However, this may be of less importance with *R. equi* than with some other pathogens, because the T-lymphocyte responses that play a significant role in immunity to *R. equi* may be less affected by maternal antibody than humoral responses.[259,260]

Several candidate vaccines have been investigated, but as yet none has been developed for widespread use. Killed virulent *R. equi* did not elicit protective immunity in mice.[261] Similarly, killed virulent *R. equi* given intramuscularly did not protect foals from experimental infection.[262] Immunization of foals with two exoenzymes produced by *R. equi*, cholesterol oxidase and phospholipase C, did not prevent the development of lung abscesses after experimental challenge, although severe clinical signs did not develop in either vaccinated or control foals in this study.[263] A number of vaccines have been evaluated for the prevention of *R. equi* under field conditions, including an inactivated *R. equi* vaccine with and without EHV-2, a preparation of soluble antigens of *R. equi* that include VapA and "equi factor" exoenzymes, and an EHV-2 subunit vaccine.[91,264,265] Although studies have suggested that these vaccines could provide some protection against *R. equi*, data are limited and further study is needed.

Infection with avirulent *R. equi* does not result in protection, suggesting that the virulence plasmid encodes antigens critical to protective immunity.[261,266] Several studies have focused specifically on the potential of VapA as an immunogen. Vaccination with VapA results in the production of VapA-specific antibodies in both horses and mice.* A study in mice demonstrated that immunization with partially purified VapA also resulted in significantly enhanced clearance of organisms from the liver and spleen after experimental challenge.[28] Other studies, however, have suggested that VapA vaccines are unable to prevent bacterial replication despite their immunogenicity.[267,268] In a study by Prescott et al.[124] on an enzootic farm, vaccination of mares and their foals with a VapA extract did not protect foals from natural infection with *R. equi* despite the presence of opsonizing antibody. Limited data from a study in pregnant mares suggest that the use of a VapA candidate vaccine could result in passive antibody-mediated protection of foals and warrants further investigation.[128]

Exposure to live virulent *R. equi* elicits protective immunity in both foals and mice. Specifically in foals, oral immunization with live virulent *R. equi* protected foals against experimental challenge, confirming that young foals can mount a highly effective protective immune response.[269,270] Foals that were orally immunized developed high concentrations of antibody specific to VapA and VapC but not to other Vap proteins, indicating that Vap A and VapC are highly immunogenic.[270] Although oral immunization with live virulent bacteria is protective, it is not considered a practical means of widespread vaccination because of the risks of developing disease in some individuals and disseminating large numbers of organisms into the environment.

Efforts to develop a safe, effective vaccine for *R. equi* are ongoing. Even at a young age, most foals are probably capable of mounting a protective immune response, as supported by the observations that the majority of foals do not develop clinical disease after natural exposure and that foals are protected after oral immunization with live virulent bacteria. An effective vaccine will most likely induce both humoral and cellular immunity and will direct the immune response to the protective phenotype. Some strategies under investigation include the development of attenuated strains of *R. equi* by transposon mutagenesis, DNA vaccination, and the use of a recombinant bacille Calmette-Guérin (BCG) vaccine expressing VapA antigen.[271-274]

PUBLIC HEALTH CONSIDERATIONS

Rhodococcus equi is an emerging pathogen in human medicine and is most often recognized as an opportunistic infection in immunocompromised patients.[46,247] The first case of *R. equi* infection in a human patient was not reported until 1967, and only about 12 additional cases were reported during the next 15 years. However, coincident with the emergence of HIV infection and advances in organ transplantation and cancer treatment, the incidence of *R. equi* in humans has greatly increased since the early 1980s. Improvements in laboratory diagnosis and enhanced awareness of the disease have also contributed to the increase in reported cases. In the past 15 years, at least 100 cases of *R. equi* infection in humans have been reported in the medical literature.[46] Approximately 85% to 90% of human patients with *R. equi* are immunocompromised, with these patients being divided between those with HIV infection and those who are otherwise immunocompromised as a result of disease, immunosuppressive medications, or both. These immunocompromised patients often have concurrent infections with other opportunistic pathogens. Only about 10% to 15% of *R. equi* infections occur in seemingly immunocompetent hosts.

Rhodococcus equi infection in human patients is thought to be acquired by inhalation, inoculation into a wound or mucous membrane, or ingestion. The soil is believed to be the most common source of infectious organisms. The possible role of other routes of *R. equi* acquisition, including human colonization and person-to-person transmission, is poorly understood. It is believed that *R. equi* does not colonize the intestine of human patients.[46,275] Because rhodococcal species other than *R. equi* are among the species that dominate the nasal microbiota of healthy adults, it has been speculated that nasal colonization with *R. equi* could occur.[46,276] Unlike in foals, where essentially all isolates from clinical cases express VapA, only 20% to 25% of isolates recovered from human patients express VapA.[46]

The clinical manifestations of *R. equi* infection in human patients are varied, and the organism has been isolated from almost every body site. As in foals, pulmonary infection, often resulting in pyogranulomatous pneumonia, is common, being recognized in approximately 84% of immunocompromised patients and approximately 42% of immunocompetent patients.[46,247] Localized infections, often associated with wounds, represent about 50% of reported cases in immunocompetent hosts.[247] Combination antibiotic therapy is the mainstay of treatment, and empiric two-drug regimens typically include erythromycin, rifampin, and/or ciprofloxacin. Vancomycin, imipenem, aminoglycosides, and a number of other antibiotics have also been recommended. Surgical drainage of abscesses in sites of poor antibiotic penetration is probably beneficial. The mortality rate among immunocompetent patients is approximately 11%, compared with rates of 50% to 55% among HIV-infected patients and 20% to 25% among non–HIV-infected immunocompromised patients.

Exposure to domesticated animals, especially horses and pigs, may play a role in some cases of *R. equi* infection in humans, although only one third of all patients have a history of exposure to horses or pigs.[46] However, it is recommended that immunocompromised patients with significant exposure to domesticated animals be cautioned regarding the possible risk of *R. equi* infection.

REFERENCES

See the CD-ROM for a list of references linked to the abstract in PubMed.

*References 28, 118, 124, 128, 267, 268.

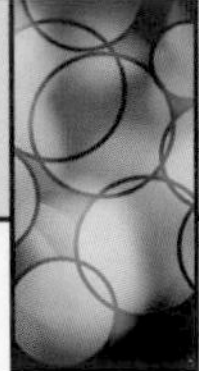

CHAPTER • 33

Mycobacterial Infections

J. Lindsay Oaks

ETIOLOGY

The mycobacteria comprise the only genus in the family *Mycobacteriaceae* and are a large group of aerobic, non–spore-forming bacterial rods. The most salient feature of this group is their ability to retain arylmethane dyes such as fuschin when mixed with phenol to allow uptake of the dye (e.g., carbolfuschin), then resist decolorization with acid alcohols or inorganic acids. This is the basis for their designation as "acid-fast." The ability to stain acid-fast results from the high cell wall content of hydrophobic mycolic acids and other complex lipids and waxes. Nutritionally, most mycobacteria are able to utilize simple substrates as sources of carbon and nitrogen, although some are fastidious and require supplemented media for growth in culture (e.g., mycobactin for *Mycobacterium avium* subspp., *paratuberculosis*). Growth in culture is generally stimulated by the presence of fatty acids, and thus many media for the culture of mycobacteria contain lipid sources such as egg yolk or oleic acid.[1]

In general, mycobacteria have long generation times and thus are slow growing compared with other bacterial pathogens. Although growth rates vary widely, most of the significant human and veterinary mycobacterial pathogens take 14 to 60 days of culture to detect visible growth.[1,2] Some, such as *Mycobacterium leprae* and *Mycobacterium lepraemurium*, the cause of human and feline leprosy, respectively, effectively remain unculturable.[3] Slow growth, groups or "complexes" of closely related organisms, and unreliable phenotypic or biochemical differentiation schemes have greatly complicated the diagnosis and taxonomic description of mycobacteria.[1,2,4] In recent years, however, genetic analysis of regions such as the 16S ribosomal ribonucleic acid (rRNA) or heat shock protein genes and biochemical analysis of fatty acids have resulted in great advances in both the identification and the taxonomy of mycobacteria.[4,5]

EPIDEMIOLOGY

Mycobacterial infections generally result in either multifocal pulmonary or disseminated granulomatous disease ("tubercles") or localized subcutaneous infections. Pulmonary or disseminated tuberculous disease is typically caused by the obligate pathogens *Mycobacterium tuberculosis* and *Mycobacterium bovis*, the classic agents of human and bovine tuberculosis.[1,6] Multifocal to infiltrative disease in ruminants is caused by another obligately pathogenic organism, *Mycobacterium avium* subsp. *paratuberculosis*, the causative agent of Johne's disease.[7] These particular mycobacteria are relatively unusual in that they are primary pathogens in mammalian hosts, and host immunodeficiency is not a prerequisite for disease.[1,6-8]

In contrast, the other mycobacteria are environmental organisms that cause sporadic and opportunistic infections. They are ubiquitous in soil and water and typically cause either disseminated disease in immunocompromised hosts or localized infections in immunocompetent hosts. The only environmental mycobacterium frequently associated with disseminated granulomatous disease in veterinary medicine is *Mycobacterium avium* subsp. *avium* (MAA), sometimes referred to as "atypical tuberculosis" or "avian tuberculosis." Pulmonary or disseminated MAA infections occur sporadically in a variety of domestic and nondomestic animals, as well as humans.[9-11] In humans, pulmonary mycobacterial infections are usually associated with underlying lung disease, and extrapulmonary disease is typically observed only in people with significant immunosuppressive conditions, most notably human immunodeficiency virus (HIV) infection.[1,6,9,12] Although MAA infections have been associated with immunosuppression in dogs and cats, in most cases of MAA disease in domestic animals, an obvious immunosuppressive condition is not recognized.[11,13] Birds are the only species in which epizootics of MAA disease occur. High challenge doses and virulence appear to play a role.[10,14] The other common form of mycobacterial disease in humans and veterinary species is localized infection that occurs opportunistically in immunocompetent hosts. These infections may be caused by a large number of environmental mycobacteria, including MAA.[1,5,15,16] Finally, many mycobacteria are entirely saprophytic and nonpathogenic. These become an issue when encountered in diagnostic samples, and caution needs to be used in ascribing significance to them.[5]

In horses, mycobacterial infections are rare. Although disease caused by *M. bovis* and to a lesser extent *M. tuberculosis* has been reported in horses, they appear to be inherently resistant based primarily on the observation that equine tuberculosis has remained uncommon even in areas where the disease is prevalent in humans and other animals.[17-19] In areas with effective control programs for *M. bovis* and *M. tuberculosis*, the incidence of these infections in horses has decreased correspondingly.[17] In areas where these diseases occur, however, cases may still be seen in horses.[20] Moreover, with the continued presence in North America and Europe of *M. bovis*, particularly in wildlife,[8] and the resurgence of *M. tuberculosis* in humans,[21] the possibility of these infections in horses should not be disregarded.

Infection with *M. avium* subspp., *paratuberculosis* (Johne's disease) can be induced experimentally in horses.[22] The recent literature also describes a single case in a Sicilian ass from North America, although the diagnosis was not confirmed by culture.[23] Consequently, naturally occurring equine Johne's disease, if it truly occurs at all, appears to be exceedingly rare.

The most common mycobacterial disease currently seen in horses is disseminated disease caused by MAA, which has been reported sporadically from North America and Europe.[13,17,24-30] These reports describe infection with MAA serotypes 1, 2, 4, 5, and 8, in some cases with multiple serotypes from a single horse. These serotypes indicate equine infections have been caused by MAA rather than the closely related *Mycobacterium intracellulare* (in human medicine often referred to as part of the "*Mycobacterium avium* complex").[1] Interestingly, in humans, MAA infections are most often associated with disseminated disease in patients immunosuppressed by HIV infections,[1,12] whereas *M. intracellulare* infections predominate in patients with pulmonary disease.[31,32] Although completely speculative, this may suggest that horses with disseminated MAA infections have an underlying immune defect that predisposes them to this disease. Other than a single case in which MAA was associated with septic arthritis,[16] all MAA infections described in horses have been disseminated disease. Although little is known about the source of equine MAA infections, the cases are very sporadic, and there is no evidence that these infections are contagious among horses. In other species, including humans, the source of infection is environmental.[6,11,15,33,34]

Localized infections with other species of mycobacteria have also been described in horses but are surprisingly rare. These include a single case of abortion caused by *Mycobacterium terrae*,[35] a recent case of fetal disseminated granulomatous disease and abortion from which a pure culture of *Mycobacterium holsaticum* was obtained from fetal tissues (Slavic D, Shapiro J, Animal Health Laboratory, University of Guelph, unpublished data), and a single case of subcutaneous infection caused by *Mycobacterium smegmatis*.[36]

PATHOGENESIS

No studies of MAA pathogenesis have been performed in horses, so information regarding the pathogenesis of this disease must be extrapolated from what is described in other species. However, because the lesions are so similar, it is reasonable to assume that at least the major features of pathogenesis in horses will be similar to other species. The predominant lesions in horses are respiratory and enteric, indicating that the entry of MAA is by aerosol or ingestion of environmental organisms, respectively. On ingestion, MAA has the ability to survive low pH conditions in the stomach and transit to the intestines.[37] Once in the intestine, MAA initially infects enterocytes, and to a lesser extent M cells, overlying intestinal lymphoid tissue. Although enterocyte infection is receptor mediated and a metabolically active process that blocks bacterial degradation in cellular vacuoles, MAA infection appears to be silent in that it elicits neither chemokine responses nor inflammation.[38]

After extrusion from the intestinal epithelium into the submucosa, MAA is scavenged by local macrophages. MAA is a facultative intracellular parasite of macrophages, and the ability to infect and replicate within macrophages is the defining characteristic of pathogenic mycobacteria. Entry of MAA into macrophages is mediated primarily by complement receptors, including CR3 (CD11b/CD18 complex) and CR1. After uptake into the phagosome of a resting macrophage, MAA selectively upregulates gene expression[39] and is able to alter a number of host cell functions to prevent bacterial degradation and facilitate survival. These include blocking phagosome-lysosome fusion and acidification of the phagosome, upregulation of enzymes used in fatty acid metabolism, expression of MAA transcriptional regulators, and facilitation of iron transport.[38,40] Replication within macrophages appears to impart to progeny bacteria increased efficiency of infecting new macrophages, possibly by utilization of alternate receptors for entry, such as β_1-integrins and transferrin, as well an enhanced ability to block macrophage activation. This process may facilitate reinfection and dissemination.[41]

The host immune response to infected macrophages results in granuloma formation by activation and recruitment of macrophages into the affected area.[42] Cell-mediated host responses that effectively activate and induce bactericidal mechanisms in MAA-infected macrophages are required to control infection. Neither CD8+ cytotoxic T lymphocytes nor specific antibodies appear to be important in control of MAA.[38,43] Key cytokines and cells involved in effective macrophage activation and anti-MAA immune responses include interferon gamma (IFN-γ) from natural killer (NK) cells and antigen-specific CD4+ T lymphocytes, tumor necrosis factor alpha (TNF-α) and granulocyte-monocyte colony-stimulating factor (GM-CSF) from macrophages, and interleukin-12 (IL-12) from macrophages, NK cells, and neutrophils.[32,38,43] TNF-α and IFN-γ in particular are key to granuloma formation.[43] TNF-α is one of the most critical cytokines for activation of bactericidal activity in infected macrophages, including production of antibacterial proteins, production of superoxide anions, inhibition of bacterial replication, and induction of apoptosis. Interference with TNF-α activity in infected mice leads to higher bacterial loads, and blocking TNF-α expression in infected macrophages is associated with increased MAA virulence.[44-46]

To maintain infection, MAA is able to counter by interfering with host antibacterial responses. MAA increases production of transforming growth factor beta (TGF-β), IL-10, and IL-6, which suppresses macrophage function and responsiveness to IFN-γ and TNF-α.[38,43] MAA may also directly interfere with IFN-γ cell-signaling pathways in macrophages.[43] The lack of phagosome acidification and suppression of co-stimulatory molecules interfere with antigen presentation and prevent infected cells from initiating proinflammatory responses.[38,47]

Clinical disease resulting from MAA is ultimately caused by organ dysfunction from infiltration and destruction of tissue by granulomatous inflammation. Weight loss is also frequently observed in MAA-infected horses. Although in many equine cases this is probably caused by intestinal involvement and malabsorption, in monkeys MAA also has the ability to cause cachexia directly by disruption of growth hormone and insulin-like growth factor regulation of metabolism.[48] In immunocompetent animals, antibacterial host responses are generally sufficient to control or eliminate infections. Because exposure is most likely ubiquitous and probably occurs routinely in all horses, the vast majority of MAA infections are eradicated subclinically. What tips the balance in some horses toward the inability to control infection is not known. Equine MAA infections are not associated with overt congenital or acquired immunodeficiency syndromes. However, more subtle defects that predispose horses to MAA infections may go unrecognized. For example, human susceptibility to disseminated MAA infections have been associated with genetic defects in IFN-γ and IL-12 immune responses.[32]

CLINICAL FINDINGS

MAA infections in horses are typically diagnosed only after disease is highly advanced, and such infections have been uniformly fatal.[13,17,24-30] As with most disseminated diseases, the clinical presentations may be quite variable depending on the organ system(s) affected and in which organ system(s) clinically significant pathology predominates. Cases of MAA have been described only in horses greater than 1 year of age. It is not known if the absence of disease in foals represents innate resistance, or if it means that MAA has a long incubation period. Interestingly however, cases do tend to occur in younger horses, with 13 of 21 horses in the series of cases reviewed being 6 years of age or younger.[13,17,24-30] There does not appear to be a gender or breed predisposition.

MAA is a chronic disease, with most affected horses having clinical disease histories of 2 to 12 months. These horses likely were subclinically infected for some time before the onset of clinically apparent disease. Horses with MAA infections usually have many of the nonspecific signs of chronic bacterial infection, including depression, intermittent fever, and weight loss. Many, but not all, infected horses have mild neutrophilia. In some cases, anemia is present. One of the most consistent clinical presentations of equine MAA infections is chronic diarrhea caused by involvement of the small intestine, cecum, or colon.* Many of these horses also have hypoalbuminemia from malabsorption and protein-losing enteropathy, which may result in ascites, pleural effusion, and edema. Although pulmonary involvement is common, overt respiratory signs such as dyspnea and coughing are uncommon. Similarly, although the liver is usually affected, and elevated liver function tests may be seen on clinical chemistries, overt liver disease is uncommon.[13,17,24-30] Thoracic and mesenteric lymphadenopathy is usually present. Involvement of the axial skeleton, particularly the cervical vertebrae, is also frequently described and results in lameness, neck or back pain or stiffness, and occasionally spinal cord signs.[17,27] Other clinical lesions reported in conjunction with disseminated MAA infection include abortion,[26] oral ulcers,[26] ocular infection,[29] guttural pouch masses and ulcers,[25] dermatitis,[13,30] abscessation, and mastitis.[17]

Localized infections with other mycobacteria are generally the result of traumatic injuries that inoculate environmental mycobacteria into lesions. Although these types of infections appear to be rare in horses, they should be suspected with nonhealing granulomatous or pyogranulomatous wound infections that do not respond to conventional drainage and antimicrobial therapy. In other animals and humans, cutaneous mycobacterial infections typically present as nodular, ulcerated, fistulous draining tracts.[49]

DIAGNOSIS

The antemortem diagnosis of MAA may be challenging because of nonspecific clinical signs. A wide array of differential diagnoses need to be considered, including other chronic bacterial infections, fungal infections, and neoplasia. If MAA is suspected, however, and the lesions are amenable to biopsy, the characteristic granulomatous lesions and presence of acid-fast organisms are diagnostic for a mycobacterial infection. The absence of visible acid-fast organisms does not rule out mycobacterial infection, however, since smears or sections from culture-positive samples may be negative.[13,16,17,28] Because of their hydrophobicity, mycobacteria generally will not stain with Gram stain or Romanowsky-type stains (e.g., Diff-Quik).[1,49] Intradermal tuberculin testing with *M. bovis* or MAA antigens appears to lack specificity, with up to 70% of apparently uninfected horses giving positive reactions.[18,50] However, although these studies do not closely examine the number of infected horses with negative reactions, a negative test may suggest that a horse is not infected. Because equine MAA infections are almost invariably fatal, there is usually an opportunity to obtain necropsy samples. The gross necropsy findings are often highly suggestive, and histopathology is generally suggestive or diagnostic of a mycobacterial infection.

Culture of tissue or fluid samples remains the "gold standard" for detection of mycobacterial pathogens. Because of the small volume of material and the scarcity of organisms in some infections, swabs are not the preferred specimen. The hydrophobicity of mycobacteria may also interfere with efficient transfer of organisms to agar plates.[1] Particular care should be taken to avoid environmental contamination of the sample because many mycobacteria, including MAA, are present in soil, tap water, feed, bedding, and the mucous membranes of normal horses.[1,5,11,34,51] Mycobacteria are environmentally hardy, and thus they can be shipped to the laboratory with only minimal precautions to prevent desiccation of the sample.[1] Samples for culture should be stored and shipped at 4° C (39° F).

When samples are submitted for culture, it is essential to inform the laboratory that mycobacteria are suspected because they require specialized media and prolonged incubation for successful isolation. Mycobacteria will not be detected with routine aerobic culture methods. It is also important to inform the laboratory of the sample type and the likelihood that the sample may be contaminated with fungi or other bacteria that may overgrow mycobacteria during prolonged incubation. Because of the inherent resistance of mycobacteria to disinfectants and other chemicals, contaminants can be selectively removed from samples with various combinations of sodium hydroxide, antibacterials, antifungals, and detergents. However, effective removal of contaminants will also reduce the numbers of mycobacteria, so pretreatment is avoided for noncontaminated samples.[1,52]

Media for isolation of mycobacteria generally contain nitrogen and carbon sources and are supplemented with lipids (e.g., egg yolk, glycerol, oleic acid) to stimulate mycobacterial growth. Most media also contain compounds to inhibit the growth of fungi and other bacteria.[1] Nonselective media usually contain inhibitors such as malachite green and are appropriate for samples from sterile sites or that have been decontaminated. Selective media additionally contain a variety of antibacterials and antifungals to further inhibit growth of contaminants, but because these media may also slow or inhibit the growth of mycobacteria, samples should be inoculated on both nonselective and selective media.[1]

Certain mycobacteria have specific nutritional requirements and require media with specific supplements, such as mycobactin for *M. avium* subspp. *paratuberculosis*.[7] A variety of broth media formulations are also used and may be required for isolation of some mycobacteria, such as *Mycobacterium genavense*.[9] Broth media also improve recovery rates and decrease the time for detection of mycobacteria and are recommended for use on all samples. Cultures are generally incubated at 35° to 37° C (95°-98.6° F) in atmospheres of 5% to 10% carbon dioxide, although some mycobacteria (e.g., *Mycobacterium marinum*, *Mycobacterium chelonae*) grow optimally at 25° to 33° C (77°-91.4° F), and wound samples should be incubated at both temperatures.[1,9] Mycobacteria generally are slow growing, but quite variable. *M. bovis* or *M. tuberculosis* require 6 to 8 weeks to detect visible growth, whereas *Mycobacterium fortuitum* or *M. smegmatis* may be visible after only 2 to 3 days.[1,9,49]

Cultured mycobacteria can be identified by a panel of phenotypic properties, such as growth rate, colony morphology and pigmentation, temperature sensitivity, and biochemical reactions.[1,2] Thin-layer, high-performance liquid and gas-liquid chromatographic analysis of mycolic acids and lipids produced by isolates has also been useful for identification.[5] MAA can generally be isolated readily with Middlebrook 7H10 or 7H11 solid formulations, which produce detectable growth in 2 to 4 weeks, or in Middlebrook 7H9 broth, which may produce detectable growth in 1 to 2 weeks.[9] Seroagglutination can be used to characterize MAA further into strains.[53]

Traditional culture methods have the disadvantage of being slow and often less than definitive for identification of mycobacteria. Fortunately, recent advances in the application of molecular biology to diagnostic mycobacteriology have greatly improved both the timeliness and the accuracy of laboratory testing.[4,54-56] A number of deoxyribonucleic acid (DNA) probes that specifically hybridize to and identify isolates of the major pathogenic mycobacteria are commercially available.[9,54] Although these probes are sensitive and specific for their mycobacterial targets, they still require that the organism first be cultured.

*References 13, 17, 24, 26, 28, 30.

DNA amplification by the polymerase chain reaction (PCR) assay is currently one of the most common molecular methods being used by veterinary diagnostic laboratories. Depending on the selection of oligonucleotide primers, PCR assays for mycobacteria may either be designed to be species specific or to amplify genes for sequencing and genetic analysis. Mycobacterium-specific PCR reactions are generally used for the more common pathogens, such as MAA.[57] Although we have not had an opportunity to use MAA-specific PCR assays in horses, we have found this to work well in other animals, including dogs, birds, and rabbits (Washington Animal Disease Diagnostic Laboratory, unpublished data). The main disadvantage to this approach is that if the test is negative, the organism is not identified. In addition, certain gene targets, such as insertion sequences, may give false-negative results if they are not present in all strains.[54]

Because of the diversity of mycobacteria that may be encountered in clinical samples, sequencing and genetic analysis of PCR-amplified genes, such as the 16S rRNA or heat shock protein, is a very powerful tool for general identification of mycobacteria. This approach uses primers to highly conserved regions of a given gene to amplify a fragment from any mycobacterial species. The fragment is then sequenced, and the unique regions are compared to genetic databases (e.g., GenBank, RIDOM). Analysis of the 16S rRNA gene has become the gold standard for bacterial phylogenetics, and analysis of this region has proved to be very useful for definitive identification of mycobacterial isolates.[4,54-56] This approach has also been used successfully for identification of veterinary mycobacterial pathogens,[58-60] including MAA in a horse.[16] PCR methods, including sequencing, also have the advantage of rapid results (2-3 days). PCR methods can be performed directly on clinical samples, eliminating the need for culture and greatly reducing the time required for a diagnosis.[57-60] In cases where fresh tissue samples are not available, PCR methods can also be used on formalin-fixed, paraffin-embedded samples[60] (Washington Animal Disease Diagnostic Laboratory, unpublished data). The primary disadvantage of direct detection of mycobacteria in clinical samples is that it precludes evaluation of biologic properties, such as antimicrobial resistance. However, susceptibility testing and other phenotypic information often are not essential for the diagnosis or treatment of mycobacterial infections.

PATHOLOGIC FINDINGS

Horses with disseminated MAA are typically thin to emaciated. The most salient gross necropsy findings in horse with disseminated MAA are multifocal to miliary nodules, ranging in size from microscopic up to about 4 cm in diameter in affected organs.[13,17,24-30] These nodules are generally solid, pale colored, firm in consistency, and often give the appearance of being neoplastic.[18,42] The center of the nodules is sometimes caseous or contains fluid, but this is not typical. Calcification or fibrosis of the nodules is rare.[10,13,42] Any portion of the gastrointestinal tract may be affected, but the cecum and colon appear to be most frequently involved.* In severe cases the large numbers of coalescing nodules may give the appearance of an infiltrative disease similar to bovine Johne's disease.[13,27] Another prominent feature of intestinal infection is the presence of ulceration or crateriform lesions in the mucosa.[24,26,28] Ulceration may also be seen when lesions are present on the skin[13,30] or other mucosal surfaces, such as the guttural pouch[25] or oral mucosa.[26]

Microscopically, the nodules are granulomatous inflammation, with the primary inflammatory cells consisting of macrophages, epithelioid macrophages, and multinucleated giant cells (Langhans' cells).[13,17,24-30,42] Variable numbers of lymphocytes, neutrophils, plasma cells, and fibrosis may also be present. Caseous or liquefactive necrosis may be observed in some nodules. With ulcerative lesions, suppurative inflammation may be seen at the ulcerated surface,[25] most likely from secondary infections by other bacteria. Acid-fast bacilli can generally be demonstrated in the cytoplasm of macrophages within lesions[13,24-27,29,30] (Fig. 33-1). However, in a significant proportion of culture-confirmed cases described in the literature, acid-fast organisms were not detectable.[17,28]

*References 13, 17, 24, 26, 28, 30.

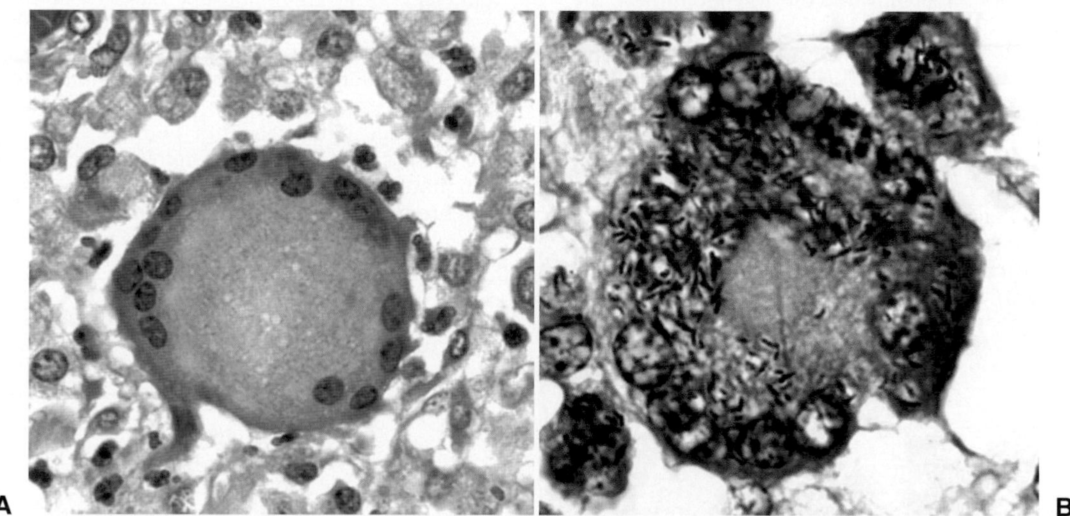

Fig. 33-1 Multinucleated giant cells from horse with *Mycobacterium avium* infection. **A**, Hematoxylin and eosin stain of multinucleated giant cell in which no organisms can be seen. **B**, Acid-fast stain of multinucleated giant cell demonstrating large numbers of acid-fast bacilli. (Courtesy Anatomic Pathology Section, Diagnostic Center for Population and Animal Health, College of Veterinary Medicine, Michigan State University.)

THERAPY AND PREVENTION

Opportunities to treat MAA-infected horses will be rare. In the previously reported cases, MAA-infected horses were presented with either very advanced or terminal disease, and treatment was not attempted.[13,17,24-30] Based on the experience with treatment of MAA-infected humans, therapy with drug combinations that are highly effective for treating *M. tuberculosis* (ethambutol, isoniazid, rifampin, streptomycin) are ineffective for treating MAA. The high failure rates have been attributed to the inherent antimicrobial resistance of MAA and the presence of underlying immunosuppressive diseases. However, the more recent incorporation of the newer macrolides *azithromycin* and *clarithromycin* into MAA treatment regimens has vastly improved the success rates.[9,32,61] These macrolides are more effective against MAA because of their low minimum inhibitory concentrations (MICs) and ability to achieve high concentrations in macrophages and tissues. However, monotherapy with macrolides is not recommended, and azithromycin or clarithromycin should be combined with other drugs, such as ethambutol or rifampin, for additive or synergistic efficacy and to prevent development of resistance.[9,61] Human patients are treated for up to 1 year after conversion to culture-negative status for MAA pulmonary disease and lifelong for disseminated MAA disease.[9]

Combinations of azithromycin (10 mg/kg every 24 hours [q24h]) or clarithromycin (7.5 mg/kg q12h) with rifampin (5-10 mg/kg q12-24h) have been used safely and successfully to treat *Rhodococcus equi* pulmonary infections in foals.[62] Toxicity was limited to mild and self-limiting diarrhea in 5% to 28% of these foals. Therefore, it may be theoretically possible to treat selected MAA-infected horses with some expectation of success. However, the long-term treatment of an adult horse with these drugs may be prohibitively expensive, and no data are available on toxicity with prolonged therapy or the actual clinical efficacy of these drugs for equine MAA infections.

Treatment of cutaneous or other localized infections caused by other environmental mycobacteria is much more likely to be successful. In the single described case in which treatment of a subcutaneous *M. smegmatis* abscess was attempted, the infection was successfully resolved with surgical debridement and 18 days of trimethoprim-sulfonamide (30 mg/kg q12h), followed by 28 days of oral enrofloxacin (5 mg/kg q12h).[36] In treatment of these types of mycobacterial infections in dogs, cats, and humans, the role of surgical debridement of deep-seated infections and removal of any associated foreign bodies is strongly emphasized for success.[9,15,49]

In general, the environmental mycobacteria most often associated with localized infections in other animals and humans—*Mycobacterium abscessus, M. chelonae, M. fortuitum, M. marinum,* and *M. smegmatis*—are predictably susceptible, as well as predictably resistant, to certain antibiotics, including amikacin, cefoxitin, clarithromycin, doxycycline, enrofloxacin, and sulfonamides.[9,15,63] Because patterns of susceptibility are characteristic for different mycobacterial species, accurate identification of isolates is necessary for selecting appropriate antimicrobials. Based on published susceptibility data for a given mycobacterium, it is usually possible to select an appropriate drug regimen empirically.[9,15,49,63] For equine cases, cost and route of administration will also likely be factors in selecting a feasible course of therapy. Acquired resistance may also occur, particularly to fluoroquinolones, and it is generally recommended that all clinically significant isolates of environmental mycobacteria be susceptibility tested.[9,15,49]

Control strategies in the form of disinfection, quarantine, or vaccination are neither required nor likely to be helpful because MAA and other environmental mycobacteria are ubiquitous in the environment, and disease in horses is not defined by exposure.[6] The exceptions would be infections with *M. bovis* or *M. tuberculosis*. Although treatment of these infections is theoretically possible and has been accomplished successfully in other veterinary species, the public health implications and poor prognosis are likely to make attempted therapy prohibitive or impractical.[8]

PUBLIC HEALTH CONSIDERATIONS

Mycobacterium bovis is a well-documented zoonotic disease that may be acquired by drinking contaminated milk or through inhalation of, or wound contamination with, infected tissues.[8] Although there appear to be no documented human cases of *M. bovis* acquired from infected horses, no theoretic reason exists why this cannot occur, and appropriate safety precautions should be observed if working with an infected horse. *Mycobacterium tuberculosis* is primarily a human pathogen that occasionally infects animals.[8,18] Human cases of *M. tuberculosis* acquired from domestic animals have not been documented, and indeed most infections in animals appear to be acquired from humans.[8] Nevertheless, if an infected horse is encountered, due caution would be prudent, and any humans who may have been the source of infection should be referred to their physician for tuberculosis screening. As eradicated or regulated diseases, detection of either *M. bovis* or *M. tuberculosis* has significant public health and agricultural implications, and these are reportable diseases in most developed countries.

MAA and other environmental mycobacteria are not regarded as zoonotic organisms. Susceptibility to disease is not defined by exposure, which for most humans and animals is continuous. Although both humans and animals develop MAA disease, molecular epidemiologic analysis of the isolates from human and animal MAA cases indicates that human cases are not acquired from animals.[5,6,9,11,15]

REFERENCES

See the CD-ROM for a list of references linked to the abstract in PubMed.

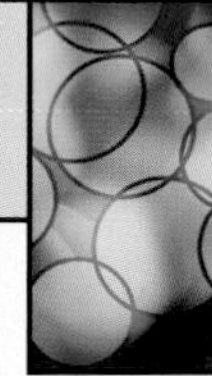

CHAPTER • 34

Leptospirosis

Melissa T. Hines

Leptospirosis is a bacterial disease of worldwide distribution caused by spirochetes of the genus *Leptospira*. The disease affects humans, domestic animals, and wildlife, including reptiles and amphibians. The first formal report of leptospirosis was in human patients by Adolf Weil over 100 years ago, accounting for the name *Weil's disease*.[1,2] Subsequently, leptospirosis was identified in dogs and livestock. The first report of naturally occurring leptospirosis in horses was in 1947 in Russia.[3] In horses the disease has most often been associated with abortion and equine recurrent uveitis; however, sporadic cases of renal and hepatic disease have also been reported.

ETIOLOGY

The order Spirochaetales includes two families of spiral bacteria, *Spirochaetaceae* and *Leptospiraceae*, which share unique morphologic and functional features[4,5] (Fig. 34-1). The genus *Leptospira* is within the family *Leptospiraceae* and includes a large number of both pathogenic and nonpathogenic bacteria. Morphologically, all the leptospires are indistinguishable and are flexible, tightly coiled, unicellular bacteria. At least one end is hook shaped, leading Stimson[6] in 1907 to name the organism initially *Spirochaeta interrogans* because of the resemblance to a question mark. The organisms are slender, with a diameter of approximately 0.1 to 3.0 μm and a length of 6 to 20 μm. The helical coil amplitude is 0.1 to 0.15 μm.

Structurally, the leptospires have a helical protoplasmic cylinder consisting of nuclear material, cytoplasm, and the cytoplasmic membrane and peptidoglycan cell wall[4,7] (Fig. 34-2). There are two axial *flagella*, or axial filaments, each attaching at opposing ends of the organism by platelike insertion discs. The distal end of each flagellum is not attached and extends toward the center of the cell, sometimes overlapping the flagellum from the opposite end. These flagella facilitate motility. As with other spirochetes, the leptospires have a double-membrane structure in which the cytoplasmic membrane and peptidoglycan cell wall are closely associated and are overlaid by an outer membrane that surrounds the protoplasmic cylinder and periplasmic flagella. This outer membrane is rich in lipopolysaccharide, the composition of which is similar to that of other gram-negative bacteria, but with less potent endotoxic activity.[8,9] Despite the gram-negative characteristics of leptospires, they do not stain well with conventional bacteriologic dyes. Therefore, other techniques, such as darkfield microscopy, silver impregnation, and immunologic staining, have been developed for identification of leptospires.

Leptospires are obligate aerobes with an optimum growth temperature of 28° to 30° C (82.4°-86° F).[4] Although slow growing, they can be isolated on artificial media, a characteristic that is unique among spirochetes. They require either long-chain fatty acids or long-chain alcohols as a primary energy source.

Order	Family	Genus
Spirochaetales	*Spirochaetaceae*	*Serpulina*
		Treponema
		Borrelia
	Leptospiraceae	*Leptospira*
		Leptonema and Turneria (nonpathogenic)

Fig. 34-1 Classification of major spirochetes of veterinary importance.

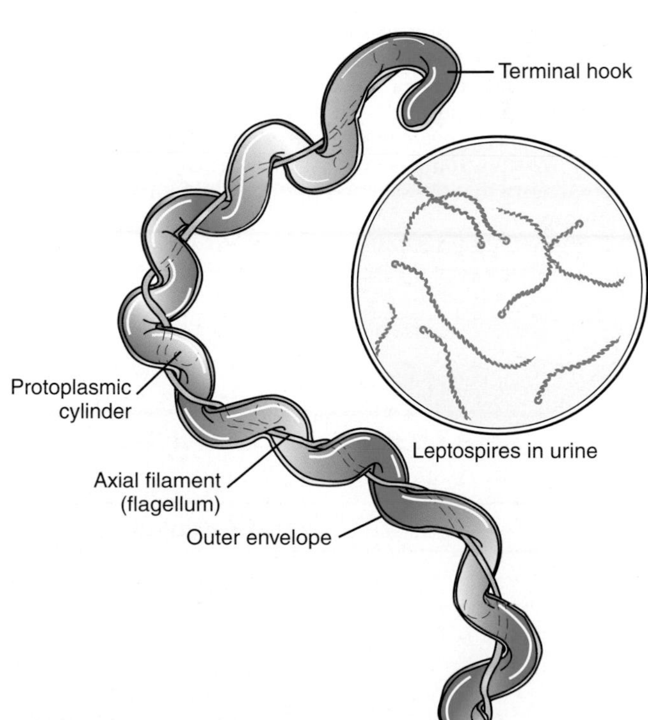

Fig. 34-2 Ultrastructure of pathogenic leptospires. (From Greene CE, editor: *Infectious diseases of the dog and cat*, ed 3, St Louis, 2006, Saunders, p 404; courtesy University of Georgia, Athens.)

The leptospiral genome is approximately 5000 kilobases (kb) in size and consists of two sections, a 4330-kb chromosome and a smaller 359-kb chromosome.[10-12] No other plasmids have been identified. Evidence suggests horizontal transfer of genetic material within the genus. The genome has been sequenced, and a number of leptospiral genes have been cloned.

Classification of organisms within the genus *Leptospira* is complex and has been undergoing revision. Currently, two separate systems of classification are used: (1) the traditional phenotypic classification system based on serotyping and (2) a genotypic classification system based on deoxyribonucleic acid (DNA) homology.

In the traditional serologic classification system, the leptospires are grouped into two species, the pathogenic species *Leptospira interrogans* and the nonpathogenic, saprophytic species *Leptospira biflexa*.[4,5,12] Within each species, the "serovars" are organized into "serogroups" based on shared antigenicity. In this system, *L. interrogans* contains at least 218 serovars organized into 23 serogroups, and *L. biflexa* contains at least 60 serovars organized into 28 serogroups.

Analysis of leptospiral DNA by DNA hybridization revealed significant genetic heterogeneity within the two phenotypic species, *L. interrogans* and *L. biflexa*, resulting in the reclassification of species based on DNA homology.[13-15] Currently, 17 "genomospecies" of *Leptospira* have been defined, and ongoing studies suggest that further taxonomic revisions are likely.[14,16-19] Serologic testing is used within the genomospecies to identify serovars (Table 34-1). The name *L. interrogans* is used to identify species in both the phenotypic and the genotypic classification systems, causing some confusion. Therefore, *L. interrogans* sensu stricto, meaning "in the strict sense," is sometimes used to denote the specific genomospecies, whereas *L. interrogans* sensu lato, meaning "in the broad sense," is used when referring to the more general phenotypic species.

The two systems of classification do not correspond. The genomospecies of a strain cannot be predicted by the serogroup or serovar, and serologically similar leptospires may belong to different genomospecies. In addition, both pathogenic and nonpathogenic serovars may occur within the same genomospecies. Within some serovars, there is sufficient genetic heterogeneity that the same serovar may be found in multiple genomospecies.

The genotypic classification system is taxonomically correct, but in part because of the lack of simple molecular identification methods, many diagnostic laboratories retain the serologic classification of leptospires. Also, in most veterinary literature published to date, leptospires are identified by the classic serologic system. Therefore, most descriptions in this chapter refer to organisms classified by serotyping.

Table • **34-1**

***Genomospecies Identified with Selected Serovars of* Leptospira**

SEROVAR	GENOMOSPECIES
Australis	*interrogans*
Autumnalis	*interrogans*
Bratislava	*interrogans*
Canicola	*interrogans*
Grippotyphosa	*interrogans, kirschneri*
Hardjo	*interrogans, borgpetersenii, meyeri*
Icterohaemorrhagiae	*interrogans, inadai*
Pomona	*interrogans, noguchii*
Sejroe	*borgpetersenii*

EPIDEMIOLOGY

Leptospirosis is maintained in nature by subclinically infected *maintenance hosts*, also known as *reservoir hosts* or *definitive hosts*.[4,5,12] These maintenance hosts, which include numerous wild and domestic animal species, serve as a source of infection for *incidental* or *accidental hosts*, including humans (Table 34-2). Specific serovars of *Leptospira* are generally found in particular maintenance host species, and epidemiologic studies suggest that these host preferences may vary both with geographic regions and over time. In the maintenance hosts the organism is considered to be host adapted, and infection is endemic. Although the host is highly susceptible to infection, the organism is usually of low pathogenicity, and disease is usually subclinical or mild. There is generally prolonged excretion of leptospires in the urine, making these maintenance hosts the primary source of environmental contamination and transmission to other species.

In contrast, *incidental hosts* typically have a low susceptibility to infection, but they are more likely to develop acute, severe disease when they do become infected. Incidental hosts generally shed organisms for relatively short periods, making them inefficient transmitters of disease. For most serovars of *Leptospira*, horses are incidental hosts. However, recent evidence suggests that as with cattle and pigs, horses may be a maintenance host for *L. interrogans* serovar Bratislava.[20-25]

The primary source of exposure to *Leptospira* is infected urine. Maintenance hosts may shed organisms in the urine for prolonged periods because of chronic infection of the renal tubules.[12,26-28] The organism can also be spread through aborted fetuses, placental tissues, uterine discharges, and milk. Contact with the organism may occur either directly or indirectly through contaminated soil, bedding, feed, or drinking water. Once in the environment, leptospires may survive for several weeks under favorable conditions, which is generally a warm, moist environment, such as stagnant or slow-moving warm water. Survival is favored by a neutral or slightly alkaline pH and inhibited by a pH of less than 6 or greater than 8. Therefore, organisms can survive only transiently in undiluted acidic urine. Ambient temperatures of 10° to 25° C (50°-77° F) favor survival, and temperatures lower than 7° to 10° C (44.6°-50° F) or higher than 34° to 36° C (93.2°-96.8° F) are detrimental. The organism is susceptible to freezing and drying. Some evidence indicates that leptospires may survive in insects or other invertebrate hosts, but the significance of this is unknown.[29,30]

Although contact with infected fluids is the most common means of direct transmission of leptospirosis, venereal and transplacental transfer have been documented in some species.[12,26,28] Leptospiral organisms have been found in the semen of infected bulls, and transmission by natural breeding or artificial insemination can occur but is uncommon. In humans, transmission through sexual intercourse during convalescence has been reported.[31] Data in horses are limited, but there are currently no reports of leptospiral transmission through semen or embryo transfer.[32] Fetal infection has been documented in foals after localization in the pregnant uterus, resulting in resorption, abortion, stillbirth, or weak neonatal foals.[20,21,33-38]

Seroprevalence

Serologic surveys to assess the prevalence of antibody to leptospiral organisms have been performed in multiple species, including horses. These studies confirm that there is widespread exposure to *Leptospira* worldwide and that exposure is significantly more common than clinical disease. Specifically, in horses, seroprevalence has varied from 1% to 95% depending on the geographic location and the serovars assessed.[20,22,23,39-60] In some studies, horses were more likely to be seropositive than other domestic animal species.[42,47,49,50] Titers to a wide variety of serovars have been reported in horses, and although there is variation between studies, in general, titers to *Leptospira interrogans* serovars Icterohaemorrhagiae, Bratislava, Pomona, Ballum, and Grippotyphosa tend to be most common. Various serovars of leptospires have also been isolated from bacteriologic surveys of horses at necropsy.[34,51,59] Studies in The Netherlands, Northern Ireland, Canada, and Kentucky suggest that at least in these regions, horses may be a maintenance host for serovar Bratislava because of the prevalence of this serovar.[20-25]

Risk Factors

Several studies have assessed risk factors for exposure to leptospirosis in horses. An early study in Australia did not find any correlation between increased moisture in the environment and seroprevalence.[60] In a Canadian study of 1923 horses in which the seroprevalence ranged from 0.8% to 94.6% depending on the serovar, age was significantly associated with the presence of titers, with the chance of being seropositive increasing by approximately 10% with each year of life.[48] In addition, horses managed individually, such as horses at a track, were about half as likely to be seropositive as those managed in groups, such as rodeo horses. Several other studies have also shown an increase in prevalence with increasing age.[25,41,61,62] Barwick et al.[61,62] evaluated sera from 2551 horses on 572 farms in the state of New York and used a multidimensional indexing system to identify risk factors associated with seropositivity to various serovars. Although findings varied somewhat depending on the specific serovar assessed, age was again identified as a risk factor, as were management practices. The density of horses turned out together was positively associated with the risk of exposure. Also, exposure to rodents, wildlife, and potentially contaminated soil and water could be associated with increased risk of seropositivity to some serovars.

Abortion, Stillbirths, and Neonatal Deaths

Well established as a cause of abortion in cattle and swine, leptospirosis has been sporadically reported as a cause of abortion in horses since the 1950s, but problems in making an accurate diagnosis have made determination of the true prevalence difficult.[36,63,64] Several recent studies indicate leptospirosis is a significant cause of abortion in mares.[35,65-70] In a study reviewing the pathology case records of 3527 cases of abortion, stillbirth, and perinatal death in horses, fetoplacental infection caused by bacteria was diagnosed in 628 cases, of which leptospirosis was identified in 78.[69] In comparison, equine herpesvirus was diagnosed in 143 cases. Related studies in Kentucky have found leptospirosis in 2.5% to 4.4% of submissions of equine fetuses, stillborn foals, and placentas.[65-67] Abortions, stillbirths, and perinatal death have also been confirmed in other geographic locations worldwide.[34,35,37,71]

PATHOGENESIS

The usual portal of entry for leptospires is by penetration of the mucous membranes and abraded or soft, moist skin. Occasionally, organisms may enter by inhalation, ingestion, or animal bites. As with most infectious diseases, the outcome of exposure to leptospires depends on the dose, virulence, and host susceptibility. After entry into the lymphatics and bloodstream, the organisms multiply and are carried to multiple organs. Bacteremia typically occurs 4 to 10 days after initial exposure. There is no apparent tissue tropism, and leptospires replicate

Table • 34-2

Selected Serovars of Leptospira Identified in Horses and Their Hosts

SPECIES: SELECTED SEROVARS	KNOWN PRIMARY RESERVOIR HOSTS	DOMESTICATED ANIMAL HOSTS	PEOPLE	WILDLIFE
***L. interrogans* Sensu Stricto**				
Bratislava	Rat, pig, cow, hedgehog, horse?	Horse, dog, cow	+	+
Pomona	Cow, pig, skunk, opossum	Horse Dog, cat, sheep, goat, rabbit, cavy	+	+
Icterohaemorrhagiae	Rat	Horse Dog, cat, cow, pig, cavy	+	+
Hardjo	Cow, occasionally sheep	Horse Dog, pig, sheep	+	+
Canicola	Dog	Horse Dog, cat, cow, pig	+	+
L. kirschneri				
Grippotyphosa	Vole, raccoon, skunk, opossum	Horse Dog, cat, cow, pig, sheep, goat, rabbit, gerbil, cavy	+	+

in many tissues, including the kidneys, liver, spleen, central nervous system (CNS), eye, mammary gland, and genital tract. The action of the axial flagella and the release of hyaluronidases may facilitate invasion, especially into the CNS and eye. Fetal infection can occur following localization in the pregnant uterus. The organism may persist, most often in renal tubular epithelial cells.

The exact mechanisms by which leptospires cause disease are not completely understood. One feature of the disease is systemic vasculitis. Studies in mice suggest that the endothelial cell membrane of small vessels is disrupted by the intercalation of a glycolipoprotein toxin that displaces host long-chain fatty acids required to maintain vascular cell wall integrity.[72] The damage to the vascular endothelium allows for further migration of spirochetes into the tissues, as well as capillary leakage and hemorrhage, with disruption of tissue architecture, ischemia, and necrosis. There is a broad spectrum of clinical signs depending on the specific tissues affected and the severity of the infection.

Clear differences exist in the virulence of different isolates of *Leptospira*, but information relative to specific virulence factors and their role in pathogenesis is limited. Several outer membrane proteins, including lipopolysaccharide (LPS), may contribute to virulence. Highly immunogenic, LPS is responsible for the serovar specificity of leptospires.[12,73] Although leptospiral LPS exhibits endotoxic activity in biologic assays, it is of low potency.[8,9,74-76] Outer membrane components may play a role in the pathogenesis of interstitial nephritis.[8,77,78] In addition, the outer envelope may have an antiphagocytic function.[79]

A number of factors in addition to the outer membrane proteins potentially contribute to the virulence of leptospires. Toxins other than LPS are produced by some pathogenic strains. Several serovars, including Pomona and Hardjo, produce hemolysins.[80,81] Protein and glycolipoprotein cytotoxins have also been identified.[12] Virulent leptospires can induce apoptosis in vitro and in vivo, and increased concentrations of inflammatory cytokines, such as tumor necrosis factor alpha (TNF-α), are found in patients with leptospirosis.[82]

Immune-mediated mechanisms may also play a role in the pathogenesis of leptospirosis in several species. This is supported in part by the observation that significant clinical disease may be present even after apparent clearance of the majority of organisms.[12] In human patients, levels of circulating immune complexes correlate with disease severity, and in patients who survived, circulating immune complex concentrations decreased concurrently with clinical improvement.[83] A number of autoantibodies, including antiplatelet antibody, have been detected in clinical leptospirosis, but their role in pathogenicity is uncertain.[12] In horses, evidence indicates that immune mechanisms may be important in some cases of equine recurrent uveitis, as discussed later.[84-88]

The humoral immune response appears to be primarily responsible for the control of infection and immunity to leptospires.[12,89,90] Antibodies, which are predominantly directed against outer envelope epitopes, are generally produced within a few days of infection. Immunity usually is specific to the inciting serovar and closely related serovars, although some broadly reactive antigens have also been described. After opsonization by antibodies, organisms are cleared by the reticuloendothelial system. However, when there is infection by a host-adapted serovar in a maintenance host, concentrations of antibody may remain low, allowing organisms to persist, primarily in the kidney. Fetal infection, especially in the third trimester, may result in a specific antibody response that can be protective. Passive immunity can be transferred by antibodies alone, but cell-mediated immune responses to leptospires also occur.[12] However, these cell-mediated responses are currently thought to have a minimal role in protection. The duration of immunity to leptospirosis is uncertain.

The pathogenesis of leptospiral-induced inflammation in equine recurrent uveitis (ERU) has not been fully elucidated despite considerable research in this area. There is evidence that both persistent infection and autoimmune mechanisms may play a role in the pathogenesis. *Leptospira* within the eye may cause direct damage, initiate a local immune response to the bacteria, or incite an autoimmune reaction through molecular mimicry. Studies investigating the cellular and cytokine response to *Leptospira*, as well as immunopathology, support a role for immune mechanisms in the pathogenesis or ERU, in particular a delayed-type hypersensitivity response.[84,91]

Horses inoculated with *L. interrogans* produce cross-reactive antibodies that bind to cornea and lens in addition to *Leptospira*.[85-88,92] After inoculation with killed leptospiral organisms, antibodies reacting with cornea have been found in tears, aqueous humor, and serum of horses.[86] In addition, horses inoculated with either killed *Leptospira* or equine cornea develop cross-reacting antibody and corneal opacity.[85] Specifically, a 90-kilodalton (kDa) leptospiral protein has been identified that shares antigenicity with a 66-kDa equine corneal protein.[93] This leptospiral protein responsible for antigen mimicry appears to be present in several serovars of *L. interrogans* sensu stricto, but it is not present in the nonpathogenic *L. biflexa* sensu stricto or in *L. borgpetersenii* serovar Tarassovis strain Perepelicin, which is pathogenic but has not been associated with ERU.[94] It has been hypothesized that persistent infection may not be necessary to induce immune-mediated ocular inflammation, because any release of inflammatory cytokines could reactivate memory T cells that react with ocular antigens.[84,95]

CLINICAL FINDINGS

Clinical leptospirosis in horses has been primarily associated with abortion and ERU, although sporadic cases of systemic disease have also been reported. After experimental induction of leptospirosis in horses, fever was the most consistent clinical sign, with anorexia, listlessness, and icterus observed in some cases.[96-98] The majority of experimentally infected horses exhibited leukocytosis and neutrophilia during acute infection, and hyperbilirubinemia was occasionally seen. Although not a consistent finding, some horses developed uveitis, generally several months after exposure.

Abortion, Stillbirth, and Neonatal Disease

Leptospiremia may lead to infection of the reproductive organs, and in pregnant animals, this may result in fetal resorption, abortion, stillbirth, or weak neonates. In an outbreak of leptospirosis associated with flooding on a farm with 70 broodmares, there were eight abortions, a stillbirth, three neonatal deaths, and a case of neonatal illness in a 6-week period.[71] Abortion has also been associated with mixed *Leptospira* and equine herpesvirus type 1 (EHV-1) infection.[67,99] Leptospiral abortions most often occur in middle to late gestation. Although affected placentas may appear grossly normal, they more frequently are thick, edematous, and hemorrhagic. The chorionic surface may appear brown and mucoid; occasionally the allantois is discolored green with adenomatous hyperplasia. Placental lesions are diffuse, consistent with placentitis secondary to leptospiremia.

Equine Recurrent Uveitis

Uveitis has long been recognized as a sequela of leptospirosis in both equine and human patients. In horses, uveitis has been described after naturally acquired infection as well as experimental infection with leptospires. Although the condition generally occurs months to years after infection, some cases may be more acute.[100,96-98,101-105] Several serovars have been associated with uveitis, with Pomona being most often incriminated. Despite the association between ERU and leptospirosis, one should remember that most exposure to leptospires does not result in uveitis, and that uveitis may have many other causes.[103,106,107]

The signs of ERU include miosis, blepharospasm, photophobia, aqueous flare, iritis, ciliary injection, and occasionally keratitis (Fig. 34-3). Chronically, there may be synechia, cataract formation, atrophy of the corpora nigra, chorioretinitis, altered iris color, and ultimately blindness. These clinical signs are nonspecific and do not distinguish cases of leptospiral uveitis from those with other causes. Interestingly, a study by Dwyer et al.[106] of 112 horses with ERU suggested that leptospiral uveitis may be more severe than ERU from other causes, because horses with uveitis that were seropositive to leptospires were 4.4 times more likely to lose vision than were seronegative horses with uveitis.

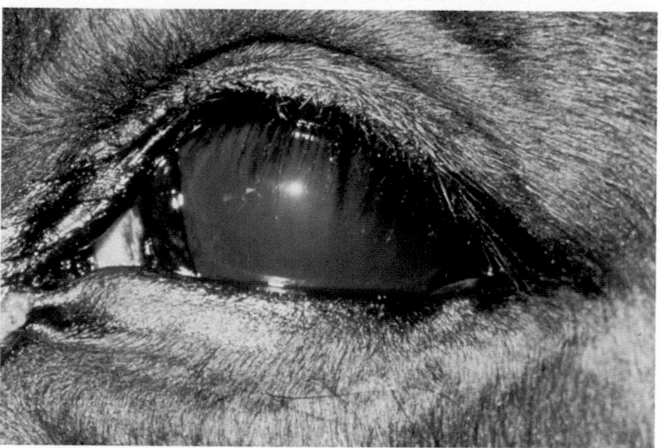

Fig. 34-3 Uveitis in equine eye characterized by miosis, aqueous flare, and corneal edema. Leptospirosis is one cause of equine recurrent uveitis (ERU); however, making a definitive diagnosis can be difficult. (Courtesy Dr. Brian Gilger.)

Systemic Disease in Adults and Foals

Although exposure to leptospires is common in the equine population, systemic disease appears to occur infrequently. However, clinical leptospirosis has been sporadically reported in horses of all ages. In several reports of leptospirosis in neonatal and premature foals, infection was most likely acquired in utero.[33,35,64,71,108] Signs included weakness and icterus, and in one foal, hematuria and dysuria were present. Leptospirosis has also been diagnosed in slightly older foals. Leptospires were isolated from the urine of a 5-week-old foal with signs of dullness and poor body condition on a farm on which multiple foals had died by 14 weeks of age.[109] Also, leptospirosis was thought to be involved in the deaths of 12 foals 4 to 12 weeks of age on one farm over a 3-year period.[24] These foals had severe respiratory distress with depression and pyrexia. Other signs included jaundice in one foal, an unsteady gait in one foal, and diarrhea in two foals. The disease was rapidly fatal, and hemorrhagic pneumonia was found in all foals on necropsy. *Leptospira interrogans* serovar Lora was isolated from the blood of one foal, two foals had high microscopic agglutination test (MAT) titers in single sera, and two others had marked increases in the MAT titers in paired sera.

Reports of leptospirosis in adult horses have described fever, anorexia, and lethargy.[107,110,133] Icterus and hepatic dysfunction have also been reported.[45,101,104] Acute renal failure associated with leptospirosis has been documented in a 7-year-old stallion, a 3-month-old filly, and a 7-month-old filly.[111-113] Common signs in these cases included anorexia and lethargy, and two of the three horses were febrile. Laboratory evaluation revealed leukocytosis with hyperfibrinogenemia, azotemia, and isothenuria. Ultrasound revealed enlarged kidneys in two of the three cases. A renal biopsy was only performed in the 3-month-old foal and confirmed tubulointerstitial nephritis.[112] All affected horses responded to antimicrobial therapy.

DIAGNOSIS

Leptospirosis should be considered as a differential diagnosis in patients with compatible clinical signs, such as abortion, uveitis, and renal or hepatic disease, especially when the history suggests exposure to contaminated urine. However, making an accurate diagnosis of leptospirosis can be problematic because of difficulty in identifying the organism and the high seroprevalence in the equine population. Therefore a number of methods for diagnosing leptospirosis have been developed, and studies are ongoing to develop simpler and more reliable methods.

Direct Detection Methods

Leptospires are difficult to visualize by standard light microscopy because they stain weakly or not at all with traditional stains. Therefore, darkfield microscopy is the most common means of microscopic identification.[4] The organisms appear as slender, silver rods with hooked end(s) and are motile if viable. The helical coils may give the organism a "beaded" appearance. Although darkfield microscopy can provide a presumptive diagnosis of leptospirosis, the technique is not highly sensitive or specific. Approximately 10^4 to 10^5 leptospires/mL are necessary for one organism to be visible per field. Other motile bacteria and filamentous cellular extrusions or fibrin strands can be mistaken for leptospires.

Several samples, such as blood, urine, cerebrospinal fluid (CSF), milk, and macerated tissue, can be examined by darkfield microscopy. Usually, however, the organism is identified in urine because relatively large numbers of leptospires can be shed in the urine of infected animals. Diuresis with furosemide appears to dislodge leptospires from the kidney, and if the patient is well hydrated, it is recommended to administer furosemide and collect midstream urine from the second urination to facilitate recovery.[114] Urine should generally be examined within 20 minutes because the organism can deteriorate rapidly, especially in highly alkaline or acidic urine. If the urine cannot be examined promptly, it is recommended to neutralize the pH or to add formalin, in which case the leptospires will be killed and nonmotile, but morphology will be maintained. Leptospires may also be demonstrated in blood during the bacteremic phase of acute illness. Usually, too few organisms are present in the CSF for detection by darkfield microscopy, but occasionally organisms will be seen. When low numbers are present, centrifugation of the sample may help to concentrate the organisms.

Immunofluorescence and immunoperoxidase staining have been used to increase the sensitivity of direct microscopic examination.[4,5] In particular, the *fluorescent antibody test* (FAT) has improved the ability to identify leptospires in fluids and tissues or tissue impression smears. Although the characteristic morphology of leptospires may be less evident when using FAT compared with darkfield microscopy, FAT is more

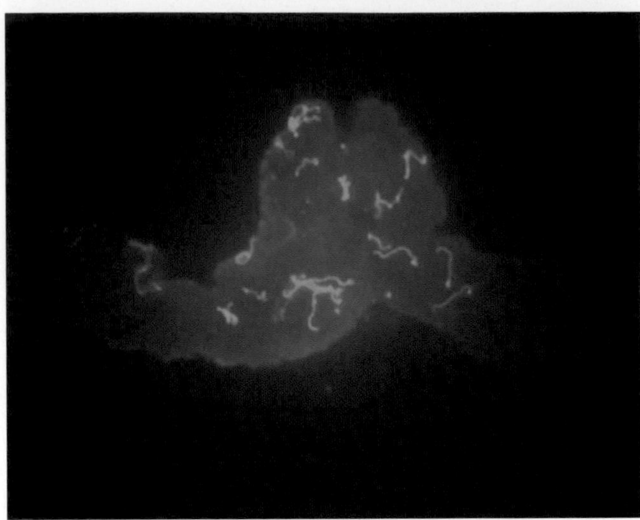

Fig. 34-4 Leptospires identified by fluorescent antibody testing (100×). (Courtesy Dr. Lindsay Oaks.)

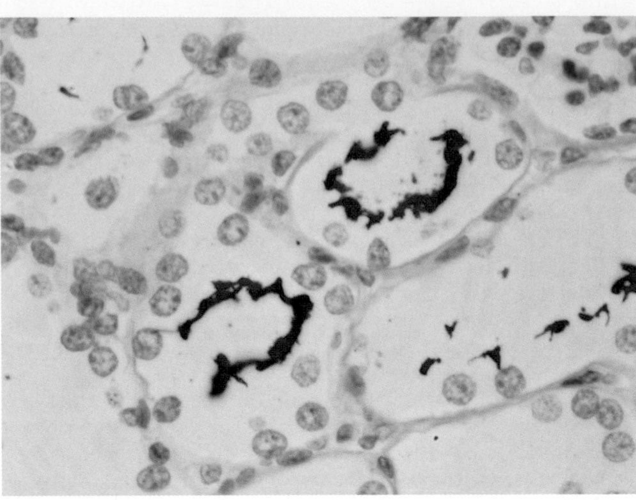

Fig. 34-5 Immunohistochemical staining demonstrating spirochetes in renal tubules aggregating along luminal borders of tubular epithelial cells. (Courtesy Dr. Tim Baszler.)

sensitive, can detect degenerated organisms, and can be serovar specific. Several other methods to detect leptospiral antigens in clinical samples have been evaluated but are not currently in widespread clinical use. These include a radioimmunoassay (RIA), an enzyme-linked immunosorbent assay (ELISA), a double-sandwich ELISA, and an immunomagnetic antigen capture assay.[12,115]

A variety of histopathologic stains have been applied to the detection of leptospires in tissues. Leptospires were first visualized using silver staining, and the Warthin-Starry stain, a modified silver stain, is widely used for histologic examination.[4,5] Dieterle's and Steiner's are other modified silver stains that have also been used. In some cases, leptospires can be seen by light microscopy in tissue sections or on air-dried smears with Giemsa stain. Both immunofluorescent (Fig. 34-4) and immunohistochemical (Fig. 34-5) methods have been useful in detecting leptospiral antigens and intact leptospires in tissue specimens.

Culture

Culture has been considered the "gold standard" for the diagnosis of leptospirosis, but the sensitivity is considered to be low.[4,5] Leptospires are fastidious, slow-growing organisms. Some serovars, such as Hardjo and Bratislava, may require incubation for 4 to 6 months. Organisms are cultured in special media, most often Ellinghausen, McCullough, Johnson, and Harris medium (EMJH), at 28° to 30° C (82°-86° F). Leptospires are readily overgrown by contaminants, and adding antibiotics or 5-fluorouracil may improve recovery. After culture, isolates can be identified using DNA profiles and serology. Occasionally, leptospires have been cultured from fluids and tissues of healthy dogs, and therefore culture may not always be diagnostic of clinical illness.[29]

Proper timing and handling of samples for culture are essential to the recovery of leptospires because of the fastidious nature of these organisms. Although leptospires have been cultured from multiple specimens, it is most common in clinical cases to culture blood and urine. Ideally, samples should be collected before the initiation of antibiotic therapy. To improve the recovery rate, the culture of multiple samples of both blood and urine may be helpful. In addition, it has been recommended to use furosemide to dislodge leptospires from the kidney before collecting urine midstream from the second urination.[114] Blood cultures are generally obtained during the first 4 to 10 days of infection, when infected animals are most likely to be leptospiremic. If indicated, CSF samples can be collected for culture in this same time frame. Urine shedding typically begins within 2 weeks of infection and may continue intermittently for prolonged periods, especially in chronic cases. Leptospires may also be cultured from tissue samples collected by biopsy or at necropsy.

Optimally, samples should be inoculated into culture media immediately. However, this is often not possible, in which case samples should be either diluted 1:10 with 1% bovine serum albumin, buffered saline, or culture media or inoculated into transport media. If not diluted immediately, blood should be anticoagulated with sodium oxalate, preservative-free heparin, or sodium polyethylene sulfonate; citrate anticoagulants should be avoided because they inhibit the growth of leptospires. Urine pH should be adjusted to neutral if necessary. When shipped, tissue and fluid samples should be kept in transport media or on ice, but not frozen.

DNA Methodology

A number of molecular techniques, including dot blotting, DNA hybridization, genomic probes, and PCR, have been applied to the identification of leptospires in various species.[12,116,117] Currently, PCR is the most frequently used of these assays in veterinary medicine. PCR has been used in urine and semen of cattle and in some studies has been more sensitive than FAT or culture for the detection of organisms.[116,118-120] However, a study using a magnetic immunocapture PCR assay for the detection of leptospires in bovine urine suggested that culture should remain the standard for the identification of leptospires because PCR did not detect organisms in 24% of culture-positive samples.[121] A study of horses with ERU concluded that PCR was more reliable than culture for detecting the presence of leptospires in the aqueous humor.[100] PCR has also been used to detect *Leptospira kirschneri* in a premature foal, and it was suggested that a

PCR assay capable of detecting *L. kirschneri* be included in routine diagnostic investigations in which *Leptospira* spp., infection is suspected.[38]

Animal Inoculation

The intraperitoneal inoculation of urine, blood, tissue suspensions, and environmental samples into weanling gerbils, hamsters, or guinea pigs has been used in the diagnosis of leptospirosis.[4] Blood samples from the inoculated animals are used to inoculate media and to assess the serologic response.

Serology

Diagnosis of leptospirosis has often been based on serology because of the difficulties in direct identification and culture of the organism. Antibodies are usually present in blood about 5 to 7 days after the onset of signs, and concentrations may remain elevated for years after exposure. Antibodies have also been detected in a variety of clinical samples in addition to blood; the most important in horses is aqueous humor.

The reference method for serologic diagnosis of leptospirosis is the *microscopic agglutination test* (MAT), in which sera are reacted with live antigen suspensions of various leptospiral serovars.[4,12,122] The MAT detects both immunoglobulin M (IgM) and immunoglobulin G (IgG) antibodies. Results are read by darkfield microscopy, with the end point being the highest dilution of serum at which 50% of the leptospires are agglutinated. It is a serogroup-specific assay, although cross-reaction may occur between some serogroups, especially in acute-phase samples. In general, the MAT has high specificity, but sensitivity may be low. In particular, infections by host-adapted strains in reservoir hosts may not be identified because antibody concentrations are often low. The MAT can be a challenging assay to implement and interpret, and there have been several modifications. In addition, a macroscopic agglutination test and agglutination assays that utilize formalinized antigens have been used.

Serologic tests must be interpreted with caution because of the widespread exposure of horses to leptospires. The MAT has been employed in most epidemiologic surveys of seroprevalence, with titers of 100 or higher being considered positive. In the diagnosis of clinical disease, serology is most useful in diagnosis of acute infections in incidental hosts, where antibody responses tend to be greater than in reservoir hosts or chronic infections. A single elevated titer, generally 800 or greater, detected in association with clinical signs is suggestive of acute infection. Detection of a fourfold change in antibody titer in paired sera obtained 2 weeks apart is considered to be stronger evidence for a diagnosis of leptospirosis. However, especially in cases of abortion or uveitis, acute infection may have occurred earlier, and there may be no change in titer. Although vaccination of horses for leptospirosis is not common, vaccination will cause a detectable antibody response that cannot be differentiated from natural exposure.

A number of additional techniques for the detection of leptospiral antibodies have been developed, including complement fixation, ELISA, indirect hemagglutination assay, and intradermal skin testing.[12,26,122-124] The most widely used of these assays in veterinary species is the ELISA, which is specific and has greater sensitivity than the MAT.[122] Either IgM or IgG can be detected by ELISA. Because IgM is the initial antibody produced, a positive IgM-specific ELISA suggests infection within the previous month.

Diagnosis of Abortion, Stillbirth, and Neonatal Deaths

Multiple *Leptospira* serovars have been associated with abortion. Among the most common is serovar Pomona type kennewicki, which was identified in 43 of 45 isolates in a Kentucky study.[67] The other two isolates in this study were identified as serovar Grippotyphosa and a serovar similar to Pomona. In Ireland, strains belonging to four serogroups—Australis, Pomona, Hebdomadis, and Icterohaemorrhagiae—were isolated.[34] In the outbreak following flooding in California, two serovars, Pomona and Hardjo, were isolated, and two mares had mixed infections with these serovars.[71] In general, aborting mares have titers to multiple leptospiral serovars, and these titers do not necessarily correspond with the cause of abortion.[25,37,70,71] In the investigation of three Kentucky horse farms, no correlation was found between the serovar that caused abortion in the previous year and the prevalence of positive titers to that serovar in horses tested on that farm the following year.[25] The level of titers observed in aborting mares varies widely, with most titers ranging from 1:100 to 1:1600, and titers of 1:204,800 and higher occasionally seen.[25,65-67,70,71]

Numerous diagnostic techniques have been used to confirm leptospirosis as the specific cause of abortion or stillbirths, including isolation of the organism; demonstration of spirochetes on histopathology, typically by Warthin-Starry staining; and a positive FAT for the organism. It is important to evaluate both fetal tissues and placenta. In addition, positive fetal antibody titers and high leptospiral titers in aborting mares are considered supportive of a diagnosis of leptospirosis. In 74 cases of leptospiral abortion in Kentucky during the 1991–1993 foaling season, organisms were isolated in 60.8% of cases (45/74).[67] The diagnosis was supported by FAT and MAT in the remaining cases. In this study the specificities of FAT on fetal tissues and mare's placenta and of MAT on fetal fluid were 100%, and the sensitivity of FAT was 98.7% and of MAT was 81.3%. In a similar study of 71 cases (51 aborted fetuses and 16 stillborn foals), spirochetes were identified in the allantochorion and/or kidney with the Warthin-Starry stain in 69 of 71 cases, 56 of 60 cases were positive using the direct FAT, and leptospires were isolated from fetal tissues in 20 of 42 cases.[70]

Several investigators have evaluated urinary shedding by mares on farms with leptospiral abortions. Bernard et al.[21] documented leptospiruria by FAT in a mare that aborted and in two of five other seropositive horses on the farm. In the California outbreak associated with flooding, leptospires were identified in the urine from three of six mares tested.[71] Donahue et al.[67] identified leptospires in the urine of 14 of 67 mares within 10 days of leptospiral abortion (20.9%). However, a study of three central Kentucky horse farms with a history of leptospiral abortions found no evidence of long-term urinary shedding of *Leptospira* by horses with high leptospiral antibody titers.[25]

Diagnosis of Equine Recurrent Uveitis

Confirming leptospirosis as the definitive cause in cases of ERU can be difficult. The significance of serum antibody is unclear because of the relatively high seroprevalence in the equine population and conflicting results from studies of ERU. Several studies have demonstrated a positive relationship between ERU and leptospiral seroreactivity.[45,106,125-127] For example, in the Dwyer et al.[106] study of 372 horses, seropositive horses were 13.2 times more likely to have uveitis than seronegative horses. However, other studies have failed to confirm a significant association between ERU and serum antibody concentrations.[100,107,128,129] A study of 30 horses with ERU and 16 control horses found no correlation between serologic results and the presence of leptospiral DNA or organisms in the aqueous humor.[100] In another study, 4 of 41 horses with ERU and positive *Leptospira* cultures in the vitreous were seronegative.[128]

Such studies have caused many investigators to conclude that serologic testing is of low sensitivity and specificity in the diagnosis of leptospiral-related uveitis.[100,107,128,129] Some suggest that the presence of antibodies to *Leptospira* in the aqueous or vitreous humor is more accurate than serology in establishing a diagnosis of leptospiral uveitis, especially with evidence of local production of antibody, as suggested by intraocular titers that exceed serum titers, or comparison with total IgG concentrations or albumin.[107,128,130-133] However, Wollanke et al.[134] concluded from a study of 242 horses with ERU and 39 control horses that even vitreous antibody titers that are four times higher than serum titers may not be a sensitive test for the diagnosis of ERU associated with *L. interrogans* infection.

Several studies have demonstrated the presence of leptospiral organisms within the eye of horses with ERU, and because many of the horses were chronically affected with uveitis, some suggested that the infection was persistent.* In the study by Wollanke et al.,[134] 38% of the 120 horses from which *Leptospira interrogans* was isolated from the vitreous had been clinically affected for longer than 1 year. In a U.S. study by Faber et al.,[100] 21 of 30 horses (70%) with ERU had leptospiral DNA in the aqueous humor detectable with polymerase chain reaction (PCR), compared with 1 of 16 control horses (6.25%).[100] Only 6 of 27 horses with uveitis (22.2%) in this study were culture positive in the aqueous humor, all of which were positive by PCR, leading the investigators to conclude that PCR was more reliable than culture for detecting the presence of leptospires in ERU. Vitreous humor samples were cultured in several European studies of ERU, and *Leptospira* was isolated in 9% to 50% of vitreous humor samples from eyes with uveitis, with the most common serogroup being Grippotyphosa.[128,130,131,134,135] The prevalence of the serogroup Grippotyphosa led to the hypothesis that although many pathogenic serovars may penetrate the eyes, only a few are able to persist.[135] In a 2-year-old filly with uveitis resulting in blindness, organisms positive to Warthin-Starry stain were found in the renal cortex, and PCR was positive in the kidney, suggesting a nonulcerative keratouveitis was caused by systemic infection with *Leptospira*.[105]

PATHOLOGIC FINDINGS

Information related to the pathologic findings associated with systemic leptospirosis in horses is limited. In general, leptospirosis is characterized by vasculitis with endothelial damage and inflammatory infiltrates composed of monocytic cells, plasma cells, histiocytes, and neutrophils.[12] Lesions can be found in multiple tissues because the organism can replicate in many sites. Icterus, pulmonary hemorrhage, glomerulonephritis, renal interstitial edema, and tubulointerstitial nephritis have been reported in horses.[24,101,112]

Gross and histologic lesions have been identified in the placenta and fetus in some cases of leptospiral abortion.[34,37,70,136] In a study of 71 cases (51 aborted fetuses and 16 stillborn foals), gross lesions were found in 80.3% of fetuses, stillborn foals, and placentas, whereas microscopic lesions were observed in 96%.[104] The lesions, which were consistent with those identified in other studies, included gross placental lesions of edema, cystic allantoic nodules, and necrosis of the chorion with necrotic mucoid exudates. Histologic placental lesions included thrombosis, vasculitis, mixed inflammatory cell infiltration of the stroma and villi, hyperplasia of allantoic epithelium, and villous necrosis and calcification. In the fetus or stillborn foal, gross abnormalities were most common in the liver, as seen in 23 cases, whereas abnormalities were identified in the kidneys of seven cases. The liver was enlarged, mottled, and pale to yellow. Histologically, there was hepatocellular dissociation, mixed leukocytic infiltration of the portal triads, and giant cell hepatopathy. The kidneys were swollen and edematous with white radiating streaks in the cortex and medulla. Microscopically, there was suppurative and nonsuppurative nephritis. Additional lesions included pulmonary hemorrhages, pneumonia, and myocarditis.

*References 100, 128, 130, 131, 134, 135.

THERAPY

Appropriate treatment for leptospirosis varies depending on the severity and duration of clinical signs as well as the site of infection. Some cases may resolve spontaneously or with only supportive therapy. However, specific antimicrobial therapy may be indicated in some patients.

Well-controlled studies related to the efficacy of antibiotic treatment for leptospirosis in any species are limited. Results have been conflicting between in vitro and in vivo studies of antibiotic susceptibility. Also, antibiotic efficacy may vary when treating patients with acute versus chronic disease. In general, antibiotics to which leptospires appear susceptible include penicillin, ampicillin, amoxicillin, cefotaxime, ceftiofur, erythromycin, and ciprofloxacin.[137-143] Whereas in vitro susceptibility to streptomycin and tetracyclines was intermediate in some studies, these drugs have been clinically effective in the treatment of leptospires.[144-146] Resistance to sulfonamides, chloramphenicol, and cephalothin has been documented for some isolates.

Currently, penicillin and doxycycline are most often recommended for treatment of leptospirosis in human patients.[12,147-151] Although the effects of these antibiotics on outcome and duration of clinical illness have been variable, a consistent finding in human studies has been the prevention of leptospiruria or a significant reduction in its duration.[147,148,150,151] Similarly, dihydrostreptomycin, tetracycline, and erythromycin have been shown to prevent urinary shedding in laboratory animals.[152-154-155] Reports on the efficacy of dihydrostreptomycin in eliminating the carrier state in cattle and swine have been variable.[146,155-157]

No specific studies have addressed antibiotic therapy for leptospirosis in horses. Some recommended antibiotics include penicillin, oxytetracycline, streptomycin, dihydrostreptomycin, and erythromycin.[20,141] In one limited study, tetracycline, penicillin, and dihydrostreptomycin did not eliminate shedding in horses, although the dosages and duration of treatment may not have been adequate.[21] Penicillin has been administered to pregnant mares with rising leptospiral titers in late gestation, with the delivery of clinically normal foals, although the significance of this is uncertain.[21] In the reported cases of acute renal failure in horses, two horses were treated with penicillin and the third with ticarcillin–clavulanic acid, all with a positive outcome.[111-113] A premature neonatal foal with hematuria and leptospiruria was successfully treated with penicillin and amikacin sulfate.[33] In all cases, appropriate adjunctive therapy, such as intravenous fluids and furosemide, was given. Because horses with clinical leptospirosis may be azotemic, it is important to consider the potential for nephrotoxicity when selecting a specific antibiotic.

Equine Recurrent Uveitis

Treatment for ERU typically consists of a combination of antiinflammatory agents and mydriatics. Recently, implantation of a sustained-release delivery system for the immunosuppressant drug cyclosporine has shown some efficacy.[158] In view of the evidence of persistent infection with *Leptospira* in some horses with ERU, more aggressive antibiotic therapy may be indicated, but to date, no controlled studies have assessed therapeutic efficacy.

Vitrectomy and replacement of vitreous with a saline solution of gentamicin has been recommended for treatment of ERU. In a study of 38 horses with follow-up of at least 6 months, owners reported no further uveitis episodes in 42 of 43 eyes.[128] Some vision was maintained in 31 of 43 eyes (72%), whereas 12 of 43 (28%) were blind. It was thought that improvement was primarily caused by removal of persistent intraocular bacteria, as well as inflammatory mediators and cells that contribute to the progression of intraocular inflammation.

Anecdotally, it has been suggested that vaccination of horses with leptospiral vaccines may either decrease subsequent episodes of uveitis or potentially worsen the disease by stimulating the autoimmune response. In a recent study, 41 horses with ERU were vaccinated with either a vaccine containing six serovars of *Leptospira* (20 horses) or a placebo (21 horses).[95] Although the vaccine appeared to decrease the days to recurrence of uveitis, it failed to slow the progression of the disease. These data do not support the use of vaccination against leptospirosis as adjunctive therapy for horses with ERU. However, there was no exacerbation of ocular disease, with only one horse developing a local injection site reaction.

The value of systemic or local antibiotics in the treatment of suspected leptospiral-induced ERU remains unclear. Persistent infection of the eye with leptospires is present in some horses with ERU.* Therefore, as previously discussed, antibiotic therapy and in particular vitrectomy, followed by replacement of the vitreous with saline and gentamicin, have been recommended for the treatment of uveitis.[117] Data on the efficacy of antibiotic therapy in ERU generally are limited, however, and further study is indicated.

PREVENTION

Limiting exposure to stagnant water and to potential carriers, such as cattle, swine, rodents, and wildlife, may help to control leptospirosis.[20,26] On one farm with leptospiral abortions, abortions ceased when horses were no longer fed by spreading feed on the ground.[67] Numerous wildlife of various species had been observed in the area during feeding. Infected animals should be isolated and contaminated areas cleaned and disinfected. For people in high-risk environments, doxycycline once weekly is effective for short-term prophylaxis.[159,160] This practice is controversial because of concerns about developing antibiotic resistance, and it has not been recommended for prevention of disease in horses..

*References 100, 128, 130, 131, 134, 135.

Vaccination against leptospirosis is common in some species. Although currently no vaccines are approved for use in horses, limited studies have assessed the response of horses to vaccination with leptospiral bacterins.[95,161-164] It appears that horses mount an antibody response after vaccination. To date, the only adverse effect documented has been infrequent local injection site reactions. Anecdotally, vaccination has been used on farms with leptospiral abortions and uveitis, but no controlled data support its efficacy. In a study by Rohrbach et al.,[95] vaccination was used in horses with preexisting ERU in an attempt to modulate the disease, but not to prevent initial infection with leptospires. For a vaccine to be effective, it would be important for the appropriate serovars to be included. There are ongoing studies to develop new vaccines for *Leptospira*, such as a DNA vaccine expressing the hemolysin-associated protein 1.[165] Potentially, some of these vaccines may be cross-protective.

PUBLIC HEALTH CONSIDERATIONS

Leptospirosis is perhaps the most widespread zoonosis in the world. Recently the prevalence has been increasing, resulting in the description of leptospirosis as a reemerging disease.[12,166-168] The incidence is greatest in geographic regions with warm climates, and within the United States the highest incidence is found in Hawaii. The spectrum of signs in human patients is broad. In most cases the disease is subclinical or mild; however, 5% to 10% of patients may develop severe icteric leptospirosis with multisystemic involvement.[12,168] The mortality in these patients typically ranges between 5% and 15%.

The source of human infection is usually either direct or indirect contact with the urine of an infected animal. Occupation has been established as a significant risk factor for humans, with farmers, especially dairy farmers, veterinarians, and abattoir workers, among those at increased risk.[12,169] Certain recreational activities, such as water sports and hunting, have also been shown to increase the risk of exposure.[12]

Personnel should be careful when dealing with infected animals to limit exposure. Latex gloves should be worn when handling urine or urine-contaminated materials. Areas contaminated with urine should be washed with detergent and treated with disinfectants, such as iodophors. Prophylactic antibiotic therapy may be indicated if exposure to urine or tissues from an infected animal has occurred. In the case of the weanling with acute renal disease caused by *L. interrogans*, personnel closely involved in the treatment of the horse were treated with doxycycline for 1 week.[113]

REFERENCES

See the CD-ROM for a list of references linked to the abstract in PubMed.

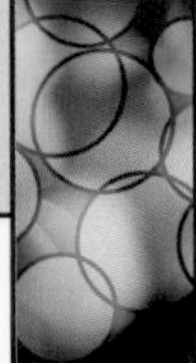

CHAPTER • 35

Lyme Disease

Thomas J. Divers

ETIOLOGY

Lyme disease is caused by at least three strains of the spirochete *Borrelia burgdoferi* sensu lato complex,[1,2] which includes several worldwide species. The North American strain is *B. burgdorferi* sensu stricto ("in the strict sense").[3] *B. burgdorferi* organisms are helical-shaped, gram-negative, unicellular spirochetes with flagellar projections.[4] *B. burgdorferi* bacteria are not free-living organisms and quickly die outside a host. They are maintained in a 2-year enzootic life cycle that involves ixodid ticks (in North America) and mammals.[4] Deer and the white-footed mouse are the most common mammals involved in maintaining the life cycle of this spirochete (Fig. 35-1).

EPIDEMIOLOGY

The seroprevalence of Lyme disease in horses in the United States is not known but is likely similar to that in humans (Fig. 35-2). The mid-Atlantic and northeastern states have a high seroprevalence, as do areas of Minnesota and Wisconsin. Seropositive horses are rare in the Rocky Mountain states, the Dakotas, and Nebraska. In one New England survey, 45% of horses had *Borrelia* antibodies.[12] In a Wisconsin study, 118 of 190 horses were serologically positive.[13]

PATHOGENESIS

Infection in horses is caused by attachment and prolonged (>24 hours) feeding of infected adult *Ixodes* spp., ticks. Female ticks are likely the competent vector and can be identified by the complete arch over the anus (see Fig. 35-1). Larvae and especially nymphs are responsible for a high percentage of infections in humans because they are small and often escape visual inspection.[5] It is not known if these stages transmit the spirochete to horses. Once feeding begins, the organism begins its complicated up-and-down regulation of genes to enhance survival in the host. Exact pathogenesis of *Borrelia* in the horse is not known. After experimental infection of ponies, the organism appears to reside mostly in skin near the tick bite, as well as in connective tissue and muscle and around nerves and blood vessels near synovial membranes.[14] A lymphocytic plasmacytic reaction may occur within these tissues, and in experimentally infected ponies, this reaction was associated with the highest concentration of the *Borrelia* organism.[14,15]

The organism lives in the tick gut and is transferred to animals during blood meals. Generally, 24 to 48 hours of attachment is required to transfer the organism successfully from the tick to the mammalian host.[5] This time may be needed for the organism to downregulate an outer membrane protein (OspA), which may be important to maintain survival in the mammalian host.[6] Conversely, other surface proteins (e.g., OspE, OspF) that are in low concentration in the tick gut are upregulated to enhance complement resistance and other methods of immune evasion in the mammalian host.[7] The changes in expression of surface proteins may be triggered by the blood meal. Other genes permit antigenic variation, ensuring survival in the host. Many other components of the agent may be important for infection or virulence, but these are poorly understood.[8] *Borrelia burgdoferi* may also survive in the host by residing in collagen and connective tissue, having no requirement for iron and by possibly forming resistant cysts within the host.[9-11]

CLINICAL FINDINGS

A wide variety of clinical signs have been attributed to *Borrelia* infection in horses, but cause and effect have been difficult to document. Clinical signs most often attributed to equine Lyme disease include low-grade fever, stiffness and lameness in more than one limb, muscle tenderness, hyperesthesia, lethargy, and behavioral changes.[21-25] Unlike human Lyme disease, joint effusion has been minimal in most Lyme-suspect horses, although it was pronounced in one horse. Muscle wasting and pain over the thoracolumbar area have been present in a few horses with high serum titers. One suspect horse the author examined had ataxia and severe lymphocytic infiltration of the meninges. There is one published report of neurologic dysfunction in a horse attributed to Lyme disease,[22] and in another report, panuveitis was reported in a pony.[26] There has been no further evidence to suggest that *Borrelia* infections are in any way associated with recurrent uveitis in the horse. The high fever and limb edema typically reported in association with *Borrelia* seroconversion are most often the result of *Anaplasma phagocytophila* infection, because many ticks are concomitantly infected with both *Borrelia* and *A. phagocytophila*.[27]

Experimental infection of ponies has caused lesions in the skin, muscle, fascia, nerves, and perisynovial tissues of some ponies, but clinical signs were not observed. The pathology has been mild in most of the experimentally infected ponies. Until clinical signs can be experimentally reproduced, the association between *Borrelia* infection and clinical disease will remain speculative. It is possible that only certain horses, possibly associated with major histocompatibility complex (MHC) types and antigen-antibody reactions, may be predisposed to develop clinical signs after infection.

DIAGNOSIS

The diagnosis of exposure to *Borrelia* is straightforward, but determining if the horse is currently infected is more difficult, and to determine whether or not clinical disease is associated with *Borrelia* is extremely difficult. Enzyme-linked immunosorbent assay (ELISA, Cornell Diagnostic Laboratory, Ithaca, New York) or immunofluorescent antibody (IFA) testing is the preferred screening test for detection of antibodies

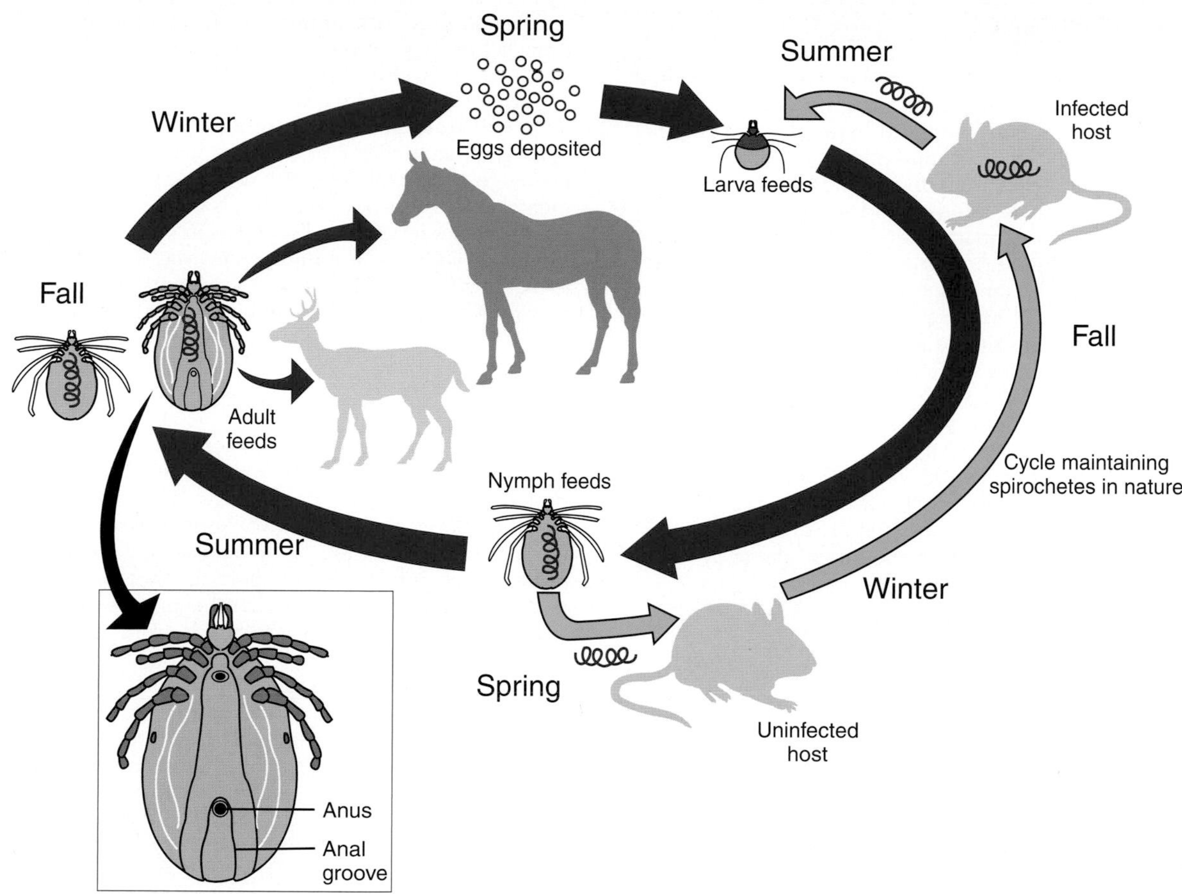

Fig. 35-1 Two-year enzootic cycle of *Borrelia burgdorferi* and distinguishing features of *Ixodes* species ticks. *Inset,* Female ventral abdomen.

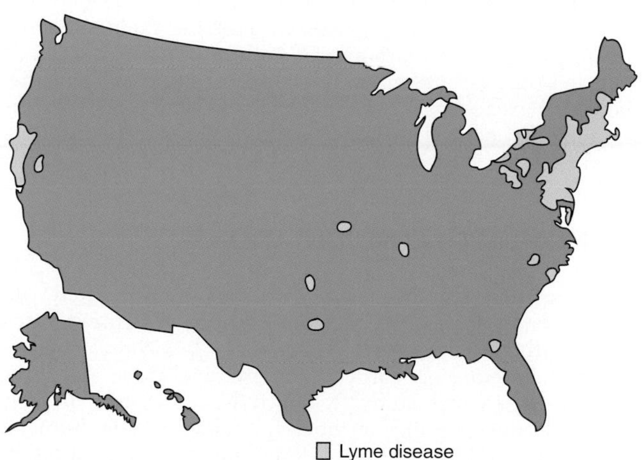

Fig. 35-2 Risk of Lyme disease in the United States. (Courtesy Centers for Disease Control and Prevention, Atlanta.)

indicating exposure. If the ELISA value is less than 110 units, it indicates nonexposure, distant exposure but no current infection, or recent infection (within 2 months).[14] A repeat sample taken in 2 months that remains less than 110 would rule out the latter.[14] Experimentally infected ponies successfully treated with antibiotics (no organisms found at euthanasia) had titers that decreased to less than 110 units 4 months after treatment was initiated.[17] Antibiotic-treated ponies that remained infected at euthanasia had some decrease in titer during antibiotic treatment, but not as low as 110, and had a rebound increase in titer after discontinuing antibiotic therapy.[17] The value of the C6 test (Snap3Dx IDEXX Laboratories, Westbrook, Maine), based on antibody to a peptide that reproduces the sequence of the invariable region 6 (an immunodominant, conserved region), has good correlation with the ELISA in horses (Drs. A. Johnson and T. Divers, Cornell University). In humans the C6 antibody cannot always be used to assess treatment outcome or the presence of active infection but has comparable sensitivity to Western blot for diagnosing Lyme disease.[18,19]

The principal value of the Western blot assay is in separating horses that are ELISA positive because of natural infection from horses that are ELISA positive because of vaccination. In experimentally infected ponies the Western blot assay was positive at 8 to 10 weeks after infection, versus 6 to 8 weeks for the ELISA.[14]

Clinical signs are not obvious in ponies experimentally infected with *Borrelia,* and a large number of apparently asymptomatic horses are seropositive; therefore, clinical diagnosis is difficult. To complicate the relationship between infection and clinical signs further, the most common drugs (oxytetracycline and doxycycline) used to treat *Borrelia* in the horse have antiinflammatory properties that may alleviate musculoskeletal pain in horses, thus preventing the use of response to therapy as a diagnostic test.[20]

PATHOLOGIC FINDINGS

Lesions in experimentally infected horses are mostly limited to a lymphohistiocytic reaction in the skin surrounding the site of the tick attachment and lymphoid hyperplasia of regional lymph nodes.[14,15] One experimental pony had a mononuclear cell reaction in cutaneous muscle and the panniculus, especially surrounding small arteries and nerves. Perivascular, perineural mononuclear inflammation is reported in human patients with Lyme disease.[16] In one pony there was a nonsuppurative synovitis with mononuclear subsynovial perivascular infiltration. Perivascular mononuclear cell aggregates also formed around small arteries adjacent to the perineurium of peripheral nerves, including the ulnar, facial, sciatic, labial, and fibular nerves and the dorsal spinal nerve roots. A perivascular mononuclear inflammation was also present in skeletal muscle in multiple areas.[15] All these changes have been reported in human patients with Lyme disease, and the association of these lesions with Lyme disease in experimental ponies is strengthened by the observation that all lesions in the one pony were most severe on the side of the body where the ticks were attached.[15]

THERAPY

The two most frequently used drugs for treatment of Lyme disease in horses are intravenous (IV) *tetracycline* and oral (PO) *doxycycline*. In experimental ponies, IV tetracycline was more effective than PO doxycycline for eradicating *Borrelia*.[17] IV tetracycline obtains much higher tissue concentrations than PO doxycycline, which has low bioavailability in the horse.[28] If blood concentrations were equal, one would expect doxycycline to be the preferred drug because of better volume of distribution. Doxycycline cannot be administered by the IV route to horses because of potential adverse effects.[29] Tetracycline should not be given orally to horses because of low bioavailability and risk of active drug reaching the colon and causing diarrhea (unlike PO doxycycline, where much of the unabsorbed drug is inactive in the colon).[30]

The exact dose and the frequency and duration of therapy with tetracycline and doxycycline in the treatment of *Borrelia* infection are not known. A common scenario in clinical practice has been to give IV tetracycline, 6.6 mg/kg every 24 hours (q12h) for 7 to 10 days, followed by PO doxycycline, 10 mg/kg q12h for at least 1 month. To consider the treatment effective, titers should decline before treatment is discontinued and should continue to decline to less than 110 ELISA units.

Although IV tetracycline (5 mg/kg q24h for 28 days) was 100% effective in eradicating *Borrelia* from experimentally infected ponies (treatment initiated 4 months after infection),[14] this same protocol has not been as effective in causing a decline in antibody in horses with naturally occurring infections. It is unknown whether this discrepancy is a result of treatment failure associated with duration of infection before beginning treatment, reinfection, and/or molecular mimicry causing a persistently high serum antibody concentration. Cyst forms may be present in some chronically infected humans, and these cyst forms are not killed by tetracycline. Metronidazole may be effective against the cyst forms but is not effective against free-living *Borrelia*.[31] In refractory cases, it may be reasonable (but with unproven efficacy) to treat with both a tetracycline (e.g., oxytetracycline, with or without doxycycline) and metronidazole.

Other classes of drugs used to treat *Borrelia* in humans have no practical advantages over tetracycline (e.g., IV or intramuscular [IM] ampicillin), or are toxic when given orally to adult horses (e.g., macrolides), or were not effective in the experimental pony study (e.g., ceftiofur; Naxcel, Pharmacia & Upjohn, Kalamazoo, Michigan).[14] Enrofloxacin (Baytril, Bayer, Shawnee Mission, Kansas), a fluoroquinolone, was tested in vitro against an equine isolate of *Borrelia* and was not effective (T.J. Divers and Y.F. Chang, personal communication, 2005).

PREVENTION

The components for prevention of Lyme disease in endemic areas may include (1) the prevention of tick exposure or prolonged (>24 hours) attachment, (2) the provision of early antimicrobial treatment after known *Ixodes* exposure, or (3) vaccination. Various insecticidal sprays can be used to prevent tick infection, but most are not approved for use in horses, and efficacy in the horse is unproven. Currently, no adverse effects are known to result from use of the more common canine tick sprays (e.g., fipronial; Frontline, Merial, Duluth, Georgia) in the horse. Permethrin-based insecticides are approved for use in horses, but efficacy against ticks is not well documented. Spraying and close observation for ticks should be performed most diligently in late summer, fall, and early winter (after fly season) because this is the most common time for adults to attach. If ticks are found on a horse, they can be examined to determine if they are *Ixodes* spp. (see Fig. 35-1), the only species of North American tick known to transmit *B. burgdorferi*.

Ponies were completely protected against experimental infection by vaccination with a recombinant OspA antigen vaccine when infected ticks were attached 92 days after the third vaccination.[15] Duration of protection in the horse, adverse effects, and efficacy of the currently available canine vaccines are unknown. Differentiation of natural exposure antibody from an OspA vaccine antibody response can be made by either Western blot testing or C6 SNAP test. Whole-cell vaccine antibody and natural exposure antibody can also be differentiated with the Western blot or C6 test.

PUBLIC HEALTH CONSIDERATIONS

There are minimal public health considerations associated with equine Lyme disease. A significant number of Lyme-infested horses with clinical signs of lameness or behavioral changes are spirochetemia or spirocheturia positive (53% and 20%, respectively, in one study[24]), but it is considered unlikely that adult ticks feeding on horses would move to humans. Seroprevalence in horses in an area might be an important sentinel for risk of human Lyme disease in the same area.

REFERENCES

See the CD-ROM for a list of references linked to the abstract in PubMed.

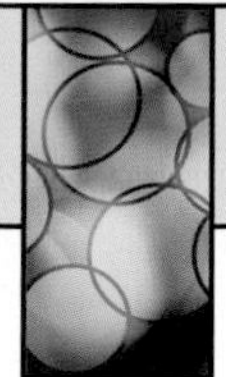

CHAPTER • 36

Lawsonia intracellularis

Jean-Pierre Lavoie and Richard Drolet

ETIOLOGY

Lawsonia intracellularis is the etiologic agent of the proliferative enteropathies of animals, variously known as proliferative enteritis, proliferative ileitis, and intestinal adenomatosis. This new bacterium, isolated and identified in the mid-1990s, is taxonomically distinct as a species.[1,2] The obligate intracellular organism does not grow on conventional bacteriologic media but can be cultivated in some specific cell lines, including a rat small intestine cell line, under an atmosphere of reduced oxygen tension. Bacteria present in host or cultured cells are gram-negative, straight to slightly curved rods, 1.25 to 2 μm long and 0.25 to 0.43 μm wide. These organisms have a wavy, trilaminated outer cell wall, contain dense cytoplasmic granules, and divide transversely by septation.[1]

Isolates of intracellular bacteria from a variety of animal species affected with proliferative enteropathy (PE), including horses, show close 16S ribosomal deoxyribonucleic acid (rDNA) similarity (>98%) to cultures isolated from pigs, the species in which the disease is most prevalent.[1]

EPIDEMIOLOGY

Proliferative enteropathy attributable to infection with *L. intracellularis* has been described in a number of animal species, including the pig, hamster, fox, dog, ferret, rat, guinea pig, rabbit, monkey, ostrich, emu, sheep, deer, and horse.[1] *L. intracellularis* has a worldwide distribution, and equine cases of PE have been reported in most American states[3-7] and Canadian provinces[8,9] and in Great Britain[10] and Australia.[11] Foals from the Czech Republic have been found to be fecal positive for *L. intracellularis* using polymerase chain reaction (PCR) analysis.[12] The source of infection has not been determined in equine cases. As with most other enteric microbial pathogens, fecal-oral spread and transmission through drinking water and food appear to be the common avenues for infection. Contact with pig manure is speculated to represent a potential source of infection for horses, but in most cases no history or evidence of direct exposure to pigs or their feces has been reported.

Because of the apparent wide host range of PE, numerous potential reservoirs likely exist. Recently, *L. intracellularis* was detected by PCR in the feces of a variety of animal species, including a red deer, red foxes, gray wolves, dogs, calves, hedgehogs, and a giraffe.[13,14] Transmission of infection in foals may be through exposure to *L. intracellularis*–infected feces from feral animals or in-contact horses.[8,11] Naturally occurring transspecies transmission of this disease has not been clearly documented, although experimental transmission from pig to hamster[15] and from pig to foal[16] has been reported with induction of disease. As observed in pigs, factors that may predispose foals to PE include weaning (age), overcrowding, lack of specific immunity, commingling of animals, and introduction of new animals on the premises.[8]

In pigs, infection and fecal shedding may persist as long as 12 weeks.[17] *L. intracellularis* can survive for at least 2 weeks in the environment.[18] The duration of bacterial shedding in feces of horses after infection has not been thoroughly determined. Similarly, the possible role of subclinical infections in the transmission of the disease between horses is not known. Subclinical PE occurs in pigs and rabbits.[19]

PATHOGENESIS

The severity of disease caused by infection with *L. intracellularis* depends on the number of organisms ingested by the host and the extent of host immunity.[20] Intestinal flora and other enteric pathogens may facilitate the development of disease,[2] and polymorphisms in equine immune response genes may predispose to *L. intracellularis* infection.[12] The pathogenesis of PE is not totally understood, and most of the information available is extrapolated from experimental observations in hamsters and pigs and from infected cell cultures.[1,2,21]

After ingestion, bacteria associate with the cell membrane of dividing intestinal crypt cells and quickly enter the enterocyte through an entry vacuole. Approximately 3 hours later, bacteria are released from the endocytic vacuole and start to multiply free in the cytoplasm. Infected cells continue to divide, even when heavily infected. PE develops as a progressive proliferation of immature epithelial cells harboring numerous intracellular bacteria.[1,2,21] The incubation period of the disease is 2 to 3 weeks in swine[21] and is estimated to be the same in foals.[16] Resolution of lesions is closely related to the disappearance of the intracellular bacteria.

Lesions of PE, when extensive, may potentially result in a significant decrease in intestinal digestive and absorptive capabilities causing diarrhea and weight loss. Hypoproteinemia is a common laboratory finding in foals affected with the disease.[5-11] This low plasma protein concentration is probably attributable to the combined effect of intestinal protein loss, malabsorption of amino acids, and increased protein catabolism. In pigs with PE, evidence suggests that hypoproteinemia results from intestinal protein loss and malabsorption of amino acids; normal protein metabolism is observed after the resolution of digestive signs.[22,23]

CLINICAL FINDINGS

Most reports of PE in foals have described isolated cases,[3-7,9,11] although multiple foals may be affected on breeding farms.[8,10] The age of affected foals varies from 3 to 13 months, but weanling foals 4 to 7 months of age are most susceptible to *L. intracellularis* infection.[8] There appears to be no gender or breed predisposition to the disease. Clinical signs are usually suggestive of the enteric location of the infection.

Depression,[3-6,8,9,11] fever,[5,8,9,11] anorexia,[3-6,8,9] weight loss,[5,6,8,10,11] diarrhea,[3-6,8,10,11] and colic[7,8] are often observed. Most of these clinical signs were also observed in a foal experimentally infected with a porcine isolate of *L. intracellularis*.[16] Weight loss may become apparent over a few days, although one yearling was presented for growth retardation of 5 months' duration.[8] Extremely poor body condition with a rough haircoat and a pot-bellied appearance is common in severely affected foals (Fig. 36-1). Diarrhea may be of varying frequency and severity, ranging from soft "cow pie" feces to black and tarry or aqueous and profuse diarrhea.[3,5,8] Similarly, colic signs, when present, are of variable severity.[7,8] Subcutaneous edema may be marked, especially when fluid therapy is administered.[6,8,9,11] However, severe hypoproteinemia may be present in absence of detectable subcutaneous edema (see following discussion). Concomitant disorders,such as upper or lower respiratory tract infection, intestinal parasitism, gastric ulcers, and dermatitis, were common findings in one study.[8]

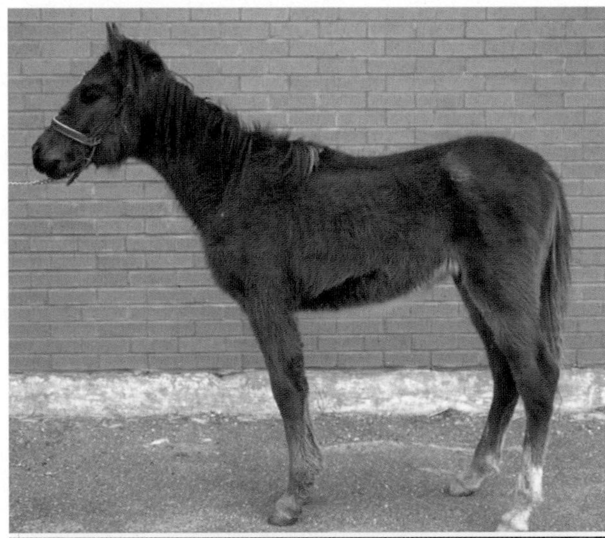

A

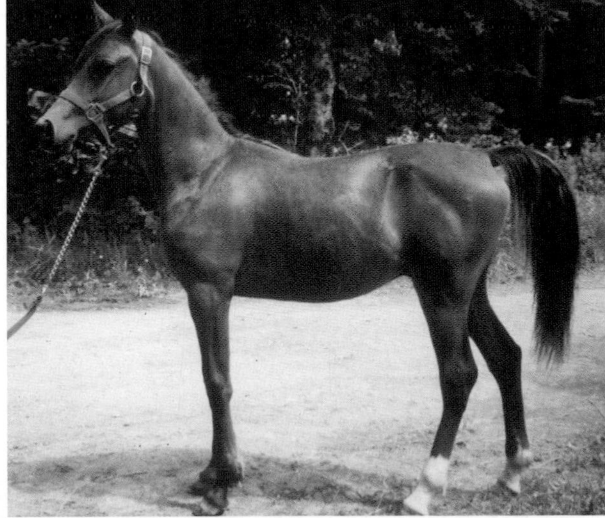

B

Fig. 36-1 Thirteen-month-old gelding with proliferative enteropathy before (A) and 4 months after (B) initiation of therapy with erythromycin.

CLINICAL PATHOLOGY

Hypoproteinemia (<5 g/dL) is the most consistent laboratory finding in foals with PE, although it is not present in all cases. Hypoproteinemia usually results from a panhypoproteinemia[5,6,8,11] and, when profound, may result in a spontaneous coagulopathy. Other frequently observed laboratory abnormalities include leukocytosis,[5,6,9,11] neutrophilia,[6,8] hyperfibrinogenemia,[5,6,8] increased creatine kinase,[6,8] hypocalcemia,[6,9] hyponatremia,[5,8,9] and azotemia.[5,9] Anemia is less often observed[6,8] but may be marked, especially in chronic cases.[8] Urinalysis, abdominal fluid cytology, and glucose and D-xylose absorption tests remain within normal limits.[5,6,8,9]

PATHOLOGIC FINDINGS

In foals, generalized emaciation and subcutaneous dependent edema are frequent nonspecific findings on gross necropsy examination. Gross lesions suggestive of PE involve various lengths of the small intestine and are characterized mainly by a marked thickening of the mucosa, giving its surface an irregular and corrugated appearance (Fig. 36-2). Although duodenal lesions have been occasionally observed, lesions are often confined to the jejunum and ileum, with the ileum more severely affected. In contrast to some other species affected with PE, lesions in the large intestine have not been reported to date in horses. Other possible gross changes include submucosal intestinal edema, muscular hypertrophy of the intestinal wall, and hypertrophy of the mesenteric lymph nodes.

Histologic examination reveals that the thickened mucosa is attributable to severe hyperplasia of crypt epithelium.

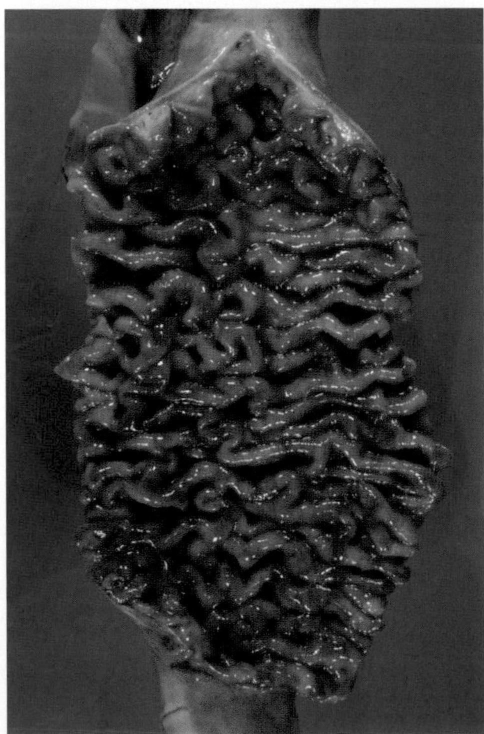

Fig. 36-2 Ileum of foal with proliferative enteropathy. The mucosa is diffusely thickened and has a corrugated appearance. (From Lavoie JP, Drolet R, Parsons D, et al: *Equine Vet J* 32: 418-425, 2000.)

Affected crypts are extremely elongated and often branched, devoid of goblet cells, and lined by immature epithelial cells. Intestinal villi may become decreased in length and lined by an immature epithelium. Mucosal inflammation and focal necrosis are additional secondary changes observed in some cases. Silver-stained sections of affected areas reveal numerous short and slightly curved bacterial rods, confined mainly to the apical cytoplasm of the immature epithelial cells (Fig. 36-3).

Electron microscopic examination of affected tissue demonstrates bacteria free in the cytoplasm of crypt enterocytes (Fig. 36-4). PCR analysis and immunohistochemistry (IHC) can more specifically confirm the presence of *L. intracellularis* in affected intestinal tissues.

DIFFERENTIAL DIAGNOSIS

The clinical signs in foals with PE may resemble those associated with common gastrointestinal diseases, including acute intestinal obstruction, sand impaction, parasitism, gastroduodenal ulcers, infiltrative bowel disease such as neoplasia (lymphoma), eosinophilic gastroenteritis, and intoxication with plants, chemicals, and pharmacologic agents such as nonsteroidal antiinflammatory drugs (NSAIDs). Many other infectious agents may be implicated in weanling diarrhea and include *Salmonella* spp. (Chapter 38), *Rhodococcus equi* (Chapter 32), *Clostridium* spp. (Chapters 44 and 45), *Neorickettsia risticii* (Chapter 43), *Campylobacter jejuni*, rotavirus (Chapter 17), and adenovirus. However, these conditions are unlikely to cause outbreaks of disease characterized by weight loss, diarrhea, colic, and severe hypoproteinemia in foals of this age group. Other causes of hypoproteinemia include malnutrition, hepatopathy, renal disease, and protein loss in the abdominal or thoracic cavities or blood loss.

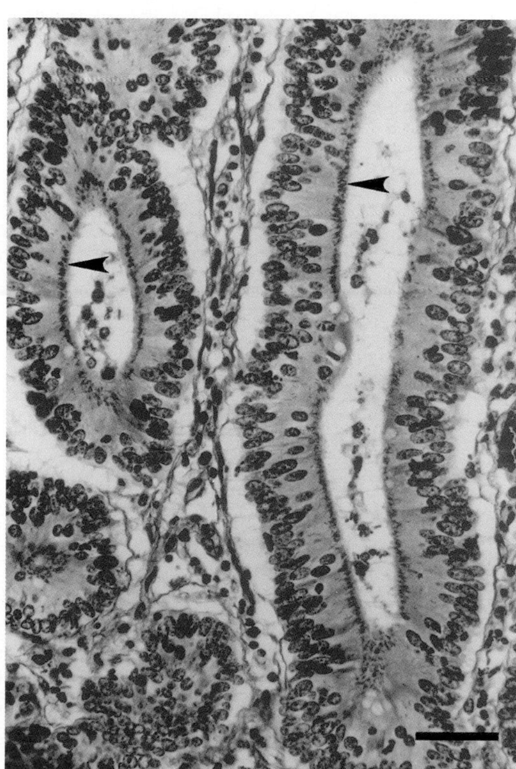

Fig. 36-3 Ileal mucosa from foal with proliferative enteropathy. Epithelial cells of hyperplastic crypts have aggregates of bacteria *(arrowheads)* in their cytoplasm. (Warthin-Starry silver stain; bar = 30 μm.) (From Lavoie JP, Drolet R, Parsons D, et al: *Equine Vet J* 32:418-425, 2000.)

DIAGNOSIS

Antemortem diagnosis of PE is based on clinical signs, hypoproteinemia, the exclusion of common enteric disorders, positive serology, and positive PCR analysis of the feces. A thickening of segments of the small intestinal wall observed on abdominal ultrasonography (Fig. 36-5) would further support the diagnosis, although this finding is not present in all cases. Isolation of the organism is not a practical means of diagnosis because *L. intracellularis* cannot be cultured in conventional cell-free media.

Experimental challenges with *L. intracellularis* in pigs indicate that the sensitivity of serology is superior to that of fecal PCR and that both techniques are highly specific.[24] Similar studies have not been performed in foals but, based on reported cases, serology also appears to be more sensitive than fecal PCR in this species.[8,10,11] Positive serology for *Lawsonia* may be observed within a few days after the clinical signs of PE are first noted, suggesting that serology may confirm exposure to this bacteria in some cases, even at the onset of the detected clinical disease. Furthermore, specific antibodies have persisted up to 6 months in foals after natural infection. Fecal excretion of *L. intracellularis*, detected by PCR, rapidly stops after the initiation of erythromycin therapy.[25] This finding suggests that PCR on feces may not be appropriate to reach a diagnosis of PE after antimicrobial therapy has begun. Antimicrobial administration before collection of feces for

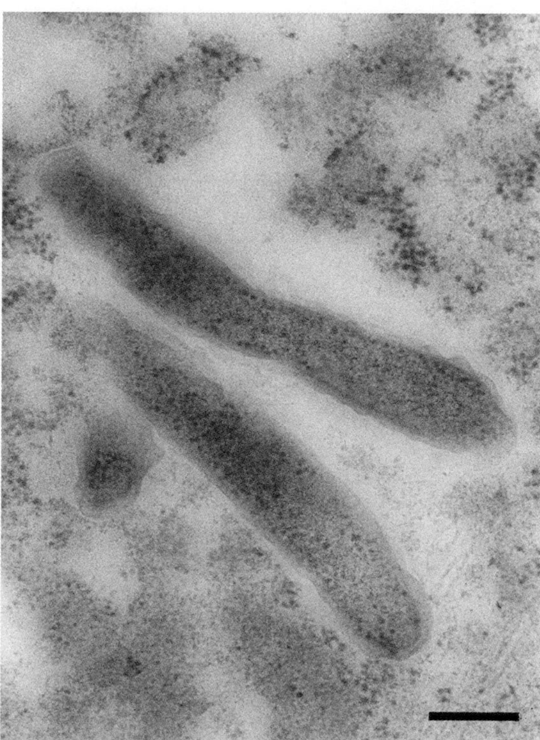

Fig. 36-4 Electron microscopic demonstration of two bacteria lying free in cytoplasm of crypt epithelial cell. (Bar = 0.3 μm.)

diagnostic purposes may have contributed to the apparent low sensitivity of fecal PCR for diagnosis of equine PE.

Diagnosis of PE is confirmed by the presence of characteristic intracellular bacteria within the apical cytoplasm of proliferating crypt epithelial cells of the intestinal mucosa using Warthin-Starry silver stain, or preferably by IHC.[24] The usefulness of histologic examination and PCR analysis of endoscopic-guided duodenal biopsies has not been investigated for the diagnosis of PE, but the diagnosis was confirmed by jejunal biopsy performed during an exploratory celiotomy in one foal.[7]

THERAPY

Antimicrobial treatment is critical for the treatment of PE in foals. Because *L. intracellularis* is an obligate intracellular bacterium, selection of an antimicrobial with good intracellular penetration is preferred. Erythromycin estolate (25 mg/kg orally [PO] every 8 hours [q8h]), alone or combined with rifampin (10 mg/kg PO q12-24 h), administered for 3 weeks or more, has been used most often in controlling the disease.[7-11] Chloramphenicol and tetracyclines may be viable alternatives to erythromycin. Disease progression has been reported to continue despite treatment with penicillin,[11] trimethoprim-sulfa combination,[9] ceftiofur,[6] and gentamicin,[11] suggesting that these antimicrobials may not be effective in equine PE. These results are in agreement with the findings that erythromycin has a low minimum inhibitory concentration (MIC) for *L. intracellularis* of porcine origin, whereas the organism is resistant in vitro to ceftiofur, gentamicin, and enrofloxacin.[26]

The dosages of antimicrobials currently used for the treatment of PE in foals are based on recommended therapies for systemic infection. However, because *Lawsonia* infection affects almost exclusively the small intestine, orally administered drugs would likely reach concentrations in the infected small intestinal enterocytes greatly exceeding the MIC for this bacterium. This might explain why in a large outbreak, foals appeared to respond to reduced dosages and less frequent administration of erythromycin than predicted from pharmacodynamic studies.[8]

Foals with severe hypoproteinemia may benefit from plasma transfusion. Additional symptomatic treatment, such as antiulcer therapy, intravenous crystalloid or colloid fluid therapy, and parenteral feeding, may be required. Appropriate therapy should be aimed at controlling concurrent medical conditions when present.

A rapid improvement in attitude, appetite, and weight gain, and a decrease in the frequency and severity of colic signs or diarrhea is observed in most foals after administration of appropriate antimicrobials, unless significant concurrent problems are present. Correction of hypoproteinemia often lags behind improvement in clinical signs. A delay of up to a month or more may be expected before a return to normal values is observed.[8]

The possibility of spontaneous recovery or prolonged subclinical infection, as reported in other species, has not been documented to date in foals, but is likely to occur. Foals treated symptomatically without administration of effective antimicrobial agents consistently fail to survive.[3,5,6,8]

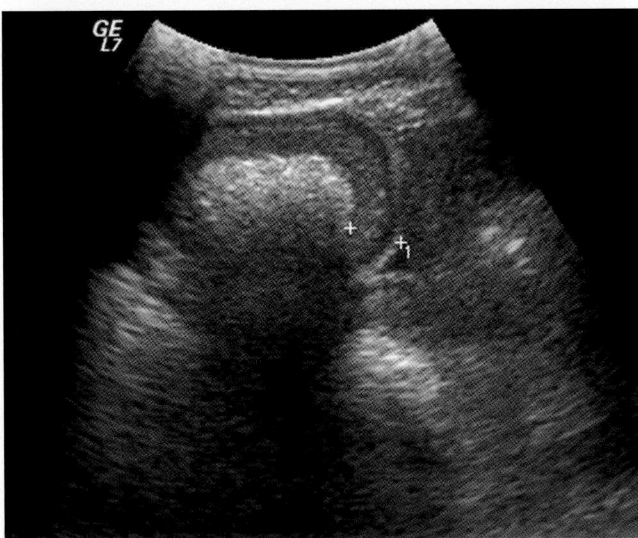

Fig. 36-5 Ultrasound image showing thickened section of small intestinal wall of 4-month-old filly with proliferative enteropathy. Note the loss of distinction between the submucosal and mucosal layers and the increased mucosal echogenicity.

PREVENTION

A better understanding of the epidemiology of equine PE is required before effective methods for the prevention of this disease in foals can be recommended. In pigs, overcrowding, ration changes, antibiotic administration, mixing, and transportation seem to be associated with the onset of the disease. These factors are also often encountered in foals after weaning and may contribute to equine PE.

When PE is diagnosed on a farm, several measures may be attempted in an effort to limit the transmission of infection within the herd. Affected foals should be isolated from other animals, ideally until they stop shedding the bacteria. Infected pigs remain carriers for up to 12 weeks,[17] and foals could also excrete the bacteria for an extended period if left untreated. Preliminary data indicate that once appropriate antimicrobial therapy is instituted, foals stop shedding the bacteria within a few days.[25] The stable should be thoroughly disinfected because *L. intracellularis* may remain infective for up to 2 weeks in feces at environmental temperatures that range from 5° to 15° C. Quaternary ammonium and povidone-iodine are the most effective disinfectants against *L. intracellularis*.[18]

An orally administered, avirulent live vaccine for *L. intracellularis* is well tolerated and protective in pigs.[27] Considering the strong homology between the equine and porcine isolates of the bacteria, the vaccine could limit the severity of the diseases in equine PE.

PUBLIC HEALTH CONSIDERATIONS

Proliferative enteropathies caused by *L. intracellularis* are reported in an ever-increasing range of host species, and the recent description of the disease in nonhuman primates certainly raises the question as to whether people are susceptible to infection.[28] Currently, however, PE is not considered a zoonotic disease.

REFERENCES

See the CD-ROM for a list of references linked to the abstract in PubMed.

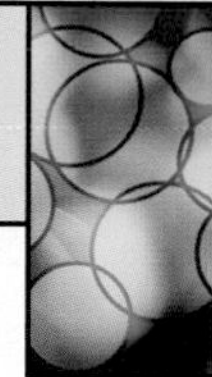

CHAPTER • 37

Endotoxemia

Katharina L. Lohmann and Michelle Henry Barton

ETIOLOGY

The clinical syndrome of endotoxemia is the result of a massive, dysregulated, and generalized inflammatory response to endotoxin, the major structural component of the outer membrane layer of the gram-negative bacterial cell wall (Fig. 37-1). Sources of endotoxin relevant to equine medicine include gram-negative pathogens, as well as gram-negative bacteria that are part of the normal intestinal, especially cecal, microflora. Endotoxemia associated with gram-negative infections may result from generalized disease, such as neonatal septicemia, or from more localized processes, such as pleuropneumonia, peritonitis, or endometritis. With localized infections, "spillover" of inflammatory mediators into the systemic circulation may occur once a critical concentration has been reached at the local site.[1]

Translocation of endotoxin from the intestinal lumen may occur on compromise of the mucosal barrier, which is most pronounced with severe inflammation, such as during acute colitis, or with ischemia, as in strangulating intestinal lesions. Other suggested causes of endotoxin translocation include severe shock states, severe trauma, malnutrition, and strenuous exercise.[2-6] Mechanisms of gut barrier compromise under these conditions may include reduced intestinal blood flow, resulting in ischemia; hypoxemia; and increased body temperature. The relevance of endotoxin translocation from these causes has not been investigated sufficiently in horses; however, these may serve to explain the occurrence of endotoxemia in compromised patients without primary infection or intestinal disease.

Endotoxin molecules have *lipopolysaccharide* (LPS) structure and consist of three distinct portions: the O-polysaccharide (or O-chain), core oligosaccharide (divided further into inner and outer core), and lipid A (Fig. 37-2). *Lipid A* represents the biologically active portion of LPS and anchors the endotoxin molecule in the cell membrane; therefore it is not available for interaction with inflammatory cells until endotoxin is released from the bacterial cell.[7] This release occurs on cell division and cell death, but also on bacterial killing from antimicrobial treatment.[8] After release from the bacterial cell, endotoxin molecules tend to aggregate and form micelles based on their amphipathic nature. In plasma, individual LPS molecules can be removed from these micellar aggregates by plasma proteins, most notably *lipopolysaccharide-binding protein* (LBP).[9] LBP then transfers LPS monomers to the surface of inflammatory cells, where the molecules bind to a specific receptor complex and elicit cell activation. Increased production and release of cytokines and other inflammatory mediators in response to this cell activation represents a crucial step in initiation and maintenance of the inflammatory cascade.

The structure of endotoxin, particularly the lipid A portion, is well conserved among pathogenic gram-negative bacteria. Research in recent years has shown that a group of "pathogen-associated molecular patterns" (PAMPs) play the role of "recognition signals" for the presence of pathogens. These PAMPs are molecules that are consistently present in certain types of pathogens and are structurally conserved. Rather than nonspecifically stimulating immune cells, PAMPs are recognized by "hard-wired"[10] receptors of the innate immune system, which as a group are referred to as "pattern recognition receptors" (PRRs). Endotoxin can be regarded as the prototypic PAMP signaling the presence of gram-negative bacteria, and *toll-like receptor 4* (TLR4) has been identified as the PRR for endotoxin.[11] In addition to TLR4, 10 other TLRs have been identified to date, and most of their ligand specificities have been identified (Table 37-1). TLR4 functions as part of a receptor complex that also

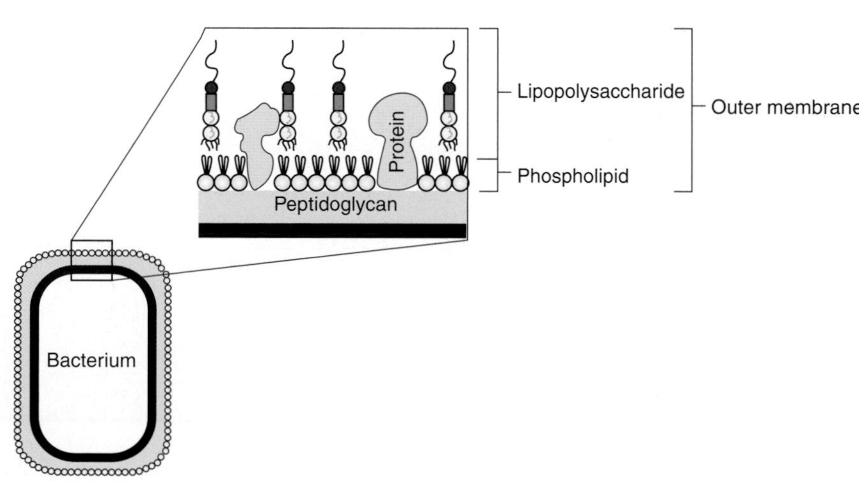

Fig. 37-1 Lipopolysaccharide (LPS, endotoxin) is the major component of the outer membrane layer of the gram-negative bacterial cell wall.

includes the *cluster of differentiation antigen 14* (CD14) and *myeloid differentiation factor-2* (MD-2), a small protein that interacts with the extracellular portion of TLR4. Although all three proteins appear to be required to provide a high sensitivity of cells to endotoxin, TLR4 is the only protein with a transmembrane domain and therefore deserves particular recognition when investigating cellular stimulation by endotoxin.

It is important to understand that the inflammatory response to endotoxin primarily serves to provide innate immunologic defense against invading bacteria, and is therefore indispensable for survival. Strict regulation of the inflammatory reaction normally ensures removal of offending organisms without harm to the host, and clinically significant endotoxemia or even shock states and organ failure only develop when the immune response becomes dysregulated and spirals out of control. Because of the signal function of endotoxin, pathophysiology and clinical findings are quite similar whether endotoxin acts alone or in combination with intact bacteria or other bacterial products to initiate the immune response.

Similarities of the inflammatory response extend to other inciting causes, such as gram-positive bacterial, viral, or fungal infection and severe trauma. The term *systemic inflammatory response syndrome* (SIRS)[12] was introduced to describe the clinical entity of an overzealous inflammatory response in the absence of an etiologic diagnosis. For the purpose of case definition in human clinical trials, SIRS is defined by the presence of at least two characteristic findings, including hypothermia or hyperthermia; tachycardia, tachypnea, or hypocapnia; and leukocytosis, leukopenia, or an increased number of immature leukocyte forms.[12] These criteria certainly apply to many horses currently diagnosed as being "endotoxemic," and therefore use of the term *SIRS* in equine medicine may be appropriate and potentially more useful.[13]

Additional definitions applicable to human patients include *sepsis* (SIRS caused by demonstrable infection, whether localized or in the form of bacteremia), *severe sepsis*, and *septic shock* (sepsis-induced hypotension, persisting despite adequate fluid resuscitation, along with the presence of hypoperfusion abnormalities or organ dysfunction).[12] *Multiple organ dysfunction syndrome* is defined as insufficiency of two or more organs, which may manifest as clinical changes or may be diagnosed based on clinicopathologic data. An adjustment of this terminology to the equine patient has not been undertaken to date but might offer advantages with respect to case definition for clinical trials as well as establishment of prognostic criteria for "endotoxemic" patients.

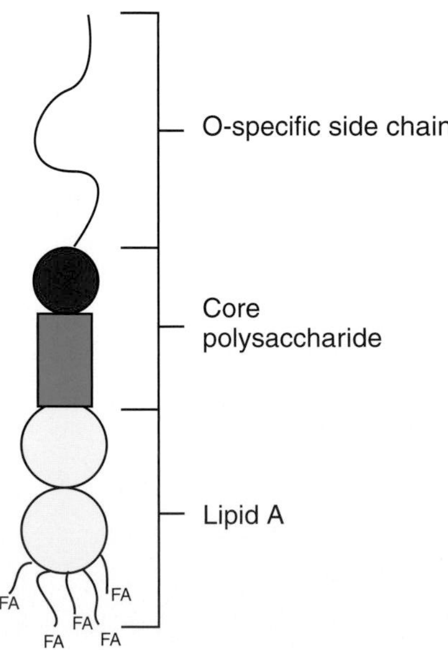

Fig. 37-2 Structure of LPS (endotoxin). *FA*, Fatty acid.

EPIDEMIOLOGY

Endotoxemia affects horses and ponies of either gender and of all breeds and ages, including neonatal foals. Studies performed at referral institutions have found that 10% to 40% of horses presented for colic[14-16] and 50% of septic neonatal foals[17] had measurable circulating endotoxin concentrations. The number of colic patients testing positive for endotoxin was increased when only horses with conditions requiring exploratory surgery were investigated.

Individual differences in the sensitivity to endotoxin, although anecdotally observed, have not been documented in horses. In other species, including humans, presence of certain gene polymorphisms has been associated with a reduced sensitivity to endotoxin challenge ("hyporesponders") and may also be associated with disease susceptibility and outcome. *Gene polymorphisms* are defined as allelic variants that exist stably in a population and occur in frequencies (>1%) not attributable to new mutations.[18] Polymorphisms most often occur as *single-nucleotide polymorphisms* (SNPs) and may affect coding as well as noncoding regions of genes.

SNPs within coding regions *(exons)* that result in altered amino acid sequence presumably affect protein function. For example, SNPs in the coding region of the human TLR4 gene are associated with impaired signal transduction in response to LPS stimulation.[19] An association between SNPs in human TLR4 and unfavorable outcome of sepsis in human patients has been suggested[20,21] and may be attributable to a reduced immune defense against infection favoring the development of sepsis. Changes in noncoding regions *(introns)* or in gene promoters may alter transcription rate and messenger ribonucleic acid

Table • 37-1

Toll-Like Receptor (TLR) Ligands

RECEPTOR	MICROBIAL AND SYNTHETIC LIGANDS
TLR1	Triacyl lipopeptides (e.g., Pam3Cys)
TLR2	Lipoproteins, lipopeptides, peptidoglycan, yeast zymosan, lipoteichoic acid, atypical lipopolysaccharide (LPS), lipoarabinomannan
TLR3	Double-stranded RNA
TLR4	LPS, taxol, viral F-protein (e.g., respiratory syncytial virus)
TLR5	Flagellin
TLR6	Diacyl lipopeptides, yeast zymosan, lipoteichoic acid
TLR7	Imidazoquinoline, loxoribine, single-stranded RNA viruses
TLR8	Imidazoquinoline, single-stranded RNA viruses
TLR9	CpG DNA, CpG oligonucleotides
TLR10	Not identified
TLR11	Ligands derived from uropathogenic bacteria

Modified from Horner AA, Redecke V, Raz E: *Curr Opin All Clin Immunol* 4:6, 555-561, 2004.

(mRNA) stability or may serve as "markers" for certain traits if they are in linkage with biologically active SNPs in other gene regions.[18]

A polymorphism in the human *tumor necrosis factor alpha* (TNF-α) gene promoter[22] may affect the magnitude of TNF-α expression on cell stimulation and is likely associated with outcome of septic shock. Polymorphisms in promoter regions of human *interleukin-6* (IL-6) and *interleukin-10* (IL-10) are associated with decreased cytokine production in vitro, although their clinical relevance has not been evaluated to date.[18] The biologic significance of SNPs in the equine TNF-α gene promoter[23] has not been determined. Investigation of gene polymorphisms currently is an area of great interest as it may provide the basis for a more individualized approach to patient assessment and therapy.

PATHOGENESIS

Inflammatory Cell Activation

Investigation is ongoing as to the exact mechanism by which endotoxin binds to its cellular receptor complex and initiates cell activation, as well as the details of intracellular signaling in response to cell stimulation. One obstacle in the evaluation of ligand-receptor interactions is the current lack of understanding of the three-dimensional structure of LPS receptor proteins and therefore the LPS-binding site(s). As mentioned earlier, at least three proteins (CD14, TLR4, MD-2) constitute the major receptor complex for LPS, and interaction of LPS with all proteins during initiation of cell signaling has been demonstrated experimentally.[24] Additional binding proteins, which may be involved in the initiation of cell signaling and cell activation, include β_2-integrins, moesin, heat shock proteins, chemokine receptors, growth differentiation factors, and intracellular nucleotide-binding oligomerization domain (NOD)1 and NOD2.[7,25-27]

CD14 was the first protein known to be essential for LPS binding and cellular activation.[28] CD14 is a 60-kilodalton (kDa) protein that is constitutively expressed on myeloid cells, including monocytes, macrophages, and neutrophils, as well as B lymphocytes and several other cell types.[7] In horses experimentally infused with endotoxin, an increase in the number of circulating CD14-expressing cells, as well as in the number of immunoglobulin M (IgM)–positive and major histocompatibility complex (MHC) class II–positive cells, correlated with changes in vital parameters.[29] In addition to membrane-bound forms (mCD14), a soluble form (sCD14) is present in plasma and may be able to transfer LPS to non–CD14-bearing cells (e.g., endothelial cells) to render these cells endotoxin responsive.[30] Conversely, high concentrations of sCD14 may have "detoxifying" effects by scavenging LPS and preventing it from interacting with inflammatory cells. This "bipolar" effect has similarly been suggested for LBP.

TLR4 in association with MD-2 represents the actual signaling portion of the LPS receptor complex.[11,31] TLR4 is a 92-kDa type I transmembrane receptor with an *interleukin-1 receptor* (IL-1R)–like intracellular domain. Similarities to IL-1R extend beyond structure, and signaling pathways in response to TLR4 stimulation or IL-1R stimulation show substantial similarity. TLR4 is expressed constitutively on neutrophils, monocytes, macrophages, and dendritic cells, but also on epithelial and endothelial cells. Expression levels vary among individuals and are regulated in a tissue-specific manner by LPS and cytokines (e.g., TNF-α). Oligomerization is required for signaling through TLRs, and MD-2 may have an effect on TLR4 aggregation on the cell surface.[32] MD-2 is a small, secreted glycoprotein that associates with the extracellular domain of TLR4 and is most likely required for proper receptor function. MD-2 may also be involved in ensuring proper glycosylation and transport of TLR4 to the cellular surface.

An interesting observation is that certain "atypical" LPS molecules, which show variation from enteric LPS in their lipid A structure, can act as endotoxin antagonists. These molecules compete for receptor binding but do not cause cell activation, and in effect they block cellular response to "agonist" endotoxin.[33] Curiously, recognition of LPS molecules as agonists or antagonists depends on the host species, which has prompted investigations into the determinants of receptor specificity. Uniformly, these studies have shown that the species origin of CD14 does not determine receptor specificity, a finding that further supports a primary role for CD14 as an endotoxin capture molecule. Conclusions concerning the relative role of TLR4 and MD-2 have been variable; some studies suggest that either TLR4 or MD-2 is the primary determinant of receptor specificity, and others suggest that both proteins play a role.[34-36] Cell transfection experiments performed in vitro suggest that the complex of TLR4 and MD-2 mediates recognition of endotoxic LPS in equine cells.[37]

Intracellular signaling pathways resulting in activation of *nuclear factor kappa B* (NF-κB) and stimulation of *mitogen-activated protein* (MAP) *kinases* are of major significance for cell activation by LPS (Fig. 37-3), although additional pathways have been suggested. In effect, cell-signaling events culminate in the translocation of transcription factors to the cell nucleus, with a resulting increase in gene transcription and protein expression. Translational and posttranslational processes may also be activated, such that the regulation of protein expression in response to endotoxin is a complex event offering multiple targets for regulation and potential therapeutic influence.

Inflammatory Mediators

The pathogenesis of endotoxemia is primarily determined by the effects of inflammatory mediators, many of which are released after inflammatory cell stimulation. Important mediators include the cytokines, prostaglandins, thromboxanes, leukotrienes, platelet-activating factor, nitric oxide, reactive oxygen species, histamine, kinins, complement components, and growth factors. Table 37-2 summarizes the origin, regulation, and biologic effects of some of the major inflammatory mediators. Cytokines play a particularly important role because they not only exert pathophysiologically relevant effects, but also regulate the release of other mediators. Primarily, proinflammatory cytokines (e.g., TNF-α, IL-1) are central to the initiation and maintenance of an inflammatory reaction, and development of SIRS has classically been attributed to an uncontrolled overproduction of these proinflammatory mediators.[1]

In recent years, however, studies have increasingly investigated cytokines with mostly antiinflammatory activity, such as IL-10, IL-4, IL-11, and *transforming growth factor beta* (TGF-β), which are produced along with their proinflammatory counterparts and may serve to contain and attenuate inflammation after an invading pathogen has been eliminated. In addition to these cytokines, downregulating effects on the inflammatory cascade are attributed to soluble cytokine receptors (e.g., soluble TNF receptor) and cytokine receptor antagonists (e.g., soluble IL-1R antagonist), which inhibit cytokine effects at the level of the inflammatory cell. The role of antiinflammatory responses in disease development is not completely understood. However, a *compensatory anti-inflammatory response syndrome* (CARS) has been described in which excessive production of antiinflammatory mediators results in immunosuppression and ultimately immune anergy.[38]

The paradigm of "immunologic dissonance," as proposed by Bone,[1] therefore provides a more comprehensive and

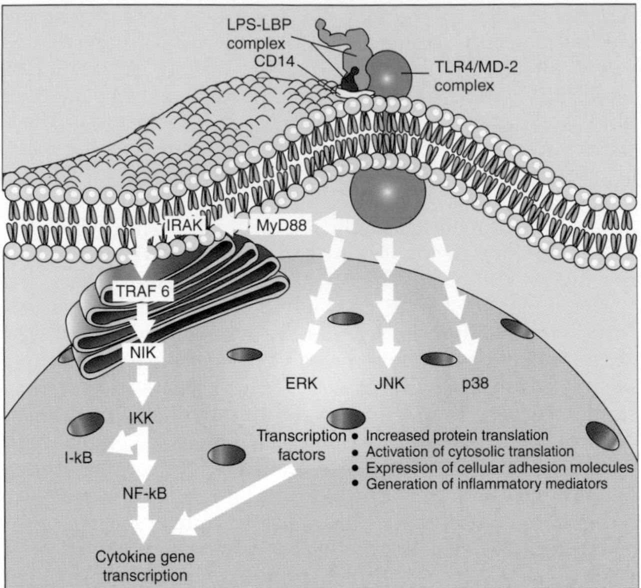

Fig. 37-3 Intracellular signaling events after endotoxin binding. Lipopolysaccharide-binding protein *(LBP)* associates with lipopolysaccharide (*LPS*, endotoxin) and transfers it to the cellular surface. LPS interacts with a receptor complex comprising CD14, toll-like receptor 4 *(TLR4)*, and myeloid differentiation factor-2 *(MD-2)*; TLR4 (but not CD14 or MD-2) possesses a transmembrane portion to allow signal transduction to the cytosol. Signaling via the mitogen-activated protein (MAP) kinases (extracellular signal-regulated kinase, *ERK;* c-*jun*-terminal kinase, *JNK;* p38) results in numerous alterations of cellular metabolism. Activation of IκB-kinase *(IKK)* via sequential phosphorylation of myeloid differentiation factor 88 *(MyD88)*, interleukin-1 receptor–associated kinase *(IRAK)*, tumor necrosis factor receptor–associated factor *(TRAF 6)*, and nuclear factor kappa B *(NF-κB)*–inducing kinase *(NIK)* leads to phosphorylation, ubiquination, and degradation of IκB and release of NF-κB. Transcription factors such as NF-κB translocate to the nucleus and promote gene transcription.

flexible view of inflammatory responses during infection and endotoxemia. According to this paradigm, every severe insult produces a response consisting of both proinflammatory and antiinflammatory components, and it is the relative balance (or lack thereof) of these components that determines outcome in the form of reestablishment of homeostasis or disease progression toward shock.

Some of the "earliest" or most "proximal" cytokines produced in response to endotoxin include TNF-α, IL-1, and IL-6. The importance of TNF-α in particular is underscored by experiments showing that TNF-α has very similar effects to endotoxin when administered experimentally,[39] and that blockade of TNF-α during early endotoxemia abrogates the development of clinical disease in laboratory animals[40] and horses.[41] In septic human patients, the magnitude of increase in TNF-α and IL-6 concentration is correlated with the severity of sepsis, whereas concentrations of IL-1 are often undetectable and show poor correlation with disease severity.[42] In horses, plasma activity of TNF-α is positively correlated with mortality in patients with acute gastrointestinal disease and in septic neonates.[14,43,44]

Eicosanoids are *arachodonic acid* (AA) metabolites and include the prostaglandins, thromboxanes, leukotrienes, lipoxins, hydroxyeicosatetraenoic acid (HETE), and epoxides.[45] The rate-limiting step in the production of eicosanoids is the liberation of AA from phospholipid pools in the cell membrane, followed by metabolism of AA through several different pathways (Fig. 37-4). The most important eicosanoids in the pathophysiology of endotoxemia are *thromboxane* A_2 (TxA_2) and the *prostaglandins* E_2 (PGE_2), I_2 (PGI_2), and $F_{2\alpha}$ ($PGF_{2\alpha}$); the significance of leukotrienes is less well understood.[46] TxA_2 promotes platelet aggregation, vasoconstriction, bronchoconstriction, and leukocyte adhesion;[47] PGE_2 and particularly PGI_2 (prostacyclin) cause vasodilation and have platelet antiaggregating effects. PGE_2 and PGI_2 also exert antiinflammatory effects by reducing cytokine production, inhibiting activation and proliferation of B cells, decreasing macrophage phagocytosis, and inhibiting neutrophil functions.[45] In horses, increased plasma concentration of TxA_2 has been associated with very early responses to experimental endotoxemia, including pulmonary hypertension, dyspnea, and hypoxemia, whereas a rise in PGI_2 occurred concurrently with clinical signs of abdominal pain, mucous membrane discoloration, prolongation of the capillary refill time, and the development of hypotension.[48]

Endothelial Dysfunction, Hemodynamic Changes, and Shock

Endotoxic shock is generally classified as "distributive shock" and is largely attributable to peripheral vascular dysfunction resulting in maldistribution of blood flow and perfusion deficits. Endotoxin exerts peripheral vasomotor effects through release of inflammatory mediators such as prostacyclin and nitric oxide, which cause widespread vasodilation and vasoplegia, leading to blood pooling in the periphery and a reduction of effective circulating volume.[49] In addition, cardiac function is compromised by decreased coronary blood flow and the release of myocardial depressant factors; circulating volume is reduced by increased vascular permeability; and tissue oxygen extraction is impaired. Initially, tachycardia and increased cardiac output as well as increases in central venous pressure and pulmonary arterial pressure (hyperdynamic phase) may have a compensatory effect.[49] However, disease progression is characterized by the development of systemic hypotension and ultimately perfusion deficits of vital organs.

In addition to its role in vascular failure, endothelial dysfunction promotes the development of microvascular thrombosis, thereby contributing to the development of organ failure. Loss of the normal endothelial surface with its antithrombotic properties favors thrombus formation by exposing subendothelial tissue factor and allowing platelet aggregation to occur. Endothelial damage is primarily neutrophil mediated by a mechanism involving neutrophil-derived enzymes (e.g., elastase), hydrogen peroxide molecules, endothelial enzymes (e.g., xanthine oxidase), and endothelial cytosolic iron. Free radicals, predominantly HO^- (hypochlorite), which are formed in endothelial cells, directly cause cell damage; neutrophil-derived matrix metalloproteinases (MMPs) and direct effects of cytokines (e.g., TNF-α, IL-1) also contribute. Constitutive production of nitric oxide (NO) may afford some protection against radical-mediated endothelial cell damage; however, overproduction of NO by the inducible NO synthase (iNOS) enzyme has detrimental effects and compounds tissue damage.

Neutrophil Activation

Neutrophil activation during bacterial infection generally serves to promote extravasation into infected tissues and increase the cells' bactericidal capacity. Activated neutrophils express adhesion molecules for interaction with endothelial cells,

Table • **37-2**

Important Mediators of the Systemic Inflammatory Response to Endotoxin

MEDIATOR	ORIGIN	EFFECTS
Tumor necrosis factor (TNF)	Macrophages Monocytes Neutrophils CD4+ T cells Natural killer cells	Synthesis of TNF, IL-1, IL-6, PGI_2, PAF, and GM-CSF Neutrophil activation Activation of coagulation and fibrinolysis Activation of complement and contact systems Catabolic state Insulin resistance Pyrogen (direct and via IL-1 induction)
Interleukin-1 (IL-1)	Activated macrophages Endothelial cells Fibroblasts Dendritic cells Lymphocytes Keratinocytes	Pyrogen via central release of PGE_2 Release of prostaglandins, leukotrienes, and PAF Neutrophil activation and chemotaxis Activation of coagulation and fibrinolysis Activation of complement and contact systems Acute-phase response Increases activity of lipoprotein lipase Mobilizes amino acids Induces muscle proteolysis
Interleukin-6 (IL-6)	Activated macrophages Fibroblasts Keratinocytes T lymphocytes	Acute-phase response Stress response Weak pyrogen
Interleukin-8 (IL-8)	Macrophages Endothelial cells	Neutrophil activation and chemotaxis
Interleukin-10 (IL-10)	T helper cells type 2 Monocytes Epithelial cells	Inhibition of macrophage activation Inhibition of synthesis and release of cytokines from T cells and macrophages Suppresses function of antigen-presenting cells
Thromboxane A_2 (TxA_2)	Platelets	Vasoconstriction Platelet aggregation
Prostaglandin E_2 (PGE_2)	Most nucleated cells	Vasodilation Platelet aggregation Pyrogen Antiinflammatory effects (e.g., inhibition of neutrophil functions)
Prostaglandin I_2 (PGI_2)	Vascular endothelial cells	Vasodilation Inhibits platelet aggregation
Prostaglandin $F_{2\alpha}$ ($PGF_{2\alpha}$)	Most nucleated cells	Vasoconstriction Luteolysis
Platelet-activating factor (PAF)	Macrophages Monocytes Platelets Neutrophils Mast cells Eosinophils Endothelial cells	Platelet aggregation Activation of macrophages and neutrophils Hypotension Increases vascular permeability Leukocyte recruitment Visceral smooth muscle contraction Negative inotrope, arrhythmogenic Ileus
Leukotriene B_4 (LTB_4)	Neutrophils Monocytes Alveolar macrophages	Chemoattractant Promotes neutrophil interaction with endothelial cells Neutrophil activation Increases vascular permeability
Leukotrienes C_4, D_4, E_4 (SRS-A)	Eosinophils Monocytes	Increase vascular permeability Bronchoconstriction Vasoconstriction

SRS-A, Slow-reacting substance of anaphylaxis.

Continued

Table • 37-2

Important Mediators of the Systemic Inflammatory Response to Endotoxin—cont'd

MEDIATOR	ORIGIN	EFFECTS
Kinins	Produced from serum precursors	Increase vascular permeability Smooth muscle contraction Pain
Complement components (C3a, C5a)	—	Neutrophil activation and chemotaxis Smooth muscle contraction Mast cell degranulation Release of histamine and serotonin Increase vascular permeability
Oxygen-derived free radicals	Macrophages Neutrophils	Cell membrane and tissue damage Enzyme inactivation
Granulocyte-monocyte colony-stimulating factor (GM-CSF)	—	Rebound neutrophilia

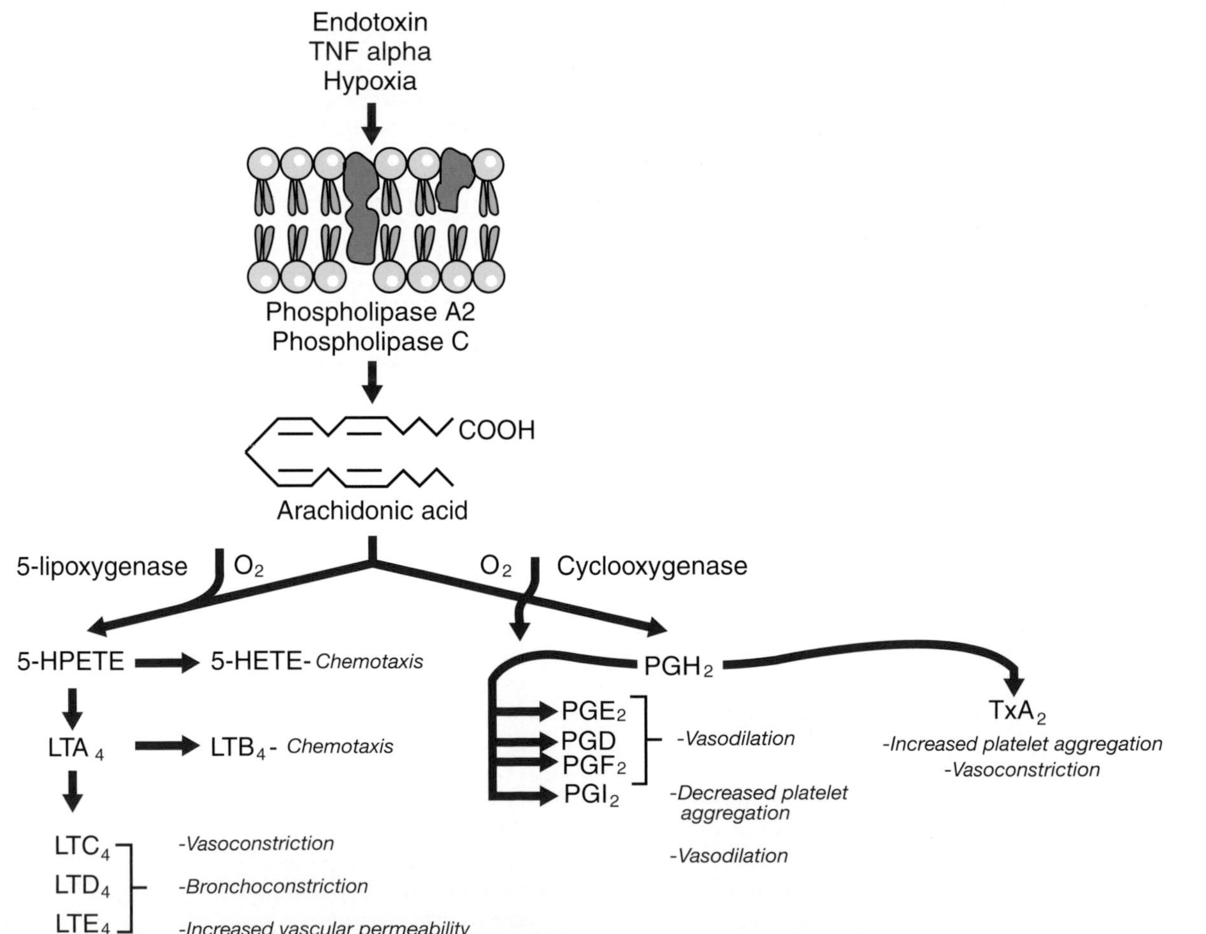

Fig. 37-4 Eicosanoid formation pathways. *TNF,* Tumor necrosis factor; *PG,* prostaglandin; *LT,* leukotriene; *Tx,* thromboxane; *HPETE,* hydroperoxyeicosatetraenoic acid; *HETE,* hydroxyeicosatetraenoic acid.

exhibit an increased capacity for phagocytosis and respiratory burst, and release lysosomal enzymes and inflammatory mediators.[50] Neutrophil margination and extravasation occur in three phases, characterized by the expression of different adhesion molecules on neutrophils and endothelial cells. The first phase of neutrophil tethering and rolling is mediated by *P-selectin* and *E-selectin* on endothelial cells, which interact with *P-selectin glycoprotein ligand-1* (PSGL-1) and sialylated Lewis-X–like structures on leukocytes. Firm adhesion of neutrophils to the endothelium during the second phase results from the interaction between endothelial *intercellular adhesion molecule-1* (ICAM-1) and neutrophil integrins *leukocyte function–associated antigen-1* (LFA-1) and Mac-1. The third phase of neutrophil transmigration depends on expression of *platelet/endothelial cell adhesion molecule-1*, located at the intercellular junction of endothelial cells.

Neutropenia is an early finding during experimental endotoxin administration and may be the only specific clinicopathologic evidence of acute sepsis or endotoxemia.[51] Neutrophil margination is observed particularly within the lung vasculature,[52] and neutrophils are important players in the development of acute lung injury after endotoxin administration. Mechanisms of neutrophil-mediated lung injury may include vascular endothelial damage, as outlined in the previous section; neutrophil migration into airways; expression of proinflammatory cytokines (e.g., IL-1, TNF-α); and oxidant-induced injury resulting in loss of epithelial integrity.[53] In some cases, these events may culminate in the development of a "shock lung,"[54] and pulmonary failure remains the leading cause of sepsis-related death in human patients.

Recent investigations using chimeric mouse models have shown that activation of circulating neutrophils by endotoxin is not sufficient to induce neutrophil sequestration within the lung. These studies have suggested that TLR4-mediated endothelial cell activation is the dominant event in the development of inappropriate leukocyte trafficking during endotoxemia.[55] On recovery from endotoxemia or infection, reentry of marginated neutrophils into the circulation leads to rebound neutrophilia; however, it is questionable whether these neutrophils exhibit normal cellular function and signify a recovery of normal immune responses. Increased release of neutrophils from the bone marrow caused by stimulation of myeloid cell proliferation by *granulocyte-macrophage colony-stimulating factor* (GM-CSF) also contributes to rebound neutrophilia.

Coagulopathy

Coagulopathy often develops during endotoxemia and has been described in horses with colic,[56-58] as well as in septic foals.[17] Coagulopathy develops because of simultaneous activation of coagulation and fibrinolysis, and in its most severe form, results in *consumptive coagulopathy* and *disseminated intravascular coagulation* (DIC).[59] Usually, however, clinical signs of coagulopathy are limited to an increased thrombotic tendency (e.g., jugular venous thrombosis) or an increased bleeding tendency (e.g., following venipuncture or nasogastric intubation). Diffuse microthrombosis may contribute to tissue ischemia and the development of organ failure. The factors that determine whether activation of procoagulant or fibrinolytic pathways predominates are poorly understood. Because an abnormal coagulation profile can be detected before the development of clinical signs of coagulopathy, evaluation of coagulation parameters is an important step in patient assessment, and abnormalities should prompt preemptive treatment to prevent further deterioration.

Activation of coagulation is by both the intrinsic and the extrinsic pathway and culminates in thrombin-mediated conversion of fibrinogen into fibrin. Endotoxin directly activates the intrinsic coagulation pathway through the contact system comprising factor XII (Hageman factor), prekallikrein, and high-molecular-weight kininogen. More importantly, however, activation of the extrinsic pathway results from exposure of subendothelial tissue factor after endothelial damage and stimulation of tissue factor expression on activated mononuclear phagocytes and endothelial cells. Increased expression of monocyte tissue factor (also referred to as "procoagulant activity") is reported to be significantly associated with poor prognosis in equine colic patients.[60] Tissue factor expression by peritoneal macrophages may favor the development of intraabdominal adhesions in colic patients undergoing exploratory laparotomy.[61] Tissue factor forms complexes with coagulation factor VIIa and subsequently activates factors X and IX. Factor Xa associates with factor Va to effect prothrombin conversion into thrombin (prothrombinase complex), whereas factor IXa in association with factor VIIIa further activates factor X activation. *Thrombin* is formed initially on tissue factor–bearing surfaces and cells and subsequently stimulates amplified thrombin production on the platelet surface.[62] Thrombin stimulates platelet adhesion and activation and activates clotting factors V, VIII, and XI. In addition, platelet aggregation is favored by increased release of TxA_2 from activated vascular endothelial cells and release of TxA_2 and *platelet-activating factor* (PAF) from activated platelets. A predominant role for PAF rather than TxA_2 in endotoxin-induced platelet aggregation has been suggested.[63,64]

Procoagulant tendency during endotoxemia is further attributable to impairment of regulatory (i.e., anticoagulant) mechanisms. For example, endothelial dysfunction leads to decreased activation of protein C as well as decreased expression of antithrombin III. *Activated protein* C (APC) is important for the anticoagulant properties of normal endothelium and acts in concert with protein S by inactivating clotting factors Va and VIIIa as well as *plasminogen activator inhibitor* (PAI).[65] Production of APC depends on thrombin interaction with thrombomodulin on the vascular endothelium, such that decreased thrombomodulin expression by damaged endothelial cells decreases APC formation. *Antithrombin III* inhibits multiple components of both the intrinsic and the extrinsic coagulation pathway, including clotting factors IIa, IXa, Xa, XIa, XIIa, VIIa/tissue factor, and kallikrein.[66]

Regulation of fibrinolysis occurs at the level of plasminogen (plasminogen activator, PAI) and at the level of plasmin, the actual fibrin-degrading enzyme (α_2-antiplasmin). Increased fibrinolysis leads to an accumulation of *fibrin degradation products* (FDPs), which inhibit platelet aggregation, thrombin formation, and fibrin polymerization and thereby enhance bleeding tendency. FDPs also play a role in increasing vascular permeability. In endotoxemia, cytokines such as TNF-α and IL-1 activate fibrinolysis by increasing expression of both *tissue-type* (tPA) and *urokinase-type* (uPA) *plasminogen activator.* These cytokines, however, also stimulate synthesis of PAI, which opposes fibrinolysis. Increased plasma concentrations of PAI were observed in horses with colic,[67,68] suggesting that inhibition of fibrinolysis and therefore further increased procoagulant tendency may be the predominant abnormality in these patients.

Coagulopathy has long been recognized as an important complication of endotoxemia requiring control to prevent the development of large vessel and microvascular thrombosis and bleeding episodes. The recognition of positive-feedback loops between coagulation and inflammatory pathways,[69] however, and the results of studies showing beneficial effects of treatment with recombinant APC in human patients with severe sepsis[70] have provided novel insights into the

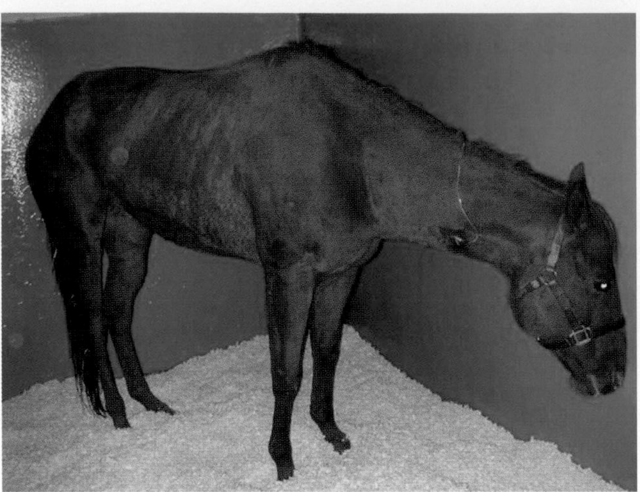

Fig. 37-5 Obtunded mentation is often observed in horses with profound endotoxemia. (Courtesy Dr. Clare Ryan.)

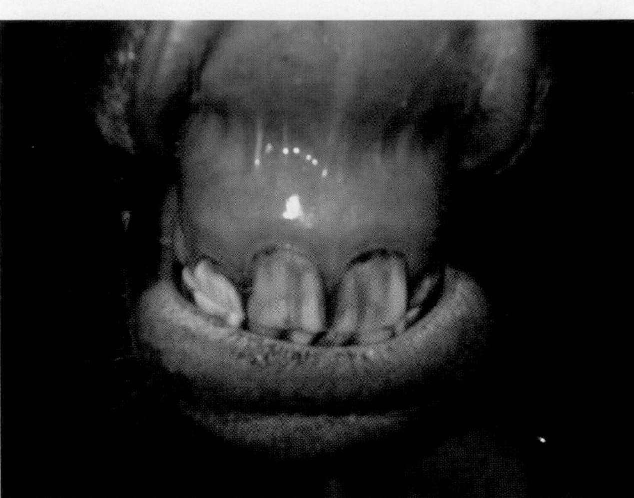

Fig. 37-6 Congested and hyperemic mucous membranes in horse with endotoxemia. (Courtesy Dr. Clare Ryan.)

pathophysiology of inflammation during sepsis and endotoxemia. It is now understood that activation of coagulation not only results in clot formation but also in endothelial cell activation and expression of inflammatory cytokines such as IL-6 and IL-8, thereby contributing to leukocyte activation and endothelial adhesion.[62,71] Proposed mechanisms for the beneficial effects of APC treatment include blockade of TNF-α production, blockade of NF-κB activation in monocytes and endothelial cells, blockade of genes upregulated during inflammation, and an increased expression of antiapoptotic genes.[62] Because of an observed increased bleeding tendency in patients treated with APC, recommendations for use in human patients are currently restricted to those with severe sepsis or septic shock.

Complement Activation

Complement activation in response to infection serves the purpose of forming a *membrane attack complex* to cause bacterial cell destruction. Endotoxin activates the complement pathway through the alternative pathway by direct interaction with complement components. Complement activation further occurs on bacterial surfaces, by acute-phase proteins, and by immune complexes.[72] Plasmin and kallikrein, produced during activation of coagulation and fibrinolysis, also activate complement components C3 and C5, which act as anaphylatoxins and cause vasodilation and increase vascular permeability by activation of mast cell degranulation. C5a further acts as a chemotaxin and increases leukocyte migration, promotes neutrophil adhesion to endothelial cells, stimulates enzyme release from phagocytic cells and superoxide anion production by neutrophils, and activates leukotriene production in neutrophils and monocytes. C5a also has inhibitory effects on neutrophil function and contributes to a procoagulant state. Blockade of C5a generation or C5a receptor blockade during the onset of sepsis improves survival in experimental models.[72]

Acute-Phase Response

During acute inflammation, production of a number of proteins by the liver is increased, possibly to counteract and contain inflammatory responses.[73] This acute-phase response is primarily initiated by IL-1 and IL-6 and is limited to the first 24 to 48 hours after an insult. Acute-phase proteins identified in horses include fibrinogen, haptoglobin, ferritin, transferrin, ceruloplasmin, coagulation factor VIII:C, serum amyloid A, C-reactive protein, α_1-acid glycoprotein, and phospholipase A_2.[74] *Fibrinogen* is the acute-phase protein most frequently evaluated in horses, and the capacity for fibrinogen production often outweighs increased fibrinogen consumption in clinical or subclinical DIC.[75]

CLINICAL FINDINGS

Clinical signs of endotoxemia depend on the severity and duration of the insult and must be interpreted in the context of the underlying disease process. If endotoxin is administered experimentally at a sublethal dose, early clinical signs include depression, anorexia, sweating, muscle fasciculations, and signs of abdominal discomfort such as yawning, pawing, or recumbency. Heart and respiratory rates increase, and intestinal sounds are decreased or absent. Mucous membranes become hyperemic, and the capillary refill time is accelerated, indicating the hyperdynamic phase.[51] Fever is frequently observed and can be attributed to the effects of pyrogenic cytokines (e.g., TNF-α) as well as central prostaglandin production.

With progression of endotoxemia, depression and anorexia typically worsen and diarrhea may develop, whereas abdominal pain usually subsides after the initial phase (Fig. 37-5). Mucous membrane color changes to brick red or purple; in addition, congestion, a periapical "toxic line," and a prolonged capillary refill time are observed[51] (Fig. 37-6). The shock phase is characterized by decreased pulse pressure and reduced venous filling (hypodynamic phase), cool extremities, diffusely gray or purple mucous membranes, and reduced body temperature. A "muddy" mucous membrane color and diffuse scleral reddening (Fig. 37-7) indicate vascular endothelial damage and increased capillary permeability.

Coagulation abnormalities may be identified as thrombosis at catheter placement sites (Fig. 37-8), petechiae or ecchymoses (Fig. 37-9), and an increased bleeding tendency (e.g., following venipuncture or nasogastric intubation). Spontaneous gross hemorrhage in the form of epistaxis may occur in severe cases.[76] Clinical signs of organ failure can vary greatly because

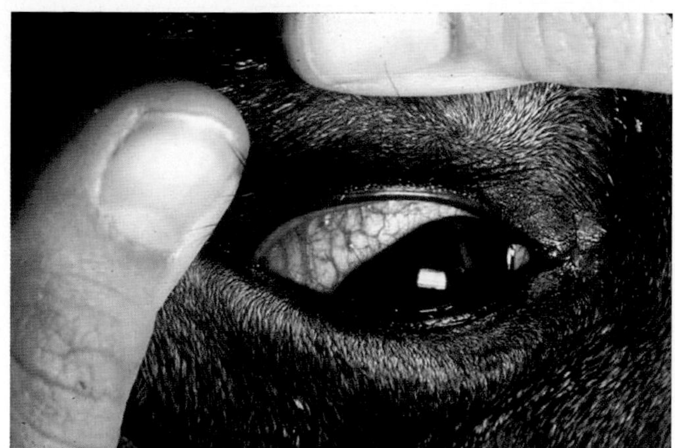

Fig. 37-7 Marked scleral injection secondary to endotoxemia. (Courtesy Dr. Clare Ryan.)

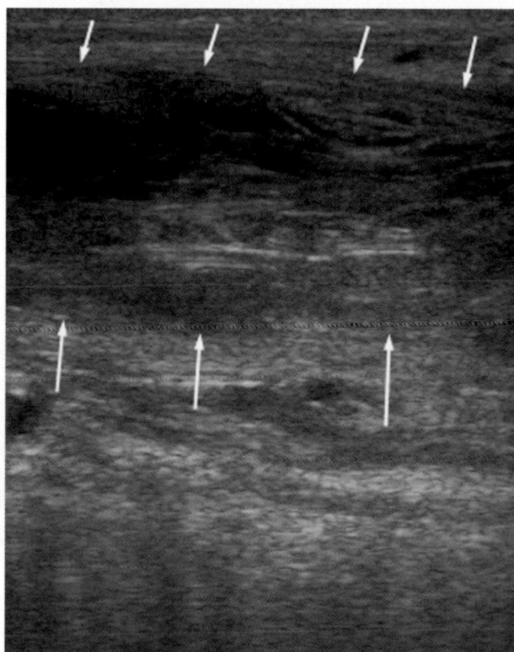

Fig. 37-8 Longitudinal ultrasonogram of jugular vein from 3-year-old Thoroughbred colt that developed septic jugular thrombosis after surgery to correct colon torsion. Three weeks after onset of signs, the large heterogenous thrombus *(between arrows)* has become very echogenic, with central linear echoes reflecting fibrosis as thrombus begins to resolve. (Courtesy Dr. Celia Marr.)

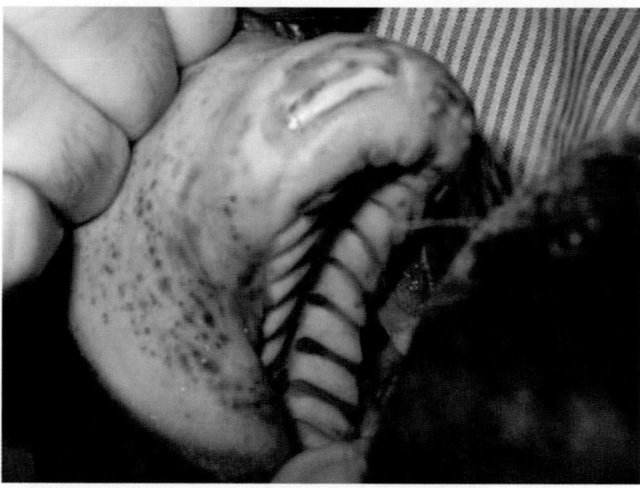

Fig. 37-9 Petechial hemorrhages of oral mucous membranes in neonatal foal with gram-negative septicemia. (Courtesy Dr. Clare Ryan.)

generally any body system can be affected; however, renal dysfunction and laminitis appear to be the most common complications of endotoxemia in horses. Renal failure is attributable to ischemic cortical necrosis and acute tubular necrosis and may result in anuria or oliguria, polyuria, and hematuria from renal infarction. Proteinuria, hematuria, and decreased concentrating ability may be detected on urinalysis. Laminitis should be suspected in horses with sudden onset of lameness, increased hoof wall warmth, bounding digital pulses, and sensitivity to hoof tester pressure, and radiographic assessment should be pursued early (Fig. 37-10). Abdominal pain and ileus can be the result of endotoxemia; however, differentiation from clinical signs attributable to the primary disease is difficult in horses presenting with colic or colitis. Infrequent manifestations of organ failure may include signs of respiratory dysfunction (dyspnea, abnormal lung sounds), hepatic disease (icterus, hepatic encephalopathy), or cardiac dysfunction (e.g., myocarditis, tachyarrhythmias). In endotoxemic pregnant mares, abortion caused by increased $PGF_{2\alpha}$ production and reduced progesterone concentration[77,78] should be anticipated as a potential complication.

DIAGNOSIS

A diagnosis of endotoxemia is usually made based on the identification of clinical signs and supportive clinicopathologic changes, as well as the recognition of risk factors, or conditions known to be associated with its development. In most cases, clinical signs of the primary disease (e.g., colic) are the reason for patient evaluation; sometimes, however, clinical signs of endotoxemia may precede the development of more distinct signs of the primary disease. In this latter clinical scenario, diagnostic efforts should be aimed at identification of common causes of endotoxemia, such as septicemia in the neonate, alimentary tract disease, and infection of the intestinal or respiratory tract, peritoneal cavity, and uterus of postpartum mares.

Although plasma endotoxin concentration can be measured by the *Limulus amebolysate* (LAL) assay,[79] use of this assay has mostly been restricted to research purposes. The LAL assay is based on the existence of an endotoxin-sensitive coagulation cascade in the hemolymph of the horseshoe crab *Limulus polyphemus* and is commercially available in form of a multisample assay kit. The assay is relatively easy to perform, but it requires specialized equipment and is rather expensive unless a large number of samples are analyzed at once. The assay's predictive value with regard to a clinical diagnosis of endotoxemia has not been fully evaluated.

Detection of leukopenia, neutropenia, a left shift, or toxic morphologic changes within neutrophils (basophilia,

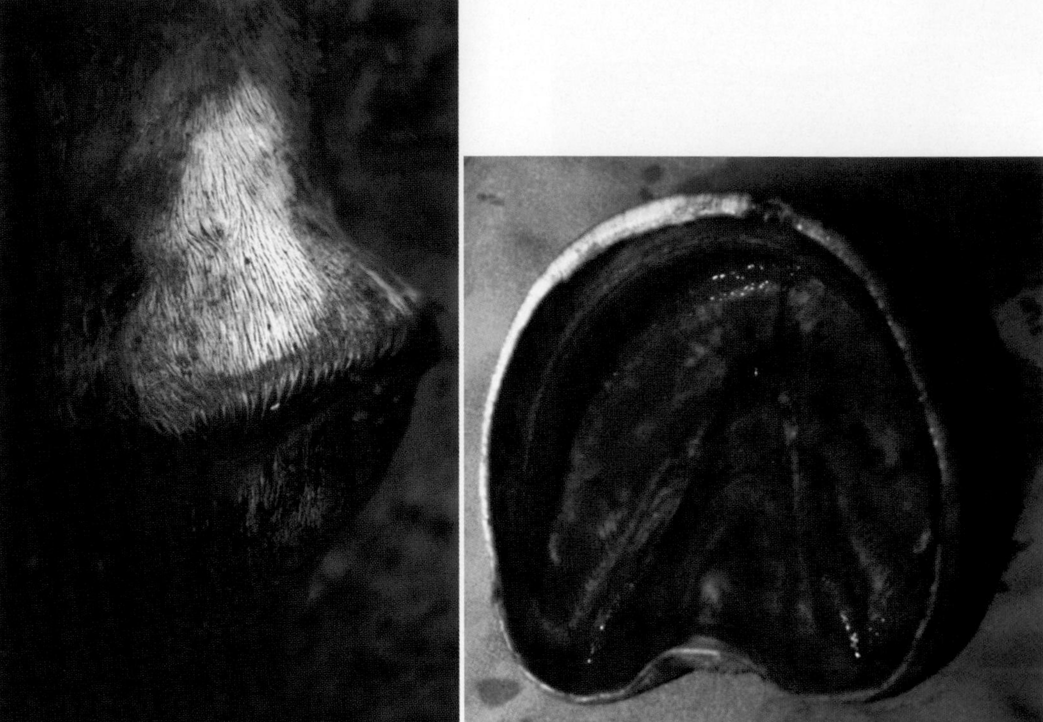

Fig. 37-10 Sloughed hoof capsule and left hind digit of 5-year-old Thoroughbred stallion that developed widespread arterial thrombosis in metatarsal region secondary to enterocolitis associated with quinidine toxicity. (Courtesy Dr. Celia Marr.)

vacuolization, Döhle bodies) should always prompt the clinician to search for a bacterial infection or other underlying diseases that result in endotoxemia. Additional clinicopathologic changes usually reflect the primary disease process and the development of organ failure. Common abnormalities include electrolyte and acid-base disturbances as well as protein loss in horses with gastrointestinal (GI) disease, increased blood urea nitrogen (BUN) and creatinine in dehydrated horses (pre-renal azotemia) or those with renal dysfunction, elevated liver enzymes, and possibly elevated muscle enzymes in colicky or recumbent horses. Fibrinogen concentration will often be increased as an indicator of the acute-phase response. A coagulation profile should be evaluated in all horses with severe endotoxemia and should include as a minimal database a platelet count, clotting times (prothrombin time [PT], activated partial thromboplastin time [aPTT]), and antithrombin III (ATIII) and FDP concentrations.

In a report of horses with acute GI disease, coagulation profiles showed abnormalities in 28 of 30 horses,[57] indicating the high prevalence of subclinical coagulopathies in endotoxemic patients. Reported abnormalities include increased concentration of FDPs and soluble fibrin monomer, prolonged PT indicating factor VII consumption, prolonged aPTT indicating factors VIII:C and IX consumption, prolonged thrombin time, decreased ATIII activity, thrombocytopenia, and decreased protein C and plasminogen activities. A diagnosis of DIC may be made if three or more coagulation parameters are abnormal; however, some clinicians prefer to reserve the diagnosis of DIC for horses with overt clinical signs of hemorrhage and thrombosis.[58] Prognostically, decreased ATIII concentration has been reported to reflect most closely the risk of death in mature horses with colic.[57] In addition, persistent abnormalities or worsening of coagulation parameters on repeated evaluation probably should be regarded as a negative prognostic indicator.

PATHOLOGIC FINDINGS

Postmortem findings typically reflect the underlying disease causing endotoxemia. Findings attributable to endotoxemia include evidence of coagulopathy (widespread petechial or ecchymotic hemorrhages and thrombi or microthrombi), shock, and multiorgan failure.

THERAPY

Given the complexity of the inflammatory cascade, the presence of feedback loops among types of inflammatory mediators, and the redundancy in the effects of many mediators, it is unlikely that interruption of the inflammatory process at one site will suffice to treat endotoxemia. A common approach is therefore to address multiple aspects of inflammation, which may include cell activation by LPS, mediator production, and mediator effects. Additional major objectives in the management of endotoxemic horses are treatment of the underlying disease process, thereby reducing the amount of endotoxin available for interaction with inflammatory cells, and general supportive care.

Lipopolysaccharide Scavengers

In the early stages of endotoxemia, removal of endotoxin from the circulation may be achieved by antiendotoxin antibodies or endotoxin-binding drugs such as polymyxin B. Antibodies that bind LPS are thought to provide steric blockade against lipid A interaction with inflammatory cells and to increase LPS and bacterial clearance by opsonization and complement activation.[80-82] A vaccine for protection against endotoxemia in horses is commercially available (Endovac-Equi, Immvac, Columbia, Missouri). Experimentally, vaccination with bacterin-toxoid vaccines prepared from "rough" mutants of *Salmonella typhimurium* and *S. enteritidis* provided protection against homologous and heterologous endotoxin challenge and carbohydrate overload.[83,84]

Despite these encouraging results, most research and clinical application have focused on passive immunization with plasma or serum products obtained from hyperimmunized horses. Antibodies against endotoxin are generally raised against the core region of LPS to ensure cross-reactivity among LPS from different sources. To expose the core region, mutant bacterial strains producing LPS with a reduced or absent O-chain, so-called rough LPS, are used. Mechanisms proposed to allow protection by anti–core LPS antibodies against smooth LPS present in natural infections include serum enzymatic factors that allow unmasking of shared antigenic sites, incomplete LPS assembly during infection, and partial disruption of bacterial cells by other host defense mechanisms and by antimicrobial treatment.[85] Lack of efficacy of antibody preparations in some studies, however, has prompted suggestions that mere transfer of passive immunity is insufficient for protection against endotoxemia, and that additional mechanisms, possibly related to cell-mediated immunity, might be required.[85]

Studies evaluating the efficacy of anti-LPS antibodies in horses have yielded conflicting results. Several authors have reported protective effects in experimental endotoxemia, clinical endotoxemia, clinical cases of enterocolitis and peritonitis, and prophylactically in foals and surgical colic patients.[86-88] Conversely, other studies failed to show beneficial effects of an *Escherichia coli* O111:B4 (J5) antiserum in an experimental endotoxemia model[89] or equine plasma containing antibodies raised against "rough" *E. coli* O111:B4 (J5) and *Salmonella minnesota* Re595 cells in a clinical study of endotoxemic foals.[85] Possible explanations for treatment failures, as provided by the authors, included failure of antigen to stimulate production of cross-protective antibodies, lack of adequate antibody production by inoculated donor horses, production of antibodies against nonprotective antigenic determinants, administration of an insufficient amount of antibody to recipients, insufficient patient numbers to show a small but significant treatment effect, and inadequate inclusion criteria of treated patients in clinical studies. Lack of a statistically significant difference between antibody-containing plasma and "nonimmune" plasma in the foal study may have been caused by a partial effect of low concentrations of antibody contained in the nonimmune plasma.[85] However, significant difference between hyperimmune and "preimmune" plasma was demonstrated in another clinical study of adult horses with endotoxemia caused by intestinal insults.[87] One experimental study in foals reported adverse effects of a *S. typhimurium* antiserum in the form of increased respiratory rates and increased serum activities of IL-6 and TNF-α after endotoxin challenge; this observation may have been attributable to a priming effect of minimal LPS contamination of the serum, as identified by the LAL assay.[90]

Currently available anti-LPS antibody products for use in horses include hyperimmune plasma obtained from horses vaccinated with a rough strain (J5) of *E. coli* (Polymune-J, Veterinary Dynamics, Templeton, California) and serum containing antibodies against a rough *Salmonella typhimurium* strain (Endoserum, Immvac). Manufacturer recommendations suggest use of Endoserum at a dose of 1.5 mL/kg body weight; for plasma, administration of at least 1 to 2 L to an average-size horse (450 kg) is proposed. Hyperimmune plasma without specific antiendotoxin antibodies is further available from several sources (Hi-Gamm Equi, Lake Immunogenics, Ontario, New York; Polymune and Polymune-Plus, Veterinary Dynamics) and may aid in treatment of endotoxemia, especially if coagulopathy is present, by providing complement components, fibronectin, clotting factors, and ATIII.

Polymyxin B is a polycationic antibiotic that is able to bind and neutralize endotoxin by interaction with the anionic phosphate substitutions of the lipid A backbone. As opposed to anti-LPS antibodies, polymyxin B binds endotoxin molecules based on their charge, such that antigenic differences among bacterial strains have less impact on the efficacy of this drug. Assuming that the underlying cause of endotoxemia can be corrected, the benefit of administering polymyxin B is likely limited to the first 24 to 48 hours of treatment, and prolonged use is not expected to provide additional advantages.[91]

Polymyxin B at doses of 1000 and 10,000 units per kg body weight (U/kg) was able to significantly reduce ex vivo TNF-α production for 3 to 6 and 12 to 24 hours, respectively, although a demonstrable effect on endotoxin binding was only observed for the higher dose.[92] In horses with experimentally induced endotoxemia, pretreatment with polymyxin B at a dose of 6000 U/kg was effective in suppressing cytokine production and clinical signs of endotoxemia.[90] In another endotoxin infusion experiment, pretreatment with polymyxin B (1000 and 5000 U/kg) as well as treatment 1 hour after the start of LPS infusion (5000 U/kg) also significantly reduced clinical signs of endotoxemia, leukopenia, and plasma TNF-α activity.[93] The dose-dependent effect observed in these studies is likely attributable to the 1:1 binding stoichiometry of polymyxin B to LPS molecules; therefore, individual clinicians may choose to vary the dose of polymyxin B depending on the perceived severity of disease.

Current recommendations suggest intravenous (IV) administration of polymyxin B at 1000 to 6000 U/kg every 8 to 12 hours.[91] Although some clinicians prefer to administer polymyxin B diluted in fluids, administration of the full dose as a slow bolus has not been reported to carry a significant risk of side effects. Because of its nephrotoxic and neurotoxic properties, caution is advised when administering polymyxin B to dehydrated, hypovolemic, or azotemic patients. Careful evaluation of the risks and benefits of using polymyxin B and adequate concurrent fluid therapy are recommended.[91] Reduced toxicity of polymyxin B may be achieved if the drug is administered as a conjugate with Dextran-70;[94] however, this product has not been fully evaluated for use in horses. The cited experimental studies have reported no adverse effects from a single bolus dose of polymyxin B, however, one study in healthy ponies reported neurologic signs (ataxia, hypermetria, apnea, head shaking) after administration of 18,000 to 36,000 U/kg every 6 hours for a total of 48 hours.[95] In human patients, increased toxicity has been reported when polymyxin B was used concurrently with aminoglycoside antibiotics or was given soon after anesthesia.[96]

Reduction of Endotoxin Release

An obvious necessity for the treatment of endotoxemia is correction of the underlying cause and thereby reduction of the amount of endotoxin available for inflammatory cell interaction. If gram-negative bacterial infection is suspected as the inciting cause, the site of infection, as well as the identity and antimicrobial susceptibility pattern of the offending organism, should be identified by clinical examination and adjunctive tests as deemed necessary. To this end, diagnostic tests may include thoracic or abdominal radiography and ultrasonography, abdominocentesis or pleurocentesis, repeated blood culture, fecal cultures for *Salmonella*, urinalysis, and urine culture. Blood culture is especially important in neonatal foals with suspected sepsis; the umbilicus (external and internal structures) and joints should further be given special consideration as potential septic foci in foals.

Therapeutically, removal of infected tissues or fluids may be helpful; in addition, appropriate antimicrobial therapy is warranted. Because endotoxin is released from the bacterial cell wall on bacterial death,[97] some suggest combining antimicrobial therapy with endotoxin-binding drugs (see earlier) during the initial treatment phase. Information derived from in vitro studies suggests that the magnitude of endotoxin release may depend on the type and dose of the antimicrobial drug.[8] Endotoxin release was inversely related to antimicrobial drug concentration, which suggests that adequate dosing based on the patient's body weight is imperative. Although endotoxin is only present in gram-negative bacteria, broad-spectrum antimicrobial treatment is frequently indicated before obtaining culture and sensitivity (C&S) results; further, gram-positive bacterial products also have the capacity to induce SIRS.

For horses in which endotoxemia results from translocation of LPS from the intestinal lumen, every effort should be made early to identify whether intestinal compromise warrants surgical exploration (e.g., strangulation obstruction) or demands medical therapy (e.g., acute colitis). In the absence of a definitive diagnosis, exploratory laparotomy is indicated in patients showing persistent abdominal pain and deterioration of cardiovascular parameters, including heart rate, pulse pressure, mucous membrane color, and capillary refill time. Resection of compromised bowel serves to limit further endotoxin translocation; however, clinical impression suggests that translocation may be transiently increased after correction of strangulating lesions and restoration of blood flow. Administration of LPS scavengers such as polymyxin B before intestinal manipulation may therefore be useful.[91]

Relatively little research has been devoted to the medical control of endotoxin translocation. In patients with primary intestinal disease, systemically administered antiinflammatory drugs, such as flunixin meglumine or dimethyl sulfoxide, may decrease intestinal inflammation and aid reestablishment of mucosal barrier function. Prokinetics such as lidocaine promote intestinal motility and may decrease contact time of endotoxin with the compromised mucosa; lidocaine also possesses antiinflammatory and analgesic properties and may inhibit cytokine production and hemodynamic changes in response to endotoxin.[98] A common regimen for lidocaine administration dictates infusion of an initial bolus (1.3 mg/kg) followed by a constant-rate infusion at 0.05 mg/kg/min. Topical medications such as bismuth subsalicylate have a coating effect and possess antiinflammatory properties; however, it is questionable whether these compounds maintain their medicinal activity by the time they reach the small intestine and especially the large intestine.

Other treatments aimed at reestablishing normal mucosal barrier function include the use of misoprostol in cases of nonsteroidal antiinflammatory drug (NSAID)–induced GI ulceration and right dorsal colitis. *Misoprostol* is a synthetic PGE_1 analog[99] and may speed intestinal healing by improving intestinal blood flow. Misoprostol decreased basal acid secretion in horses;[100] however, its effectiveness in treating colonic disease has not been evaluated. Important side effects of misoprostol, including colic, diarrhea, and abortion in pregnant mares, need to be taken into account before administration.

Experimentally, glutamine and acetylcysteine have shown promise in reestablishing intestinal mucosal integrity[101,102] and may therefore be able to reduce endotoxin translocation from the intestinal tract.

Nonsteroidal Antiinflammatory Drugs

Interference with the production and effects of inflammatory mediators probably represents the mainstay of treatment of endotoxemia in equine medicine. NSAIDs are used frequently in the treatment of colic as well as for septic and inflammatory conditions, with the goals of suppressing prostanoid production, reducing fever and inflammation, and relieving pain. Additional beneficial effects—which only maybe achieved, however, at doses high enough to increase the risk of side effects—include iron chelation and scavenging of oxygen-derived free radicals.[103] All NSAIDs exert their effects by inhibiting *cyclooxygenase* (COX) and reducing eicosanoid production, and beneficial effects in endotoxemia have been demonstrated for NSAIDs often used in horses, including phenylbutazone[104] and ketoprofen,[105] and for eltenac.[106]

Flunixin meglumine, however, remains the most frequently used NSAID for treatment of endotoxemia in horses. Numerous studies evaluating the effects of flunixin meglumine have found that it improves clinical signs, reduces cytokine release, improves blood pressure and maintains tissue perfusion, prevents hypoxemia and lactic acidosis, reduces endothelial damage, reduces the risk of pregnancy loss in mares, and increases survival in experimental endotoxemia.[78,104,107-112] A dose-dependent effect of flunixin meglumine on eicosanoid production has been demonstrated, and a reduced dose of the drug (0.25 mg/kg every 8 hours) decreased cytokine and lactate production in experimental endotoxemia.[113,114] Clinical studies comparing the two dosing regimens have not been performed; however, a survey among internists and surgeons with an equine emphasis showed that low-dose administration of flunixin meglumine is used widely.[115] Until further studies are performed, choice of the "full" dose (1.1 mg/kg once or twice daily) or a reduced dose may depend on the individual case and clinician preference. With regard to adverse side effects, including GI ulceration and renal papillary necrosis, flunixin meglumine has been shown to range between phenylbutazone and ketoprofen, although doses higher than those generally used in clinical cases were evaluated.[116]

Corticosteroids

The rationale for using corticosteroids in the management of shock, including septic shock, has been based on their global antiinflammatory action involving multiple pathways and cell types and their ability to maintain homeostasis and organ function. Clinical studies on the use of corticosteroids at antiinflammatory "high" doses (>30 mg/kg of methylprednisolone or 2-4 mg/kg of dexamethasone daily) in human patients, however, failed to show significant survival benefit in most patients with sepsis and septic shock.[117] More recently, relative adrenal insufficiency and peripheral corticosteroid resistance have been identified in septic human patients, resulting in recommendations to use "low-dose" corticosteroids (e.g., 200-300 mg hydrocortisone daily) in the treatment of septic shock.[117] In addition to replacement therapy, low doses of corticosteroids in human patients with septic shock promote shock reversal and reduce shock mortality.

A limited number of studies have evaluated corticosteroid use in equine endotoxemia. In horses with experimentally induced endotoxemia, dexamethasone (2 mg/kg) and prednisolone (10 mg/kg) were less effective than flunixin meglumine in reducing cytokine production, hemoconcentration, and hemodynamic changes.[107,118] Dexamethasone did inhibit TNF-α production by LPS-stimulated equine peritoneal macrophages in vitro; however, the required concentration was much higher than that achieved by currently recommended doses.[119] Dysfunction of the hypothalamic-pituitary-adrenal axis has not been evaluated in endotoxemic horses. Therefore, based on the currently available information, corticosteroid treatment cannot be recommended for use in endotoxemic equine patients. An additional caveat is the suggested association between corticosteroid use and development of laminitis.

Antioxidants

The most commonly used antioxidant in horses is *dimethyl sulfoxide* (DMSO), and surveys show that it is frequently used in the treatment of endotoxemia.[115] Antioxidants may reduce tissue damage by scavenging reactive oxygen radicals that are released from activated neutrophils and other cell types. In horses with colic, antioxidants have further been suggested for treatment of reperfusion injury after periods of bowel ischemia. However, experimental studies have failed to show beneficial effects of DMSO treatment,[120-122] and the role of oxidative processes in the development of ischemia and reperfusion injury in the equine colon has been questioned.[123] Because mucosal loss was increased when large-colon ischemia and reperfusion were treated with a higher dose (1 g/kg) of DMSO,[122] a lower dose (0.1 g/kg) has been proposed and is used by many clinicians. DMSO is typically administered intravenously as a 10% solution in fluids, however, administration by nasogastric tube as a 10% to 20% solution is also possible.

Allopurinol exerts antioxidant effects by inhibiting xanthine oxidase, an enzyme produced from xanthine dehydrogenase during periods of ischemia, which catalyzes formation of superoxide radicals on reperfusion.[124] Experimentally, allopurinol afforded protection against endotoxin challenge in horses,[125] although a protective effect against reperfusion injury was not observed.[121]

Other Mediator-Directed Therapies

Several studies have addressed the approach of selectively suppressing the production or biologic effects of specific inflammatory mediators. Experimentally in horses, beneficial effects have been demonstrated for PAF receptor antagonists,[126] inhibitors of TNF-α production, and antibodies directed against TNF-α.[41] Despite its ability to inhibit TNF-α activity in vitro, however, a polyclonal anti–TNF-α antibody was unable to improve clinical and hematologic parameters when given shortly after an in vivo endotoxin infusion.[12] Clinical studies on the use of these drugs in equine patients are lacking; clinical studies in septic human patients have led to the conclusion that targeted mediator suppression does not offer an overall survival benefit.[72]

Pentoxifylline is a methylxanthine derivative and phosphodiesterase inhibitor that can alter neutrophil function and inhibit production of various cytokines, including TNF-α and IL-6, as well as interferons, thromboxane B_2 (TxB_2), and thromboplastin.[128] Experimentally in horses, pentoxifylline reduced the effect of endotoxin infusion on rectal temperature and respiratory rate at individual time points, but had no effect on cytokine production, heart rate, or blood pressure.[129] Added benefit may be achieved by combining pentoxifylline with flunixin meglumine.[130] Current dosage recommendation for pentoxifylline in horses is 8 mg/kg orally every 8 hours. Because of its rheologic properties, that is, its ability to increase red blood cell deformability and improve microvascular blood flow, pentoxifylline may further be useful for the treatment of horses with or at risk for laminitis.

Supportive Care

Supportive care is a crucial aspect of the management of endotoxemic and septic patients. Important considerations include hydration, maintenance of electrolyte and acid-base homeostasis, pain control, and nutrition.

General principles of fluid therapy apply; rapid resuscitation may be necessary in patients presenting in septic or endotoxic shock. For resuscitation, large volumes (10-20 mL/kg/hr) of isotonic solutions (e.g., lactated Ringer's solution) or hypertonic saline (7.5% sodium chloride) at a dose of 4 mL/kg may be used. Hypertonic saline administration transiently increases plasma osmolality and results in fluid shifting from the interstitial space into the vasculature, thereby restoring circulating volume. Hypertonic saline should be administered intravenously as a rapid bolus over several (10-15) minutes and must be followed with crystalloid solutions to restore total body fluid volume. In horses administered endotoxin experimentally, treatment with hypertonic saline increased cardiac output and decreased total peripheral resistance and was superior to administration of an equal volume of normal saline.[131] Because of the possible risk of hypernatremia and hyperchloremia, serum electrolyte concentrations should be monitored in horses given hypertonic saline, especially if renal excretion may be compromised. Heart rate, pulse quality, mucous membrane color, and capillary refill time can be used to monitor patient response to fluid therapy; measurement of blood pressure is indicated in shock patients but is often not practical. Failure of dehydrated horses to urinate once fluid volume has been restored should prompt careful evaluation of renal function.

Hypoproteinemia and *hypoalbuminemia* are frequent concerns in patients with significant intestinal inflammation, but also in horses with effusive pleuritis and peritonitis, as well as in patients with acute renal failure. In addition to gross protein losses, endotoxin-induced vascular endothelial damage may result in leakage of fluid and protein into the interstitium, leading to tissue edema formation and contributing to organ dysfunction and fluid losses. After initial resuscitation, fluid therapy should therefore be tailored to the individual patient, and administration of plasma and synthetic colloids should be considered. Colloids help to maintain plasma colloid osmotic pressure and reduce edema formation; as discussed earlier, plasma may have the additional benefit of providing antiendotoxin antibodies and coagulation factors. Administration of plasma to maintain serum total protein concentration above 4.2 g/dL has been suggested;[132] however, large volumes of plasma required to achieve this goal may sometimes be unavailable or prohibitively expensive.

Of the synthetic colloids, *hetastarch* (hydroxyethyl starch) is most often used in horses and is commercially available as a 6% solution in 0.9% sodium chloride (Hespan, Hextend). In hypoproteinemic horses given hetastarch at a dose of 8 to 10 mL/kg, a significant colloid oncotic effect was maintained for 24 hours.[133] Hetastarch should be administered at 5 to 15 mL/kg by slow IV infusion and should be accompanied by an equal or greater volume of isotonic crystalloid fluids.[134,135] Possible adverse effects of hetastarch treatment include the development of coagulopathies, and its use in horses with established coagulation parameter abnormalities should be preceded by careful evaluation of the risks and benefits. In one study in horses, effects of hetastarch on coagulation parameters were evident at higher doses (20 mL/kg) and appeared to be caused by a decrease in von Willebrand factor:Ag activity,[136] whereas another study did not report the occurrence of bleeding abnormalities.[137] In human patients, hetastarch use has been associated with prolonged aPTT, decreased factor VIII activity, and decreased serum fibrinogen concentration.[138]

Inotropic and vasopressor support should be considered in patients with evidence of inadequate tissue perfusion after restoration of circulatory fluid volume. For human patients with septic shock, current recommendations include the use of norepinephrine or dopamine as the vasopressors of choice and dobutamine to increase cardiac output.[139] Norepinephrine has been evaluated in hypotensive critically ill foals and was found to increase mean arterial pressure and urine output at a dose of up to 1.5 µg/kg/min concurrently with dobutamine.[140] Doses for dobutamine of 1 to 2 (up to 5) µg/kg/min as a continuous infusion are recommended for use in horses.[141] Monitoring parameters for horses or foals treated with vasopressors and inotropes should include heart rate and rhythm as well as blood pressure.

Coagulopathies

Successful management of the underlying disease process is likely the most appropriate way to prevent and treat coagulopathies. In the horse with severe endotoxemia or sepsis, however, treatments specifically directed at interruption of coagulation and fibrinolytic cascades may be useful. Because most coagulopathies in septic or endotoxemic patients are subclinical, management and monitoring must be based on the evaluation of coagulation parameters (see Diagnosis). Abnormalities may indicate a predominantly procoagulant state or increased fibrinolytic activity, although mixed abnormalities reflecting activation of both coagulation and fibrinolysis may also be present. In many cases, therefore, treatment will include anticoagulants as well as clotting factor replacement strategies.

Common anticoagulants for use in horses include heparin and aspirin. The effects of *heparin* depend on adequate concentration of ATIII and include inhibition of thrombin; facilitation of ATIII-mediated inhibition of clotting factors IX, X, XI, and XII; release of tissue-factor pathway inhibitor; and inhibition of platelet activation.[142,143] Because of the need for adequate ATIII concentrations, administration of heparin in plasma may be useful, especially if endogenous ATIII concentration is low. One study evaluating DIC in horses with colic found no significant survival benefit if horses were treated with heparin alone;[75] however, patient numbers in this study were relatively small. The recommended dosing regimen for heparin includes an initial administration of 80 to 100 U/kg, followed by 40 to 80 U/kg three times daily or a continuous infusion of 5-25 U/kg/hr.[132,143] Horses treated with heparin should be monitored for increased bleeding tendency; in addition, heparin may result in thrombocytopenia and anemia from erythrocyte agglutination. Use of low-molecular-weight heparin to avoid these complications has been recommended;[144] suggested doses for horses are 50-100 U/kg subcutaneously for dalteparin and 40-80 U/kg subcutaneously for enoxaparin.[143,145] At a dose of 50 U/kg once daily in colic patients, dalteparin elicited fewer side effects than unfractionated heparin, which was associated with jugular vein changes, transiently decreased hematocrit, and prolonged clotting times.[146]

Aspirin (acetylsalicylic acid) irreversibly inhibits COX activity in platelets, thereby preventing platelet aggregation and reducing the occurrence of microthrombosis. The currently recommended dose is 10 to 30 mg/kg orally every 48 hours. Increased bioavailability after rectal administration has been reported recently, and lower doses may be adequate if the drug is administered by this route.[147] An oral dose of 300 mg acetylsalicylic acid in healthy horses[148] resulted in prolonged bleeding time and reduced blood viscosity. However, the benefit of aspirin treatment in endotoxemic horses has been questioned after findings that aspirin did not inhibit endotoxin-induced platelet aggregation in vitro.[63,64] These studies suggested that PAF rather than TxA_2 is an important activator of platelet aggregation during endotoxemia.

Fresh-frozen plasma products can be used to replenish coagulation factors and ATIII; platelet-rich plasma may further be indicated in patients with thrombocytopenia. As an alternative to commercially available products, collection of platelet-rich plasma using platelet collection kits and two-speed centrifugation techniques has been suggested.[143] The volume of plasma administration depends on the severity of coagulation abnormalities; however, a minimum of 1 to 2 L should probably be administered to an adult horse.

Organ Dysfunction or Failure

Organ failure caused by severe inflammation, refractory cardiovascular compromise, and widespread endothelial dysfunction is the most dreaded sequela of endotoxemia and often results in treatment failure and ultimately euthanasia. In the human literature, as defined earlier, the term *multiple organ dysfunction syndrome* (MODS) was introduced to stress the continuum of organ dysfunction during sepsis and SIRS rather than focusing on its result, organ failure.[1] Acute renal failure and laminitis appear to be the most common complications of endotoxemia in horses; interestingly, however, the pathophysiologic role of endotoxin in the development of laminitis remains poorly understood. Because of the poor prognosis associated with laminitis and renal failure in horses, a proactive approach to these conditions is of utmost importance. The reader is referred to other sources for more detailed discussion of prevention and management.[149-151]

In addition to renal failure and laminitis, the potential for failure of any organ must be considered during the evaluation and treatment of endotoxemic patients. Abnormalities that may be detected during physical examination and routine clinicopathologic evaluation include respiratory compromise (dyspnea, coughing, abnormal lung sounds), cardiac compromise (tachycardia, murmurs, arrhythmias), GI dysfunction (ileus, colic, diarrhea), liver failure (icterus), and neurologic disease (severe depression, seizures). Although some of these signs may also be associated with the primary disease process, clinicians should be alert to the development of further endotoxemia-induced organ compromise. Prognostically, development of any of these complications, especially if the horse is unresponsive to appropriate therapy, must probably be regarded as an indicator of poor outcome.

Future Therapeutic Directions

Antagonists of endotoxin interaction with receptors on inflammatory cells are under investigation and may soon be available for use in human patients.[152,153] Because of findings that a natural endotoxin antagonist in human cells, LPS from *Rhodobacter sphaeroides*, acts as an agonist in equine cells and stimulates cytokine production in vitro as effectively as *E. coli* LPS,[154] use of these products in horses without further species-specific studies must be discouraged. Recognition of *R. sphaeroides* LPS in equine cells depended on the TLR4/MD-2 complex,[37] and additional research concerning the details of endotoxin-receptor interaction and cell stimulation may provide insights into the structural requirements for use of an endotoxin antagonist in horses.

Inhibitors of apoptosis have shown beneficial effects in experimental models of sepsis; specifically, inhibition of lymphocyte apoptosis, which may contribute to immunosuppression, and intestinal epithelial cell apoptosis, which may promote endotoxin and bacterial translocation, improved survival in animal models.[155,156] The observed increase in apoptosis of these two cell types during sepsis may be caused by an acceleration of physiologic processes[156] and may be mediated by cytokines such as TNF-α.[72] Interestingly, increased lymphocyte apoptosis was observed in septic as well as critically ill, nonseptic human patients, thereby suggesting that noninfectious mechanisms may be operative, and that apoptosis may be one mechanism by which critically ill patients are predisposed to sepsis.[156] In addition to a reduction of available immune cells, apoptosis may indirectly induce immune tolerance, because phagocytosis of apoptotic cells increased release of antiinflammatory cytokines while it suppressed production of proinflammatory mediators.[157,158] Conversely, necrotic cells had immunostimulatory effects. This immunomodulating effect of apoptotic and necrotic cells, respectively, may be mediated by interferon gamma (IFN-γ).[156]

PREVENTION

Prevention of endotoxemia has two aspects: prevention of the inciting cause (i.e., release of endotoxin into the circulation) and prevention of the uncontrolled activation of the inflammatory cascade. Early diagnosis and appropriate treatment of conditions known to be associated with endotoxemia are therefore of utmost importance.

To prevent the development of a systemic inflammatory response, patients at risk for endotoxemia must be identified early, and proactive treatment must be initiated before the development of clinical signs. For example, polymyxin B or plasma products aimed at scavenging LPS, as well as antiinflammatory medications aimed at reducing mediator release, may be useful in high-risk patients, such as colic patients undergoing surgery or horses with acute grain overload or retained placenta. However, the time window for successful prevention of cell activation and mediator release is likely very small, and many patients may not be presented for treatment until inflammatory reactions have progressed beyond the initial stages. In experimental studies, significant release of cytokines and inflammatory mediators has been demonstrated soon after administration of endotoxin. This fact alone probably explains why therapies directed against LPS itself or specific mediators so often appear promising in experimental trials of controlled endotoxemia, but fail to provide detectable benefit in the clinical scenario.

Omega-3 fatty acids (FAs) have been evaluated for their potential to alter composition of cell membrane phospholipids and alter production pathways of inflammatory mediators. Omega-3 FA incorporation into cell membranes reduces the availability of arachidonic acid (an omega-6 FA) for cleavage by COX and shifts eicosanoid production from the 2-series prostaglandins and 4-series leukotrienes to their 3- and 5-series equivalents.[159] These latter mediators have reduced biologic activity and therefore may reduce the severity of inflammatory responses. In addition, omega-3 FAs may be able to reduce LPS-induced cellular activation by preventing upregulation of CD14 on monocytes by endotoxin.[160] Experimentally, IV infusion of omega-3 FAs was able to alter cell composition of membrane phospholipids,[161] and endotoxin-induced expression of tissue factor, TxB_2, and TNF-α in vitro was reduced significantly in horses fed omega-3 FAs in the form of linseed oil for several weeks.[162,163] However, no significant clinical benefit was observed in horses on an omega-3 FA–rich diet when they were given endotoxin in vivo.[164]

As noted earlier, a vaccine directed against endotoxin is commercially available (Endovac-Equi, Immvac) but appears to be used mostly for vaccination of donor horses in the production of hyperimmune plasma. Stimulation of anti–lipid A antibody production using a murine monoclonal anti–idiotypic antibody that shares an epitope with lipid A in horses has further been demonstrated.[165] Benefits of vaccination against endotoxin have been demonstrated experimentally;[83,84] however, the potential protective effect against naturally occurring disease has not been evaluated.

REFERENCES

See the CD-ROM for a list of references linked to the abstract in PubMed.

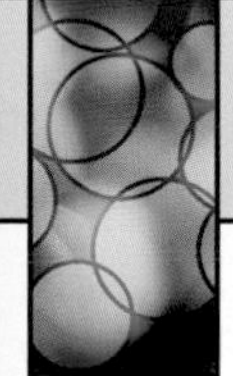

CHAPTER • 38

Salmonellosis

Josie L. Traub-Dargatz and Thomas E. Besser

ETIOLOGY

Salmonellosis is disease caused by an enteric or systemic infection with a bacterium of the genus *Salmonella*. This genus contains two species, *Salmonella enterica* and *Salmonella bongori*. To the authors' knowledge, *S. bongori* has never been reported as the cause of equine salmonellosis. *S. enterica* includes six subspecies with more than 2000 serovars.[1] All these species and subspecies are potentially pathogenic, but the virulence of many is undefined; the vast majority of clinical cases are associated with a single subspecies, *S. enterica* subsp. *enterica*. The National Veterinary Services Laboratory (NVSL) annually provides a valuable summary report of the frequency of clinical and nonclinical serovars by host species of origin; these data show that relatively few serovars of *S. enterica* subsp. *enterica* consistently account for a large percentage of clinical isolates.[2-6]

In horses the most frequently occurring serovars isolated from clinical cases vary somewhat from year to year, but *Salmonella* Typhimurium, Newport, Anatum, and Agona are consistently among the most frequent isolates from equine salmonellosis cases in the United States. The relative ranking of these common serovars undergoes periodic shifts as epidemic strains emerge

Table • 38-1

Frequently Occurring Equine Salmonellosis Serotypes: Number (Percent) of All Equine Serotypes

SEROVAR	2003-2004	2002-2003	2001-2002	2000-2001	1999-2000	1998-1999
Typhimurium	259 (31.4)	207 (21.8)	134 (17.7)	264 (25.8)	327 (37.5)	244 (44.0)
Newport	139 (16.8)	146 (15.4)	128 (16.9)	211 (20.6)	76 (8.7)	29 (5.2)
Agona	40 (4.8)	126 (13.3)	135 (17.8)	210 (20.5)	118 (13.5)	50 (9.0)
Anatum	24 (2.9)	83 (8.8)	46 (6.1)	32 (3.1)	50 (5.7)	55 (9.9)
All others	364 (44.1)	386 (40.7)	314 (41.5)	308 (30.1)	370 (42.4)	176 (31.7)
Total	826	948	757	1025	872	554

Data from U.S. Animal Health Association *Salmonella* Committee, National Veterinary Service Laboratories, 1998 to 2004.

and disappear. For example, in the mid 1990s, *Salmonella* Typhimurium was relatively predominant, reflecting the global epidemic of the pentaresistant Typhimurium strain DT104. During the past 5 years (as of 2006), however, *Salmonella* Newport has increased in relative frequency, with the emergence of the North American *cmy*-2 cephalosporinase-producing strains (Table 38-1).[2-6]

Certain different *Salmonella* serovars produce distinct clinical syndromes that result in their classification as "host adapted" or "non–host adapted." Serovars with strong host specificity and with clinical similarity to human *Salmonella typhi* infections are considered host adapted, whereas non–host-adapted serovars show minimal host specificity and a different clinical presentation. Host-adapted serovars produce systemic infections characterized by bacteremia, fever, and systemic signs. In host-adapted salmonellosis, diarrhea is not observed or, if present, is a relatively minor component.[7] The equine host-adapted serovar, *Salmonella* Abortus-equi, causes a disease with bacteremia and infectious abortion as its principal manifestations.[8] In contrast, non–host-adapted serovars typically produce localized infections of the intestine and colon with enterocolitis and diarrhea as the predominant components.[7] *Salmonella* Abortus-equi is common in many tropical countries but does not occur in the United States; there have been no reports since at least 1978 (K.E. Ferris, personal communication). Where *Salmonella* Abortus-equi is not present, the principal manifestation of equine salmonellosis (the United States at present) is enterocolitis. Nevertheless, even non–host-adapted serovars can produce septicemic disease (although generally accompanied by enterocolitis) in highly susceptible hosts such as neonates.

For some purposes, strain-specific identification of *Salmonella* isolates within serovars is useful to identify potential nosocomial and other common-source outbreak strains and to investigate the epidemiology of *Salmonella* infection. *Salmonella* strain typing can be accomplished by different methods, including phenotypic procedures such as phage typing and antimicrobial resistance typing.[9] *Phage typing* is a highly reproducible and discriminatory method, but this procedure is not widely available.[10] More recently, genetic typing with *pulsed-field gel electrophoresis* (PFGE) after chromosomal digestion with infrequent-cutting restriction endonucleases has been increasingly used as a means of identifying strain types of *Salmonella* infection.[11] Both phage typing and PFGE typing may be insufficiently discriminatory to identify subtypes within disseminated clonal types of *Salmonella* spp. For example, isolates of the epidemic type *Salmonella* Typhimurium DT (phage type) 104 obtained from widely distant sites around the world are frequently homogenous by these tests. Even more discriminatory tests, such as analysis of *variable-number tandem repeat* (VNTR) deoxyribonucleic acid (DNA) sequences, have proved useful to differentiate epidemiologically linked isolates of highly conserved strains such as DT104.[12]

EPIDEMIOLOGY

Source of Infection

The source of infection in individual horses and even in outbreaks of salmonellosis in groups of horses is often not definitively identified. Unless surveillance for infection is ongoing, the source of infection may be difficult to identify because it may no longer exist. For example, contaminated feed has been consumed, or there may be extensive environmental contamination and many infected animals, such that the incident case or original single source is no longer obvious even if an epidemiologic investigation is conducted.

The primary route of exposure is likely oral intake of the organism; thus there are multiple potential sources of infection for equids (Fig. 38-1). These include consumption of contaminated water or feed and oral contact with the feces of infected animals, with contaminated environmental surfaces, or with animal care worker's contaminated hands or equipment. It is unknown what percentage of *Salmonella* infections in equids are caused by these various potential sources. Aerosol exposure to the agent has been proposed in other animal species.[30,31] Although evidence of this route of exposure in horses is lacking, it theoretically could occur.

The most frequently reported outbreaks of equine salmonellosis have been among hospitalized patients. At least some of these outbreaks are associated with nosocomial spread of a given serotype of *Salmonella* spp. The source of the organism in these outbreaks is often not definitively determined. Multiple potential sources that culture positive for the agent, such as the equipment or hands of health care workers or environmental surfaces, are identified through outbreak investigations.[32,33] However, which of these potential sources play the major role in a specific nosocomial infection is not always determined, and a different source may be involved for various patients during an outbreak.

Clinically normal horses shedding *Salmonella* in their feces potentially pose a risk to animals with which they have direct contact and can contaminate the environment, which serves as a source of the organism to susceptible animals.[34] A larger

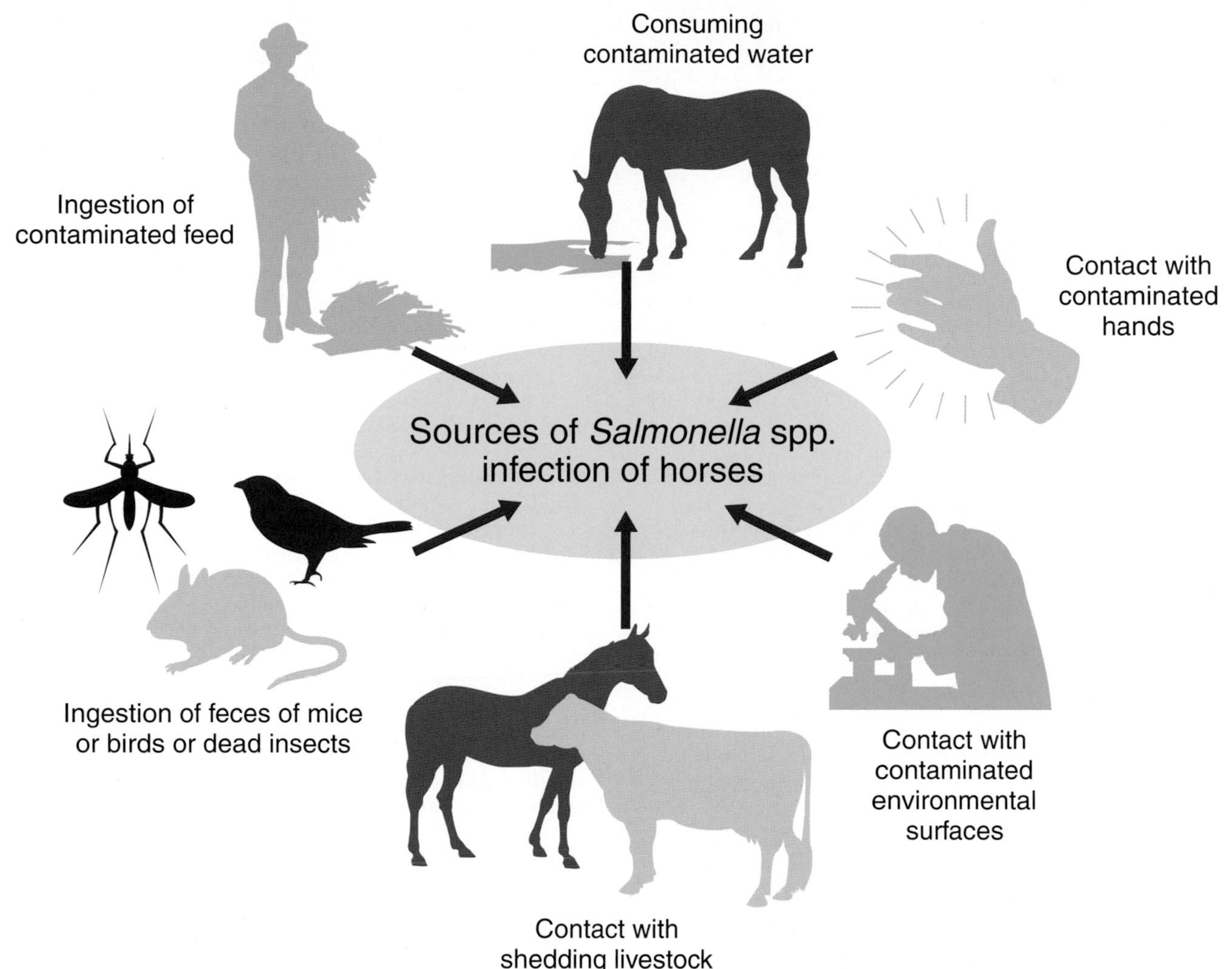

Fig. 38-1 Examples of the multiple potential sources for *Salmonella* exposure to equids.

percentage of horses appear to shed the organism in summer than in winter months.[35-37] Other livestock could also be a source of *Salmonella* for horses. Through surveillance of all large animal hospital patients, cattle (specifically dairy cattle) have been found to shed *Salmonella* spp., more than equids or other large animal patients.[38]

Salmonellae can persist in the environment in fecal matter for months to years depending on the serotype, moisture content, and temperature conditions.[39,40] In one study, *Salmonella* Dublin persisted in dried bovine feces for up to 5 years.[41] In another study, *Salmonella* Cholerasuis was more persistent when feces were in the dried (13 months) versus wet form (3 months).[39] In veterinary hospitals, where most outbreaks of equine salmonellosis have been described, environmental contamination with potential persistence of the organism may be a source of infection for susceptible animals, as are fomites and contaminated hands of hospital workers.

Feed is a potential source of *Salmonella* for horses. Most commercial equine feeds are manufactured using good manufacturing procedures (GMP), but none is certified to be *Salmonella* free. A National Animal Health Monitoring System (NAHMS) survey estimated that 0.4% of grain or concentrate that was the primary feed source for horses was positive for *Salmonella* spp., and that the serotypes detected were not those typically associated with clinical disease in horses.[37] Thus it would appear from this study that concentrate source is rarely positive for *Salmonella* spp., on most equine operations. However, contaminated feed given to broodmares who then shed the organism in their feces was implicated as a cause of an outbreak of salmonellosis among neonatal foals in California. The serotype implicated was *Salmonella* Ohio, and biochemical profiles, restriction endonuclease analysis, and ribotyping demonstrated that feed and poultry isolates, most of which were in geographic proximity to the broodmare farm, were indistinguishable from the outbreak isolates.[42] One report identified maize silage as containing *Salmonella* Typhimurium that resulted in fatal diarrhea and colic in horses to which it was fed.[43] Pelleting likely decreases the number of salmonellae in contaminated feed, depending on the temperature used in the processing procedure.[44]

Apparently, components of livestock feed could be contaminated with *Salmonella* spp. In September 1990 the Food and Drug Administration Center for Veterinary Medicine (FDA-CVM) announced a goal of having zero salmonella contamination of animal feed ingredients and finished feed. One step in the process toward this goal was for FDA to perform a monitoring program of animal feeds. FDA conducted a survey in 1993 of processors manufacturing either animal or vegetable protein products used in animal feeds to determine the prevalence of *Salmonella* spp.[45] The findings of the study represented 4530 individual samples. *Salmonella* was detected in 56.4% of animal protein samples and 36% of the vegetable protein products. In an FDA report, 34% of animal protein–derived feed samples were positive for salmonella in 2002 and represented 27 serotypes.[46] In a 2-year study of *Salmonella* Typhimurium DT 104 on cattle farms, feed and grain sources remained contaminated throughout the study.[47] An evaluation of inoculated swine feed and meal found a difference in survival of various salmonellae serotypes.[48] For example, *Salmonella* Anatum persisted for 429 days in ground feed and 299 days in meat and bone meal, *Salmonella* Infantis was present at 723 days in feed and at 588 days in meal, and *Salmonella* Enteritidis survived approximately the same amount of time in feed and meal (728 days in feed and 750 days in meal).[48] It was speculated that these non–host-adapted strains survived longer than host-adapted types evaluated, such as *Salmonella* Typhisuis and Cholerasuis.[48]

Equine feed sources such as grain or other concentrate sources also could become contaminated after processing once at the equine premises. Potential sources of contamination include the feces of rodents and birds or bodies of insects. Rodents have been proposed as a reservoir for *Salmonella* spp.,[44,49] and have been determined to carry the same strain as was involved in an equine salmonellosis outbreak.[32] Insects such as flies can become contaminated with *Salmonella* spp.[50] when they contact infected feces or surfaces and then carry *Salmonella* to susceptible animals, which may either ingest the insect when eating or the insect may come into contact with the horse's oral surfaces.

Pastures could become contaminated with *Salmonella* spp., if organic fertilizers or bone meal are used, if runoff occurs from surrounding animal holding facilities, or if contaminated water supply is used for irrigation or sprinkling. Feces passed by infected animals being housed on the pasture or from wildlife that may have access to the pasture (e.g., birds, wild mammals) could contaminate a pasture. Soils have been reported to remain positive for *Salmonella* spp., for a variable period from 120 to 280 days.[51] Also, hay sources could become contaminated by these same means and then, when harvested, could act as a source of *Salmonella* to susceptible horses.

The role that contaminated water sources play in equine salmonellosis is unknown. Surface water (e.g., creeks, irrigation ditches, ponds or lakes) could be contaminated with the organism. In a national study of equine health and management, 10% to 33% of equine operations used surface water as the primary water source for equids.[52] No testing of these water sources was performed as part of this study. *Salmonella* survives in pond water for 115 days.[51] This likely varies with the serotype of *Salmonella* and environmental temperature, as well as other characteristics of the water (e.g., pH, salinity). Freezing reduces the total number of organisms, but survivors may remain viable and infective for months.[51]

Many studies that have lead to the detection of *Salmonella* spp. in feed, water, and the environment have been based on a qualitative outcome (i.e., detected or not detected); thus the method of sample collection and method used to determine the presence of the organism likely affected the outcome. Whether all the previously cited potential sources of *Salmonella* contain an infective dose of the organism is often not known.

Prevalence

The wide range in the reported prevalence of salmonellosis in equids results from several factors, which must be considered when reviewing the literature. These include the population of equids being studied, the method used to detect the *Salmonella* isolate (direct culture, culture after enrichment, PCR test), the number of samples tested per animal, the season of the year as well as the region, and the varied definition of salmonellosis.

The definition of salmonellosis includes infection with the organism as well as the occurrence of detectable disease signs secondary to infection,[53] although some reports on equine salmonellosis also include animals shedding the organism without signs of disease.[34,35] This is likely in part a result of the transition from early investigations focusing only on animals with clinical disease to the current interest in surveillance of the general population or overall hospital population for shedding of the organism. Therefore, all these factors need to be considered when describing *Salmonella* infection or shedding by equids. It has been proposed that three types of salmonella-infected horses may exist: carrier without fecal shedding, carrier with fecal shedding, and shedder with clinical disease.[35] Also, there could be a "pass-through phenomenon" in which the horse is not infected (carrier) but instead ingests the organism and passes it through the gastrointestinal (GI) tract without any recognition of the agent's presence (no serologic or local GI response to the organism).

In describing prevalence, the first distinction to make is whether the prevalence being reported is for a population of ill equids, the entire equine hospital population, or the general equine population on their home premises. If one assumes that salmonellosis equates to some clinical disease associated with the infection, it is thus distinct from the prevalence of equids shedding the organism in their feces. Therefore the horses with clinical disease or salmonellosis would be a subset of the total number of horses that shed the organism in their feces.

The prevalence of clinical salmonellosis in the general equine population is unknown. During outbreaks of salmonellosis on a given farm or in a given veterinary hospital, the attack rate is variable, and there are few reports of the actual prevalence of clinical cases; instead, the number of cases is reported, but the number of animals at risk is usually not provided. In the hospital setting this may be the case because by the time the outbreak is recognized, the number of patients or patient days at risk is not available retrospectively. The prevalence of *Salmonella* infection as a cause of disease among horses with diarrhea has been evaluated in a Dutch study.[54] During 1990 and 1991, 380 fecal samples were collected from horses that were referred for treatment of diarrhea. Most horses had a single fecal sample collected from the rectum, or if they died soon after arrival, samples were collected at necropsy. Of these samples, 18% (69/380) were positive for *Salmonella* spp. The most common serotype identified was *Salmonella* Typhimurium (43/69). Other serotypes identified less frequently included *Salmonella* Hadar (3/69), Arizona (2), Enteritidis (2), Virchow (1), Blockley (1), and Bareilly (1).

It is also important to distinguish whether the method used to determine the animal's shedding status is direct plating, plating on several different agars after an enrichment process, or a polymerase chain reaction (PCR) test. Generally, the likelihood of detection of the organism would increase from direct plating to enrichment with subsequent plating and then PCR testing. The population tested will impact the prevalence of shedding reported (e.g., hospitalized equids with enteric disease versus the general equine population).

The prevalence of fecal shedding in a national study of the general horse population sampled while on their home premises, based on a single sample per animal, was 0.8%. The prevalence of fecal shedding by horses in this study was higher in the summer months (1.1%) than in the winter months (0.2%) and in the southern region (1.4%) than in the northern region (0.2%) of the United States.[37] A total of 16 different serotypes were identified, with the most common serotype being Muenchen, followed by Newport, Schwartzengrund, and Typhimurium.

One of the first studies of the prevalence of fecal shedding among the general hospitalized equine population was conducted as a surveillance program at a university teaching hospital in the late 1970s. A total of 1451 horses were sampled, with a reported 3.2% prevalence of fecal shedding of *Salmonella*.[35] The serotypes identified included Typhimurium, Typhimurium var Copenhagan, Infantis, Montevideo, Meleagridis, and Drypool, as well as untypeable isolates. Seasonal variability was marked in detection of fecal shedding, with the highest incidence in the late summer and early fall and the lowest in the spring. Of the 46 horses shedding *Salmonella* in this study, 18 had diarrhea, and seven deaths were attributed to salmonellosis. Since this early report, many more reports on the prevalence of shedding *Salmonella* by hospitalized equids have been published. In a study of the general equine hospitalized population (anticipated hospital stay ≥3 days, 246 horses), the prevalence of fecal shedding was 7%, with serotypes identified including Oranienberg, Newport, and Arizona, in descending order of frequency, followed by Newington, Drypool, Anatum, Thompson, and Meleagridis, each represented by single isolates.[55] Only 3 of the 18 culture-positive horses in this study were admitted for diarrhea.

Some reports on the prevalence of fecal shedding of *Salmonella* spp., were based on a subset of the hospital population, for example, patients admitted for colic or needing intensive care. The prevalence of fecal shedding among colic patients (246 horses, with an average of three samples per horse) at a veterinary teaching hospital was 9%.[56] The serotypes were Typhimurium, Infantis, Muenchin, and Anatum, in descending order of frequency, followed by a similar number with Oranienburg, Montevideo, and Thompson, all with the same frequency. In a second study of colic patients (based on culture of feces or rectal swab samples) the prevalence was 13% (100 horses, with an attempt to collect five samples per horse, unless it died before day 5), and the most common serotype identified was Senftenberg, followed by Typhimurium, then London and Agona.[57] Senftenberg was also the most frequently isolated serotype from horses "without colic" in this report. In a survey of equids admitted to a veterinary teaching hospital intensive care unit over a 4-year period (1583 horses, with daily collection of fecal samples for culture), the overall prevalence of shedding was 5.5%, and the most common serotypes identified were Typhimurium and Krefeld; other types identified included Anatum, Agona, Enteriditis, Heidelberg, Muenster, Newington, Oranienberg, Poona, and Tennessee.[58]

The prevalence of carrier horses that are not shedding the organism in their feces as detectable by culture is difficult to determine. There are few studies of long-term, repeated fecal culture and sampling of mesenteric lymph nodes and other sites that *Salmonella* spp. may reside. In one study of 85 equids undergoing necropsy for various causes other than salmonellosis in England, 20% had *Salmonella* spp. isolated from one or more sites, with the mucosa of the cecum and large colon being the most common sites harboring the organism. No details on culture method or sampling method were included in this report.[59] A culture survey at one equine slaughter plant showed a 70% prevalence of carrier horses.[60] In a second slaughter plant study the prevalence of isolation was 27%.[61]

In a study of 102 horses that underwent necropsy between April and December 1994 at a veterinary teaching hospital, only two foals had *Salmonella* spp., recovered from the mesenteric lymph nodes.[62] These authors concluded that the results of cross-sectional studies using culture to determine *Salmonella* infection should be interpreted with caution because the results of prevalence from a single facility may not reflect the prevalence of infection in the general population. In one of the slaughter plant surveys the authors speculated that the horses were becoming infected while at the slaughter plant because the serotype of *Salmonella* identified was similar to that obtained from birds sampled from corrals where the horses were housed before slaughter.[63]

The prevalence of fecal shedding by horses as determined by a PCR test can be quite different from prevalence determined by culture. It is important to recognize that PCR results vary depending on which primers are used,[64] so when describing the prevalence of shedding of *Salmonella* by horses, it is important to distinguish if prevalence for shedding was detected by bacterial culture or by PCR test as well as what primers were used in the PCR test. For example, 71 of 110 horses tested positive using a PCR test with the *hisJ* gene on feces, whereas only 11 of these same horses were positive based on fecal culture.[65] From this example, therefore, the prevalence of fecal shedding based on PCR would obviously be much higher than that based on culture of fecal samples. At this time, most prevalence data reported for shedding are based on culture rather than PCR results.

The prevalence of serotypes identified among *Salmonella* isolates of equine origin is reported annually at the U.S. Animal Health Association *Salmonella* Committee meeting by the NVSL staff[2-6] (see Etiology for annual statistics).

Risk Factors

The ability to infect horses with *Salmonella* and the subsequent development of clinical disease depend on multiple factors (Fig. 38-2). Age may be a risk factor for development of clinical illness, with foals more likely to develop disease than adults.[79,80] Stress may be a predisposing factor for initiating equine salmonellosis, and horses may be carriers of *Salmonella* and may not shed the organism in their feces until stressed.[35] Stress is difficult to define, and what may predispose one animal to disease if infected may not predispose the next. Various factors have been associated with increased prevalence of salmonellosis or the shedding of the organism in feces by equine populations, including transportation or shipping,[14,56,81,82] surgery,[14,83] feed withdrawal,[14] change in feed,[55] antimicrobial treatment,[57,84-86] deworming,[87] colic,[57] and diarrhea.[56] Some of these factors may be an outcome of the infection rather than predisposing factors, such as the association with diarrhea.

One of the first reports of salmonellosis in hospitalized horses was in 1969.[83] Since that time, most outbreaks of equine salmonellosis occurred at veterinary teaching hospitals.[32,33,54,88-91] The development of large equine veterinary hospitals in the twentieth century brought major advances in the health care available for equids, but also the congregation of horses with different levels of susceptibility to infectious disease agents and the likelihood for exposure to these agents.[74] Hospitalized horses may be subjected to one or more of the factors associated with salmonellosis, including transportation to the hospital, altered diet, feed withdrawal before anesthesia, surgery, and treatment with antimicrobials.[92] In addition to these stresses, hospitalized horses are often from multiple sources, and thus without existing biocontainment protocols, pathogens could be shared between animals from different sources. The occurrence of salmonellosis was a major driving

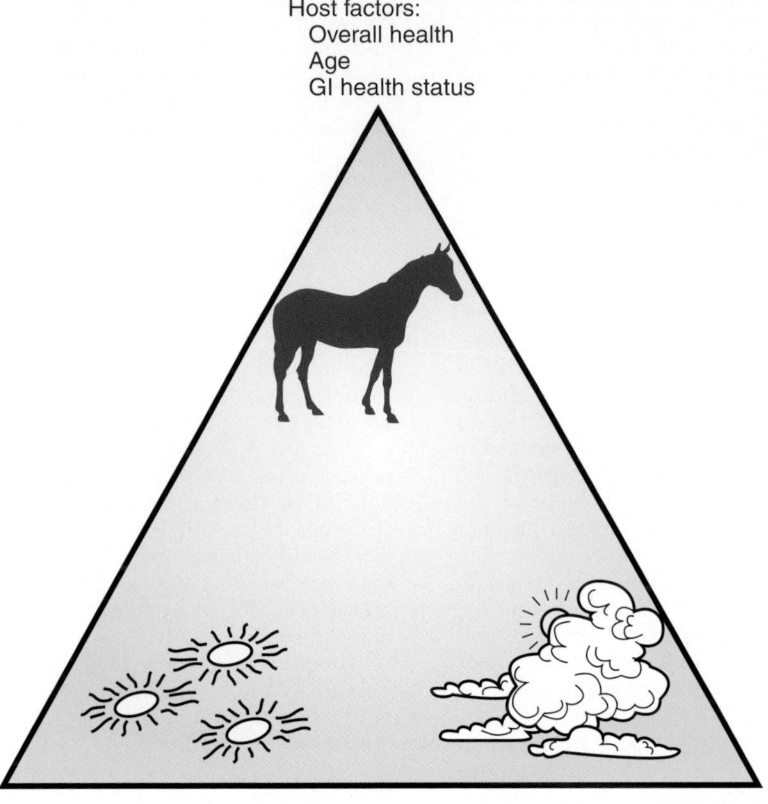

Fig. 38-2 Triad of disease factors resulting in *Salmonella* infection. Disease results when multiple risk factors come together, including those associated with the *host* (e.g., age, antimicrobial treatment), the *agent* (e.g., virulence, infective dose), and the *environment* (e.g., heat stress).

force in the recognition of the need for infectious disease control programs in equine hospitals.[74]

Normal intestinal flora and motility likely make horses more resistant to colonization with *Salmonella* spp.[93] Challenge studies that vary the doses of *Salmonella* organisms in horses subjected to feed change or restriction or to different antimicrobial regimens that may alter GI flora have not been reported. Fasting and diet change could alter the normal bacterial flora. Both stress and antimicrobial treatment may alter the normal flora in horses and thus predispose to colonization and eventually to disease associated with *Salmonella* infection.[94] The barrier effect of the indigenous intestinal flora that prevents establishment and multiplication of potentially pathogenic bacteria is called *colonization resistance*.[95] Although little is known about the complexity of interactions among indigenous microflora of the intestine in the horse, disturbances of the normal flora may predispose to colonization and multiplication of pathogenic bacteria.[96] A syndrome of antibiotic-associated diarrhea is often associated with proliferation of different enteric pathogens, such as *Salmonella* spp., *Clostridium difficile*, and *Clostridium perfringens*.[97]

In one of the few experimental studies of the impact of various stressors on experimentally infected equids, Owen et al.[14] reported that transportation of experimentally infected ponies resulted in reactivation of the *Salmonella* infection. Details regarding the duration and method of transportation are lacking in this report, and during transport the ponies also had feed deprivation as an additional stressor. The authors noted that treatment with oxytetracycline resulted in prolonged fecal shedding of *Salmonella* spp., in treated ponies. In another study of risk factors associated with isolation of *Salmonella* Saintpaul from hospitalized horses, those horses receiving antimicrobials were at increased risk for shedding the organism.[98]

Factors associated with hospitalization of equine patients were associated with salmonellosis decades ago.[99] Factors associated with increased likelihood for nosocomial infection with *Salmonella* among horses hospitalized in an intensive care facility included large colon impaction, number of days on bran mash, duration of treatment with potassium penicillin, number of days that other horses were shedding the organism in the hospital, and mean ambient environmental temperature of 80° F (26.6° C) or more compared with 60° F (15.5° C).[58] Factors associated with a reduced risk of infection included withholding feed. An increase in ambient temperature may increase risk of infection by favoring survival and multiplication of the organism in the environment, but also by compromising the immune response of the host.[100] Most outbreaks of equine salmonellosis reported in the literature have occurred in summer months, reinforcing the concept that heat stress may make horses more susceptible to infection. However, the roles of environmental contamination and host resistance have not been evaluated separately. House et al.[58] proposed that withholding of feed might reduce the risk of oral exposure to the organism by eliminating the possibility of consuming contaminated feed or feeding from contaminated surfaces.

PATHOGENESIS

Salmonella bacteria are transmitted by the fecal-oral route. In experimental studies, most animals require oral administration of very high numbers ($\geq 10^8$) of *Salmonella* organisms to cause disease.[13] Before establishing colonization of the ileum and colon, ingested *Salmonella* cells must survive a series of host-derived obstacles, such as salivary bactericidal enzymes, stomach acid, intestinal proteases, lysozymes, antimicrobial peptides and bile salts, complement, and phagocytes, as well as interference by the normal bacterial flora, including nutrient competition and bacteriocins.[7] Anything that interferes with the activity of these nonspecific responses is likely to decrease greatly the infectious dose of *Salmonella* required to cause disease, a process termed *facilitation*. For example, oral antacid preparations or administration of drugs that decrease gastric acid secretion increases the risk of salmonellosis, presumably from increased passage of viable bacterial cells into the intestinal tract.[14,15] Similarly, antimicrobial treatment that disrupts the normal intestinal or colonic flora increases the risk of salmonellosis, along with several other causes of infectious enteritis.[14] Many of the stress factors that predispose to salmonellosis, including transportation, sudden feed changes, spoiled feedstuffs, and other illnesses, probably act at least in part by affecting the innate resistance of the horse through the mechanisms previously described, for example, by disrupting the natural GI bacterial flora, reducing GI motility, or reducing the stomach acid or other natural barriers to colonization.

Invading cells that reach the target organs must penetrate the epithelial mucous layer and attach to the epithelial cell surface (Fig. 38-3). This attachment is mediated principally by bacterial fimbriae with specific receptor-ligand interactions with the epithelial cell surface.[16] Genetic analysis and whole-genome sequencing of *Salmonella* Typhimurium revealed the presence of more than 10 different fimbrial systems.[17] Most of these fimbriae are not expressed in culture but are activated in vivo. The multiple fimbrial systems probably work in concert, and the redundancy of fimbriae may be a strategy for *Salmonella* spp. to avoid immune responses directed at a single system.[18]

Salmonella spp. invade the intestinal epithelial cells by a process called *bacterial-mediated endocytosis*, which involves a rearrangement of the epithelial cell cytoskeleton triggered by proteins secreted by the attached bacterium, resulting in the epithelial cell membranes enveloping and internalizing the bacterial cell.[19] However, invasion of epithelial cells may not be required for the pathogenesis of enteric salmonellosis. Most of the key events of salmonellosis, including neutrophil recruitment, intestinal inflammation, and increased fluid secretion into the intestinal lumen, are now known to be induced by *Salmonella* spp. through the actions of a "type 3 secretion system" (T3SS). Type 3 systems are molecular "syringes" that inject bacterial effector proteins directly into the host-cell cytoplasm and do not require internalization of the bacterial cell for their activity.[20] The T3SS encoded in the "*Salmonella* pathogenicity island 1" (SPI1) plays a central role in bacterial-mediated endocytosis, and *Salmonella* isolates that lack T3SS-SPI1 are unable to induce the actin rearrangements that result in the internalization of *Salmonella* into the epithelial cells. In addition to invasion of epithelial cells, *Salmonella* cells also may traverse the epithelium by following phagocytes[21] or may enter the submucosa directly through the disrupted epithelium characteristic of the villous tip where normal cell sloughing occurs.

During attachment and invasion, *Salmonella* T3SS-SPI1 effectors induce a massive recruitment of neutrophils. An important mediator of this process is the cytokine interleukin-8 (IL-8, now also termed CXCL8), secreted by epithelial cells in response to *Salmonella* infection. The specific trigger for IL-8 secretion is thought to result from an interaction of *Salmonella* flagellin with the toll-like receptor 5 at the epithelial basolateral cell surface.[22] Flagellin may reach the basolateral cell surface along with invading *Salmonella* cells, but the proinflammatory effects of flagellin are also caused by its interaction with the T3SS-SPI1 effector SopE2.[23] IL-8 and other chemoattractant molecules mediate the recruitment of neutrophils to the submucosal space. The subsequent diapedesis of neutrophils to penetrate the tight junctions between epithelial cells to reach the apical surface occurs in response to another chemoattractant whose secretion is triggered by T3SS-SPI1 effectors, the eicosanoid hepoxilin A_3.[24,25]

Neutrophil chemotaxis to the apical epithelium, followed by degranulation and the release of inflammatory mediators, is largely responsible for the epithelial cell destruction and loss of epithelial barrier functions that elicit the clinical signs of salmonellosis.[25-27] Release of inflammatory mediators by large numbers of activated neutrophils has long been considered central to the inflammation associated with salmonellosis.[26,27] This inflammation results in massive epithelial damage, including sloughing of large areas of the epithelium with subsequent pseudomembrane formation. Inflammation and epithelial necrosis result in loss of serum protein into the lumen, with resultant hypoproteinemia typical of severe salmonellosis. Damage to the intestinal epithelium and the presence of invading salmonellae in the submucosa also result in release of endotoxin into the circulation, with the well-known subsequent effects on cardiac function, fever, leukopenia, hemoconcentration, lactic acidosis, coagulopathies, and hypotension (see Chapter 37).

In addition to their roles in epithelial invasion and neutrophil chemotaxis, T3SS-SPI1 effectors trigger increased fluid secretion at the site of infection. The increased fluid secretion is caused by increased chloride ion secretion, mediated in part by increases in the concentration of inositol polyphosphates (IPs) triggered by one or more T3SS-SPI1 effectors, likely including SopB. SopB contains motifs that are homologous to other IP-stimulating proteins and produces this effect on IPs in vitro.[28,29]

The hallmarks of host-adapted *Salmonella* serovar pathogenesis, including that of *Salmonella* Abortus-equi, are invasion, bacteremia, and disseminated disease, primarily without enteritis. On reaching the submucosa, these strains are internalized in macrophages and disseminate through lymphatic and blood circulations, resulting in bacteremia and colonization of the target organs (e.g., placenta, testicle) typical of this agent.

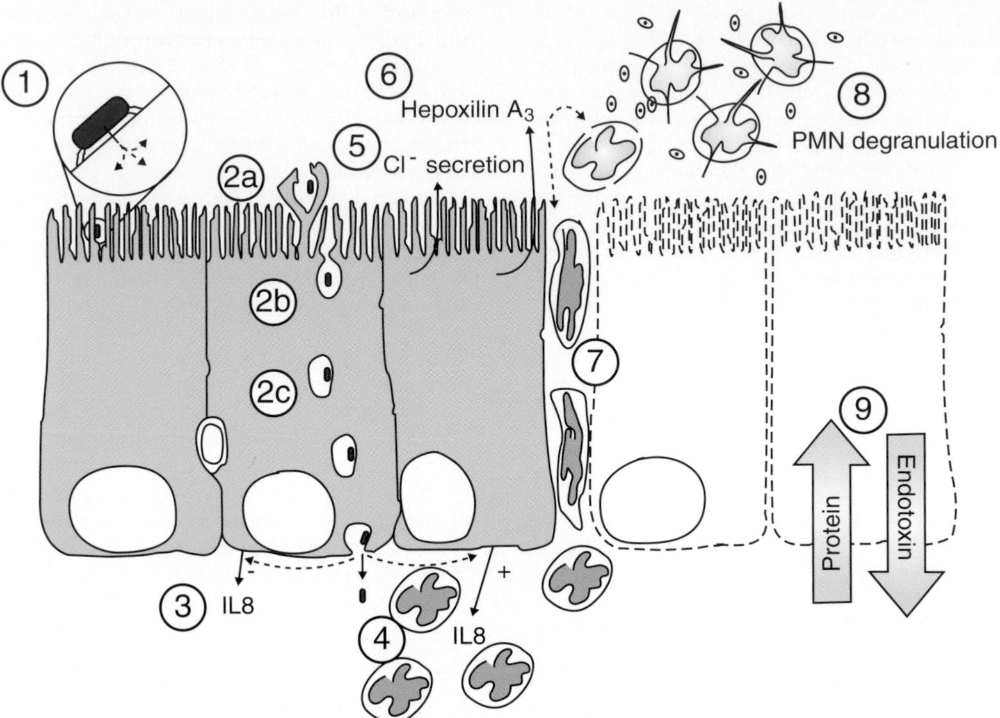

Fig. 38-3 Schematic of events in pathogenesis of *Salmonella* enterocolitis. *1*, *Salmonella* bacteria penetrate the intestinal mucous layer and bind to epithelial cells with one or more fimbrial adhesions. The type 3 secretion system, *Salmonella* pathogenicity island 1 (SPI1), is activated, and effectors are injected into the epithelial cells. *2*, *Salmonella* SPI1 effectors trigger actin rearrangements, resulting in bacteria-mediated endocytosis *(a)*, internalization *(b)*, and eventually transcytosis *(c)* of *Salmonella* bacteria. *3*, *Salmonella* SPI1 effectors trigger transcytosis of bacterial flagellin, which interacts with toll-like receptor 5 at the basolateral cell surfaces, triggering a cascade of cellular signals and resulting in release of interleukin-8 *(IL8)* and other chemotactic molecules. *4*, Interleukin-8 and other chemotaxins attract large numbers of polymorphoneutrophil leukocytes (PMNs) to the epithelial basolateral cell surface. *5*, *Salmonella* SPI1 effectors trigger increased chloride *(Cl^-)* secretion from the epithelial cells, probably mediated through increased inositol polyphosphate concentrations within the epithelial cells. *6*, *Salmonella* SPI1 effectors trigger release of hepoxilin A_3 at the apical surface. *7*, Hepoxilin A_3 acts as a chemoattractant, drawing PMNs through the intercellular spaces and through the tight junctions to reach the intestinal lumen. *8*, Polymorphoneutrophil *(PMN)* degranulation is triggered at the epithelial cell apical surfaces, releasing inflammatory mediators and causing necrosis of the epithelial cells. *9*, Loss of the epithelial barrier functions results in increased leakage of protein-rich fluid into the intestinal lumen and increased absorption of bacterial endotoxin.

CLINICAL FINDINGS

Horses infected with *Salmonella* may show a range of clinical signs, from inapparent shedding of the organism to peracute death.[34,101] Multiple factors may influence the resultant clinical signs in exposed equids, including the virulence of the *Salmonella* sp., exposure dose, and host resistance.

Inapparent Infection

Inapparent infections with *Salmonella* include horses that are "silent carriers" (those with infection but not shedding the organism) and those with fecal shedding but no signs of clinical disease.[34] Horses with fecal shedding but no detectable clinical signs of disease could have subclinical infection. An example would be a horse with some local intestinal or serologic response to the agent but no detectable signs of disease. Alternatively, the organism could pass through the GI tract with no bodily response to the agent.

Mild Infection

A mild form of infection has been described in which the horse is febrile, has reduced feed intake, and is mildly obtunded.[34,35] Some of these horses may have slightly loose, "cow pie" feces. These mild infections are often self-limiting. A major differential diagnosis is viral respiratory disease, in which the only clinical signs may be a fever and loss of appetite. Horses with this form of disease can shed the organism during and after the illness. This syndrome has been reproduced in horses experimentally challenged with *Salmonella* spp.[102] These horses will often be neutropenic, and a complete blood count (CBC) may help differentiate a viral respiratory infection from this syndrome.

Severe Acute Diarrhea

The form of the disease most often associated with salmonellosis involves severe diarrhea. At the onset of disease, horses may have fever, colic, anorexia, and neutropenia, often with a left shift. The neutropenia is not specific for salmonellosis and occurs with other causes of endotoxemia.[34] The diarrhea associated with this form of the disease can be quite voluminous with a high water content. This makes containment of the fecal material very difficult. Feces are sometimes but not always malodorous. It is rare for feces to contain gross evidence of blood in adult horses with salmonellosis. Tremendous fluid and electrolyte losses can occur with the diarrhea, resulting in dehydration and electrolyte abnormalities. Protein loss from the serum can also occur.

Horses with this form of the disease often have an increase in packed cell volume (PCV) associated with dehydration, with a normal to low serum total protein (TP) concentration and concurrent electrolyte abnormalities. This makes replacement fluid therapy a challenge both from a volume and a content standpoint. It is important in managing such horses to assess electrolyte and acid-base status as well as PCV/TP frequently during the course of the disease. Thrombocytopenia may also be seen.[34] Subsequent liver and kidney damage may occur with this form of the disease and would be reflected on a biochemistry profile. Laminitis may also be observed as a sequela of severe acute diarrhea caused by salmonellosis.

Septicemia

Septicemia is the presence of bacteria or their toxins in the blood and can occur with salmonellosis. Bacteremia (presence of bacteria in the blood) caused by salmonellosis is rare but can occur in adult horses and is usually associated with signs of severe colitis. Sites of infection include the liver, mesenteric lymph nodes, and kidneys. Septicemia in foals is more common and can occur without overt signs of enterocolitis concurrent with or preceding the septicemia.[34] Localized sites of infection in foals with *Salmonella* include lungs, joints, and physes.

Abortion

Equine salmonellosis caused by *Salmonella* Abortus-equi is called *equine paratyphoid*. The disease is manifested as abortion with other signs, including fistulous withers, orchitis, septicemia, and arthritis. This agent is isolated from approximately 100 horses annually in an endemic area in Japan.[103,104] An outbreak of abortion in mares attributed to *Salmonella* Abortus-equi was reported in 1997 in Europe.[105] This agent is reportedly no longer identified in the United States.[106]

Other Possible Signs or Syndromes

Salmonellosis may manifest as gastric dilation and ileus syndrome in horses.[107] It has been the authors' experience that occasionally, horses with mild fever and ileus with gastric reflux may have positive cultures for *Salmonella* spp. The gastric reflux is generally not of large volume. Occasionally this reflux contains blood and is malodorous. In at least one case the authors were able to isolate two different serotypes of *Salmonella* spp. at necropsy from culture of intestine. Whether *Salmonella* was the cause of the disease or the horse became colonized because of the illness is difficult to determine. Clinicians should take precautions with the disposal of gastric reflux from such horses and use barrier precautions when managing such cases (see Chapter 66).

Chronic diarrhea, defined as diarrhea that has persisted for at least 4 weeks, is not a typical feature of equine salmonellosis.[34] Although some horses may have diarrhea for weeks associated with the severe form of salmonellosis, this diarrhea eventually resolves in most horses and typically does not recur. If *Salmonella* is isolated from the feces of horses with chronic diarrhea, it may be simply colonizing the patient because of altered GI function as a result of another disease process rather than causing disease. In a review of chronic diarrhea in horses, Merritt[108] mentions *Salmonella* shedding as a possible occurrence in some horses with chronic diarrhea, and many of these horses have a deficiency in both IgG and IgA on a radioimmunodiffusion test. Some of these patients have responded to immunostimulant and enrofloxacin treatment, thus suggesting a cause-and-effect outcome for this intervention.[108]

In other species and in horses, impaction of the small colon has been associated with salmonellosis.

DIAGNOSIS

A working case definition of salmonellosis is an illness of variable severity manifested by diarrhea and abdominal pain. Inapparent infections may occur, and the organism may occasionally cause extraintestinal infections. Laboratory confirmation of this diagnosis currently requires the isolation of *Salmonella* from a clinical specimen from the suspected case. Both false-positive and false-negative diagnoses are possible with this definition. False-positive diagnoses, where the clinical signs result from a cause other than *Salmonella*, may occur because it and related organisms may frequently be found in the environment, and passive shedding of these environmental source organisms may occur in feces of noninfected animals. False-negative diagnoses may result from failure to detect *Salmonella* in the feces of an infected horse due to shedding of low numbers or the presence of bacterial competitors in the diagnostic specimen that interfere with the identification of the agent.

Clinical Pathology

A variety of hematologic and clinical chemistry findings are consistent with, but not diagnostic for, equine salmonellosis, depending on the severity of the infection and stage of the disease.[94] Hematologic findings may include neutropenia with left shift early in the disease course as a result of the intense neutrophil efflux into the affected intestinal tissues. Later in the disease course, a mature neutrophilic leukocytosis may result as the animal responds to demand. Endotoxemia may exacerbate the neutropenia because of increased margination of neutrophils and may cause sequestration of platelets in the lung and liver (see Chapter 37).

Clinical chemistry abnormalities associated with salmonellosis are also variable but can include hypoproteinemia, hypoalbuminemia, hyperglycemia or hypoglycemia, and pre-renal azotemia.[94] Electrolyte abnormalities can include hyponatremia, hypochloremia, and hyperkalemia. Metabolic acidosis is frequently present.

Detection of the Organism

Bacterial isolation is the most definitive means of establishing the presence of *Salmonella* organisms. With the use of selective enrichment and multiple selective plating agars, bacterial isolation is a highly sensitive method.[109] Nevertheless, false-negative cultures are thought to occur frequently because of low concentration of the organism in the feces at particular stages of the disease. Multiple serial bacterial cultures are frequently recommended to increase the sensitivity of culture,[34,57,110] despite the increased likelihood of false-positive results caused by detection of passive shedding. Because of the number of enrichment steps required, detection in culture of *Salmonella* when the organism is shed at low concentrations may take a week or more from the onset of culture.[64,109]

Bacterial isolation is required for determining the serotype and the antimicrobial resistance of the infecting *Salmonella* spp.

and thus aids establishing appropriate treatment and an accurate prognosis. In addition, comparative phenotypic or genetic analyses of *Salmonella* isolates, critically important in the epidemiologic investigation of potential outbreaks of disease, require the availability of viable bacterial isolates.

Fecal culture methods for detection of *Salmonella* spp. are poorly standardized and vary greatly from laboratory to laboratory. The most sensitive fecal culture methods include selective enrichment using one or preferably two different parallel or sequential broths. Subcultures of these enrichment broths should be made to two or more different selective differential agar plates to identify candidate colonies.[109] *Salmonella* serovars differ greatly in their tolerance for the various selective media in common use, so use of several different media with different degrees of selectivity will significantly increase the frequency of *Salmonella* isolation.

Fecal specimens (at least 1 g) are most often used for bacteriologic culture of *Salmonella*. Although enrichment cultures of larger volumes of fecal specimens tend to increase the likelihood of isolating *Salmonella*, practical limits are imposed by the volumes of media required, and multiple small samples may be a more rewarding approach. However, rectal mucosal biopsies have also been used and in at least some situations may provide more sensitive diagnosis than feces.[111] Unlike the situation with host-adapted serovars, enteric salmonellosis is not typically associated with bacteremia, and blood cultures are unrewarding in equine salmonellosis except in neonatal foals. Bacteremia is thought to occur most frequently in salmonellosis affecting young animals (1-6 months) or foals with failure of passive transfer, and blood culture would be warranted in these patients.

Postmortem specimens for bacteriologic culture should include cecal and colonic contents, mesenteric lymph nodes, liver, and spleen, as well as any other sites where clinical history or gross lesions indicate localization of the infection. Cultures of these necropsy specimens may be positive even when repeated fecal cultures are negative, and whether or not antimicrobial therapy has been administered.

Polymerase chain reaction (PCR) and other molecular biologic techniques that detect the presence of *Salmonella*-specific genes have been reported to aid in the diagnosis of equine salmonellosis. These techniques offer the potential of much faster detection compared with conventional bacteriologic culture, although enhanced sensitivity also requires cultural enrichment preceding the application of PCR.[64,112-115] Numerous *Salmonella*-"specific" genes are targeted by these methods; however, comparative studies demonstrate that the amplified genes may not be entirely specific to the target organism, raising the possibility of false-positive diagnoses with this method.[116] In addition, as with all PCR reactions, false-positive reactions may result from laboratory contamination by the amplification products of previous testing. Published comparisons between conventional microbiology and PCR-based tests for *Salmonella* applied to replicate specimens from clinical cases have produced results ranging from nearly perfect agreement between the two methods to a large excess of PCR-positive diagnoses.

PCR-positive, culture-negative cases should be interpreted with great caution because false-positive reactions are possible, caused either by laboratory contamination or by the unexpected occurrence of the target genes in nontarget organisms in the diagnostic specimens. Most PCR reactions are checked for specificity by application to a panel of bacterial species known to occur frequently in feces. However, anaerobic species tend to be greatly underrepresented in these in vitro specificity tests. Nonculturable bacteria are not represented at all despite their presumed occurrence in large numbers in feces. Either group of agents could potentially carry genes capable of being amplified by PCR primers. For PCR test results to be useful in clinical decision making, it is important to ensure that the primers used have been confirmed to be specific to *Salmonella* spp.[116] Also, test results should correlate closely with sensitive bacteriologic culture methods in comparative studies on equine feces.[64,112,117]

In investigating and implementing infection control measures with a known or suspected outbreak of salmonellosis, it is often useful to assess the degree and nature of environmental contamination. More information about the approaches to identifying environmental *Salmonella* contamination is available elsewhere.[32,118-120]

Serologic Testing

Serologic testing for exposure to *Salmonella* antigens is possible but is not widely available. Seropositive animals are not necessarily actively infected, and actively infected animals may be seronegative early in the infection. Antigenic differences between some infecting strains and some serologic tests may also result in false-negative results.

PATHOLOGIC FINDINGS

The gross pathologic findings in horses with salmonellosis are typically those of enteritis or enterocolitis. The predominant necropsy lesion is typically that of diffuse fibrinous or hemorrhagic inflammation of the cecum and colon. The mucosa may show superficial necrosis, and grayish pseudomembranes may adhere to the mucosa. Circumscribed focal mucosal ulcers underlain by edematous submucosa may develop in more chronic cases. The mesenteric lymph nodes are enlarged and may exhibit hemorrhage and edema.

Elsewhere in the GI tract, the stomach may be hyperemic with edema and focal hemorrhages. Small intestine changes may vary from simple congestion to a mucoid or hemorrhagic exudate. Histologically, the most severe lesions are also typically found in the cecum and colon. Hemorrhage and superficial coagulative necrosis with a predominantly mononuclear cell infiltrate are the principal findings. Fibrinocellular exudates may be attached to the necrotic epithelium. The capillaries of the lamina propria are frequently occluded by fibrin thrombi. "Paratyphoid nodules," small foci of hepatic necrosis that may be associated with aggregations of inflammatory cells, are not always present but are suggestive of salmonellosis when observed.

THERAPY

Antimicrobial Treatment

The use of antimicrobials for treatment of adult horses with salmonellosis is controversial.[94] Generally, antibiotic treatment of adult horses with salmonellosis is avoided, although some cases may warrant such treatment.[93]

Treatment of inapparent *Salmonella* infections with antimicrobial drugs has not proved to be an effective means of eliminating the carrier state. Because there is a paucity of information on the benefits versus disadvantages of antimicrobial treatment of equine salmonellosis, it is difficult to make definitive recommendations on the use of antimicrobials to treat adult horses with enterocolitis caused by *Salmonella* infection.[34] Horses that develop diarrhea while receiving antimicrobial treatment should have discontinuation of that antimicrobial drug(s).[121]

It has been suggested that antimicrobial treatment of adult horses with enterocolitis caused by *Salmonella* infection does not alter the course of the enterocolitis[94] or duration of shedding of the organism in feces.[34,94] Use of antimicrobials may be justified in some patients because of the risk for septicemia from severe neutropenia or persistent fever, the translocation of bacteria across the injured epithelium of the bowel, the presence of an indwelling intravenous catheter, or the presence of widespread endothelial damage.[94,121] Most clinicians decide on a case-by-case basis whether or not to institute antimicrobial treatment in adult horses with enterocolitis suspected or confirmed to be caused by salmonellosis. The choice of antimicrobials should be individualized based on the antimicrobial susceptibility pattern of the isolate from the patient or from past experience with isolates from that farm, hospital, or geographic region. A lipid-soluble drug would be optimal because *Salmonella* spp. can be intracellular bacteria. Combinations of gentamicin and a beta-lactam drug are often administered to horses with colitis of undetermined origin and to horses with confirmed salmonellosis, but this regimen has the disadvantage of poor intracellular penetration and the risk of renal toxicity (gentamicin).[94]

Papich[93] has suggested that, if antimicrobials are used, the drug of choice for treatment of salmonellosis in horses is a *fluoroquinolone*. This drug was selected because it has an injectable form (enrofloxacin at 5-10 mg/kg IV q24h), favorable pharmacologic features (intracellular penetration), bactericidal activity, and minimal effect on the anaerobic intestinal flora. Fluoroquinolones should not be administered to young foals because of concerns about their adverse effect on cartilage. For foals with salmonellosis, Papich[93] suggests a β-lactam drug such as an extended-spectrum cephalosporin or ampicillin-sublactam alone or in combination with an aminoglycoside (gentamicin or amikacin). Oral ciprofloxacin was associated with colitis in four Standardbred horses in part because of poor absorption after oral administration, and Weese et al.[122] suggest that because this drug does not reach therapeutic levels after oral administration and may cause colitis, the oral route should be avoided in horses.

Because some isolates of *Salmonella* from horses, especially those with clinical illness, can be multidrug resistant, choice of an antimicrobial before the availability of an antibiogram on the isolate is even more challenging. In addition, the use of some antimicrobials may apply selection pressure toward enhanced ability of multidrug-resistant *Salmonella* spp. to colonize equine patients.[123]

In neonatal foals bacteremia is more likely, so antimicrobial therapy is indicated, especially if there is an associated bone or joint infection.[121] Choice of antimicrobial should be based on antibiogram of the isolate if possible. Joint lavage and limb perfusion may also be considered in patients with bone or joint infection.[124-126]

Merritt[108] proposed using enrofloxacin and an immunostimulant in the treatment of horses with chronic diarrhea that are shedding *Salmonella* in the feces, implying a favorable outcome to treatment.

Fluid and Colloidal Therapy

Initial assessment should include determination of hydration status, plasma electrolyte concentration (sodium, potassium, chloride, calcium, magnesium), acid-base status (venous blood gas or total CO_2), serum glucose, and osmolality.[127] Generally, large volumes of polyionic intravenous (IV) fluids are required for treatment of adult horses with severe enterocolitis caused by salmonellosis. Goals of fluid therapy include replacement of fluid and electrolyte losses and maintenance of fluid, electrolyte, and acid-base balance after replacement has occurred. Frequent measurement of serum electrolytes, assessment of acid-base status, and PCV/TP monitoring are indicated because a wide variety of abnormalities may occur in horses with salmonellosis.[34] *Systemic inflammatory response syndrome* (SIRS), such as occurs with endotoxemia and sepsis, often results in increased vascular permeability, reduced vascular responsiveness, and myocardial depression (see Chapter 37). Hypoalbuminemia is common and results in decreased oncotic pressure.[128] These factors predispose to reduced circulating volume and inadequate perfusion. The need to augment replacement or maintenance fluids is based on repeated evaluation of serum electrolytes.[127]

In patients with complications such as hypovolemic shock, significant ongoing fluid losses, and hypoalbuminemia, IV administration of colloidal solutions may be indicated. Small-volume colloidal administration may be accomplished over a short time to expand the intravascular volume by osmotic redistribution from the extracellular fluid. Several commercially available colloids are available, including plasma and hydroxyethyl starch (HES). Experimental studies have shown HES to be superior to plasma for treatment of endotoxic shock in attenuation of endotoxin-induced vascular permeability. Hypertonic saline (HYS) may be indicated as an adjunct to intravascular resuscitation. In hypovolemic shock, HYS may be important in stabilization of the cardiovascular system. It is important that isotonic replacement fluids be given with HYS. HYS is contraindicated in patients with renal failure, cardiac arrhythmias, hypernatremia, hypokalemia, thrombocytopenia, or coagulopathies.[127]

Clinicians should pay careful attention to catheter selection, placement, and maintenance in horses with enterocolitis and endotoxemia because such patients are at increased risk of venous thrombosis. Although more expensive, polyurethane catheters may prove to be more economical because they can be left in place longer than catheters made of alternative materials and may reduce the risk of thrombosis in horses with severe GI disease.[127] Any signs of heat, pain, swelling, or thickening of the vein should prompt immediate catheter removal, and if sepsis is suspected, the catheter should be submitted for bacterial culture.

For further information on fluid treatment of diarrheic equine patients, the reader is referred to in-depth reviews on the subject.[127,128]

Treatment of Endotoxemia and Inflammation

There are five principal goals of treatment for endotoxemia: (1) prevention of movement of endotoxin into the circulation; (2) neutralization of endotoxin before it interacts with inflammatory cells; (3) prevention of synthesis, release, or action of inflammatory mediators; (4) prevention of endotoxin-induced cellular activation; and (5) general supportive care with IV fluids or colloids and inotropic agents (as previously addressed).[129]

Prevention of movement of endotoxin into the circulation needs to be addressed at the bowel level. Ditrioctahedral (DTO) smectite (Biosponge; Platinum Performance, Buellton, California) is a natural, hydrated aluminomagnesium silicate containing chelated macrominerals and microminerals available for use in horses.[129,130] Although the mechanism remains speculative, DTO reduced the duration of diarrhea and the frequency of defecation in horses with experimentally induced colitis.[131] Further controlled studies to determine the in vivo efficacy of DTO in horses with salmonellosis are needed.

Neutralization of toxin before activation of inflammatory cells can be attempted in two ways: administration of antiendotoxin antibodies or administration of polymyxin B, which forms a stable complex with lipid A. The conclusions of various studies of serum or plasma products enriched with *antiendotoxin antibodies* have been variable. Additional controlled studies need to be performed using strict entrance criteria and in which antiendotoxin antibodies or nonspecific immunoglobulins are administered early in the course of the disease.[129] With the recent report of fatal serum hepatitis associated with commercial plasma transfusion in horses, the benefit of this treatment must be weighed against the risk of this potential, although rare, complication.[132] *Polymyxin B* has been evaluated in several experimental studies and is currently used in clinical cases for the treatment of endotoxemia in horses.[133,134] It is optimal to initiate polymyxin treatment (1000-6000 units/kg q8-12h) as early in the course of endotoxemia as possible.[134] Use of polymixin B should be avoided in horses with renal compromise.

Preventing or reducing the synthesis, release, or effect of inflammatory mediators secondary to endotoxemia includes treatment of horses with nonsteroidal antiinflammatory drugs (NSAIDs) such as *flunixin meglumine*. The NSAIDs have been the main means of treatment of horses with endotoxemia for decades. These drugs inhibit cyclooxygenase and thus the formation of arachidonic acid metabolites. Another class of drug used for treatment of horses with endotoxemia is *pentoxifylline* (8 mg po q8h).[129] During in vitro experimental studies, this drug reduced production of cytokines, thromboxanes, and expression of tissue factor while increasing plasma concentration of prostaglandin I_2. However, during in vivo experiments in horses, pentoxyfylline had limited benefit.[135] Other drugs are being explored for the treatment of endotoxemia through inhibition of the production, release, or effect of inflammatory mediators, but most of these are not available for clinical use. Corticosteroids are likely contraindicated in treatment of salmonellosis because of their immunosuppressive effect.[94,129]

New treatments are being developed and tested for their ability to interfere with endotoxin-induced cellular activation.[129] These new treatments seek to modulate proinflammatory and antiinflammatory mediators in response to endotoxin.

A detailed discussion of the pathogenesis, diagnosis, and treatment of endotoxemia and SIRS is presented in Chapter 37.

Colonic Flora Modulation

No benefit was demonstrated with the use of two commercially prepared probiotic products on the prevalence of fecal shedding of *Salmonella* in the postoperative period of equine colic patients.[56,136] Possible reasons for failure of these products include lack of viable organisms in the product, failure of the organisms to remain viable in the GI tract, and inappropriate organisms to provide an intestinal flora barrier to colonization with *Salmonella* spp.[130] A recent study demonstrated the potential benefit of *Lactobacillus pentosus* WE7. This organism is acid and bile tolerant and moderately inhibitory to growth of *Salmonella* spp. in vitro.[137] A randomized masked placebo study of the efficacy of this organism on the shedding of *Salmonella* in high-risk equine patients is warranted.

Other Treatment Considerations

All horses with diarrhea should be isolated from other animals, and barrier precautions should be used to minimize the exposure of other animals and human handlers to the feces of diarrheic horses during treatment (see Chapters 66 and 67). These horses should be housed in an area where insect, rodent, and bird control is optimal.

Horses with severe disease should be kept as comfortable as possible. An effort should be made to keep the horse's coat and skin clean of feces; surfaces such as the perineum may require frequent cleaning, and topical application of skin protection products is warranted. Affected horses should be protected from extremely cold or hot and humid environmental conditions. These horses should be housed on a stall surface that is cleanable with plenty of bedding in case they want to lie down. The stall should be kept reasonably clean by frequent removal of soiled bedding and replacement with fresh bedding. A cushioned stall floor is ideal because these horses are prone to laminitis. If cushioning of the stall with mats is not an option, then application of hoof support with padding using various materials cut to fit over the sole of the hoof and attached with tape is indicated.

All horses with diarrhea should have access to fresh water unless gastric dilation and ileus are a part of the disease process. Some horses will consume electrolyte solutions orally, which may reduce the amount of IV supplementation required; therefore, offering an electrolyte bucket along with access to plain fresh water is indicated.

Special attention to diet is warranted for horses with diarrhea. Efforts should be made to provide clean feed (not contaminated with diarrheic feces) in small amounts several times a day to encourage consumption and to adequately monitor feed intake. The horse should be offered several options of types of feed to enhance feed consumption if appetite is reduced. Feeds that are low bulk and low in soluble carbohydrate are ideal, such as complete pelleted rations, good-quality grass hay, or judicious amounts of alfalfa hay. Small amounts of fresh grass may stimulate anorectic horses to eat, but large amounts of lush pasture should be avoided. If the horse is hypoproteinemic, provision of a complete pelleted ration or alfalfa hay will provide a source of protein in the diet. If the horse is unwilling or unable to eat for an extended time, addressing protein and calorie malnutrition is warranted through parenteral nutrition. Equine patients prone to hyperlipemia or those that are underweight require nutritional support more quickly than horses in optimal body condition. A detailed description of parenteral nutrition is beyond the scope of this chapter, and the reader is directed to other sources of information on this topic.[138]

It is important in any horse with diarrhea to monitor vital signs and select laboratory tests frequently to determine the need for and most appropriate change in therapy. Monitoring horses with enterocolitis for early signs of laminitis is very important so that treatment for laminitis can be promptly implemented. For more information on the pathogenesis, treatment, and prevention of laminitis, the reader is referred to reviews on this topic.[139,140]

If the horse is showing signs of abdominal pain that is refractory to management with NSAIDs such as flunixin meglumine, consideration should be given to administration of more potent analgesics on an as-needed basis. Options for pain management would include administration of xylazine, potentially in combination with butorphanol or detomidine. In some horses with enterocolitis, a constant-rate IV infusion of butorphanol may be necessary. Other sources of information on management of abdominal pain in horses are available.[141,142]

PREVENTION

Options for prevention of salmonellosis in equids can be separated into two broad categories: (1) prevent or minimize exposure and (2) optimize host resistance if exposed.[92] *Salmonella* spp. are ubiquitous enough that avoiding all exposure is likely not feasible; however, means are available to minimize both frequency and dose of exposure. The level of risk aversion of the horse owner or veterinarian will dictate which, if any, of the options for reducing exposure are feasible. Most methods of reducing exposure to infectious agents come with an associated cost, often in increased time and effort dedicated to implementing biosecurity and biocontainment steps in management of the horses either on the farm or in the veterinary hospital. Clearly, no single "silver bullet" can easily prevent 100% of equine salmonellosis cases.

Reducing Exposure to *Salmonella* Species

Exposure of horses to *Salmonella* spp. can be minimized by reducing chances of oral exposure to the organism. This can be accomplished by using biosecurity and biocontainment strategies on the farm and in veterinary hospitals (see Chapter 66). The following overview of options for reducing risk of exposure to *Salmonella* provides selected examples to illustrate the preventive measures.

New arrivals to the farm or resident horses returning to the farm from high-risk situations, such as from veterinary hospitals, should be isolated from the resident equine population for 14 to 21 days to reduce the chances of exposing the resident horse population to the organism. Housing horses in veterinary hospitals based on risk level may reduce cross-contamination between patients. For example, colic patients could be kept stalled separately from elective orthopedic cases.

Providing horses on farms with access to pastures that are well maintained can reduce the bacterial load. Avoiding overcrowding and overgrazing will decrease the fecal load on pastures as well as keep grasses longer and allow horses to avoid grazing where other horses have defecated. Avoiding common-use turnout areas for hospitalized horses will minimize exposure. If grazing of hospitalized horses is desirable, providing grass in raised beds or hydroponically produced grass should be considered.

Using feeds that are manufactured using good manufacturing procedures and that do not contain animal protein sources may reduce the likelihood of feed-related exposure to *Salmonella* spp. Pelleted feeds may be less likely to contain live bacteria because of the heating process. Horse feeds should be stored so that rodent and bird fecal contamination is minimized. Storing concentrate sources in rodent-proof containers and keeping lids closed can reduce contamination of feeds stored on the farm or in veterinary hospitals.

Although challenging, control of insect, rodent, and bird access to equine housing areas should be considered, especially in the areas where horses are fed. Open rafters in barns can be blocked off using wire mesh nailed to the rafters to reduce bird roosting above horse stalls and in areas where feed may be stored. Keeping the quantity of available feed to a minimum will reduce rodent and bird populations. Insect control can be accomplished by keeping livestock fecal material removed from stalls and disposing of feces away for horse housing areas. Performing a walk-through of the facility with personnel specially trained in insect, rodent, and bird control can provide valuable information on options for a given farm or veterinary hospital.

Water sources for horses should be tested for quality assurance purposes, unless the source is regularly tested because it is for human consumption, such as municipal water supplies. Most water testing includes bacterial counts. Optimally, these would be identified as enteric bacteria, and if present, there is increased potential of exposure to *Salmonella* spp. For example, if horses have access to irrigation ditches, creeks, or ponds, these water sources should be tested.

Regular removal of livestock feces from stalls and pastures reduces the load of enteric bacteria in the horse's environment. Disposal sites for feces should be distant from the equine housing area and pastures. Runoff from fecal disposal sites into horse pastures or stall areas should be prevented. It is important to consider the cleanability of surfaces when designing and building equine housing. For example, it is impossible to clean and disinfect dirt-floored stalls thoroughly. Serious consideration should be given to drainage systems used in horse barns so that the materials going down the drains do not run off onto horse pastures, paddocks, or feeding sites.

In one outbreak of salmonellosis in neonatal foals, mares were suspected to be shedding *Salmonella* Ohio in their feces at the time of foaling. Control measures included cleaning and disinfection of the surfaces in the foaling barn, thorough bathing of mares immediately after foaling, frequent removal of mare's feces from the stall, and giving the newborn foal colostrum from a bottle before suckling from the udder. These measures appeared to prevent further cases.[143]

Monitoring of fecal shedding by horses and the environmental contamination in high-risk areas (e.g., veterinary hospitals) can allow for rapid intervention to control spread of *Salmonella* spp.[144] The most appropriate monitoring program would depend on the risk aversion of the facility director, the available funding and the type of facility, and patient load. In a survey of U.S. veterinary teaching hospitals, most had some form of infection control program that focused on reducing the risk of nosocomial spread of infectious diseases, with an emphasis on control of salmonellosis.[74]

Cleaning and disinfection of equipment used on equine patients between uses or use of dedicated equipment for high-risk patients is important in controlling spread of *Salmonella* between hospitalized patients. For example, cleaning and disinfection of stomach tubes between equine patients is important in reducing the spread of multiple types of nosocomial agents. Use of dedicated thermometers also reduces the risk of fecal-oral spread of bacteria.

Environmental control measures for prevention of salmonellosis include designing hospital facilities to allow for thorough cleaning and disinfection and keeping equine housing areas cooled during hot and humid weather conditions to reduce the risk of *Salmonella* overgrowth in the environment and reduce susceptibility of ill horses to severe salmonellosis if exposed.[74] *Salmonella* spp. can persist and perhaps even multiply in the environment; thus, hygiene practices that reduce the bacterial load likely are important, especially in areas where high-risk animals are housed, such as veterinary hospitals or foaling barns. Hygiene efforts can be more focused if there is ongoing surveillance as part of a hospital infection control program.[144] Disinfection is one of the most important means to control certain infectious equine diseases, especially the enteric pathogens such as *Salmonella*.[145] The stall and surrounding areas for any known *Salmonella*-positive animal should be considered contaminated and appropriate barrier precautions taken. Once the horse has left the facility, cleaning and disinfection should be implemented and the effectiveness of these procedures monitored.

When determining the best means of reducing or eliminating *Salmonella* from the environment, considerations include the type of surfaces, the associated organic material, and the agent involved. It is important to emphasize cleaning the environmental surfaces as part of the process. Virtually all equine infectious disease agents are associated with some organic material, such as feces, pus, or blood. Physically removing these materials by cleaning is an important first step. Basic concepts include cleaning from top to bottom and farthest from a drain toward the drain and cleaning from the least toward the most contaminated areas. It is important to emphasize the safety of personnel in the cleaning and disinfection process to reduce their exposure to a potentially zoonotic pathogen (*Salmonella* spp.) and to potentially toxic chemicals.[145] In choosing a disinfectant, the infectious agent, the ambient temperature, organic mater present, Environmental Protection Agency (EPA) rules, type of surfaces, likely damage to surfaces with long-term repeated use, and pH of the disinfectant solution must all be considered. For details regarding disinfection of equine facilities, the reader is directed to Chapters 66 and 67 and recent reviews.[38,145]

Unlike patient care for humans and small animals, it is nearly impossible to provide veterinary care for hospitalized horses without footwear contacting the patient's fecal material. Because this fecal material could contain pathogenic bacteria, attention to foot traffic in high-risk areas is very important. Use of footbaths or mats with disinfectant is a common measure to control trafficking of pathogenic microorganisms in livestock operations and veterinary hospitals.[38] Alternative approaches include use of dedicated footwear in a particular facility or area in the hospital (e.g., isolation facility, colic aisle way). Often a combination of these methods is used. The reader is referred to several publications on disinfectants and their efficacy in equine facilities.[38,120,145]

An important part of optimal patient care includes the regular use of effective hand hygiene. It is important to wear gloves when examining high-risk patients. However, because fecal shedding of *Salmonella* can occur in normal-appearing horses, use of hand hygiene between all patients is indicated. Hand hygiene is one of the most important parts of an infection control program. The product type to be used should be considered as well as the regular implementation of the methods by hospital personnel. Several veterinary hospitals are now using not only handwashing but also disinfectant hand gels as part of their infection control strategies.[146]

Optimizing Resistance

Vaccination to stimulate specific immunity is one option often undertaken in control of infectious diseases.[92] However, no commercial vaccine is currently on the market for prevention of salmonellosis in horses. If immunization against salmonellosis is considered as an approach to control, the timing and the selection of appropriate horses to receive vaccination need to be considered. For example, a horse with colic that requires hospitalization could rarely be anticipated, so vaccination may need to be implemented as part of a routine program for all horses or perhaps for broodmares on farms with a known problem with neonatal salmonellosis.

Development of vaccines depends on the potential marketability, and thus the marketplace needs to be explored for such a vaccine along with determination of the best way to vaccinate against the disease. An intranasal vaccine has undergone experimental investigation in ponies with some promising results, but to the authors' knowledge, progress toward development of a vaccine for commercial use in horses has not occurred. The intranasal vaccine contained a Δcya Δcya-pabA mutant (MGN-707) of *Salmonella* Typhimurium.[147] In this particular study the vaccine isolate stimulated a mucosal and serologic immune response. Intestinal immune response was stimulated by administration of this isolate intranasally, with no detectable shedding in the feces after vaccination. The migration of B cells from equine nasal-associated lymphoid tissue (NALT) in the nasal mucosa to distant mucosal sites may explain the intestinal immune response to this vaccine.

Recently, a conditionally licensed *Salmonella* Newport bacterial extract vaccine for use in cattle has become available. The vaccine is based on induction of antibodies to purified siderophores and porins (SRPs), and the manufacturer suggests there would be cross-protection across serotypes of *Salmonella* spp. This vaccine is produced specifically for use in cattle (Salmonella Newport Bacterial Extract, AgriLabs, St. Joseph, Missouri). It would be important to determine how well horses tolerated the adjuvant and the overall vaccine before any off-label use in horses or foals was considered.

Other options for improving resistance of horses to salmonellosis include reducing stress when possible (see earlier discussion on host resistance). Feasible options for reducing stress and maintaining normal GI flora that may act as a barrier to colonization by *Salmonella* include judicious use of antimicrobials and gastric ulcer medications, minimizing dietary changes, and keeping the environmental temperature cool during hot and humid weather conditions.

Supplementation with probiotics in the limited number of studies conducted to date did not reduce the fecal shedding of *Salmonella* by hospitalized equine colic patients.[56] Competitive exclusion has shown some promise in increasing the resistance of poultry to pathogenic *Salmonella* spp.[148,149] Further investigation into a probiotic treatment for use in high-risk equine patients may lead to dietary additives that improve resistance to *Salmonella* at the GI barrier level.[137]

PUBLIC HEALTH CONSIDERATIONS

Salmonellosis is an important zoonotic disease estimated to cause more than 1 million cases of diarrheal disease, 15,000 hospitalizations, and 400 human deaths annually in the United States.[66] The economic costs of salmonellosis are considered the largest single contributor to the overall burden of human acute bacterial enteric disease, which was estimated at almost $8 billion in 1989.[67]

Although it is generally assumed that most cases of human salmonellosis result from food-borne exposure, other important routes of infection exist. The prevalence of contamination of horsemeat with *Salmonella* at slaughter plants is of concern from a public health perspective because horsemeat is exported from the United States to some countries for human consumption. Contamination of horsemeat and food-borne transmission of *Salmonella* by horsemeat have been reported.[68,69] In some countries, horsemeat is consumed raw as steak tartare. A link between contaminated horsemeat and an outbreak of human illness in France caused by multidrug-resistant *Salmonella* Newport has been reported.[69] Because horsemeat consumption is rare in the Untied States, a more significant route of infection is transmission by direct or indirect contact with infected animals. Direct contact with infected horses is a significant risk factor for zoonotic transmission of *Salmonella* spp.[70,71] This risk is presumably greater for contact with clinically ill animals with salmonellosis. Indirect animal contact may also result in significant exposure to *Salmonella*; household environmental contamination of workers exposed to a veterinary *Salmonella* outbreak is quite common.[72] Although direct contact transmission from horses to humans does occur, such reports appear to be infrequent[73,74] (J.L. Traub-Dargatz, Colorado State University, personal communication).

The global epidemiology of *Salmonella* spp. can be strongly affected by the epidemic dissemination of specific strains.[75] Recent examples of this process include *Salmonella* Typhimurium DT104 in the 1990s and the *cmy-2*–positive *Salmonella* Newport since 2000. DT104 was first detected in psittacine birds in England in the mid-1980s. Interestingly, direct-contact infections of humans were reported almost simultaneously with these first reported avian cases. However, the epidemic of DT104 assumed large-scale status in the early 1990s, with increasing reports from humans and a wide variety of animal species. As the scale of the DT104 problem was recognized, retrospective studies in numerous countries worldwide led to the recognition that DT104 had emerged as a major epidemic globally at about the same time. Before application of high-resolution typing methods (e.g., phage typing, PFGE), the emergence of DT104 was largely recognized as an increase in the frequency of chloramphenicol resistance among *Salmonella* Typhimurium, because DT104 was the earliest, widely distributed chloramphenicol-resistant strain within the serotype. Subsequently it was recognized that the shift in antimicrobial resistance among *Salmonella* Typhimurium at this time was essentially caused entirely by the epidemic of this single strain type. Furthermore, its appearance in at least some regions appeared to be unrelated to local antimicrobial drug use practices.[76] In the late 1990s, *Salmonella* Typhimurium DT104 diminished considerably in frequency, much as previously epidemic *Salmonella* Typhimurium strain types diminished in frequency with the appearance of DT104.

More recently, North America has seen the emergence of a new epidemic, multidrug-resistant serovar, *Salmonella* Newport.[77] This new epidemic *Salmonella* is of particular concern from a public health viewpoint because of its *cmy-2*–encoded decreased susceptibility to extended-spectrum cephalosporin drugs, including ceftriaxone and ceftazidime and the veterinary drug ceftiofur. These cephalosporin drugs are considered the drugs of choice for childhood *Salmonella* infections that require antimicrobial therapy when fluoroquinolone drugs are contraindicated. This *Salmonella* Newport strain has been reported as the cause of significant problems with equine nosocomial infection and raises concerns about direct-contact transmission to veterinary hospital staff and clients.[78]

REFERENCES

See the CD-ROM for a list of references linked to the abstract in PubMed.

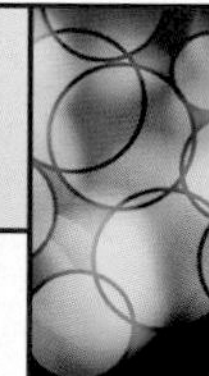

CHAPTER • 39

Glanders

Paul L. Nicoletti

Glanders is one of the oldest recorded plagues among perissodactyls (odd-toed ungulates) and may have been originally described by early Greek and Roman writers.[1] Three forms of glanders are generally recognized: cutaneous (farcy), nasal, and pulmonary. Pulmonary glanders is an extension of the nasal form. The common etiology of these diseases was first demonstrated by Viborg at the end of the eighteenth century.[1] The etiologic agent, now known as *Burkholderia mallei*, was isolated in 1882 by German and French scientists.[2] The mallein test for diagnosis of glanders was developed in 1890.[2]

By the second half of the nineteenth century, glanders was widespread in horses in North America, and a major epidemic of disease occurred in association with movement of horses during and after the Civil War.[2,3] During World War I, *B. mallei* was used as a biologic warfare agent against the horses of the Allied forces, and currently it is considered significant as a potential agent of bioterrorism today (category B, U.S. Centers for Disease Control and Prevention).[4,5] Disease caused by *B. mallei* must be reported to the World Organization for Animal Health (formerly the Office International des Epizooties [OIE]) in Paris.

ETIOLOGY

Burkholderia mallei (formerly *Pseudomonas, Bacillus, Pfeiferella, Loefflerella, Malleomyces, Actinobacillus, Corynebacterium,* and *Mycobacterium*) is a short, rod-shaped, gram-negative, aerobic, facultative intracellular, nonmotile and non–spore-forming bacterium. The organisms survive outside the host for varying times depending on many factors. Relatively little is known about virulence factors of *B. mallei*. Capsular polysaccharide is essential for virulence in hamsters and mice.[6] An acapsular mutant of *B. mallei* failed to induce disease in experimentally infected horses.[7] Disease caused by *B. mallei* must be reported to the World Organization for Animal Health.

EPIDEMIOLOGY AND PATHOGENESIS

Although occasional cases of glanders occur in cats, dogs, goats, sheep, and camels, the principal hosts are horses, donkeys, and mules. Carnivores, such as lions, may be infected from ingestion of contaminated meat. Mice and guinea pigs can be experimentally infected. Chronically infected equids are the only known reservoir for *B. mallei*. Human infections can occur by aerosol transmission from infected animals and are frequently fatal if untreated (see Public Health Considerations).

Glanders is restricted geographically to Eastern Europe, Asia, and North Africa and is considered endemic in countries such as Iraq, Turkey, Pakistan, India, Mongolia, and China,[8-12] where reported outbreaks appear to be increasing in the last 10 to 20 years. Reports of recent outbreaks in Brazil and the United Arab Emirates have appeared in the veterinary literature[13] and on the OIE website. Glanders has been eradicated from Europe, Australia, and North America by a rigorous policy of culling animals that are positive by complement fixation test, serum agglutination test, or the mallein test (see Diagnosis). An accidental human infection occurred in a laboratory worker in 2000,[14] but there have been no naturally occurring cases of glanders in North America for more than 60 years. The last case in animals in the United States was in 1942.

Burkholderia mallei is a host-adapted pathogen that does not persist in the environment outside of its equine host.[7] The organisms are thought to gain entrance through mucous membranes; common water and feed are likely the main source of infection. The disease can be spread by subclinically infected horses. Poor sanitation, crowding, and immunosuppression from parasitism are considered risk factors. The incubation period varies from a few days to several months. Some workers have suggested that the disease is more severe in donkeys and mules than in horses.[9] The disease has been the target of eradication efforts for many decades because of its clinical effects in *Equidae* and its public health implications.

CLINICAL FINDINGS

In the cutaneous form of glanders, also known as *farcy*, nodules develop into crater-shaped ulcers with exudation (Fig. 39-1). The subcutaneous tissues and lymph nodes are affected. Lymphatic vessels become swollen and corded with development of "farcy buds," swellings that enlarge, ulcerate, and drain.

In horses with the nasal form of glanders, small nodules on the nasal septum develop into ulcers called *stellate* (starlike) *scars* (Fig. 39-2), with a purulent unilateral or bilateral discharge (Fig. 39-3). These lesions degenerate into deep ulcers with raised, irregular borders that may ultimately obstruct the oropharynx, resulting in extreme dyspnea. There is an accumulation of necrotic cells with kayorrhectic nuclei.[9] Submaxillary and other lymph nodes are enlarged and edematous. There may be severe congestion of the spleen and liver. Orchitis may be present (Fig. 39-4).

In the acute pulmonary form of disease, horses have a high fever (41° C [106° F]), septicemia, and bronchopneumonia (Fig. 39-5). There are small, tubercle-like nodules with caseous or calcified centers in the lungs (Fig. 39-6). The mortality for untreated horses with acute disease is very high.

Horses with glanders either die rapidly or live for several years with chronic abscessation. They may have varying degrees of respiratory difficulty with no fever. Other possible clinical signs in infected horses include mild depression, decreased food intake, and infrequent defecation.[7]

Acute neurologic dysfunction was described in horses experimentally infected with *B. mallei*.[7] Small numbers of *Streptococcus equi* subsp. *zooepidemicus* were cultured from the brains of these horses at necropsy, suggesting that the blood-brain barrier was compromised.

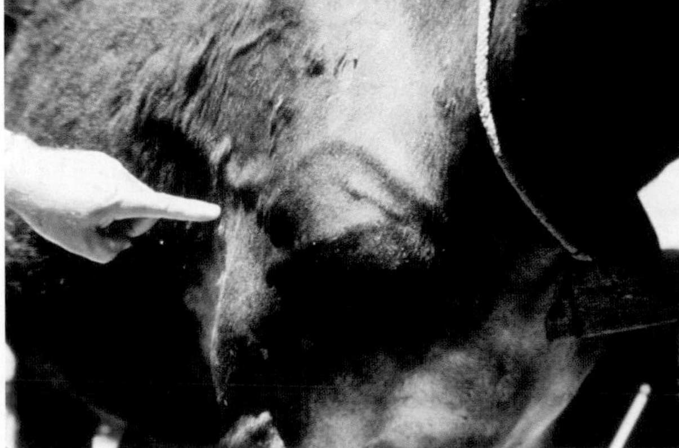

Fig. 39-1 *Top* and *bottom*, Nodules, swollen cutaneous lymphatic vessels, and drainage typical of horses with glanders.

DIAGNOSIS

Glanders must be differentiated from other bacterial infections, including meliodosis (*Burkholderia pseudomallei*) or disease caused by members of the genera *Streptococcus, Rhodococcus, Pasteurella*, or *Mannheimia*. Confirmation of the diagnosis requires one or more test procedures.

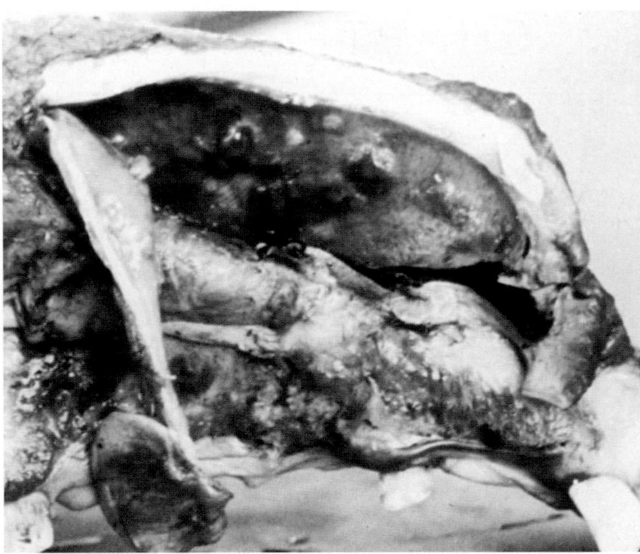

Fig. 39-2 Granulomas and ulcers (stellate scar) in nasal septum of horse with glanders.

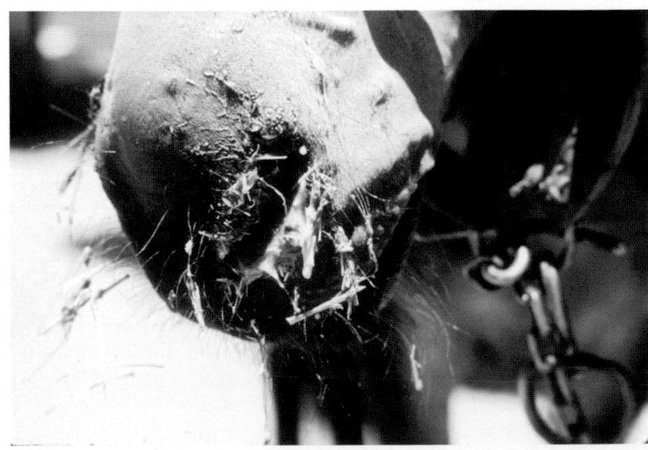

Fig. 39-3 Nasal exudate in horse with glanders.

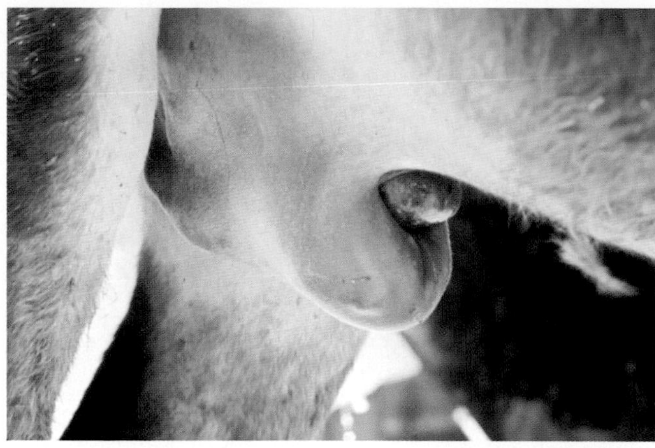

Fig. 39-4 Swollen sheath in horse with orchitis caused by glanders.

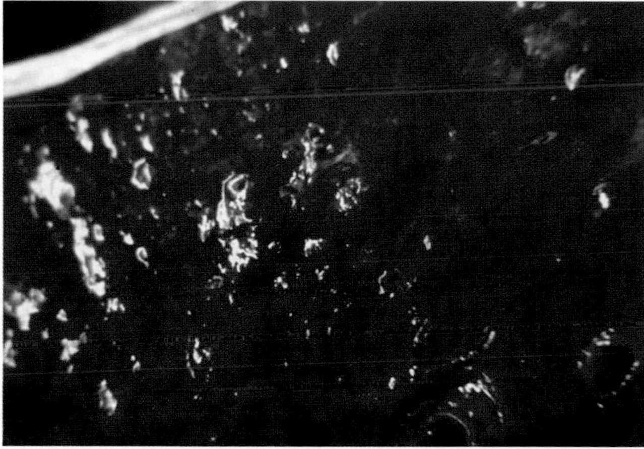

Fig. 39-5 Pulmonary granulomas and marked congestion observed at necropsy of horse with glanders.

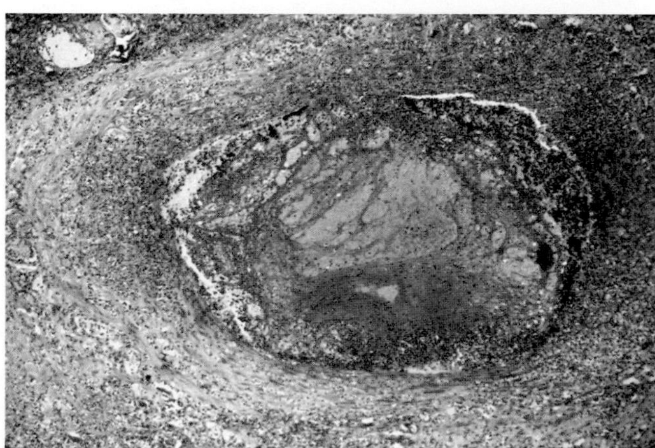

Fig. 39-6 Photomicrograph of typical nodule from horse with glanders.

Historically, the diagnostic test for suspected glanders and the test required before international movement of horses has been the *mallein test:* intradermal injection of 0.2 mL of mallein in the neck (cervical) or eyelid and subsequent observation for hypersensitivity. Mallein is a heat-killed, primarily lipopolysaccharide (LPS), extract of *B. mallei.*[15] The reagent may also be used as an antigen in serologic tests. Criteria for a positive reaction include a rectal temperature greater than 40° C (104° F), local swelling of 35 mm in diameter after 48 to 72 hours, and lacrimination[9] (Fig, 39-7). The immunologic basis for the test is primarily a stimulation of memory T cells. Anergy may result in a false-negative reaction. False-positive reactions may also occur. In negative horses, mallein may induce antibodies that are detectable for up to 6 weeks after injection.

Several serologic tests and other diagnostic techniques are now available for glanders diagnosis, including complement fixation, agglutination, indirect hemagglutination, enzyme-linked immunosorbent assay (ELISA), counter immunoelectrophoresis, and competitive ELISA (cELISA).[15] A relatively large number of false-positive and false-negative results can arise from these tests. These problems are thought to result from the use of crude preparations of whole cells as test antigens.[16] Culture and immunohistochemical staining for bacterial antigen may be used. Although rarely used, guinea pigs are highly susceptible, and an acute purulent orchitis occurs in a few days after inoculation of material (Strauss test). A lack of sensitivity of this procedure and culture has been reported.[9] Recent advances in our understanding of *B. mallei* and the increasing availability of molecular diagnostic tools may soon result in a new generation of more sensitive and specific diagnostic tests for glanders in horses.[16]

THERAPY

Euthanasia and slaughter of equids with glanders are strongly recommended and may be mandatory in some countries. Although there are relatively few studies of antimicrobial susceptibility patterns of *Burkholderia mallei*, it appears that this organism is resistant to many antimicrobial drugs, including

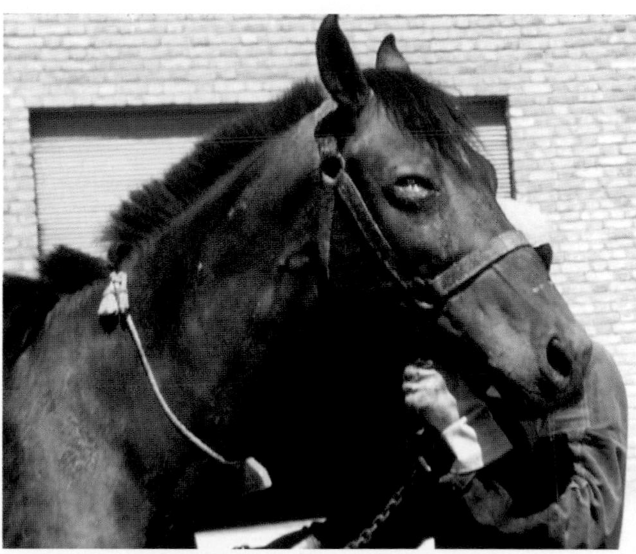

Fig. 39-7 Positive ocular reaction to mallein.

beta-lactam antibiotics.[17-20] A recent study examined the antimicrobial susceptibility patterns of 15 isolates of *B. mallei* to 35 antimicrobial agents.[20] The most effective drugs in vitro included ticarcillin-clavulanate, cefotaxime, imipenem, chloramphenicol, doxycycline, rifampicin, and erythromycin. There were no obvious differences in susceptibility patterns among human, animal, and environmental isolates. Experimental glanders is reported to respond to treatment with trimethoprim-sulfonamide antimicrobial therapy.[19]

PREVENTION

Glanders has been successfully eliminated from most countries through rigorous slaughter of mallein test–positive animals. Quarantine of infected animals and pretesting of animals in commerce are necessary components of disease control. A wide variety of national and international regulations exist, and glanders is a reportable disease for the OIE and many countries.

There is no vaccine for prevention of glanders in animals. Some research efforts are focused on development of a vaccine for people in case the organism becomes an instrument of bioterrorism.

PUBLIC HEALTH CONSIDERATIONS

Glanders is a rare but serious zoonotic disease. Most human cases are ultimately traced to direct contact with *B. mallei* through exposure to infected animals or laboratory exposure to the organism.[14,21,22] The organism often enters via cutaneous exposure through the hands or arms. The incubation period is estimated to be a few days to several weeks. Local suppuration and regional lymphadenopathy with fever and lethargy are often the first symptoms.[14] Dissemination of infection occurs 1 to 4 weeks after lymph node involvement becomes apparent. Systemic effects may include abscesses in the liver, spleen, lungs, pleura, subcutis, and muscles.[14,22] Mortality in acutely affected people with untreated disease approaches 95% within 3 weeks. As previously mentioned, several antibiotics have reliable activity against *B. mallei*.[14,17-20] In a recent report of glanders in a laboratory worker, treatment with imipenem and doxycycline for 2 weeks, followed by azithromycin and doxycycline for 6 months, was successful (in vitro susceptibility testing did not support the use of azithromycin).[14] Glanders in human patients may be confused with a variety of other diseases, including typhoid fever, tuberculosis, syphilis, erysipelas, lymphangitis, pyemia, yaws, and meliodosis.

REFERENCES

See the CD-ROM for a list of references linked to the abstract in PubMed.

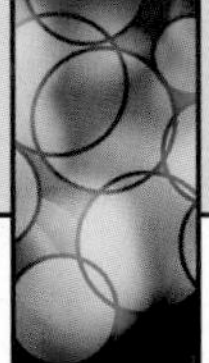

CHAPTER • 40

Brucellosis

Paul L. Nicoletti

In 1897, Bang[1] described *Bacillus abortus*, the agent of infectious abortion of cattle. In 1920, Meyer and Shaw[2] placed the organism in the genus *Brucella*. *B. abortus* was first associated with fistulous withers of horses in 1929, although descriptions of that disease significantly predate the correlation with *B. abortus* infection.

Chromosomal DNA analysis supports the use of the natural host species as a valid phenotypic characteristic for species classification of the genus *Brucella*.[3,4] Infections in horses usually involve the cattle pathogen *B. abortus*, although infections with *Brucella suis* have also been reported. Equine infection with *B. abortus* is associated with septic supraspinous bursitis ("fistulous withers"),[5-7] atlantal bursitis ("poll evil"),[7] other bursal infections,[8] septic arthritis,[9] vertebral osteomyelitis,[10] and abortion.[11,12] *B. suis* has been isolated from horses with septic bursitis, aborted equine fetuses, and the internal organs of a mare with no external signs of disease.[13,14] Because infection of horses with *B. abortus*, although rare, is more common than infection with *B. suis*, this chapter focuses on brucellosis caused by *B. abortus* unless otherwise indicated.

ETIOLOGY AND EPIDEMIOLOGY

Brucellosis in horses is caused by infection with species of the genus *Brucella*, especially *B. abortus* and *B. suis*. There are no reports of successful natural or experimental infection of horses with *Brucella melitensis* or *Brucella canis*.[15] *Brucella* spp., are nonmotile, aerobic, intracellular gram-negative cocci or short rods that are usually arranged singly or less frequently in pairs, short chains, or small groups.[3] They require complex media for growth in culture, and many strains require supplementary carbon dioxide (CO_2) for optimal growth on primary isolation. On clear media, colonies are transparent, raised, and convex with a smooth, shiny surface. They appear as a pale honey color by transmitted light.[3] The optimum temperature for growth is 37° C (98.6° F), but growth occurs between 20° and 40° C (68°-104° F).[3]

Brucella abortus infections have been reported worldwide but have been effectively eradicated from several European countries, Japan, and Israel. Cattle are the most common natural hosts for *B. abortus*, but the organism has also been isolated

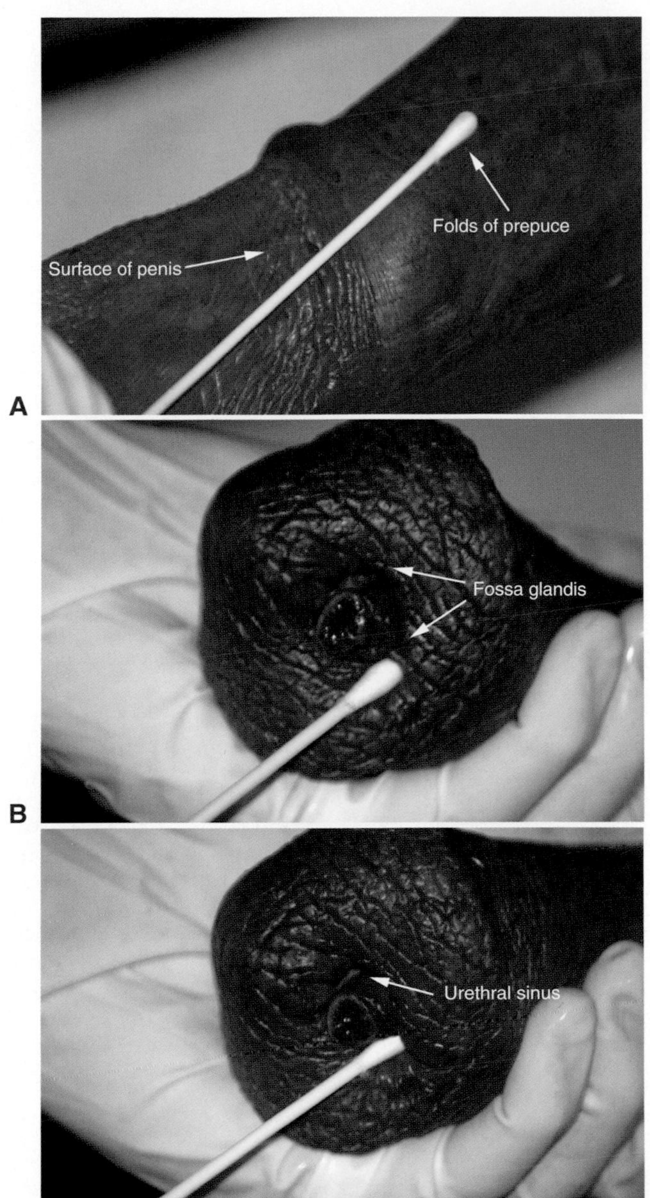

Fig. 41-3 Locations in stallion for culture of **A,** surface of penis and folds of prepuce; **B,** fossa glandis; and **C,** urethral sinus.

tetracycline, and trimethoprim-sulfamethoxazole.[16,17] U.S. Department of Agriculture (USDA) guidelines for treatment of CEM-infected mares and stallions are the same as the prophylactic treatment schedule outlined for routine testing for CEM. For an infected mare, the clitoral sinuses are flushed with a cerumenolytic agent and 0.2% nitrofuracin solution and packed with 0.2% nitrofurazone ointment. The clitoral sinuses and fossa are subsequently scrubbed for 4 more days with 4% chlorhexidine gluconate and packed with 0.2% nitrofurazone ointment. The external genitalia of infected stallions are scrubbed for 5 days with 4% chlorhexidine and packed with 0.2% nitrofurazone ointment. Both treated stallions and treated mares are retested for CEM no less than 21 days after completion of treatment, as previously described.

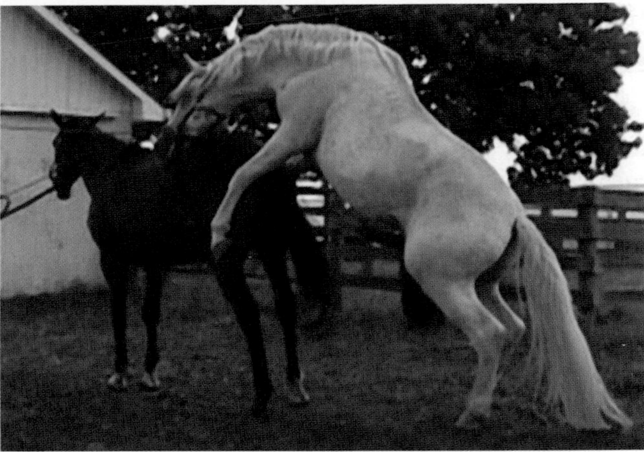

Fig. 41-4 Stallion mating the first of two test mares.

USDA treatment protocols are not always effective, and a more aggressive combination of both topical and systemic antibiotics is required to treat some CEM-positive stallions and mares.[5,18,19,20] A treatment regimen with either oral trimethoprim-sulfamethoxazole, 30 mg/kg twice daily (Mutual Pharmaceutical, Philadelphia), or an antibiotic choice based on sensitivity, along with cleaning of external genitalia (as previously described) and packing with 1% silver sulfadiazine cream (Theremazene, Kendall, Mansfield, Mass), is recommended.[18] The addition of local antibiotics to the uterus of an infected mare could also be beneficial.

PREVENTION

CEM remains a clinically and economically important disease of horses.[21] The estimated annual worth of export of horses from the U.S. is $300 million. The reintroduction of CEM into the U.S. would be costly for horse breeders and would severely reduce annual revenues of this industry.[21] Although national and international control procedures have reduced the incidence of CEM,[11,22] the disease has been detected in many countries and was recently isolated in Turkey for the first time.[23] Stringent control methods and regulations for equine movement remain necessary to minimize and control the spread of CEM.

REFERENCES

See the CD-ROM for a list of references linked to the abstract in PubMed.

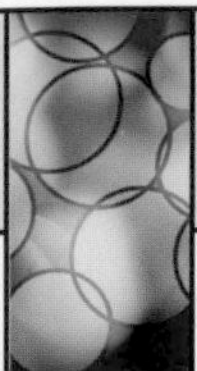

CHAPTER • 42

Anaplasma phagocytophila

Nicola Pusterla and John E. Madigan

ETIOLOGY

Anaplasma phagocytophila (also *A. phagocytophilum*, formerly *Ehrlichia equi*) is the etiologic agent of *equine granulocytic ehrlichiosis* (EGE). *A. phagocytophila* has recently been classified based on genetic analysis in the genus *Anaplasma*, with *Anaplasma marginale*, which causes infectious anemia in cattle by infecting erythrocytes, and *Anaplasma platys*, which causes canine cyclic thrombocytopenia by infecting platelets.[1]

Because 16S ribosomal ribonucleic acid (rRNA) gene sequences differ only up to three bases (99.1% homology) among former *E. equi*, *Ehrlichia phagocytophila* (cause of tick-borne fever in Europe), and the recently discovered *human granulocytic ehrlichiosis* (HGE) agent, these organisms are now all considered strains of *A. phagocytophila*. *E. equi*, *E. phagocytophila*, and the HGE agent are also closely related on the basis of morphology, host cell tropism, and antigen analysis by indirect fluorescent antibody tests.[2] The deoxyribonucleic acid (DNA) sequences of the 16S rRNA gene from the peripheral blood of naturally infected horses in Connecticut and California are identical with those of the HGE agent.[3] Moreover, blood derived from HGE patients causes typical EGE when injected into horses. In turn, the blood from these horses can transmit disease to other horses. The HE agent also induces protection in horses to subsequent challenge with *E. equi*.[4,5] These data suggest that the agent of EGE and HGE are conspecific. *A. phagocytophila* has been cultured in vitro using the tick-embryo cell line IDE8[6] and a human promyelocytic leukemia cell line HL60.[7]

Anaplasma phagocytophila is found in membrane-lined vacuoles within the cytoplasm of infected eukaryotic host cells, primarily neutrophilic and eosinophilic granulocytes. These inclusion bodies consist of one or more coccoid or coccobacillary organisms approximately 0.2 μm in diameter as well as large granular aggregates called *morulae*, which are approximately 5 μm in diameter. Organisms are visible under high, dry, or oil-immersion objective with light microscopy. They stain deep blue to pale blue-gray with Giemsa or Wright-Leishman stains. Electron microscopy reveals loosely packed, ovoid to round *A. phagocytophila* organisms in several membrane-lined vacuoles of equine granulocytes. The size of vacuoles ranges from 1.5 to 5 μm in diameter.

EPIDEMIOLOGY

Equine granulocytic ehrlichiosis occurs during late fall, winter, and spring. The horse represents an aberrant host, and it seems unlikely that infected horses could serve as effective reservoirs of *A. phagocytophila*, because the presence of the organism in an affected animal is limited to the acute phase of the disease. Horses of any age are susceptible, but the clinical manifestations are less severe in horses younger than 4 years.[8] Horses from endemic areas have a higher seroprevalence of antibody to *A. phagocytophila* than horses from nonendemic areas, suggesting the occurrence of subclinical infection in some animals.[9] Further, horses introduced into an endemic area are more likely to develop EGE than native horses.

Persistence of *A. phagocytophila* has not been demonstrated in naturally or experimentally infected horses. The disease is not contagious, but infection can be transferred readily to susceptible horses with transfusion of as little as 20 mL of blood from horses with active infection. Most often, one infected horse is observed in a group of horses in the same pasture. The disease, first reported in the late 1960s in the foothills of northern California, has since been reported in horses in Washington, Oregon, New Jersey, New York, Colorado, Illinois, Minnesota, Connecticut, Florida, Wisconsin, and outside the United States, in Canada, Brazil, and northern Europe.

In recent years, EGE has been experimentally transmitted by the western black-legged tick *(Ixodes pacificus)*[10] and the deer tick *(Ixodes scapularis)*.[11] Further, an epidemiologic study in California showed that the spatial and temporal pattern of EGE cases closely paralleled the well-characterized life history and distribution of *I. pacificus*, but not other ticks typically associated with horses.[12] In the eastern and midwestern United States, *I. scapularis* is the vector of granulocytic ehrlichiosis, and small rodents such as white-footed mice, chipmunks and voles, as well as the white-tailed deer, are potentially important reservoirs.[13] In California, white-footed mice, dusky-footed wood rats, cervids, lizards, and birds have been proposed as reservoirs.[14] In Europe, where granulocytic ehrlichiosis is transmitted by the sheep tick *(Ixodes ricinus)*, the reported reservoir hosts are wild rodents, deer, and sheep.[15]

PATHOGENESIS

The pathogenesis of EGE is poorly understood. Clearly, after entering the dermis by tick-bite inoculation and spread, presumably through lymphatics or blood, ehrlichiae invade target cells of the hematopoietic and lymphoreticular systems. Ehrlichiae replicate within vacuoles of professional phagocytes. Whether or how these granulocytic ehrlichiae directly injure cells is not known, despite clear evidence of cytolytic activity in vitro.[7] Granulocytic ehrlichiae are suspected to initiate a cascade of localized pathologic inflammatory events after invading organs such as spleen, liver, and lungs. Subsequent tissue injury is thought to be mediated locally by accumulating inflammatory cells and systematically by induction of proinflammatory responses.[16] The mechanism by which sufficient cells are removed to cause pancytopenia is unknown. However, the presence of normal cellularity or diffuse hyperplasia of bone marrow, combined with hemophagocytosis in spleen and lymph nodes, and the presence of infected granulocytes in spleen and lung support peripheral sequestration, consumption, and destruction of normal blood elements as the major mechanisms for ehrlichia-induced pancytopenia.[16]

Granulocytic ehrlichioses caused by *A. phagocytophila* are diseases that trigger dysfunction or suppression of host defenses.

It is well established that horses infected with *A. phagocytophila* are predisposed, as are humans and sheep, to develop opportunistic infections and secondary infections with bacteria, fungi, and viruses.[17] These animals develop defects in both humoral and T-cell–mediated immunity and abnormalities in normal neutrophil phagocytic and migratory functions.[18]

Immunologic studies with *A. phagocytophila* indicate both a cell-mediated and a humoral immune response to clinical infection. Horses that recover from experimental infections develop these responses by 21 days after infection.[19] In naturally infected horses, antibody titers peak 19 to 81 days after the onset of clinical signs. Immunity persists for at least 2 years and does not appear to depend on latent infection or carrier status.[20,21]

CLINICAL FINDINGS

The incubation period after experimental exposure of horses to infected ticks is 8 to 12 days and after needle inoculation of infectious blood, 3 to 10 days. The incubation period for natural infection is believed to be less than 14 days. This estimate is based on the time of onset of clinical signs in horses that had presumptive exposure to ticks while on a trail ride before returning to a nonendemic area for EGE.

The severity of clinical signs of EGE varies with the age of the horse and the duration of the illness.[8] This can make clinical recognition of EGE difficult at the first examination. Adult horses over 4 years of age generally develop characteristic progressive signs of fever, depression, partial anorexia, limb edema, petechiation, icterus, ataxia, and reluctance to move. Clinically and experimentally, it appears that horses less than 4 years old tend to develop milder signs, including moderate fever, depression, moderate limb edema, and ataxia. In horses less than 1 year old, clinical signs may be difficult to recognize, with only a fever present. During the first 1 to 2 days of infection, fever is generally high, fluctuating from 39.4° to 41.3° C (102.9°-106.3° F). Initial clinical signs are reluctance to move, ataxia, depression, icterus (Fig. 42-1), and petechiation of nasal septum mucosa (Fig. 42-2). Weakness and ataxia can be severe, to the point that horses will sustain fractures after falling. Staggering is often seen, and the tendency to assume a base-wide stance suggests proprioceptive deficits. Partial anorexia develops in most affected horses. Limb edema (Fig. 42-3) and more severe signs of disease develop by day 3 to 5, with fever and illness lasting 10 to 14 days in untreated horses. Heart rate is often modestly high (50-60 beats/min). Rarely, there is cardiac involvement with development of cardiac arrhythmias. Ventricular tachycardia and premature ventricular contractions have been observed with the usual clinical signs. The clinical course of the disease ranges from 3 to 16 days. The disease is normally self-limiting in untreated horses; fatalities can result from secondary infection and from injury secondary to trauma caused by incoordination. Abortion has not been observed in pregnant mares, and laminitis has not been reported as part of the clinical syndrome.

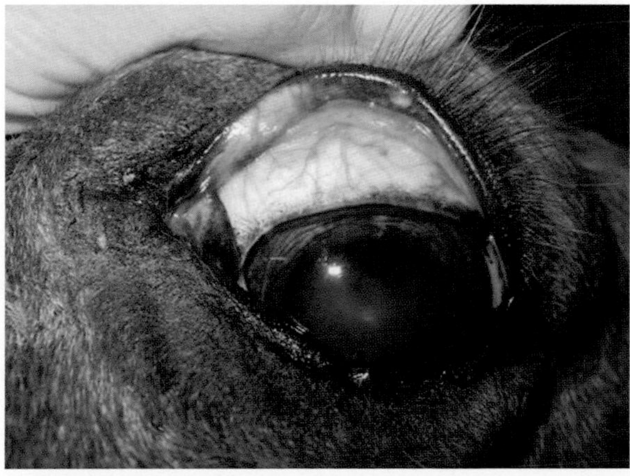

Fig. 42-1 Horse infected with *Anaplasma phagocytophila* showing icteric sclera.

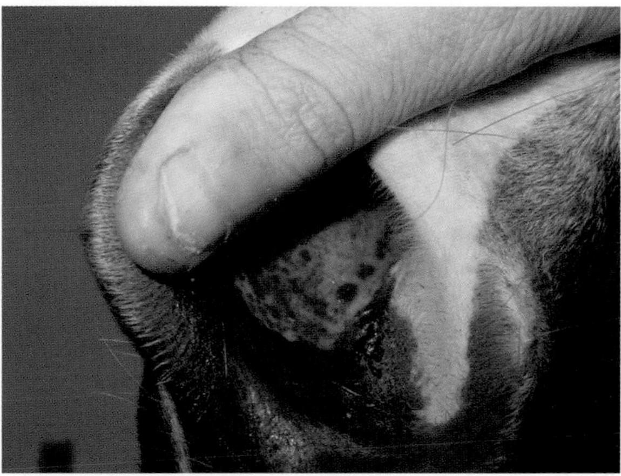

Fig. 42-2 Horse infected with *A. phagocytophila* showing petechiation of nasal septum mucosa.

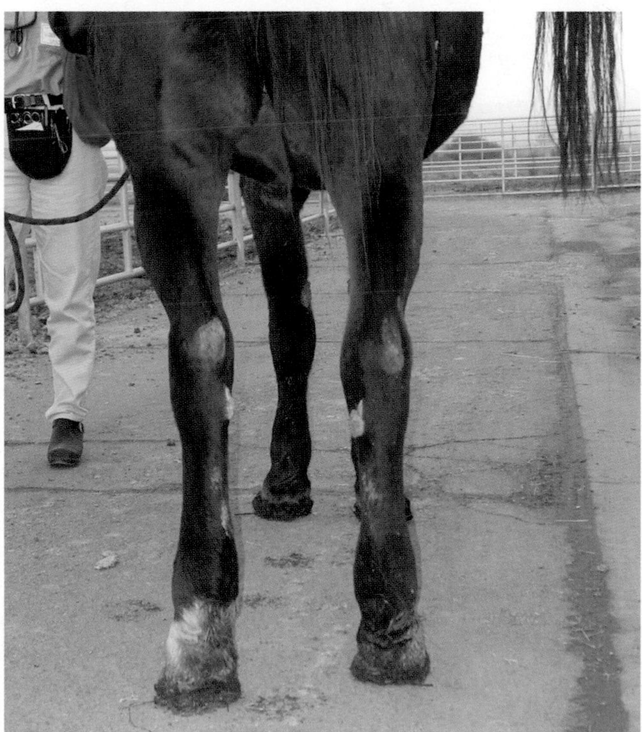

Fig. 42-3 Horse infected with *A. phagocytophila* showing distal limb edema.

The initial stage of the disease is characterized by the development of a fever and may be mistaken for a viral infection. The differential diagnoses for EGE include purpura hemorrhagica, liver disease, equine infectious anemia, equine viral arteritis, and encephalitis.

Laboratory abnormalities in horses affected with EGE may include leukopenia, thrombocytopenia, anemia, icterus, and characteristic inclusion bodies (morulae) in neutrophils and eosinophils. The morulae are pleomorphic, blue-gray to dark blue in color, and often have a spoke-wheeled appearance.

DIAGNOSIS

Diagnosis is based on awareness of geographic area for infection, typical clinical signs, abnormal laboratory findings, and visualizing characteristic morulae in the cytoplasm of neutrophils and eosinophils in a peripheral blood smear stained with Giemsa or Wright's stain (Fig. 42-4). Because affected horses are leukopenic, a greater percentage of neutrophils can be examined by use of the buffy coat preparation and subsequent staining.

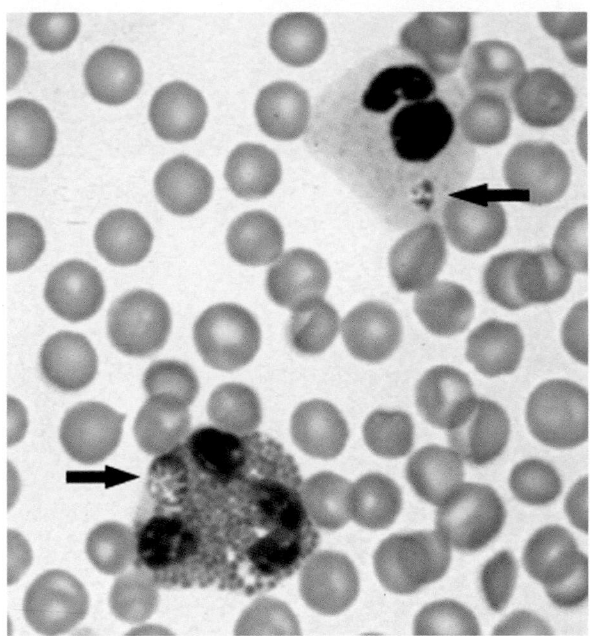

Fig. 42-4 *Anaplasma phagocytophila* inclusions *(arrows)* in neutrophilic and eosinophilic granulocyte of horse with equine granulocytic ehrlichiosis (buffy coat smear, Giemsa stain, 1000×).

The number of cells containing morulae varies from less than 1% of cells initially to between 20% and 50% of neutrophils by days 3 to 5 of infection. However, more than three ehrlichial inclusion bodies need to be seen on a blood smear to consider the diagnosis definitive.

Culture is rarely attempted for horses infected with *A. phagocytophila*. Alternatively, an indirect fluorescent antibody test is available, and paired-titer testing with a significant (fourfold or greater) rise in antibody titer to *A. phagocytophila* can be performed to confirm recent exposure retrospectively.[9] However, because inclusion bodies are always visible during the midstage of the febrile period, antibody testing is not usually required to make a definitive diagnosis.

Recently, several polymerase chain reaction (PCR) assays have been developed for members of the *A. phagocytophila* genogroup and are considered to be highly sensitive and specific.[22,23] PCR analysis is useful for the diagnosis of EGE, particularly during early and late stages, when the number of organisms may be too small for diagnosis by microscopy (Fig. 42-5).

PATHOLOGIC FINDINGS

The characteristic gross lesions observed in experimentally infected horses are hemorrhages, usually petechiae and ecchymoses, and edema. Edema is observed in the legs, ventral abdominal wall, and prepuce. Hemorrhages are most common in the subcutaneous tissues, fascia, and epimysium of the distal limbs. Histologically, there is inflammation of the small arteries and veins, primarily those in the subcutis, fascia, and nerves of the legs, as well as in the ovaries, testes, and pampiniform plexus.[17] Vascular lesions may be proliferative and necrotizing, with swelling of the endothelial and smooth muscle cells, cellular thromboses, and perivascular accumulations, primarily of monocytes and lymphocytes but also, to a lesser extent, neutrophils and eosinophils. Mild inflammatory vascular or interstitial lesions have also been reported in the kidneys, heart, brain, and lungs of animals necropsied during the course of the disease.[16] The ventricular tachycardia and premature ventricular contractions occasionally observed in affected horses are thought to be associated with myocardial vasculitis. Further, horses with a chronic bacterial infection may develop an exacerbation of the preexisting lesion (bronchopneumonia, arthritis, pericarditis, lymphadenitis, cellulitis).[17]

THERAPY

The intravenous administration of oxytetracycline at 7 mg/kg body weight once daily for 5 to 7 days has been an effective treatment for EGE.[8] Prompt improvement in clinical

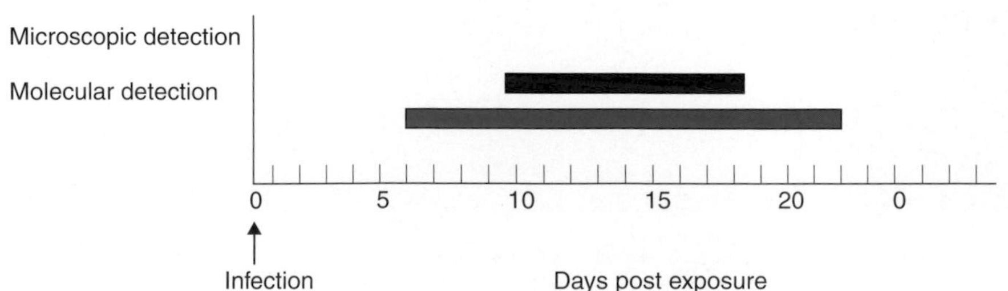

Fig. 42-5 Microscopic and molecular detection time of *A. phagocytophila* in blood of horse experimentally infected with *Ixodes scapularis.*

appearance and appetite and decrease in fever are noticed within 12 hours of treatment. Indeed, a failure of defervescence within 24 hours would strongly indicate another cause for illness. On rare occasions, horses treated for less than 7 days relapse within the following 30 days. When untreated, the disease can be self-limiting in 2 to 3 weeks if no concurrent infection is present, but weight loss, edema, and ataxia are of increased severity and duration. In treated horses, ataxia will persist for 2 to 3 days, and limb edema may persist for several days. Inclusion bodies generally are difficult to find after the first day of treatment and are no longer present within 48 to 72 hours. Supportive measures are recommended in severe cases, including fluid and electrolyte therapy, supportive limb wraps, and stall confinement of severely ataxic horses to prevent secondary injury. The prognosis in EGE is considered excellent in uncomplicated cases, in sharp contrast to some of the differential diagnoses.

PREVENTION

At present, no vaccine is available against EGE, and prevention is limited to the practice of tick control measures, such as the use of permethrin repellent products.[24]

REFERENCES

See the CD-ROM for a list of references linked to the abstract in PubMed.

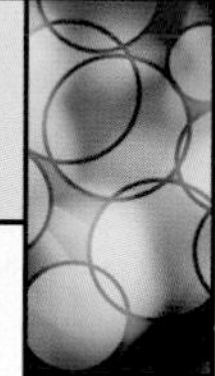

CHAPTER • 43

Neorickettsia risticii

Nicola Pusterla and John E. Madigan

ETIOLOGY

Neorickettsia risticii (formerly *Ehrlichia risticii*) is the etiologic agent of *Potomac horse fever*, also called "equine monocytic ehrlichiosis" or "equine ehrlichial colitis." *N. risticii* has recently been classified based on genetic analysis in the genera *Neorickettsia* among three other species: *Neorickettsia sennetsu* (human agent of Sennetsu fever), *Neorickettsia helminthoeca* (agent of salmon poisoning in the dog), and an ehrlichia-like bacterium present in the metacercarial stage of the fluke *Stellantchasmus falcatus* (SF agent).[1] Based on sequence analysis of the 16S ribosomal ribonucleic acid (rRNA) gene, *N. risticii* shares 98.9% homology to *N. sennetsu*, 94.8% to *N. helminthoeca*, and 99.1% to the SF agent. Strain variance has been determined among 11 *N. risticii* strains, with a maximum divergence of 0.7%.

Neorickettsia risticii is a gram-negative coccus and stains dark blue to purple with Giemsa stain and Romanowsky's stain, red with Macchiavellos stain, and pale blue with hematoxylin and eosin. The organism tends to occupy one side of the cytoplasm rather than being symmetric and is generally round. *N. risticii* divides by binary fission and is found in membrane-lined vacuoles within the cytoplasm of primarily macrophages and glandular epithelial cells in the intestine of the horse. The organism is rarely observed in peripheral blood monocytes. In cell culture or host cells, *N. risticii* occurs in two different forms, either singly or in groups *(morulae)*, the former being 0.8- to 1.5-µm electron-lucent and the latter 0.2- to 0.4-µm electron-dense bodies. *N. risticii* has been successfully cultured in human histiocytic lymphoma cells and in canine, equine, and murine monocytes.

EPIDEMIOLOGY

Potomac horse fever (PHF) was recognized originally in 1979 along the Potomac River in the state of Maryland.[2] PHF is known to occur in 43 of the United States, three Canadian provinces (Nova Scotia, Ontario, Alberta), South America (Uruguay, Brazil), Europe (The Netherlands, France), and India. Isolation or detection of the causative agent from clinical cases of the disease using conventional cell culture or molecular detection by polymerase chain reaction (PCR) has only been reported from 13 states (California, Illinois, Indiana, Kentucky, Maryland, Michigan, New York, New Jersey, Ohio, Oregon, Pennsylvania, Texas, Virginia), Nova Scotia, Uruguay, and Brazil.

The epidemiology of *N. risticii* has been the subject of intensive research efforts for more than 20 years. The disease typically occurs near freshwater streams, rivers, and on irrigated pastures, mainly during middle to late summer (May to November). The seasonal incidence of the disease, the geographic distribution of PHF, and the experimental transmission by the intradermal route implied the involvement of a blood-sucking arthropod as a vector. The historical connection between other ehrlichial agents and tick vectors prompted many to regard ticks as prime candidates for the transmission of *N. risticii*. Therefore, many studies focused on identifying an arthropod vector for PHF. Despite intensive investigation, however, no evidence was found for spread of the disease by arthropod vectors such as ticks.[3]

The causative organism is present in the feces of experimentally infected horses and can be experimentally transmitted by the oral route using feces from infected horses. These findings, together with the close serologic and molecular relationship between *N. risticii* and *N. helminthoeca* isolated from flukes, suggest that the vector of *N. risticii* may not be an arthropod but instead a helminth closely associated with aquatic habitats. Barlough et al.[4] provided strong evidence that *trematodes*, which use operculate freshwater snails as intermediate hosts, may be involved in the life cycle of *N. risticii*. This theory was confirmed when deoxyribonucleic acid (DNA) of *N. risticii* was detected by nested PCR in operculate snails (*Pleuroceridae: Juga* spp.) collected from stream waters in a northern California pasture where PHF is endemic. The results of sequencing

PCR-amplified DNA from a suite of genes (16S rRNA, groESL heat shock operon, and 51-kDa major antigen genes) indicated that the source organism was clearly related to the type strain of *N. risticii*. The PCR-amplified product is associated with the presence of virgulate cercariae in the snail secretions[5] (Fig. 43-1). The number of snails harboring the trematode stages varied from 3.3% to 93.3%, and the number of PCR-positive snails (3.3%-20%) appears to depend on the size of the snails, the month of collection, and geographic origin.

In northern California the species of snail incriminated in the life cycle of *N. risticii* is *Juga yrekaensis*, a common pleurocerid snail, which inhabits fresh or brackish stream water in the northwestern United States (Fig. 43-2). Additionally, DNA from *N. risticii* has been detected in virgulate cercariae in lymnaeid snails (*Stagnicola* spp.) from northern California, in virgulate xiphidiocercariae isolated from pleurocerid snails (*Elimia livescens*) in central Ohio, and from pleurocerid snails (*Elimia virginica*) in central Pennsylvania, suggesting that other types of snails may also harbor infected trematodes.[5-7] This type of trematode is known to become encysted in the second intermediate host. *N. risticii* DNA has been detected by PCR in mesocercariae and metacercariae in various aquatic larval, nymphal, and adult insects such as caddisflies, mayflies, damselflies, and dragonflies in northern California and in central Pennsylvania[7,8] (Fig. 43-3). PCR investigations suggest that the prevalence of aquatic insects harboring *N. risticii* varies from 10% to 80%.

Recently, two potential helminth vectors, *Acanthatrium* spp. and *Lecithodendrium* spp., both infected with *N. risticii*, were found in the intestine of bats and birds collected in northern California and Pennsylvania[9,10] (Fig. 43-4). These trematodes belong to the *Lecithodendriidae* family, common parasites of bats, birds, and amphibians in North America, which use pleurocerid freshwater snails as first intermediate hosts and aquatic insects as second intermediate hosts. Additional trematodes, members of the *Lecithodendriidae* or other families, may also act as vectors of *N. risticii* in other endemic regions of the United States.

Since *N. risticii* was first identified, no definitive reservoir host of the organism has been proposed. Seroepidemiologic studies have revealed the presence of antibody titers specific to *N. risticii* in domestic and wild animals such as dogs, cats, coyotes, pigs, and goats from regions in which PHF is endemic.[11] A variety of nonequine mammalian species, such as mice, dogs, cats, and cattle, are susceptible to *N. risticii*.[12-14] Based on vertical transmission of *N. risticii* in the trematode *Acanthatrium oregonense* and detection of *N. risticii* DNA in the blood, liver, or spleen of bats and swallows, it is speculated that these insectivores act as both definitive host of the helminth vector and natural reservoir of *N. risticii*.

The biologic activity of *N. risticii* in infected vectors has been recently investigated by the inoculation of PCR-positive trematode stages into horses and mice. Horses injected subcutaneously with *N. risticii* PCR-positive trematode stages (virgulate cercariae and sporocysts) collected from *J. yrekaensis* snails developed clinical signs and hematologic changes consistent with PHF.[15] Furthermore, *N. risticii* was transmitted to mice using PCR-positive metacercariae isolated from caddisfly

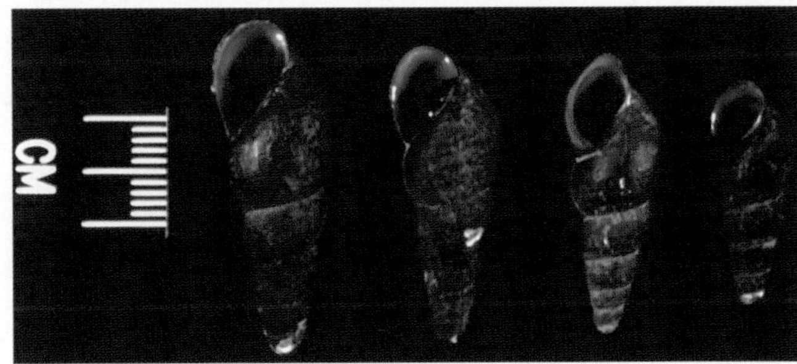

Fig. 43-2 *Juga yrekaensis* pleurocerid snails collected from Potomac horse fever (PHF)–endemic region in northern California (bar = 1 cm).

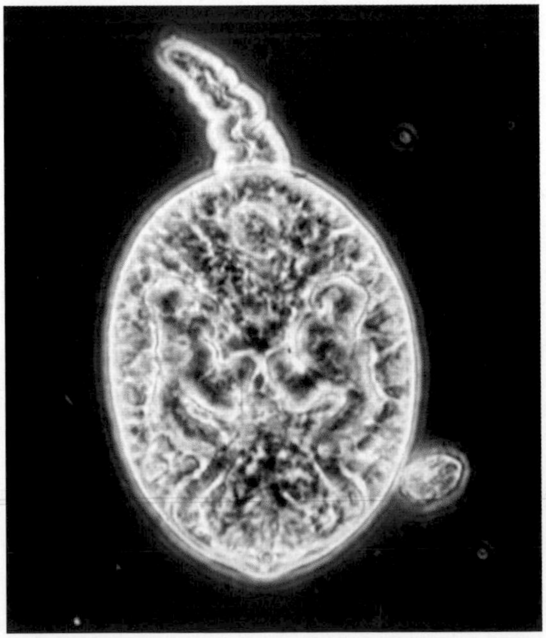

Fig. 43-1 Photomicrograph of virgulate cercaria released by pleurocerid snails of genus *Juga* (bar = 0.01 mm).

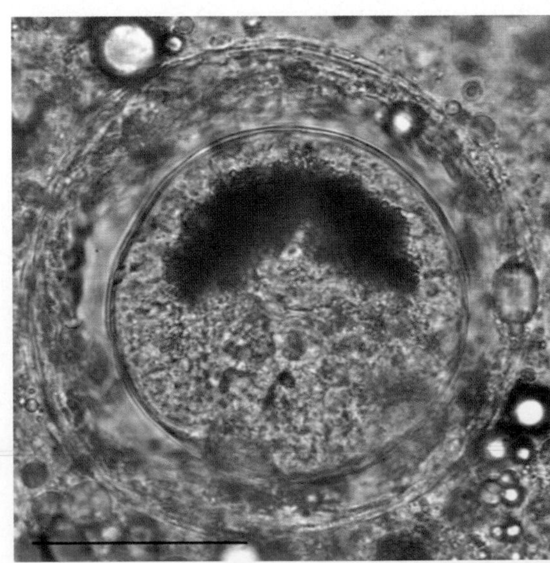

Fig. 43-3 Photomicrograph of metacercaria collected from caddisfly larva (bar = 0.2 mm). (From Madigan JE, Pusterla N: *Vet Clin North Am Equine Pract* 16:487, 2000.)

larvae (*Dicosmoecus* spp.).[8] These data confirm that *N. risticii* is associated with a helminth vector and illustrate the value of PCR technology as a screening method for epidemiologic studies.

PATHOGENESIS

The mode of transmission of *N. risticii* has remained one of the greatest mysteries of PHF. *N. risticii* has been successfully transmitted by the intravenous, intramuscular, subcutaneous, intradermal, and oral routes using whole blood from naturally infected horses or with infected cell culture material.[16-20] In light of recent epidemiologic discoveries concerning the vector of *N. risticii* and its helminth hosts, horses could conceivably be exposed to *N. risticii* through skin penetration by infected cercariae or by consuming infected cercariae in water or metacercariae in a second intermediate host such as an aquatic insect. One horse fed adult caddisflies *(Dicosmoecus gilvipes)* in northern California[21] and two horses fed adult caddisflies *(Cheumatopsyche campyla, Hydropsyche hageni)* or a mixture of adult caddisflies and mayflies *(Leucrocuta minerva)* in central Pennsylvania developed PHF.[7] These studies attempted to mimic the natural route of infection with *N. risticii* and showed that oral transmission using infected aquatic insects was not only possible, but also that the clinical disease produced was similar to that seen in naturally infected horses. Aquatic insects, such as caddisflies and mayflies, represent a likely source of infection because of their abundance in the natural environment, their high infection rate with *N. risticii* as determined by PCR, and the mass hatches regularly observed during summer and fall. Under natural conditions, horses grazing near rivers or creeks will ingest adult insects along with grass (adult insects live near water and are likely to die there) or consume adult insects trapped on the water surface. Horses also may consume insects that are attracted by stable lights and subsequently accumulate in feed and water (Fig. 43-5). A serosurvey performed at two Ohio racetracks in 1986 reported that cases of PHF were associated with certain barns as well as specific stalls in those barns.[22] Aquatic insects might have been present in larger numbers in those locations, perhaps attracted by specific lighting, and were accidentally ingested by the horses in their food.

After natural or experimental transmission in horses, *N. risticii* infects blood monocytes. Although the pathogen is readily phagocytized by monocytes, it appears to elude the host's defense mechanisms by inhibiting lysosomal fusion with phagosomes.[23] *N. risticii* can be isolated by cell culture from the peripheral blood monocytes of infected horses as early as 6 days after ingestion of adult aquatic insects harboring the organism, and bacteremia can persist up to 2 weeks after

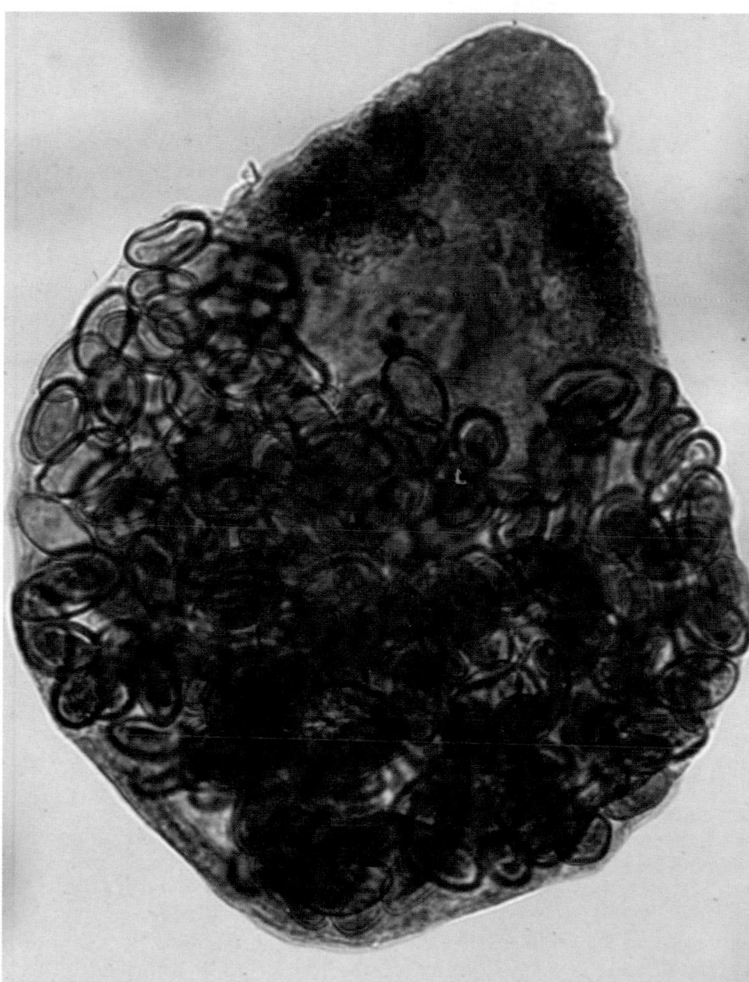

Fig. 43-4 Photomicrograph of adult *Acanthatrium* trematode collected from intestine of *Myotis yumanensis* bat (bar = 0.5 mm). (From Madigan JE, Pusterla N: *Vet Clin North Am Equine Pract* 16:487, 2000.)

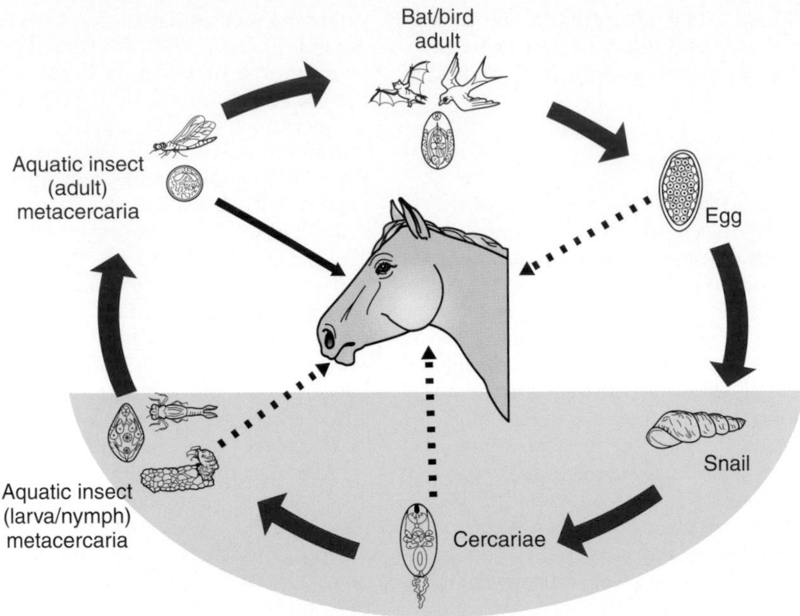

Fig. 43-5 Life cycle of helminthic vector of *Neorickettsia risticii* and natural route of transmission. Solid balck arrow represents demonstrated route of transmission with adult aquatic insects. Dashed black arrows represent possible routes of infection with trematode eggs, free cercariae, or larval/nymphal aquatic insect stages.

spontaneous resolution of clinical signs.[7] *N. risticii* also has a predilection for the intestinal wall, especially that of the large colon. Colonic epithelial cells, mast cells, and tissue macrophages are the targets of infection. Lesions are confined to the gastrointestinal tract. The resultant diarrhea is thought to be caused by loss of epithelial cell microvilli, reduction in electrolyte transport, and increase in intracellular cyclic adenosine monophosphate in infected intestinal cells. All these mechanisms contribute to the reduced luminal absorption of electrolytes (sodium and chloride) and increased water losses in the large and small colon.[24]

Neorickettsia risticii causes significant immune depression in mice and detectable alterations of the immune system in horses. Whether a clinically significant immune depression occurs in horses is unclear. Recovered horses are resistant to development of clinical disease by rechallenge for a least 20 months. Humoral and cell-mediated immune responses appear to have significant roles in conferring protection against *N. risticii*. Antibodies can be protective when they block the pathogen's attachment to or penetration of host cells. This occurs by several mechanisms, such as blocking ehrlichial binding to its specific receptor, by inhibiting ehrlichial metabolism, or by conferring antibody-dependent cell-mediated cytotoxicity. However, the presence of antibodies does not always correlate with clearance of ehrlichial organisms and presence of protective immunity. This has been shown with horses that have been vaccinated with a killed *N. risticii* vaccine and subsequently developed clinical disease after natural exposure.[25] Antibodies induced by a killed vaccine may not be effective, because protective antigens may only be expressed during cell invasion or replication. Cell-mediated immunity likely plays a dominant role in protecting the host from *N. risticii* infection, as shown for other rickettsial infections.

CLINICAL FINDINGS

The incubation period for *N. risticii* infection in horses is approximately 1 to 3 weeks. In two recent studies, horses fed aquatic insects harboring *N. risticii*–infected metacercariae developed clinical signs 9 to 15 days after oral challenge.[7,21] The clinical features of PHF have been extensively reported over the years. Naturally occurring cases of PHF are typified initially by an acute onset of mild depression and anorexia, followed by a biphasic increase in body temperature ranging from 38.9° to 41.7° C (102° to 107° F). At this stage, decreased intestinal sounds can be auscultated.

Within 24 to 48 hours, moderate to severe diarrhea ranging from "cow pie" to watery consistency develops in approximately 60% of affected horses. The onset of diarrhea is often accompanied by mild abdominal discomfort. Some horses develop severe toxemia and dehydration, which result in cardiovascular compromise characterized by increased heart rate and respiratory rate and congested mucous membranes. Subcutaneous edema along the ventral abdomen has also been observed in horse with PHF. Laminitis can supervene as a severe complication of PHF in as many as 40% of affected horses. Laminitis may progress, despite resolution of other clinical signs. Interestingly, laminitis has only been reported in naturally infected horses and probably reflects as-yet undetermined pathophysiologic mechanisms related to the natural route of transmission. It should be emphasized that a horse with PHF may present with all or any combination of these clinical signs.

Case-fatality rates vary from 5% to 30% and depend mostly on the strain involved. Fatalities are associated with toxemia and severe laminitis. Long-term problems appear to be related to sequelae such as laminitis. To date, no evidence exists that

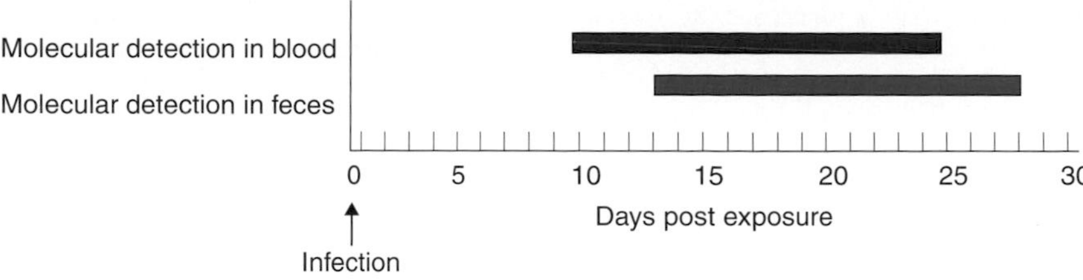

Fig. 43-6 Molecular detection time of *Neorickettsia risticii* by real-time polymerase chain reaction (PCR) in blood and feces of horses with PHF.

N. risticii infection results in chronic disease. Attempts to isolate *N. risticii* by culture or PCR after clinical signs have abated have been unsuccessful.

Transplacental transmission of *N. risticii* has been reported in natural and experimental infections, and the organism may induce abortion or resorption of the fetus or produce weak foals, which require extensive neonatal care. Pregnant mares, which exhibit clinical signs of PHF, can subsequently abort around 7 months of gestation, regardless of the severity of infection.[26] In mares experimentally infected at 90 to 120 days of gestation, abortion occurred at 65 to 111 days after inoculation.[27] Abortions are spontaneous with a fetus in fresh condition. Gross findings of the fetuses include meconium staining and petechiation of external surfaces.

Hematologic findings vary in the early stage of PHF from a transient leukopenia (white blood cell count <5000/μL), characterized by a neutropenia and a lymphopenia, to a normal hemogram, despite evidence of systemic toxicity.[28] A common finding in cases of PHF is a marked leukocytosis (>14,000/μL), usually observed within a few days of disease onset. Increases in both packed cell volume and plasma protein concentration secondary to dehydration and hemoconcentration can occur. A transient nonregenerative anemia and thrombocytopenia may develop and can be profound in some horses. Horses often present with evidence of a hypercoagulable state, characterized by significant changes in plasma fibrinogen, fibronectin, factor VIII, and plasminogen. In contrast to the tick-borne *Anaplasma phagocytophila* infection (see Chapter 42), visual observation of *N. risticii* in peripheral blood monocytes is rarely successful.

DIAGNOSIS

A provisional diagnosis of PHF is often based on the presence of typical clinical signs and the seasonal and geographic occurrence of the disease. A definitive diagnosis of PHF, however, should be based on the isolation or detection of *N. risticii* from the blood or the feces of infected horses. Serologic testing using indirect fluorescent antibody or enzyme-linked immunosorbent assay test formats is of limited value as a diagnostic tool because antibody levels to *N. risticii* may not be detectable for some time after infection. Paired serum tiers must be evaluated; single titers are useless for confirmatory testing of PHF. The reliability of the indirect immunofluorescence technique for antibody detection has been questioned because the test yields a high percentage of false-positive results.[29]

Isolation of the agent in cell culture from the peripheral blood of affected patients, although possible, can take from several days to weeks of culture before detection is successful and is not routinely available in many diagnostic laboratories. The recent development of *N. risticii*–specific PCR assays has greatly facilitated and hastened the diagnosis of PHF.[30,31] In experimentally and naturally infected animals, PCR performed on feces and peripheral blood was more sensitive than culture.[32] Conventional PCR assays, however, are time-consuming and prone to contamination. Real-time PCR platforms associated with automated nucleic acid extraction allow the detection of *N. risticii* DNA within the same day of sample receipt, making this technology a much more practical assay for routine diagnostic testing.[33] To enhance the chances of detection of *N. risticii*, the assay should be performed on blood as well as fecal samples, because the presence of the organism in blood and feces may not necessarily coincide (Fig. 43-6). Another routine application of PCR is the detection of *N. risticii* DNA in fresh or formalin-fixed and paraffin-embedded colon tissue, allowing postmortem diagnosis.

Differential diagnoses should include peritonitis and any clinical syndrome of enterocolitis, such as salmonellosis, clostridial diarrhea, or intestinal ileus secondary to displacement or obstruction. Diagnostic tests specific to ruling out these diseases should be concurrently pursued.

PATHOLOGIC FINDINGS

Gross necropsy findings in the acute stage of PHF disease include distended large colon and cecum filled with watery contents. Mucosal hyperemia and ulceration and areas of necrosis and hyperplasia of lymphoid follicles and lymph nodes may also be observed. Microscopic changes include areas of moderate to severe lymphohistiocytic infiltration of the submucosa and lamina propria of the cecum and large colon.[24] Lack of severe lesions and absence of neutrophil infiltration are important in the differential diagnosis of PHF. Both silver stain and immunoperoxidase procedure using a specific antibody to *N. risticii* can demonstrate rickettsial organisms in intestinal epithelial cells and macrophages in paraffin-embedded tissue specimens. Although not routinely done, electron microscopy can be used to detect *N. risticii* infection during disease.

Changes in fetuses aborted because of *N. risticii* infection are consistent, unique, and diagnostic of this abortion syndrome. Fetuses have increased volume of feces within the small and large intestine and liver discoloration. Microscopic findings include lymphohistiocytic enterocolitis, periportal hepatitis, lymphohistiocytic myocarditis, and severe splenic inflammation characterized by both intense lymphohistiocytic infiltration and lymphoid necrosis.[26,27] *N. risticii* can be recovered by cell culture from bone marrow, spleen, lymph node, colon, and liver of aborted fetuses.

THERAPY

Horses with PHF can be treated successfully by the intravenous (IV) administration of oxytetracycline at 6.6 mg/kg twice a day, when given early in the clinical course of the disease. A response to treatment is usually seen within 12 to 24 hours, associated with a decrease in rectal temperature followed by an improvement in demeanor, appetite, and borborygmal sounds.[34] The disease does not progress after initiation of treatment. If therapy is begun early in the course of PHF, clinical signs frequently resolve by the third day of treatment. No more than 5 days of antimicrobial therapy are usually needed. Whether treatment of clinically affected broodmares during the diarrheal stage of disease prevents subsequent abortion remains unknown. In horses exhibiting signs of enterocolitis, IV administration of polyionic fluids is extremely important to prevent hypovolemia and shock. Addition of calcium, magnesium, and potassium to fluids may be necessary in horses with prolonged anorexia and fluid losses. Concurrent use of nonsteroidal antiinflammatory drugs (NSAIDs) such as flunixin meglumine (0.25 mg/kg IV or PO q8h) or phenylbutazone (2.2-4.4 mg/kg IV or PO q12h) is indicated. Horses developing severe protein-losing enteropathy associated with decreased albumin concentrations may benefit from plasma transfusion. Preventive measures for laminitis, the most common potentially lethal sequela of PHF, should be implemented as well. Although no specific therapy is universally recognized to prevent laminitis, the authors recommend stall confinement of affected horses, use of foot support (deep bedding, padded support), ice for the feet, and administration of NSAIDs as previously described.

PREVENTION

Several inactivated, whole-cell vaccines based on the same strain of *N. risticii* are commercially available and have been used in endemic areas for several years to protect horses from PHF. Vaccination has been reported to prevent all clinical signs except fever in 78% of experimentally infected ponies.[35] Protection conferred by this vaccine appears to be much shorter in duration than protection after natural infection, which can last up to 2 years. For unexposed horses, considering the time required to develop immunity after vaccination, the short-lasting humoral immunity, and the existence of antigenic variations in the field, it is questionable how much benefit the vaccine will provide under field conditions. Vaccine failure has been reported and attributed to antigenic and genomic heterogeneity among *N. risticii* isolates.[25] Vaccine failure may also be caused by lack of protection at the site of exposure, because the natural route of transmission seems to be the oral route. An improved vaccine for PHF is strongly desired in the future.

If vaccination of horses is performed using inactivated vaccines, the primary series should include two vaccines given 4 weeks apart. A third dose should be given if the patient is a foal that received the first dose at less than 5 months of age. Thereafter, boosters should be administered at 4- to 6-month intervals. *N. risticii*–induced abortion is not prevented by vaccination.

The ingestion of aquatic insects carrying infected trematodes is probably the only means of transmission of *N. risticii* under natural circumstances. In endemic regions, control measures should limit access of susceptible horses to freshwater streams, ponds, and irrigated pastures during peak incidence.

REFERENCES

See the CD-ROM for a list of references linked to the abstract in PubMed.

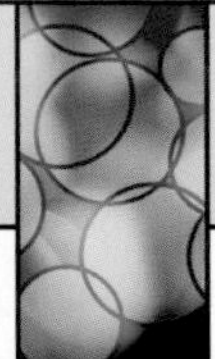

CHAPTER • 44

Enteric Clostridial Infections

J. Scott Weese

ETIOLOGY

The genus *Clostridium* comprises a diverse group of gram-positive, anaerobic, spore-forming bacteria (see Chapter 27), many of which have been implicated as pathogens of a variety of body systems in different animal species. In particular, *Clostridium difficile* and *Clostridium perfringens* are important enteropathogens and in some areas are the most frequently identified causes of colitis in horses.[1-7]

Clostridium difficile is the most commonly diagnosed cause of antimicrobial-associated and nosocomial diarrhea in humans.[8] (Figs. 44-1 and 44-2). It has received increasing attention over the past few years because apparent changes in the incidence and severity and large outbreaks of nosocomial disease have been reported.[9,10] In horses, a variety of studies have implicated *C. difficile* as a cause of enterocolitis in adult horses and foals,[1,2,4-7,11-13] and disease has been reproduced experimentally in immunocompetent foals.[14] *C. difficile* can be found throughout the environment in veterinary hospitals and horse farms.[15-17] Outbreaks of *C. difficile*–associated disease (CDAD) have been reported in an equine hospital and on farms.[5,6,18]

Although of lesser importance than *C. difficile*, *C. perfringens* is a recognized cause of nosocomial and antimicrobial-associated diarrhea in humans[19] (Fig. 44-3). It is a leading cause of food poisoning through production of an enterotoxin in improperly stored foods.[20] *C. perfringens* is commonly found in the intestinal tracts of a variety of animal species and in the environment, and it has been described as being the most widely occurring pathogenic bacterium.[21] It is also a recognized cause of enteric disease in horses of all ages.[3,4,7,22-25]

A variety of other clostridia, including *Clostridium sordellii* and *Clostridium septicum* may also be involved in equine colitis;[26,27] however, minimal information is currently available. *Clostridium spiroforme* and *Clostridium colinum* are causes of enteric disease in other species, but their role in equine disease, if any, is unknown.[21] Implication of other clostridia in equine diarrhea is hampered by limitations in specific diagnostic tests

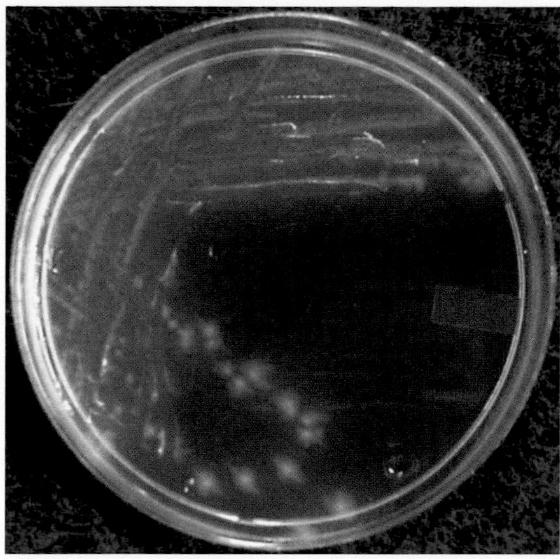

Fig. 44-1 Colony morphology of *Clostridium difficile* on cycloserine-cefoxitin fructose agar (CCFA), a selective and differential culture medium used for isolation of *C. difficile*.

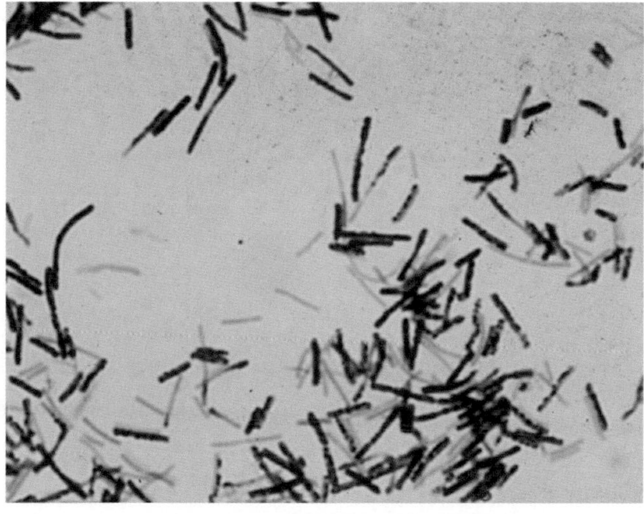

Fig. 44-2 Gram stain morphology of *Clostridium difficile*. Note the long, thin rods. The variable staining appearance (pink to purple) may be encountered in cultures after 48 hours or longer.

and difficulties in determining whether a clostridial species is part of the normal microflora, has overgrown in response to flora disruption from diarrhea of another etiology, or is the primary etiologic agent.

EPIDEMIOLOGY AND PATHOGENESIS

Clostridium difficile

The pathogenesis of CDAD in horses presumably occurs from proliferation of toxigenic strains of *C. difficile* in the intestinal tract, with subsequent toxin production and development of enterocolitis. *C. difficile* can produce a variety of toxins.

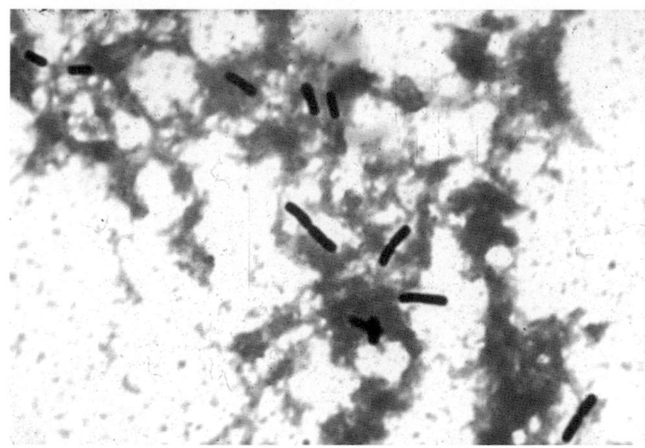

Fig. 44-3 Gram stain appearance of *Clostridium perfringens*, demonstrating the characteristic appearance of short, thick, gram-positive (purple) rods.

Table • **44-1**

Classification of* Clostridium perfringens *Isolates Based on Production of Toxins

	TOXINS					
TYPE	ALPHA	BETA	EPSILON	IOTA	BETA-2	ENTEROTOXIN
A	×				±	±
B	×	×	×		±	±
C	×	×			±	±
D	×		×		±	±
E	×			×	±	±

Toxin A, an enterotoxin, and *toxin B*, a cytotoxin, have been evaluated most extensively and are believed to work synergistically to cause disease (Table 44-1). The vast majority of toxigenic *C. difficile* isolates produce both these toxins; however, a small percentage of isolates from humans are toxin A negative and toxin B positive but are able to produce disease.[28] A toxin A–negative, B–positive strain was recently isolated from a horse with duodenitis and proximal jejunitis (L. Arroyo, personal communication). Some isolates, including those from horses, also produce a binary toxin (CDT), but the role of this toxin in disease is currently unclear.[29,30] Not all strains of *C. difficile* are able to cause disease; approximately 13% of equine isolates cannot produce any known toxins and are clinically irrelevant.[31]

A small percentage of normal horses may carry toxigenic strains of *C. difficile* without adverse effects, although the prevalence of subclinical carriage in normal adult horses is quite low (0%-1%).[2,7,15,16] Antimicrobial therapy may influence colonization rate, as demonstrated by the more frequent isolation of *C. difficile* from horses after penicillin treatment and experimental inoculation compared with nontreated horses.[32] Age also apparently influences colonization rates. Baverud et al.[16] reported subclinical colonization in 29% of foals less than 14 days of age, but in less than 1% of older foals.

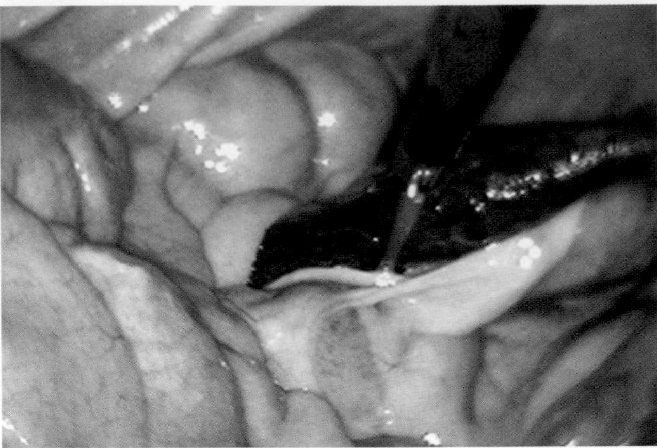

Fig. 44-4 Exploratory laparoscopy in horse with duodenitis and proximal jejunitis. Note the hyperemic small intestine.

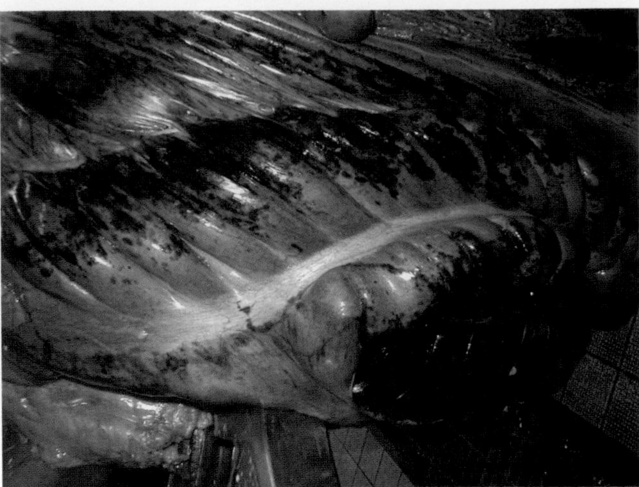

Fig. 44-5 *Clostridium difficile* colitis. Note the widespread petechial and ecchymotic hemorrhages consistent with disseminated intravascular coagulation.

Antimicrobial therapy is the main risk factor for development of CDAD in humans.[8] Penicillins, cephalosporins, and clindamycin are considered the highest-risk antimicrobials in humans;[33,34] recent evidence suggests that fluoroquinolone administration may also be an important risk factor.[35] Antimicrobial therapy is presumably also an important risk factor for development of CDAD in horses. Initial studies linking antimicrobial therapy and CDAD in horses involved identification of colitis in mares whose foals were being treated with erythromycin. It was presumed that mares were being exposed to low levels of erythromycin during treatment of their foal.[1] Subsequently, CDAD was reproduced experimentally with low-dose erythromycin administration, supporting the observational association of CDAD with erythromycin.[36] Another study reported that all affected horses had been treated with beta-lactam antimicrobials;[2] however, the risks of certain antimicrobials have not been objectively evaluated. The use of proton pump inhibitors (PPIs) is an important risk factor for CDAD in hospitalized humans.[37] The relative risk of omeprazole administration in development of CDAD in horses has not been evaluated.

The role of clostridia in small intestinal disease of horses is less well understood, but recent evidence suggests that *C. difficile* may be a cause of duodenitis and proximal jejunitis (anterior enteritis; Fig. 44-4)[38] (L. Arroyo, personal communication).

Clostridium perfringens

Unlike *C. difficile, C. perfringens* is a normal inhabitant of the equine intestinal tract and can be found in a large percentage of normal horses. Tillotson et al.[39] isolated *C. perfringens* from 19% to 35% of broodmares and more than 90% of 3-day-old foals. Although *C. perfringens* is commonly found in healthy horses, it can be a pathogen. The pathogenesis of disease is unclear, and the reason that some horses develop disease likely relates to a combination of host and bacterial factors. A study evaluating foal management practices associated with *C. perfringens* diarrhea identified housing in a stall or drylot for the first 3 days of life; the presence of other livestock on the premises; delivery of dirt, sand, or gravel; and feeding of small amounts of hay and grain to the mare postpartum as risk factors for development of *C. perfringens* enteritis in foals.[40] Antimicrobial treatment is likely a risk factor as well in adult horses and foals.

The type of *C. perfringens* is also a very important determinant of disease. *Clostridium perfringens* isolates are classified into different types based on production of four major toxins; alpha, beta, epsilon, and iota (see Table 44-1). In addition, a variety of other toxins may be produced, including beta-2 (β_2) toxin and enterotoxin.[7,41,42] While β_2 toxin and enterotoxin are not classified as major toxins, they may be the most important toxins clinically and both have been independently associated with diarrhea in adult horses and foals.[3,4,7,38,43] Type A is the predominant type in normal and diarrheic horses.[39,43] All type A strains produce alpha toxin in varying amounts, although the role of alpha toxin alone in production of disease is questionable. While type A strains have been associated with disease in horses,[44] this may be based on production of β_2 toxin or enterotoxin by some strains,[43] not because of inherent pathogenicity of all type A strains. A correlation between the presence of β_2 toxin and fatal enterocolitis has been reported.[42] Although less common, type C strains have been associated with enterocolitis horses, particularly severe disease in foals.[23,39,45] There are limited reports of disease caused by type B[46,47] and D strains.[48]

CLINICAL FINDINGS

The "classic" presentation of clostridial enteric disease is acute colitis. However, the clinical presentation will vary depending on a variety of factors, including the area of the gastrointestinal tract that is affected. It is impossible to differentiate CDAD from *C. perfringens*–associated diarrhea or clostridial diarrhea from other infectious causes of enterocolitis, because all the major pathogens can cause highly variable diseases, and there are no pathognomonic clinical or clinicopathologic abnormalities.

If the large colon is affected, diarrhea with varying degrees of depression, dehydration, toxemia, colic, anorexia, and pyrexia may be present. The clinical condition can be highly variable, ranging from mild diarrhea to peracute, rapidly fatal, necrohemorrhagic colitis (Fig. 44-5). In some horses, death may occur before diarrhea is passed.

If only the small intestine and cecum are affected, diarrhea may not be observed because of the tremendous absorptive capacity of the large colon. In these horses, colic, depression, pyrexia, hypoproteinemia, toxemia, and leukopenia may be present. If the proximal small intestine is involved, gastric reflux may develop.

Mortality rates are highly variable. With acute CDAD, mortality rates of up to 42% have been reported, with adult horses more likely to die than foals. Mortality of adult horses with acute CDAD is higher than for colitis of other etiologies.[7] Similar data are not available for *C. perfringens;* however, certain strains of *C. perfringens* may be important causes of severe, fatal enterocolitis.[42]

Complications such as laminitis and thrombophlebitis frequently develop in horses with colitis of any etiology. Although it is likely that the integrity of the intestinal mucosa is often compromised, clinically relevant bacterial translocation is infrequently identified. In some patients, thrombosis of major intestinal vessels, presumably because of disseminated intravascular coagulation (DIC), will result in rapid deterioration, with ischemic necrosis, severe pain, abdominal distention, and death.

DIAGNOSIS

Clostridium difficile

The "gold standard" for diagnosis of CDAD is detection of toxin B in feces using the cell cytotoxicity assay.[49] However, this test is time-consuming, expensive, and not readily available commercially. Clinically, diagnosis typically requires identification of *C. difficile* toxin A or B or both in fecal samples.[49,50] A variety of immunoassays are available and are widely used; however, none has been specifically validated for use in horses, and the sensitivity and specificity of the different tests are unclear. In human studies, sensitivities of different immunoassays range from 65% to 95%, with specificities between 70% and 100%.[49,51] Care should be taken to determine which antigens an immunoassay is identifying. Some tests detect *glutamate dehydrogenase* (GDH), sometime referred to as "common antigen," which is present in toxigenic and nontoxigenic strains. Detection of GDH can be used as a screening test, particularly because inexpensive and rapid tests are available, but cannot be used for a diagnosis of CDAD.[51] At present, detection of toxins in feces by *enzyme immunoassay* (EIA) should be the clinical standard for diagnosis, either as the sole test or after a positive GDH screening EIA. *C. difficile* toxins are stable for prolonged periods in fecal samples refrigerated or frozen,[52] and high temperatures should be avoided during sample storage and submission.

Culture for *C. difficile* can be performed but is not diagnostic by itself (see Fig. 44-1). Inherent problems exist with culture-based diagnosis. Because some *C. difficile* isolates are nontoxigenic and clinically irrelevant, culture alone is not useful. Culture combined with further testing (e.g., PCR) to determine whether isolates are able to produce toxins is more useful, but questions linger about the diagnostic value of this methodology in the absence of detection of toxins in feces. *C. difficile* is also difficult to isolate by a laboratory with little experience dealing with this fastidious organism. At this point, it appears that culture is best reserved for epidemiologic analysis and evaluation of antimicrobial susceptibility, if antimicrobial resistance is a concern. Direct polymerase chain reaction (PCR) analysis of feces has also been evaluated as a diagnostic test for clostridial disease.[53] However, concerns remain regarding the sensitivity of direct fecal PCR and basing a diagnosis solely on detection of toxigenic isolates.

Clostridium perfringens

Diagnosis of *C. perfringens* enteritis is more complicated because it is a commensal organism that is commonly present in normal animals, including the majority of horses with diarrhea not associated with *C. perfringens* enterotoxin. Isolation of *C. perfringens* from feces is not diagnostic, nor is quantitative culture of *C. perfringens* or enumeration of bacterial spores in fecal smears.[7] Genotyping of *C. perfringens* isolates may be useful, particularly if testing for β_2 toxin and enterotoxin is performed. Genotyping is likely most useful when strains are identified that are uncommon in normal horses and highly associated with severe disease (e.g., type C). Detection of specific *C. perfringens* toxins in feces would be the preferred method of diagnosis. Two types of enterotoxin assay are currently available: EIA and *reverse passive latex agglutination* (RPLA) test.[24] The RPLA has questionable specificity and is not frequently used. A commercial EIA is more often used, but an objective evaluation of the sensitivity and specificity is lacking and would aid in test interpretation. A recent study in humans reported low sensitivity but high specificity for a commercial enterotoxin EIA.[54]

Other Clostridia

Diagnosis of other clostridia as causes of enteric disease is difficult. General anaerobic culture could be performed, but it would be difficult to ascribe disease to a certain bacterial species in the absence of organized research studies because of the variability in the equine microflora and the relatively poor overall knowledge of the equine clostridial microflora. This was highlighted by a report of experimental lincomycin-induced colitis.[55] *Clostridium cadaveris* was initially implicated as the cause, but this was subsequently refuted.

TREATMENT

Supportive care is the most important component of a treatment plan for clostridial enteritis of any presentation or etiology. Specific treatments may be useful adjunctively. Although often used, there is little evidence to support broad-spectrum systemic antimicrobial therapy in adult horses with colitis. The goal of systemic antimicrobial therapy in horses with colitis is the prevention or treatment of *bacterial translocation*, or migration of bacteria across the compromised intestinal mucosa. Scant evidence exists to suggest that bacterial translocation is a significant clinical problem in adult horses, and antimicrobial therapy could further disrupt the already-perturbed intestinal microflora. However, the real risks and benefits have not been adequately evaluated, and some clinicians choose to treat certain horses with systemic antimicrobials. In adult horses, systemic antimicrobial therapy is sometimes used in those with severe neutropenia, marked toxic changes in white blood cells, hemorrhagic diarrhea, or persistent or intermittent pyrexia. Broad-spectrum antimicrobial therapy is probably indicated in all neonatal foals with colitis.

Specific antimicrobial therapy directed against enteric clostridia may be useful and is widely used clinically, although objective data are not available. In humans with uncomplicated antimicrobial-associated diarrhea, withdrawal of antimicrobial therapy is often the first treatment,[8] with specific antimicrobial therapy reserved for nonresponsive or more severe cases, or in compromised or otherwise high-risk individuals. Antimicrobial sensitivity testing of enteric clostridia is rarely performed by diagnostic laboratories, and treatment choices are usually based on historical information on antimicrobial sensitivity and response to treatment.

Metronidazole is widely used for the treatment of colitis in horses and has been reported to be effective in the treatment of idiopathic colitis.[56] Studies evaluating the efficacy of metronidazole in clostridial colitis in horses have not been reported, but the author's clinical impression is that metronidazole is an important and useful treatment. Metronidazole resistance among equine C. *difficile* isolates is rare but has been reported.[5] Less information is available regarding the antimicrobial susceptibility of equine C. *perfringens* isolates, although metronidazole appears to be an appropriate choice. The author currently uses an empiric dosing regimen of 15 mg/kg orally (PO) every 8 hours (q8h) for horses of all ages; a dose of 10 mg/kg PO q8-12h has also been recommended for neonates.[57]

Zinc bacitracin has been evaluated as a treatment of colitis in horses.[58] This antimicrobial is effective against C. *perfringens* in vitro, but almost universal resistance among C. *difficile* isolates has been reported.[7,31] Zinc bacitracin is perhaps best used as a second-line therapy when there has been poor response to metronidazole or when metronidazole is contraindicated (e.g., pregnant mares).

Vancomycin is often used for the treatment of refractory CDAD in humans.[8] Although reasonable from a pharmacologic standpoint, however, serious consideration should be given to the equine use of drugs such as vancomycin that are of critical importance in human medicine, particularly without objective evidence of necessity and efficacy.

Adsorption of clostridial toxins in the intestinal tract might be a useful means of decreasing the severity of disease. Further, adsorption of endotoxin that is normally present in the intestinal tract could reduce clinical signs of endotoxemia that result when endotoxin is absorbed across a compromised mucosal barrier. *Ditrioctahedral smectite* (BioSponge, Platinum Performance, Bellton, Calif.) adsorbs C. *difficile* toxins A and B, C. *perfringens* enterotoxin, and endotoxin in vitro.[59] Clinical studies evaluating this product for the treatment of colitis have not been reported, but the clinical impression among some clinicians is positive.

Saccharomyces boulardii is a yeast that is effective in the treatment of recurrent (but not initial) CDAD in humans and for the prevention of β-lactam–associated diarrhea.[60-62] There are anecdotal reports of its use in horses, but neither safety nor efficacy has been established. Probiotics are often recommended as adjunctive treatments in equine colitis; however, there is currently no evidence of efficacy.

Preliminary studies in people suggest that immunoglobulin therapy might be useful in intractable or severe CDAD.[63] Immunotherapy for C. *perfringens*–associated disease has not been reported. The author is not aware of any studies that have evaluated immunotherapy for clostridial disease in horses.

PREVENTION

Four aspects of disease prevention need to be considered: prevention of sporadic disease, prevention of transmission of disease from affected to other horses, management of outbreaks, and prevention of zoonotic transmission.

Prudent use of antimicrobials is likely one of the most important means of preventing clostridial diarrhea.[64] Antimicrobials should only be used when necessary, and drugs associated with a higher risk of colitis should be avoided unless other options are not available. Antimicrobials that have not been properly evaluated in horses should not be administered. Infection control methods to reduce infectious diseases, in general, should be used to reduce the overall incidence of infectious disease and potentially reduce the need for antimicrobials. Care should be taken to reduce accidental ingestion of erythromycin by mares when their foals are being treated for *Rhodococcus equi* pneumonia.[64] Ideally, foals should be treated outside the stall and their mouths washed after treatment. Because low but potentially dangerous concentrations of erythromycin can be found in feces, stalls of housed mares and foals should be cleaned frequently during the day.

Affected horses should be isolated. Barrier precautions (overboots or dedicated boots, specific barrier gown or other item to protect underlying clothing and skin, and gloves) should be used whenever these horses are handled or their environment is entered (see Chapters 66 and 67).

Because they are spore-forming bacteria, clostridia can persist in the environment for prolonged periods. Even C. *difficile*, which is exquisitely sensitive to aerobic environments, can persist for years as spores resistant to environmental effects and disinfectants. C. *perfringens* is present in a large percentage of normal horses and consequently in the horse's environment.[39] Elimination of all clostridia from the environment is neither reasonable nor practical; however, measures should be taken to reduce high-level environmental contamination by affected horses and to reduce the overall environmental clostridial burden. If clostridial diarrhea is suspected, all in-contact items should be disinfected, including all medical instruments, buckets, shovels, wheelbarrow, and bowls. Many items are difficult, if not impossible, to disinfect. Similarly, the stall and pasture environments are virtually impossible to disinfect. In these situations the goal should be to reduce the environmental burden. This can be achieved with careful cleaning, removal of all organic debris, and application of an appropriate disinfectant (see Chapter 67). There is evidence that bleach cleaning can reduce nosocomial CDAD in humans,[65] and bleach can be an effective disinfectant on horse farms and equine hospitals in some situations; however, bleach is readily inactivated by organic debris and will be ineffective unless used properly. Accelerated hydrogen peroxide *(not regular hydrogen peroxide)* and peroxygen disinfectants are also effective against clostridial spores[66,67] and may be more useful in equine practice. Regardless of the disinfectant used, proper disinfection requires careful cleaning before the disinfectant is applied.[68] Frequent handwashing by personnel in contact with infected horses is important, even if gloves are used. Hand hygiene and the use of gloves reduce nosocomial CDAD in humans.[69]

Outbreaks of clostridial diarrhea can occur on farms and in veterinary hospitals.[6,18] Judicious perioperative antimicrobial use and proper environmental cleaning are important for prevention and control of these outbreaks. On farms, outbreaks seem to be more common in foals on large breeding farms. Outbreaks tend to accelerate over the foaling season, and the incidence of disease can be quite high in late foals. Outbreaks are less common in adult horses but can occur. If an outbreak of clostridial diarrhea is encountered, an investigation of potential antimicrobial contamination of feed is warranted. Mass treatment (metronidazole) of unaffected animals is not recommended.

Vaccines are available for prevention of C. *perfringens*–associated disease in other species. These vaccines are designed to protect against types C and D, not enterotoxin or β_2 toxin. Although there are anecdotal reports of use of these vaccines in horses, particularly vaccination of mares during outbreaks in foals on breeding farms, vaccination with ruminant vaccines is not recommended because of the anecdotally high incidence of adverse effects (muscle irritation, abscess formation), lack of relevant strains, and lack of evidence of efficacy.

Probiotics are widely available commercially, and some are marketed for the prevention of diarrhea, particularly during antimicrobial therapy. There is currently no evidence that commercial probiotics are effective at prevention of clostridial enteritis in horses. It has been generally accepted that probiotics are, at worse, harmless; however, a recent study reported that probiotic therapy was associated with development of disease in foals.[70]

PUBLIC HEALTH CONSIDERATIONS

Both *C. difficile* and *C. perfringens* are recognized enteropathogens in people, but public health risks associated with equine clostridial infections have not been adequately explored. A recent study reported that approximately 20% of clinical *C. difficile* isolates from horses were indistinguishable from isolates from humans with CDAD.[71] Although this does not confirm interspecies transmission, it suggests that this could occur. Potential risks associated with other clostridial infections are unclear.

Regardless of the public health risks associated with clostridial infection, all horses with enteritis should be treated as infectious because of the possibility of *salmonellosis*, an important zoonotic pathogen. General infection control measures should be equally effective at reducing the risk of zoonotic transmission of clostridia or *Salmonella* spp. Infection control protocols as described earlier should be useful at decreasing the risk of zoonotic transmission. Additionally, people who may be at higher risk for contracting a zoonotic bacterial enteric disease, such as very young or very old persons, immunosuppressed patients, and possibly those being treated with antimicrobials, should be restricted from contact with affected horses, with their environment, and with potentially contaminated items.

REFERENCES

See the CD-ROM for a list of references linked to the abstract in PubMed.

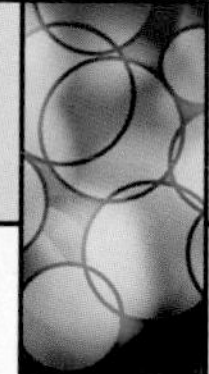

CHAPTER • 45

Systemic Clostridial Infections

CLOSTRIDIAL MYONECROSIS

Simon F. Peek

Etiology

Clostridial myonecrosis in horses is most often caused by infection with *Clostridium perfringens*,[1,2] although sporadic cases have been described in association with other *Clostridium* species, including *C. septicum*,[1,3,4] *C. chauvoei*,[1,2,5] *C. novyi*,[1,6] *C. ramosum*, *C. sporogenes*,[1] and *C. fallax*.[7] The majority of cases in the literature have been single-species infections, but mixed infections have been reported.[1,3] These highly pathogenic clostridial organisms are gram-positive, spore-forming, anaerobic bacilli that can elaborate numerous potent exotoxins. Vegetative growth of these clostridial species is accompanied by production of dermonecrotizing and vasoactive toxins that lead to gas production, extensive tissue damage, and necrosis, as well as rapidly developing, life-threatening systemic toxemia.

Epidemiology

The prevalence of clostridial myonecrosis is low, and although the disease is sporadic, more cases appear to occur in certain regions. Many cases reported in the literature are from the northeastern[1,2,4] and midwestern[1,5,8] areas of the United States, but the disease may occur anywhere in the United States,[3] Canada,[9] Europe,[10] and the Southern Hemisphere.[7,11] Although species such as *Clostridium perfringens* can frequently be cultured from the environment and soil wherever livestock are found, the means by which spores or vegetative organisms gain access to areas of affected soft tissue is not fully understood. Some of the species involved, including the most frequently isolated species, *C. perfringens*, can also be found within the gastrointestinal tract, in both the vegetative and the spore form, and some strains may be regarded as commensals. Spores of some clostridia (e.g., *C. sporogenes*, *C. histolyticum*) can be found in healthy equine muscle tissue, which suggests that after creation of appropriate anaerobic conditions, these spores may vegetate and begin exponential growth.[12] However, spores of species typically isolated from clinical cases of equine myonecrosis have not, as yet, been identified dormant within muscle tissue.

Most cases of equine myonecrosis temporally occur soon after parenteral injection of pharmacologic or biologic agents (≤48 hours) in the affected area of the body.[1,2,9] The condition is more common in the cervical musculature,[1-4,8,9] but occasional cases involving the gluteal muscles[1,8,9] and rarely the caudal thigh musculature[1] have been reported. Cervical and throatlatch lesions are sometimes encountered secondary to inadvertent perivascular leakage of pharmacologics intended for intravenous (IV) administration.[1] Traumatic wounds have rarely been associated with the condition.[1,9] A wide array of pharmacologic and biologic preparations have been incriminated as inciting causes of clostridial myonecrosis, including nonsteroidal antiinflammatories,[1,2,4,8,9] antihistamines,[1,2,9] multivitamins,[1,2,9] antipyretics,[1,7,13] dewormers,[2,9,14] vaccines, diuretics,[1] and synthetic prostaglandins.[13] The most frequently reported pharmacologic agent associated with the development of clostridial myonecrosis is *flunixin meglumine*, with the most cases occurring in the cervical region.[1-11,13,14]

Pathogenesis

Most information regarding the pathogenesis of clostridial myonecrosis comes from rodent models of infection. Because identical species of clostridia, specifically *C. perfringens* and *C. septicum*, are the most commonly recognized causes of human clostridial myonecrosis, it is reasonable to assume that etiologic-specific pathogenic factors are comparable. During vegetative growth of *C. perfringens*, the primary toxin implicated in the disease process is alpha (α) toxin, a dermonecrotic toxin with both phospholipase C and sphingomyelinase activity.[15] The definitive role that α-toxin plays during myonecrosis has been well established using controlled vaccine protection studies in which mice immunized against the C-terminal domain of the α-toxin were protected against lethal intramuscular (IM) doses of the organism, whereas unvaccinated controls were not.[16] Deletional mutants of *C. perfringens* in which the structural α-toxin gene has been removed are nonpathogenic, and virulence is restored by recombination with a plasmid expressing the wild-type gene.[17] Other toxins that can be produced during vegetative growth by *C. perfringens* and other clostridial species include theta toxin (perfringolysin), kappa toxin (collagenase), and mu toxin (hyaluronidase).[15,18] Although other exotoxins elaborated by *C. perfringens* (and also other species) have highly potent and pathogenic effects extracellularly, no compelling evidence exists that they are required for lethal disease, as is the alpha toxin.

Many of the signs of systemic toxemia, cardiovascular collapse, and multiorgan dysfunction observed clinically in horses with clostridial myonecrosis can similarly be explained by observations made in rodent and rabbit models of gas gangrene. Alpha toxin directly suppresses myocardial contractility in vivo,[19] whereas theta toxin is a potent reducer of systemic vascular resistance.[20] Theta toxin has demonstrable ability to dysregulate polymorphonuclear/endothelial cell interactions, promoting leukostasis and interfering with normal cellular host responses to tissue injury at the active site of infection.[21]

Clinical Findings

Horses with clostridial myonecrosis demonstrate rapid soft tissue swelling, subcutaneous and deeper soft tissue emphysema, and rapid toxemia that may progress to circulatory collapse and multiorgan failure over just a few hours.[1-3] Clinicopathologic data from horses that have died acutely corroborate multiorgan failure and diffuse intravascular coagulation as two major pathologic processes that occur in terminally ill horses with clostridial myonecrosis.[1,2,8] Some horses that develop clostridial myonecrosis have a recent history of colic, resulting in the administration of IM analgesics, with subsequent myonecrosis in the region of the injection.[1,2,8,9] Some authors have postulated that colic may truly be a prodromal sign of equine clostridial myonecrosis,[4] drawing comparisons with the nausea and abdominal pain that are early symptoms of clostridial myonecrosis in human patients.[22,23]

Occasionally, horses with clostridial myonecrosis will develop hemolytic anemia/crisis after several days to 1 or 2 weeks of therapy.[1,24] This appears to be a distinct entity to the life-ending, diffuse intravascular coagulation that other horses develop in the early stages of the disease. It is not certain whether hemolytic events are a direct effect of the clostridial infection. Some clostridia (e.g., *C. septicum*) can elaborate one or more exotoxins with in vivo hemolytic activity.[22,23] Alternatively, hemolysis may be a potential immunologic complication of penicillin or other drug therapy.

Diagnosis

Clostridial myonecrosis may be presumptively diagnosed in any horse that develops acute-onset, rapidly progressive soft tissue swelling accompanied by emphysema in the area of a recent parenteral injection. Clostridial myonecrosis associated with penetrating traumatic wounds appears to represent a rare subset of cases.[1,9] Acute-onset cellulitis without emphysema should be viewed as suspicious for the disease, but confirmed by cytologic evaluation and Gram stain before aggressive fasciotomy or debridement is performed (Fig. 45-1). Ultrasonography of areas of postinjection cellulitis should be performed to identify areas of deeper emphysema and gas production that may not yet be palpable in the immediate subcutis. Definitive etiologic confirmation can be achieved by Gram stain and anaerobic culture of fluid aspirates from an affected soft tissue area. Numerous, characteristic gram-positive rods, sometimes with endospores present, can be easily visualized on air-dried smears, particularly from the periphery of an area of soft tissue emphysema. Speciation after anaerobic culture by genetic or fluorescent antibody techniques provides definitive confirmation and may guide prognosis.[1,25]

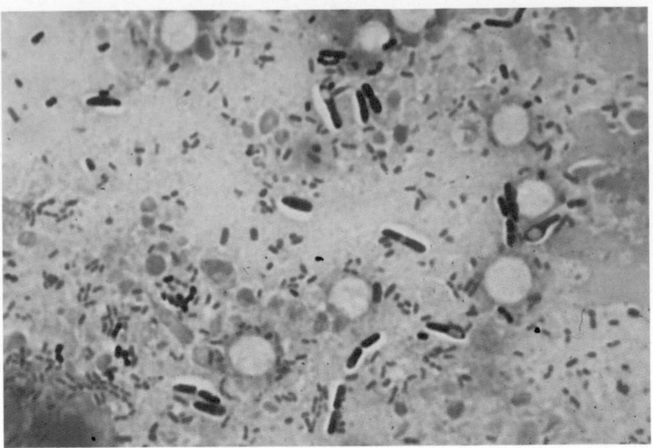

Fig. 45-1 Gram stain of aspirate from subcutaneous tissues of horse with acute clostridial myonecrosis. Notice the numerous, large, gram-positive rods.

Therapy

Higher survival rates are associated with aggressive combinations of medical and surgical treatment.[1,2,4] Barotherapy has become a component of the approach to treatment of human cases of clostridial myonecrosis, but hyperbaric oxygen chambers are only beginning to become available for use in large animal veterinary medicine. Rapid therapeutic intervention with high doses of IV crystalline penicillins should be considered as soon as a presumptive diagnosis is made. Potassium penicillin at doses as high as 88,000 IU/kg every 2 hours (q2h) have been used, and conventional doses of 22,000 IU/kg q6h should be viewed as the minimum required dose, expense permitting.[25] Oral metronidazole (25 mg/kg q6h) is often included in therapy but is unlikely to reach the high tissue levels that may be achieved with IV penicillin.

Intensive fluid, electrolyte, and cardiovascular support are indicated in the acute stages of clinical disease because dehydration and systemic toxemia can be life threatening at this time.[1-3,25] Many affected horses become hypotensive, with diminished cardiac output and renal function, complicated by substantial myoglobin release and the potential for pigment nephropathy. Fenestration of affected soft tissues appears to be an important part of therapy, and clinicians are advised to be aggressive in incising areas of subcutaneous emphysema, extending the incisions into deeper tissues and adjoining areas of healthy tissue (Fig. 45-2). Because of the obtunded mentation of many affected horses and the rapid progression of tissue necrosis in affected areas, these procedures can usually be performed under sedation without

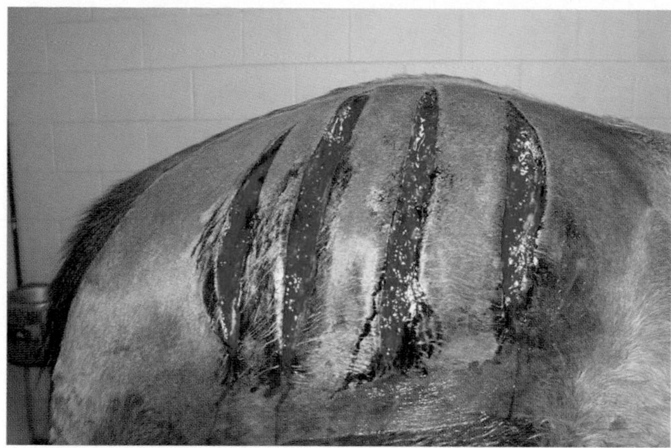

Fig. 45-2 Fasciotomy/myotomy incisions in gluteal region of 2-year-old Quarter Horse filly that developed clostridial myonecrosis secondary to vaccination at the site. (Courtesy Dr. Susan Semrad.)

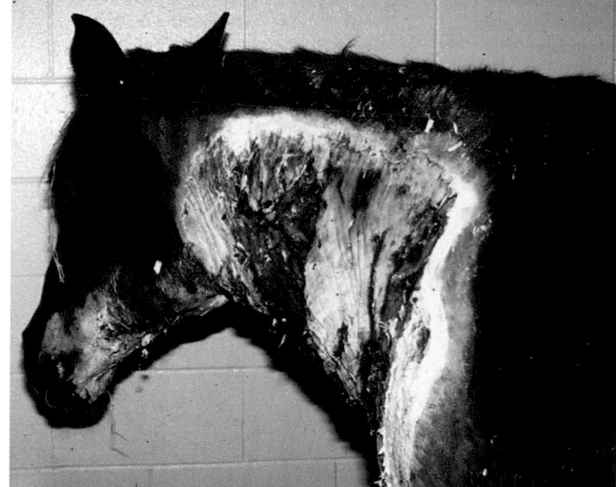

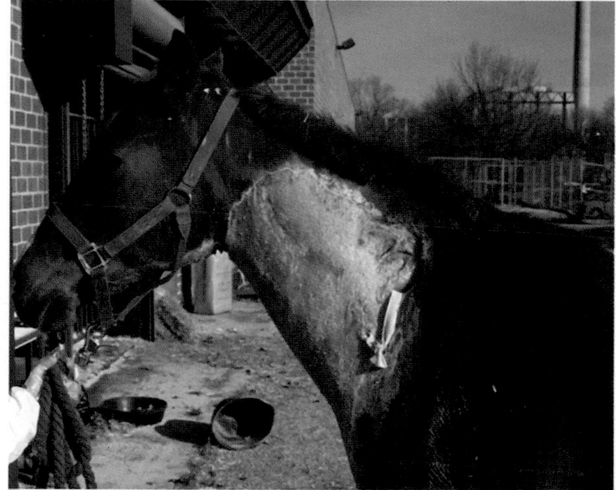

Fig. 45-3 **A,** Mature Quarter Horse gelding showing skin and muscle sloughing 2 weeks after surgical fenestration of an area of clostridial myonecrosis in the cervical region. **B,** The same horse approximately 30 days after surgical fenestration showing near-complete granulation bed in prior area of clostridial myonecrosis.

the need for local anesthesia.[25] Frequent reevaluation of the horse for signs of spreading emphysematous cellulitis, necessitating repeated incisions and debridement, is advised. Local infusion of penicillin into tissue at the margins of debrided muscle may have some benefit in limiting the spread of the infection.

For horses that survive the acute stages of disease, prognosis will improve significantly. However, veterinarians should warn owners of the significant soft tissue and skin sloughing that will likely ensue over coming days to weeks (Fig. 45-3). Long-term wound care will often be needed, with many cases taking weeks to months before granulation and second-intention skin healing are complete. Cosmetically, some horses may heal with pigmentation changes and significant cicatrix formation (Fig. 45-4), but the visual appearance of healed wounds is often normal.[25]

Prognosis appears to vary according to the species of *Clostridium* involved. A much better prognosis is afforded to horses with soft tissue lesions associated with *C. perfringens* than to those with *C. septicum* or *C. chauvoei* infections.[1] The largest retrospective study published to date reported an overall survival rate of 73% for horses with clostridial necrosis when they were treated with a combination of aggressive medical and surgical therapy in a referral hospital setting. Horses with *C. perfringens* infection had a survival rate of 81%.[1] There was no gender predilection observed in that study, but the disease did appear disproportionately to affect Quarter Horses. Previous studies have demonstrated much higher case-fatality rates,[2,8,9] and therefore clinicians and owners should be mindful of the need for prompt, aggressive, and potentially expensive therapy if horses are to have the best chance of survival. The majority of horses that die will succumb within the first few days.

Prevention

Although bacterin-toxoids should be in common use for prevention of disease caused by *Clostridium tetani* in all horses (see Chapter 47) and *Clostridium botulinum* in susceptible and at-risk foal populations (see Chapter 46), there is no standard vaccination practice for the prevention of clostridial myonecrosis in horses. Current preventive methods focus on appropriate injection technique, particularly with respect to the location of IM administration of pharmacologic and biologic preparations. No protective effect appears to be gained from skin disinfection, hair clipping, or disinfection of the top of multidose vials before IM injection in preventing clostridial myonecrosis.[26] When administering IM injections, however, particularly in the neck, where the disease most often occurs, it is prudent to ensure appropriate needle placement. When administering potentially irritant substances, particularly if lay people are responsible for injecting flunixin meglumine, it may be prudent to encourage use of the larger, better-vascularlized, caudal thigh musculature.

TYZZER'S DISEASE

Debra C. Sellon

In 1917, Ernest Edward Tyzzer[27] described an infectious syndrome of gastrointestinal and hepatic disease in Japanese Waltzing mice that came to be known as Tyzzer's disease. He isolated and characterized the etiologic agent and reproduced the disease experimentally in mice. The etiologic agent

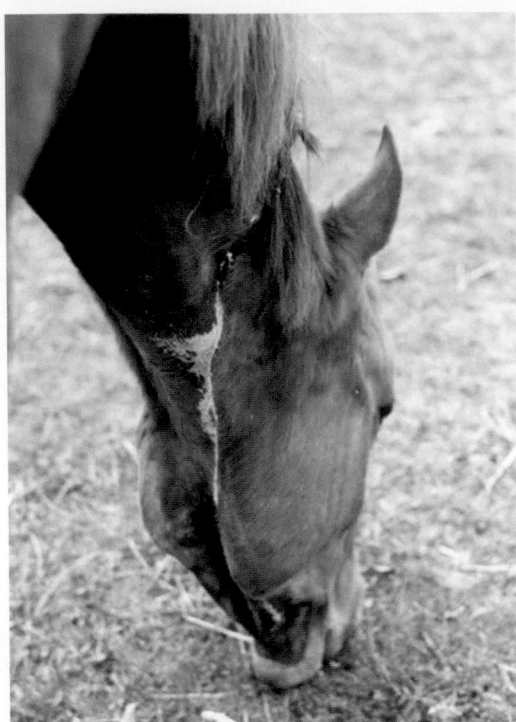

Fig. 45-4 Scarring and skin depigmentation in a healed area of clostridial cellulitis and myonecrosis in throatlatch region associated with perivascular injection. (Courtesy Dr. Susan Semrad.)

was originally named *Bacillus piliformis*. However, in 1994, Duncan et al.[28,29] demonstrated that the organism was more closely related to clostridial bacteria than to the *Bacillus* genus, and it was renamed *Clostridium piliformis*. In 1973, Swerczek et al.[30] described focal bacterial hepatitis in foals in Kentucky attributable to infection with *Clostridium (Bacillus) piliformis*.

Etiology

Clostridium piliformis (also *C. piliforme*) is a motile, pleomorphic, gram-negative, spore-forming, obligate intracellular bacterium. It is classified as an organism that is "extremely oxygen sensitive" (EOS) and is gram positive only if fixation and staining are performed under strictly anaerobic conditions.[31,32] *C. piliformis* does not grow in cell-free media but can be propagated in the yolk sac of chick embryos or some types of cell culture. *C. piliformis* stains poorly with routine hematoxylin and eosin stains of formalin-fixed tissue samples. Silver impregnation or Giemsa stains facilitate visualization of the organism (Fig. 45-5). The large vegetative form of *C. piliforme* ranges from 8 to 40 mm in length. This vegetative phase is quite labile; in contrast, spores may survive for up to 1 year in soiled bedding at room temperature or for 1 hour at 56° C (133° F).

Epidemiology and Pathogenesis

Infection with *C. piliformis* has been reported in a variety of laboratory, wild, and domesticated mammalian species, including the horse,[30,33-49] cow,[50,51] dog,[52-55] cat,[56] rat,[57-63] mouse,[58,59,64-69] hamster,[69-71] gerbil,[72-74] guinea pig,[75-79] rabbit,[80-82] muskrat,[83-85] wombat,[86] red panda,[87] coyote,[88] snow leopard,[89] gray fox,[90] raccoon,[91] and serval.[92] Among laboratory animals, clinical disease is most common in rabbits, gerbils, hamsters, and guinea pigs. Infections of mice and rats are more likely to

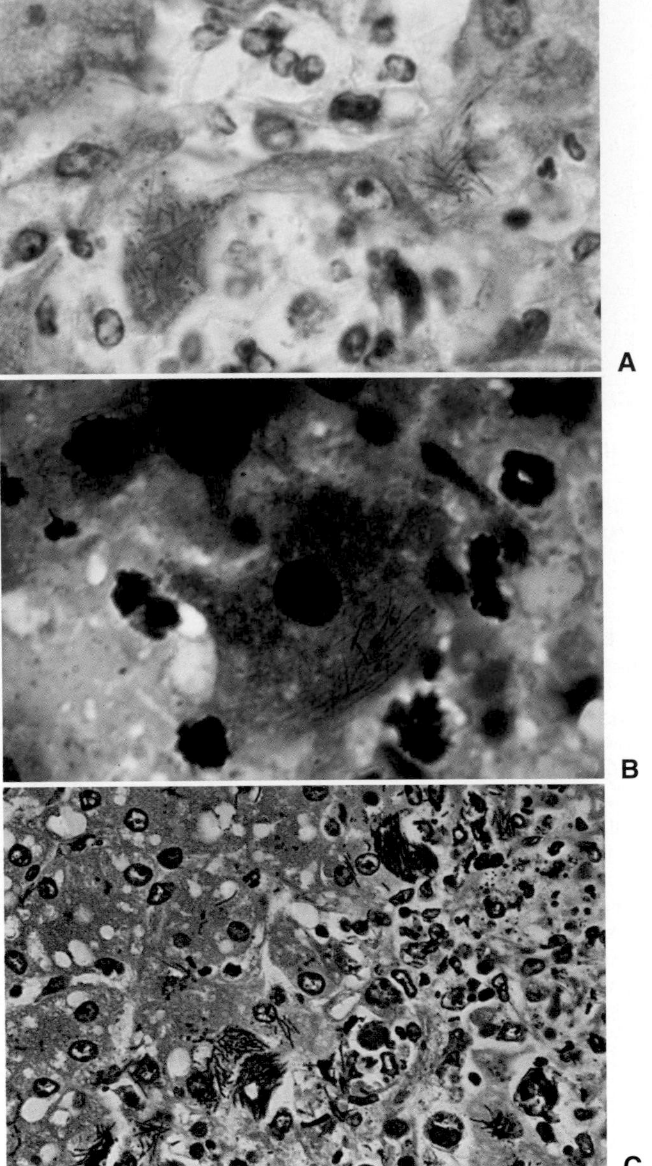

Fig. 45-5 Photomicrographs of the liver of foals with Tyzzer's disease. Note the thin, filamentous bacilli visible within hepatocytes. **A**, Giemsa stain, 400×. **B**, Diff-Quik stain, 400×; imprint from liver of affected foal. **C**, Warthin-Starry (silver) stain, 160×. (Courtesy Dr. Charles Leathers.)

be subclinical.[62] There is one report of infection in a severely immunocompromised person.[93] There have been a few reports of infection in avian species.[94,95] Disease has been reported in horses in many parts of the world, including North America, Australia, Europe, and Africa.

The natural route of infection of horses with *C. piliformis* is unknown, but the most likely route of exposure is by ingestion of spores from the environment. This theory is supported by the distribution of lesions in affected animals[30,35,96] and experimental reproduction of disease in foals by oral transmission. Experimental infection of adult horses results in fecal shedding of the organism, and coprophagia may contribute to the likelihood of infection in foals.[46] The sporadic nature of the disease in foals suggests that direct transmission is unlikely.[50,97,98] However, clusters of disease may be observed on specific horse premises.[30,37,46,47]

Serologic studies suggest that there is widespread exposure of horses to *C. piliformis*.[98] Approximately 23% of horses tested had antibodies to the flagellar antigens of an equine *C. piliformis* isolate, 14% had antibody to epitopes of a rat isolate, and 5% had antibody to epitopes of a hamster isolate. This variability in seropositive rates between isolates suggests the possibility of multiple strains of bacteria that cause disease in horses.[99,100] However, shared epitopes among strains have also been identified,[99] making it difficult to determine whether only certain strains may cause disease in animals or whether individual strains may be restricted to specific host species.

In a study of affected and unaffected Thoroughbred foals on a farm in California, several risk factors for Tyzzer's disease were identified.[37] Data from nine affected foals from a population of 322 foals were examined. In the final multivariable logistic regression analysis, foals born between March 13 and April 13 were 7.2 times as likely to develop Tyzzer's disease as those born at other times; foals of nonresident (visiting) mares were 3.4 times more likely to be infected than resident foals; and foals of mares less than 6 years of age were 2.9 times as likely to develop disease as foals born to older mares. Seasonal risk may reflect management, environmental, or climatic factors that influenced disease incidence. The increased risk observed for foals born to nonresident mares and foals born to younger mares suggests that colostrum may be important for passive immunity in foals.[37] Hook et al.[98] have demonstrated colostral transfer of antibodies to *C. piliformis*.

Very little is known about the pathogenesis of infection with *C. piliformis* in horses or other animals. Murine susceptibility to Tyzzer's disease varies with host strain, age, and immune status. Depletion of neutrophils or natural killer cells in experimentally infected mice increases the severity of disease, but macrophage depletion does not alter the course of disease.[101] In rodents and lagomorphs, outbreaks of disease are characterized by fatal diarrhea, with pathology predominantly observed in the gastrointestinal tract.[102]

Clinical Findings

Tyzzer's disease affects foals between 7 and 42 days of age.[37,43,47,48,98] Clinical signs include severe depression, fever, icterus, diarrhea, dehydration, and seizures. Some foals are found dead with no recognizable premonitory clinical signs. Almost all affected foals die; the overall course of disease is usually less than 48 hours from onset of clinical signs until death. Clinicopathologic abnormalities frequently include hemoconcentration, metabolic acidosis, hypoglycemia, hyperbilirubinemia, and increased hepatic enzyme activities.[37,43] Ultrasonographic examination of the abdomen of affected foals may reveal hepatomegaly with an increased vascular pattern.[43]

Diagnosis

Tyzzer's disease should be considered as a differential diagnosis for foals between 7 and 42 days of age with compatible clinical signs and laboratory evidence of hepatitis. The likelihood of this diagnosis is increased if previous cases of *C. piliformis* infection have been confirmed on the premises. Currently, no reliable antemortem laboratory tests are available to confirm a diagnosis of Tyzzer's disease in foals. Diagnosis is confirmed on postmortem examination by observation of typical gross and histopathologic lesions and observation of intracellular bacteria at the periphery of lesions when liver sections are stained appropriately (see Fig. 45-5).

Pathologic Findings

At postmortem examination, affected foals have a grossly enlarged liver with multifocal, light-colored areas in the liver capsule and parenchyma.[97] These light-colored areas correspond with areas of severe, random, diffuse acute to subacute hepatic necrosis.[45] Intracellular filamentous bacilli can be observed in parallel or random arrangements in hepatocytes at the periphery of these lesions if sections are silver-stained (Warthin-Starry stain). Occasionally, lesions consistent with enterocolitis or myocardial infection may be observed.[39,41,103]

Therapy

The prognosis for foals with Tyzzer's disease is poor. Three foals with presumptive *C. piliformis* infection did survive.[37,43] These foals received appropriate supportive care and antimicrobial therapy rapidly after they developed clinical signs. Because of difficulties cultivating *C. piliformis* in vitro, there is relatively little information regarding antimicrobial susceptibility patterns for this organism. The only available data are based on in vitro studies using embryonated eggs in which penicillin, tetracycline, erythromycin, and streptomycin were considered effective. Treatment of laboratory animals with either sulfonamides or corticosteroids can induce active Tyzzer's disease in carrier animals.[104] A 10-day-old foal that survived presumptive Tyzzer's disease was treated with sodium penicillin and trimethoprim-sulfadiazine.[43] In addition, the foal received intensive IV fluid therapy with dextrose, sodium bicarbonate, and potassium chloride solutions. Seizure activity was controlled with IM xylazine. Nutritional needs were met with IV parenteral nutrition. Additional supportive therapy included IV dimethyl sulfoxide and antiulcer prophylaxis. Clinical improvement was observed within 24 hours of initiation of therapy. Antimicrobial and antiulcer therapy was continued for approximately 3 weeks.

Prevention

No vaccines are available for prevention of Tyzzer's disease in foals. Because *C. piliformis* is most likely transmitted by a fecal-oral route, good farm hygiene may be beneficial for decreasing the likelihood of disease. Maintaining foals in well-grassed paddocks has been proposed as a preventive measure to decrease exposure to contaminated soil.[45] It is also recommended that all foals receive adequate passive transfer of immune globulins soon after birth. High-risk foals[37] should be closely monitored for the earliest signs of disease and treated aggressively as soon as these are recognized. Spores are reported to be sensitive to disinfection with 0.3% sodium hypochlorite;[105] however, this disinfectant is readily inactivated in the presence of organic matter and may not be an effective disinfectant for use in barns.

PUBLIC HEALTH CONSIDERATIONS

There is a single report of human infection with *C. piliformis* in a severely immunocompromised patient.[93]

REFERENCES

See the CD-ROM for a list of references linked to the abstract in PubMed.

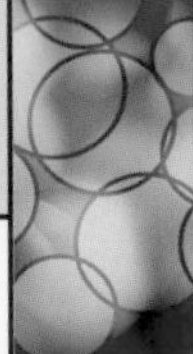

CHAPTER • 46

Botulism

Pamela A. Wilkins

Botulism is a neuromuscular disorder of horses and other mammals caused by neurotoxins of *Clostridium botulinum*; similar disease has been described resulting from toxins produced by a few strains of *Clostridium baratii* and *Clostridium butyricum*. The first published reports of botulism in horses appeared in the early 1950s.[1] Disease characterized by flaccid paralysis may occur in adult horses or in foals, where it has been termed "shaker foal syndrome."[2-4]

Botulinum toxin is considered to be one of the most potent toxins known.[5] Although it has medicinal uses in the treatment of specific disorders,[5,6] clinical botulism is a serious, frequently fatal disease. The exotoxin causes paresis and paralysis by interfering with acetylcholine release at the neuromuscular junction.[6,7] Death is usually attributed to respiratory failure. Because of the pathogenicity of botulinum toxin, especially for humans, it has been placed on the list of select agents to facilitate control of dangerous biologic agents and toxins. Botulism can result from the ingestion of preformed botulinum toxin or the growth of *C. botulinum* in anaerobic tissues, with subsequent in vivo elaboration of toxin. Outbreaks of botulism resulting from consumption of contaminated feed can be devastating, with high morbidity and mortality.

ETIOLOGY

Clostridium botulinum is a gram-positive, saprophytic, spore-forming, anaerobic rod-shaped bacterium. Eight neurotoxins isolated from *C. botulinum* (A, B, Ca, Cb, D, E, F, and G) are distinguished by neutralization of biologic activity with type-specific serologic reagents and are classified in seven serogroups designated A through G. Bacterial strains are usually identified on the basis of the type of toxin produced. Although all types of botulinum toxin produce an identical clinical disease, determination of the toxin type is important if antitoxin is used for treatment. Clinical botulism in horses has been attributed to *C. botulinum* types A, B, C, and D.

Clostridium botulinum spores are highly resistant to heat, light, and drying. Germination occurs under anaerobic conditions at temperatures of 15° to 45° C (59°-113° F). Toxin may be released from vegetative cells by cell lysis or by diffusion through the cell wall within several days of germination. After release, the single-chain toxins are inactive until cleaved by bacterial or tissue proteases to the active dichain neurotoxin. All serotypes of botulinum toxin are composed of a heavy chain with a molecular weight of approximately 100 kDa and a light chain of 50 kDa connected by a single disulfide bond.

EPIDEMIOLOGY

Equine botulism is most frequently observed in Kentucky and the Mid-Atlantic region of the eastern United States, although the disease had been reported worldwide.[3,8] In the United States, horses are most often affected with type B or C botulism, although type A botulism has been confirmed in adult horses and foals.

Type B *C. botulinum* spores can be isolated from the soil of most geographic regions of the United States, but they are most common in the soil of the northeastern and Appalachian regions. In contrast, *C. botulinum* type A spores are more common in the soil in the western United States. The frequency of occurrence of types A and B food-borne botulism in humans parallels the distribution of these types in the soil.[9] A similar correlation between frequency of environmental isolation of a specific serotype of *C. botulinum* and the frequency of disease caused by that serotype is observed in horses in North America. Type B botulism is most often seen in the Mid-Atlantic states and Kentucky, type C occurs mainly in Florida, and type A has been observed predominantly in the western United States.

PATHOGENESIS

Equine botulism may occur after ingestion of preformed botulinum toxin in contaminated feed *(forage poisoning)*,[10-14] ingestion of spores with elaboration of toxin within the gastrointestinal tract *(toxicoinfectious botulism)*,[15] or contamination of wounds with *C. botulinum* and subsequent in vivo toxin production *(wound botulism)*.[16] Ingestion of preformed botulinum toxin in decaying vegetable matter (grass, hay, grain, spoiled silage) or carcasses is the most common type of botulism observed in adult horses.[3,8] An outbreak of botulism type C was associated with bird droppings and a horse burial site.[17] Toxicoinfectious botulism is most common in foals 1 to 3 months of age, although it has been observed in foals as young as 7 days of age. Toxicoinfectious botulism may also be the cause of "grass sickness" in horses in Europe.[18-20]

Clostridial toxins are dichain structures with a molecular weight of approximately 150 kDa that are synthesized as single chains and posttranslationally cleaved into heavy (H) and light (L) chains. They are metalloproteinases that are structurally similar to tetanus toxin and that prevent the spontaneous or action potential–induced presynaptic release of acetylcholine at the neuromuscular junction.

Botulinum neurotoxin (BoNT) consists of a light chain that functions as a zinc-dependent endopeptidase and a heavy chain with two functional domains of approximately the same size. The N-terminal section of the H chain is the translocation domain that forms ion channels spanning endosomal membranes to facilitate translocation and activation of light chains. The C-terminal section of the H chain is the ganglioside-binding domain to facilitate binding and internalization of the toxin at the cholinergic neuron.[21]

Botulism intoxication occurs by a multistep process, involving each of the functional domains of the toxin, and can be summarized as the outcome of three distinct stages: (1) binding to the target cell and internalization, (2) translocation, and (3) inhibition of neurotransmitter release.

Binding to cholinergic nerve terminals is thought to require gangliosides and a protein receptor, possibly synaptotagamin for BoNT types A, B, and E.[22,23] Once bound to the cell surface, BoNT is internalized into an acidic compartment by endocytosis that is temperature and energy dependent. After internalization, the toxin cannot be neutralized by antitoxin.

Translocation is thought to involve a pH-dependent structural rearrangement of BoNT inside an acidic compartment within the cell, possibly synaptic vesicles or the endosomal compartment.[24,25] The active light chain is translocated to the cytosol, where it interacts with, and eventually cleaves, SNARE proteins. SNARE proteins are a group of proteins that are critical for exocytosis of neurotransmitters from the cell and include synaptobrevin (VAMP family), syntaxin, and SNAP-25.[21] The specific SNARE protein cleaved and the site of cleavage vary with the specific serotype of botulinum toxin. BoNT types B, D, F, and G cleave members of the VAMP family of SNARE-complex proteins, whereas types A, C, and E cleave SNAP-25. BoNT type C also has the capacity to cleave syntaxin.

BoNT prevents exocytosis of acetylcholine at the neuromuscular synapse by the cleavage of SNARE proteins involved in the fusion of synaptic vesicles with the plasma membrane. Cleavage of SNARE proteins creates a nonfunctional complex where coupling between calcium ion (Ca^{++}) influx and synaptic vesicle fusion is disrupted.[26] The cleavage of the SNARE proteins allows docking of the synaptic vesicle but prevents exocytosis. Increasing intracellular Ca^{++} can partially overcome the effects of BoNT type A.[21,27]

The extended duration of activity of BoNT at the neuromuscular junction is the root of the clinical problem and the reason for its recent application as a therapeutic tool in human medicine. Specific BoNT serotypes vary in their duration of action. For example, BoNT type A induces long-term inhibition (months) of neurotransmission, whereas BoNT type E induces a comparatively short-term inhibition (weeks).[28,29] The reasons for these differences have not been fully elucidated but may relate to the half-life of the light chain in the cytosol and to persistence of SNAP-25 fragments in the SNARE complex.

CLINICAL FINDINGS

Clinical signs in horses with botulism are related to inhibition of acetylcholine release at the neuromuscular junction and resultant generalized lower motor neuron and parasympathetic dysfunction.[8,30] This includes dysphagia; flaccid paralysis; diminished pupillary reactivity; decreased eyelid, tongue, and tail tone; and progressive flaccid tetraparesis and tetraplegia.[3,8,31] The time to onset of clinical signs after exposure to toxin varies from 12 hours to several days. Sudden, unexplained death of one or more horses may be the initial signal of the onset of an outbreak. Decreased eyelid, tongue, and tail tone may be observed early in disease. Horses that walk may have a stilted, short-strided gait without ataxia. Muscle trembling and weakness may be apparent, particularly in foals. Pupillary dilation with sluggish pupillary light reflexes is common. There is normal cutaneous sensation with depressed spinal reflexes. Pharyngeal paralysis is frequently observed in adult horses with botulism and may be confirmed by endoscopic examination of the upper airway.

Clinical signs may rapidly progress to recumbency. Tachycardia may occur, particularly in foals. Foals may appear or become constipated and dysuric. Signs of colic may be associated with diminished gastrointestinal (GI) motility. Dyspnea and cyanosis may be present initially or terminally. Death is generally attributed to respiratory failure secondary to respiratory muscle paralysis.

DIAGNOSIS

Diagnosis of botulism is primarily made on the basis of history and clinical signs after exclusion of other diagnostic possibilities.[3,8,31] Differential diagnoses include but are not limited to severe electrolyte imbalance (hyponatremia), tick paralysis, and postanesthetic myasthenic syndrome. Routine laboratory work, including complete blood count, serum biochemical profile, and urinalysis, is generally unremarkable unless secondary problems (e.g., infection, dehydration) have developed. Although characteristic electromyographic changes have been described in association with infant botulism and toxicoinfectious botulism in foals, electromyography (EMG) is not uniformly available, and most veterinarians are not trained to interpret this test properly.[32]

Definitive diagnosis is usually based on detection of toxin in serum, feces, GI contents, or feed. A variety of tests, including enzyme-linked immunosorbent assay (ELISA), radioimmunoassay (RIA), passive hemagglutination, and polymerase chain reaction (PCR), have been described for identification of botulinum toxin; however, the diagnostic test of choice remains *mouse inoculation*. Serum or an extract of feed, feces, or GI contents is injected into the peritoneal cavity of mice, which are observed for classic clinical signs of botulism. The specific serotype of botulinum toxin present in a sample is determined by co-injection of mice with suspect samples and specific antisera. If appropriate antiserum is present, clinical signs will not occur. Although serum samples are occasionally positive for botulinum toxin by mouse inoculation assay, the quantity of circulating toxin is usually too small for detection.[3] Isolation of *C. botulinum* or its toxin from feedstuffs, feces, or GI contents or from lesions or wounds in the patient is strong circumstantial evidence of infection.[3,8]

PATHOLOGIC FINDINGS

No pathologic findings are directly attributable to the effects of botulinum toxin. Pressure sores and regions of self-trauma may be seen in recumbent horses, and all patients, old or young, may have aspiration pneumonia secondary to dysphagia (Fig. 46-1). Gastric ulceration reported at postmortem examination in foals in the past may have been a reflection of the severity and progression of the disease rather than an inciting event. Gastric ulceration has been reported in association with severe illness in foals, but as intensive care techniques have improved, the incidence of gastric ulceration in nonsurviving patients at necropsy has decreased.[33]

In human infants, the large intestine is thought to be the site of colonization with *C. botulinum* and toxin-induced infection.[34]

If "grass sickness" is confirmed to be a form of toxicoinfectious intestinal botulism in adult horses, as it appears currently, specific lesions would include degenerating neurons in peripheral autonomic ganglia, as well as in intramural intestinal ganglia, that stain positive for synaptophysin, a SNARE protein.[20]

THERAPY

The efficacy of early administration of antitoxin in improving survival and decreasing length of hospital stay has been clearly demonstrated for humans and horses and is the mainstay of therapy.[3,8,31,35-40] Before the use of botulinum antitoxin in affected foals, the disease was almost uniformly fatal within 12 to 72 hours of the onset of clinical signs, except in very mildly affected horses.[31] Currently, equine-origin polyvalent (anti-B and anti-C) botulism antitoxin (Botulism Laboratory, New Bolton Center, Kennett Square, Pennsylvania) and monovalent (anti-B) botulinum antitoxin (Veterinary Dynamics, Templeton, California) are commercially available.

Respiratory failure is almost uniformly the proximate cause of death in both adults and foals with botulism. Adults and foals with mild respiratory failure (normal pH and mild to moderate increase in arterial carbon dioxide tension [$Pa{CO_2}$]) can frequently be treated with intranasal oxygen insufflation, positioning in sternal recumbency, and repeated arterial blood gas (ABG) monitoring to detect worsening respiratory failure. Close ABG monitoring is required for the first 24 to 48 hours of treatment because administration of botulinum antitoxin does not remove toxin already bound to receptors within the terminal neuromuscular junction of the axon, and the equine patient may deteriorate further during this period. ABG analysis should also be performed if the patient's condition appears to change; these horses may suddenly alter their respiratory rate and pattern as respiratory failure worsens. Increased nostril flare, decreased chest excursion, and restlessness may be physical indicators of worsening respiratory failure.

Foals with botulism and respiratory failure can be mechanically ventilated successfully.[40] Mechanical ventilation can ameliorate ABG abnormalities and allow time for the patient to recover cholinergic neuromuscular control. Volume-cycled ventilators tend to be better tolerated by foals. In SIMV mode, a minimum breath rate is set, along with a predetermined tidal volume and inspiratory flow rate, resulting in flow-controlled, volume-cycled mandatory breaths.[41] The sensitivity, related to the inspiratory effort the patient must generate to trigger a breath, should be set low in these horses. This is in recognition of their primary problem, botulism, and the muscular weakness associated with the disease.

Antimicrobial administration, although not required for treatment unless wound botulism is suspected, is frequently employed in an effort to prevent or reduce some of the complications of the disease, such as aspiration pneumonia caused by dysphagia. Antimicrobial choice in botulism is influenced by the disease process being treated. Antimicrobial drugs that might potentiate neuromuscular blockage (e.g., procaine penicillin, aminoglycosides, tetracyclines) should be avoided.[42-44]

Nutritional management must be considered in horses with botulism and can generally be achieved in foals by feeding milk or milk replacer via indwelling nasogastric or nasoesophageal tubes* as small, frequent meals (every 2 hours). In adult horses, periodic nasogastric intubation of slurry meals can be provided. In prolonged cases, it may be beneficial to consider commercially available liquid diets. Parenteral nutrition is generally not necessary. Intravenous fluid support may be required until patients are able to drink water safely.

Nursing care is an important part of treatment, and equine patients should be protected as much as possible from development of decubital ulcers, corneal ulcers, and inadvertent aspiration. Frequent turning and slinging of adult horses are arduous tasks and require skill and persistence (Fig. 46-2). Ocular examination should be performed at least daily and ocular lubricant ointments used to prevent exposure keratitis. Care should be taken to ensure the "down" eye is protected.

Survival rate for botulinum neurointoxication in appropriately treated foals less than 6 months of age is greater than 90%. Approximately 50% of affected foals will require some form of ventilatory support, ranging from intranasal oxygen insufflation to mechanical ventilation, and all affected foals should have repeated ABG analysis performed during the first 48 hours of treatment (Fig. 46-3). Mechanical ventilation can ameliorate ABG abnormalities and allow time for the patient to recover cholinergic neuromuscular control. Foals recovering from botulism are not protected after specific immunoglobulin G (IgG) from antitoxin is depleted, and they should be vaccinated.

Adult horses with botulism that remain standing have a good prognosis for recovery; however, it may require several weeks to months before affected horses regain sufficient

*Kangaroo, 12-French, 43-inch enteral feeding tube, Sherwood Medical, St. Louis, MO 63103.

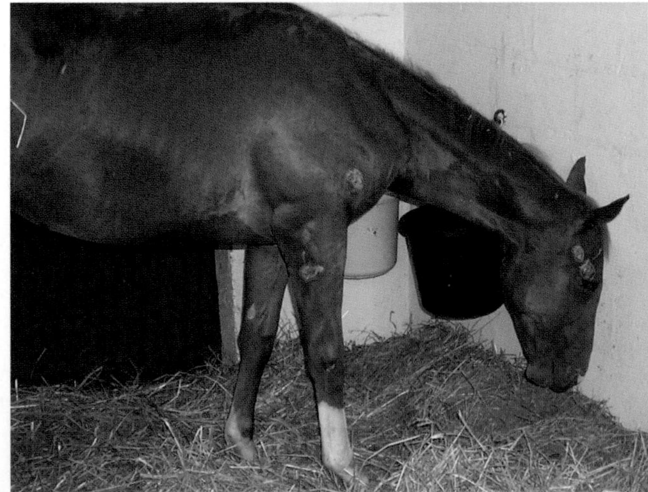
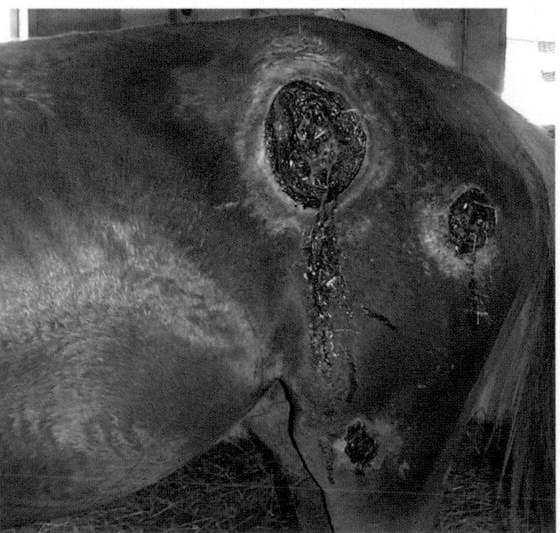

Fig. 46-1 A, Mild pressure sores associated with recumbency in horse, caused by neurologic disease other than botulism. B, The same horse with severe pressure sores. (Courtesy Dr. Amy Bentz, Chadds Ford, Penn.)

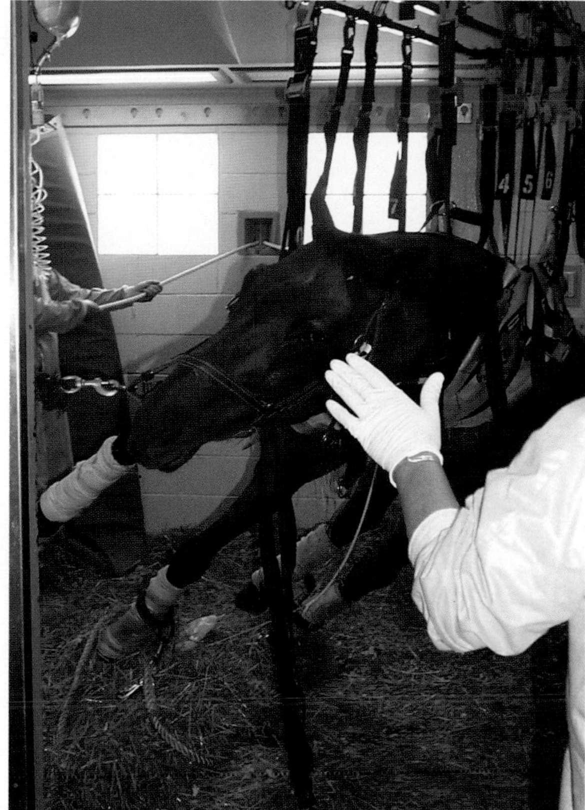

Fig. 46-2 "Slinging" a horse. The sling used here is the Anderson sling; the horse is not yet upright. Slings can be used to support horses in a standing position or can be used as an aid to change recumbency in "down" horses. This horse has neurologic disease, not botulism, but botulism cases would be similarly handled. (Courtesy Dr. Amy Bentz, Chadds Ford, Penn.)

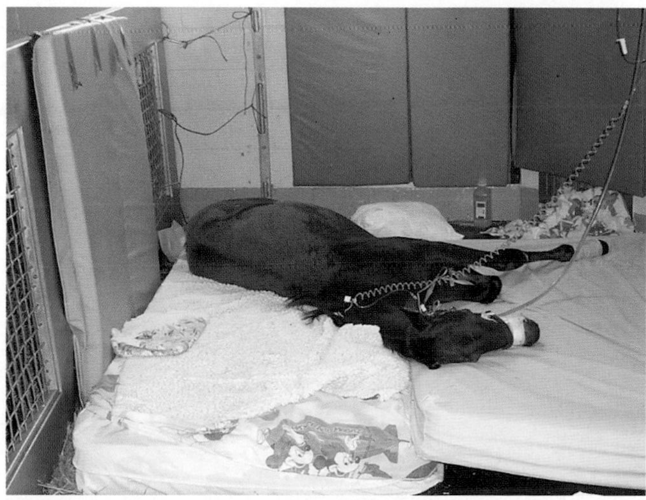

Fig. 46-3 Weanling with botulism maintained in lateral recumbency on mattresses. Note intravenous line (coil) for fluid support and oxygen line providing intranasal oxygen insufflation. Two twin mattresses were required for this foal, and synthetic sheepskin was used to protect the body from pressure sores and skin maceration associated with prolonged recumbency. This weanling also received antitoxin and survived. (Courtesy Dr. Amy Bentz, Chadds Ford, Penn.)

strength to return to work. Horses that become recumbent have a poorer prognosis even with antitoxin administration and excellent nursing care. This is related in part to their size and the secondary effects of prolonged recumbency. The degree of respiratory compromise can be severe, and long-term (days) mechanical ventilation of adult horses is a difficult undertaking.

PREVENTION

Appropriate vaccination (*Clostridium botulinum* type B toxoid, Neogen, Tampa, Florida) is thought to be almost 100% protective in adult horses[3,8] (Box 46-1). However, foals born to vaccinated dams can present with botulism, suggesting that reliance on passive transfer of immunity for protection of foals may be inadequate in endemic areas.[31] Failure of transfer of specific immunity to botulinum toxin can originate from failure of passive transfer of immunity. However, foals less than 2 weeks old with adequate blood concentration of IgG (>800 mg/dL) have also been diagnosed with botulism. In these cases the dose of toxin may have overwhelmed the available antitoxin, or the dam may not have produced

Box • 46-1

Botulism Vaccination Protocol

Adult Horses

Broodmare: Initial three-dose series at 30-day intervals, with last dose 4 to 6 weeks before anticipated parturition date. Annually thereafter, 4 to 6 weeks prepartum.

Other adult horses: Should consider vaccination, particularly if in endemic regions. Initial three-dose series, then annual booster.

Foals

From vaccinated mares: Three-dose series of toxoid at 1-month intervals, starting at 2 to 3 months of age.

From unvaccinated mares: Foal may benefit from (1) toxoid at 2, 4, and 8 weeks of age; (2) transfusion of plasma from vaccinated horse; or (3) antitoxin (efficacy needs further study).

Table • 46-1

Mammalian Species Affected by Each Type of Botulinum Toxin

BOTULINUM TOXIN	MAMMALIAN SPECIES AFFECTED
A	Horse, human, cattle, ferret, mink
B	Horse, human, cattle
C	Horse, cattle, sheep, dog, cat, mink, ferret
D	Horse, cattle, sheep, dog
E	Human, mink, ferret
F	Human
G	—

sufficient specific antibody in response to the vaccination to provide adequate protection to the foal through colostrum. Older foals from vaccinated dams may have lost specific passive immunity by the time of their exposure to the toxin and before their own vaccination. In humans, plasmapharesis of patients no longer responding to botulinum toxin administered for medicinal purposes can return them to responder status, most likely by decreasing available specific IgG.[45]

PUBLIC HEALTH CONSIDERATIONS

There is no zoonotic potential with equine botulism.

REFERENCES

See the CD-ROM for a list of references linked to the abstract in PubMed.

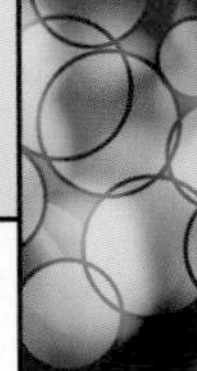

CHAPTER • 47

Tetanus

Robert J. MacKay

Tetanus was first described in Egypt more than 3000 years ago and was familiar throughout the ancient world.[1,2] In 1890, von Behring and Kitasato[3] demonstrated that rabbits produced neutralizing antibodies in response to the administration of small doses of tetanus toxoid. Two years later, von Behring immunized sheep and horses against tetanus toxin to produce commercial quantities of antitoxin, and equine antitoxin was used extensively in injured soldiers during World War I. In 1927, Ramon and Zoeller[4] developed a vaccine from tetanus toxin; a similar vaccine for horses was first used in the 1940s.

ETIOLOGY

Tetanus is caused by exotoxins produced by *Clostridium tetani*, a motile, anaerobic, gram-positive bacillus. *C. tetani* is a ubiquitous soil inhabitant and can be isolated from feces of domestic animals, including horses.[5] Endospores are formed that give the sporulating organism a drumstick appearance.[1] They are not completely destroyed by boiling but can be eliminated by autoclaving at 115° C (239° F) for 20 minutes.[6] Toxin may account for 5% of the mass of the organism during proliferative growth.[7] It has been estimated that the lethal dose for humans is 500 pg/kg.[8] Among animals, the horse is considered most sensitive to tetanus toxin.[9]

The most common route of infection is inoculation of wounds with *C. tetani* spores (Fig. 47-1). Puncture wounds contaminated by manure, soil, or rusty metal are especially likely to cause tetanus. In 18 horses with tetanus after known wounding, nine had lesions of the lower limb, six had punctures in the solar surface of the hoof, and two had wounds on the face.[10] Contaminated surgical sites, the postpartum uterus, injection abscesses, and infected umbilical structures are also potential sites for C *tetani* infection. Causative wounds were not found in 2 of 20 horses with tetanus[10] and reportedly are not found in 15% to 30% of human cases.

EPIDEMIOLOGY

Tetanus occurs in all parts of the world but is most likely in closely settled areas that are intensively farmed. Although the disease is rare in developed countries, tetanus is still important worldwide. In 1992, more than 1 million human deaths were still caused by tetanus, more than half of which were in neonates.[11]

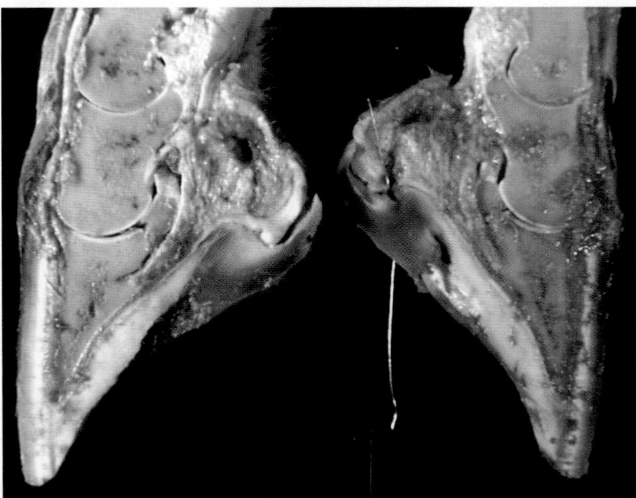

Fig. 47-1 Sagittal section of equine hoof. A wire has been placed through the area of subsolar abscessation responsible for introduction of *Clostridium tetani*. Subsequent exotoxin elaboration resulted in clinical signs seen in Figures 47-3 and 47-4. (Courtesy Dr. Robert Mealey.)

PATHOGENESIS

The clinical signs of tetanus are caused by exotoxins encoded on a 75-kilobase plasmid.[12] Two toxins are produced: tetanolysin and tetanospasmin.[13] *Tetanolysin* damages viable tissue, lowering the redox potential and creating favorable conditions for expansion of the anaerobic infection.[14] *Tetanospasmin* is produced as a single, inactive, 150-kilodalton polypeptide comprising three linked domains: L, H_N, and H_C. The peptide is activated by posttranslational, single-site proteolysis into active, heavy (H) and light (L) chains connected by a single disulfide bond. After its production by proliferating organisms, active tetanospasmin diffuses locally and circulates in the bloodstream to peripheral nerve terminals throughout the body. Tetanospasmin does not enter the central nervous system (CNS) directly, except at the fourth ventricle. At nerve endings, the lectinlike H_C domain binds to membrane gangliosides GD_{1b} and GT_{1b}. The toxin is then internalized and transported retrograde in axons at 75 to 250 mm/day.[15] After 1 to 14 days the toxin enters the CNS, traverses the synaptic cleft, and binds irreversibly to presynaptic inhibitory interneurons.[2] Following H_C-mediated binding to membranes, the entire toxin is internalized by a process requiring H_N. Within the endosome, the disulfide link is reduced, and the L chain is released into the cytosol. The L chain is a zinc metalloproteinase that cleaves synaptobrevin, a protein necessary for exocytosis of neurotransmitter vesicles.[13,16] In inhibitory interneurons, the light chain thus prevents release of the inhibitory neurotransmitters glycine and gamma-aminobutyric acid (GABA).[17] This results in the sustained excitatory discharge of alpha motor neurons, evident clinically as muscle rigidity and muscle spasms.[14]

Preganglionic autonomic neurons in the lateral column of the gray matter and parasympathetic centers are affected by a similar mechanism, but with delayed kinetics compared to somatic motor neurons.[18] Autonomic dysfunction therefore occurs days after spasms begin, probably because of relatively slow transport of toxin in the autonomic nerves.[2] There is both a basal increase in sympathetic activity and episodes of intense hyperactivity ("autonomic storms") involving both α-adrenergic and β-adrenergic receptors. During autonomic storms the concentration of circulating catecholamines increases up to tenfold. The resulting sympathetic overactivity causes hemodynamic instability and is an important cause of death in ventilated patients with tetanus.

The tetanus toxin also acts at the neuromuscular junction to cause muscle paralysis.[19] This botulinum-like effect causes the facial paralysis characteristic of the rare cephalic form of tetanus; however, any paralysis usually is overridden by spasmogenic effects at the inhibitory interneuron. Tetanospasmin also has been shown in experimental animal studies to have a cortical convulsant effect.[20] Whether this contributes to tetanic spasms in horses is unknown.

Neuronal binding of toxin is thought to be irreversible.[21] Recovery requires growth of new nerve terminals, a process that is completed in weeks to months.

DIAGNOSIS

The diagnosis of tetanus is presumptive and is based on clinical signs in the context of a history of poor or absent vaccination against tetanus. An early and sensitive diagnostic test in the horse is transient prolapse of the nictitans provoked by stimulation around the head. Typically, this response is induced by lightly tapping the skin beneath the eye. Differential diagnoses to rule out include myopathy, meningitis, colic, pleuritis, hyperkalemic periodic paralysis, trauma, epilepsy, and laminitis.

CLINICAL FINDINGS

The time from wound inoculation by *C. tetani* to development of first clinical signs can range from 1 day to more than 60 days, but usually is 7 to 10 days. In a series of 18 horses with tetanus, signs were first seen 2 to 21 days after wounding, with an average *incubation period* of 9 days.[10] The *period of onset* (time from first sign to first spasm) has not been reported for equine cases but probably is similar to the 1 to 7 days reported for humans.[1]

Generalized, localized, and cephalic forms of tetanus are described in humans. By far the most commonly recognized form in horses is *generalized tetanus*. Neonatal tetanus is always of this type. Probably because cranial somatic nerves are shorter than nerves to the limbs, the first signs of tetanus are associated with rigidity of muscles around the head and neck. Increased tonus of the masticatory muscles (trismus), rigidity of facial expression (risus sardonicus), and neck stiffness are typical presenting signs[10,22-27] (Fig. 47-2). Prolapse of the nictitans begins during this phase[9] (Fig. 47-3). The head and neck are held in an extended position, and the face has a fixed, anxious expression. Often, the mouth is clamped shut, and the jaws cannot be pried apart manually (lockjaw). Hyperthermia (usually <39.1° C [102.5° F]) occurs in some horses during the early stages, and rectal temperature may rise further after tetanic convulsions.[9]

In mildly affected horses, signs may be restricted to the head and neck (Box 47-1). Moderately affected horses exhibit signs of dysphagia because of pharyngeal involvement, and rigidity extends to the muscles of the limbs, trunk, and tail. These horses also adopt a "sawhorse" posture, with rigid extension of the neck, back, and limbs and elevation of the tailhead[10,26,27] (see Fig. 47-2). The gait appears stiff and stilted. In severe tetanus, affected animals are recumbent, and respiratory muscles are affected.

In all cases of generalized tetanus, tonic spasms develop within days of the onset of rigidity (Fig. 47-4). These can be initiated by external tactile, visual, emotional, or auditory stimuli or by voluntary movements. The dramatic responses to even minor stimuli can make a horse with tetanus appear hyperresponsive or hyperesthetic. When the face is touched,

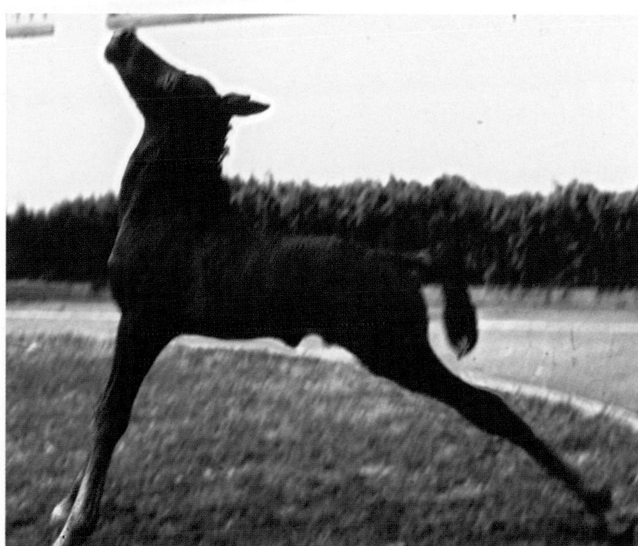

Fig. 47-2 Extensor rigidity observed in foal with tetanus secondary to umbilical abscess. (Courtesy Dr. John Barnes.)

there is reflex retraction of the eye and prolapse of the nictitans.[9] Attempts to chew or suckle set off rounds of masseter contraction that are easily visible under the skin. Reflex spasms may prevent an affected horse from reaching to the ground for food or water. Even if the horse is able to move ingesta to the pharynx, reflex pharyngeal and laryngeal spasms result in nasal regurgitation and stridor.

Because there is no reflex inhibitory control of movement, antagonistic flexor and extensor muscles contract simultaneously and with full power. The force of these contractions may cause rhabdomyolysis, intramuscular hemorrhage, tendon avulsion, and fracture of long bones or vertebrae. Efforts to stand may provoke cycles of violent muscle contraction of the limbs and trunk that pitch the horse back into recumbency. Even during apparent convalescence, muscle spasms can be disabling enough to cast an adult horse onto the floor of a stall.[24,28] Once down, it is extremely difficult for a horse with tetanus to regain its feet.[9]

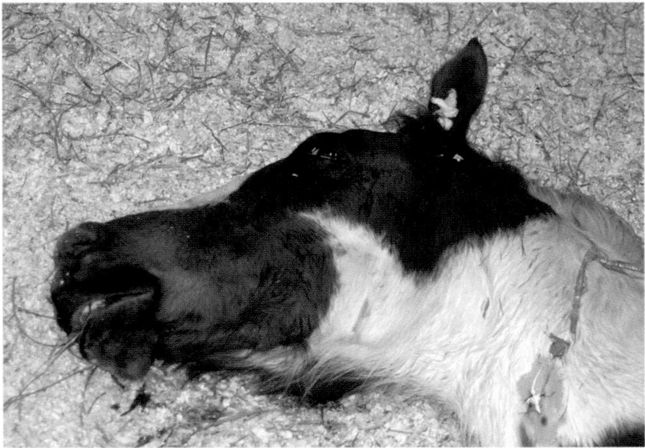

Fig. 47-3 Clinical signs of tetanus in 8-year-old Paint Horse mare with tetanus secondary to subsolar abscess. Note the muscle rigidity around the nostrils and muzzle and the partially prolapsed nictitans. (Courtesy Dr. Debra Sellon.)

Tetanus presents in a local form in approximately 2% of human cases.[2] *Local tetanus* probably also occurs in horses, although it has not been documented in the literature. This form usually is associated with low toxin load and partial humoral immunity. Rigidity and spasms are restricted to muscles adjacent to the inciting wound. *Cephalic tetanus* usually begins with asymmetric facial paralysis, although any cranial nerve can be affected. Signs frequently progress to generalized tetanus with high mortality.

Disturbances of autonomic function may occur after several days of muscle spasms. There may be increased or fluctuant heart rate, increased or fluctuant blood pressure, and profuse sweating. These signs of sympathetic overactivity are usually overlooked until after muscle spasms have been controlled. It is reported that hypersalivation, increased respiratory secretion, and late-onset hypotension occur because of parasympathetic overactivity.

Death usually results from euthanasia of recumbent horses with uncontrollable paroxysmal muscle contractions or from

Box • 47-1

Classification of Clinical Severity of Equine Tetanus

Mild
- Anxious expression
- Prolapsed nictitans
- Trismus
- Extended head

Moderate
- *As for **mild**, plus:*
- Dysphagia
- Hyperresponsiveness
- Muscle spasms
- Tailhead extension
- "Sawhorse" stance
- Stiff gait

Severe
- *As for **moderate**, plus:*
- Lateral recumbency
- Frequent, severe spasms
- Respiratory difficulties
- Cardiovascular instability

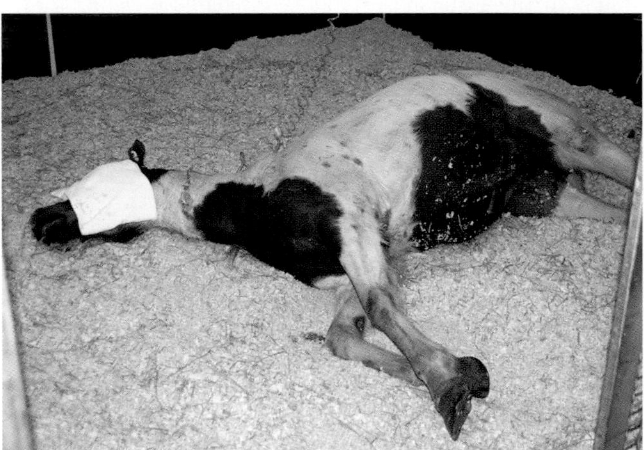

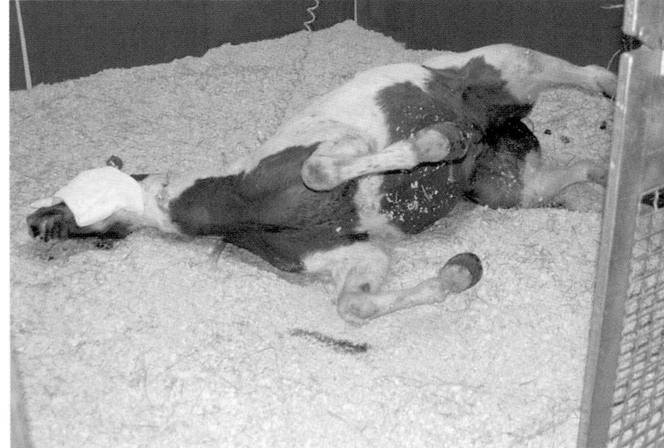

Fig. 47-4 Tonic-clonic spasms in horse with tetanus. (Courtesy Dr. Debra Sellon.)

associated musculoskeletal injuries. Spontaneous deaths usually are attributed to compromised respiration. This may be caused by laryngeal spasm and asphyxia; contractions of the chest wall, diaphragm, and abdomen; accumulation of excessive respiratory secretions; and aspiration pneumonia. Long-bone fractures may occur during muscle spasms or result from accidental falls. In humans and possibly horses, sudden death may occur because of cardiac or other effects of autonomic dysfunction.

Reduced intestinal borborygmi, infrequent defecation, colic, and dehydration are frequent nonneurologic signs of tetanus.

THERAPY

Treatment for tetanus should have the following objectives: (1) provision of a safe, quiet environment; (2) elimination of *C. tetani* and unbound toxin; (3) sedation and muscle relaxation (Table 47-1); and (4) general support.

Horses should be moved carefully to a large, well-bedded stall. All possible external stimuli, including light and noise, should be minimized. Feed and water should be hung so that the horse does not need to lower its head.[29] Horses in danger of falling may be maintained in a body sling,[29] tackle and girdle,[30] or stocks.

If a recent wound or other infection can be identified, it must be opened, cleaned, debrided, and flushed. *Tetanus antitoxin* (TAT) can be infiltrated into the tissues around the lesion. Penicillin traditionally has been administered to kill remaining *C. tetani* organisms; however, the drug has been found to have potential anti-GABA and proconvulsant activities.[31] *Metronidazole* now is considered the antimicrobial of choice[1,32] and may be administered at 20 to 30 mg/kg orally (PO) every 12 hours (q12h) for 3 to 5 days. If the horse's condition precludes oral medication, give 40 to 60 mg/kg per rectum or 10 to 20 mg/kg intravenously (IV) q6-8h (neonates).

Although some evidence suggests that massive parenteral doses of TAT reduce mortality in experimental tetanus in mice, active toxin that is already bound is not accessible to serotherapy. By the time a horse shows clinical signs, circulating toxin is not detectable.[10] To ensure neutralization of any residual unbound toxin, give 10,000 to 50,000 IU of TAT IV, intramuscularly (IM), or subcutaneously (SC), and repeat daily for 3 to 5 days. Because TAT does not cross the blood-brain barrier, large doses have been given intrathecally to patients with tetanus. The results of intrathecal therapy, as reported in small case series in horses, have been inconclusive;[10,30] however, meta-analysis of the major human studies has not revealed any survival advantage for this route of TAT administration.[33] Administration of TAT has been associated with acute hepatic necrosis in horses. The first clinical signs of this potentially fatal adverse reaction may appear 4 to 10 weeks after administration of TAT and has been reported in horses that received TAT for treatment of clinical tetanus.

Sedatives and muscle relaxants are used for control of muscle spasms and rigidity. The traditional approach in humans has been the combination of a phenothiazine-based ataractic sedative such as chlorpromazine with a GABAergic agent such as diazepam or phenobarbital.[2] In horses, chlorpromazine[10,22,29,34] is the most common such treatment, although acepromazine,[24,26] promazine,[27] and propionyl promazine[30] have also been used. In moderately affected horses, obvious muscle relaxation occurs within minutes of treatment and lasts for hours. Chlorpromazine additionally has α-adrenergic antagonist and anticholinergic actions that may help suppress autonomic overactivity.[1] Pentobarbital sodium is sometimes recommended for additional muscle relaxation in horses but must be titrated very carefully to avoid recumbency.[10,29] Phenobarbital likely would be effective, but oral administration may be difficult in a patient with trismus. Large doses of diazepam are effective for short-term control of muscle rigidity in humans, and the drug (in combination with xylazine) appeared effective for treatment of severe signs in two horses.[10] Diazepam may be given IV to horses and repeated as necessary to control muscle spasms. Because of potential accumulation of diazepam and respiratory or CNS depression, however, diazepam may be inappropriate for long-term treatment. Midazolam does not

Table • 47-1

Drugs for Sedation or Muscle Relaxation in Horses with Tetanus

DRUG	ACTION(S)	DOSE (mg/kg)	INTERVAL (h)	ROUTE
Acepromazine	S, MR, AA	0.02-0.1	6-12	IV, IM
Chloral hydrate	S	5-10 mg/kg	PRN	IV
Chlorpromazine	S, MR, AA	0.4-1.0	6-12	IV, IM
Dantrolene sodium	MR	2-8	24	PO
Diazepam	S, MR, AA	0.1-0.2	PRN	IV
Glyceryl guiacolate*	MR	To effect	PRN	IV
Methocarbamol	MR	10-50	6-12	IV
$MgSO_4$	MR, AA	25-50, then 5-20/h	CRI	IV
Midazolam	S, MR	0.1-0.2/h	CRI	IV
Morphine	S, AN	0.05-0.1	PRN	IV, IM
Pentobarbital Na*	S, MR	1-3	6-12	IV
Phenobarbital Na	S, MR	10-20, then 2-10	12-24	IV, PO
Promazine	S, MR, AA	0.4-1.0	6-12	IV, IM
Xylazine	S	0.25-1	PRN	IV, IM

S, Sedative; *MR*, muscle relaxant; *AA*, adrenergic antagonist; *AN*, analgesic; *PRN*, pro re nata (as needed); *CRI*, constant-rate infusion; *h*, hour; *IV*, intravenous; *IM*, intramuscular; *PO*, oral.
*Serious risk of recumbency during treatment.

accumulate and can be used as a constant infusion, but it is too expensive for use in adults. Additional strategies under study to increase GABA in patients with tetanus include pyridoxine (vitamin B_6),[35] intrathecal baclofen,[36] and sodium valproate.

Methocarbamol,[25] glycerol guiacolate,[26] mephenesin, and *d*-tubocurarine[37] have all been used for muscle relaxation in horses with tetanus but have not found wide application. The direct muscle relaxant dantrolene is used in horses for prevention of myopathy[38] and might have application to the treatment of tetanus. This drug has been used successfully in human tetanus.[39]

In developing countries, *magnesium* has recently become the treatment of choice as sole agent for tetanus of children.[2] Magnesium has multiple potentially useful actions against spasms and autonomic dysfunction and is inexpensive. It blocks neuromuscular transmission, interferes with catecholamine release from nerves and the adrenal medulla, reduces receptor responsiveness to released catecholamines, and is an anticonvulsant and vasodilator. Interestingly, electromyographic studies show that magnesium tends to spare the respiratory muscles, which is a marked advantage. Because parenteral magnesium sulfate ($MgSO_4$) is used widely and safely in horses for treatment of cardiac arrhythmia[40] and is recommended for hypoxic-ischemic encephalopathy of neonates,[41] it seems reasonable to try $MgSO_4$ in horses with tetanus. Signs of toxicity have been reported in horses given large amounts of enteral $MgSO_4$, so treatment should be monitored closely.[42]

Various approaches have been used for treatment of autonomic overactivity in human patients with tetanus.[1] These have included reserpine, clonidine, angiotensin-converting enzyme (ACE) inhibitors, α-blockers (chlorpromazine, phentolamine), β-blockers (propranolol, esmolol, labetalol), atropine, and intrathecal bupivacaine. Treatment has not been particularly successful and, with the exception of chlorpromazine, has little obvious application in the horse.

Intensive supportive therapy during at least the initial few days of signs is essential. In horses that cannot eat or drink, intravenous fluids and nutrition may be provided.[23] Enteral nutrition may be given via an indwelling nasogastric or esophagostomy tube. Because muscle rigidity and spasms reportedly are extremely painful in humans with tetanus, analgesia should be provided in well-hydrated horses with a nonsteroidal antiinflammatory drug (e.g., flunixin meglumine or equivalent) or narcotic (e.g., morphine, fentanyl patches, or butorphanol). Full paralysis and mechanical ventilation of a severely affected foal are theoretically possible. Except for the need for paralysis with a drug such as pancuronium, management would be similar to that used for botulism of foals[43] and likely would require 1 to 3 weeks of ventilation.

PROGNOSIS

The case-fatality rate is at least 50% in most reports[28] and was 75% in the most recent North American series.[10] In that study, all horses that subsequently died were recumbent by 24 to 48 hours after admission. In surviving horses, signs are usually stabilized in 2 to 7 days, with gradual recovery over the next several weeks.[10,22,24,27,28] However, one horse reportedly remained stiff at 6 months but was normal at 9 months after onset of signs.

Based on various prognostic scoring systems used for human tetanus[1] and the few small equine series published, negative prognostic indicators are incubation period less than 7 days, period of onset (time from first sign to first spasm) less than 2 days, umbilical or uterine entry site, no vaccination within the previous year, and presence of comorbid disease. Severe signs at presentation, recumbency, and initially rapid progression of clinical signs all are predictive of poor outcome.

PREVENTION

Tetanus has long been preventable by vaccination with inexpensive toxoid preparations. Nonvaccinated horses should be given an initial two-dose series of tetanus toxoid administered 3 to 6 weeks apart. Protective responses are usually attained within 2 weeks of the second dose. Booster doses should be given annually thereafter or additionally at the time of injury or surgical procedure.[44] Broodmares should be revaccinated 4 to 6 weeks before foaling to provide for colostral transfer of immunity to their foals. Passively transferred antibody suppresses the IgG response of foals to toxoid vaccination at 3 months but not 6 months of age.[45] Therefore, it is recommended that foals from vaccinated mares be given a three-dose initial series at 6, 7, and 8 to 9 months of age.[44] Foals from nonvaccinated mares are vaccinated at 3 to 4 and 4 to 5 months of age. Tetanus antitoxin is produced by hyperimmunization of donor horses with tetanus toxoid. Administration of one vial of antitoxin (1500 IU) to a nonvaccinated horse provides immediate protection that lasts for 2 to 3 weeks. Antitoxin is indicated in foals from nonvaccinated mares and in any horse that has not been vaccinated within the previous year. In these cases, antitoxin and toxoid should be administered concurrently, with separate syringes at separate sites. Because the use of antitoxin is associated with hepatic necrosis (serum hepatitis) in a small number of horses, antitoxin should not be given in horses that are adequately covered by toxoid vaccination.[46]

REFERENCES

See the CD-ROM for a list of references linked to the abstract in PubMed.

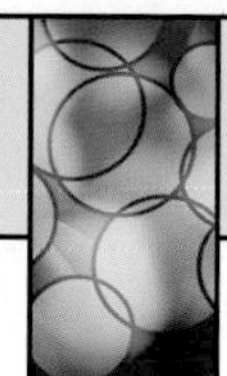

CHAPTER • 48

Miscellaneous Anaerobic Infections

J. Lindsay Oaks

Obligately anaerobic bacteria, referred to here as "anaerobes," are common opportunistic pathogens. Veterinary clinicians and microbiologists have historically been aware that these organisms can cause significant pathology, often requiring specific antimicrobial therapy. Traditionally, little effort has been devoted to specific detection or identification of these bacteria. Anaerobes usually require specialized equipment to culture and have been inherently difficult to identify accurately once isolated. Historically, identification of an anaerobe did not alter therapy because anaerobes were, and in most cases remain, predictably susceptible to many of the antibiotics already being used to treat concomitant infection with facultatively anaerobic or aerobic bacteria. (The facultative anaerobe group, which includes most of the common veterinary bacterial pathogens, and the obligately aerobic bacteria are typically referred to as "aerobes," and this colloquial nomenclature is used in this chapter.)

More recently, innate or acquired antimicrobial resistance in anaerobes has been observed in human isolates, providing more incentive to detect and identify these pathogens. Studies in human hospitals investigating the value of anaerobic microbiology show both medical and financial benefits.[1] Although such economic analyses are not available for equine medicine, the specific detection and treatment of anaerobic bacterial infections improve clinical outcome in equine cases. To realize these benefits, it is incumbent on veterinary diagnostic laboratories to provide accurate and clinically timely results of anaerobic testing. This chapter addresses nonenteric infections caused by obligately anaerobic bacteria. Enteric and systemic/myonecrotic diseases caused by *Clostridium* spp., are discussed in Chapters 44 and 45, respectively.

ETIOLOGY

The anaerobic bacteria are a large and taxonomically diverse group of bacteria that are unable to survive in the presence of free oxygen concentrations greater than about 5 μM.[2] Sensitivity to molecular oxygen results from their inability to detoxify reactive oxygen molecules formed as a byproduct of either respiratory metabolism or exposure to ambient levels of atmospheric oxygen. Bacteria that are tolerant of oxygen or that utilize oxygen metabolically (obligate aerobes and facultative anaerobes) typically possess enzymes such as catalase, superoxide dismutase, and peroxidases to detoxify reactive oxygen molecules.[3] These enzymes are generally absent in anaerobes because the detoxification reactions of catalase and dismutase result in formation of more molecular oxygen. To avoid the production of oxygen, the predominant metabolic pathways for obligately anaerobic bacteria are fermentative, and they utilize organic molecules as electron acceptors in energy production. The metabolic end products of carbohydrate and amino acid fermentation include volatile fatty acids, alcohols, indole, and sulfur compounds that are foul smelling, one of the hallmark clinical signs of anaerobic infections.[4]

Anaerobes have limited protection from exposure to oxygen by alternate detoxification pathways such as superoxide reductase. This enzyme produces hydrogen peroxide, which is detoxified into water by reductase and rubrerythrin pathways.[3,5] Aerotolerance is also quite variable among what are classified as obligate anaerobes, and growth of some obligate anaerobes such as *Bacteroides* may even be enhanced by low levels of oxygen (about 300 nM). Some obligate anaerobes may metabolically utilize, and detoxify, oxygen with cytochrome oxidase systems and oxygen-dependent respiratory chains.[2,3] These features may allow *Bacteroides*, as well as other obligate anaerobes with similar systems, to colonize mucous membranes or establish infections without prior colonization of and reduction of oxygen by facultatively anaerobic bacteria such as *Escherichia coli*.[2]

The taxonomy of anaerobic bacteria is complex and currently undergoing major revisions; this trend is likely to continue for the foreseeable future.[6-9] Although these taxonomic revisions are primarily of academic interest, they do reflect the difficulty in obtaining accurate identification of anaerobic isolates and may complicate the optimal selection of appropriate antimicrobial therapy. This also makes it difficult to compare the results of older studies to newer studies. The primary basis for this ongoing taxonomic reorganization is the use of nucleotide sequence-based phylogenetic analyses, particularly of the 16s ribosomal deoxyribonucleic acid (rDNA) gene, in place of the previously used, less reliable analyses based on phenotypic and biochemical characteristics.[7,9]

For the aerobic and facultatively anaerobic bacteria, taxonomy based on phenotypic and biochemical characteristics correlate relatively well with genetic analyses. However, for anaerobes, schemes based on phenotypic and biochemical characteristics result in much greater discrepancies, including misclassification of organisms with regard to highly fundamental traits such as Gram-staining properties, morphology, aerotolerance, and spore formation.[6,7,9] Despite the dramatic changes in the classification of anaerobes and the great diversity of this group of bacteria, most of the clinically significant anaerobic pathogens of humans and other mammals, including horses, belong to a limited number of genera[7-16] (Table 48-1).

EPIDEMIOLOGY

Anaerobic bacteria are ubiquitous members of the normal flora of the skin and mucous membranes of all mammals,[7,12,17] and the major genera found as normal flora of horses appear to be similar to the clinically significant and normal flora anaerobes of humans and other mammals. It may seem somewhat counterintuitive that obligately anaerobic bacteria are found in high numbers at sites that are exposed to ambient air, such as the skin or oral cavity. However, in addition to the inherent aerotolerance that some obligate anaerobes possess, anaerobic microenvironments are created in these areas by the presence of facultatively anaerobic bacterial flora (including many of the other bacteria familiar to clinicians, such as

Table • 48-1

Clinically Significant Obligately Anaerobic Bacteria of Humans, Horses, and Other Mammals

ORGANISM GROUP	GENERA
Gram-negative rods	*Bacteroides*
	Campylobacter
	Capnocytophaga
	Fusobacterium
	Porphyromonas
	Prevotella
	Selenomonas
	Wolinella
Gram-negative cocci	*Veillonella*
Gram-positive rods	*Actinomyces*
	Bifidobacterium
	Clostridium
	Eubacterium
	Lactobacillus
	Mobiluncus
	Propionibacterium
Gram-positive cocci	*Gemella*
	Peptostreptococcus

staphylococci, streptococci, pasteurellas, actinobacilli, and members of the Enterobacteriaceae) that consume free oxygen.[18] Anaerobes are also frequent opportunistic pathogens that cause infections when these bacteria gain access to anaerobic conditions in tissue, usually resulting from the presence of necrotic tissue and co-infection with facultatively anaerobic bacteria. Although anaerobes may cause infections by themselves, in most cases anaerobic infections are polymicrobic, with multiple obligately anaerobic bacteria as well as facultatively anaerobic bacteria.

Although most of the clinically significant anaerobes can be found on most sites of the body, certain genera are more common in certain sites. In humans the genera that predominantly colonize a given site are also those most likely to be found in infections associated with those anatomic areas, and detection of certain genera in the blood can predict the part of the body where the infection originates. Although this association has not been well demonstrated for horses, this most likely reflects the lack of information about normal equine anaerobic flora and routine anaerobic blood culturing rather than lack of such a correlation.

The most clinically important equine infections caused by obligately anaerobic bacteria are pneumonia and pleuropneumonia (see Chapter 1). Anaerobes that are reported from the equine oral and respiratory tracts include *Bacteroides*, *Clostridium*, *Eubacterium*, *Fusobacterium*, *Peptostreptococcus*, and *Veillonella*, as well as a number of other, unidentified anaerobic gram-positive rods and cocci.[10,19,20] In one series of studies, 37% to 68% of lower respiratory tract infections had involvement of anaerobes, usually *Bacteroides*; 68% to 81% were mixed with facultative anaerobes such as streptococci, pasteurellas, actinobacilli, and Enterobacteriaceae; and 85% had multiple anaerobes.[14,15,21,22] The most frequently reported anaerobes from cases of equine respiratory disease include *Bacteroides*, *Clostridium*, *Eubacterium*, *Fusobacterium*, *Peptostreptococcus*, and *Veillonella*.[10,14,15,20-27] The clinical significance of the anaerobic component of these infections is suggested by studies that found the presence of anaerobes was associated with decreased survival,[14,15,22,26] and horses treated with metronidazole showed improved clinical responses and survival rates.[15,24] The anaerobic bacteria involved in equine respiratory infections most likely arise from aspiration of normal oral flora, because most of the respiratory anaerobic pathogens are also found on the pharyngeal tonsillar surfaces.[10] Anaerobes are also often associated with a variety of paraoral infections, including submandibular abscesses, mandibular osteomyelitis, sinus infection, and dental abscesses. The predominant anaerobes involved in these infections are very similar to those found in respiratory infections and as normal flora of pharyngeal tonsillar surfaces,[10] and they presumably arise by extension from normal flora opportunistic infections.

Anaerobes are also common flora of the equine reproductive tract (see Chapter 8). In normal stallions, 96% of samples collected from the urethra, urethral fossa, smegma, and preejaculatory fluid contained *Bacteroides*, *Clostridium*, *Fusobacterium*, *Peptococcus*, and *Peptostreptococcus*. In normal mares, 100% of clitoral swabs, 24% of endometrial swabs, and 40% of endometrial washes contained *Bacteroides*, *Clostridium*, *Fusobacterium*, *Peptococcus*, and *Peptostreptococcus* spp.[28] Anaerobes, including *Bacteroides*, *Clostridium*, *Fusobacterium*, and *Peptostreptococcus* spp., can also be isolated from uterine samples from mares with cytologic evidence of acute endometritis. Presumably, anaerobes may contribute to uterine pathology during active infection, but the ability to culture anaerobes from clinically normal mares illustrates the difficulty in interpreting the significance of anaerobic bacteria identified in mucosal samples.

Anaerobic bacteria are also frequently associated with intraabdominal infections, such as abscesses and cholangiohepatitis.[29-31] The genera of anaerobic bacteria associated with these infections are similar to those found as normal flora in the equine colon and include *Bacteroides*, *Bifidobacterium*, *Clostridium*, *Eubacterium*, *Lactobacillus*, and *Peptostreptococcus*.[32-35] A variety of other opportunistic infections, including orthopedic,[18] mammary, cutaneous, and muscular infections,[36] may involve anaerobes. As a general rule, any wound or sterile site, especially when infection is caused by contamination with bacteria from the skin or mucous membranes, may potentially involve anaerobic bacteria.

PATHOGENESIS AND CLINICAL SIGNS

Although it is uncommon for anaerobic bacteria to be the primary or sole pathogen in an infection, when this is the case, they contribute significantly to the pathology and clinical signs. Any infection in which the source of bacteria is skin or mucosal flora may be complicated by anaerobic involvement under appropriate conditions. The presence of necrotic tissue and co-infection with facultatively anaerobic bacteria are the two main predisposing factors.[18,37] Necrotic tissue will have a compromised blood supply and thus decreased levels of oxygen. Facultatively anaerobic bacteria will reduce the oxygen tension sufficiently through aerobic metabolism to allow anaerobes to proliferate. Concomitant infection with the obligately anaerobic bacteria benefits survival of facultative anaerobes by providing nutritional or growth factors, suppression of antibacterial responses such as leukocidins, suppression of neutrophil chemotaxis, suppression of phagocytosis, and impairment of opsonization.[18,38] This mutually beneficial relationship likely explains the high frequency of co-infection with both obligate and facultatively anaerobic bacteria.

Anaerobic infection, once established, results in extensive tissue necrosis and pus formation. Although a very diverse group, many of the pathogenic anaerobes have similar types of virulence factors. Many anaerobes produce a number of potent exotoxins, including collagenases, proteases, DNases, heparinases, and leukocidins, that result in necrosis of tissue and localization of leukocytes.[18,39] Other important virulence factors are structural molecules, including the presence of a polysaccharide capsule, pili, and endotoxin. Capsule formation is classically associated with *Bacteroides fragilis* but may also be found with other anaerobic bacteria.[38,39] Capsules on bacteria may increase tissue adherence and may be chemotactic for neutrophils, which favors abscess formation, and capsular material from *B. fragilis* has been shown to be able to induce abscess formation in the absence of any viable organism.[18,38-40] The increased recruitment of neutrophils does not necessarily result in clearance of the bacteria because these encapsulated bacteria are also more resistant to killing by neutrophils.[18,38] In addition, the gram-negative anaerobes also produce endotoxin.[39]

No clinical signs or lesions definitively differentiate infections with anaerobic bacteria from infections with, or infections that include, facultative bacteria. Moreover, because most anaerobic infections are co-infected with facultative bacteria, most anaerobic infections will have the typical suppurative and inflammatory lesions that are associated with bacterial infections in general. However, two products of the fermentative metabolism utilized by most anaerobic bacteria, foul-smelling compounds and gas, produce clinical signs that, when present, are highly suggestive of anaerobic involvement. As previously mentioned, many of the metabolic end products of carbohydrate and amino acid fermentation are foul smelling,[4] and clinical samples from anaerobic infections will have a foul odor. In one study of equine pleuropneumonia, 62% of horses with anaerobic involvement had putrid breath or pleural samples.[22] Putrid-smelling breath and clinical samples are also frequently noted in other reports of equine anaerobic respiratory infections.[14,24,26] Free-gas echoes detected by ultrasound within pleural or abscess fluids have also been shown to be a sensitive and specific indicator of anaerobic infections.[26]

DIAGNOSIS

The diagnosis of anaerobic infections is made primarily by culture and identification. Gram-stained cytology slides may assist in making a presumptive diagnosis of anaerobic involvement, although the morphology of anaerobes is not generally unique enough to be able to differentiate them definitively from other types of bacteria. However, the visualization of multiple types of bacteria in a suppurative lesion, with isolation of fewer types of bacteria on aerobic culture, may suggest the presence of anaerobes. Gram-negative rods with tapered ends may suggest *Fusobacterium* spp.

The primary requirement for the isolation of anaerobic bacteria is the ability to create an oxygen-free environment. This is usually accomplished with either anaerobic chambers for large caseloads or benchtop jars or bags for smaller-scale use. Initial isolation is made on a variety of nonselective and selective agar-based media formulations. Subsequent identification is usually based on phenotypic and biochemical characteristics. However, accurate identification to the species level is often difficult. Fortunately, for clinical purposes, identification to the genus level is generally sufficient to document anaerobic involvement or to make decisions regarding antimicrobial therapy or the need for antimicrobial susceptibility testing. If further identification is required, this may be done by analysis of short-chain fatty acid profiles, using liquid chromatography or capillary electrophoresis, or by molecular methods, such as 16s rDNA sequencing.[7,41] Because many anaerobes are fastidious and relatively slow growing, identification even to the genus level generally takes 4 to 7 days, and clinicians should be aware that anaerobic culture results will take longer than those for most facultative or aerobic bacteria.

One of the greatest challenges for the clinician in the diagnosis of anaerobic infections is to maintain the viability of these bacteria in clinical samples between collection and receipt by the laboratory. Anaerobic bacteria in general are fragile and highly susceptible to inactivation by adverse environmental conditions; thus proper sample collection, storage, and transportation are essential to obtain good results from the laboratory. The first priority is to prevent exposure of the bacteria in the sample to oxygen. During collection, the length of time that the sample is exposed to ambient air should be minimized. As a general rule, tissue samples with a volume of 1 cm^3 or greater, or fluid samples with a volume of 1 mL or greater, submitted in a sterile, airtight container will effectively maintain an anaerobic environment and anaerobe viability for several hours.[42] However, larger volumes greater than 2 cm^3 or 2 mL are optimal. Smaller samples should be collected into anaerobic transport systems that are designed to maintain a low oxygen tension and prevent desiccation. Although there are anaerobic transport systems designed for use with swabs, another important general rule to observe whenever possible is that samples of tissue or fluid are preferable to swabs because of the larger volume of material available for culture, as well as the improved ability to prevent exposure to ambient air. Samples for anaerobic culture should be submitted to the laboratory as quickly as possible; even with properly collected samples in anaerobic transport systems, the recovery rates begin to drop after 24 hours.[43] The optimal temperature at which to hold and transport samples is room temperature.[42] Samples should not be frozen or refrigerated (4° C) because this will decrease recovery rates.[44]

Proper sample selection and collection is also very important for interpretation of laboratory results. Samples for anaerobic culture should be collected from normally sterile sites. Because of their ubiquitous presence and very high numbers (up to 10^9-10^{12} bacteria per gram), it is generally inappropriate to request anaerobic cultures from sites that have normal anaerobic flora, such as the skin, oral cavity, nasopharyngeal cavity, genital mucous membranes, feces, or intestinal lumen.[42] When sample collection requires bypassing areas with normal flora, such as with bronchoalveolar lavage, great care should be taken to avoid contaminating the sample with normal flora. Because most anaerobic infections are acquired from normal flora, any degree of contamination will potentially result in misleading results.[10,22] A number of anaerobic pathogens, including *Bacteroides*, *Clostridium*, *Fusobacterium*, and *Peptostreptococcus*, are present in the lungs of dead horses without respiratory disease.[20] This indicates that, as with interpretation of other types of microbiology findings, anaerobic bacteriology results must be interpreted with regard to other clinical and laboratory evidence that supports a diagnosis of infection.

THERAPY

Treatment of anaerobic infections is similar to that of other bacterial infections, with *debridement* and *antimicrobial drugs* being the most important components of therapy.[21,45,46] Removing necrotic debris by either surgical debridement or drainage of pus is crucial for increasing blood supply and oxygen tension, improving host antibacterial immune responses, and improving the access and function of antimicrobials at the site of infection.[45]

A number of antibiotics have good activity against obligate anaerobes, including penicillins, cephalosporins, carbapenems, chloramphenicol, lincosamides, metronidazole, macrolides, glycopeptides, tetracyclines, and the newer quinolones (which does not include the earlier quinolones labeled for veterinary use, such as enrofloxacin).[45,47,48] Many of these antimicrobials are not used routinely in horses for reasons of safety (lincosamides) and expense (carbapenems, macrolides, glycopeptides, quinolones). Consequently, the drugs most often used in the treatment of anaerobic infections in horses are penicillins, cephalosporins, chloramphenicol, metronidazole, and tetracyclines. In human medicine the resistance of a number of anaerobes, including *Bacteroides*, *Fusobacterium*, *Prevotella*, and *Porphyromonas*, to penicillins, cephalosporins, and tetracyclines is reported to be increasing.[17,47,49] Accurate or recent comparative data on the prevalence of antimicrobial resistance in veterinary medicine in general, and equine medicine in particular, are lacking.[50] However, even older equine literature reports significant rates of resistance of *Bacteroides* spp., to penicillins (18%-68% of isolates), cephalosporins (17%-62% of isolates), and tetracyclines (2%-36% of isolates), indicating that these drugs should not be regarded as predictably effective against anaerobic infections.[14,48,50,51] Lower rates of resistance to penicillins and tetracyclines are also reported for *Fusobacterium*, *Prevotella*, and *Porphyromonas*.[14,51] More recent literature examining human isolates of these organisms indicates that their rate of resistance to tetracyclines is much higher (33%-50%).[17] The variable susceptibility of multiple anaerobic bacteria to these antimicrobials indicates that their use should always be based on susceptibility testing.

At present, the drug that remains a good empiric choice for treatment of anaerobic infections is *metronidazole*. Metronidazole is able to reach plasma levels above the 90% minimal inhibitory concentration for anaerobes when given intravenously, orally, or rectally. It also appears to be safe and improves survival in equine patients with pleuropneumonia.[22,24,27,52] Resistance to metronidazole remains rare in human medicine[17,47,49,53] and equine medicine but has been reported for up to 10% of *Prevotella* spp., and 17% of *Bacteroides tectum* isolates.[14] Metronidazole resistance is also reported in an approximately 10% to 15% of *Sutterella* spp.,[17] organisms that have not been reported from horses.

Although there are safety concerns for humans who handle *chloramphenicol*, this antibiotic also remains a good empiric choice that is predictably effective against most of the common anaerobic pathogens, including *Bacteroides* spp.[50,51] Trimethoprim-sulfamethoxazole is reported to have good in vitro activity against anaerobes; however, its activity in vivo may be limited by the presence of purulent material, and clinically it does not appear to be highly effective in the treatment of lower respiratory tract infections.[15,23,54] Because most anaerobic infections are polymicrobic, antimicrobials directed against facultative bacteria are also usually required, especially when using metronidazole, which does not have activity against aerobic or facultatively anaerobic bacteria.

PUBLIC HEALTH CONSIDERATIONS

There are no public health concerns with the anaerobic bacteria, because none of these bacteria are regarded as zoonotic pathogens.

REFERENCES

See the CD-ROM for a list of references linked to the abstract in PubMed.

SECTION • IV
Fungal Diseases

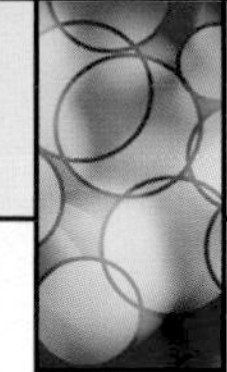

CHAPTER • 49

Laboratory Diagnosis of Fungal Diseases

Barbara A. Byrne

INTRODUCTION TO FUNGI

Fungi are eukaryotic organisms, unlike prokaryotic bacteria. Fungi are characterized by cellular organelles, such as a nucleus; however, they have several important differences from mammalian eukaryotic cells. Fungi have a cell wall that contains the sterol ergosterol and many carbohydrates, such as glucan and galactomannan. The metabolic pathways for synthesis of these unique structures are the primary targets of antifungal therapy.

Fungi have a variety of morphologic structures and forms in vivo and in vitro. The terminology describing fungal morphology and taxonomy can be complex. Additionally, fungal names and structures will vary depending on whether asexual or sexual reproduction is being observed; the asexual forms most often are clinically relevant. Box 49-1 provides a primer for fungal terminology.

Whether opportunistic or primarily pathogenic, fungi occur as yeasts (e.g., *Candida* spp.) or molds (e.g., *Aspergillus* spp.). *Yeasts* generally exist as single-celled organisms that multiply through budding. *Molds*, or *filamentous fungi*, form hyphae or elongated structures that may or may not be septate. Reproduction of filamentous fungi can occur through several mechanisms. Dermatophyte hyphae within the host may fragment to become *arthroconidia*, which are easily spread to other animals and the environment. Hyphomycetes, such as *Aspergillus* spp., can form complex asexual reproductive forms often called *fruiting structures*. Zygomycete asexual reproduction occurs through sporangium that contains *sporangiospores*. Fruiting structures and sporangiospores are rarely found within tissues unless exposed to air, such as in the sinus or guttural pouch. These reproductive structures can occasionally be observed histologically and are essential to fungal identification in culture. Other fungi, such as *Coccidioides immitis* or *Sporothrix schenkii*, are dimorphic, having different structures in vivo (e.g., spherules or yeasts) and in vitro (hyphae).

This chapter provides the clinician with the necessary information regarding basic sample collection, culture techniques, morphology, identification, and antifungal susceptibility testing to ensure optimal sampling for fungal culture and accurate interpretation of results.

Host Susceptibility

Fungal infections, with the exception of dermatophytosis, are generally rare in equine species, but they still represent important pathogens. Disease caused by fungal infection depends on many factors, primarily host susceptibility, pathogenicity of the fungal species, and dose of fungal organisms. Fungal infections such as candidiasis can be observed in neonatal foals that are often immunocompromised through failure of passive transfer, have increased susceptibility because of alterations in normal flora from antibiotic use that decreases colonization resistance, and may have poor physical defenses resulting from indwelling medical devices and wounds or abrasions. These foals illustrate the major host factors contributing to fungal infection.

Sources of Fungal Pathogens

Most fungal infections are *opportunistic* and originate from the environment, transient contamination, or normal flora. Fungi that survive and reproduce in the environment are termed *saprophytes;* they can be opportunistic pathogens. Some fungi utilize host substances without causing harm; these are *commensal* fungi. Many saprophytic fungi can be found on body surfaces without causing damage or utilizing host substances; these are termed *transients*. Some fungi require an animal host for survival, cause host damage, and are considered *obligate* pathogens; for example, the zoophilic dermatophytes require an animal host but are transmissible from animal to animal and to humans.

Knowledge of the source of agents can be important for interpretation of fungal culture results. Because most fungal infections arise from the environment, they can be a frequent contaminant in samples collected for fungal culture. Samples such as skin can have a large number of transient fungal species that can be detected in the laboratory. Transient fungal organisms are also common in the upper respiratory tract, where spores are filtered from inspired air by nasal turbinates and mucus. Feeds such as hay and alfalfa will often have high numbers of molds, which can easily contaminate the nasal passages and upper trachea. Many saprophytes will grow on conventional agar used to isolate and identify fungi, leading to false-positive results on fungal culture.

Laboratory Safety

Although safety is an important concern when working with any infectious agent, fungal pathogens require special consideration, especially in the laboratory. Filamentous fungi cultured in the laboratory produce millions of conidia, that are easily aerosolized when a culture plate is opened. This leads to widespread contamination of the laboratory that can be introduced into other cultures and expose laboratory personnel to large numbers of infectious fungi. Even saprophytic fungi can cause disease in healthy adults if sufficient numbers of conidia are present. The systemic dimorphic fungi such as *Coccidioides immitis* are generally not infectious from the patient but are highly infectious when they are in mold form in the laboratory (see Chapter 51). *C. immitis* is one of the most common and dangerous of laboratory-acquired infections.

Box • 49-1

Definitions of Common Terms Used in Mycology

Arthrospore Asexual spore formed by fragmentation of the hyphae, usually found in vivo; often seen in dermatophytosis; arthrospores are a type of conidium.
Chromoblastomycosis Fungal infection of the skin and subcutaneous tissue characterized by brown sclerotic bodies; also caused by dematiaceous fungi such as *Fonsecaea.*
Conidium Asexual reproductive cell formed from hyphae or phialides by budding or division; an infectious unit; plural *conidia.*
Dematiaceous Descriptive term for fungi with melanin pigment that gives hyphae a brown or black color.
Dermatophytosis Infection of the hair and superficial skin by fungi of the genera *Microsporum* and *Trichophyton* in animals.
Dimorphic Structural term for fungi that can convert between two different morphologies (e.g., yeasts and molds); temperature is one factor that triggers the conversion; examples include *Coccidioides immitis* and *Blastomyces capsulatum.*
Ectothrix Arthrospores that are outside the hair shaft in dermatophytosis.
Endothrix Arthrospores that are inside the hair shaft in dermatophytosis.
Fungus Eukaryotic cell (or groups of cells) with cell walls that are nonmotile and do not photosynthesize.
Hyalohyphomycosis Fungal infection caused by any mold that forms colorless, septate hyphae (e.g., seen with *Aspergillus*).
Hyphae Elongated filaments seen in molds; can be septate or nonseptate; singular *hypha.*
Hyphomycete Filamentous fungus with uncolored hyphae; asexual reproduction occurs through formation of conidiophores, phialides, and conidia; hyphae are frequently septate; examples include *Aspergillus* and *Acremonium.*
Macroconidia Large, multinuclear conidia that form from hyphae; seen only in culture, not in animal; basis for identification of many fungi, particularly dermatophytes.
Microconidia Small, single-celled conidia that form directly off hyphae.
Molds Multicellular fungi that can form mycelium; they are a subset of fungus.
Mycelium Grossly visible mat or accumulation of hyphae; plural *mycelia.*
Mycetoma General term for a tumorlike lesion that has granule-containing pus; granules of a *eumycotic* mycetoma contain fungi; an *actinomycotic* mycetoma is caused by bacteria such as *Actinomyces* and *Nocardia.*
Phaeohyphomycosis Fungal infection caused by dematiaceous fungi (e.g., *Phaeoacremonium parasiticum, Alternaria*); usually found in the skin or subcutaneous tissues, but infection can also be internal or disseminated.
Phialide Cell that produces and pushes out conidia.
Pseudohyphae Filamentous elongation of budding cells (e.g., *Candida*) that do not separate to form chains; generally the pseudohyphae narrow at the point of attachment.
Septae Divisions between hyphae or cross-walls of hyphae.
Spherule Saclike structure that contains many endospores; characteristic of *Coccidioides immitis* in vivo.
Spore Infectious unit that results from sexual reproduction in fungi; often used improperly when referring to conidia.
Vesicle Oval structure bearing phialides and conidia (e.g., seen in *Aspergillus*).
Yeasts Unicellular fungi that do not produce mycelia and reproduce by budding.
Zygomycete Filamentous fungus that has asexual reproduction through sporangia and sporangiospores; generally considered a lower form of fungi; hyphae are frequently nonseptate; examples include *Rhizopus* and *Mucor.*
Zygomycosis Fungal infection caused by a zygomycete (e.g., *Rhizopus, Mucor*).

Consequently, manipulation of all fungal cultures should be carried out in a biosafety hood, and plates should be sealed to prevent aerosolization of hyphae and conidia. The clinician should *always* inform the laboratory when a fungal infection is suspected, especially the dimorphic fungi.

SPECIMEN COLLECTION AND TRANSPORT

Aspirates, tissues, and hair or scales can be appropriate for fungal culture. Fungal organisms do not withstand extreme heat or cold and should be protected appropriately during storage and transport to the laboratory. Almost all samples can be collected as they would for bacterial culture (see Chapter 27). Because some pathogenic fungi may be present in small numbers within a tissue, a swab does not provide an adequate sample size for optimal detection of fungi. A biopsy sample or fluid aspirate is preferred. In general, samples do not require refrigeration if they are to be placed on culture media within a few hours. If transportation to the laboratory for primary culture will take longer, they should be stored and shipped at 4° C (39° F) to prevent overgrowth by bacteria and by contaminating fungi.[1]

Skin

The skin has many fungi on its surface, and cleaning with 70% ethanol before sample collection can help to remove these superficial contaminants (see Chapters 7 and 54). Hair and scales from a suspected ringworm lesion should be collected using forceps or by skin scraping. The leading edge of the lesion is best for culture because it will contain the most fungal elements. Collected specimens should be placed in a dry container for transport to the laboratory. It is not necessary to store skin scrapings and hair at cool temperatures as long as the sample can be inoculated on fungal culture media within 72 hours. If a deeper infection is considered likely, a punch biopsy is a preferred sample.

Eye

Fungal infections of corneal tissue are common, particularly in neonatal foals or as a complication of corneal ulceration (see Chapter 10). As for bacterial culture, the cornea should be scraped gently. Scrapings should be placed in a sterile container and can be left on the instrument used for scraping. A sample should be placed immediately on a slide for cytologic examination.

Blood

The lysis-centrifugation method or broth medium for blood culture can be used for fungal culture (see Chapter 27). The pellet resulting from centrifugation or media from the blood culture broth should be inoculated to the appropriate fungal culture medium.

Fluids

Fluids collected by aspiration are appropriate for fungal isolation and identification. The volume collected should be enough to represent the lesion present and should allow for inoculation of multiple media and for cytologic examination. If the sample also contains bacteria, such as a transtracheal aspirate, it should be kept cold (4° C) and shipped on wet ice to minimize overgrowth of the bacteria.

Tissue

Ideally, a biopsy of affected tissue should be collected for fungal culture and cytologic examination. Swabs may be used for diagnosis of oral lesions of suspected candidiasis (see Chapter 53).

DIRECT EXAMINATION

Cytology and histopathology are essential components for diagnosis of fungal disease. Fungal elements can be rare and localized within a lesion, so samples submitted for culture may not contain fungal organisms. Thus, cytologic and histolopathologic examination may increase sensitivity of testing for fungal organisms. It will also allow detection of unculturable agents or those that are very difficult to isolate. Unfortunately, a specific etiologic diagnosis usually cannot be made from fungal elements observed, with the exception of the typical capsule of *Cryptococcus* spp. Culture of the organism or use of molecular techniques will be necessary for definitive identification of the causative agent.

Fungal infection is almost always accompanied by inflammatory cells. In most tissues, granulomatous inflammation along with some suppuration is typically seen. One exception is infection caused by *Cryptococcus* spp. Often, minimal to no inflammation is present, most likely because of the antiinflammatory effect of the fungal capsule.

Potassium Hydroxide Treatment

Potassium hydroxide (KOH) can be used on clinical specimens to clear cellular material and better visualize fungal elements. This method is used most often when examining skin scrapings or flakes and hair for the presence of hyphae and arthroconidia in suspected dermatophyte infections, but KOH can be used on many sample types (see Chapter 54). The specimen is placed in a few drops of 10% to 20% KOH and incubated for 5 to 10 minutes; gentle heating can clear samples more quickly. A coverslip is placed over the KOH-digested sample and the slide examined microscopically without staining. Alternatively, a variety of stains can be used after KOH treatment. In dermatophytosis, arthrospores develop and form as hyphae break apart and appear as a linear chain of small, round to rectangular, highly refractile structures. *Ectothrix*, when arthrospores are present on the outside of the hair shaft, is consistent with most animal dermatophyte infections. When arthrospores are found within hairs, it is termed *endothrix*.

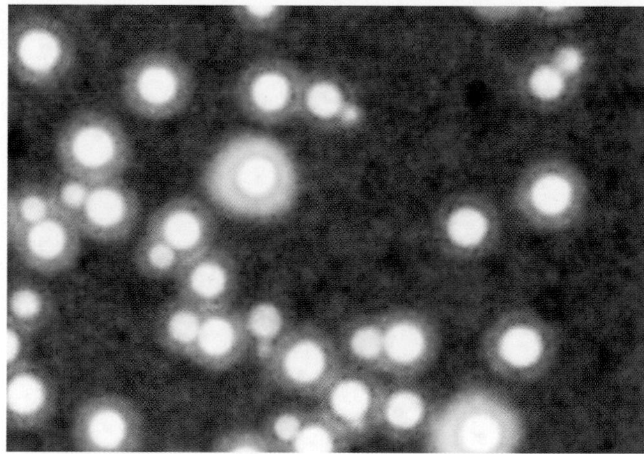

Fig. 49-1 India ink stain of *Cryptococcus neoformans*. The unstained halo around the yeast is capsular material consistent with this yeast. Budding organisms are present. (600×.)

India Ink

India ink is most useful for identification of *Cryptococcus neoformans* in fluids or tissues (see Chapter 57). A drop of India ink is placed on a slide with a drop of water and then the fluid or tissue is added. The ink will stain the background dark, leaving the abundant capsular material unstained (Fig. 49-1). The appearance is pathognomonic for *C. neoformans*.

Gram Stain

The Gram stain is very good for demonstrating the presence of yeasts. The yeast organisms will stain dark blue/purple, and budding will be easy to detect. Other fungal structures, such as hyphae, may stain variably or even poorly with Gram stain.

Some of the structures seen during a direct microscopic examination include hyphae when a filamentous fungus is present, yeasts, and spherules in the case of coccidioidomycosis. Occasionally, when a filamentous fungus is present in a body space where there is free air or oxygen, a conidial head may form with phialides and conidia. Otherwise, this structure is usually only observed when the fungus is cultured in vitro.

The fungal features present can help to narrow the list of possible fungal species present. Colorless septate hyphae branching at 45-degree angles with parallel walls and septae are suggestive of *Aspergillus* (Fig. 49-2). Broad (5-20 μm) hyphae with few to no septae and walls that are not parallel are most consistent with zygomycosis. Septate hyphae that are black or brown color are most likely a dermatiaceous fungal species that contains melanin as a component of the fungal cell wall. This condition is called *phaeohyphomycosis*. The presence of sclerotic bodies that appear brown with both horizontal and vertical septations is most similar to *chromoblastomycosis*.

Yeasts can be partially differentiated on the basis of size, shape, and budding characteristics. *Candida* are round to

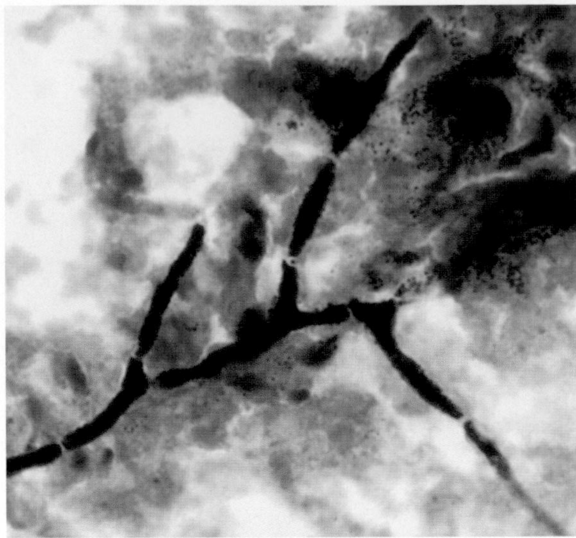

Fig. 49-2 Gram stain of fungal hyphae in clinical specimen, *Aspergillus* spp. (1000×.)

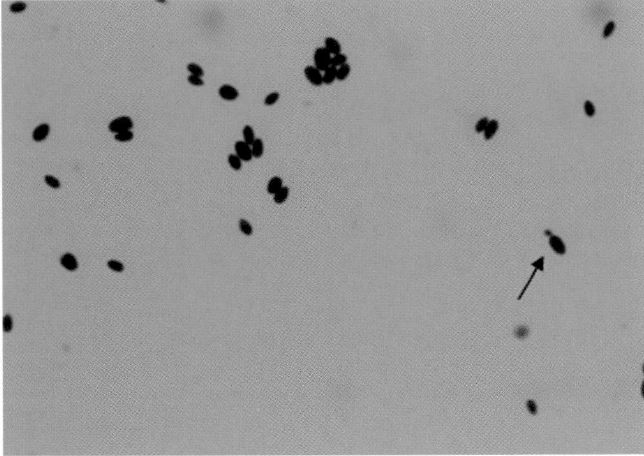

Fig. 49-3 Gram stain of *Candida* spp. The arrow points to a budding yeast. (1000×.)

oval (Fig. 49-3); they can form pseudohyphae in tissues. Pseudohyphae are an elongated outgrowth from the yeast cell and tend to narrow at the cellular divisions. *Cryptococcus*, in addition to its abundant capsule, exhibits narrow-based budding; *Cryptococcus neoformans* can stain somewhat poorly, and can have a stippled appearance (Fig. 49-4). *Coccidioides immitis* forms spherules within the host tissue. These are large, 10 to 100 mm in diameter, containing multiple round endospores. *Sporothrix schenckii* organisms are oval yeasts that have elongated or cigar-shaped budding.

Artifacts can occur with the Gram stain. Linear strands of fibrin or degenerate cells will stain pink and can appear similar to fungal hyphae.

Other Stains

Two common stains used to identify fungi in clinical specimens are Gomori's methenamine silver (GMS) and periodic acid–Schiff (PAS). The GMS stain is very useful for detection

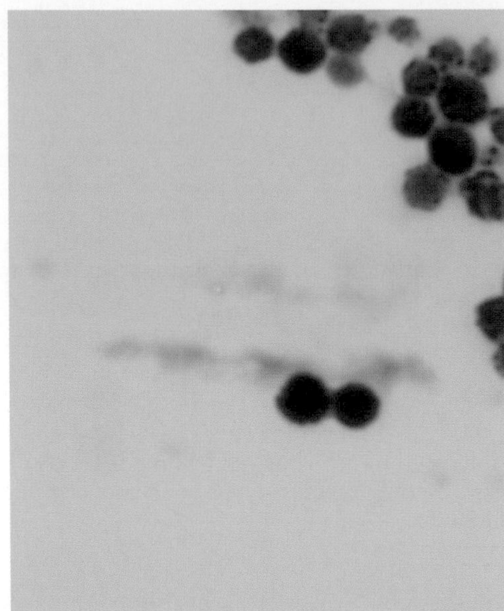

Fig. 49-4 Gram stain of *Cryptococcus neoformans*. The yeast can have stippled staining. Note very narrow ("wasp-waist") budding. (1000×.)

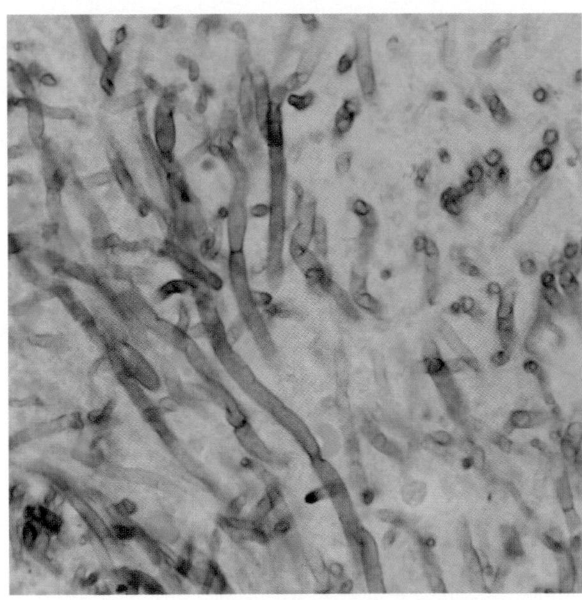

Fig. 49-5 Gomori's methenamine silver stain of biopsy from ethmoid turbinate of horse. The hyphae stain gray-black. *Aspergillus* was isolated from the sample. (1000×.)

of both yeasts and filamentous fungi, but it is generally reserved for histology laboratories and fixed-tissue sections because the staining procedure is specialized. GMS stains fungi gray or black (Fig. 49-5). PAS stains the fungal cell wall, and fungi appear pink. The PAS stain is very useful for detection of yeasts and hyphae.

Many other staining techniques are available, including methylene blue, Giemsa, and calcofluor white stains. Methylene blue can be useful to identify the intracellular yeast *Histoplasma capsulatum*. Calcofluor white staining is rapid but requires

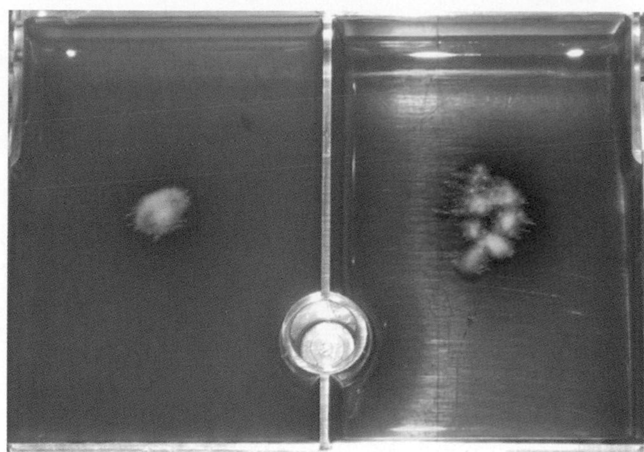

Fig. 49-6 Inoculated rapid sporulation media *(left)* and dermatophyte test media (DTM, *right*) on split plate. The DTM medium has turned red, with growth of *Microsporum gypseum*.

a fluorescent microscope for viewing, and artifacts can make interpretation difficult.

CULTURE AND IDENTIFICATION

Specialized media are required for fungal isolation and identification; consequently, fungal culture should be specifically requested when samples are submitted to the microbiology laboratory. Some fungi may grow on conventional blood agar plates used in bacteriology; this method is not reliable for identification, however, and fungal growth should be subcultured to appropriate fungal culture medium. All cultures should be incubated at 30° C (86° F); if no suitable equipment is available, samples should be cultured at room temperature (about 25° C [77° F]). Culture plates should be sealed to minimize evaporation but allow air exchange. Agar plates should be examined every few days for 4 weeks before considering them as negative for fungal growth. Growth of yeasts usually occurs within a few days to 1 week. Growth of molds can take days to weeks.

Dermatophyte Culture

Collection of hair or scales from suspected dermatophytosis lesions and culture probably represent the most common and easiest fungal detection method used by equine practitioners (see Chapter 54). Hair and scales should be placed on suitable media, such as dermatophyte test medium (DTM) or dermatophyte identification media, and incubated in the dark at room temperature. DTM contains chloramphenicol, gentamicin, and cycloheximide to inhibit bacteria and some saprophytic fungal growth. Dermatophytes will turn the media alkaline, resulting in a color change to red. Some type of medium that encourages sporulation (e.g., rapid sporulation medium) should be inoculated at the same time because dermatophytes grown on DTM may not have adequate conidia production for identification. DTM cultures should be examined daily for fungal growth and color change; the red color should appear before or when fungal growth is evident to be consistent with a dermatophyte (Fig. 49-6). Some saprophytic fungi will grow on DTM and may cause a red color. Regardless of the color change, the mold should be examined for macroconidia and microconidia to confirm the isolate as a dermatophyte rather than a saprophytic contaminant (Fig. 49-7).

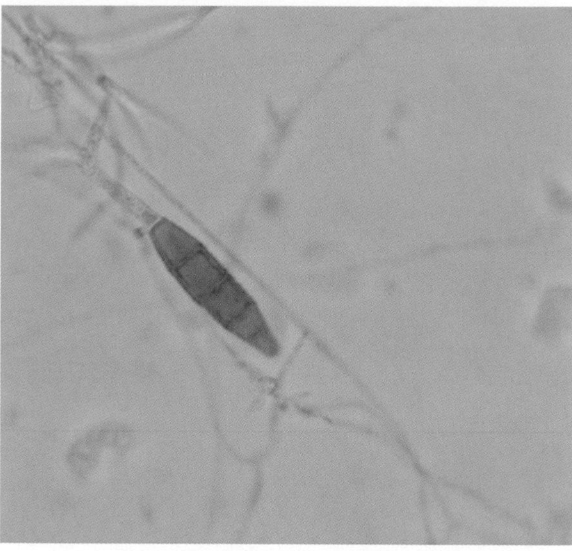

Fig. 49-7 Tape preparation of fungal growth of *Microsporum gypseum* stained with lactophenol analine blue. The large structures are macroconidia. The rough outer wall of the macroconidia and few (or no) microconidia are consistent with the genus *Microsporum*. (600×.)

Culture of Fluid or Tissue

Any fluid samples, such as urine, bronchoalveolar lavage (BAL), or transtracheal aspirate (TTA), should be centrifuged and the resulting pellet used to inoculate media. Tissue samples should be macerated with a tissue grinder or stomacher to release fungal elements. Generally, samples will be plated initially on some type of fungal agar. If the sample is likely to have bacteria, it will be cultivated on a medium containing antibiotics, such as *inhibitory mold agar* (IMA), which contains chloramphenicol. If no contaminants are expected, the sample can be inoculated onto a noninhibitory medium, such as Sabouraud dextrose agar or potato dextrose agar. Although the IMA will inhibit growth of contaminating bacteria, many molds will not have their characteristic gross and microscopic morphology, necessitating subculture to a noninhibitory medium and delaying definitive identification. Some fungi will grow on blood agar used for bacterial isolation and identification, but will also need subculture to a noninhibitory fungal agar for identification.

Identification of Fungal Species

Identification of the fungal species causing an infection is both art and science. Much of identification is based on fungal morphology in vitro but also can rely on biochemical testing. The first step in identification depends on the morphologic differentiation between yeast and mold; often this can be done based on the initial direct examination of the submitted sample.

Yeasts will appear as regular colonies on inoculated plates and as single-celled organisms with budding on Gram stain. Their shape and budding characteristics can be used for preliminary identification of the genus. Definitive identification will depend on additional biochemical testing. Kits are available for identification of many pathogenic yeasts, including the API Microbial Identification Strips 20C AUX, Yeast (bioMérieux Vitex, Hazelwood, Missouri), and RapID yeast plus panel (Remel Labs, Lenexa, Kansas). Additionally, selective agar that produces a characteristic color change

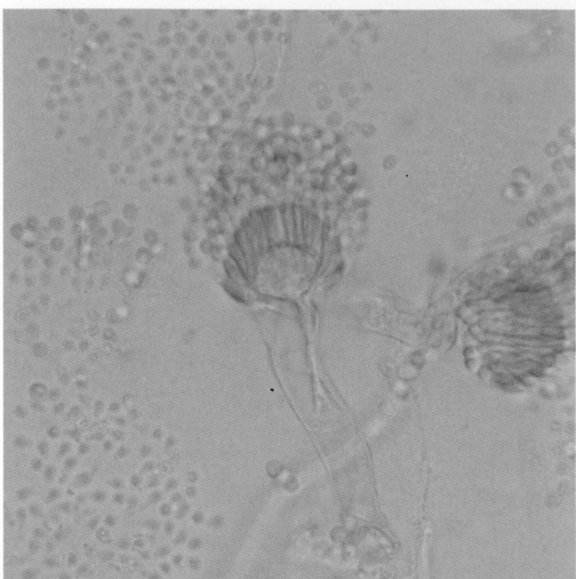

Fig. 49-8 Tape preparation of fungal growth of *Aspergillus* spp. stained with lactophenol analine blue demonstrating characteristic fruiting structures. (600×.)

(CHROMagar Candida) can be used for both genus and species identification of *Candida*. Although identification to the genus level is often sufficient for treatment, many yeasts, particularly certain species of *Candida* (e.g., *C. glabrata*), have shown resistance to common antifungal agents. Thus, speciation can aid selection of the appropriate drug for treatment.[2]

Molds are identified based on macroscopic appearance, such as color, rapidity of growth, and diffusible pigment in the agar, and microscopic features, such as hyphal morphology, with or without septae and asexual reproductive structures. Algorithms are available for fungal identification.[3] When microscopic morphology does not allow definitive identification, molecular techniques can be used for species identification. As for yeasts, definitive identification of molds to the species level can be helpful for choosing the most appropriate treatment, particularly with *Aspergillus* spp. (Fig. 49-8), because some species have known resistance to certain antifungal drugs.[2,4]

Pneumocystis carinii (P. jirovecii)

Pneumocystis carinii is an organism with uncertain taxonomic position; it has frequently been categorized as either a fungus or a protozoon (see Chapter 50). Ribosomal ribonucleic acid (rRNA) sequencing suggests that *P. carinii* is most closely related to fungi, particularly *Saccharomyces cerevisiae*.[5] This agent does not grow in routine bacterial or fungal cultures. Consequently, it is detected using a variety of stains. A Giemsa or Papanicolaou stain demonstrates abundant foamy material in BAL or alveolar spaces. *P. carinii* is better visualized with a GMS stain or immunohistochemical staining to detect *Pneumocystis* antigen. Alternatively, molecular methods can be used to detect *Pneumocystis* deoxyribonucleic acid (DNA).[6]

INTERPRETATION OF CULTURE RESULTS

Interpretation of a positive fungal culture from a site that is often contaminated with saprophytic fungi can be difficult. Therefore, it is important to include a cytologic or histologic examination of the tissue to document the presence of fungi, such as yeasts or hyphae, in the tissue. Isolation of common saprophytic fungi that are often not pathogenic, such as *Mucor* or *Rhizopus*, is more consistent with contamination. Furthermore, inflammation almost always accompanies fungal infection and would help to support the interpretation.

Probably the most common samples from which fungi are isolated are TTAs and skin scrapings or biopsies. Isolation of an opportunistic fungus must always be interpreted cautiously because these sites frequently have transient fungi that can contaminate the sample. The patient should have other clinical, cytologic, or histologic evidence that a fungus is present before interpreting the isolate as a true infecting agent.

Finally, because fungi can be found in small numbers within lesions, samples submitted to the laboratory may not contain fungal elements that are sufficiently viable for isolation. Consequently, a negative fungal culture does not rule out the presence of a fungal infection.

MOLECULAR DIAGNOSIS OF FUNGAL INFECTIONS

General molecular methods used to identify pathogenic organisms are described in Chapter 27. This section identifies specific fungal organisms for which molecular methods could be used for diagnosis and addresses issues that apply directly to fungal pathogens.

The *polymerase chain reaction* (PCR) is the most common method used to detect fungal DNA in samples. Primers can be designed to recognize fungi at many levels of identification. For example, universal primers detect virtually all species of fungi; genus-specific primers identify fungi belonging to a single genus, such as detection of all *Aspergillus* spp., and species-specific primers may be used for detection of a single species. Most PCR tests used for fungal detection are directed toward rRNA genes or the spacer regions between the genes. PCR using universal fungal primers can be helpful when the histologic examination suggests a fungal infection, but no fungal elements are present and isolation was not successful. However, this test should be used only on samples that do not have any chance of saprophytic contamination, or a false-positive result will be obtained. If a sample is positive, further testing (e.g., sequencing of PCR product, DNA probe) can be used to identify the genus and species present.

PCR can also be used to identify a fungus after growth is observed in the laboratory. Because morphologic identification can take days to weeks, PCR amplification can provide a rapid result and lead to more rapid, definitive treatment.

Molecular methods for detection exist for many fungi. Most frequently these techniques are used to detect *Aspergillus* spp., *Cryptococcus* spp., and *Candida* spp.[7,8] PCR methodology is also available for diagnosis of *Pythium insidiosum*[9] (see Chapter 55).

One disadvantage of using molecular methods for diagnostic testing is that fungal cells can be scarce in infected tissues, making detection difficult. Thus a negative result does not mean that a fungal infection is not present. Molecular methods should not replace primary culture, isolation, and identification, but rather supplement these standard diagnostic techniques to provide the quickest and most accurate diagnosis.

FUNGAL ANTIGEN DETECTION

Testing for fungal antigen is available to aid diagnosis of fungal infections in humans and animals. The most frequently used methods are latex agglutination and enzyme immunoassay (EIA) for detection of *Cryptococcus* spp. capsule. Large amounts of capsule are released into the systemic circulation; this allows detection of fungal antigen in serum or exudate from the site of suspected infection. The result is reported as a "titer" but is a measure of *antigen*, not antibody. Because this test is quantitative, it can be used during treatment to evaluate response. A declining antigen titer indicates a positive response to treatment.

Several tests exist to detect *Aspergillus* spp. infection in humans. These methods most often use EIA to measure *galactomannan*, a component of the fungal cell wall, in body fluids or serum.[10] These tests have not been validated in horses to diagnose aspergillosis. Another, but less specific, cell wall component measured to detect fungal infection is (1→3)-beta-D-glucan.[11] This substance is present in several fungi, including *Aspergillus* and *Candida*.

ANTIFUNGAL SUSCEPTIBILITY TESTING

Testing of fungal isolates for susceptibility to antifungal drugs is becoming more widely available, and many human and veterinary laboratories will perform testing on yeasts. Determination of a minimum inhibitory concentration (MIC) for filamentous fungi is more difficult to perform and standardize; consequently, this testing is limited to a few laboratories. Traditionally, few equine isolates are tested for antifungal drug susceptibility because many antifungal drugs are prohibitively expensive for use in large species. However, as more drugs become available in the less expensive generic formulations, use of these drugs to treat horses will become more widespread. An understanding of the advantages and limitations of antifungal sensitivity testing is important for the equine clinician to ensure optimal use of antifungal drugs.

The Clinical and Laboratory Standards Institute (CLSI), formerly the National Committee for Clinical Laboratory Standards (NCCLS), has standardized testing of antifungal drugs against yeasts since 1997 and molds since 2002.[12,13] Standardization of methodologies is necessary for reproducibility and comparison of results within and between laboratories and assessment of the clinical utility of this testing. Establishment of an MIC or zone of inhibition of growth to indicate that an organism is susceptible or resistant to a particular drug is in its infancy and is only available for a few drugs and fungal species.

The usefulness of antifungal drug susceptibility testing is the ability to use the result to predict clinical outcome. In general, the clinician should remember that (1) in vitro measurement of susceptibility does not guarantee clinical success, (2) finding an organism to be resistant in vitro should predict therapeutic failure, and (3) host factors can be the most important component for a positive clinical outcome.[14] Interpretation of an MIC as susceptible or resistant depends on two criteria: (1) whether the MIC measured in vitro meets or exceeds the drug concentrations found within the animal and (2) reliable clinical data that demonstrate successful treatment of the respective fungal infection at or below the MIC.[14] Interpretive criteria are best established for yeasts, particularly *Candida* spp., with the antifungal drugs amphotericin B and the azole class. Unfortunately, few data exist in the human literature for mold susceptibility interpretations, and few to no studies have been performed in common veterinary species such as the horse. Thus the use and interpretation of MIC values for fungi are controversial.[15]

However, a number of yeast and mold isolates have demonstrated both in vivo and in vitro resistance to common antifungal drugs. Some of these species, such as *Aspergillus terreus, Aspergillus fumigatus, Paecilomyces lilacinus, Candida* spp., and *Cryptococcus neoformans*, do cause infections in veterinary species.[2,4,16] Consequently, more laboratories are using fungal susceptibility testing.

The two major methods for antifungal susceptibility testing are *agar diffusion* using either disks or E-test (an antifungal imprenant strip that allows determination of fungal MIC on agar media) and *broth dilution*. Most testing evaluates the ability of the drug to inhibit fungal growth (80% reduction), rather than determining fungicidal activity.[17]

Although all laboratories do not currently offer antifungal susceptibility testing, several commercial broth-based systems are available for yeast MIC determinations. The Sensititre Yeast One Colorimetric Antifungal Panel (Trek Diagnostic Systems, Westlake, Ohio) has a fairly wide range of drug concentrations and has at least 85% agreement with reference methods.[18]

SEROLOGY

Serologic testing can be used to confirm fungal infection in horses, although its use has been limited. Serology for *Aspergillus* infection has been done for horses using agar gel immunodiffusion, immunoblot, or enzyme-linked immunoassay (ELISA).[19,20] This testing has been helpful in diagnosing systemic aspergillosis but has had variable results in detecting *A. fumigatus* infection of the guttural pouch. The ELISA test does not seem to differentiate normal from diseased horses, but detection of antibody directed toward two *Aspergillus* proteins of 22 and 26 kilodaltons did identify diseased horses in immunoblot tests.[20]

Serology has helped to identify horses with coccidioidomycosis (see Chapter 51). Only 4% of normal horses have a positive titer, and this titer remains stable or decreases with time.[21] Thus a positive test result should be highly suggestive of infection and can be used prognostically.[22]

REFERENCES

See the CD-ROM for a list of references linked to the abstract in PubMed.

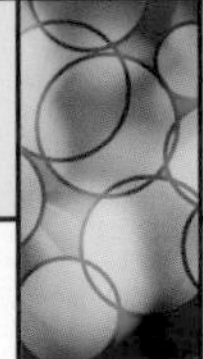

CHAPTER • 50

Pneumocystis Infections

Maureen T. Long

Pneumocystis carinii is a pathogenic fungus that most frequently causes lung disease in the immunocompromised host. Because *P. carinii* is an uncultivable agent, its biology and life cycle and concepts of general pathogenicity have been difficult to elucidate. Recent molecular advances have improved knowledge of *P. carinii* pathogenesis in immunodeficient and immunologically normal individuals.[1] These observations may lead to a better understanding of *P. carinii*–induced disease in the horse.

ETIOLOGY

Pneumocystis organisms are a group of pathogenic fungi, some of which are host adapted.[1] The organism was initially classified as a parasite closely related to the trypanosomes because of the presence of several morphologic forms and similarities in life cycle.[2,3] There is a thin-walled, "trophozoite-like" form with a single nucleus, as well as a typical thick walled, cystlike organism with multiple (usually eight) inner bodies. The procyst is considered either a product or a subtype of the trophozoite stage. Knowledge of the life cycle of *Pneumocystis* has been determined by electron microscopy; the organism cannot be cultured in vitro, and the complete natural history of *Pneumocystis* remains elusive. At present, *Pneumocystis* is evolutionarily placed between the sister groups of fungi, Ascomycota and Basidiomycota.[4] The Ascomycota are the very large group of fungi that vary from the sexual *Saccharomyces* to the asexual *Aspergillus* and *Candida*. The Basidiomycota include the edible and inedible mushrooms, rusts, and pathogens such as *Cryptococcus*.

In the absence of the ability to culture *Pneumocystis* in vitro and confirm species by cross-mating of isolates, a trinomial nomenclature evolved in which *forma specialis* (f. sp.) is used to designate each type or variety until formally designated. Sequence analysis of mitochondrial deoxyribonucleic acid (DNA) now clearly demonstrates heterogeneity between isolates and the presence of multiple species of *Pneumocystis*.[5-7] *Pneumocystis carinii* f. sp. *hominis* is now recognized as *Pneumocystis jirovecii* and is thus far the only *Pneumocystis* species that has been found in humans.[8] Each "type" or species demonstrates variability between isolates, facilitating molecular epidemiologic studies of spread and persistence of strains.[8,9] The human genosequence *Pneumocystis* has never been demonstrated in nonhuman primates. The primate sequences demonstrates more variability than what appears to be present in the human-adapted species.[9] *Pneumocystis carinii* f. sp. *carinii*, or *P. carinii*, is the host-adapted species for the rat.[10] A specific subtype associated with equine infection was identified by sequencing of the mitochondrial ribosomal ribonucleic acid (rRNA) gene. Samples from four foals were sequenced and demonstrated 85%, 84%, and 78% agreement with human and ferret, SCID-mouse, and rat sequences, respectively.[11] Species identification and alignment are an ongoing process as the genomic analysis of this organism proceeds.

EPIDEMIOLOGY

Historically *P. carinii* infection and disease have been considered a problem primarily in immunocompromised hosts. However, recent evidence supports the hypothesis that this organism is either a component of normal respiratory flora or a primary upper respiratory pathogen of immunocompetent animals.[1,12] Seroepidemiologic studies show a positive correlation between age and presence of serum antibodies in humans.[13] Exposure to the organism is apparently widespread, indicating that it is ubiquitous in the human environment.

Based on genetic studies, it is now recognized that human exposure and infection with *Pneumocystis* occurs during childhood, often during the neonatal period.[14] Vaginally delivered rat pups are DNA positive by oral swab after delivery, indicating lateral transmission soon after birth (as from environmental and maternal respiratory secretions).[15] Upper respiratory secretions of women are more likely to be DNA positive by the third trimester of pregnancy.[16] In serologic studies, between 70% and 85% of children demonstrate seroconversion to *Pneumocystis* during childhood.[17,18]

The syndromes associated with *Pneumocystis* infection in immunocompetent children include asymptomatic infection, mild upper respiratory infection, and bronchiolitis. Several studies suggest an association between this organism and sudden infant death syndrome.[19-22] Because these associations were made using molecular methods, questions remain regarding the causal relationship between *Pneumocystis* spp. infection and primary disease in the immunocompetent host. The presence of this organism may be related to an underlying disease process not yet identified.

With genetic sequencing, carriage of *Pneumocystis* in samples from the upper respiratory tract or by bronchoalveolar lavage (BAL) has been confirmed in asymptomatic animals and people with no identifiable immunologic risk.[16,23-25] In one study, 20% of asymptomatic, immunocompetent people carried *Pneumocystis* in their respiratory tract.[24] Similarly, 24% of health care workers treating human immunodeficiency virus (HIV)–infected patients are *Pneumocystis* carriers.[25] Subtle differences in these populations that might affect immune status may still be identified. For example, some of these carriers may have chronic lung disease. Pregnancy, concomitant medications (not classified as immunosuppressive agents), or undiagnosed immune compromise may have affected the frequency of detection of *Pneumocystis* DNA in these studies. Asymptomatic *Pneumocystis* infection has also been demonstrated in mice, rats, and ferrets.[23,26-28]

Evidence from environmental, animal, and human molecular epidemiologic studies suggests that the fulminant syndrome, *Pneumocystis carinii* pneumonia (PcP), may not be the result of reactivation of a latent infection that was acquired earlier in life, as previously believed.[29] Environmental monitoring casts doubt on whether *Pneumocystis* can propagate independent of a host. Clustering of infections has been reported since World War II. Initial infections likely originate from direct transmission of the organism from an immunocompetent carrier to an immunocompromised individual.[30] Transmission of *Pneumocystis* genotypes occurs from HIV-infected mothers to their children, as does lateral transmission from immunocompromised patients to normal people.[7,18,26,27,30-33] Air samples from hospital rooms of HIV-infected patients demonstrate identical strains of organisms.[34] These types of investigations on horse farms would be of value to determine the epidemiology of PcP in equids.

Pneumocystis infections have been detected in many other animals. Immunodeficient dogs die from overwhelming *Pneumocystis* infections, and the organism has been detected sporadically in dogs with interstitial pneumonia.[13,15,35-46] The organism has been detected sporadically in dogs with interstitial pneumonia. Young swine develop a fatal interstitial pneumonia and can be concomitantly infected with *P. carinii*.[40,43,47-49] Cattle, goats, and sheep have reportedly been infected with *P. carinii;* infected goats and sheep are likely to have a pneumonitis type of disease.[4,43]

PATHOGENESIS

Pneumocystis infection is associated with two disease conditions in horses: acute, fulminant PcP and secondary infections with pulmonary fibrosis (pneumocystosis).[50] When an overwhelming alveolar infection occurs in the immunocompromised host, the ensuing PcP is life–threatening, and the organism is readily found in the alveoli of the lung.[47,50-52] It resides extracellularly in alveolar spaces, adhered to alveolar type I cells, and causes a severe exudative disease process. The tissue reaction is moderate and characterized by lymphocyte and plasma cell localization within the alveoli and mild thickening of the interstitium surrounding the alveoli. Foals with *severe combined immunodeficiency* (SCID) develop classical PcP in which alveoli are packed with *P. carinii* (Figs. 50-1 and 50-2). The alveolar spaces become moderately thickened with inflammatory cells. Severe accumulations of proteinaceous debris create dyspnea and hypoxia.

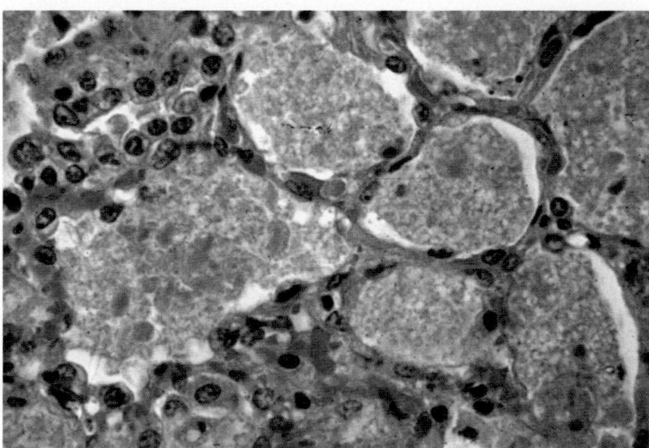

Fig. 50-1 Photomicrograph of section of lung, stained with hematoxylin and eosin, from foal with severe combined immunodeficiency (SCID). The alveoli are moderately thickened and contain small numbers of mononuclear inflammatory cells with occasional neutrophils. The alveoli are lined with epithelium that is cuboidal, consistent with pneumocyte type I hyperplasia. The alveoli are filled with pink-staining, granular fluid (highly proteinaceous). Distinct areas along the alveoli do not pick up stain.

Pneumocystis infections in immunocompetent humans and horses with normal numbers of CD4+ T cells have been described. However, the requirement of CD4+ T cells for protection against disease has been demonstrated in murine models and in human patients with acquired immunodeficiency syndrome (AIDS).[7,13,57-59] Loss of CD4+ cells and susceptibility to disease can be reversed by interferon-gamma (IFN-γ).[60,61] Cytotoxic CD8+ T cells are an end-effector cell that mediates clearance after antigen-specific activation by CD4+ helper cells. Nonspecific CD8+ effector cells actually increase lung injury.[62] Macrophages are considered important in the killing of *Pneumocystis* organisms; however, these cells must be augmented by T cells, IFN-γ, and granulocyte colony-stimulating factor (G-CSF).[63] Other effector molecules are likely also important and have yet to be identified.

Localization of *Pneumocystis* to the alveoli results in accumulation of a proteinaceous fluid, causing severely impaired oxygenation.[64] This condition has been compared to a disease called *alveolar proteinosis*. Pulmonary alveolar proteinosis is characterized by insidious onset of exercise intolerance and dyspnea. The proteinaceous material is thought to be alveolar secretions consistent with surfactants. In idiopathic disease, lack of clearance rather than overproduction of proteinaceous fluid is considered the pathogenesis. Granulocyte-macrophage colony-stimulating factor (GM-CSF) is necessary for activation of pulmonary macrophages and removal of the pulmonary surfactant. The exact pathogenesis of proteinaceous accumulations in PcP is not known.

In many animals and humans with signs or symptoms of pulmonary disease, *Pneumocystis* organisms have been detected with BAL. Many of these reports describe the presence of chronic fibrosing lung pathology.[33,50] In these cases, *Pneumocystis* may not be the inciting cause of pulmonary disease[53-56] but may have colonized the compromised lung secondary to another disease process. This condition is referred to as *pneumocystosis* to differentiate it from acute, overwhelming PcP as previously described. Pneumocystosis in immunocompetent humans and rabbits has been associated with severe malnutrition.[7,65,66]

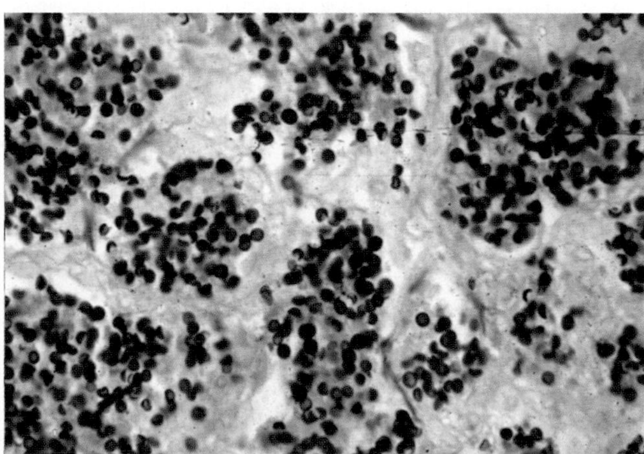

Fig. 50-2 Photomicrograph of section of lung, stained with Gomori's methenamine silver (GMS), from foal with SCID. The alveoli are filled with approximately 6-μm organism that pick up GMS stain (black refractile bodies), consistent with *Pneumocystis*.

CLINICAL FINDINGS

Immunodeficient Horses

The primary immunodeficiency of horses associated with PcP is the SCID syndrome in which Arabian foals are born without functional B cells and T cells.[57] This infection is one of several respiratory pathogens to which these foals may succumb as their maternal antibody levels wane over 3 to 6 months of life. Adenovirus and *Rhodococcus equi* infections are the most common concomitant infections of these foals and increase the severity of the initial presentation. Onset of PcP is insidious, with foals presenting in moderate to poor body condition with other systemic signs such as anorexia and depression. These foals usually have intermittent fever and nasal discharge that may initially respond to antibiotic therapy. Foals become increasingly dyspneic, with persistent fever, tachycardia, and tachypnea. On auscultation, foals have bilateral crackles and moist rales in the trachea. Eventually an abdominal breathing pattern ensues, and foals exhibit signs of respiratory compromise and hypoxemia. These foals frequently develop infections of other body systems (e.g., joint ill, diarrhea), which may also ultimately result in their demise.

Immunocompetent Horses

Pneumocystis has been isolated from presumably immunocompetent foals (4 months to 1 year of age) and adult horses with severe, atypical interstitial pneumonia.[52,54-56,67,68] Affected animals present in acute respiratory distress with exceptional abdominal effort. Usually these animals are persistently febrile. Lymphadenopathy may be present. A dry, harsh cough is common, and wheezes and crackles are audible over both thoracic cavities. Therapy is unrewarding, and horses often die within 1 week. Sudden collapse and death have also been described. Whether or not there is an underlying acquired or other immunodeficiency in affected equids is unknown; however, when investigated, most of these horses have either normal lymphocyte or CD4+ T cells.

Pneumocystosis and splenic lymphoid hypocellularity were described in a Paso Fino foal; no other assessment of this foal's immune system was reported.[69] Immunoglobulin (Ig) concentrations were normal in a 3-month-old Swiss Warmblood foal with pneumocystosis.[67] CD3 cells were detected in fixed sections, but immunophenotyping was not pursued. In a report of pneumocystosis in three Quarter Horse foals, one foal had decreased gamma-globulin levels, and the other two were treated with corticosteroids before the onset of clinical signs.[70] In a report of five Thoroughbred foals affected with pneumocystosis, no immunologic testing was pursued.[11,71] Five of the foals in a Florida study were Arabians, but SCID was not a reported feature of the clinical syndrome of these animals.[50] Recently, an adult Paso Fino mare was reported to have a syndrome consistent with common variable immunodeficiency: decreased IgM and IgA with decreased expression of major histocompatibility complex (MHC) class II antigens.[68,72] This horse also had proliferative pneumonia attributable to *Pneumocystis* infection.

DIAGNOSIS

Clinical testing for *Pneumocystis* infection is similar to that described for other types of respiratory infection, including complete blood count, serum biochemistry, transtracheal wash (TTW), and BAL. Abnormalities of leukocyte counts are not consistent unless animals have the SCID defect, in which case a lymphocyte count of less than 1000 cells/μL is present. Immunocompetent animals may have decreased, normal, or increased white blood cell counts, characterized predominantly by changes in neutrophil numbers. Serum biochemical analysis may be normal or may demonstrate hypergammaglobulinemia unless there is a concomitant gastrointestinal disorder allowing loss of protein or horses are SCID and have minimal gammaglobulin production. Hyperfibrinogenemia is also common. Affected foals may be severely hypoxemic and hypercapneic.

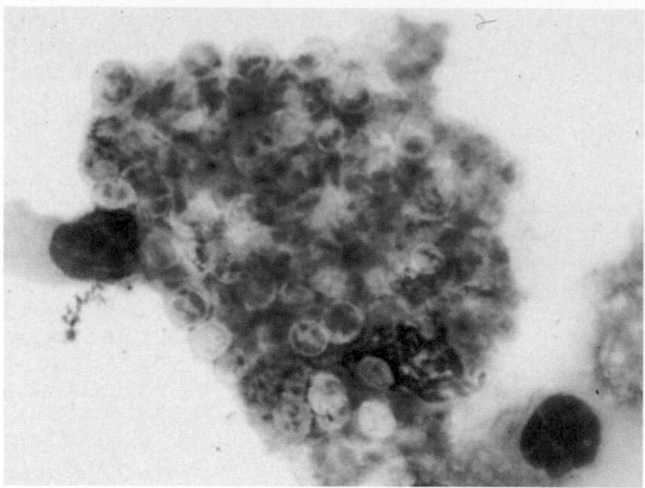

Fig. 50-3 Wright-Giemsa–stained slide of bronchoalveolar lavage (BAL) fluid sample from horse in respiratory distress. The many clusters of round, negatively stained organisms approximately 6 μm in diameter demonstrate the ring stage of the fungus *Pneumocystis*. (250×.)

Transtracheal washes usually reveal the presence of increased mucin and neutrophils. Fungal elements may or may not be observed; usually the *Pneumocystis* organism is not detected in these samples. Bacteria are frequently observed and isolated by culture. In human and equine infections with *Pneumocystis*, BAL is essential for detection of fungal elements. Cellular analysis of the BAL is more consistently mononuclear than observed with TTW samples, consisting of macrophages and giant cells. Areas of negative staining are frequently observed within the foamy eosinophilic background (Fig. 50-3). Staining of these specimens with Gomori's methenamine silver (GMS) demonstrate the oval to crescent-shaped organisms in the areas that were originally negatively stained (Fig. 50-4).

Foals with *Pneumocystis* infection have a mixed alveolar and interstitial pattern on thoracic radiography (Fig. 50-5). The interstitial pattern in these foals has been described as a reticulonodular pattern.[52] Air bronchograms indicate the presence of an alveolar pattern. The presence of abscessation is highly associated with concomitant *R. equi* infection. Ultrasound evaluation reveals consolidation characterized by a "comet tail" appearance of the parietal pleura throughout all lung fields. Abscesses identified concomitantly with this modality also indicate *R. equi* infection.

Molecular diagnostic techniques performed on respiratory secretions are considered confirmatory for a diagnosis of *Pneumocystis* infection in an animal with compatible respiratory signs and appropriate cellular responses. These molecular techniques primarily consist of polymerase chain reaction (PCR) performed on either BAL samples, fresh lung tissue, or fixed lung tissue.[34] PCR performed on nasal swabs is of value for epidemiologic purposes; positive results obtained from the secretions of the lower respiratory tract indicate pulmonary colonization with *Pneumocystis*.

Infections with *Pneumocystis* or other opportunistic pathogens should prompt investigation of the immune status of the affected horse. This should include quantification of Ig classes, immunophenotyping of circulating lymphocytes, and in

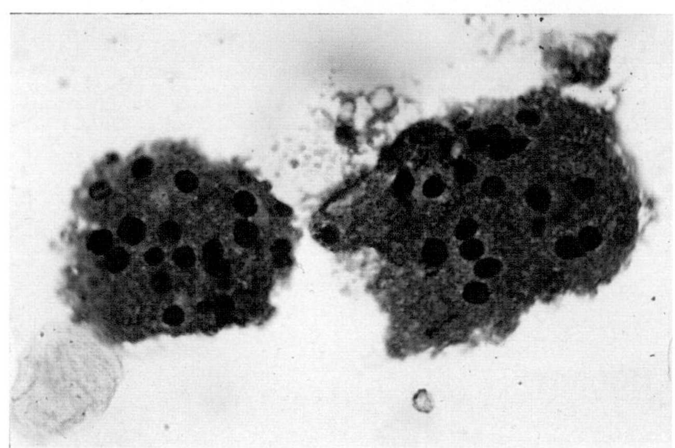

Fig. 50-4 BAL fluid obtained from horse in respiratory distress. BAL was centrifuged, and cells stained with GMS demonstrate many organisms approximately 6 µm in diameter, consistent with the fungus *Pneumocystis*.

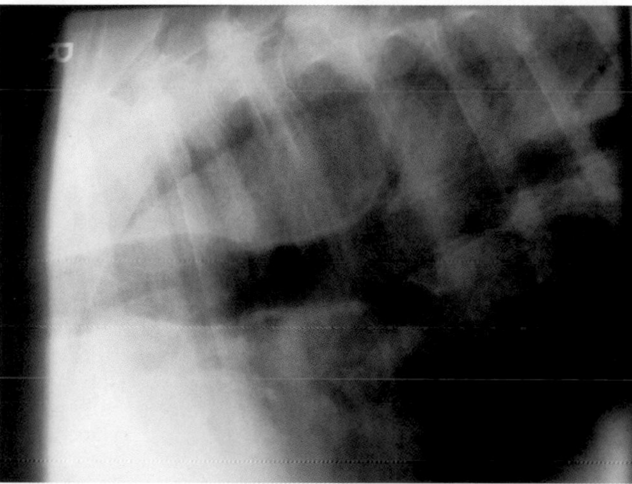

Fig. 50-5 Thoracic radiograph of horse with atypical interstitial pneumonia. BAL revealed organisms consistent with the fungal pathogen *Pneumocystis*. The changes are consistent with a severe alveolar pattern. Large air bronchograms are present within the dorsal lung fields, and the trachea is distended (ballooning).

situ evaluation of cell phenotypes in lymphoid organs. Immune function tests, such as lymphocyte blastogenesis testing, may be considered.

PATHOLOGIC FINDINGS

Grossly, the lungs of affected horses are firm and dark red (hepatized).* Fluid may run from cut surfaces. Histopathology associated with alveolar infection of immunocompromised horses is similar to that of other species. Alveolar changes consist of proliferation of the alveolar epithelia resulting from type II pneumocyte hyperplasia. Within the alveoli, there is accumulation of pink or acidophilic cellular fluid. This edema fluid frequently fills the alveolar space and has a "honeycomb" appearance with accumulations of karyorrhectic nuclei, neutrophils, and giant cells. Neutrophils may be increased in the bronchi and bronchioles. Where the alveoli are not completely occluded, the "trophozoite-like," thin-walled form resides. The walls of the alveoli are only moderately thickened and contain infiltrates of plasma cells and lymphocytes. GMS staining demonstrates the organism within tissue sections (see Fig. 50-5). "Cysts with parenthesis-like bodies" are considered diagnostic for *Pneumocystis* infection.

When associated with atypical interstitial pneumonia, the primary lesion is a severe histiocytic, proliferative interstitial pneumonia.[54] Neither an etiologic agent nor an immune deficiency has previously been associated with this condition. A toxic etiology has been proposed, with pyrrolizidine alkaloid plants containing the possible agent. Although not as severe as the lung lesions, changes may occur in the liver of affected horses compatible with exposure to pyrrolizidine alkaloid–containing plants.[50]

*References 50, 51, 54, 55, 67, 70, 73.

THERAPY

Limited reports of successful treatment of *Pneumocystis* infection in horses are available. One horse with a transient CD4+ and CD8+ lymphopenia responded to traditional therapy with potentiated sulfonamides (trimethoprim-sulfamethoxazole, 30 mg/kg every 12 hours for 30 days). This foal was also treated with interferon-alpha (100 units) orally every 24 hours for 5 days. Dapsone (3 mg/kg orally every 24 hours), a sulfone antimicrobial that inhibits folic acid, has been used as a follow-up treatment in a foal with acute *Pneumocystis* infection.

A short course of corticosteroid therapy may be considered for affected horses. There is evidence of increased survival with the use of corticosteroids in children and AIDs patients with PcP.[74] This course of corticosteroid therapy is used in children regardless of immune status.

PREVENTION

Because of the sporadic nature of PcP and pneumocystosis, preventive strategies are not available. The cause of underlying pulmonary fibrosis is not known, although viral infection has been suggested as a cause. Thus, immunoprophylaxis of foals, horses, and broodmares against respiratory pathogens should be performed to minimize herd respiratory disease. Second, control of dust and ammonia within the environment will contribute to overall respiratory health. Third, exposure to plants containing pyrrolizidine alkaloids should be minimized. Exposure to plant or environmental toxins has been proposed as a cause for underlying interstitial pneumonia in horses (see Chapter 1). The stall of any immunocompromised horse should be disinfected, and environmental decontamination with sodium hypochlorite is advised.

PUBLIC HEALTH CONSIDERATIONS

Because of the recent identification of a host-adapted species of *Pneumocystis*, previous designation of these infections as "zoonotic" is questioned.[6,8] However, because the organism may be capable of infecting humans, personal protection consisting of gloves, boots, gown, and possibly mask is recommended when performing necropsies, handling respiratory secretions, or performing invasive pulmonary techniques. This will minimize inadvertent exposure when handling at-risk animals.

REFERENCES

See the CD-ROM for a list of references linked to the abstract in PubMed.

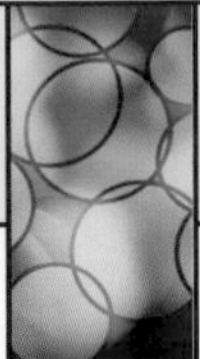

CHAPTER • 51

Coccidioidomycosis

Demosthenes Pappagianis and Jill Higgins

Coccidioidomycosis is an infectious disease caused by the mold/fungus *Coccidioides immitis*. (Recently, a second species, *Coccidioides posadasii*, has been proposed for the genus.[1]) *C. immitis* resides in the soil and causes disease in mammalian hosts after being inhaled or rarely through transcutaneous introduction.

Many animal species have been infected with *C. immitis*, including many equids (Boxes 51-1and 51-2). Because human patients have more clinically recognized coccidioidal infections than other species, much of the knowledge about the disease derives from infections of *Homo sapiens*.

The first reported case of coccidioidomycosis was described in a person in Argentina by Posadas[2] in 1892. In 1894, Rixford[3] reported a human case in California, the forerunner of thousands of additional cases occurring in the southwestern United States. Both Posadas and Rixford carried out experiments involving injection of *C. immitis* into experimental animals (not including equids).

Naturally occurring coccidioidomycosis in nonhuman mammals was reported in cattle by Giltner[4] in 1918. The disease was not reported in equids until the 1940s, according to Maddy.[5] Wilding et al.[6] alluded to the disease in burros. The earliest infections recognized in horses included those reported by Maddy. Thirteen of 22 horses raised near Phoenix and a burro near Mesa, Arizona, were reactive to intracutaneously injected coccidioidin, indicating prior infection with *C. immitis.*

Deliberate infection of horses by intravenous injection of live *C. immitis* was carried out by Smith et al.[7] to induce antibodies that could serve as standardized serologic controls (particularly for the diagnosis of coccidioidomycosis in humans). Neither the size of the inoculum (i.e., how many viable *C. immitis* cells were injected) nor the clinical outcome was described, although serum from these horses was satisfactory as an antibody-positive serologic control. Cases of equine coccidioidomycosis were reported by Zontine,[8] Rehkemper,[9] and Crane.[10]

Box • 51-1

Equids with Naturally Acquired Coccidioidomycosis

Burro *(Equus assinus)*
Horse, domestic *(Equus caballus)*
Horse, Przewalski's *(Equus przewalski)*
Kiang *(Equus hemionus kiang)*
Onager *(Equus hemionus onager)*
Zebra, Grevy's *(Equus grevyi)*
Somali wild ass *(Equus africanus somaliensis)*

ETIOLOGY

Coccidioides immitis is a mold/fungus that is diphasic and pleomorphic; its (saprobic) growth phase in nature or in usual laboratory culture differs morphologically from the (parasitic) growth phase usually seen in the tissues of an infected host (Fig. 51-1). The saprobic form consists of filaments (hyphae) 2 to 3 μm in diameter, some of which can differentiate into a chain of thick-walled arthroconidia ("spores"). These conidia can be barrel shaped or cylindrical, 2×5 μm in size, and often alternate with empty, degenerate "disjunctor" cells that readily fracture, permitting airborne dispersion of the arthroconidia.

The arthroconidia are highly infectious. Clinicians who suspect the presence of C. immitis *in material submitted to the laboratory must inform laboratory personnel of the potential hazard of handling such samples.*

When inhaled or otherwise introduced into the tissue of a mammalian host, the arthroconidia become rounded and enlarge to become spherules (20-100 μm in diameter), which undergo internal division of cytoplasm and nucleus. This results in the production from a single cell (arthroconidium) of hundreds of endospores in one generation. Each released endospore can then enlarge to become a spherule, which releases more endospores. The conversion from arthroconidia to spherules is influenced by elevated (body) temperature, increased carbon dioxide (CO_2) and perhaps surface-active agents; in vivo the process appears to be influenced by presence of inflammatory leukocytes (Fig. 51-2). The released endospores evoke a polymorphonuclear leukocyte (PMN) response, whereas the spherules evoke a macrophage response. Thus, mixed suppurative-granulomatous inflammation is characteristic of coccidioidal lesions. In chronic lesions, caseation and hyalinization (fibrosis and collagen deposition) are seen.[11]

The wall of *C. immitis* contains the polysaccharides chitin, glucan, and mannosyl (proteins);[12] these impart toughness to the exterior. During the growth of the spherule-endospore phase, enzymes such as chitinase, glucanase, and proteases likely participate in changing the cellular structure during the morphologic changes. With the maturation of the spherule and its release of endospores, chitinase is released.[13] This enzyme is the antigen to which the infected host responds by production of immunoglobulin G (IgG, complement-fixing antibody).[14]

EPIDEMIOLOGY AND EPIZOOTIOLOGY

Coccidioides immitis resides in soils of the Western Hemisphere. The areas affected extend from 40 degrees south latitude (Argentina) to 40 degrees north latitude (California, Northeastern Utah) (Fig. 51-3). Thus, areas of South, Central, and North America harbor *C. immitis*. The fungus is indigenous to California, Arizona, Utah, Nevada, New Mexico, Texas, and adjacent areas of Mexico.[15]

Persistence of this fungus in the soil and arrival of previously uninfected individuals (human and nonhuman) ensure continued occurrence of coccidioidomycosis. Many, but not all, of the areas to which the organism is endemic correspond to the Lower Sonoran Life Zone, characterized by hot, dry summers, relatively mild winters, and moderate rainfall. The number of cases of coccidioidomycosis is influenced by rainfall in at least two ways: (1) rainfall wetting the soil can reduce dust and airborne arthroconidia, suppressing the number of infections, or (2) rainfall, by moistening the soil, can lead to growth of the hyphal/arthroconidial form, increasing the subsequent risk of exposure to infectious arthroconidia and therefore more cases. In the late summer and in the fall, there is usually a progressive increase in the number of cases until the rainy season begins. In Arizona, a dry period is followed by summer "monsoon" rains, then followed by another dry season, resulting in essentially two annual seasons of coccidioidomycosis.

Coccidioides immitis does not appear uniformly distributed throughout endemic areas; rather, it exists in scattered pockets of soil. The characteristics of the soils have not provided a specific, clear reason for the restricted distribution and persistence of the organism. The soil often is alkaline, may contain ash from the ancient campsites of Native American Indians, and often contains concentrations of certain salts, such as calcium,

Box • 51-2

Animal Species with Naturally Acquired Coccidioidomycosis

Aardvark[1] *(Orycteropus aferi)*
Armadillo, nine-banded[2] *(Dasypus novemcinctus)*
Baboon[1] (*Papio* spp.); mandrill (*Mandrillus* spp.)
Badger[1] *(Taxidea taxus)*
Bear, Malayan sun[1] *(Ursus malayanus)*
Binturong,[1] a civet *(Arctitis binturong)*
Burro *(Equus assinus)**
Cat, domestic *(Felis catus)*
Cattle, domestic *(Bos taurus)*
Cheetah[1] *(Acinonyx jubatus)*
Chimpanzee[1] *(Pan troglodytes)*
Chinchilla[1] *(Chinchilla lanigera)*
Coyote[1,2] *(Canis latrans)*
Deer, white-lipped[1] *(Cervus albirostris)*
Dog *(Canis familiaris)*
Dog, Cape or African hunting[1] *(Lycaon pictus)*
Dolphin, Pacific bottle-nosed[2] *(Tursiops gilli)*
Ferret[1] (*Mustela* spp., *Mustela putoris furo*)
Gazelle *(Gazella thomsonii)*
Genet[1,3] *(Genetta felina)*
Gorilla: mountain[1] *(Gorilla gorilla beringeri)*;
  lowland[1] *(Gorilla gorilla gorilla)*
Horse
  Domestic *(Equus caballus)**
  Przewalski's[1] *(Equus przewalski)**
Human *(Homo sapiens)*
Impala[1] *(Aepyceros melampus)*
Jackrabbit[2] *(Lepus californicus)*
Kangaroo[1] *(Macropus rufus)*
  Wallaroo[1] (*Macropus robustus* or *M. erubescens*)
Kiang[1] *(Equus hemionus kiang)**
Kit fox[2] *(Vulpes velox)*
Lemur: ringtail[1] *(Lemur catta)*; red ruffed[1]
  (*Varecia variegata* v. suber)
Lion, mountain[1] *(Felis concolor)*
Lion, transvaal[1] *(Panthera leo krugeri)*
Llama[1] *(Lama glama)*
Makhor, turkomen (*Capra megaceros* or *C. falconeri*)
Monkey[1]
  Tropical American *(Cebus hypoleucus)*
  Spider[3] (*Ateles* spp.)
  Wooley[3] (*Lagothrix* spp.)
  Colobus *(Colobus guereza)*
  Sooty mangabey *(Cerocebus atys)*
  Guenon DeBrazza *(Cercopithecus neglectus)*
  Bonnet macaque *(Macaca radiata)*
  Celebes macaque *(Macaca maurus)*
  Lion tail macaque *(Macaca silenus)*
  Rhesus *(Macaca mulatta)*
Okapi[1] *(Okapia johnstoni)*
Onager[1] *(Equus hemionus onager)**
Otter: river[1] *(Lutra canadensis)*; sea[2] *(Enhydra lutris)*
Rhinoceros: northern white[1] *(Ceratotherium simum
  cottoni)*; black *(Diceros bicornis)*
Rodents[2]
  Pocket mouse *(Perognathus baileyii, P. penicillatus,
    P. intermedius)*
  Grasshopper mouse *(Onchyomys torridus)*
  Kangaroo rat *(Dipodomys merriami)*
  Ground squirrel *(Citellus harrisi)*
Sea lion[1,2] *(Zalophus californianus)*
Sheep *(Ovis aries)*
  Barbary *(Ammotragus lervia)*
  Bighorn *(Ovis canadensis nelsoni)*[2]
Skunk, hog-nose[1,3] (*Mephitis* spp.)
Snake, Sonoran Gopher[2] *(Piticophis melanoleucus affinis)*
Swine *(Sus scrofa)*
Tapir[1] *(Tapirus terrestris)*
Tiger,[1] Bengal and Sumatran *(Panthera tigris)*
Wild ass *(Equus africanus somaliensis)**
Wisent *(Bison bonasur)*
Zebra,[1] Grevy's *(Equus grevyi)**

This compilation includes cases detected by Raymond Reed, DVM, and Kathryn Orr, DVM; data also from various publications.
*Equids.
[1]Zoo or captive animals.
[2]In the wild.
[3]Species name uncertain.

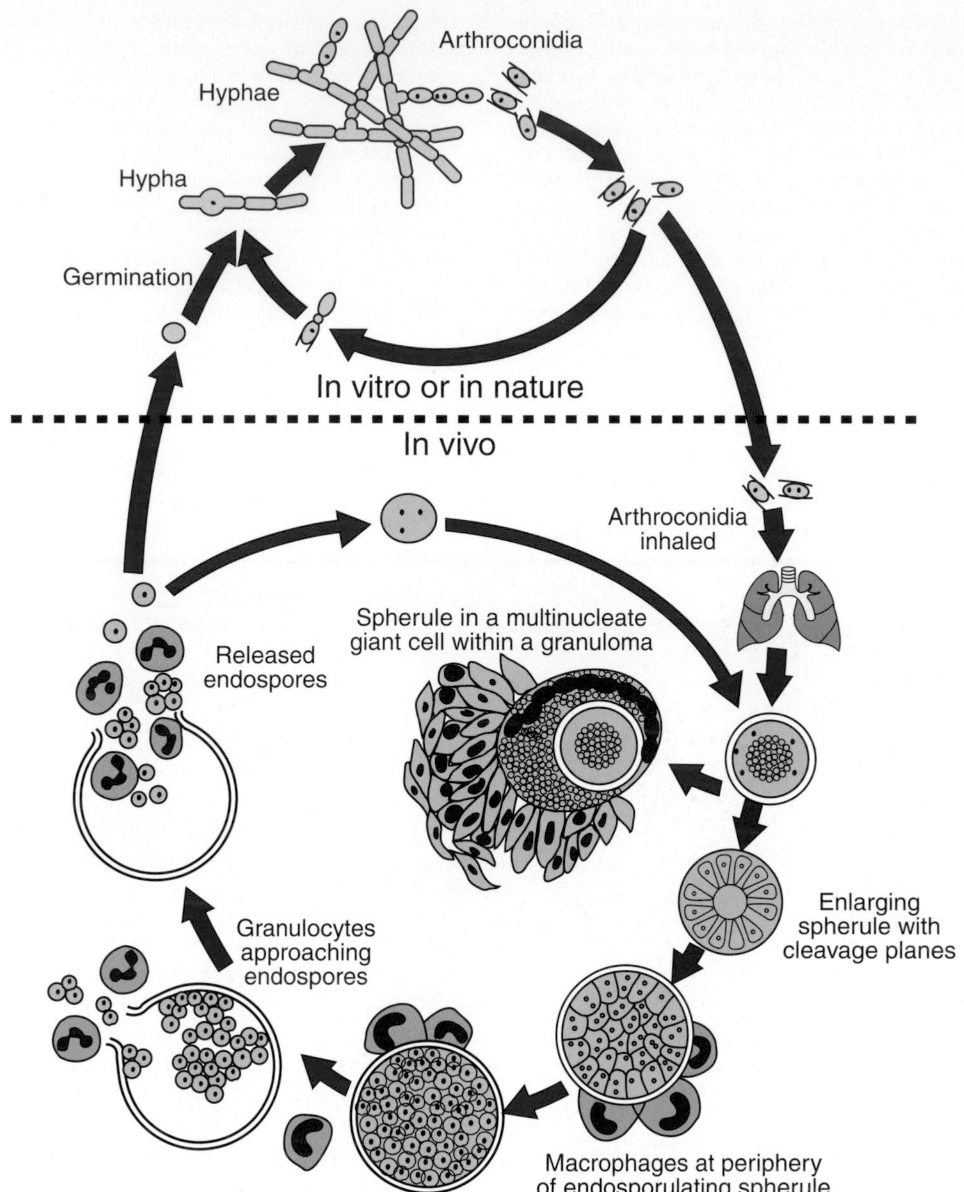

Fig. 51-1 Life cycle of *Coccidioides immitis*. (Modified from Collier L, et al, editors: *Topley & Wilson's microbiology and microbial infections*, ed 9, London, 1998, Hodder Arnold.)

sulfate, and sodium chloride, which can inhibit microorganisms that can compete with (or inhibit) *Coccidioides*. These competing organisms probably decrease as the soil water evaporates, increasing the concentrations of salt but still permitting survival of *Coccidioides*.

Equine cases of coccidioidomycosis have been reported from the southwestern United States, although in some cases, equid acquisition of *C. immitis* may have occurred at some location remote from the home area. Indeed, horses not residing in coccidioidal areas may be exposed to products (e.g., alfalfa, grass hay) exported from endemic areas. For example, a man who resided in London was exposed when unpacking pottery from Arizona, through finely shredded packing material,[16] and a man in North Carolina was exposed to *C. immitis*–contaminated cotton from California. Sporadic cases of coccidioidomycosis in horses are usual. However, several cases occurred at the same site in a compound holding several Przewalski horses.[17] It has been proposed that the herd of young males, intimidated by more dominant adult males, may have been stressed, increasing their susceptibility to develop clinically apparent coccidioidomycosis.

Transmission from one host to another does not ordinarily occur, except rarely from a mother to a fetus[18,19] or from an infected organ donor to organ recipient (see Prevention and Public Health Considerations).

PATHOGENESIS

Inhaled arthroconidia can be deposited in large or small airways. The arthroconidia shed an outer wall layer that is antiphagocytic and, under the influence of leukocytes, increased

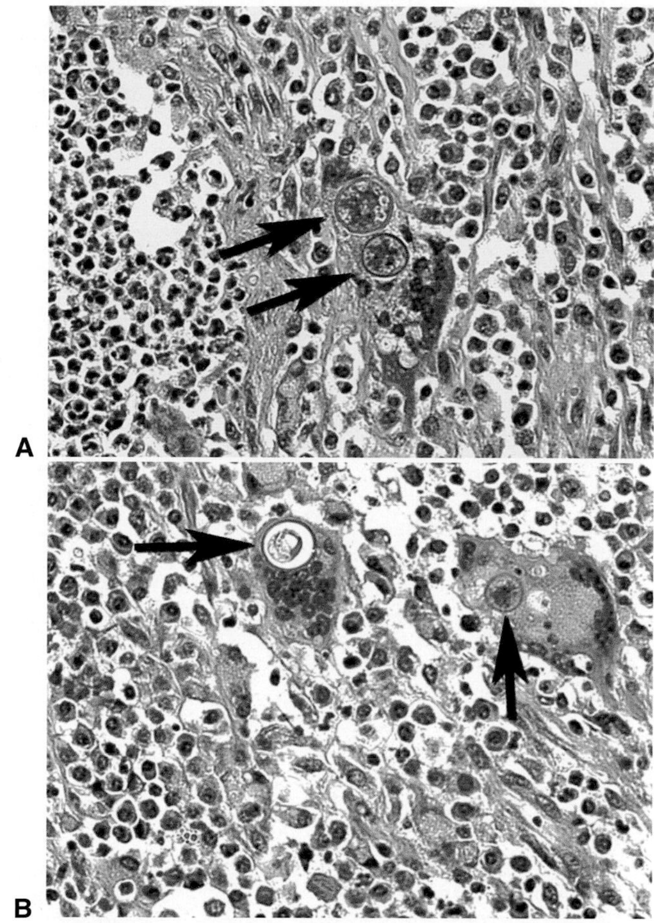

Fig. 51-2 Histopathologic appearance of *Coccidioides immitis* in an equine spleen. **A,** Two endosporulating spherules *(arrows)* in area containing plasma cells, lymphocytes, and portion of multinucleated giant cell near abscess containing abundant neutrophil granulocytes. **B,** Two nonendosporulating spherules *(arrows)* in multinucleated giant cells. (Courtesy Suzanne Johnson, PhD.)

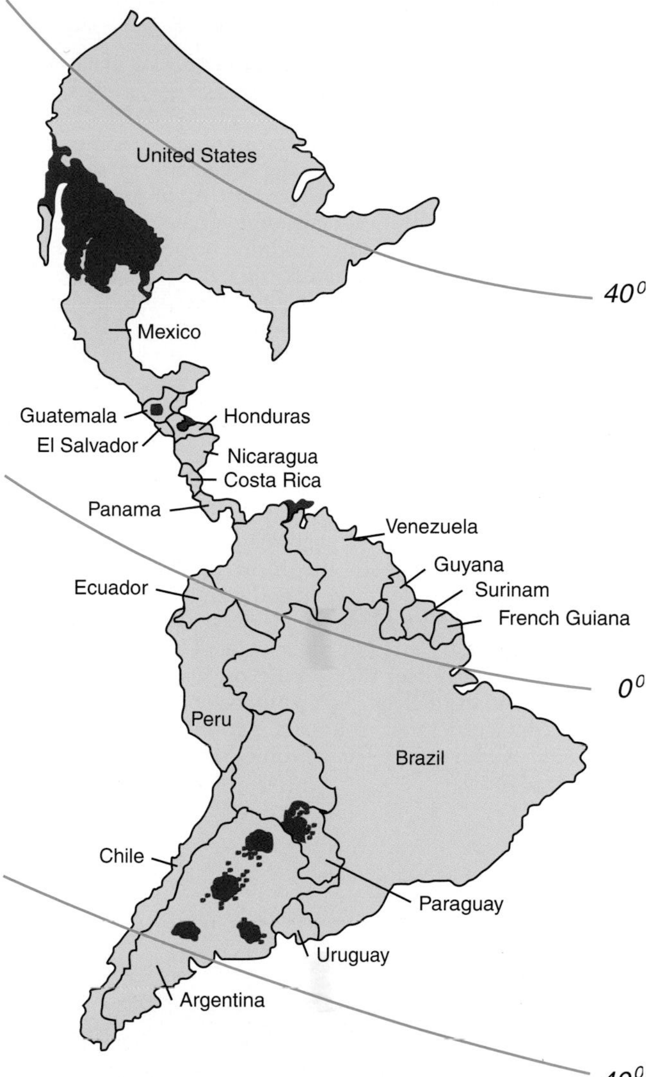

Fig. 51-3 Geographic distribution of *Coccidioides immitis* sites where coccidioidomycosis is usually acquired. (Modified from Pappagianis D. In Stevens D, editor: *Coccidioidomycosis*, New York, 1980, Plenum.)

CO_2, elevated (body) temperature, and surface-active agents, become rounded and enlarge to produce the spherule. Enzymes such as serine and aspartyl proteases, urease, alkaline phosphatase, and chitinase are released during the morphologic evolution of *Coccididoides*. At least some of these enzymes may contribute to the pathogenesis. Urease is reported to alkalinize the phagosome of leukocytes, thereby impairing phagocytic destruction of the fungus.[20] Proteinases may exert damaging effects on the host tissue components or leukocytes. Chitinase, a potent antigen,[13] may contribute to pathogenesis through formation of antigen-antibody complexes.[14]

The usual respiratory route of infection can lead to asymptomatic, subclinical infection (60% of infected people). The symptomatic infection (40% of infected people) can be variable. Most infected individuals recover after weeks to months. Complete recovery leads to immunity against a second "primary" (pulmonary) infection. From 5% to 10% of symptomatic human patients will have a residual pulmonary lesion (e.g., cavity, solitary nodule). Approximately 5% to 7% of symptomatic patients have the disease spread (disseminate) outside the thorax; this is influenced by innate factors, including racial derivation, presence of certain human leukocyte antigen (HLA) tissue markers, and blood group B. Dissemination also is increased by certain acquired states: immunosuppression by human immunodeficiency virus (HIV) or medication for organ transplantation and by pregnancy.

Early infection is endobronchial or pneumonic, often accompanied by hilar lymphadenopathy. Extrathoracic dissemination can involve virtually any tissue or organ, an exception being the rare involvement of the mucosal surface of the alimentary tract or of the endocardium.

A broad range of animals (over 64 different species) have been infected with *Coccidioides* (see Box 51-2). The spectrum of the disease varies among and within species. Dogs appear to fit a clinical range similar to that of humans. Cattle and sheep, on the other hand, are resistant, rarely exhibiting illness despite coccidioidal lesions in the thoracic lymph nodes. The equids that have been infected included domestic and wild species (see Box 51-1).

CLINICAL FINDINGS

Multiple manifestations of coccidioidomycosis have been reported in horses, with a wide range of severity and effect on survival. Various anatomic sites are affected (Fig. 51-4). Once thought to be a universally devastating disease, some forms of coccidioidomycosis may now be amenable to successful treatment or even spontaneous recovery. As in other species, equine exposure usually occurs through inhalation of airborne arthroconidia. Because of this common exposure route, the disease often affects the respiratory tract; however, lymphohematogenous dissemination can occur, leading to foci of infection in various organs, such as bone, skin, and abdominal viscera.[21,22] Rarely, inoculation is thought to occur percutaneously, leading to localized subcutaneous infections.[23] The multiple clinical syndromes have been described as miliary or interstitial pneumonia[24-26] (Fig. 51-5), pneumonia with pleural effusion[21] (Fig. 51-6), osteomyelitis,[27,28] mastitis,[29] abortion,[18,19] and various sites of superficial or internal abscessation.[22] An obstructive nasal coccidioidal granuloma in an Arabian gelding was excised[30] and recurred 5 years later.[31]

Clinical signs vary with the form of disease; however, common signs include fever, significant weight loss, and current or historical respiratory signs (adventitial lung sounds, increased respiratory rate, coughing, evidence of pleural fluid). Other signs may reflect the specific organ system involved, including musculoskeletal pain with osteomyelitis, abortion with placental infection, colic and peritoneal effusion with abdominal involvement, or chronic draining tracts with peripheral lesions.

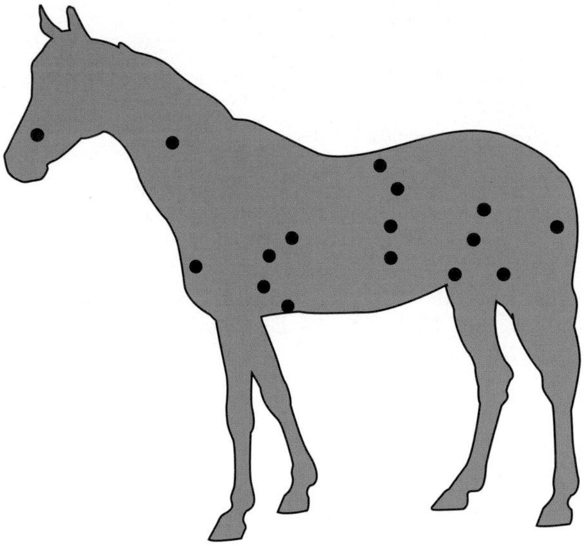

Fig. 51-4 Anatomic locations of coccidioidomycosis reported in the horse.

In horses with pulmonary coccidioidomycosis, thoracic ultrasound may identify "comet tail" artifacts consistent with pleural roughening, areas of pulmonary consolidation, and accumulations of pleural fluid. Common thoracic radiographic abnormalities include diffuse interstitial/miliary pattern (see Figs. 51-5 and 51-6) consistent with a granulomatous

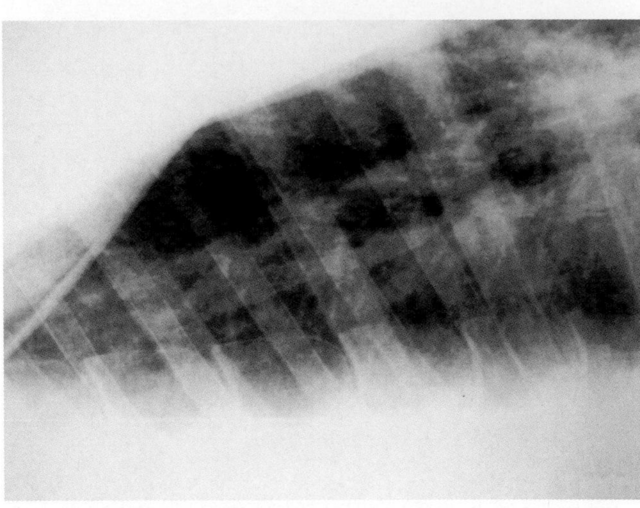

Fig. 51-5 Radiograph showing multiple small nodular lesions in lung of horse with coccidioidomycosis.

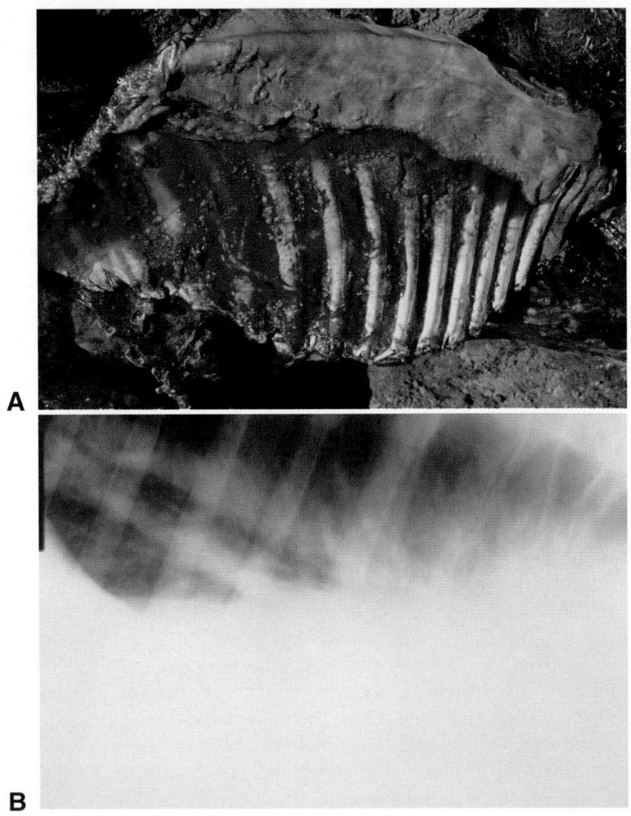

Fig. 51-6 A, Parietal pleura with granulomata in horse with coccidioidomycosis. B, Radiograph indicating pleural effusion in horse with coccidioidomycosis. (Courtesy Richard Mansmann, VMD, PhD.)

pneumonia, pleural fluid lines, dorsal displacement of large airways by hilar lymphadenopathy, and large mass lesions in the mediastinum or small focal abscesses throughout the lung field.[22,26]

Hematologic abnormalities in horses with coccidioidomycosis include an inflammatory leukogram with hyperfibrinogenemia, leukocytosis with mature neutrophilia and hyperglobulinemia, as well as mild anemia.[22]

A recent retrospective study showed different survival trends for different clinical syndromes.[26] For example, all six mares that aborted an infected fetus had a low serum coccidioidal IgG titer by quantitative immunodiffusion (≤8) and showed no signs of systemic infection. All survived, and one mare reportedly had several healthy foals subsequent to the abortion. Conversely, the disease in horses with massive dissemination or pneumonia with thoracic effusion (mean serum titer of 176 and 332, respectively) was overwhelmingly fatal (19/21) despite treatment in some cases. Serologic data have recently confirmed that subclinical infection with natural resolution occurs in horses living in endemic areas (previously associated also with positive skin tests[5]), further supporting the wide spectrum of infection and disease exhibited in horses.[32] Prognosis should be assessed individually for each horse on the basis of chronicity of infection, severity of clinical signs, organ systems involved, dynamics of titer over time, initial response to treatment, and immune status of patient.[26]

Some trends have been identified regarding the signalment of affected horses. They tend to be young to middle aged when presented, 6.3 years in one retrospective study[22] and 8.1 years in another.[26] Serologic data suggest that horses in endemic areas are exposed to the pathogen at a young age.[32] Older horses likely were previously exposed to the fungal pathogen and have overcome the infection. Those that develop clinically apparent disease will likely do so at the initial exposure. Coccidioidomycosis does not appear to be a disease of older or debilitated horses; this is similar to trends reported in dogs[33] and people[34] (mean age of 5 and 40.3 years, respectively). Females have been overrepresented (66%[26] and 76%[22]) among affected horses in both equine retrospective studies. Pregnancy has been postulated to have an effect on severity of clinical signs in mares, as it does in humans.[35] However, no conclusion has been made as to whether this contributes to the overrepresentation of clinical female equine patients. Arabians were significantly overrepresented as clinical patients in one retrospective study[22] and made up a high proportion of healthy horses carrying a positive titer.[32] However, numbers are still too small to ascribe a greater susceptibility to this breed. A seasonal trend has been identified, with 72% of clinical cases presenting from late fall into winter (October through March), possibly following exposure during the dry, dusty months of late summer and early fall.[26] Heightened awareness is appropriate for diagnosticians during this time of year.

Nondomestic horses display a range of clinical presentations. Although disseminated coccidioidomycosis was reported to have a high incidence in Przewalski's horses,[17] seropositive, apparently healthy Przewalski's horses have also been detected. A Grevy's zebra in southern California had disseminated coccidioidomycosis affecting the cervical vertebrae and internal organs.

DIAGNOSIS AND PATHOLOGIC FINDINGS

Confirmation of coccidioidomycosis requires laboratory support. However, diagnosis depends on suspicion and awareness of the provenance (residence and travel) history of the horse, appreciation of the varied clinical patterns of disease, estimation of the time of onset of illness, and the usefulness of laboratory tests.

Direct demonstration of *Coccidioides* in tracheobronchial washings, exudates, or tissues, as stained by hematoxylin and eosin (H&E) and periodic acid–Schiff (PAS), Papanicolaou, or calcofluor white for detection of chitin in the fungal wall, can secure the diagnosis promptly (see Chapter 49). Potassium hydroxide digestion of host cell tissue components is withstood by the *C. immitis* cell. Detection of an unequivocal endosporulating spherule establishes the diagnosis. Usually the coccidioidal cells are visible in H&E-stained tissue (see Figure 51-2), but cells can be sparse and are more readily visualized with PAS or methenamine silver stains that can detect the polysaccharides of fungal cell walls. Occasionally, clinicians may not observe the pathognomonic endosporulating spherules (20-100 μm in diameter) but will see immature spherules with rather thick, double-contour walls (15-50 μm) that can be confused with other fungi (e.g., *Blastomyces dermatitidis*).

Attempts to recover the fungus by culture should be made for confirmation of the diagnosis and, should it become necessary during treatment, for the assay of the susceptibility to antifungal agents. Culture of infected tissues or exudates on conventional culture media (blood agar, Sabouraud glucose agar) or media containing cycloheximide (to inhibit nonpathogenic fungi) and chloramphenicol or other antibacterial antibiotics can enhance recovery of *Coccidioides*. Mycelial growth can become visible in 2 to 3 days and can yield a sufficient amount of the organism to permit application of the Hybridization Protection Assay (Gen-Probe) for specific identification of ribonucleic acid (RNA) of a suspected *C. immitis* isolate within hours (Fig. 51-7). Inoculation of mice with the unknown culture usually requires growth of the organism for approximately 1 week to yield sufficient cells of the organism to replicate in the animal and to produce the characteristic endosporulating spherules.

Even while attempting to recover and identify the infecting organism, serum samples should be tested for antibody.[14] In general, a consistent, sequential serologic response occurs after infection with *Coccidioides*: early, there is an immunoglobulin M (IgM) response, and later, an IgG antibody response (IgA can also be detected, but its usefulness has not been clearly established). The IgM is produced in response to polysaccharide/peptide antigen, and the IgG is induced by chitinase (Fig. 51-8).

Various tests can be used to detect IgM, IgG, or both. Screening for antibody can be carried out by immunodiffusion (ID), enzyme immunoassay (EIA), or antigen-coated latex particle agglutination (LPA). The role of EIA or LPA in equine serology is unknown. Because of false-positive reactions for IgM by EIA or LPA, reactive sera should be tested for confirmation by ID (Table 51-1). Careful observation reveals that in ID, some equine sera produce a confusing line of reaction with human serum. Once a qualitative test is positive for coccidioidal antibody, usually little is gained by repetition of the qualitative tests. However, because a recognized correlation exists between the titer (concentration) of IgG and the severity and extent of coccidioidal disease, quantitative serologic tests (complement fixation or quantitative ID) should be performed to obtain a titer of antibody. By experience, titers greater than 1:16 have been associated with possible metapulmonary disseminated coccidioidomycosis. Testing sequential sera, initially at 1-month intervals (later at longer-spaced periods), permits comparison of titers. A rising titer is usually indicative of worsening disease, whereas a falling titer indicates improvement.

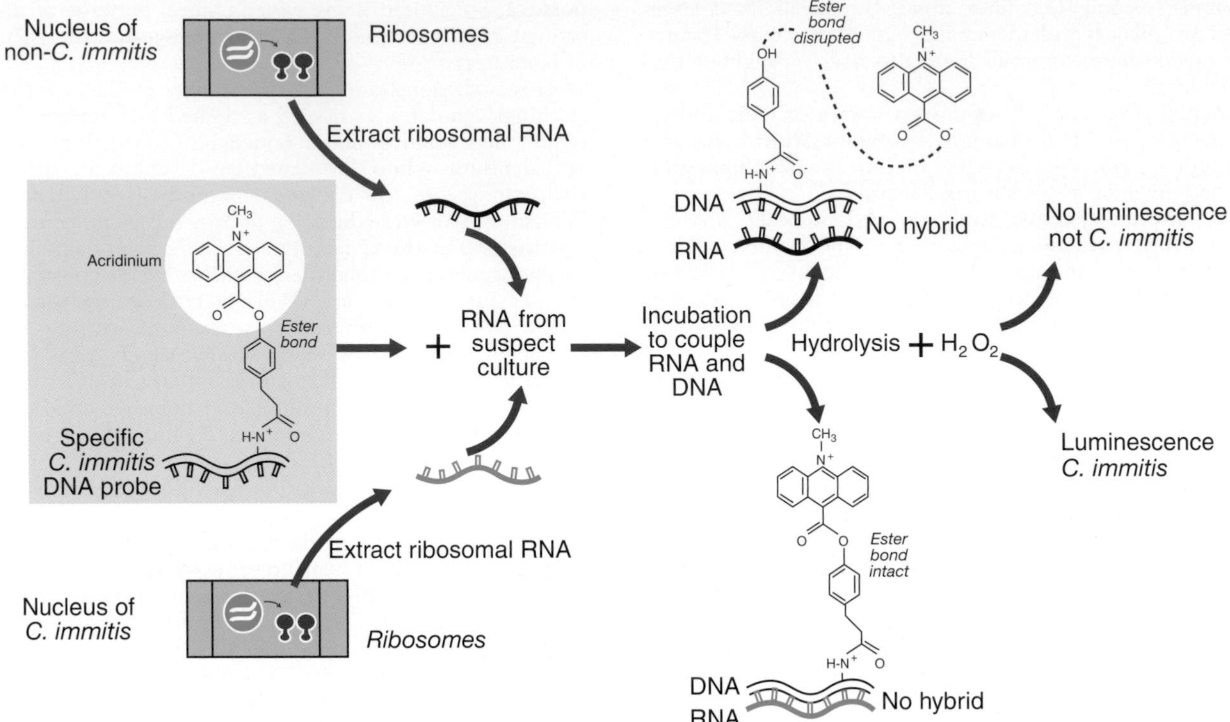

Fig. 51-7 Hybridization Protection Assay (Gen-Probe) for *Coccidioides immitis*. (Modified from Pappagianis D, National Foundation of Infectious Diseases, 1996.)

Presence of antibody in the serum of horses usually indicates past or current coccidioidomycosis.[14] However, the authors have recently detected coccidioidal antibody in the serum of a 2-day-old foal that did not have coccidioidomycosis, but the dam was known to be seropositive. Apparently, the antibody in the foal was derived from milk (colostrum). In humans, transplacentally transferred antibody can be detected in newborn infants without coccidioidomycosis, but whose mothers had coccidioidomycosis.

Detection of coccidioidal antigen[36] or deoxyribonucleic acid (DNA)[37] may allow infection to be detected earlier than antibody, but these tests have not yet achieved clinical utility.

THERAPY

Therapy of coccidioidomycosis can be conservative (supportive), surgical, medical, or a combination of medical/surgical modalities, depending on the extent of the disease and the intent of the owners. Coccidioidomycosis can be chronic, necessitating treatment lasting for months or years. Systemic antifungal therapy in horses is expanding as newer and generic agents have become available and financially feasible for many horse owners. Therapy that was considered cost prohibitive because of the price of drugs and duration of treatment is now considered a reasonable option.

The conservative approach may be attempted for mild forms of the disease (e.g., placentitis, abortion) or other forms that are accompanied by a low titer (<8) and mild clinical signs. A small proportion (4.1%) of healthy horses in endemic areas may carry a titer of up to 8 at a given time.[32] These horses are subclinically infected and may not require treatment. Because of the possibly devastating nature of disease, however, all cases should be monitored closely (clinically, serologically, and hematologically) to allow for early detection of disease progression and to institute antifungal therapy before disease has become too severe. In horses with a low titer, a decision for antifungal medical intervention should be based on hematologic evidence of inflammation, weight loss, clinical signs of active infection (e.g., fever), and a rising IgG titer over time.[32]

Surgical therapy can be applied to various tissues. If the disease is limited to peripheral and cutaneous tissues, excision could be curative. Limited osseous disease can be approached surgically, but this is appropriately carried out with accompanying systemic antifungal medication.

Medical therapy can include parenteral or oral medications. Currently, two main classes of antifungal medications are used to treat coccidioidomycosis: polyenes and azoles.

Amphotericin B (AMB) and its lipid formulations are administered parenterally, particularly by intravenous (IV) or intrathecal route. The *polyenes* interact adversely with ergosterol in the fungal cell membrane. The increased availability of azole antifungal agents has resulted in a decrease in the use of AMB both because of ease of administration and because of the nephrotoxic, hematopoietic toxic, and vasculopathic effects of AMB. In some cases, however, such as rapidly progressing coccidioidomycosis, AMB may remain the first-choice antifungal.

Ketoconazole and the triazoles itraconazole, fluconazole, and voriconazole are currently available to treat fungal infections. These drugs are usually administered orally, although

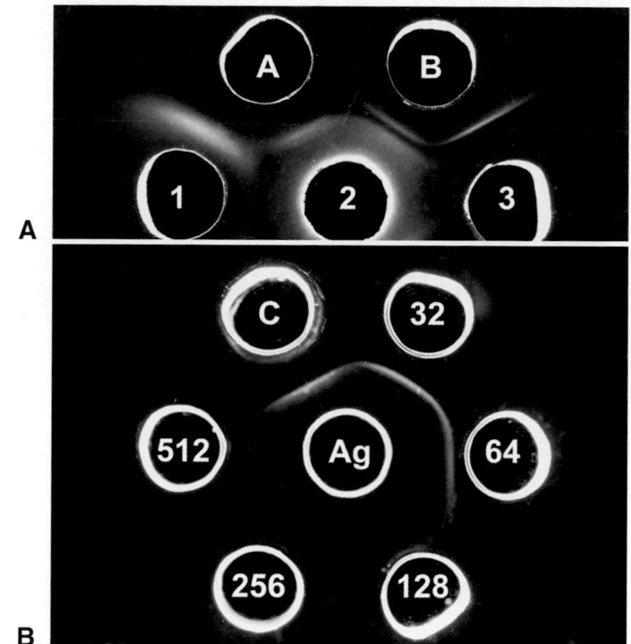

Fig. 51-8 Immunodiffusion serologic test for coccidioidomycosis. **A,** Qualitative test with serum from horse with coccidioidomycosis in central well. Left well contains control human serum positive for IgM. Right well contains control human serum positive for IgG. Left upper well contains coccidioidal antigen (heated) reactive with IgM. Right upper well contains coccidioidal antigen (unheated) reactive with both IgM and IgG. The equine serum was positive for both IgM and IgG. **B,** Quantitative test in which center well contains coccidioidal antigen. Left upper well contains control (human) serum positive for IgG. Right upper, right middle, right lower, and left lower wells contain equine pleural fluid diluted 1:32, 1:64, 1:128, and 1:256, respectively. The line of antigen-antibody precipitation indicates that the titer is 1:128.

Table • **51-1**

Current Application of Serologic Tests in Coccidioidomycosis

TEST	DETECTION OF IgM	DETECTION OF IgG
Immunodiffusion (ID)	Yes	Yes
Enzyme immunoassay (EIA)	Yes*	Yes†
Complement fixation (CF)	No (rare‡)	Yes
Latex (antigen-coated) agglutination	Yes*	No

*These tests, intended for detection of IgM, have a substantial proportion of false-positive reactions.
†Occasionally, EIA positive for IgG has only IgM demonstrable by ID.
‡Rarely, serum positive by CF contains only IgM detectable by ID.

some IV preparations are available. The *azoles* inhibit the synthesis of ergosterol, leading to faulty sterol in the fungal cell membrane. Toxicity of the azoles is relatively greater for fungal cells than for the mammalian cells. Oral ketoconazole is poorly absorbed in the horse[38] and usually requires co-administration of an acidifying agent to enhance alimentary absorption. Fluconazole and itraconazole are practical for long-term oral administration, but with a possible side effect of dose-dependent hepatotoxicity. There is a report of successful treatment of coccidioidal osteomyelitis in a horse with oral itraconazole[28] and a recent report of two horses with pulmonary coccidioidomycosis treated successfully with fluconazole.[24] Fluconazole possesses a superb pharmacokinetic profile in horses, with a high oral bioavailability, a high volume of distribution, and a long elimination half-life.[39] Thus, fluconazole should be considered as a favorable agent to treat equine coccidioidomycosis. Because of its long half-life, fluconazole may show a cumulative effect, and therefore therapeutic drug monitoring throughout the course of treatment is warranted to facilitate adjustment of the dose if necessary.[24] Periodic blood tests to monitor hepatic parameters is also recommended.

Previously reported dosing regimens for mycotic infections in the horse include fluconazole at a loading dose of 14 mg/kg orally (PO), followed by 5 mg/kg PO once daily;[24,39] itraconazole at 2.6 mg/kg PO twice daily;[28] and amphotericin B intravenously daily or every other day to a cumulative dose of 12 mg/kg over 1 month,[40] or a cumulative dose of 6.75 mg/kg over 5 weeks.[41]

Sufficient duration of treatment is often a dilemma when treating any horse with coccidioidomycosis. In the recent cases of pneumonia, discontinuation of treatment at 5 to 6 months was based on complete resolution of signs and hematologic abnormalities, as well as a decreasing IgG titer.[24] In both these horses, clinical signs resolved within 2 weeks of initiation of treatment; however, chronic inflammation evidenced by leukocytosis and hyperfibrinogenemia persisted for 2 to 4 months after resolution of signs. Serial titers should be used to follow response during the course of treatment and for early detection of relapse in the posttreatment period.[14] Long-term, intermittent serologic testing of recovered horses may be indicated until their titers have become low, 1:2 to 1:4, but clinical assessment should be foremost.

PREVENTION AND PUBLIC HEALTH CONSIDERATIONS

Minimizing exposure to soil dust containing C. *immitis* in endemic areas may reduce the risk of infection. Efficacious experimental vaccines (thus far effective in mice and monkeys, but not in people) may be forthcoming.[42,43]

Horses and other species acquire coccidioidal infections by inhalation of arthroconidia (rarely through the skin). Horse-to-horse and horse-to-human (or human-to-human) transmission, in general, does not occur. However, following a report of (ultimately fatal) coccidioidomycosis in a veterinarian who was present during a necropsy of a horse with disseminated coccidioidomycosis,[44] some owners and veterinary personnel became concerned that the disease might be acquired by proximity to an infected horse. (The veterinarian may have been exposed not only during the necropsy, but also through contaminated artifacts, including the mane and tail of the index infected horse.) Natural transmission of the spherule/endospore phase (which would be the usual morphologic form expressed in the infected host) from host to host has not been demonstrated, except from infected organ donors to organ recipients.[45,46]

An interesting interhuman transmission of C. *immitis* (other than maternal to fetus) has been reported.[47] A patient with coccidioidal osteomyelitis of the right knee and left ankle underwent curettage and irrigation of the wounds. Plaster casts were applied to immobilize the limbs. Windows cut in the plaster casts permitted placement of dressings in the wound sites. Subsequently, several medical personnel, who were near or involved in removing dressings, developed coccidioidomycosis. The exudates from the infected limbs contaminated the plaster casts on which *C. immitis* grew in the hyphal/arthroconidial form and became aerosolized when the dressings were changed.

In the laboratory the infectious arthroconidia are produced in about 5 days. Therefore, *Coccidioides*-containing body fluids, exudates, or dressings used to cover lesions should be changed in less than 48 hours. Moistening dressings before removing them will help to minimize the risk of formation and aerosolization of the infectious arthroconidia. Contaminated dressings and body fluids should be treated with bleach disinfectant (0.5% sodium hypochlorite) for at least 30 minutes before discarding. The arthroconidia are also readily killed by heating at 60° C (140° F) for 30 minutes.

There is a theoretic risk that exudates (or an infected placenta) deposited in the soil of a corral or paddock could contaminate the soil with *C. immitis*. In an endemic area, however, infectivity of the environment already exists for the human owners and horses. If a horse has acquired the infection while in an endemic area, but is then transported to a nonendemic area, it is unlikely that conditions would be suitable for the propagation of *C. immitis* in the soil in the new location.

In the performance of a necropsy on a horse with putative or proven coccidioidomycosis, it would be prudent to wear gown, gloves, and mask and to decontaminate the postmortem site with 0.5% sodium hypochlorite.

ACKNOWLEDGMENTS

Spencer Jang, University of California, Davis, provided the discussion on histology. We are grateful to Linsey Jordan for preparation of the typescript.

REFERENCES

See the CD-ROM for a list of references linked to the abstract in PubMed.

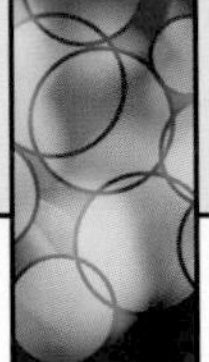

CHAPTER • 52

Sporotrichosis

Robert J. MacKay

Sporotrichosis is a chronic, progressive, lymphocutaneous infection of horses and other animals caused by *Sporothrix schenckii*. The disease in horses and mules was first described in 1909.[1]

ETIOLOGY

Sporothrix schenckii is a dimorphic fungus, growing in a yeast form in tissue and in culture at 37° C (98.6° F) but as a filamentous fungus at 30° C (86° F).[2,3] The mycelial form has fine, septate, branching hyphae that carry ovoid roseate conidia. The organism converts to the yeast form at 37° C when grown on blood agar in 10% carbon dioxide. Yeast colonies are cream colored, moist, and smooth. *S. schenckii* is a common saprophyte of decaying plant material but also can live on sphagnum moss and other living plants.

EPIDEMIOLOGY AND PATHOGENESIS

Sporotrichosis is an uncommon disease of people, horses, and other animals.[4,5] The organism and disease occur worldwide but are more common in tropical and subtropical climates.[2] Disease occurs when the fungus is traumatically inoculated into the dermis. Although infection can theoretically be passed between animals, no case of horse-to-human transmission has been reported.[2] After 3 to 5 weeks,[2] the infection establishes in the skin and subcutis and can spread in lymphatics to other parts of the skin, with resultant lymphangitis. Proximal lymph nodes may become involved in this manner, and rarely the infection can disseminate to other organs. Virulence factors are not well understood but may correlate with thermotolerance in culture.[5] Agglutinins to the yeast form occur during infection and are detected in various diagnostic tests.[6]

CLINICAL FINDINGS

Lesions most often begin on the distal limb, although the face, neck, or torso can also be the initial site of infection[3,6-9] (Fig. 52-1). There are single to multiple, firm, well-demarcated (0.5-5 cm in diameter), nonpruritic, nonpainful cutaneous nodules. Lesions enlarge slowly and usually ulcerate and drain a creamy red-brown to yellow purulent discharge. The infection may stay localized or spread along lymphatics (see Fig. 52-1). The lymphatics appear corded and are interrupted by indurated nodules that ulcerate and drain. Linearly arranged lesions thus may have a "beads on a necklace" appearance. Cycles of healing and recurrence of lesions may occur over months or even years.

DIAGNOSIS

The finding of ulcerative lymphangitis is highly suggestive of the diagnosis of sporotrichosis.[3,7] Other diagnostic considerations are undifferentiated bacterial lymphangitis, glanders *(Pseudomonas mallei)*, epizootic lymphangitis *(Histoplasma farciminosum)*, ulcerative lymphangitis *(Corynebacterium pseudotuberculosis)*,

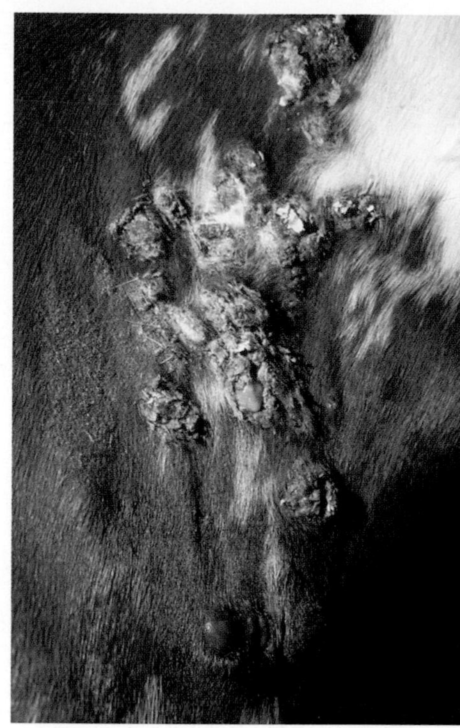

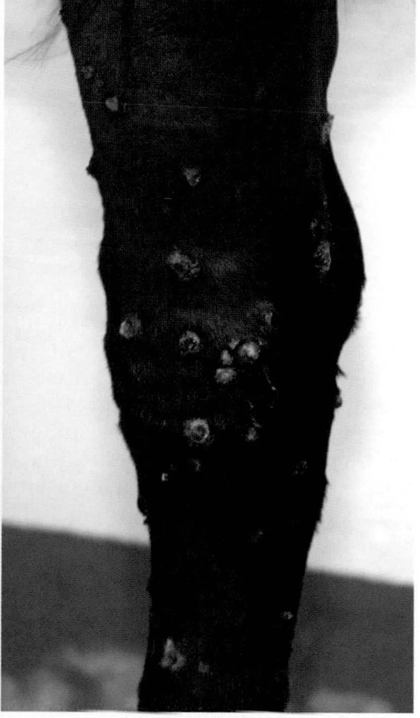

Fig. 52-1 A, Typical subcutaneous nodules with ulceration and cording of lymphatics in shoulder of 16-year-old Paint Horse mare with sporotrichosis. **B,** Sporotrichosis on distal limb of horse. (*A* courtesy Dr. Debra Sellon; *B* courtesy Dr. Bonnie Rush.)

and leishmaniasis. Supportive evidence for the diagnosis is the finding of characteristic budding, spherical to cigar-shaped yeast bodies in exudate, tissue fluid, or biopsies.[2,3,6] Organisms can be found either extracellularly or within neutrophils, macrophages, or multinucleate giant cells.

In horses, organisms are sparse, so diagnosis by cytology and histology may be difficult. Predigestion with diastase and staining with periodic acid–Schiff, methenamine silver, Gridley's, or Giemsa stains may improve sensitivity of these techniques. Immunostaining of cytologic or histologic preparations allows differentiation of *S. schenkii* from other parasitic yeasts.[6] Definitive diagnosis is by culture of the organism on Sabouraud agar at 30° C or room temperature.[2] Final identification of the organism requires demonstration of either mycelium-to-yeast conversion in culture or pathogenicity for mice.[10] Slide latex agglutination and tube agglutination tests for serum antibodies against *S. schenckii* are available. Titers of 8 are supportive of the diagnosis.

THERAPY, PROGNOSIS, AND PREVENTION

Iodine is the treatment of choice.[6-9] Regimens that have been used successfully in horses include sodium iodide (20-40 mg/kg intravenously daily as a 20% solution, then orally at the same dose), potassium iodide (10 mg/kg orally once or twice daily) and ethylenediamine dihydroiodide (EDDI; 20 mg/kg orally once or twice daily). Lesions typically resolve over a period of weeks.

To prevent relapses, it is recommended that treatment continue for 4 weeks beyond the resolution of clinical signs. Iodide should not be given to pregnant mares and should be discontinued in any horse with signs of iodism, such as fever, anorexia, coughing, lacrimation, nasal discharge, nervousness, or cardiovascular dysfunction.

Ketaconazole, itraconazole, fluconazole, and amphotericin B have been used in horses for treatment of other fungal infections and may have efficacy in the treatment of sporotrichosis.

The prognosis for full recovery from sporotrichosis is good to excellent.

Because of the potential for transfer of infection to humans, gloves should be worn during handling of an infected horse.

PUBLIC HEALTH CONSIDERATIONS

S. schenckii is pathogenic to humans although horses are not considered a source of infection. Human disease is characterized by skin infections (rose handler's disease) and can rarely progress to lymphangitis. This infection is especially dangerous for immunocompromised people, and laboratory infections have occurred.[11]

REFERENCES

See the CD-ROM for a list of references linked to the abstract in PubMed.

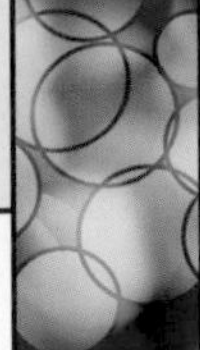

CHAPTER • 53

Candidiasis

Natalie Ann Carrillo

ETIOLOGY

Members of the genus *Candida* are dimorphic fungi that belong to the family *Cryptococcaceae;* they are small (2-6 μm), thin-walled, ovoid yeasts that reproduce by asexual multilateral budding.[1,2] They are ubiquitous, are found on many plants, and are considered part of the normal flora of the alimentary tract, upper respiratory tract, and genital mucosa of mammals. *Candida* species are opportunistic pathogens, and *Candida albicans* is by far the most common species isolated from healthy and diseased people and animals (Fig. 53-1). Other common *Candida* species include *C. tropicalis*, *C. glabrata*, *C. parapsilosis*, and *C. famata*.

EPIDEMIOLOGY

Candida is first acquired by neonates during passage through the birth canal, subsequently colonizing the mucosal and mucocutaneous surfaces of the gastrointestinal (GI), respiratory, and genitourinary tracts.[1] Opportunistic infections and life-threatening pathology can occur in neonatal and adult patients whose immune defenses have been altered by disease or various interventional strategies.[2]

Risk factors for candidiasis include prolonged broad-spectrum antibiotic therapy;[1,3-5] disruption of cutaneous or mucosal barriers by burns, surgery, cytotoxic agents, or trauma;[1] prolonged immunosuppression by disease states such as sepsis;[5] and administration of drugs such as glucocorticoids.[1,2,4] Other risk factors identified are low birth weight[5] (e.g., in premature foals), long-term placement of indwelling intravenous and urinary catheters,[1,3,5] long-term endotracheal tubes,[1,5] prolonged parenteral nutrition,[1,3,5] persistent neutropenia,[1,2] and severe primary immunodeficiency (e.g., agammaglobulinemia, selective IgM deficiency) and acquired immunodeficiency (e.g., failure of passive transfer).[6]

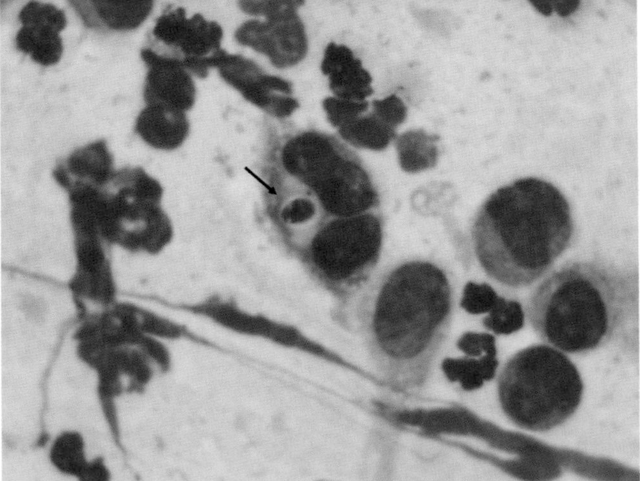

Fig. 53-1 Binucleated, macrophage-engulfing yeast *(arrow)*, latter identified as *Candida albicans*. Sample was taken from the left tibiotarsal joint of a neonatal foal. (Courtesy Heather L. Wamsley, Department of Clinical Pathology, University of Florida, College of Veterinary Medicine.)

PATHOGENESIS

Under most circumstances, overgrowth of *Candida* spp. is inhibited by the normal microflora of the GI and respiratory tracts, genitalia, and skin. When the mammalian host is compromised by any of the previously mentioned risk factors, *Candida* can readily become pathogenic. Local proliferation in wounds or mucosal surfaces is often the first step in spread of infection.[1] The organism often invades through breaks in the skin or mucosa; electron microscopic studies have implicated mechanical as well as enzymatic factors in the invasion of the oral epithelium.[4]

Once in the body, circulating neutrophils appear to be an important determinant of further spread of candidal infection.[1,2,4] Immunosuppressed patients and those with persistent neutropenia are at risk for developing candidiasis.

The microcirculation of tissues (e.g., lung, kidneys, joints, eyes, liver, brain, myocardium) acts to filter and clear the blood of pathogens. When systemic candidiasis is present, this activity results in embolic colonization and microabscess formation at these sites,[1] leading to the different presentations of candidal disease.

Candida albicans appears to have a number of virulence factors that promote successful parasitism, such as rapid germination upon seeding of tissue from the bloodstream, protease production to help invade tissues, surface integrin-like molecules for adhesion to extracellular matrix proteins, phenotypic switching and surface variation to avoid clearance by the immune system, and hydrophobicity.[2] *Candida* also has several mechanisms by which it can develop resistance to several antifungals, thereby increasing its pathogenicity.

CLINICAL FINDINGS

Thrush

Thrush is a local overgrowth of *Candida* spp. in the oral mucosa and tongue that manifests as white plaques on these areas (Fig. 53-2). Oral colonization with infection is the most common presentation in immunosuppressed human patients, especially those with human immunodeficiency virus (HIV) infection. This is likely the most common presentation in horses as well, although epidemiologic studies are lacking.[8] Mucocutaneous forms of candidiasis such as thrush are often related to defects in cell-mediated immunity, whereas systemic spread is generally associated with neutropenia.[2] Oral candidiasis is a clear indication for initiation of antifungal therapy and pursuit of further diagnostic testing to determine systemic involvement.

Systemic Candidiasis

Clinical manifestations of systemic candidiasis are often nonspecific, with unresolved fever the only clinical sign in many cases.[9] Hematogenous candidiasis can occur after colonization of the oral mucosa or GI tract or can be acquired through the introduction of venous (and urinary) catheters. Administration of total parenteral nutrition is a risk factor for human patients, and this association appears likely in the foal.[1,3,5,8]

The hematogenous spread of *Candida* can lead to meningitis, omphalophlebitis,[5] pneumonia,[5,6] and arthritis.[3,5,6,10] Systemic candidiasis with fungal keratitis and panophthalmitis has been reported in a foal with systemic candidiasis.[5] In human patients, endophthalmitis is considered pathognomonic for systemic candidiasis.[11]

Septic arthritis caused by *Candida* spp. can present as two clinical syndromes: (1) an isolated monoarthritis caused by direct intraarticular inoculation of commensal fungi, by means of an injection, laceration, or during surgery, or (2) a monoarthritis or polyarthritis from hematogenously disseminated candidiasis.[10] In either case, treatment is difficult, and prognosis is guarded. Clinical signs of septic arthritis caused by *Candida* spp. are clinically indistinguishable from those of infectious arthritis caused by other, more common bacterial pathogens.[10,12] Affected foals present with synovial effusion with or without lameness and fever (Fig. 53-3). Nucleated cell counts in synovial fluid of human patients with *Candida* arthritis more often resemble noninfectious inflammatory arthritis than acute bacterial arthritis, and routine culture does not readily detect these organisms.[12]

The role of *Candida* spp. in the pathogenesis of gastric ulcers remains to be determined. In one study, however, *Candida* spp. colonized the keratinized layers of gastric mucosa surrounding ulcers in foals that died or were euthanized because of gastric rupture. This finding suggests that this pathogen plays a predisposing role in the pathogenesis of gastric ulcers in some foals.[4]

Fungal endometritis is present in 1% to 5% of mares diagnosed with endometritis.[13] Repeated iatrogenic invasion of the reproductive tract, decreased ability to clear fluid and organisms, pneumovagina, poor conformation, and administration of progesterone may be involved in the pathogenesis (see Chapter 8). Because yeasts are considered commensal organisms of the urogenital tract, the presence of *Candida* is insufficient to support a diagnosis of fungal endometritis. Concurrent evidence of an inflammatory response must be obtained on cytology or biopsy.[13]

DIAGNOSIS

A diagnosis of candidiasis is supported by isolation of the organism from appropriate clinical samples, such as blood cultures, synovial fluid, surgically resected umbilical structures, and cerebrospinal fluid (CSF). Caution must be exercised when *Candida* spp. are isolated from transtracheal washes and uterine biopsies because of the commensal nature of these organisms in the more external portions of the respiratory and urogenital tracts, respectively.

THERAPY

Antifungal Therapy

Polyenes

Amphotericin B is an antifungal agent produced by *Streptomyces nodosus*. This drug targets the membrane of the fungal cell by binding to ergosterol (principal sterol in cell membrane), increasing membrane permeability, allowing leakage of intracellular contents, and causing cell death. The in vitro spectrum of activity includes *C. albicans*, *Mucor* spp., and *Aspergillus fumigatus*. Other *Candida* spp., *Fusarium*, and other *Aspergillus* spp. are resistant to amphotericin B.[9] Amphotericin B deoxycholate has been available for more than 40 years, but its clinical usefulness is limited by nephrotoxicity and infusion-related toxic effects. The agent binds to sterols on the cholesterol-rich lysosomal membranes of the distal renal tubular cells, with resultant increased cell permeability and cell death.

Renal vasoconstriction also plays a role in renal toxicity of amphotericin B by a mechanism that is not fully understood.[16] Infusion-related toxic signs in horses include anorexia, depression, anemia, elevation of body temperature,[16] and thrombophlebitis.[11] Dose reduction to ameliorate adverse effects can lead to treatment failure.[9] The dose recommended for treatment of adult horses and foals is 0.1 to 0.5 mg/kg administered in a 5% dextrose solution intravenously (IV) over 30 minutes, three times per week.[14] One report described

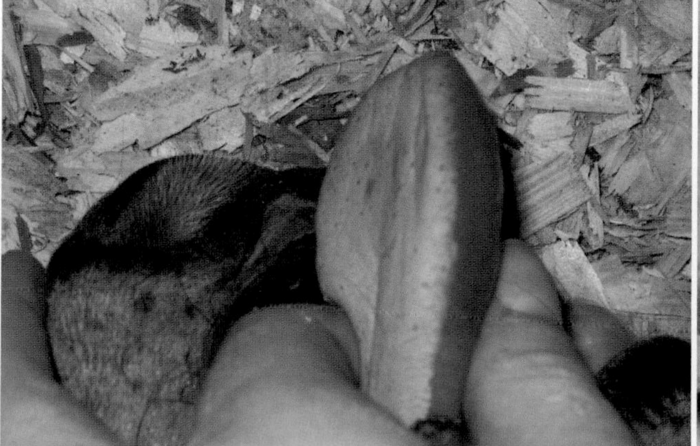

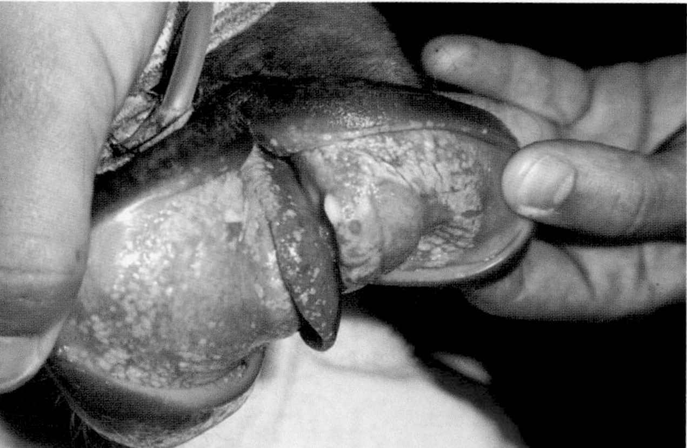

Fig. 53-2 Foal with thrush. Note the white plaques on the tongue (**A**) and mucous membranes (**B**). (Courtesy Dr. Clare Ryan and Dr. Steeve Giguére, Department of Large Animal Clinical Sciences, University of Florida, College of Veterinary Medicine.)

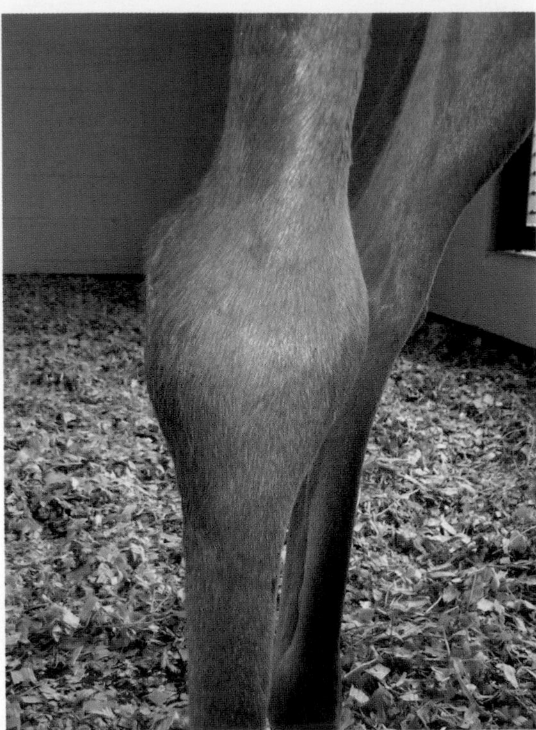

Fig. 53-3 Left hock with effusion, from foal with *Candida albicans* arthritis. (Courtesy Dr. Steeve Giguére, Department of Large Animal Clinical Sciences, University of Florida, College of Veterinary Medicine.)

daily administration of 0.1 mg/kg for 30 days to an adult horse without serious side effects.[15]

Amphotericin B is also available in several lipid-based formulations, including amphotericin B lipid complex (ABLC), amphotericin B colloidal dispersion (ABCD), and liposomal amphotericin B (L-AB). These formulations are less nephrotoxic and are associated with fewer infusion-related toxic events.[9] To the author's knowledge, use of these drug formulations has not been reported in horses.

Azoles

Azole antifungal agents target the membrane of the fungal cell by inhibiting cytochrome P-450 enzymes necessary for the biosynthesis of ergosterol, a main component of the fungal cell membrane structure.[9] *Ketoconazole* was the first available azole antifungal agent. Oral bioavailability in the horse is poor but can be increased to approximately 23% when the drug is acidified with hydrochloride (HCl).[17]

Fluconazole is active against *Candida* spp. and *Cryptococcus*, but molds such as *Aspergillus* and dimorphic fungi such as *Histoplasma* and *Blastomyces* are usually resistant. The pharmacokinetics for fluconazole outlined in the horse demonstrate that it is well absorbed after oral administration and distributes well into CSF, synovial fluid, aqueous humor, and urine, obtaining concentrations similar to those found in serum.[18] A loading dose of 8 mg/kg orally (PO) is recommended, followed by 4 mg/kg every 12 to 24 hours. Fluconazole is considered the drug of choice for treatment for equine candidiasis, but some strains of *C. albicans* and many other *Candida* spp. may be resistant to fluconazole in human patients.[8,9,19]

Itraconazole has been reported as successful for treatment of several horses at a dose of 3 mg/kg for mycotic rhinitis caused by *Aspergillus* spp. and *Conidiobolus*.[22] Preliminary studies suggest that *itraconazole* in suspension form is not well absorbed by horses and better absorption with no adverse effects was observed in horses that received capsules at a dose of 3 or 5 mg/kg (Steeve Giguere, personal communication). One foal was treated orally with itraconazole capsules at 6 mg/kg. No adverse effects were noted, and the peak serum concentrations exceeded the minimum concentration required to inhibit 90% of an *Aspergillus* spp. (MIC_{90}) that was cultured from a mare's placenta. Itraconazole has been successfully used in combination with dimethyl sulfoxide (DMSO) to treat fungal keratitis.[23] Recent work demonstrates that local treatment of keratitis with chelating agents enhances in vitro sensitivity of itraconazole against Candida albicans.[24]

The triazole antifungal agent *voriconazole* is effective against both yeasts and molds[9] in human patients, with approximately 96% oral bioavailability. CSF concentrations are reportedly approximately 50% of plasma concentrations. The recommended dose in people is 4 mg/kg for children and 3 mg/kg for adults PO or IV every 12 hours. Voriconazole was administered at the same dose and regimen IV and as regional limb perfusion to a foal with *C. albicans* septic arthritis. Peak plasma concentrations were similar to those reached in people, and no adverse effects were observed in the foal after administration of the drug by any of the routes.[20,23]

Other antifungal agents, such as posaconazole and micafugin, have been studied in humans and mice and as yet have not been investigated in horses.[25,26]

Supportive Therapy

In addition to targeted antifungal therapy, affected foals and adult horses should receive appropriate supportive therapy. Treatment of septic arthritis caused by *Candida* spp. must be aggressive and should include successive joint lavages with at least one arthroscopic flush to facilitate physical removal of accumulated fibrin. This fibrin will hide and harbor the organism and potentially perpetuate the infection.

References

See the CD-ROM for a list of references linked to the abstract in PubMed.

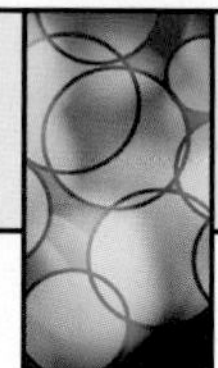

CHAPTER • 54

Dermatophytosis

Rosanna Marsella

Dermatophytosis ("ringworm") is a common superficial cutaneous fungal infection caused by keratinophilic fungi that are able to invade the stratum corneum of the skin and other keratinized structures. Several dermatophytes are reported to induce cutaneous disease in horses. Clinically, dermatophytosis presents as a crusting and scaling disease, similar to bacterial folliculitis.

ETIOLOGY

Trichophyton equinum is the most common causative agent of dermatophytosis of horses.[1,2] Two varieties of *T. equinum* have been reported, *T. equinum* var. *equinum* and *T. equinum* var. *autotrophicum*. Other, less common agents are *Trichophyton verrucosum*, *T. mentagrophytes*, *Microsporum equinum*, *M. canis*, and *M. gypseum*.[3-5] In one study, *T. equinum* var. *autotrophicum*, *M. canis*, and *M. equinum* were reported to be restricted to racing horses only, whereas *M. gypseum* occurred in racing, riding, and breeding horses.[6]

EPIDEMIOLOGY

Dermatophytes are highly contagious. Transmission occurs by either direct contact between horses or through contact with contaminated equipment. Infection can be readily transmitted, particularly by infected saddle-girths, on which the fungus can survive for 12 months.[7] Insects are also reported to play a role in the transmission of disease.[8,9] The source of infection varies depending on the dermatophyte. Some dermatophytes are zoophilic, and the source of infection may be another infected animal, such as a horse (e.g., *T. equinum*), a cat (e.g., *M. canis*), cattle (e.g., *T. verrucosum*), or a rodent (e.g., *T. mentagrophytes*). Other dermatophytes are geophilic (e.g., *M. gypseum*), and the source of infection is infected soil.

The prevalence of ringworm varies greatly depending on geographic location and husbandry conditions. In one epidemiologic study conducted in Egypt, 42% of horses with skin disease were positive for dermatophytes.[10] Horses less than 2 years old were more susceptible to infection. Fourteen species belonging to nine genera of keratinophilic and cycloheximide-resistant fungi were recovered from collected specimens. *Trichophyton* was the dominant genus, and *T. equinum* was the most frequently identified dermatophyte.

In a study of 200 horses in Italy, only 9% of horses were positive for *T. equinum*.[11] Although the clinical diagnosis of "ringworm" is quite common, many cases that clinically resemble ringworm may be bacterial folliculitis. At the University of Florida, only 5% of all the horses with skin disease that have cultures for dermatophytes are confirmed to have ringworm. The majority of horses that clinically appear to have ringworm are instead diagnosed with bacterial infections, either *Staphylococcus* or *Dermatophilus*.

PATHOGENESIS

Exposure to dermatophytes does not always result in clinical disease in horses. The outcome after exposure depends on the virulence of the dermatophyte, the conditions of the skin, environmental conditions, and the immune status of the host.

Virulence Factors

Dermatophytes produce enzymes such as keratinases that enable invasion of the hair and the stratum corneum and facilitate establishment of infection.[12,13] *T. equinum* produces urease, gelatinase, protease, hemolysins, and keratinase.[14] Some differences in enzyme production have been found between *T. equinum* and *T. mentagrophytes*. *T. mentagrophytes* may have stronger enzymatic properties, which, clinically, lead to more inflammatory reactions. Hemolytic activity and the ability to induce hypersensitivity reactions are also important virulence factors, especially for *Trichophyton* species.[15,16]

Host Factors and Immune Response

The conditions of the skin and immune system of the host play a crucial role in determining whether infection is established and how readily it is eliminated. Any impairment of the barrier function of the skin may foster establishment of infection. In particular, abrasions can facilitate the development of lesions and prolong the recovery period; abrasions are an important risk factor for infections in the girth area.[6,7]

Young horses (<3 years of age) are at increased risk for developing dermatophytosis.[6,7] Stress, such as training, also predisposes to the development of ringworm. In one study, 32% of horses in training were clinically affected, whereas only 1.1% of breeding horses were affected with pathogenic dermatophytes.[6] Concurrent diseases that may compromise the immune response can predispose to the development of dermatophytosis.[17]

Immunity is acquired by active infection. Both nonspecific and specific immune responses are important for clearing dermatophyte infections. Serum inhibitory factors deprive dermatophytes of iron, which is an essential nutrient. Both humoral and cell-mediated immune responses are elicited, but cell-mediated immunity appears to be most important for resolution of infection.[18,19] The development of cell-mediated immunity correlates with the development of an inflammatory response and is associated with clinical cure, whereas the lack of or a defective cell-mediated immunity predisposes the host to chronic or recurrent dermatophyte infection.[20] The inflammatory reaction also promotes keratinocyte proliferation, which facilitates the elimination of the fungus from the skin surface.

Horses that self-clear dermatophyte infections develop immunity and rarely experience recurrence of infection. Some horses, because of either a defective immune response or a concurrent illness, fail to develop long-term immunity and are prone to recurrent infection, unless the dermatophyte is completely eliminated from their environment.

Environmental Factors

Environmental conditions, such as high temperature, humidity, and insect exposure, also play a role in pathogenesis of dermatophytosis.[15,21] Interestingly, bedding and hygiene do not correlate with dermatophytic infections of the hooves.[22]

CLINICAL FINDINGS

Primary lesions of dermatophytosis consist of follicular papules and pustules. Individual lesions may present as spreading circular patches of alopecia (Figs. 54-1 and 54-2), surrounded by erythema and scaling (epidermal collarettes). Urticaria-like lesions can be observed in early stages of the disease. As the infection progresses, crusting and scaling (seborrhea) develop.

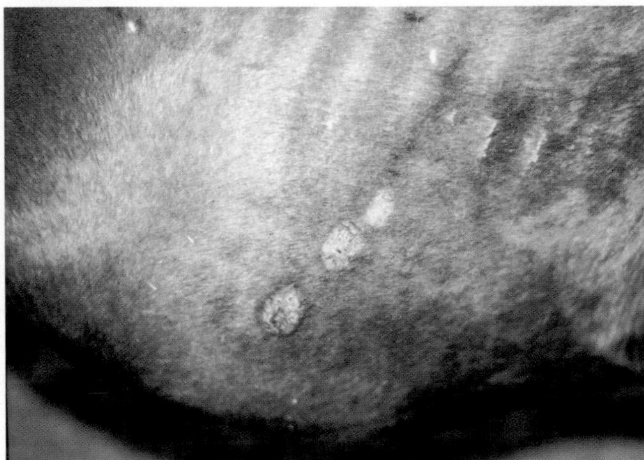

Fig. 54-1 Circular patches of alopecia caused by *Trichophyton equinum* on shoulder of horse. In this case, pruritus was present and lesions were excoriated.

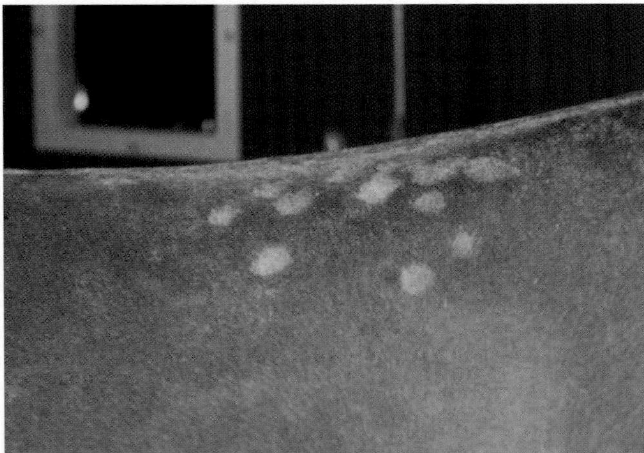

Fig. 54-2 Circular patches of alopecia on back of horse, most likely caused by contaminated saddle pad. Lesions showed minimal inflammation. No pruritus was present.

Pruritus is usually absent but may be present in some cases. Hair is epilated easily in affected areas. In some horses, nodular lesions can develop as the result of ruptured follicles (furunculosis), which elicits a strong inflammatory response, intense erythema, and suppurative exudate.

The most frequently affected sites are the girth and the shoulder area, usually from use of contaminated equipment. A survey of 568 horses in training and 2535 horses on breeding farms showed that the majority of lesions on racing horses were located on the girth areas.[6] Other frequently affected areas are the muzzle and the pastern region.

Dermatophytosis is overdiagnosed when only clinical signs are used to make the diagnosis. Differential diagnoses should include other, more common causes of folliculitis, such as bacterial infections (e.g., staphylococcal pyoderma, dermatophilosis). Therefore, cytology should be done in all suspected cases. Cytology allows assessment for the presence of bacteria and yeast and diagnosis of secondary bacterial infections. Although not as common, parasitic diseases should also be considered. Skin scraping should be performed in all cases. Although a negative scraping does not always rule out the possibility of parasitic infections, it may provide information regarding the presence of *Demodex* and other mites.

Other diseases that may present with crusting and scaling include contact allergy, sarcoids, and autoimmune diseases such as pemphigus foliaceus or systemic lupus erythematosus.[23] Importantly, acantholytic cells can be found on cytology in horses with dermatophytosis.[24] This is caused by the severe inflammatory response triggered by dermatophytes and the release of enzymes that may break desmosomal attachments between keratinocytes. Therefore the identification of acantholytic cells on cytology should not be considered pathognomonic for pemphigus foliaceus, and a definitive diagnosis should be made only after histopathologic evaluation. This is of particular importance because the therapy for pemphigus foliaceus (e.g., glucocorticoids) would be highly contraindicated in horses with dermatophytosis. In older horses, neoplastic diseases such as mycosis fungoides should also be considered as differential diagnoses for patches of alopecia and scaling. In these cases as well, biopsies are necessary for a definitive diagnosis.

DIAGNOSIS

Wood's Lamp

Examination with a Wood's lamp is not recommended as a diagnostic tool for equine dermatophytosis because only a few strains of dermatophytes show positive fluorescence. To complicate the assessment further, topical therapy may cause false-positive reactions.

Direct Examination of Hair

Arthrospores can be detected by direct examination of hair. This test requires experience and is time-consuming. Positive results have been reported in approximately half of affected horses; therefore direct examination is not considered a sensitive diagnostic test.[25]

Culture

Fungal culture is the most reliable diagnostic test for dermatophytosis. The area should be gently swabbed with alcohol to decrease contamination by saprophytic fungi. After the alcohol has evaporated, hairs should be plucked, ensuring that the roots are included. *Dermatophyte test medium* (DTM) is often used, although demonstrated to be inferior to Sabouraud dextrose agar.[26] It is important to note that *T. verrucosum* may not grow on DTM, requiring Sabouraud dextrose agar for a positive diagnosis.[27] At the optimum incubation temperature of 27° C (80.6° F), a color change to red can be observed in DTM only a few days after inoculation with infected hairs (Fig. 54-3). This color change requires approximately 3 days with *M. canis*–infected hairs, 4 days with *T. equinum*, and 5 days with *T. mentagrophytes*.[28]

Dermatophytes are positively identified by morphologic and biochemical characteristics.[29,30] *Trichophyton equinum* is identified by its morphology, dependency on nicotinic acid, hair perforation, and enzyme production. The type of culture medium influences growth and appearance of the *T. equinum* colonies. On solid Sabouraud media, two types of colonies may be observed. Colonies with characteristic radial folds and grooves in the paracentral zone and umbilical elevation in the center are the most common. Typical features of *T. equinum* include dark-red pigmentation of the reverse side of the colony in the culture on solid Sabouraud medium with glucose, and yellow-orange pigmentation on the same medium with no glucose.[31] Importantly, *T. equinum* strains cannot grow in the absence of vitamins, whereas they reveal rapid growth when nicotinic acid is added.[32] Most of the organic nitrogen sources are stimulatory for spore germination, which occurs within 24 hours.[33] Isolates of *M. equinum* produce typical macroconidia, are negative in the hair perforation test in vitro, and are urease positive.[34]

It is important to note that false-positive results with DTM can also occur. In specimens obtained from horses, a high contamination rate (36%), mostly from molds, was found with a cycloheximide-supplemented medium, making the examination of these cultures for the growth of dermatophytes impossible.[35] For this reason, it is important to use alcohol before plucking hairs to submit for culture. Also, it is important to realize that some animals may be carriers of dermatophyte organisms without associated clinical signs. Culture results should always be interpreted in conjunction with history and clinical signs.

Histology

Biopsy findings consistent with a diagnosis of dermatophytosis include luminal folliculitis and pyogranulomatous furunculosis. Biopsy can be helpful in cases when the culture results are equivocal. The presence of follicular arthrospores in conjunction with an inflammatory reaction is proof of clinically relevant infection. Superficial perivascular dermatitis with neutrophilic exocytosis and pustule formation is also often present. Palisading crusts are similar to those observed with dermatophilosis. As previously mentioned, acantholysis can be observed in some cases.

THERAPY

Because most horses spontaneously resolve dermatophyte infections, many treatments have been advertised as a "cure" for dermatophytosis. Very few controlled studies have been performed to assess scientifically the efficacy of these therapies. As a general rule, therapy is aimed at reducing contagion to the environment and facilitating the resolution of lesions, usually with topical therapy.

Animal

Topical Therapy

Topical therapy should be considered for all horses with dermatophytosis. A variety of such treatments have been recommended. A natamycin-based suspension successfully eliminated the disease within 4 weeks.[36] The reported mycologic clearance rate was 97%. This study was not controlled, so final conclusions regarding the relevance of these results cannot be made.

Povidone-iodine, thiabendazole ointment, and captan have also been reported to give satisfactory results for treatment of *T. equinum*, whereas aqueous washes containing 0.5% hexetidine or 0.3% chloramine-T did not prevent fungi isolation from lesions for up to 7 days after treatment.[37] Because a control group was not included in this study, conclusions cannot be made regarding the findings.

Currently, one of the most frequently used treatments in clinical practice is 2% lime sulfur (LymDyp).[38,39] Disadvantages of this treatment include the smell and the temporary yellow discoloration of white areas. Lime sulfur can also permanently

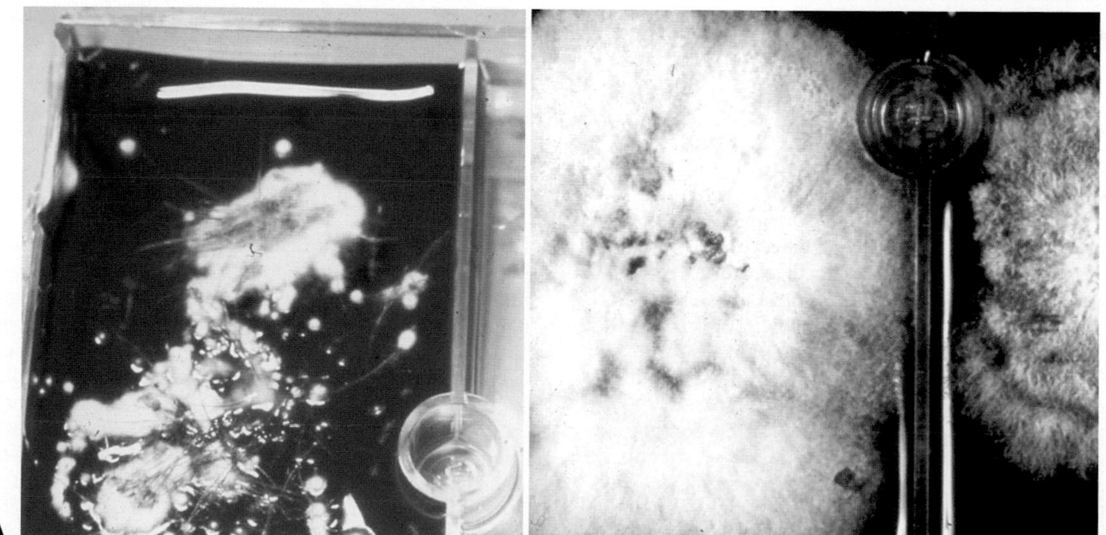

Fig. 54-3 **A,** Dermatophyte test medium (DTM) plate demonstrating red color change in conjunction with growth of *Trichophyton*. **B,** Nondermatophyte fungal growth on DTM agar.

damage jewelry and clothes. Rinses of 0.2% enilconazole, although not approved for use in horses, are reported to be effective for treatment of equine dermatophytosis when used once or twice weekly.[40] Shampoos are less desirable than rinses because of the lack of residual activity. Commonly used ingredients for "antifungal" shampoos include miconazole, ketoconazole, and chlorhexidine (e.g., Nizoral, KetoChlor). No controlled studies have evaluated the efficacy of these products in equine dermatophytosis.

All animals in contact with horses with dermatophytosis should receive topical therapy because they may be carriers without any evidence of cutaneous lesions. Treatment of large numbers of horses should be primarily aimed at reducing the spread of infection. In clinically affected horses, hair regrowth should not be used as an indication of cure because regrowth can occur while animals remain infected. It is therefore important to reculture the animal and demonstrate a lack of dermatophyte growth. Horses with low numbers of arthrospores on their coat may fluctuate between positive and negative cultures, so three consecutive negative cultures at 2-week intervals are recommended for confirmation.

Systemic Therapy

Although various dosages of griseofulvin have been recommended for the treatment of equine dermatophytosis, no published studies support this drug's efficacy and appropriate dose. Similarly, there are no studies on the pharmacokinetics and efficacy of other systemic antifungal treatments (e.g., ketoconazole, itraconazole, fluconazole, terbinafine). The lack of information together with the cost of treatment prevents the recommendation of these therapies.

Environment

Environmental control relies mostly on the use of diluted bleach (1:40) and elimination of infected tack. An enilconazole-based product (Clinafarm EC) available for use in poultry hatchery facilities may be considered for use in highly contaminated barns, although is not specifically approved for this use. All animals must be evacuated during treatment.

PREVENTION

Vaccine

Vaccines have been used in the past in small and large animals to manage endemic dermatophytosis.[41-43] Immunity obtained after vaccination appears to be cross-reactive.[44] Currently, however, there are no commercially available vaccines for prevention of equine dermatophytosis in the United States.

PUBLIC HEALTH CONSIDERATIONS

Equine dermatophytosis can be contagious to humans, as documented by several case reports.[45-47] Infection is caused by direct contact with affected horses, including bareback riding.[48] Infections in humans are either self-limiting or responsive to antifungal treatment.[49]

REFERENCES

See the CD-ROM for a list of references linked to the abstract in PubMed.

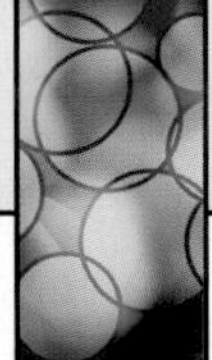

CHAPTER • 55

Pythiosis and Zygomycosis

Amy M. Grooters

Although the oomycete *Pythium insidiosum* and the zygomycetes *Conidiobolus* spp. and *Basidiobolus ranarum* fall into two taxonomically distant groups of organisms, they are typically grouped together by equine clinicians and pathologists because they share similar clinical and histologic characteristics. Both cause cutaneous lesions characterized by pyogranulomatous and eosinophilic inflammation associated with broad, sparsely septate hyphae. Because of these similarities, pythiosis and zygomycosis have been referred to collectively as "phycomycosis." Despite remaining a convenient label for cases without a definitive, culture-based diagnosis, "phycomycosis" is no longer an appropriate taxonomic designation and should be replaced in current literature with the more specific terms *pythiosis* and *zygomycosis*. Clinically, differentiating between these infections is important because of differences in epidemiology, choice of therapy, and prognosis.

PYTHIOSIS

Pythiosis, a pseudofungal infection caused by the oomycotic pathogen *Pythium insidiosum*, is best known as a cause of cutaneous and subcutaneous disease in horses[1] and of gastrointestinal or cutaneous disease in dogs.[2] It has also been described as an uncommon cause of cutaneous and subcutaneous lesions in cats and calves[3,4] and of arteritis, keratitis, or periorbital cellulitis in humans.[5,6] In older literature, *P. insidiosum* has been referred to using the now-outdated synonyms *Hyphomyces destruens*,[7] *Pythium destruens*,[8] *Pythium* spp.,[9] and *Pythium gracile*.[10]

Clinical manifestations of pythiosis have been recognized in horses for more than a century and variably referred to as "kunkers," "Florida horse leeches," "bursatti," and "swamp cancer," as well as "phycomycosis." The disease was first noted in the mid-nineteenth century when British veterinarians working with horses in India observed a chronic granulomatous cutaneous disease that they termed "bursautee." A fungal etiology for this disease was suspected on the basis of histologic findings in the late nineteenth century,[11] and the pathogen was isolated as early as 1901 by Dutch investigators working with horses in Indonesia.[12] However, it could not be induced to sporulate using standard fungal media and was thus assumed to be a sterile zygomycete or "phycomycete" fungus based on the morphologic characteristics of its vegetative hyphae. It was not until 1974 that Austwick and Copland[13] were able to produce biflagellate zoospores from isolates obtained from horses in New Guinea, identifying the pathogen as an oomycete that was likely a member of the genus *Pythium*. The species name *Pythium insidiosum* was introduced in 1987 by de Cock,[14] who was able to produce sexual reproductive structures from pathogenic isolates, and who found the morphologic characteristics of several isolates from horses and dogs to be identical.

Etiology and Epidemiology

The causative agent of pythiosis is the aquatic oomycete *Pythium insidiosum*, a member of the kingdom Stramenopila that is more closely related to algae than to true fungi.[15] The taxonomic differences between oomycetes and fungi are reflected on the cellular level by differences in cell membrane and cell wall composition. Ergosterol, an essential component of the fungal cell membrane and a common target of antifungal drugs, is not a principal sterol in the oomycete cell membrane.[16] In addition, oomycetes generally lack chitin, which is an important structural component of the fungal cell well.

The infective stage of *P. insidiosum* is thought to be the biflagellate zoospore, which is released into warm-water environments and swims in a helical pattern as part of a complex homing sequence that allows it to locate, move toward, and encyst on specific host tissues.[17] *P. insidiosum* zoospores are attracted to animal hair, as well as to cut edges of skin, and likely cause infection by encysting in damaged skin or gastrointestinal (GI) mucosa.[18] Although many infected horses have a history of recurrent exposure to standing fresh water,[19,20] other risk factors for the development of pythiosis have not been identified. Affected animals are immunocompetent and otherwise healthy. Given the affinity of *P. insidiosum* zoospores for damaged skin, it seems likely that animals with cutaneous wounds or parasite-induced injury to GI mucosa would be more likely to become infected. However, documented epidemiologic evidence to support this assumption is lacking. The presence of a traumatic wound before the development of cutaneous pythiosis has been reported in a small number of canine and equine cases. Because traumatic incidents are rarely observed by the owner, however, it is often difficult to determine whether lesions noted early in the course of disease resulted from trauma or from early infection.

In the United States, pythiosis is encountered most often in the Gulf Coast states but has been recognized in animals living as far north as New Jersey, Virginia, North Carolina, southern Illinois, southern Indiana, and Kentucky and as far west as Oklahoma, Missouri, and Kansas. Although GI pythiosis has recently been documented in dogs living in Arizona and northern California, no reports of equine pythiosis have been made from these regions to date. Globally, pythiosis is most often encountered in Southeast Asia (especially Thailand and Indonesia), eastern coastal Australia, New Zealand, and South America (especially Brazil and Costa Rica), but it has also been recognized in Korea, Japan, and the Caribbean (Haiti).

Clinical Findings

Pythium insidiosum infection in horses most often causes large, ulcerative, proliferative granulomatous lesions involving cutaneous or subcutaneous tissues of the distal limbs (generally below the knee and hock), ventral abdomen (Fig. 55-1), ventral thorax, or face.[1,7,21,22] Less frequently affected areas include the dorsum and external genitalia.[20] Solitary lesions are most common,[21] but multiple lesions have been reported.[7,20,21,23] Intense pruritus is typically associated with cutaneous pythiosis and often results in self-mutilation of the affected tissues. Lesions typically appear as circular masses that are rapidly expanding, ulcerative, and necrotic and that contain multiple fistulous tracts that drain a serosanguineous, hemorrhagic, or mucopurulent fluid.[1] In addition, a characteristically stringy, viscous fluid may be observed hanging in strands from ventral abdominal lesions (Fig. 55-1) or matting the hair around extremity lesions.

Sinus tracts in *P. insidiosum* lesions contain multiple, 1-mm to 10-mm, tan to yellow, branching, coral-like firm masses or coagula that are commonly referred to as "kunkers" or "leeches" (Fig. 55-2). Histologically, these kunkers are composed of hyphae, inflammatory cells (especially eosinophils), collagen, and necrotic debris, and they are especially prevalent deep to the junction of the ulcerated portion of the lesion and the intact epidermis.[24] Kunkers are often extruded from draining tracts and may be found in bandage material. Other diseases that can cause similar cutaneous lesions in horses include cutaneous habronemiasis, excessive granulation tissue, bacterial granulomas, sarcoid, squamous cell carcinoma, and zygomycosis. Both habronemiasis and zygomycosis can produce tissue grains, but in habronemiasis they are usually smaller and lack the typical coral-like shape of kunkers associated with pythiosis.[24,25]

Although most *P. insidiosum* lesions are confined to cutaneous and subcutaneous tissues, long-standing infections may sometimes invade deeper tissues. Extension of pythiosis through fascial planes resulting in infection or inflammation of an underlying tendon sheath, joint, or bone has been described in horses with extremity lesions present for longer than 2 months.[23,26,27] Horses with bone involvement are often presented with lameness (which may be non–weight bearing) and edema of the affected limb. Radiographic findings are characterized by extensive, disorganized bony proliferation with variable osteolysis and cortical erosion.[26-28] Bones in which infection has been observed include the phalanges, the third metacarpal and metatarsal bones, and the proximal

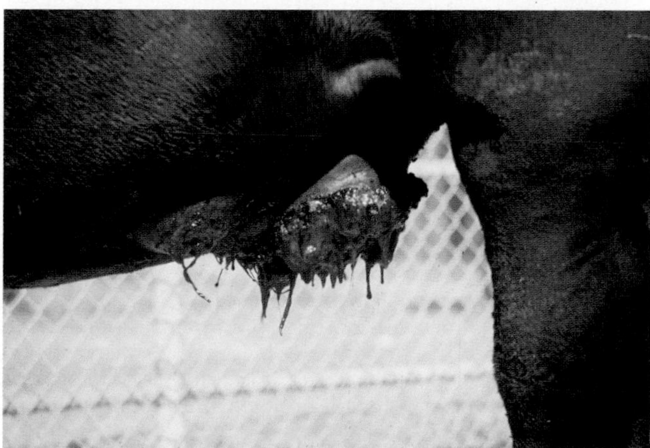

Fig. 55-1 Large, ulcerative, draining granulomatous lesion caused by *Pythium insidiosum* infection on ventrum of mare. Note the presence of a stringy, viscous fluid hanging in strands from the surface of the lesion.

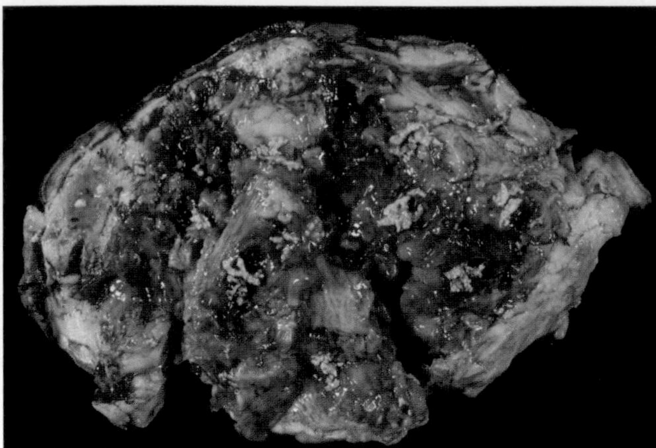

Fig. 55-2 Necropsy photograph of large subcutaneous lesion caused by *Pythium insidiosum* infection in horse. Note the presence of multiple, tan to yellow, branching, coral-like masses, commonly referred to as "kunkers." (Courtesy Dr. Corrie Brown, University of Georgia.)

sesamoid bones. Periostitis resulting from adjacent soft tissue infection may cause significant periosteal proliferation without actual invasion of the periosteum; therefore, in cases with radiographic changes that are limited to proliferative changes of the periosteum, differentiation between periostitis and osteomyelitis cannot be made without a biopsy.[28]

In addition to local invasion of deeper tissues, dissemination of chronic cutaneous *P. insidiosum* infection to regional lymph nodes and lung has been reported in a small number of horses. Infection of an inguinal lymph node has previously been described in four horses with cutaneous hindlimb lesions.[24,29] Likewise, pulmonary lesions have been described in three horses with preexisting cutaneous lesions.[1,30,31] In one of these cases, however, the organism was not isolated, and the gross and microscopic characteristics of the lesions were not described.[31]

Intestinal granulomas similar to the enteric lesions found in dogs with GI pythiosis have been described in four horses.[32-35] Clinical signs in these horses included colic, and in each case a jejunal mass was detected during abdominal exploratory (three horses) or necropsy (one foal). Two of these horses had no recurrence of pythiosis after resection of the jejunal lesion; a third horse was euthanized at surgery because of extensive jejunal infarction thought to have resulted from prolonged intestinal distention.[35]

Diagnosis

The clinical manifestations of equine pythiosis were recognized for more than a century before the pathogen itself was conclusively identified; the definitive diagnosis of pythiosis has historically been challenging because of difficulties associated with isolation and morphologic identification of the pathogen. As a result, a presumptive diagnosis is often made on the basis of typical clinical and histologic findings. However, a number of recently developed serologic, immunohistochemical, and molecular-based tools are likely to make the definitive diagnosis of pythiosis possible in a greater number of affected animals, even when culture is unsuccessful.

Although cytologic and histologic findings may be supportive of a diagnosis of pythiosis, they do not allow differentiation of pythiosis from infections caused by the zygomycetes *Conidiobolus* and *Basidiobolus*, which have similar histologic and cytologic characteristics.

Cytology

Cytologic examination of exudate from draining tracts often reveals pyogranulomatous, eosinophilic, and suppurative inflammation. Hyphal structures are not usually visualized in exudate. However, macerated tissue fixed in 10% potassium hydroxide (KOH) for 30 minutes may be examined microscopically for the presence of typical, wide, sparsely septate, branching hyphal elements.

Culture

Isolation of *P. insidiosum* from infected tissues is not difficult when appropriate sample-handling and culture techniques are employed. However, because these techniques are fairly specific, it is important to use a laboratory with expertise in the isolation of pathogenic oomcyetes. Kunkers are more likely than tissues to provide a positive culture and are the preferred source of inoculum.[36] For best results, unrefrigerated kunkers should be wrapped in a sterile, saline-moistened gauze sponge and shipped at ambient temperature to arrive at the laboratory within 24 hours of collection. However, when samples cannot be processed for more than 2 to 3 days after collection, they should be shipped with ice packs, stored in the refrigerator, or stored at ambient temperature in an antibiotic solution to decrease proliferation of bacterial contaminants.[36]

The use of selective media significantly increases the likelihood of isolating pathogenic oomycetes, especially from lesions with secondary bacterial infection. The author routinely uses vegetable extract agar[37] amended with streptomycin (200 μg/mL) and ampicillin (100 μg/mL) for the isolation of *P. insidiosum*. As a commercially available alternative, Campy blood agar (Remel, Lenexa, Kansas), which contains trimethoprim, vancomycin, polymyxin B, cephalothin, and amphotericin B, is also effective. Small pieces of fresh kunkers should be placed directly on the surface of the agar and incubated at 37° C (98.6° F); growth is typically observed within 24 hours.

Although the identification of oomycetes is generally based on morphologic features of sexual reproductive structures such as oogonia and antheridia, isolates of *P. insidiosum* rarely produce these structures in vitro. Therefore, identification of *P. insidiosum* should be based on colonial and hyphal characteristics; growth at 37° C; production of motile, reniform, biflagellate zoospores; and, if possible, specific polymerase chain reaction (PCR) amplification or ribosomal ribonucleic acid (rRNA) gene sequencing. Colonies on vegetable extract or Sabouraud dextrose agar are typically submerged, white to colorless, and have an irregular radiate pattern.[14,38] Microscopically, hyphae are broad (4-10 μm in diameter), hyaline, sparsely septate, and tend to branch at right angles. Zoospores can be readily produced by placing boiled grass blades on the surface of a 1- to 2-day-old colony growing on 2% water agar, incubating at 37° C for 18 to 24 hours, and then placing the infected grass blades in a dilute salt solution.[39-41] After 2 to 4 hours of incubation at 37° C, terminal vesicles from which zoospores are released can be visualized extending from the cut edges of the infected grass blades. Although the production of zoospores is an important supporting feature for the identification of pathogenic oomycetes, it is not specific for *P. insidiosum*. It does, however, rule out zygomycosis.

Serology

Both immunoblot[42] and enzyme-linked immunosorbent assay (ELISA)[43,44] have been used successfully to demonstrate the ability of sera from *Pythium*-infected horses to recognize soluble mycelial antigens of *P. insidiosum*. Unfortunately, the only assay currently available to practicing veterinarians has not been tested for specificity using serum from horses with basidiobolomycosis or sporotrichosis, or from healthy horses that are regularly exposed to nonpathogenic oomycetes in pasture environments; therefore its rate of false-positive results is unknown. In the author's experience, the specificity of immunoblot serology for the diagnosis of pythiosis in horses is not as high as in dogs and cats; occasional false-positive results are observed in horses with other types of fungal as well as nonfungal inflammatory diseases.

Molecular Assays

To circumvent the difficulties associated with obtaining a culture-based diagnosis of pythiosis, a *P. insidiosum*–specific PCR assay was recently developed.[45] This assay can be applied to deoxyribonucleic acid (DNA) extracted from either cultured isolates or appropriately preserved, infected tissue samples.[46] In addition, the author has successfully applied this technique to DNA extracted from paraffin-embedded tissue sections.[47] The major advantage of this assay is its high specificity.

Immunohistochemistry

Immunohistochemical (IHC) techniques using polyclonal antibodies, developed first by Brown et al.[48] and later by Patton et al.,[49] have previously been used as confirmatory tests for pythiosis. These techniques have the advantage of being applicable to paraffin-embedded tissues. However, at least one of these antibodies has demonstrated cross-reactive staining of *Conidiobolus* and *Lagenidium* hyphae in canine tissue.[50,51] Therefore the specificity of this antibody for the IHC diagnosis of pythiosis is questionable. A new polyclonal anti–*P. insidiosum* antibody raised in chickens and adsorbed with sonicated *Lagenidium* and *Conidiobolus* hyphae appears to be highly specific for the IHC detection of *P. insidiosum* hyphae in both equine tissues (Fig. 55-3) and canine tissues,[52] but it is not commercially available.

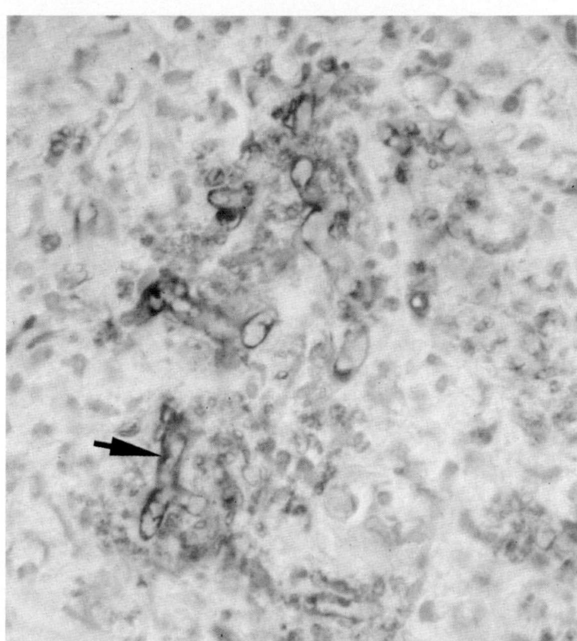

Fig. 55-3 Photomicrograph showing immunohistochemical stain of tissue excised from cutaneous lesion in horse with pythiosis. Note the presence of multiple, broad *Pythium insidiosum* hyphae *(arrowhead)* with nonparallel walls and rare septation. (Avidin-biotin-peroxidase method with polyclonal anti–*P. insidiosum* antibody; Mayer's hematoxylin counterstain; 40×.)

Pathologic Findings

Histologic findings associated with pythiosis are characterized by eosinophilic granulomatous to pyogranulomatous inflammation with necrosis and fibrosis. Infected tissues typically contain multiple foci of necrosis or coagula that contain amorphous eosinophilic material, hyphae, collagen, and degenerate eosinophils and are surrounded and infiltrated by neutrophils, eosinophils, and macrophages.[24] Some of these coagula are organized and large enough to be grossly visible as kunkers. Discrete eosinophilic granulomas may also be observed. The area between the necrotic foci or discrete granulomas is characterized by granulomatous and granulocytic inflammation and often contains epithelioid macrophages, lymphocytes, plasma cells, and mast cells. Vascular changes, including vessel wall invasion, vasculitis, thrombosis, and intimal changes, are variably present. In chronic lesions, fibrosis becomes more predominant, and the number of inflammatory cells is reduced.

Hyphal structures are usually found within areas of necrosis or at the center of discrete granulomas. Although *P. insidiosum* hyphae are difficult to visualize on hematoxylin and eosin (H&E)–stained sections, they may be identified as clear spaces ("hyphal ghosts") surrounded by a band or sleeve of eosinophilic material. Hyphae are easily visualized in sections stained with Gomori's methenamine silver (GMS) but not with periodic acid–Schiff (PAS). They are broad (mean, 4 μm; range, 2-7 μm), rarely septate, and occasionally branching.[24]

Therapy

Current recommendations for the treatment of equine pythiosis include surgical removal of as much infected tissue as possible, combined with immunotherapeutic injection of *P. insidiosum* antigens. In horses with nonresectable lesions, immunotherapy alone may be curative or may cause the lesion to regress to a size that is amenable to resection. Because the success of either surgery or immunotherapy depends on initiating therapy early in the course of disease, biopsy should be performed without delay in horses that develop lesions suggestive of pythiosis. Unfortunately, lesions caused by pythiosis (especially those that have been present for several months before diagnosis) may not resolve despite aggressive surgical and immune therapy.

Surgery

Complete surgical resection of infected tissues provides the best opportunity for cure of equine pythiosis. Whenever feasible, surgical excision of *P. insidiosum* lesions should be performed with 2- to 3-cm margins.[1] Unfortunately, the location (e.g., distal limb), size, and invasiveness of lesions often make complete removal of infected tissue difficult and necessitate leaving the incision open to heal by second intention.

Laser photoablation has recently been recommended as an adjunctive tool for reducing the risk of postsurgical recurrence in horses with cutaneous or subcutaneous pythiosis.[53,54] By inducing collateral thermal necrosis, photoablation acts to kill hyphal organisms that may have infiltrated surgical tissue margins. Photoablation with carbon dioxide (CO_2) or neodymium:yttrium-aluminium-garnet (Nd:YAG) lasers has previously been used in human patients for adjunctive therapy after partial resection of bacterial and neoplastic lesions.[55-57] Sedrish et al.[54] described the use of a Nd:YAG laser to photoablate the tissue bed after mass removal in two horses with cutaneous pythiosis. A defocused beam of 80 W, continuous power, and a noncontact fiber was used in a cross-hatch pattern, resulting in an energy density of 300 to 500 J/cm^2. Because Nd:YAG lasers create greater thermal damage, they may be more effective than diode or CO_2 lasers for postoperative photoablation treatment of *P. insidiosum* infection. Surgeons using laser photoablation for the treatment of cutaneous pythiosis should keep in mind that the laser plume is a potential vector for transmitting infectious materials[58] and should strictly adhere to laser safety protocols.

Immunotherapy

Immunotherapy, in the form of parenteral administration of water-soluble antigens extracted from an isolate of *P. insidiosum*, has been used successfully for more than 20 years for the treatment of equine pythiosis. The effectiveness of this form of treatment is likely related to stimulation of changes in the cell-mediated immune response to infection. Because immunotherapy with *P. insidiosum* antigens is not effective in horses with zygomycosis or other cutaneous diseases, a definitive diagnosis based on culture or molecular identification of the pathogen, in addition to histopathology, is needed before initiating treatment.

A therapeutic *P. insidiosum* vaccine consisting of killed, sonicated mycelium was first developed by Miller[59] in the early 1980s and was found to be effective in resolving pythiosis in approximately 50% of equine patients. Cure rates were even higher when vaccination was used in conjunction with surgical debridement. In animals that responded favorably to the vaccine, signs of improvement (decreased exudate, resolution of pruritus, stabilization of lesion size) were first noted 5 to 10 days after the first of three or more weekly injections. Epithelialization, closure of draining tracts, and reduction in inflammation and lesion size were observed 14 to 28 days after initiation of immunotherapy. Adverse effects associated with immunotherapy using this vaccine preparation included development of a severe, local tissue reaction, with pain, edema, and sterile abscesses at the injection site. Two patients with extremity lesions developed osteitis and septic arthritis despite apparent resolution of the *P. insidiosum* infection.[59,60]

A second type of *P. insidiosum* vaccine, developed by Mendoza, consisted of secreted antigens of *P. insidiosum* precipitated from broth culture medium.[61] When evaluated in 41 *P. insidiosum*–infected horses from Costa Rica, Mendoza's vaccine was found to have efficacy similar to that achieved with Miller's vaccine, but with less severe tissue reactions at the injection site. Mendoza also found that lesion duration was an important factor in predicting response to immunotherapy, with cure rates of 100% in horses with lesions that had been present for 15 days or less, but no cures in horses with lesions present for more than 2 months. In addition, the stability of the exoantigen vaccine preparation was reported to be superior to Miller's sonicated mycelial preparation, allowing Mendoza's vaccine to be stored at 4° C (39° F) for up to 18 months without loss of efficacy. Further work with both types of vaccines by Newton and Rosa[62] in the early 1990s supported Miller and Mendoza's findings.

More recently, another therapeutic vaccine that contains both secreted antigens and soluble mycelial antigens was described by Thitithanyanont et al.,[63] who used it successfully to treat *P. insidiosum* infection causing arteritis in a young boy in Thailand. Subsequently, Mendoza[64] evaluated the efficacy of this vaccine for the treatment of equine pythiosis and found that it effectively resolved *P. insidiosum*–induced lesions in 13 of 18 horses that had failed to respond to surgical and medical therapy. The protocol for immunotherapy using this vaccine consists of an initial intradermal administration of 0.1 mL of a 2-µg/mL antigen preparation, followed by subcutaneous administration of a second dose 15 days later. If a poor clinical response is observed, the vaccine is readministered on a weekly basis for up to 2 months. The local inflammatory response of the patient to the initial injection appears to be an important prognostic factor; animals that produce a large (>30 mm) wheal with erythema and edema are more likely to be cured eventually than those that have a minimal local response. This vaccine product is available through Pan American Veterinary Laboratories (pavlab.com, 800-856-9655).

Medical Therapy

The administration of traditional antifungal drugs such as amphotericin B, ketoconazole, and iodides is typically ineffective for the treatment of pythiosis. For amphotericin B and the azoles, this is likely because ergosterol is not an important component of the oomycete cell membrane. However, there are sporadic reports in the equine veterinary literature of response of *P. insidiosum* lesions to systemic treatment with amphotericin B, sodium iodide, or potassium iodide.[1,31] In addition, topical therapy with either amphotericin B or a combination of ketoconazole and dimethyl sulfoxide (DMSO) has been recommended for adjunctive therapy, although information regarding efficacy is largely anecdotal.[1] In general, medical therapy is not recommended for the treatment of pythiosis in horses except as an adjunct to surgical resection and immunotherapy.

ZYGOMYCOSIS

The term *zygomycosis* refers to infections caused by fungi in the class Zygomycetes, including the genera *Basidiobolus* and *Conidiobolus* in the order Entomophthorales, and the genera *Rhizopus, Absidia, Mucor, Saksenaea*, and others in the order Mucorales. In human and veterinary patients, the Mucorales fungi tend to cause acute, rapidly progressive disease in debilitated or immunocompromised individuals, whereas the Entomophthorales fungi typically cause chronic localized infections in subcutaneous tissue or nasal submucosa of immunocompetent patients.[65,66] Culture-confirmed infections caused by pathogens in the order Mucorales have not been well documented in equine patients, with only three case descriptions in the literature to date. However, *Basidiobolus ranarum* and *Conidiobolus* spp. have been well documented in horses as causes of cutaneous and nasopharyngeal lesions, respectively.

Etiology and Epidemiology

Basidiobolus ranarum (previously *B. haptosporus*), *Conidiobolus coronatus*, *C. incongruus*, and *C. lamprauges* are saprophytes that are widely distributed in nature. Both *Conidiobolus* and *Basidiobolus* species are found in soil and decaying plant matter, and *Basidiobolus* spp. are also frequently isolated from insects and from the feces of amphibians and reptiles.[65] Cutaneous infection with *Basidiobolus* or *Conidiobolus* spp. likely occurs by percutaneous or submucosal inoculation of soil-borne spores through minor trauma or insect bites. Infection may also result from inhalation or ingestion of spores. Affected animals are typically immunocompetent. Zygomycosis caused by the Entomophthorales occurs most often in tropical and subtropical regions of the world, with most human cases reported from Africa and Asia.[65] In veterinary patients, basidiobolomycosis and conidiobolomycosis have been encountered throughout the southeastern United States, as well as eastern and northern coastal Australia.

Clinical Findings

Basidiobolomycosis

Basidiobolus ranarum infection in horses causes cutaneous and subcutaneous lesions that are grossly similar to those caused by pythiosis, but are most often found on the lateral aspects of the head, neck, chest, or trunk[21] (Fig. 55-4). This distribution may reflect a higher likelihood for these areas to come into contact with spore-containing soil or organic material when the animal lies on the ground.[67] Lesions are single, roughly circular, ulcerative, granulomatous masses with an edematous and hemorrhagic surface[68,69] (Fig. 55-5). As with pythiosis, these lesions are pruritic and often associated with self-trauma. Kunkers are often present but are smaller than those associated with pythiosis (usually <2 mm)[67] and lack the discrete, coral-like shape of *P. insidiosum* kunkers.[24]

Conidiobolomycosis

In horses, sheep, dogs, humans, and other mammalian species, conidiobolomycosis occurs most often as a nasopharyngeal infection with or without local dissemination into tissues of the face, retropharyngeal region, retrobulbar space, or cerebrum.[2,65,70-72] Infected equine patients typically exhibit multiple ulcerative granulomas or lobulated to pedunculated nodules involving the external nares, nasal cavity, or nasopharynx[21] (Fig. 55-6). Lesions may be either unilateral or bilateral and may extend into maxillary sinuses. Thickening of the nasal septum and narrowing of the nasal passages often lead to dyspnea and noisy respiration, and blood-tinged mucopurulent nasal discharge is a common historical finding. Exudate-containing kunkers may accumulate in the guttural pouches.[73] As with basidiobolomycosis, the kunkers associated with conidiobolomycosis are typically smaller than those associated with pythiosis and are of no particular shape. In an unusual presentation, a mare with harsh respiratory sounds and bilateral nasal discharge was found to have multiple tracheal granulomas caused by *Conidibolus coronatus* infection, but no lesions in the nasal passages.[74]

Mucormycosis

Absidia corymbifera has been described as a cause of mucormycosis in three horses. One of these horses presented with an extensive left forelimb lesion consisting of an ulcerative, granulomatous mass that contained draining tracts.[75] Culture of distilled water flushed through the draining tracts yielded *A. corymbifera*. Treatment with amphotericin B administered parenterally as well as topically was unsuccessful. In two other horses kept in the same paddock, *A. corymbifera* was diagnosed on the basis of IHC staining of tissues with a

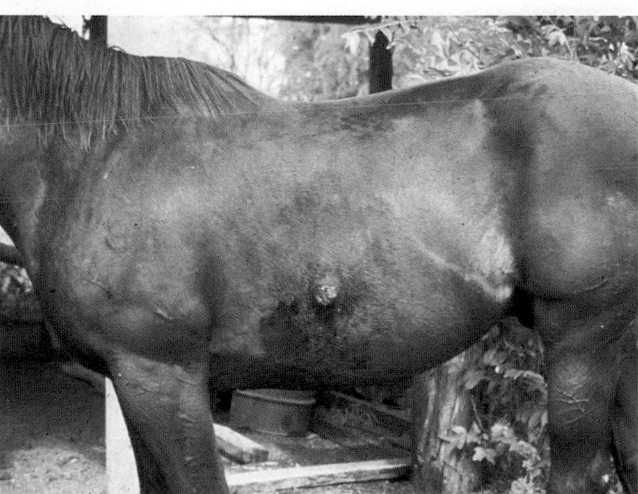

Fig. 55-4 Ulcerative cutaneous lesion on trunk of horse caused by *Basidiobolus ranarum* infection. (Courtesy Dr. Carol Foil, Louisiana State University.)

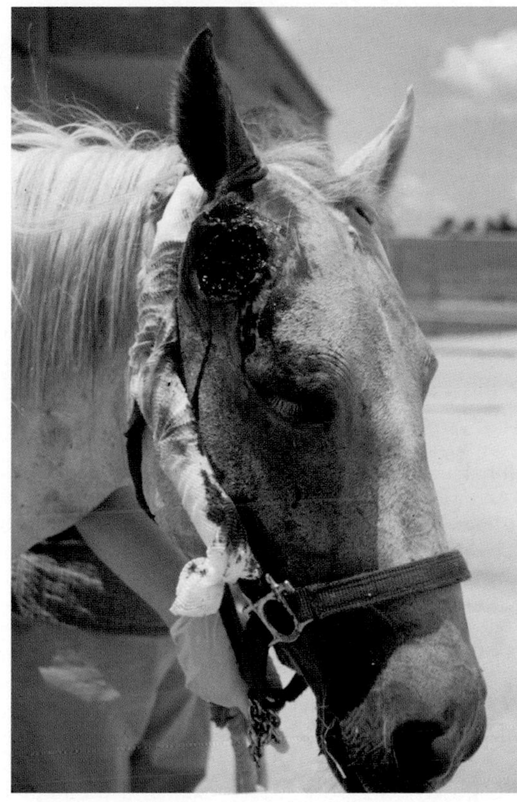

Fig. 55-5 Large, circular, ulcerative lesion caused by *Basidiobolus ranarum* infection on head of 19-year-old mare.

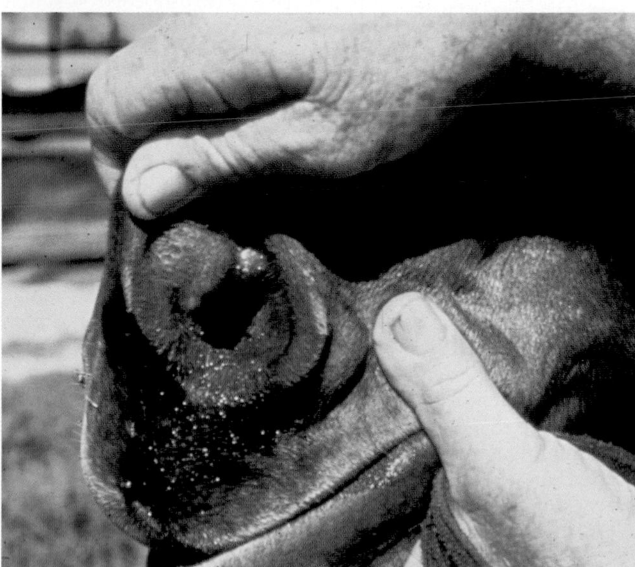

Fig. 55-6 Nasal polyp caused by conidiobolomycosis in a horse. (Courtesy Dr. Carol Foil, Louisiana State University.)

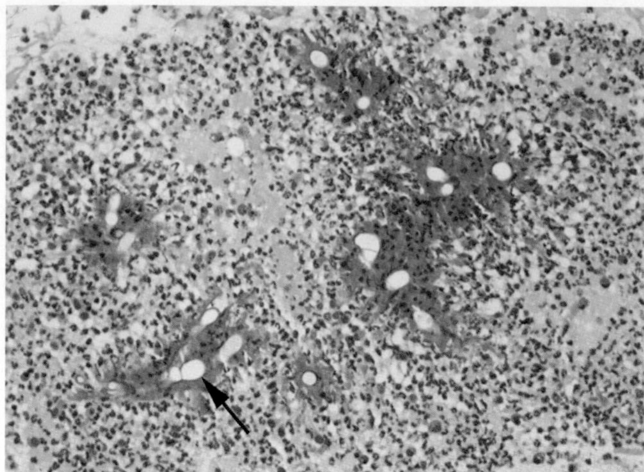

Fig. 55-7 Photomicrograph of tissue excised from basidiobolomycosis lesion shown in Figure 55-5. Note the presence of large, sometimes bulbous hyphae *(arrrow)* surrounded by a thick eosinophilic sleeve. (Hematoxylin and eosin stain; 20×.)

monoclonal antibody.[76] One of these horses had disseminated disease, with lesions in the stomach, intestine, lungs, and brain. In the second horse, only skin lesions were noted, characterized as large ulcers that initially developed as erythematous indurated areas, with subsequent central necrosis. Lesions were located on the muzzle, nostrils, lips, knees, and hocks.

Pathologic Findings

The histologic features of zygomycosis are similar to those associated with pythiosis.[24] Distinct eosinophilic and necrotic foci centered on hyphal structures and surrounded by pyogranulomatous and eosinophilic inflammation are typically observed (Fig. 55-7). Large, well-organized coagula of eosinophils and hyphae can be seen grossly as kunkers. Multinucleated giant cells, plasma cells, lymphocytes, and mast cells are common in the granulomatous tissue surrounding the eosinophilic foci. Lesions associated with mucormycosis are more likely to demonstrate vascular changes (e.g., thrombosis, vascular invasion by hyphae, infarction) than those associated with entomophthoromycosis.

On GMS-stained sections, hyphae appear broad, thin walled, and occasionally septate. The histologic hallmark of zygomycosis is the presence of a wide (2.5-25 μm) eosinophilic sleeve surrounding the hyphae and making them easily located on H&E-stained sections (Fig. 55-7). This finding helps to differentiate zygomycosis from pythiosis, in which eosinophilic sleeves tend to be thin or absent. In addition, the hyphal diameter tends to be significantly larger for *Basidiobolus* spp. (mean, 9 μm; range, 5-20 μm) and *Conidiobolus* spp. (mean, 8 μm; range, 5-13 μm) than for *P. insidiosum* (mean, 4 μm; range, 2-7 μm).[24]

Diagnosis

Because serologic and IHC techniques are not currently available for the diagnosis of zygomycosis in veterinary patients, a definitive diagnosis must be based on isolation and identification of the pathogen. The Entomophthorales fungi typically grow well on media routinely used for the isolation of pathogenic fungi, such as Sabouraud dextrose agar, potato flakes agar,[77] potato dextrose agar, and cornmeal agar. The author routinely uses potato flakes agar amended with ampicillin (100 μg/mL) and streptomycin (200 μg/mL) for initial isolation of *Conidiobolus* and *Basidiobolus* spp.

Identification of zygomycetes in the laboratory is generally based on morphologic characteristics of asexual reproductive structures (conidia) and sexual reproductive structures (zygospores).[78] *Conidiobolus* isolates on potato flakes agar or half-strength cornmeal agar readily produce primary conidia that are forcibly discharged and can be visualized on the underside of the Petri dish lid. Primary conidia of *Conidiobolus coronatus* are spherical, 40 μm in diameter, and have a prominent basal papilla. Because *C. coronatus* is a heterothallic species, zygospores are not observed in clinical isolates. *Conidiobolus incongruus*, however, is a homothallic species that produces large (15-25 μm), round, smooth, thick-walled zygospores without beaks. Reproductive structures of *B. ranarum* are readily produced after 3 to 5 days of incubation on half-strength cornmeal agar. Zygospores are easily identified as large (20-50 μm), thick-walled, round intercalary structures with beaklike protuberances that represent the remains of copulatory tubes. Primary conidia (often with a hyphal tag still attached), secondary conidia (morphologically similar to primary conidia but often smaller), and capilliconidia (oval to elongate spores with a terminal adhesive knob that develops at the end of a thin supporting hypha) may all be visualized on the inside of the Petri dish lid.

Therapy

Because it causes locally invasive lesions that rarely disseminate, the treatment of choice for cutaneous and subcutaneous zygomycosis is complete surgical resection of infected tissues. However, because lesion location and extent often preclude complete surgical excision, medical therapy with *potassium iodide* is often used either alone or in conjunction with surgical debulking of the lesion. Although the mechanism for the antifungal activity of iodides is unknown, they have been used with variable success for the treatment of both basidiobolomycosis[69] and conidiobolomycosis[70,74] in horses and have the advantage of relatively low expense. Iodides are typically administered orally as potassium iodide (10-40 mg/kg orally [PO] every 24 hours [q24h]) or organic iodide (1-2 mg/kg PO q24h). Parenteral sodium iodide (20% solution at 20-40 mg/kg intravenously q24h for 7-14 days) may be used in combination with oral iodide therapy for the first 1 to 2 weeks of treatment. Patients should be monitored for signs of iodide toxicity, which include excessive lacrimation, nonpruritic generalized alopecia with scaling, anorexia, depression, serous nasal discharge, cough, salivation, and nervousness.[79] If signs of iodism occur, medication should be stopped until signs resolve, then restarted at a lower dose. Administration of iodides to pregnant mares is not recommended.

Theoretically, as true fungi, zygomycetes should be more likely than *P. insidiosum* to respond to antifungal medications that target ergosterol, such as amphotericin B, itraconazole, ketoconazole, and fluconazole. *Amphotericin B* has been administered with variable response as an intralesional injection with DMSO or as part of a topically applied solution that also contains DMSO and ketoconazole.[1,80] McMullan et al.[31] reported resolution of suspected nonresectable nasal conidiobolomycosis after intralesional injection of amphotericin B (50 mg in 10 mL 5% dextrose administered four times at 5-day intervals) combined with topical application of amphotericin B in DMSO.

The use of oral *ketoconazole* to treat zygomycosis in horses has not been reported. However, because ketoconazole has poor absorption from the GI tract and may need to be administered by nasogastric tube,[81] its usefulness is limited. *Itraconazole* was used unsuccessfully at a dose of 3 mg/kg PO q12h to treat one horse with nonresectable nasal conidiobolomycosis.[82] Although the lesion showed a 50% reduction in size after 12 weeks of therapy, it relapsed 2 weeks after medication was discontinued, and the horse was euthanized. However, because serum levels of itraconazole were undetectable in this horse, treatment failure may have been partly caused by inadequate dosage.

Fluconazole is one of the few antifungal drugs for which detailed pharmacokinetic data are available for horses. Its bioavailability after oral dosing is high, and a long-term oral treatment protocol consisting of a loading dose of 14 mg/kg followed by 5 mg/kg q12h maintains plasma and body fluid concentrations greater than 8 μg/mL.[83] Fluconazole has been used successfully to treat nasal conidiobolomycosis in two mares in which pregnancy precluded the use of iodide therapy.[84] One mare received 2 mg/kg PO q12h for 8 weeks, and the other received a loading dose of 14 mg/kg PO followed by 5 mg/kg q12h for 6 weeks. Nasopharyngeal signs improved within 2 weeks of initiating treatment in both mares, and lesions were not detectable by endoscopic examination in either mare when treatment was discontinued. Unfortunately, long-term follow-up for potential recurrence of lesions after discontinuation of therapy was not reported.

Regardless of the choice of therapy, owners of horses with zygomycosis should be warned that the prognosis for response to therapy is guarded, and recurrence of lesions is common. Animals treated early in the course of disease are more likely to have a successful outcome. Therefore, pursuing appropriate diagnostic testing soon after lesions are detected is imperative.

REFERENCES

See the CD-ROM for a list of references linked to the abstract in PubMed.

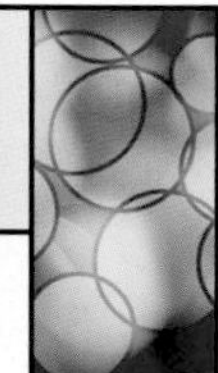

CHAPTER • 56

Aspergillosis

Catherine Kohn

Aspergillus species are among the most common fungal organisms. These saprophytes are widely distributed in the environment in soil, decaying vegetation, and organic debris. The members of this genus are opportunistic invaders of animal tissues, and healthy animals are resistant to infection unless exposed to a massive number of conidia or mycelia. Risk of disease caused by *Aspergillus* spp. is thought to be increased in immunodeficient horses and in horses with concurrent, severe enterocolitis or hematopoietic neoplasia. Transmission is usually by aerosol; guttural pouch mycosis and pulmonary disease are recognized manifestations of *Aspergillus* infection in horses. Pulmonary lesions are characteristically granulomatous. Keratomycosis caused by *Aspergillus* spp. is also common in horses.

ETIOLOGY

The classification and identification of *Aspergillus* species are based primarily on morphologic characteristics of the organism in culture. The genus *Aspergillus* is in the family *Trichocomaceae* of the order Eurotiales in the class Plectinomycetes of the phylum Ascomycota.[1] Fungi of the phylum Ascomycota are characterized by telomorphic (sexual) reproduction. Some textbooks[2] classify *Aspergillus* in the phylum Deuteromycota (fungi imperfecta), probably because this phylum contains anamorphic organisms, for which sexual reproduction has not been identified. The sexual state is found in very few species of *Aspergillus*, and the anamorphic (asexual) state is usually encountered in cultures from clinical patients.

Morphologic characteristics of *Aspergillus* spp. vary in culture. In general, *Aspergillus* spp. spread rapidly over the medium, forming a mycelium of flat to aerially branching and interlacing hyphae and conidiophores. The mycelium may be powdery white, greenish yellow, brown, or black.[1] The hyphae are nonpigmented and septate. Conidiophores (stalks) are characterized by a vesicle at the tip. The vesicle bears papillae (phialides) that give rise to unicellular conidia (cells produced by asexual reproduction) that are arranged in chains (Fig. 56-1). The characteristic shape of the conidiophore and spore heads is responsible for the name *Aspergillus*, which was conferred on the organism by an eighteenth-century priest who noted the resemblance of this pattern to that of

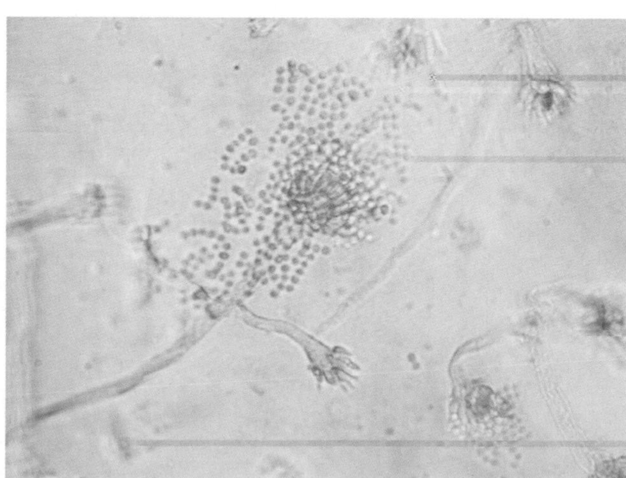

Fig. 56-1 Photomicrograph of *Aspergillus* conidiospores. (Courtesy Dr. Joseph Kowalski, The Ohio State University College of Veterinary Medicine.)

a holy water sprinkler ("Aspergillum").[1] Conidia may be colorless or darkly pigmented.

Approximately 180 species of *Aspergillus* are currently recognized, of which about 40 species have been identified in opportunistic infections of humans. Clinical studies of aspergillosis in horses usually report the presence of *Aspergillus* spp., and many do not identify the particular species involved. *Aspergillus fumigatus* is the most common species identified. *Aspergillus niger*[3,4] and *Aspergillus versicolor*[5] have also been reported to cause disease in horses. One case of keratomycosis caused by *Aspergillus oryzae* has been reported.[6] Mycotoxins produced by *Aspergillus flavus* cause equine aflatoxicosis.[7]

Virulence Factors

Because of their small size (2-3 μm in diameter), conidia of *Aspergillus* spp. remain in suspension in air for a long time, and these respirable particles can efficiently penetrate to the alveoli.[8] *Aspergillus* spp. are ubiquitous. The environment of the horse and particularly the "breathing zone" are almost continually rich in hyphae and conidia of *Aspergillus*, and people and horses constantly inhale fungal elements. In healthy horses and persons, fungi are cleared from the respiratory tract by pulmonary defense mechanisms (mucociliary clearance, phagocytosis by pulmonary macrophages). *Aspergillus* spp. are thermotolerant. The organisms thrive at 37° C (98.6° F), are able to grow at 55° C (131° F), and are reported to survive at temperatures up to 75° C (167° F).[9] These fungi are thus able to grow rapidly in body tissues of immunoincompetent hosts.

Aspergillus spp. survive in the bloodstream and tissues by being able to find and assimilate essential growth nutrients in these alien environments. The ability of these organisms to sense nitrogen sources in the environment and to regulate nitrogen utilization is essential to their survival.[10] Other fungal attributes that support the acquisition of essential nutrients include siderophores, phosphatases, and phospholipases. Fungal organisms require iron for growth, and blood is "fungistatic" because most iron is bound to transferrin.[9] *Aspergillus fumigatus* produces at least six siderophores that are able to remove iron from transferrin in vitro.[8,9] *A. fumigatus* has a high phosphate requirement. Phospholipases and phophatases allow the organism to recover phosphate from environments that are not phosphate rich, such as blood, and to utilize inorganic phosphates.

Aspergillus spp. may act as allergens. Allergic bronchopulmonary aspergillosis, allergic rhinosinusitis, asthma, and aspergilloma have been reported in immunocompetent human patients.[8] Inhalation challenge with extracts of *A. fumigatus* in horses with recurrent airway obstruction can induce signs of this disease.[11]

Gliatoxin and other toxins are putative virulence factors produced by *A. fumigatus*.[12] These factors may have direct toxic effects on tissues, and many are immunosuppressive.

A number of fungal characteristics assist *Aspergillus* spp. in evading host immune responses. Melanin pigment on the surface of conidia can neutralize reactive oxygen species and protect the organisms against attack by macrophages and neutrophils.[9] *Aspergillus* spp. have extensive antioxidant capabilities and many efflux pumps to facilitate export of toxins. Hydrophobins form part of the external layer of the cell wall of the conidia and may protect them from destruction by alveolar macrophages.[9] In vitro, conidia and hyphae may be phagocytosed by endothelial cells and tracheal or alveolar epithelial cells.[8] In theory, fungi sequestered in these cells could evade immune surveillance. Some investigators speculate that *Aspergillus* organisms may be able to "direct" their phagocytosis by these "nonprofessional" phagocytic cells during times of environmental stress.[8] This ability to invade endothelial and epithelial cells may be a mechanism that facilitates angioinvasion and thrombosis by *Aspergillus* spp. in vivo.[8]

EPIDEMIOLOGY

Aspergillus spp. are ubiquitous in the environment of horses, as previously discussed. In one study, 67.8% of the fungi recovered from air and surface samples taken in three stables in the winter were *Aspergillus* spp.[13] Fungal contamination can be reduced by management changes; more environmental fungi were recovered from stables with wooden stalls, dirt floors, and straw bedding than from hospital stalls with masonry walls, synthetic flooring, and bedding composed of wood shavings.[14] Not surprisingly, *Aspergillus* spp. may be encountered in the conjunctiva[15-18,20] (50% of 43 horses sampled in one study[19,20]) and in airway fluid samples obtained by transtracheal aspiration of healthy horses.[21] Conidia may be found free in the transtracheal wash fluid or within large mononuclear cells. *Aspergillus* can also be routinely cultured from the ingesta,[22] the skin, and the caudal reproductive tract, including the external genitalia.[23]

Universal exposure of horses to *Aspergillus* and other fungi confounds attempts to document that these agents are the cause of disease. It is important to demonstrate the presence of conidia or hyphae in diseased tissues to substantiate the diagnosis. Body fluid samples and culture plates may be easily contaminated with aspergilli or other fungi.

Mycotic Keratitis (Keratomycosis)

Aspergillus spp. are the most common cause of keratomycosis in horses. Case review studies have shown that this organism can be isolated from 33% to 77% of horses with keratomycosis[24-27] and 2% to 22% of eyes from horses with external eye disease.[17] *Fusarium* spp. are also encountered frequently (10 of 39 horses [26%] with keratomycosis in one study[28]), whereas *Alternaria, Cladosporium, Pseudallescheria, Geotrichum, Scedosporium* spp., *Stemphylium* spp., *Penicillium, Cylindrocarpon, Scytalidium*, and *Torulopsis* are infrequently reported.[25,28] Nonseptate filamentous fungi such as *Mucor* and yeasts such as *Candida* may also be associated with mycotic keratitis. The mycology of keratomycosis may vary with the geographic region. Mycotic keratitis is thought to be rare in the United Kingdom, although a recent report documented six cases (1998–2002).[29]

Although mycotic keratosis may occur more frequently during the summer and fall in some regions, cases are seen year-round in Florida, where the majority of cases are reported to occur October through January.[28] No apparent age, breed, or gender predisposition exists for mycotic keratitis.

Endometritis and Placentitis

The most common causes of mycotic endometritis are *Aspergillus* spp. and *Candida* spp.[23,30] Mycotic infections account for 1% to 5% of cases of endometritis in mares.

Aflatoxicosis

Aspergillus flavus and *A. parasiticus* produce toxic metabolites known as *aflatoxins*. Corn, peanuts, peanut meal, and cottonseed meal are the most frequently contaminated sources of aflatoxins. The toxins are also found in other nuts (pecans, walnuts, almonds, hazelnuts).[7] Ambient temperatures between 78° and 90° F (25.5°-32° C), drought stress, and high relative humidity or grain moisture favor production of aflatoxins.[31] Factors that reduce protection of the seed or damage the seed coat, such as shortened husks or insect damage, also enhance the risk of aflatoxin production.

PATHOGENESIS

The virulence of *Aspergillus* organisms is usually a function of the immune incompetence of the host, rather than the presence of specific virulence factors intrinsic to the fungus.[9] Because this fungus is ubiquitous, it is frequently inhaled, ingested, or contacted directly (e.g., corneal surface) by potential hosts. Those hosts with weakened innate or acquired immune responses are at risk for colonization by this opportunistic organism. Invasive aspergillosis has become an important disease in patients with acquired immunodeficiency syndrome (AIDS) and in other human patients who are severely granulocytopenic because of their disease or immunosuppressive treatment with anticancer drugs or corticosteroids. Invasive aspergillosis has been reported to occur in 70% of patients who remain granulocytopenic for 34 or more days.[32] A CD4 lymphocyte count less than 50 cells/mm^3 is a risk factor for invasive aspergillosis in AIDS patients.[32] Leukopenia and neutropenia are often associated with enterocolitis and typhlitis in horses.

In horses, immune incompetence is assumed to be an important risk factor for invasive aspergillosis, an otherwise uncommon disease. Pulmonary aspergillosis has been reported in a horse treated for ill thrift and intestinal malabsorption with corticosteroids[22] and in another with dysfunction of the pars intermedia of the pituitary.[33] Hyperadrenocorticism in horses with hyperplasia of the pars intermedia may be immune suppressive.[34] Invasive aspergillosis has been reported in four horses with hemolymphatic neoplasia (three with myelomonocytic leukemia and one with disseminated hemangiosarcoma).[22,35,36] Several investigators have noted an association between invasive aspergillosis and antecedent enterocolitis.[4,22,34,37-39] In one study, pulmonary aspergillosis developed in a mean of 11 days after enterocolitis in 16 horses (14 with salmonellosis).[22] In another study, 25 of 29 horses with pulmonary aspergillosis had evidence of primary or secondary disease that caused loss of the integrity of the bowel wall; 12 of these horses were leukopenic.[34] Loss of integrity of the bowel mucosa likely provided a portal for absorption of fungi from the bowel lumen, allowing embolic spread of the organisms to other organs, particularly the lungs, but also kidney and brain.[4,40] Broad-spectrum antibiotic therapy may contribute to the problem by destroying symbiotic bacteria that balance the gastrointestinal flora, preventing growth of potential pathogens.

Aspergillosis is occasionally reported in immunocompetent horses.[3,41,42] Fatal pneumonia caused by *Aspergillus niger* and *Rhizopus stolonifer* was diagnosed in two young horses recently moved to an unused, unclean stable.[3] The organisms were recovered from the lungs of affected horses and from the stable bedding. A third case of fatal invasive pulmonary aspergillosis was reported in an immunocompetent horse housed in a bank barn.[41] These authors hypothesize that affected horses were exposed to overwhelmingly large aerosol doses of fungi. *Aspergillus* spp. were isolated from a large, well-encapsulated mediastinal mass at the base of the heart in an otherwise healthy horse.[42]

Antigens of *Aspergillus fumigatus* have been implicated in the pathogenesis of recurrent airway obstruction (RAO) in horses. Inhalation challenge with an extract of *A. fumigatus* induced increased pulmonary resistance in horses with RAO[43] and caused signs of airway obstruction in RAO-affected horses in remission, but not in healthy control horses.[11] Serum allergen-specific immunoglobulin E (IgE) concentrations suggest that horses with RAO are more often sensitized to some allergens associated with *A. fumigatus* than are healthy control horses.[44] In addition, bronchoalveolar lavage fluid concentrations of IgE and IgG directed against antigens of *A. fumigatus* were greater in RAO-affected horses than in control horses,[45] and extracts or whole preparations of *A. fumigatus* induced greater in vitro histamine release from degranulating mast cells of RAO-affected horses than from healthy horses.[46] RAO has been extensively reviewed elsewhere.[47,48]

Keratomycosis

Aspergillus spp. are destructive pathogens in the eye. The propensity for horses to develop mycotic keratitis may be related to the fact that *Aspergillus* spp. and other fungi are usually among the commensal conjunctival flora, and horses are constantly exposed to fungi in fodder, bedding, and stable dust. A warm, humid environment (e.g., heated barn, ambient conditions) may predispose horses to fungal keratitis. Frequent treatment of bacterial keratitis with topical antibiotics may reduce the numbers of nonpathogenic bacteria while favoring multiplication of pathogenic bacteria and fungi.[15,49] The use of ophthalmic antibiotics is associated with a shift in the population of ocular flora from predominantly gram positive to gram negative.[50] Commensal flora of healthy eyes may produce antimicrobial substances that limit the population of pathogenic organisms.[14,15,49] For example, *Streptomyces natalensis*, a conjunctival commensal organism in healthy horses, produces the antifungal natamycin.[14,51] In one study, affected eyes of 32 of 39 horses with fungal keratitis (82%) were treated intensively with topical ophthalmic antibiotics before entry into the study, suggesting that this treatment may have been a risk factor for developing keratomycosis.[26]

Topical corticosteroids may enhance fungal replication and reduce corneal tissue resistance to fungal invasion, resulting in enhanced penetration of the cornea.[25,52] However, Andrew et al.[26] documented prior treatment with topical corticosteroids in only 6 of 39 horses with keratomycosis, whereas 5 of 23 affected horses had prior treatment with topical corticosteroids in another study.[53] These findings collectively suggest that, although treatment with corticosteroids increases the risk of keratomycosis, other factors are likely important in the pathogenesis.

The equine eye is prominent, and the cornea has a large surface area, putting this structure at risk for trauma. Any epithelial defect can provide entry for fungi into the deeper layers of the cornea, or penetrating trauma may seed deeper layers of the cornea with fungi. Fungal replication and dead fungal hyphae induce a severe polymorphonuclear neutrophil (PMN, leukocyte) inflammatory reaction. Local release of proteases from fungi, leukocytes, and keratocytes destroys stroma.[26,51,54] Once established in the corneal stroma, fungi tend to burrow toward Descemet's membrane, where they are poorly responsive to medical treatment.[51] Corneal avascularity and the absence of corneal lymphatics may slow the response to deep infection. Healing depends on neovascularization arising from the limbus. Stromal abscesses may result from penetrating corneal wounds that seed the deeper corneal tissues, although other factors may be important, particularly where clusters of cases are identified.[51] A breach in Descemet's membrane by a penetrating wound or fungal-induced inflammation may allow *Aspergillus* organisms access to the anterior chamber, resulting in endophthalmitis.

Deficiencies in the immunoprotective qualities of tear film and the cornea in some horses may predispose them to keratomycosis.[28] Gliatoxin and other putative fungal virulence factors may inhibit corneal vascularization, reduce PMN cell infiltration, suppress cell-mediated phagocytosis, reduce cytolytic T-cell proliferation and activation, and decrease leukocytic antifungal proteinase activity.[51] *Aspergillus* and *Fusarium* isolates from equine patients with keratomycosis inhibited angiogenesis in an in vitro model where fungi inhibited differentiation of capillary-like tubules from human umbilical vein endothelial cells.[55] Corneal healing in horses depends on neovascularization by endothelial budding and subsequent corneal invasion of limbal vessels. Inhibition of this process could impair corneal healing.

Endometritis and Placentitis

Common factors that increase uterine exposure to the ubiquitous aspergilli include frequent uterine lavage (which may introduce fungal organisms), poor vaginal conformation, pneumonvagina, cervical adhesions, and urine pooling (see Chapter 8). Increased exposure to *Aspergillus* organisms increases the risk of infection.

Aflatoxicosis

Of the four types of aflatoxins, B_1 is the most abundant.[31] Aflatoxins are metabolized in the liver by mixed-function oxidases. One of the metabolites is a highly reactive oxide that binds with deoxyribonucleic acid (DNA), messenger ribonucleic acid (mRNA), and proteins, impairing protein synthesis and inducing cancer in some species.[31] Impaired protein synthesis results in necrosis, particularly in the liver, and improper antibody formation. Acute intoxication with large doses of aflatoxin leads to liver damage and death. Chronic exposure to sublethal doses may be asymptomatic in horses or may induce immune suppression and ill thrift with poor feed conversion.[56] Cumulative exposure increases the risk of liver and lung cancer in humans.[56] Dietary deficiencies in protein, selenium, and vitamin E increase susceptibility to aflatoxicosis.[31]

CLINICAL FINDINGS

Despite *Aspergillus* spp. being opportunistic organisms, they have been reported to cause a diverse array of clinical disease in horses, including keratomycosis, nasal plaques, guttural pouch mycosis, RAO, pneumonia, pulmonary or mediastinal masses, placentitis, endometritis, endocarditis, vasculitis and cerebral infarction, and aflatoxicosis.

Mycotic Keratitis

Aspergillus spp. may colonize corneal erosions, producing lesions ranging from superficial abrasions with associated pain, miosis, blepharospasm, epiphora, and photophobia[54,57,58] to severe interstitial keratitis of varying depths.[57] These lesions usually develop rapidly, although indolent infections may occur.[59] Focal or diffuse corneal opacity and edema may be present (Fig. 56-2). Ulcers may appear raised and are often characterized by roughened borders, with surrounding radiating lines of leukocyte infiltration.[59] As fungi proliferate, dry, white to grayish, fluffy lesions may be observed, and the corneal surface may appear slightly green.[59] As the fungi invade the corneal stroma, neovascularization, microabscesses, and stromal malacia may be observed. Secondary anterior uveitis with aqueous flare will ensue, and corneal rupture and endophthalmitis may be sequelae.[59] Reliable signs that indicate healing of mycotic keratitis include clearing of the corneal edema, progressing from the periphery toward the lesion, in association with abundant, deep stromal vascularization that extends to the margin of the opacified stroma.[24] As the stromal opacification decreases in size, it may become more dense because of fibrosis.

Corneal stromal abscesses are characterized by a yellow-white opacity deep to intact (non–fluorescein-staining) corneal epithelium or a relatively small corneal defect[51,58] (Fig. 56-3). Satellite lesions are often observed, and associated corneal edema may be prominent.

Mycotic keratitis should be suspected in corneal lesions that respond poorly or worsen during antibiotic therapy and in those that show improvement followed by deterioration when treated with topical corticosteroids.[60] Differential diagnoses include bacterial keratitis (especially caused by *Pseudomonas* spp. and β-hemolytic streptococci), equine recurrent uveitis, bacterial stromal abscesses, viral keratitis, corneal dystrophies or degeneration, and indolent ulcers.[59]

Pulmonary Aspergillosis

In the early stages of infection, clinical signs of respiratory disease may be absent or mild.[40] Advanced or extensive pulmonary disease may be associated with nasal discharge, nasal plaques, abnormal breath sounds (crackles, wheezes, pleural friction rubs), tachypnea, dyspnea, and pleural hemorrhage.[34,40] A history of vague respiratory signs that respond poorly to antibiotic therapy should suggest the possibility of fungal infection. In one retrospective study, 4 of 29 horses with pulmonary aspergillosis had a history of intermittent treatment with moderate doses of corticosteroids, and 23 of 29 (79%) had been previously treated with antibiotics.[34]

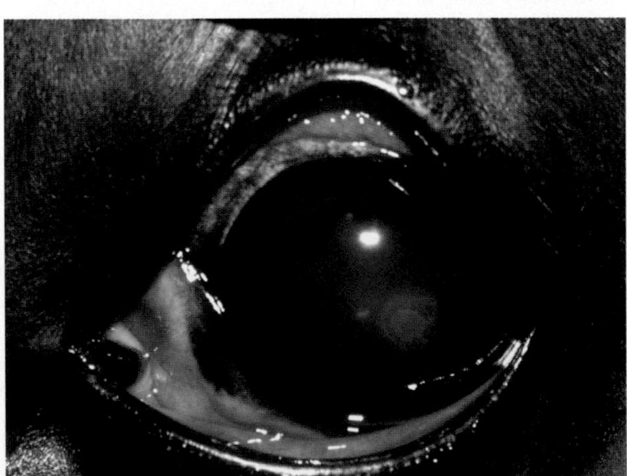

Fig. 56-2 Keratomycosis in a horse. (Courtesy Dr. Anne Metzler, The Ohio State University College of Veterinary Medicine.)

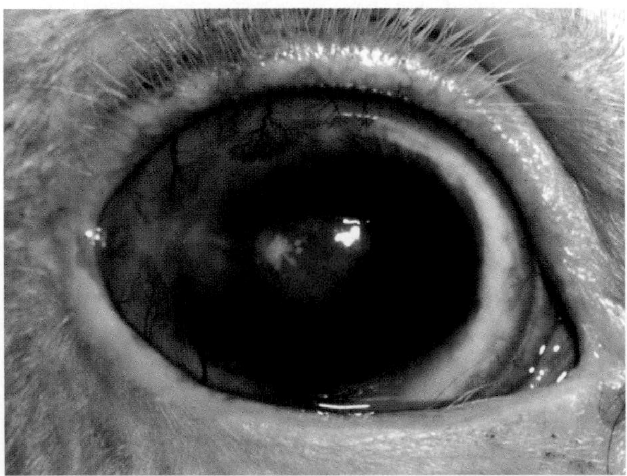

Fig. 56-3 Mycotic stromal abscess in a horse. (Courtesy Dr. Anne Metzler, The Ohio State University College of Veterinary Medicine.)

Nasal or Sinus Aspergillosis

Mycotic plaques caused by *Aspergillus* spp. may occasionally occur on the mucosa of the nasal passages in the absence of *Aspergillus* infection elsewhere, or these plaques may be present in horses with concurrent pulmonary aspergillosis. Three horses with unilateral aspergillosis of the middle meatus had unilateral, foul-smelling nasal discharge and intermittent epistaxis, and two of three had submandibular lymphadenopathy.[61] Affected horses may have multiple mycotic plaques, and nasal discharge may be continuous or intermittent. In a retrospective and prospective study of 277 cases of sinonasal disease, 13 horses had intranasal mycotic lesions, mycotic sinusitis, or mycotic lesions at the sinonasal ostium.[62] Most of these lesions were caused by *Aspergillus fumigatus*. Lesions of the nostrils were often ulcerative granulomas.[63] An ulcerated mycetoma at the commissure of the upper lip of one horse was caused by infection with *Aspergillus versicolor* that extended through to the buccal mucosa.[5]

Central Nervous System Aspergillosis

Aspergillus niger caused necrotizing vasculitis with cerebral infarction in an 18-year-old Morgan mare with a 10-day history of diarrhea.[4] The mare was depressed, incoordinated, and dysphagic and died after 4 days of treatment with fluids and trimethoprim-sulfamethoxazole and pyrimethamine.

Endometritis and Placentitis

Mares with fungal endometritis typically have a white to gray vaginal discharge. The uterus contains variable amounts of fluid that may induce distention and flaccidity.[23,64] *Aspergillus* has also been reported to cause severe focal placentitis, resulting in abortion.[65]

Aflatoxicosis

Ingestion of aflatoxin (500-1000 parts per billion [ppb]) by mature horses decreased feed intake, with resultant weight loss and induced liver damage.[7] In other horses, ingestion of feed containing 900 ppb or more than 6500 ppb of aflatoxin caused death, with brain, liver, kidney, and heart damage in affected horses.[7] Aflatoxins, fed at doses greater than 2 mg/kg, were uniformly fatal in weanling ponies.[66] Aflatoxin B_1 was found at a concentration of 114 μg/kg in corn fed to horses that died (three) or became ill.[67] Chronically affected horses show a spectrum of clinical signs, including weight loss, behavioral changes (somnolence, yawning, aggression, head pressing, circling, blindness) associated with liver impairment, or death.[7]

DIAGNOSIS

The diagnosis of aspergillosis must be based on identification of the organism in tissue, such as the cornea. The organism grows well on most commercially available fungal culture media.[2] Isolation of fungi from the conjunctiva, proximal airway, or other tissues that could collect environmental contaminants is not sufficient to establish a definitive diagnosis. Culture as well as cytologic evaluation of infected tissue or exudates should be attempted. Specimens should be obtained from several areas of the lesion, including deeper tissues, to maximize the possibility of finding fungal organisms if they are present.

Serology

Attempts to diagnose invasive aspergillosis based on serology have been unrewarding. Anti-*Aspergillus* antibodies can be detected in healthy as well as diseased horses, likely because of constant environmental exposure to these fungi.[34,42] Counter immunoelectrophoresis and enzyme-linked immunosorbent assay (ELISA) using complex antigenic mixtures did not discriminate between healthy and diseased horses.[68] However, immunoblotting analysis based on reactivity to low-molecular-mass antigens, was positive in diseased horses but not in healthy horses of the same study. This assay is not commercially available.

Real-Time Quantitative Polymerase Chain Reaction

A recently developed, real-time (RT) quantitative polymerase chain reaction (PCR) test evaluates the number of copies of DNA from fungi in corneal tissues of horses with mycotic keratitis.[69] Horses with confirmed fungal disease had a significantly greater number of copies of fungal DNA than horses with healthy eyes. Four of five horses with fungal keratitis had more than 1000 copies/25 ng of DNA, whereas healthy horses had 5 to 321 copies/25ng of DNA in their corneal tissue.[69] This assay is commercially available at the author's institution. This approach to diagnosis holds promise for quantifying fungal load and may prove useful to monitor response to therapy.

Culture

Confirmation of identification of the genus and species of the fungus requires culture of tissue or fluid samples. *Aspergillus* spp. will grow readily on most fungal media.[2] Although cultures may be positive in as little as 3 days, an average of 25 days was required to identify the isolates in one study.[70] It is not practical to wait for culture results before beginning treatment.

Susceptibility Testing

Antifungal susceptibility testing (measuring the inhibitory activity of the tested antimicrobial agent) and correlations between in vitro susceptibility and clinical outcome of invasive fungal diseases in human patients have been the subject of intensive research.[70] Many factors other than susceptibility of the etiologic agent to the chosen drug affect clinical outcome, including host immune status, location of the infection, duration of the infection, drug pharmacokinetics, and patient compliance.[71] Standardized methods of assessment of in vitro susceptibility of yeasts and filamentous fungi to some common antifungal drugs have been developed.[72] Tentative "breakpoints" for fluconazole, itraconazole, and 5-fluorocytosine against *Candida* spp. have been established, and breakpoint values for fluconazole and flucytosine are useful in predicting clinical outcome.[72] Meaningful correlations between in vitro susceptibility test results and clinical outcome for most filamentous fungi and yeasts have not been established.[71-74]

Current recommendations to physicians managing patients with fungal diseases are to (1) identify a fungal isolate at the genus and species level if possible; (2) perform in vitro susceptibility testing (using approved methods) only for fluconazole and flucytosine susceptibility of *Candida* isolates from sterile sites; (3) attempt susceptibility testing for *Candida* spp. and amphotericin B; *Cryptococcus neoformans* and fluconazole, flucytosine, or amphotericin B; and *Histoplasma capsulatum* and fluconazole for patients in whom initial antifungal therapy has failed; and (4) select therapy for all other fungal isolates based on guidelines or survey data.[72,75]

Antifungal sensitivity testing is difficult to obtain in the veterinary clinical setting,[20] and results of in vitro susceptibility testing often do not correlate well with clinical response to treatment.[28] In particular, fluconazole may demonstrate low activity with in vitro test systems, but high activity in vivo, possibly due in part to the drug's excellent tissue solubility.[76]

Troke et al.[77] demonstrated that fluconazole was 15-fold more potent than ketoconazole in a model of vaginal candidiasis in mice, despite being 80-fold less active in vitro. The value of in vitro antifungal susceptibility testing in veterinary medicine is unproven.

Currently, determination of fungicidal activities of antimicrobial agents against yeasts and molds holds promise for the development of clinically relevant correlates of in vitro susceptibility. In vitro studies employing minimum fungicidal concentration (best assessed in animal models) or "time-kill" methods (ability of antimicrobial agent to kill fungal isolate over time) have predicted in vivo response.[78] To date, these methods have not yet been standardized, and their use in the veterinary setting has not been explored.

Biopsy

Aspergillus organism are readily identifiable in infected tissues. Typical hyphae in tissue are 2-5 μm in diameter and branch dichotomously at 45-degree angles (Fig. 56-4). Hematoxylin and eosin (H&E) stain will identify the hyphae, although periodic acid–Schiff (PAS) and silver stains, such as Gomori's methenamine silver (GMS), are reported to be particularly useful in demonstrating the organisms.[23,40]

Immunohistochemical Techniques

Immunofluorescent techniques using genus-specific conjugates have been described to identify *Aspergillus* spp. in tissues.[40] These techniques do not allow speciation. A three-layer indirect enzyme immunohistochemical technique uses polyclonal rabbit antibodies raised against somatic antigens of *A. fumigatus*, *A. flavus*, and *A. niger* in a peroxidase-antiperoxidase system.[4] This latter technique distinguished *A. niger* in brain tissue of an affected horse.

Mycotic Keratitis

Cytologic Examination

Identification of fungal hyphae in corneal scrapings is considered diagnostic (Fig. 56-5). In one study, 86% of 36 corneal scrapings from horses with keratomycosis were positive for fungal hyphae.[70] If the cornea has reepithelialized, deeper scrapings must be carefully obtained because fungi tend to invade deeply, and examination of scrapings of superficial layers of the cornea may yield false-negative results. Histology of corneal tissue obtained by keratectomy may be helpful in establishing a diagnosis.

Culture

Brooks et al.[28] found that 84.6% of 39 horses with keratomycosis had positive cultures. From 30% to 50% of horses with keratomycosis are reported to have concurrent bacterial keratitis. In healthy equine eyes, gram-positive cocci and rods predominate on the conjunctiva, although gram-negative organisms may be present.[58] In one study, 90% of bacterial isolates from horses with keratomycosis were gram-positive organisms,[70] whereas a second study showed gram-positive organisms in 5% to 45% of isolates and gram-negative organisms in 2% to 45% of isolates from affected eyes.[58] Topical antibiotic treatment induces a shift from a predominance of gram-positive to an increasing proportion of gram-negative organisms.[27] Antimicrobial sensitivity patterns of bacterial agents may change during treatment, and secondary cultures may be necessary to guide adjustment of therapy.[27]

Corneal Biopsy and Staining

Examination of corneal biopsies was diagnostic in all six horses with keratomycosis in one study.[28] Histopathologic examination revealed edema, loss of epithelialization, necrosis of the corneal collagen, interstitial keratitis, and fungal organisms that tended to penetrate toward Descemet's membrane.[70]

Multifocal punctate corneal erosions may be caused by *Aspergillus* spp. but may be mistaken for viral lesions. Fungal microerosions may not take up fluorescein stain but will be visible with rose bengal staining.[79]

Pulmonary Aspergillosis

Antemortem diagnosis of pulmonary aspergillosis may be difficult. In one study, of 29 horses subsequently shown to have pulmonary aspergillosis at necropsy, only one horse was diagnosed antemortem.[34] Pulmonary ultrasonography and radiography may be useful. Radiographs may demonstrate a diffuse interstitial and peribronchiolar pattern,[39] and ultrasonography may reveal a pleural effusion. The presence of many characteristic fungal hyphae in fluids obtained by transtracheal aspiration, bronchoalveolar lavage, or thoracocentesis supports the diagnosis of pulmonary aspergillosis. Positive cultures of these fluids also support the diagnosis, particularly

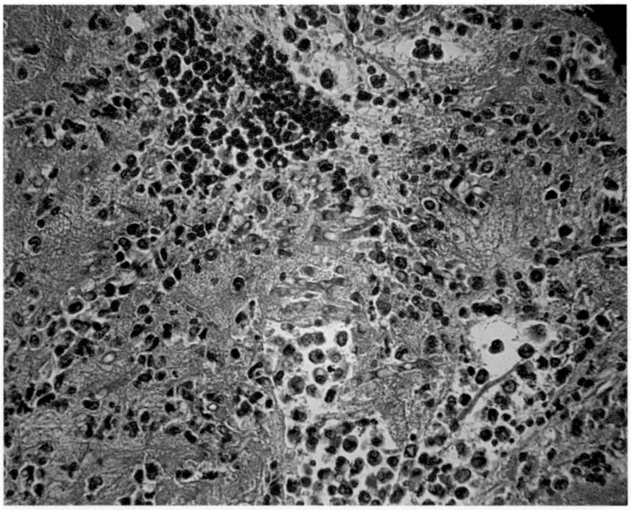

Fig. 56-4 Photomicrograph of branching hyphae of *Aspergillus* in kidney of horse with disseminated aspergillosis and hemolytic anemia.

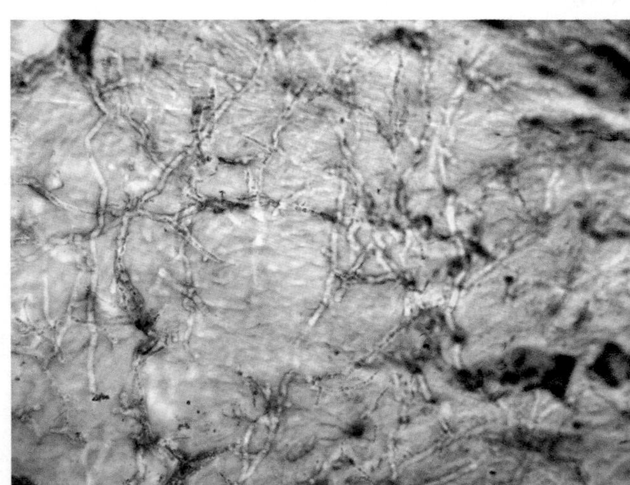

Fig. 56-5 Fungal hyphae in corneal scraping from equine eye. (Courtesy Dr. Anne Metzler, The Ohio State University College of Veterinary Medicine.)

when positive results are obtained on several occasions or when growth is rapid and exuberant and the predominant or only organism present is *Aspergillus*. Nevertheless, because healthy horses may harbor *Aspergillus* organisms in the airways, results of cytologic examination and culture of airway fluids should be corroborated by positive cultures of affected tissues. Lung biopsy may provide tissue for culture.

At necropsy, pulmonary pathology is characterized by fibrinonecrotic, hemorrhagic pneumonia with congestion or edema. Lesions are often found around large blood vessels. In more chronic cases a miliary distribution of nodules (granulomas) and fibrosis may be identified.[34,39,40] Histologically, multiple, septate, branching hyphae are found in pulmonary lesions (Fig. 56-6). *Aspergillus* organisms are angioinvasive, with hyphae possibly found radiating from the center of blood vessels,[34] and are associated with extensive vasculitis and thrombosis.[3,4]

Nasal and Sinus Aspergillosis

Endoscopy usually provides the diagnosis, although in some horses, endoscopy with the patient under anesthesia may be required to see the lesion. Radiographs of the skull and surgical exploration of the affected sinus are useful in defining the extent of nasal or sinus aspergillosis. Disease caused by plaques of *Aspergillus* spp. in the guttural pouch is described in Chapter 1.

Central Nervous System Aspergillosis

The diagnosis of central nervous system (CNS) aspergillosis is often made at necropsy. In one case report the horse's right cerebral cortex had a malacic focus 2.5 cm in diameter, with extensive hemorrhage predominantly involving gray matter.[4] Histologically, the lesion was characterized by fibrinoid necrotizing vasculitis and thrombosis with many fungal hyphae. The cecum and large colon showed large foci of severe necrosis and hemorrhage. No fungal hyphae were found in the bowel tissues; however, systemic infection likely resulted from translocation of fungi from the bowel lumen. Acute focal coagulation necrosis of the cortical white matter with hemorrhage and intralesional aspergillus hyphae were observed in a 4-month-old Morgan colt with a 1-week history of hypoproteinemia and hemolytic anemia (Fig. 56-7).

Endometritis and Placentitis

Aspergillus organisms can be identified by cytologic evaluation of uterine fluid obtained with guarded culture swab, in cultures of uterine fluid, and in appropriately stained biopsy tissue from the uterus or placenta. An accompanying inflammatory response should also be identified.

Aflatoxicosis

Clinical signs and associated serum chemistry abnormalities consistent with liver disease (increased hepatic enzyme activities and concentrations of bile acids and ammonia) suggest the possibility of aflatoxicosis. Feed should be tested to confirm the presence of aflatoxins. Aflatoxins exhibit bright–greenish yellow fluorescence, best observed in damaged grain under ultraviolet light. Thin-layer chromatography, among other techniques, can be used to identify the aflatoxin.[31]

At necropsy, acute aflatoxicosis is characterized by centrilobular hepatic necrosis and hemorrhage with ascites. In subacute cases, hepatic lipidosis may be present. Histologic abnormalities of the liver include hepatocyte degeneration and necrosis, lipidosis, bile duct proliferation, and fibrosis.[31]

THERAPY

Except for dermatomycosis and mycotic keratitis, fungal diseases in horses are relatively uncommon. Chemical, biochemical, and pharmacologic aspects as well as practical uses of antifungal agents for treating animals have been recently reviewed.[80-82] Studies of the pharmacokinetics of antifungal agents in horses are limited, and meaningful studies of treatment and outcome are lacking. The choice of a drug for treating fungal diseases in horses is largely guided by personal opinion informed by anecdotal accounts reported in the literature regarding treatment of a small number of equine patients and inferred from the literature concerning fungal diseases of humans. Fungal diseases have become increasingly common in human patients with cancer or AIDS, and the literature pertaining to treating mycoses in human patients is vast.

The systemic antifungal drugs most often used in horses include the polyene agent amphotericin B and the azole agents: the imidazole derivatives miconazole, enilconazole,

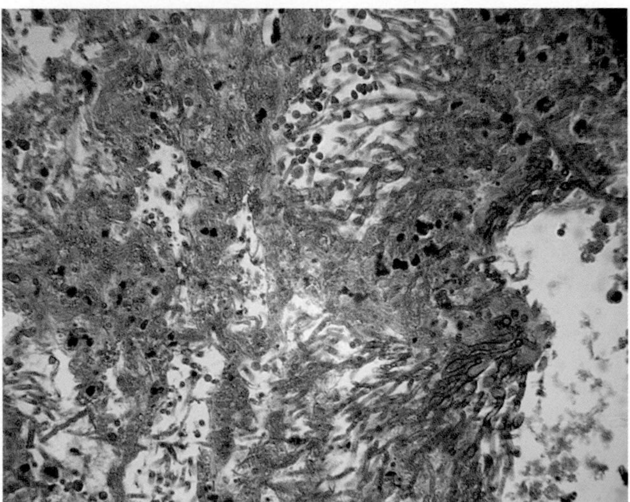

Fig. 56-6 Photomicrograph of branching *Aspergillus* hyphae in a radiating pattern typical of invasive aspergillosis in lung of horse with large-colon volvulus, diarrhea, and *Aspergillus* pneumonia.

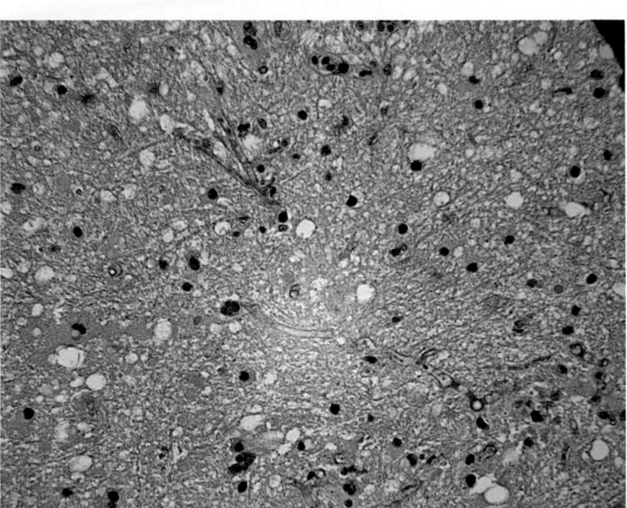

Fig. 56-7 Photomicrograph of *Aspergillus* hyphae in brain of 4-month-old Morgan colt with ileus, hypoproteinemia, hemolytic anemia, and focal necrosis of cortical white matter.

and ketoconazole and the triazole agents itraconazole and fluconazole. Dosage recommendations for systemic therapy in horses vary (Table 56-1), based on empiric experience, limited pharmacokinetic data, or extrapolation from recommendations for treating humans. Recommendations for ophthalmic therapy are discussed separately (Table 56-2).

Polyene Antifungal Drugs

Amphotericin B (AMB) is a product of the soil actinomycete *Streptomyces nodosus*. The drug is insoluble in water, is poorly absorbed after oral administration, and is administered intravenously (IV) or topically. AMB exerts its antifungal effect by binding to ergosterol in the fungal cell wall. Ergosterol is not a component of mammalian cells. Binding results in increased porosity of the fungal cell membrane, resulting in loss of essential intracellular substances and eventually cell death.[83] Reactive forms of oxygen also play a part in the lethal or cellulytic action of AMB.[80] One mechanism proposed is the autooxidation of AMB, resulting in the formation of free radicals.[84,84a] The spectrum of action of AMB is reported to include *Histoplasma capsulatum, Blastomyces dermatitidis, Cryptococcus neoformans, Candida* spp., *Aspergillus fumigatus*, and *Aspergillus flavus*.[85] Fungicidal or fungistatic activity depends on the concentration of the drug at the site of infection.[80] There are reports of successful use of AMB to treat systemic candidiasis in foals,[85] candidal arthritis,[86] fungal pneumonia,[87] phycomycosis,[88-90] pulmonary cryptococcosis,[91] and pulmonary histoplasmosis.[92] Long-term treatment with AMB failed to cure one horse with cryptococcal meningitis.[93]

Resistance to AMB among fungal isolates from animals and humans is relatively rare.[94] Some intrinsic resistance is observed among *Pseudallescheria boydii* and many *Aspergillus* spp.[80] The nephrotoxicity of this drug has limited its systemic use in horses. Adverse reactions reported in horses treated with AMB include depression, fever, lethargy, restlessness, tachycardia, tachypnea, polyuria, anorexia, collapse, phlebitis, weight loss, anemia, and uremia.[95]

Lipid-encapsulated formulations of AMB have been developed to reduce the drug's toxicity in human patients. In the clinical setting, these formulations are at least as effective as the deoxycholate conjugate of AMB.[96] Lipid-encapsulated AMB has not been evaluated in horses, and the expense will likely preclude its use, except possibly in foals. Of more practical interest are recent studies demonstrating that mild heating of AMB (70° C [158° F] for 20 minutes) reduces the toxicity of the drug to human and pig cells in vitro and to mice in vivo.[97-99] Reduced toxicity resulted in a larger therapeutic index for AMB, allowing administration of a higher dose of the drug to experimental mice with cryptococcal or candidal infections. Reduced toxicity was not associated with a reduced effectiveness of heat-treated AMB in prolonging survival of mice with experimental cryptococcosis or candidiasis.[98]

Azole Antifungal Drugs

The azole antifungal drugs act by reducing ergosterol biosynthesis. Drugs of this class variably inhibit mammalian oxidative drug-metabolizing enzymes, and therefore the metabolism of concurrently administered drugs may be affected.[100] The imidazoles have a higher affinity for mammalian cytochrome P-450 enzymes than the triazoles.[100] Drug interactions with H_2 blockers, proton pump inhibitors, phenytoin, rifampin,[101] and sulfamethoxazole[80] have been described in humans. The azoles also variably reduce gonadal and adrenal steroidogenesis.[95] This effect is most prominent for the imidazole derivatives miconazole, enilconazole, and ketoconazole, particularly miconazole, and is negligible for the triazole fluconazole. All the azole drugs except fluconazole are immunosuppressive in people, especially with respect to lymphocyte function.[102] This attribute may reduce the host inflammatory response to fungi but may also limit the efficacy of these antifungal drugs. Antifungal drugs should be used only when evidence of fungal infection is strong.[51] This issue has not been studied in horses.

In general, the azoles are active against *Candida albicans, Cryptococcus neoformans, Blastomyces dermatitidis, Histoplasma capsulatum, Coccidioides immitis*, and dermatophytes.[95] *Aspergillus* spp. are often less susceptible to ketoconazole.[95]

Miconazole (MICON) is poorly soluble in water. Oral MICON has poor bioavailability, and the topical form does not penetrate tissues well.[80] Poor bioavailability and an anecdotal report of anaphylactic reactions after systemic administration[51] limit MICON to topical use in horses. MICON is reported to be fungistatic for *Aspergillus* and the mycelial phase of *H. capsulatum*.[80] One horse with nasal plaques caused by *Pseudallescheria boydii* was successfully treated with MICON.[103]

Topical *enilconazole* (ENIL) was used successfully to treat a case of guttural pouch mycosis caused by *Aspergillus* spp. When nebulized, ENIL, in combination with oral ketoconazole, was successful in the treatment of a horse with *Scopulariopsis* pneumonia.[104]

Ketoconazole (KETO) is a lipophilic imidazole derivative. Systemic absorption is reported to be poor in horses after oral administration of 30 mg/kg every 24 hours (q24h) (serum concentrations of the drug were undetectable).[105] Oral absorption of KETO depends on gastric acidity, and concurrent administration of 0.2-N hydrochloride (HCl) (q12h) resulted in detectable levels of the drug in serum in the same study. The bioavailability of KETO was 23% in one horse. Successful treatment of one horse with oral KETO (in combination with nebulized ENIL) for *Scopulariopsis* pneumonia has been reported.[104] Oral KETO therapy failed to cure three horses with coccidioidomycosis in one study.[106] KETO should not be administered to pregnant mares.[95]

Itraconazole (ITRA) is a lipophilic triazole that is well absorbed and provides high tissue concentrations in human patients after oral administration. The pharmacokinetics of ITRA have not been established for horses. ITRA has a wider spectrum of activity than KETO and is effective against *C. albicans, Aspergillus, B. dermatitidis, C. immitis, C. neoformans*, and *H. capsulatum*.[85] Oral and topical ITRA has been used successfully to treat two horses with nasal aspergillosis,[107,108] one horse with guttural pouch aspergillosis (concurrently treated with topical ENIL),[108] and one horse with osteomyelitis caused by coccidioidomycosis.[109] One horse with guttural pouch aspergillosis was treated successfully with ENIL, using an indwelling catheter.[110]

Fluconazole (FLUC) is a newer triazole that is water soluble. In horses, FLUC is rapidly and well absorbed after oral administration (systemic availability of 101 ± 28%).[76] The harmonic mean elimination half-life was 37.8 hours after oral administration. Using the recommended dosing regimen (see Table 56-1), plasma FLUC concentrations are maintained at greater than 8.0 μg/mL, and FLUC is detectable in cerebrospinal fluid (CSF), synovial fluid, aqueous humor, urine,[76] vitreous, choroids, retina, iris, conjunctiva, cornea, and lung tissues[110a] of healthy horses.[76] FLUC is excreted primarily in the urine, and the dose should be adjusted in horses with renal compromise. In vivo responses of fungal pathogens to FLUC may be good despite a poor response in vitro.[77,80] *Aspergillus* spp. and other molds are reported to have some intrinsic resistance to FLUC.[80] Foals with systemic candidiasis have been treated successfully with oral FLUC.[85,111] Few adverse effects of FLUC treatment are reported in humans.[80]

Table • **56-1**

Systemic Antifungal Therapy in Horses

DRUG	DOSE	ROUTE	DURATION	INDICATION	OUTCOME*	REF
Amphotericin B (AMB) deoxycholate	Day 1: 0.1-0.3 mg/kg, then ↑0.1-0.5 mg/kg daily or EOD	IV or IA in 5% dextrose over 1-4 hours	Variable; several weeks	Systemic candidiasis in foals	S	85
				Fungal pneumonia	S	87
				Candida arthritis	S	90
AMB	100 mg, then ↑50 mg/day, up to 200-250 mg/450 kg	IV (?) Intrathecal		Cryptococcal meningitis	F	93
AMB	0.1-1.5 mg/kg EOD			Phycomycosis	S	88
				Phycomycosis	S	89
				Candida arthritis	S	86
AMB		Topical, intra-lesional		Phycomycosis		88
AMB		Intra-lesional		Conidiobolomycosis		132
AMB (mg/kg)	Day 1: 0.3 Day 2: 0.45 Day 3: 0.6 Days 4-7: none Days 8-30: 0.6 EOD	IV, diluted		Pulmonary histoplasmosis	S	92
AMB (mg/kg)	Days 1-3: 0.35 Days 4-5: 0.4 Days 6-31: 0.6 3 g total dose	IV diluted Pretreat with flunixin meglumine	31 days	Pulmonary cryptococcosis	S: 1 case	91
Miconazole	5 g q12h, 2% solution	Topical	4 weeks	Nasal *Pseudallescheria boydii*	S: 1 case + Na iodide IV + K iodide PO	103
Enilconazole (ENIL)	33.3 mg/mL 60 mL	Topical	2 weeks	Guttural pouch aspergillosis	S: + ITRA PO	109
ENIL	0.9% or 1.7% solution q24h	Topical	9-13 days	Atypical guttural pouch mixed mycosis, including *Aspergillus*	S: 3 cases + debride	133
ENIL		Nebulized		*Scopulariopsis* pneumonia	S: + KETO	104
Ketoconazole (KETO)	3.6 mg/kg q24h	PO		Coccidioidomycosis	F	106
KETO	30 mg/kg q24h	PO		Pharmacokinetics: undetectable in blood and tissues		105
KETO	30 mg/kg + 0.2-N HCl q12h	PO	5 doses	Pharmacokinetics: 23% bioavailability		105
Itraconazole (ITRA)	3 mg/kg q12h	PO	3-4.5 months	Nasal aspergillosis	S: 2/2 cases + surgery for 1 case	107
ITRA	q12h	Topical	14 days	Nasal aspergillosis	S	108
ITRA	5 mg/kg q24h	PO	3 weeks	Guttural pouch aspergillosis	S: 1 case + topical ENIL	109
ITRA	2.6 mg/kg q12h	PO		Osteomyelitis, coccidioidomycosis	S: 1 case	110
Fluconazole (FLUC)	9-11 mg/kg loading dose 4-55 mg/kg q24h	PO		Systemic candidiasis (foals)	S	85
				Disseminated candidiasis	S	111
FLUC	14 mg/kg loading dose 5 mg/kg q24h	PO		Pharmacokinetics		125

EOD, Every other day; *IV*, intravenous; *IA*, intraarterial; *PO*, oral; *q12h*, every 12 hours; *Na*, sodium; *K*, potassium; *HCl*, hydrochloride.
**S*, Successful treatment; *F*, failure of treatment.

Table • 56-2

Common Topical Antifungals Used to Treat Keratomycosis in Horses

ANTIFUNGAL DRUG	TOPICAL FORMULATION AND FREQUENCY
Natamycin	5% every 6 hours
Miconazole	1% every 6 hours
Itraconazole	1% with 30% dimethyl sulfoxide (DMSO) every 6 hours
Fluconazole	0.2% every 6 hours
Ketoconazole	Not available
Amphotericin B	0.15% every 6 hours
Povidone-iodine	2% solution every 12 hours
	0.1% solution every 2-4 hours*
	7% solution to cauterize after corneal scraping*
Silver sulfadiazine†	Dermatologic cream 1% q 12 hrs*

Data from Brooks DE: *Vet Clin North Am Equine Pract* 20:345, 2004.
*Data from Barton MH: *Compend Equine Pract* 14(7):936, 1992.
†Efficacy against *Candida* spp. but not recommended for use in horses.

Use of FLUC in the management of fungal diseases of horses is likely increasing, although reports evaluating clinical efficacy are lacking.

Voriconazole is a second-generation azole antifungal drug that is effective against *Aspergillus* spp. isolated from people and in the treatment of some patients with invasive aspergillosis.[101,112] Voriconazole can be given IV or orally in human patients, for whom the oral bioavailability is excellent. A single oral dose of 4 mg/kg resulted in a mean concentration of 0.86 ± 0.22 μg/mL in the aqueous humor of four healthy horse eyes.[113,114] No adverse effects were noted. Pharmacokinetic studies of voriconazole in adult horses are ongoing.[115]

Chitin Synthesis Inhibitors

These newer antifungal drugs inhibit the synthesis of chitin, an important component of the cell wall of many fungi but not of mammals. Chitin synthase inhibitors have a narrow spectrum of antifungal action.[116]

Lufenuron, a nonspecific chitin synthase inhibitor, was administered by the intrauterine route at a dose of 540 mg in 60 mL of sterile water in four mares with mycotic endometritis.[64] Based on empiric observations, the authors concluded that lufenuron contributed to the recovery of these mares. In contrast, lufenuron had no effect on the in vitro growth of *Aspergillus* and *Fusarium* spp. isolated from the corneas of horses with keratomycosis.[117] In the same study, 21 healthy adult horses were given lufenuron orally at dosages of 5 mg/kg q24h for 3 days, 20 mg/kg q24h for 3 days, or 60 mg/kg q24h for 1 day. Blood concentrations of lufenuron were lower than the ineffective concentrations achieved in vitro. Lufenuron was detected in blood samples from 20 of 21 horses. Currently, minimal data support the efficacy of lufenuron in the treatment of fungal diseases in horses.

Nikkomycin Z is a competitive inhibitor of chitin synthase. In experimental models of fungal infection, this drug has poor antifungal activity against many opportunistic fungi, including *Aspergillus fumigatus*.[112] In vitro, nikkomycin Z is synergistic with ITRA against *Aspergillus flavus* and *A. fumigatus*.[84,118] This drug has not been evaluated for use in horses.

Mycotic Keratitis

The goals of therapy are to sterilize the cornea, control secondary anterior uveitis, maximize retention of vision, speed corneal healing, and control ocular pain. Initial choice of an antifungal agent is largely based on clinical signs, results of cytologic evaluation of corneal scrapings, and knowledge of the epidemiology of fungal keratitis in the locale where the affected horse is living. Because most reported cases of fungal keratitis in horses are caused by *Aspergillus* spp., initial treatment for this organism is recommended. Delaying therapy until culture results are reported is not in the patient's best interests because of the long time frame required to obtain results. Treatment should be suitably modified when culture results are available. Antifungal sensitivity testing may be useful in horses that respond poorly to initial antifungal therapy (see previous discussion).

A limited number of antifungal drugs are available for ocular use. These include the polyene antifungal drugs natamycin and AMB; the azoles MICON, ITRA, and FLUC; the antibiotic heavy metal combination drug silver sulfadiazine (as a 1% cream); 2% povidone-iodine solutions; and an ophthalmic ointment containing 1% ITRA and 30% dimethyl sulfoxide (DMSO).[119]

Corneal penetration of the antifungal drug is a key factor in the success of treatment. The concentration of drug in the cornea depends on the molecular mass of the drug, route of administration, ability of the drug to penetrate the corneal tissues, and duration of contact with the cornea.[102] Larger compounds such as AMB and natamycin barely penetrate the intact corneal epithelium after topical administration. ITRA is lipophilic and readily penetrates cell membranes. Contact time with the cornea can be increased by frequent application of drugs (hourly or q2h), by constant infusion via a subpalpebral lavage system, or by superficial keratectomy. Application of occlusive ointments also increases contact time. When the corneal epithelium is no longer intact, these factors may be less influential in the success or failure of topical treatment.[102] Long-term treatment is usually necessary to resolve the fungal infection and the attendant inflammatory reaction. Appropriate systemic antifungal therapy in conjunction with topical antifungal treatment may be beneficial in many cases.

Polyene Antifungal Drugs

Natamycin is fungicidal and available in an ophthalmic preparation for topical use. It is the least irritating of the polyene antibiotics. Natamycin has poor solubility and is administered to human and equine patients as a 5% suspension that adheres well to ulcerated corneal tissues.[59,102] Recent studies have shown that the drug penetrates the cornea well after topical application.[102] It is a broad-spectrum antifungal with favorable activity against *Fusarium* and *Aspergillus*, but it is expensive. A formulation for systemic use is not available.

Amphotericin B, also fungicidal, can be used topically in the eye as a 0.15% solution (prepared with sterile water and refrigerated in a dark bottle). AMB generally has poor corneal penetration after topical or systemic administration and is irritating. AMB has been demonstrated experimentally to impair reepithelialization of defects in rabbit corneas when applied topically as a 1% solution,[120] and it may be toxic to corneal tissue,[102] although 0.15% solutions are well tolerated by human and equine patients. AMB is reported to be irritating if used at concentrations above 0.3%,[58,121] and subconjunctival administration of more than 125 to 300 mg may induce tissue necrosis and ulceration.[58] An ophthalmic preparation of AMB is not available commercially.

Nephrotoxicity of AMB has limited its systemic use in horses. This drug can be used when other antifungal agents have failed or are suspected to be ineffective. AMB is antagonistic to MICON, and the two drugs should not be used concurrently.[50] Recently developed lipid formulations of AMB have greatly reduced toxicity in humans; however, these have not yet been studied in horses and at present are prohibitively expensive. Heat-treated AMB is less toxic than other formulations and may be useful in horses, although it has yet to be studied in this species. AMB is light sensitive and requires refrigeration for storage.[58]

Azole Antifungal Drugs

Clotrimazole is one of the first imidazole derivatives developed for topical, broad-spectrum antifungal therapy. In vitro, clotrimazole is active against dermatophytes, *Candida* spp., *Aspergillus* spp., *C. immitis*, and *C. neoformans*.[80] Three of six horses with keratomycosis were successfully treated with topical clotrimazole in the United Kingdom.[29] The use of clotrimazole to treat keratomycosis in horses is seldom reported, however, and the efficacy of the drug in the clinical setting is unknown.

Miconazole has a broad spectrum of antifungal activity that includes *Aspergillus*. In a rabbit model, topical MICON was reported to produce corneal concentrations of 10 μg/g in undebrided corneas and 93 μg/g in debrided corneas, suggesting that topical use could be effective in the treatment of keratomycosis.[102,122]

Ketoconazole is reported to induce high corneal concentrations after experimental topical administration. Although corneal toxicity is not associated with topical use, a topical formulation of this drug is not available.[102]

After oral administration in people, ITRA produces lower corneal concentrations than those induced by oral FLUC or KETO.[102] Some success in treatment of keratomycosis in horses with oral ITRA in conjunction with topical natamycin has been anecdotally reported, although approximately 50% of these equine patients required surgical treatment of their ocular fungal diseases.[123] Topical use of ITRA may also be associated with poor corneal penetration. Recently, an ointment containing 1% ultramicronized ITRA and 30% DMSO has been shown to induce equine corneal ITRA concentrations of 7.9 ± 0.33 μg/g, a value that is approximately seven times greater than that achieved by topical administration of ITRA alone.[123,124] Brooks et al.[28] showed that 64% of all fungal isolates and all nine *Aspergillus* isolates in one study were susceptible to ITRA.

Fluconazole is minimally protein bound and highly water soluble, and it distributes well in body tissues and fluids. FLUC readily penetrates all ocular tissues and fluids in rabbits after oral administration[102] and reaches concentrations of 11.39 ± 2.83 μg/mL in the aqueous humor of healthy horses after oral administration.[76] Corneal concentrations are reported to be highly correlated with serum concentrations.[102] FLUC also achieves relatively high corneal concentrations after topical administration in rabbits,[102] but it is undetectable in equine corneas after 10 days of oral treatment (14-mg/kg loading dose, then 5 mg/kg q24h).[125] FLUC has a wide therapeutic margin of safety, and this broad-spectrum antifungal agent is fungicidal for *Aspergillus* spp.[27] In one study, however, all nine *Aspergillus* isolates were resistant to FLUC, and 21 of 22 total fungal isolates were resistant to the drug.[28] The authors recommended against the use of FLUC for mycotic keratitis in horses based on its demonstrably poor in vitro activity against equine ocular pathogens. Despite these findings, there are numerous anecdotal reports of good response of horses with keratomycosis to treatment with FLUC.[58]

Topical voriconazole, administered as 0.5% and 1.0% solutions to four healthy equine eyes, penetrated the corneas and induced mean aqueous humor concentrations of 1.43 ± 0.37 μg/mL and 2.35 ± 0.78 μg/mL, respectively.[113,114] Topical 3.0% solutions caused blepharospasm, epiphora, and chemosis. Clinical experience with this promising antifungal agent in the treatment of fungal keratitis of horses is currently limited. There are anecdotal reports of limited success in treating equine keratomycosis with topical voriconazole and oral FLUC (Cutler T: personal communication). Approximately 50% of the horses treated with this combination of antifungal drugs required surgical intervention for the management of their ocular disease.

Silver Sulfadiazine

Available as a cream, silver sulfadiazine is a combination sulfonamide and heavy metal that functions as a heavy metal donor.[125] Liberated silver binds to microbial DNA and prevents replication but does not interfere with epithelial cell regeneration.[102] The drug is effective against *Aspergillus, Fusarium*, and yeasts.[59] An isolated report suggested that silver sufadiazine has broad antifungal activity and is useful for the treatment of human keratomycosis.[126,127] An in vitro study showed that silver sulfadiazine was fungistatic and fungicidal for six *Aspergillus* spp. and 11 other fungal isolates from diseased eyes of horses.[126] The drug is inexpensive and has been used for the treatment of equine keratomycosis, although it is not labeled for ophthalmic use.[27] Topical application four to six times daily may be useful as initial therapy for a penetrating corneal injury with suspected plant contamination, when fiscal issues limit therapeutic options, and for follow-up treatment after intensive therapy has been completed.[58] The efficacy of silver sulfadiazine for the treatment of equine keratomycosis has been questioned.[51]

Povidone-Iodine Solution

Dilute (0.1%[59] or 2%[51]) povidone-iodine solutions may be used topically for treatment of equine keratomycosis. The efficacy of these solutions is not documented. More concentrated solutions or Lugol's iodine solution (2%-7%) should be reserved for cauterizing the cornea after corneal scraping.[59]

Thiabendazole

This thiazolyl benzimidazole anthelmintic is reported to have fungistatic and fungicidal properties and has broad-spectrum in vitro activity against many pathogenic fungi.[127,128] Some studies showed no correlation between in vitro activity and clinical outcome.[80] Washing skin lesions caused by *Trichophyton equinum* with a thiabendazole suspension did not prevent subsequent isolation of fungi from the lesions.[81,129] This compound has been available as a 14.29% paste for deworming pigs. Joyce[128] reported treatment with thiabendazole paste of 11 horses with nonulcerative keratitis of presumed mycotic origin. Five horses treated twice daily for 30 days recovered and had no recurrence of disease for 12 months. Thiabendazole caused no ocular irritation in any of the 11 treated horses. This modality of therapy is inexpensive, but of unproven efficacy.

Choice of Antifungal Medication

Aggressive treatment of equine keratomycosis should begin immediately (before culture results are available).[60] Topical administration of MICON, FLUC, or ITRA is reported to be successful in treating mycotic keratitis in horses.[51] Topical ITRA and 30% DMSO resolved keratomycosis in 8 of 10 equine eyes (four were positive for *Aspergillus* spp.), with a mean duration of treatment of 34.6 days (range, 16-53 days).[119] The addition of systemic antifungal therapy may be beneficial.

Brooks et al.[28] reported susceptibility patterns based on minimum inhibitory concentration (MIC) and 50% inhibitory concentration (IC_{50}) for *Aspergillus* spp. isolated from equine cases of keratomycosis. Breakpoints for determining susceptibilities were provided. In this study, all nine *Aspergillus* isolates were resistant to FLUC, and seven of nine were resistant to KETO. All nine isolates were susceptible to ITRA, MICON, and natamycin, and the authors recommend the use of MICON or natamycin, but recommended against the use of FLUC, for horses with *Aspergillus* keratitis.

Unfortunately, in vitro susceptibility information may correlate poorly with the clinical response of patients to treatment, and these relationships require further study.[17,77,102] Standard methods for susceptibility testing of filamentous fungi have been developed recently but are not universally employed or accepted.[72] In addition, criteria for determining susceptibility are often not reported. Choice of antifungal therapy for keratomycosis in horses is often based on personal preference of the attending clinician and expense of the available drugs (see Tables 56-1 and 56-2).

Duration of Therapy

Medical treatment must provide a long duration of exposure of the cornea to antifungal drugs to promote resolution of fungal infection.[51] The mean duration of successful treatment in two studies was 27 (range, 12-82) days and 48 (range, 31-192) days.[26,59] When clinical signs have improved, the frequency of treatment may be decreased. Signs of improvement include healing of the corneal epithelium (no fluorescein uptake) and diminished signs of uveitis (absence of aqueous flare, reduced ocular pain resulting in absence of blepharospasm and photophobia). Deep stromal neovascularization changes in color from deep red to pale pink or white,[51] and the corneal scar becomes more dense from fibrosis as the lesion contracts during healing. Antifungal therapies may be fungistatic rather than fungicidal, and intact fungi may remain indolent in corneal tissue. Evidence of worsening of clinical signs should prompt return to aggressive, frequent medical treatment.

Surgical Treatment

Deep or rapidly progressing corneal infections, especially those characterized by keratomalacia or that respond poorly to medical treatment, and stromal abscesses that do not respond to medical treatment in 48 to 72 hours usually require surgical intervention.[26,51,129a] Necrotic corneal tissue and associated fungal organisms are debrided. Cytologic examination and culture of material obtained by surgical debridement may provide a definitive diagnosis. Debridement and keratectomy increase drug penetration into infected corneal tissue and reduce collagenolysis.[53] Subsequent application of a flap or graft improves corneal integrity and supplies vascular access to fungal ulcers or stromal abscesses. The use of conjunctival pedicle grafts, bridge grafts, hood grafts, island grafts, and full-thickness penetrating keratoplasty has been reported.[17,26,51] Postsurgical corneal scarring may be extensive; however, early surgical intervention may speed recovery and improve the prognosis for saving the globe and for sight.[26,51]

Medical therapy should continue for several weeks after surgery, depending on clinical signs.[17] Six to 8 weeks after placement of a conjunctival flap, the limbal attachment may be severed.

Other Treatments

Atropine sulfate and flunixin meglumine for control of uveitis and ocular pain, topical antiproteinase therapy, and prevention of collagenolysis have been recently reviewed.[51] *Flunixin meglumine* may reduce the rate of corneal vascularization and therefore impair healing.[51,130] Nonsteroidal antiinflammatory drugs (NSAIDs) that reduce iridocyclitis and anterior uveitis, potentially blinding complications, must be employed in the context of careful assessment of the rate of corneal vascularization. *Phenylbutazone* may have a less negative effect on corneal vascularization than flunixin meglumine and may be a good choice when corneal vascularization is proceeding slowly.[51,130] Bacterial keratitis may complicate keratomycosis, and concurrent topical antibiotic therapy is recommended.[20,26,53,54,59]

Fibrosis and scar formation after successful treatment of mycotic keratitis may reduce vision and can be aesthetically unappealing. *Cyclosporin A*, an agent that inhibits proliferation of fibroblasts and increases fibroblast apoptosis, may be useful to reduce corneal scarring, although this treatment modality has not been studied in horses.[51] Topical antibiotic-steroid therapy at this time may help to reduce vascularization and corneal scarring,[17] although treatment with corticosteroids is risky if viable fungi remain in the cornea.[51]

Corticosteroid Treatment Contraindicated

Corticosteroid drugs should never be employed by any route in the treatment of equine keratomycosis.

Prognosis

Potential complications of keratomycosis include corneal scarring and pigmentation, iris prolapse, uveitis, synechia, cataract formation, rupture of the eye, endophthalmitis, phthisis bulbi, and blindness.[59] After medical treatment, 43% to 56% of horses have some vision, approximately 10% have a nonvisual eye, and 25% to 48% require enucleation.[58] The prognosis can be substantially improved by a combination of intensive medical treatment and timely surgical intervention. In one study, 63% of horses treated with combined medical and surgical therapy were "visual";[53] in a second study, 92% of treated horses retained sight.[26]

Pulmonary Aspergillosis

There are no reports in the literature of successful treatment of pulmonary aspergillosis in horses. Invasive pulmonary aspergillosis represents a serious therapeutic challenge in human patients as well.[131] *Aspergillus* spp. are often sensitive to ITRA and are variably sensitive to AMB and FLUC.[95] Voriconazole is likely to be effective,[101] but to date, clinical experience in horses with this second-generation azole is lacking, and its expense may preclude use.

The prognosis for horses with pulmonary aspergillosis is extremely poor. The disease was fatal for all 29 affected horses in a retrospective study,[34] as well as for all affected horses in other reports.[3,37-39] The poor prognosis may reflect the difficulty in making an early diagnosis of pulmonary aspergillosis and the severity of other concurrent disease. The ability to diagnose this disease reliably in its early stages may improve success in treatment. Real-time PCR may permit earlier diagnosis; however, the methodology has not yet been validated in this clinical setting.

Nasal and Sinus Aspergillosis

Three horses with nasal aspergillosis responded to topical treatment with natamycin (25 mg/100 mL sterile water) followed by insufflation of natamycin powder, although the condition did recur in one horse.[61] Lavage with 1% natamycin solution after transendoscopic removal of large mycotic plaques was successful in treating 10 of 11 horses with mycotic sinonasal disease.[62] Debulking facilitates medical management.

When the lesions of nasal aspergillosis represent focal disease, the prognosis for recovery is good with aggressive therapy, usually a combination of surgical debulking and topical antifungal drugs. Horses with nasal and pulmonary aspergillosis have a poor prognosis because of the devastating nature of the pulmonary disease.

Endometritis and Placentitis

Treatment of endometritis caused by *Aspergillus* spp. has included copious lavage of the uterus followed by instillation of AMB (in sterile water or saline), clotrimazole, nystatin, or FLUC; lavage with dilute iodine solutions; and intrauterine plasma.[23,30] Results of treatment are often suboptimal. Iodine solutions may cause irritation and fibrosis. Systemic treatment with FLUC has also been suggested for mares that do not respond to repeated uterine lavage and topical antifungal therapy.[23] In one study, intrauterine lufenuron showed promise for the treatment of fungal endometritis,[64] although the efficacy of lufenuron in this clinical setting has not been critically evaluated.

The prognosis for recovery from fungal endometritis is poor. Fungal endometritis and frequent lavage, particularly with iodine solutions, may result in adhesions of the uterus, vagina, or cervix.[30] Fertility may be reduced.

Aflatoxicosis

No specific antidote exists for acute aflatoxicosis, and supportive therapy (fluids, analgesics, sedatives as needed) should be instituted. In subacute intoxication, gastrointestinal absorption of aflatoxins can be reduced by oral administration of sodium calcium aluminosilicate, an agent that adsorbs aflatoxins.[31] Supplementary vitamin E and selenium may be beneficial. Prevention of ingestion of contaminated grains is imperative.

REFERENCES

See the CD-ROM for a list of references linked to the abstract in PubMed.

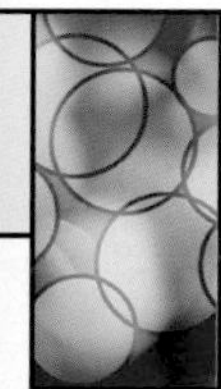

CHAPTER • 57

Miscellaneous Fungal Diseases

Catherine Kohn

BLASTOMYCOSIS

Blastomycosis is an extremely rare disease in horses. Fatal disseminated infection has been reported in two horses and a miniature horse, and fatal subcutaneous infection was reported in a third horse. *Blastomyces dermatitidis* is not contagious or zoonotic. Clusters of cases occur in persons and dogs as a result of exposure to a common environmental source of the fungi. The ecology of this fungus is still incompletely understood.

Etiology

The thermally dimorphic ascomycete *Blastomyces dermatitidis* is the cause of all manifestations of blastomycosis. Conidia, measuring 2 to 10 μm in diameter, are the infectious agents. The yeast form is thick walled and usually 8 to 15 μm in diameter, although yeasts as large as 30 μm have been reported.[1] In tissues, yeast cells display characteristic broad-based buds.

Virulence Factors

Several factors contribute to the virulence of *B. dermatitidis*.[2] In tissues the organism converts to a yeast form that is more resistant to phagocytosis and killing than are conidia. The yeast cell wall may have antiphagocytic properties, and cell wall phospholipids may contribute to virulence.[3] The *BAD1* antigen (formerly called WI-1), a cell wall surface antigen, is an important factor for the adherence of yeasts to macrophages and to lung tissue. Loss of the antigen results in impaired binding and entry into macrophages and in diminished capacity of the yeast to adhere to the lung. A strain of *B. dermatitidis* experimentally deprived of this antigen by gene deletion was avirulent in mice.[4] *BAD1* has other antiinflammatory effects that include influencing the profile of proinflammatory cytokines, such as suppressing tumor necrosis factor alpha (TNF-α) release by host macrophages.[5]

Epidemiology

The ecology of the filamentous form of *B. dermatitidis* in nature has proved challenging to define, and the organism is difficult to isolate from environmental sources. Based on environmental isolates in two outbreaks of human and canine disease, the mycelial form of *B. dermatitidis* is thought to be a saprophyte found in moist soil of acid pH and high organic content, usually in wooded areas near water.[1,2] Optimal conditions for growth of the mycelia in its natural microenvironment may be short lived, and the organism may be present in large numbers only transiently. *B. dermatitidis* is endemic in the Mississippi, Missouri, and Ohio River watersheds, the Great Lakes regions of the United States and Canada, and the St. Lawrence River Valley[1,2] (Fig. 57-1). The disease is also found in Africa, but is seldom reported from other parts of the world.

Blastomycosis has been reported in many species, most often in dogs and humans,[6] and rarely in horses. Dogs are considered sentinel animals for human infections. Blastomycosis is not contagious or zoonotic among infected persons or animals. The disease occurs sporadically, although clusters of cases have been described and are likely associated with an increase in infective conidia in an environment that is transiently optimal for mycelia growth. *B. dermatitidis* was isolated from soil on the banks of a beaver pond near a camp in Wisconsin; 48 people who visited the camp developed blastomycosis.[7]

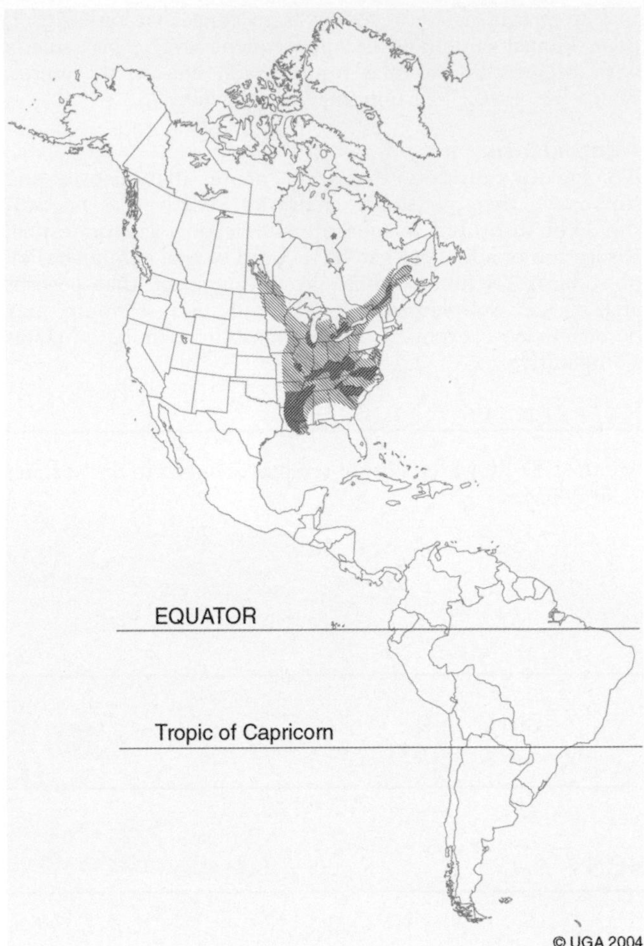

Fig. 57-1 Shading indicates area of endemic blastomycosis. Darker shading indicates areas of higher incidence. (From Greene C: *Infectious diseases of the dog and cat*, ed 3, Philadelphia, 2006, Saunders.)

Most infections occur during cooler and wetter months of the year. Agricultural workers, hunters, campers, and their canine companions are particularly at risk for infection.[1]

The prevalence of asymptomatic pulmonary infections is unknown. Spontaneous recovery from an identified blastomycosis infection in humans is uncommon, and mortality rates in untreated persons with chronic blastomycosis may be as high as 60%.[2] *B. dermatitidis* organisms are not among the flora of healthy persons. These findings suggest that the incidence of asymptomatic infection may be low.

Pathogenesis

Blastomycosis is a disease of immunocompetent persons and is relatively infrequently reported as an opportunistic infection in immunocompromised patients.[2] In patients with acquired immunodeficiency syndrome (AIDS), the neurologic form of blastomycosis is more common, and the disease is more severe and more often fatal than in immunocompetent patients.[8] Infection most often occurs by inhalation of aerosolized conidia. In the lungs the conidia are phagocytized by neutrophils, monocytes, and alveolar macrophages. Macrophages may inhibit the conversion of conidia to yeasts, but conidia that remain viable in tissues rapidly transform into the more resistant yeast. A robust cellular immune response is crucial in the host's defense against the organism. *B. dermatitidis* has a predilection for bone and skin and may reach these organs by dissemination from the lungs. Infection may also occur by direct inoculation through the skin.

Intravenous inoculation of one horse with *B. dermatitidis* caused chronic inflammatory foci in the lungs.[9] Subcutaneous inoculation did not produce disease. No further details of these studies are available.

Clinical Findings

Clinical signs in human patients with blastomycosis are variable and often nonspecific; weight loss, fever, malaise, and fatigue are common to many diseases. The onset is usually insidious, and the clinical course is often chronic. Pulmonary, cutaneous, osseous, genitourinary, and central nervous system abnormalities, as well as sporadic disease of almost any organ, have been reported in humans.[2] Forty percent of dogs with blastomycosis have ocular lesions.[6] Misdiagnosis is common in human patients, possibly because the index of suspicion for this disease is low, but also because blastomycosis can mimic many other diseases. For example, pulmonary manifestations of blastomycosis can be easily confused with bacterial pneumonia, tuberculosis, or neoplasia.[2]

Three equine cases have been reported in the literature,[10-12] and the author has seen one additional case. Two horses had cutaneous manifestations of blastomycosis. One had chronic subcutaneous abscesses, initially in the perianal and perivulvar region and progressing over several months to involve the perineum, udder, and ventral midline.[10] Multiple abscesses were noted, and abscess maturation, spontaneous decompression, resolution, and appearance of new abscesses became a constant cycle as the disease steadily worsened. A partial necropsy showed that the inflammatory process was locally aggressive. The diagnosis was based on the histopathologic identification of the typical yeasts in tissue sections showing associated pyogranulomatous inflammation. Fungal cultures were not attempted.

A miniature horse had a 6-month history of chronic subcutaneous infections in the cervical and pectoral regions, complicated by acute onset of dysphagia.[12] An open, draining wound communicated with a tract extending toward the caudal deep cervical lymph nodes; a mediastinal mass identified by ultrasonography appeared to connect by a tract to the nodes. There were abscesses in the right lung, and a bilateral pleural effusion was present. At necropsy, pyogranulomatous inflammation was found in the left kidney and the right lung. Multiple pleural abscesses and peritonitis were also present.

Two horses have had fatal disseminated blastomycosis without cutaneous disease.[11,13] Lethargy, weight loss, and cough were historical clinical signs. Both horses had pyogranulomatous pleuritis and peritonitis. Lung, mediastinum, liver, squamous stomach, large intestinal serosa, and diaphragm were affected in one horse,[13] whereas most abdominal viscera and the thoracic cavity were affected in the other.[11] In both horses, adhesions of pulmonary abscesses to the diaphragm were associated with disease on the corresponding abdominal surface of the diaphragm, suggesting extension of the inflammation from one body cavity to the other. In these cases, typical yeasts were seen in peritoneal and pleural fluid antemortem and in tissues at necropsy. *B. dermatitidis* was identified in culture, and in one horse the identification of the organisms in culture was confirmed by molecular techniques.[11]

In this small case series, blastomycosis in horses tended to be a disseminated or locally aggressive and fatal disease. Two of the affected horses resided in the Ohio River Valley (a region where blastomycosis is endemic), and a third was

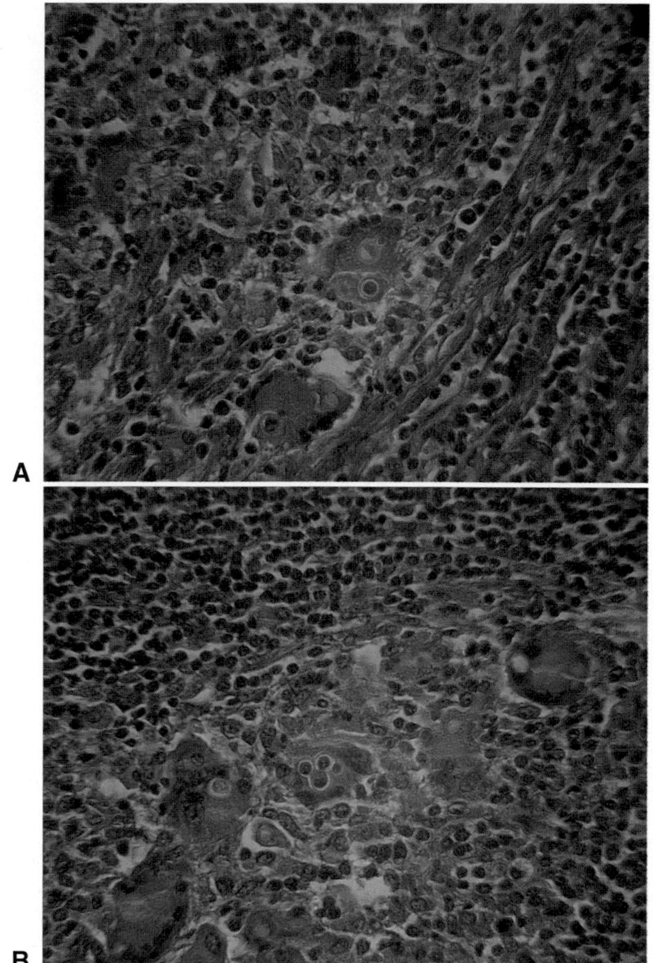

Fig. 57-2 Photomicrographs of *Blastomyces dermatitidis* in lymph node of the horse described by Toribio et al.[11] **A,** Note broad-based bud. **B,** Note multiple giant cells.

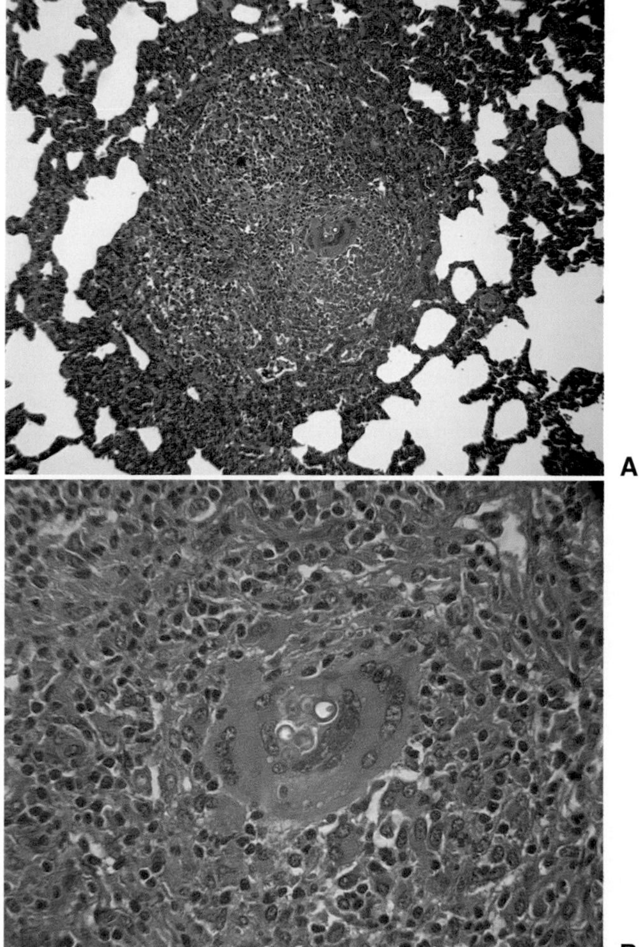

Fig. 57-3 Photomicrographs of *Blastomyces dermatitidis* in the lung of 3-year-old Rocky Mountain mare with disseminated blastomycosis. **A,** 30×. **B,** 40×.

from eastern Pennsylvania. Although rare, blastomycosis should be considered a differential diagnosis for horses with pneumonia, pleuritis, peritonitis, or skin disease that is poorly responsive to antibiotic therapy, particularly if the affected horse resides in a region where blastomycosis is endemic.

Diagnosis

Chest radiography and ultrasonography of the pulmonary and thoracic cavities are helpful in determining the location and extent of abscesses caused by *B dermatitidis*. Evaluation of the hemogram, serum chemistry profile, and serum fibrinogen aid in evaluating the systemic effects of infection.

Cytology

Cytologic examination of body fluids (transtracheal aspirate, bronchoalveolar lavage, pleural, peritoneal) often allows identification of typical, thick-walled yeasts that are 8 to 15 μm in diameter with broad-based budding.[1] The sensitivity of cytologic examination for diagnosis of blastomycosis in human patients was 93% in one study.[14]

Biopsy

In biopsies of tissues from affected humans, epithelioid granulomata, pyogranulomatous inflammation, necrosis, and fibrosis may be seen.[1] Yeasts are usually plentiful in infected tissues (Figs. 57-2 and 57-3). The thick-walled yeast cells are generally of uniform size (8-15 μm in diameter), although large cells (20-30 μm) have been described. Broad-based budding is the identifying feature and must be seen to have strong evidence of the presence of *B. dermatitidis*. The yeast wall may not stain with hematoxylin and eosin (H&E), and the cytoplasm may shrink away from the wall, leaving a space.[1] The sensitivity of histopathologic testing for the diagnosis of blastomycosis in persons in one study was 81.5%.[14]

Culture

Samples of infected body fluids or tissues usually produce characteristic yeasts within 2 to 4 weeks in cultures incubated at 37° C (98.6° F).[2] Culture is still considered the "gold standard" for the diagnosis of blastomycosis in human patients, although the sensitivity of this test in one study was 66.4%.[14]

On Sabouraud dextrose agar incubated at 25° C (77° F), the growth rate of the filamentous fungi is variable and slow, and cultures should be held for 2 months or more.[1] Colonies may be flat and glabrous (described as "skinlike") or may be fluffy white to brownish tan, sometimes with concentric rings. The appearance of the conidia is not distinctive, and identification of *B. dermatitidis* depends on observing the characteristic yeasts that appear within days to weeks when subcultures are incubated at 37° C.[1]

Molecular Identification of Yeasts

Molecular techniques for identification of the yeast form of *B. dermatitidis* in culture and fixed tissues are commercially available.[15] The application of deoxyribonucleic acid (DNA) amplification techniques to samples of body fluids or fresh tissues from clinical patients requires further study.

Serology

Antibody Detection. Serology has not proved to be a sensitive or specific method of diagnosing blastomycosis in humans. Immunocompromised persons may produce low concentrations of antibodies. A comparison of results from enzyme-linked immunosorbent assay (ELISA), complement fixation (CF), and immunodiffusion (ID) tests for antibody to *B. dermatitidis* in persons with documented blastomycosis showed that the assays had diagnostic sensitivity of 80%, 40%, and 65%, respectively.[16] Cross-reactions with other fungi (particularly *Histoplasma capsulatum*) are common.[2] An agar-gel immunodiffusion (AGID) test currently used in the diagnosis of canine blastomycosis has a sensitivity and specificity of greater than 90%. However, positive serologic testing alone is not considered sufficient to establish the diagnosis.[6]

When purified WI-1 *(BAD1)* antigen was used in a radioimmunoassay (RIA) to detect serum antibodies to *B. dermatitidis*, 85% of 68 persons known to have the disease were identified.[17] The RIA also detected 3% of patients with histoplasmosis, coccidioidomycosis, sporotrichosis, or candidiasis. All healthy persons had negative tests. In another study, anti–WI-1 serologic testing identified 75% of 32 human patients with blastomycosis.[18] Testing by RIA detected anti–WI-1 antibodies in 92% of infected dogs,[19] and RIA titers declined during treatment, suggesting that the RIA might be useful in monitoring the progress of therapy in affected dogs. AGID detected antibodies against the A antigen of *B. dermatitidis* in 41% of dogs with blastomycosis.[19]

Antigen Detection. Detection of *B. dermatitidis* antigen in the urine of persons and dogs with blastomycosis has been reported. Durkin et al.[14] used antibodies to mold antigens in an immunoassay and showed that the sensitivity of the test in patients with blastomycosis was 92.9% and the specificity 79.3%. Cross-reactions occurred in 96% of patients with histoplasmosis, 100% of those with paracoccidioidomycosis, 2.9% of those with cryptococcosis, and 1.1% of patients with aspergillosis. Shurley et al.[19a] used a competitive-binding inhibition ELISA test with antibodies raised against yeast-phase lysates and detected antigen in the urine of 100% of 36 dogs with blastomycosis. Unfortunately, cross-reactivity with *H. capsulatum* and elements in urine from healthy dogs were observed in this study. The sensitivity and specificity of tests for antigen determination should be optimized before these assays can be used reliably in the clinical setting. These tests may be useful in combination with results of physical examination, cytology, and culture in patients with suspected blastomycosis.

Therapy

Antifungal treatment of horses with blastomycosis has not been attempted.

Recommendations for treatment of humans with blastomycosis are based on limited data.[2] *Amphotericin B* (AMB) (0.5-0.6 mg/kg/day until the disease is controlled) is the treatment of choice in patients with life-threatening disease. After the disease has been controlled, an oral azole drug can be substituted for AMB. *Itraconazole* is the drug of choice for patients who have non–life-threatening disease that does not involve the central nervous system (CNS). Ketoconazole can be used for pulmonary infections that are not life threatening, although there are reports of CNS blastomycosis in patients who were successfully treated with ketoconazole for chest disease.[2] Ketoconazole distributes poorly to the CNS. Fluconazole is reported to have efficacy comparable to ketoconazole, is less toxic, and achieves good concentrations in the CNS. Fluconazole is an alternative in patients who cannot tolerate itraconazole.

Prevention

Recent studies have demonstrated that mice can be protected from an intrapulmonary challenge of *B. dermatitidis* by subcutaneous injection of a mutant strain of the fungus.[5] The mutant strain lacks the *BAD1* gene and therefore the *BAD1* cell surface antigen, previously shown to be a virulence factor. Mouse protection was characterized by the induction of a strong cell-mediated immune response.

Because blastomycosis occurs rarely in the horse, it is unlikely that development of an effective vaccine would be warranted for this species. However, for persons or horses in endemic regions, vaccination might be a consideration in the future.

CRYPTOCOCCOSIS

Cryptococcosis is an uncommon disease in horses, although the incidence of asymptomatic infection is unknown. Among approximately 40 horses reported to have cryptococcal infection, respiratory and CNS diseases were the most common clinical manifestations. *Cryptococcus* is not contagious, and cases occur sporadically. Clustering of cases in Australia may be related to the fact that ubiquitous eucalyptus trees are known to harbor cryptococci. Few horses with cryptococcosis have been treated, and there is little information in the literature to guide judgments on prognosis (usually considered to be poor) and therapy.

Etiology

Cryptococcus neoformans and *Cryptococcus gattii*, formerly known as *C. neoformans* var. *gattii*,[20] are the cause of virtually all cryptococcal disease in mammals.[21] Because of the recent change in classification of *C. gattii*, most of the literature refers to this organism as a variant of *C. neoformans*. Consequently, in this chapter, unless otherwise stated, comments regarding *Cryptococcus neoformans* can be taken to refer also to *C. gattii*. *C. neoformans*, classified in the phylum Basidiomycotina, is a spherical to ovoid, budding yeast 3 to 25 µm in diameter[22] that possesses a capsule 1 to 30 µm in thickness composed of at least three heteroglycans.[23] The heteroglycan composition of the capsule is the basis for distinguishing the many species of *C. neoformans*, of which two (in addition to *C. gattii*) are the cause of most diseases: *C. neoformans* var. *grubii* and *C. neoformans* var. *neoformans*. In animal tissues and fluids the yeast reproduces by typically narrow-based budding.[23]

Virulence Factors

Cryptococcus neoformans has three genetically controlled characteristics largely responsible for its virulence: the ability to produce a capsule, melanin formation, and the ability to grow at 37° C.[24]

Capsule. The distinctive polysaccharide capsule of the yeast affords several modes of protection from the host's immune response. The capsule blocks phagocytosis, masks ligands on the fungal cell surface to which antibodies might bind, reduces the respiratory burst of phagocytes, downregulates production of protective cytokines (T helper cell type 1 [Th1] response), and upregulates production of Th2 cytokines.[21,24] Mutant cryptococcal organisms that have deficient capsules are less virulent than their parent strains, and increases in virulence have been associated with structural changes or increased thickness of the capsule.[24,25] The capsules of the yeast may enlarge during infection.[24,26] Circulating solubilized capsular polysaccharide antigens in human patients with disseminated cryptococcosis may inhibit leukocyte migration to the site of cryptococcal infection.[27]

Melanin. *Cryptococcus* organisms are efficient producers of melanin through the enzyme phenol oxidase.[25] Melanin scavenges oxygen free radicals derived from leukocytes, and this antioxidant effect contributes to virulence.[24,27] Melanin also impairs antibody formation, depresses lymphoproliferation, and downregulates TNF-α production.[21] Because it contributes to the negative charge of *C. neoformans*, melanin may also impair phagocytosis of the organism.[27]

Thermotolerance. The ability to live and replicate at mammalian body temperature (37° C) is a characteristic of invasive fungal pathogens in general. Temperature-sensitive mutant strains of *C. neoformans* are avirulent in mammalian models of cryptococcal disease. The ability to grow at high temperature is under the control of multiple genes in *C. neoformans*.[24]

Epidemiology

Cryptococcus neoformans is an opportunistic, saprophytic yeast that is ubiquitous worldwide. Bird manure, particularly pigeon droppings, and bat guano harbor *C. neoformans* var. *grubii* and *C. neoformans* var. *neoformans*, which can remain viable for up to 2 years in fecal material.[1] Purines, urea, and creatinine are present in high concentrations in bird excreta and readily used by the yeast as substrates for metabolism.[28,29] The pigeon may be the most important vector for dispersing *C. neoformans* and maintaining it in the environment.[1] *C. neoformans* is also found in rotting wood, and *C. gattii* has been associated with flowering red and river gum trees (species of *Eucalyptus* trees) in Australia, Columbia, India, and southern California.[23] The prevalence of eucalyptus trees in the environment may explain the relatively frequent occurrence of cryptococcosis in horses and other species in western Australia.[30,31] *C. gattii* is endemic in Australia.[20] Admixture of soil with contaminated feces or rotting material from trees results in a reduction in numbers of organisms, possibly because of ingestion by soil amebae.[1] The yeast can also be isolated from ripe fruits, rotting vegetables, and dairy products.[1] High humidity fosters growth of *C. neoformans*, whereas exposure to direct sunlight can kill the yeast.[1]

Disease caused by *C. neoformans* usually occurs sporadically. Outbreaks comprising multiple cases of affected persons or animals, presumably exposed to the same source of the organism, are infrequently reported, and transmission of disease among affected animals or humans has not been described.[25] A large outbreak of *C. gattii* in persons, dogs, cats ferrets, llamas, and porpoises was reported in British Columbia.[32] Vancouver Island was found to be heavily colonized with *C. gattii*, an organism formerly thought to be restricted to warm and tropical climates. The worldwide distribution of this pathogen may be changing.[20] Although *C. neoformans*, and particularly *C. gattii*, cause disease in immunocompetent people, these yeasts are primarily opportunistic pathogens, and most affected humans and animals are immunocompromised, such as from human immunodeficiency virus (HIV) infection, corticosteroid treatment, chronic leukemia, lymphoma, sarcoidosis, and Cushing's disease.[1,24,25] Men are more frequently infected than women, and most cases occur in postpubertal persons.[25] *C. neoformans* infection has also been associated with pregnancy in women.[1]

Although *C. neoformans* is an opportunistic pathogen, it can be recovered from healthy persons on the skin or in sputum, where it may be an incidental or transient colonizer.[1] Most adults possess antibodies to this organism,[24] and the incidence of asymptomatic infection is unknown. In a preliminary study, 3% of 61 healthy horses in New South Wales had serum antibodies to *C. neoformans*, suggesting previous exposure to or latent infection with cryptococci.[31,33]

Pathogenesis

Cryptococcal disease in healthy people or animals may result from exposure to a large dose of the yeast or to a particularly virulent strain.[25] Initial exposure to the organism occurs by ingestion, contact through abraded skin or mucous membranes, or most often, inhalation of either desiccated yeast cells or (more likely) basidiospores. Basidiospores are produced in the environment by the sexual form of the *C. neoformans*, *Filobasidiella neoformans*, or from monokaryotic hyphae that develop under appropriate conditions, in the absence of mating.[27] Desiccated, poorly encapsulated yeast cells usually have a diameter greater than 2 μm (too large to be easily aerosolized and readily respirable) and reduced viability, whereas basidiospores, with a diameter of 2 μm, are small enough to reach the distal airways when inspired[27] and are resistant to desiccation. Mucociliary responses clear healthy airways of most inhaled infectious fungal propagules, and those that reach the alveoli are controlled by local host inflammatory responses, resulting in elimination of the fungi by alveolar macrophages, lymphocytes, neutrophils, and activated T cells. A robust cell-mediated immune response is essential to successful host defense against cryptococci, and Th1 immune responses are important for protective immunity.[24]

Antibodies to *C. neoformans* may be detected in human patients with early or focal infections.[8] During active disseminated infection, antibodies are usually not detectable, perhaps as a result of forming complexes with circulating capsular cryptococcal antigens or inhibition of antibody synthesis by these antigens.[8,25] In some human studies, antibody titers increase as capsular antigen titers decrease, and the patient improves clinically.[33] The presence of antibody in the serum of infected persons may be an indication for an improved prognosis.[8,33]

Yeasts that are not destroyed by the immune inflammatory response are segregated by a chronic inflammatory process that produces granulomas. The presence of a large granuloma reflects a robust cell-mediated immune response to cryptococcal organisms.[31,34] In one study, three of seven horses with *C. neoformans* infection had large granulomas in the dorsocaudal lung.[30] The same three horses had evidence of exercise-induced pulmonary hemorrhage (EIPH), and the investigators suggested that EIPH may predispose affected lung to colonization by inhaled cryptococci.[30] The dorsocaudal region of the lung receives air through the terminal ramifications of the principal bronchus and is a likely site for deposition of inhaled particles.[30,35] In addition, this is a common site in which to find evidence of EIPH.

In immunocompetent persons, *C. neoformans* may persist indefinitely in a latent state within a granuloma.[24] In theory, subsequent reactivation of latent infection may be associated with immune suppression or concurrent disease and may result in a disseminated cryptococcal infection, without evidence of recent infection.

In immunocompromised hosts, particularly those with CD4+ T-cell deficiency, cryptococcal infection disseminates within the lung, is translocated across the gastrointestinal wall after ingestion of infectious propagules or swallowing of infected nasal or pulmonary secretions, and disseminates hematogenously to other tissues, with a predilection for the leptomeninges and CNS. Dissemination from the lung may take weeks or months in human patients.[8] The reason this organism favors the CNS has not been documented. Infection of the nasal cavity and the maxillary and frontal sinuses in the horse could result in meningitis and CNS invasion by direct extension through the cribriform plate.[30,36] Hematogenous dispersion to the CNS has also been suggested.

Cryptococcal endometritis may be associated with chronic yeast colonization of the clitoral sinus.[37]

The pathogenesis of cryptococcal infections in human patients has been reviewed.[21,24,25,27]

Clinical Findings

A review of 40 cases of cryptococcosis in horses reported since 1902 showed that 16 horses had pneumonia or pleuritis,[28,30,31,38,39] 10 had upper respiratory tract infections (nasal plaques, sinus infections),[28,40] 10 had CNS disease,[28,36,41-43] three had abdominal disease,[28,30,44] two had endometritis,[37,38] and one had a locally aggressive subcutaneous mass.[45] One horse had both pneumonia and CNS disease,[43] and another had a nasal granuloma and jejunal lesion.[44]

Onset of disease is often insidious, with a slow progression characterized by vague signs. Purulent nasal discharge often creamy white in color, cough, and weight loss were common signs in horses with respiratory disease. Two foals aborted by mares with cryptococcal placentitis or endometritis had cryptococcal pneumonia.[46] Violent dementia, head tilt, ipsilateral weakness, unilateral blindness, ataxia, and weight loss were clinical signs of the neurologic form of cryptococcal disease. A pregnant mare with a large, abdominal cryptococcal granuloma had weight loss and poor fetal growth.[30] Another horse had colic resulting from an intraluminal jejunal cryptococcal granuloma within an intussusception.[28] A jejunal lesion was an incidental finding in a horse with a cryptococcal nasal granuloma.[44] One horse had a large, nonhealing skin lesion that extended into the subcutaneous tissues, invading through several intercostal spaces to the pleura.[45]

All except two of the affected horses died or were euthanized because of extensive disease, the poor prognosis, or the expense of treatment. The survivors included one pony treated successfully with AMB for a large pulmonary cryptococcal granuloma[31] and a horse with surgical resection of a jejunal intussusception involving an intraluminal cryptococcal granuloma.[28]

Diagnosis

Endoscopy

Endoscopic examination of the nasal passages permits close evaluation of cryptococcal lesions in the upper airways. The nasomaxillary ostia and the ethmoturbinate regions should be carefully examined. Tissue for cytology, culture, and histopathology can often be obtained endoscopically. Tracheoscopy may be useful to observe exudates, and bronchoscopy may help to localize the lesions and to obtain samples through bronchoalveolar lavage (BAL).

Radiography and Computed Tomography

The extent of cryptococcal infection in the nasal passages, the maxillary and frontal sinuses, and the ethmoid region should be evaluated radiographically. Computed tomography (CT) may be useful to define these lesions further, although it remains to be determined if CT will provide more information than radiography, which has the advantage of ready availability in the standing horse.

Cytology

Cryptococci can be seen in clinical specimens (cerebrospinal fluid [CSF], abdominal or pleural fluid, transtracheal aspirates, BAL fluid, aspirates from infected lesions) when stained with new methylene blue, Gram stain, or Romanovsky-type stains[23,30] (Fig. 57-4). Wright's stain is frequently used but may distort the capsule and shrink the organism.[47] India ink preparations demonstrate the capsule and may be especially useful for samples of CSF. A drop of the specimen is deposited on a drop of India ink on a slide and then covered with a coverslip.[48] The yeast (unstained) is silhouetted against a black background, and the capsule appears as a large, transparent halo[47] (Fig. 57-5). In wet preparations the cell wall is refractory, and the capsule varies in thickness from a few micrometers to a diameter greater than that of the yeast cell.[25] Yeast cells are spherical and may appear with a single bud, attached by a thin connection. Care should be taken in examining India ink preparations. When budding is not seen, lymphocytes, fat droplets, and aggregated droplets of India ink may be mistaken for yeasts.[8,47,49] Inability to visualize yeasts in cytologic preparations does not rule out infection. Yeast cells with small capsules or present in small numbers are easily overlooked.[47]

Biopsy

Impression smears from biopsy specimens can be rapidly evaluated by cytology. In tissues the yeast capsule does not stain well with periodic acid–Schiff (PAS), Gomori's methenamine silver (GMS), or Masson-Fontana stains that show encapsulated yeast cells (often distorted or collapsed) with a thin cell wall, surrounded by apparently empty space[25,47] (Fig. 57-6). Mayer's mucicarmine, which stains the capsule rose-red and the cell pink, is the best choice and does not stain other fungal organisms that might be confused with cryptococci, such as *Blastomyces* or *Coccidioides*.[47] The associated inflammatory response may be minimal or granulomatous.[25]

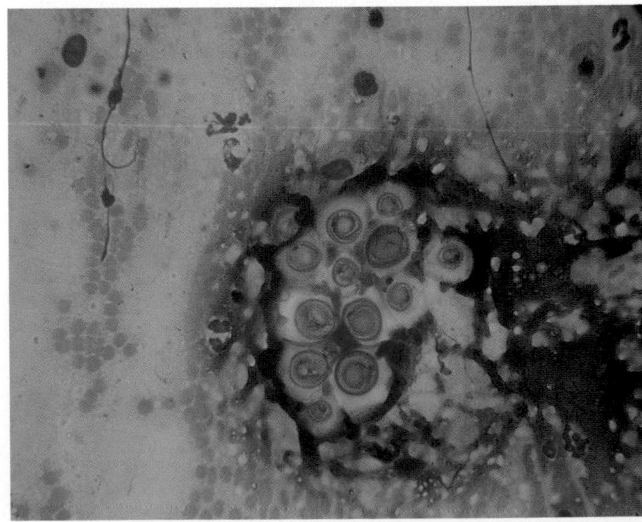

Fig. 57-4 Photomicrograph of cryptococci in exudates from infected maxillary sinus in horse.

Culture

Cryptococcus neoformans is easily cultured on standard fungal media that do not contain cycloheximide. Large, cream to yellow-colored colonies appear in 3 to 5 days when the yeast is cultured on Sabouraud dextrose agar.[23] Encapsulated colonies are mucoid.[47] Mycelia are rarely observed in culture. Colonies produce urease, assimilate D-proline, and grow readily at 37° C.[23] A generous inoculum may increase the likelihood of a positive culture. Sedimentation of 15 to 20 mL of CSF is reported to facilitate culturing cryptococci in other species,[47] and collecting such a large sample from an adult horse would be feasible.

Cryptococcus neoformans can be distinguished from most other species of *Cryptococcus* by its ability to produce melanin through phenol oxidase. When cultured on Staib's birdseed agar, colonies acquire brown to black pigment.[25] Several commercial methods are available to identify the species of the isolate. For epidemiologic studies, individual strains of *C. neoformans* can be biotyped or fingerprinted.[25]

Cultures may require several weeks for a positive result and thus are not helpful in the immediate management of clinical patients. A rapid urease test is used for expedient identification of *C. neoformans* in human patients.[25]

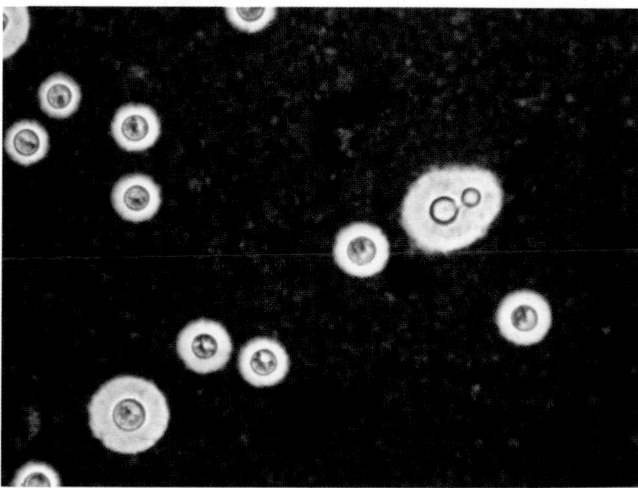

Fig. 57-5 Cryptococci in India ink preparation. The infected material was obtained from a cat. (Courtesy Dr. Joe Kowalski, The Ohio State University College of Veterinary Medicine.)

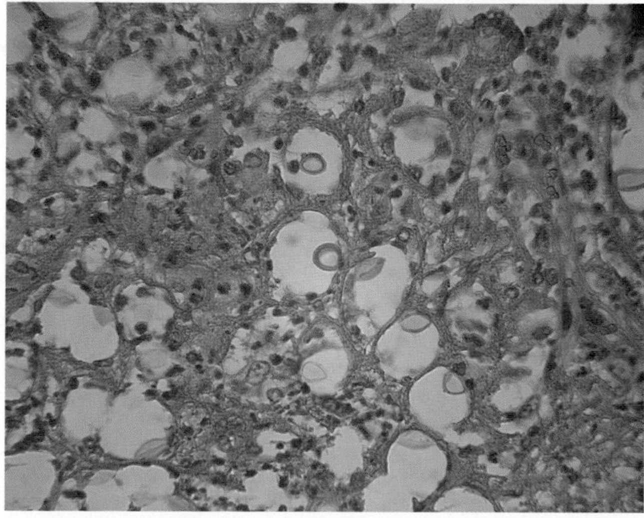

Fig. 57-6 Photomicrograph of cryptococci in meninges of horse. Note the clear halo of the unstained capsule surrounding the yeast cell. (40×.)

Serology

Assays for Cryptococcal Antigens. In persons and cats with cryptococcosis, the capsular polysaccharide antigen glucuronoxylomannan is not rapidly cleared from circulation and may be identified by a latex agglutination assay that utilizes specific rabbit hyperimmune immunoglobulin coating the latex particles.[8] Five immunodiagnostic kits for identification of cryptococcal antigen are commercially available in the United States.[25,47] Depending on the particular kit, these tests can detect as little as 10 ng of capsular polysaccharide.[25] Elimination of most interfering substances can be accomplished by digesting the test serum or CSF with pronase.[25,50] In humans a positive agglutination at a dilution of 1:4 is strongly suggestive of cryptococcal infection, whereas a titer of 1:8 is usually an indication of active infection.[25] Infected cats may display very high dilution titers (1:10,000), and a titer greater than 1 is considered positive.[47] Antigen detection is more sensitive (about 95%) than culture (about 75%) or India ink preparation in people[25] and is reported to have a sensitivity of 95% and a specificity of 100% in the cat.[51] False-positive tests may result from rare cross-reactions with antigens from other microorganisms (e.g., *Trichosporon asahii*, formerly *T. beigleii*) or contamination with agar or agarose.[8,25] False-negative tests may arise as a result of low levels of antigen, interfering immune complexes, a prozone effect (high titers of antigen), or infection with a strain that is poorly encapsulated or unencapsulated.[25] Pretreatment of the sample with pronase eliminates the immune complexes, and the effect of antigen excess is ameliorated by dilution.[8]

Changes in capsular antigen titer have proved useful in monitoring response to treatment in cats and humans.[25,47] Successful treatment is associated with a reduction in antigen titer, although decreases in antigen titer may lag behind clinical response.[47] Because results from test kits may vary, it is important to use the same methodology for successive tests.

In the few reports of measurement of serum cryptococcal antigen titers in horses, this test appears to be useful in the diagnosis and management of cryptococcal disease in this species. Serial evaluation of serum cryptococcal antigen concentrations using latex agglutination titer methodology[33] (Wampole Crypto LA, Wampole Laboratories, Cranbury, NJ) during successful treatment of a pony for cryptococcal pneumonia showed that the initial titer was 1:4096. When recovered, the pony's titer was 1:256.[31] The pericardial fluid cryptococcal antigen titer was 1:1024 in a foal with cryptococcal pneumonia.[37]

Enzyme immunoassays (EIAs), employing monoclonal antibodies for recognition of serotypes, have been developed to detect cryptococcal capsular polysaccharide antigen and anticryptococcal antibodies. EIAs have several advantages over latex agglutination tests; EIAs are less subjective, are unaffected by prozone reactions, are more sensitive, may detect antigen earlier, and may have fewer false-positive results.[25] EIAs should not be used for urine.[8] To date, use of EIA has not been reported in the diagnosis of cryptococcosis in horses.

Molecular typing and immunocytochemistry were used to identify one isolate from a horse as *Cryptococcus gattii*.[31]

Antibody Detection. In other species, anticryptococcal antibodies are not usually detected during active infection, and assessment of serum antibody concentrations is not useful for diagnosis. Serial assessments of serum antibody concentrations may be useful in monitoring therapy because the appearance of serum anticryptococcal antibodies may be a good prognostic sign. Antibody has been detected in healthy horses that were previously infected or were sequestering a latent infection.

Pathologic Findings

Cryptococcus neoformans causes both focal and disseminated disease in horses. Although clinical signs referable to one organ system may be prominent, widespread pathologic lesions may be discovered at necropsy. Histologically, typical lesions are characterized by a "soap bubble" appearance resulting from aggregation of many cryptococcal organisms with unstained capsules[52] (Fig. 57-7). Cellular reaction is usually minimal and characterized by relatively small numbers of variably degenerated macrophages, neutrophils, and lymphocytes. Other, likely more chronic lesions may be granulomatous, with multinucleate giant cells and epithelioid cells, and fibrous tissue surrounding the yeast cells.

Upper Respiratory Tract

Gross lesions may vary from nodular and granulomatous to gelatinous. Endoscopically, the lesions appear as fleshy, firm, yellowish, discrete or lobulated masses of irregular contour, sometimes associated with yellow mucinous exudate. The lesions may invade adjacent bone.

Lower Respiratory Tract

Gross lesions vary from discrete nodules to large, caseous masses that may replace a major portion of the lung. Few or many nodules may be present and widely disseminated in the lung. Calcium deposition may be evident in some nodules, and hemosiderin deposition may be obvious. In more severely affected horses the lung may be swollen or diffusely consolidated with many viscous, mucopurulent abscesses. The caseous material may be yellow and gelatinous.[53] When the cryptococcal capsules are large, the lesions may have a grossly mucinous texture.[52] Variously extensive fibrosis may be present in other areas of the lungs. Hilar lymph nodes may be enlarged and reactive or caseous. Pleuritis and pleural effusion may be present.

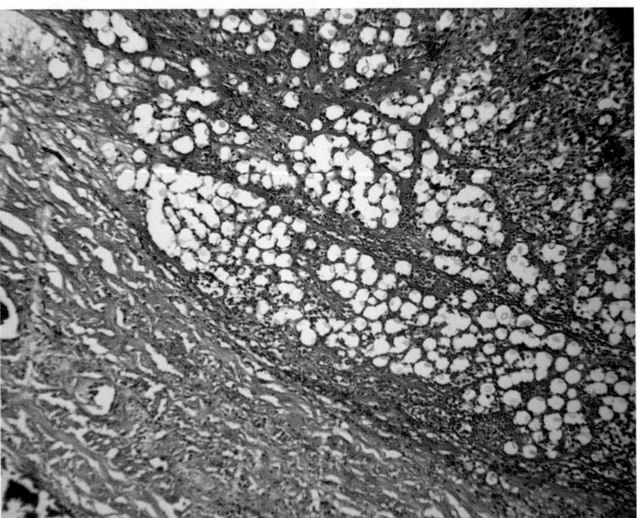

Fig. 57-7 Histologically, typical lesions from *Cryptococcus neoformans* are characterized by a "soap bubble" appearance resulting from aggregation of many cryptococcal organisms with unstained capsules.

Central Nervous System

Cryptococcus has a predilection for the meninges in horses, although lesions in the brain and spinal cord have also been observed.[36,41,54] Gross lesions may appear as discrete gelatinous foci with thickening of the meninges or as cystlike cavitations in brain tissue. Histologic examination of the tissues is often required to identify lesions because they may not otherwise be apparent.[52]

Gastrointestinal Tract

Gastrointestinal localization of cryptococcal organisms is rarely reported in horses. One of the three horses reported to have abdominal manifestations of cryptococcal infection had large cryptococcal abscesses of mesenteric lymph nodes that were adherent to adjacent segments of large colon, duodenum, ileum, and uterus.[30] Another horse had a polypoid cryptococcal granuloma attached by a narrow stalk to the mucosal wall of the jejunum at the site of an intussusception.[28] The third horse had a small, intramural cryptococcal granuloma in the jejunum that was an incidental finding at necropsy.[30]

Reproductive Tract

Two mares were reported to have cryptococcal placentitis and endometritis. Placentitis was characterized by diffusely distended stroma of the allantochorion, with associated yeasts and mild infiltration of neutrophils on the chorionic surface.[37,46] Two mares that aborted foals with cryptococcosis had endometrial biopsies characterized by clusters of giant cells within the stratum spongiosum and individual multinucleate giant cells within the stratum compactum. Giant cells contained cryptococci.[46]

Subcutaneous Tissue

An extensive ulcerating cryptococcal mass involving the skin and subcutaneous tissues was found at necropsy adherent to the parietal pleura and adjacent lung.[45]

Therapy

Treatment of horses with cryptococcal disease has been infrequently attempted and has been unsuccessful with the exception of two cases: an apparently isolated jejunal lesion successfully resected[28] and recently a pony mare treated for cryptococcal pneumonia.[31] The decision not to treat affected horses is often made because of the expense of therapy, the invasive and frequently extensive nature of cryptococcal lesions, and the poor prognosis.

Successful treatment of a large cryptococcal pulmonary granuloma was accomplished using intravenous (IV) AMB (Fungizone).[31] The minimum inhibitory concentration (MIC) of the yeast for AMB was 0.25 mg/L. This value was obtained by a method in 89% agreement with the standard broth microdilution test, according to the U.S. Clinical and Laboratory Standards Institute (CLSI, formerly National Committee for Clinical Laboratory Standards, NCCLS) Document M27-A guidelines.[55] The MIC for the yeast was within the in vitro minimum fungicidal range reported for *C. neoformans*.[56]

The initial dose of AMB was 0.35 mg/kg diluted in 1 L of 5% dextrose in water (D_5W) and infused over 1 hour. Muscle tremors, tachycardia, and pyrexia followed the second dose, and thereafter the mare was pretreated with flunixin meglumine, 100 mg intravenously (IV). On day 4 the dose of AMB was increased to 0.4 mg/kg, and on day 6, to 0.5 mg/kg IV. On day 8 the IV dose of flunixin meglumine was reduced to 50 mg. The pony was treated daily for 31 days, receiving a cumulative dose of 3 gAMB. During treatment, the urine specific gravity decreased to 1.005-1.006; no attempt was made to examine the urinary sediment, and the pony was not uremic. Ten months after treatment, the urine specific gravity remained decreased at 1.016. Despite some evidence of renal toxicity, the pony tolerated the AMB treatments well and did not experience other drug reactions when pretreated with flunixin meglumine. The pony recovered very well and returned to athletic use.

The results in this case of severe focal pulmonary cryptococcosis suggest that more aggressive attempts at treating this infection in horses may be warranted. Although cryptococcal organisms may display high MICs for fluconazole, as did the isolate in this case (8 mg/L), other isolates may be susceptible to fluconazole, for which the pharmacokinetics in horses have been well described.[57] Combination antifungal therapy may also be useful.

HISTOPLASMOSIS

Histoplasmosis is an uncommon disease of horses, although serologic studies suggest that in endemic areas, many horses have been exposed to the pathogen *Histoplasma capsulatum*. The fungus can cause disease in immunocompetent animals and people, particularly after exposure to a large, usually inhaled, amount of fungus. In immunocompromised persons a life-threatening, disseminated manifestation of infection is common. Reports of histoplasmosis in horses are too limited to warrant drawing conclusions about epidemiology, treatment, or prognosis in this species, except with respect to *Histoplasma farciminosum*.

Etiology

Three varieties of the dimorphic ascomycete *Histoplasma capsulatum* are identified: (1) *H. capsulatum* var. *capsulatum*, the cause of histoplasmosis in animals and humans; (2) *H. capsulatum* var. *duboisii*, the cause of a distinct variant form of disease in humans, African histoplasmosis; and (3) *H. capsulatum* var. *farciminosum (HCF)*, the agent causing enzootic lymphangitis in horses in Africa, the Middle East, and parts of Asia. Only *H. capsulatum* var. *capsulatum* is found in North America. *H. capsulatum* var. *farciminosum* is discussed in a separate section following this discussion of *H. capsulatum*. In nature, *H. capsulatum* var. *capsulatum* (hereafter referred to as *H. capsulatum*) is a filamentous fungus. It colonizes moist soil with high nitrogen content and is found in bat and bird guano, particularly the excreta of chickens and starlings.

In culture on Sabouraud dextrose agar the fungus grows in 2 to 3 weeks as white or brown colonies.[8] The mycelia produce macroconidia (8-16 μm in diameter) and microconidia (2-5 μm in diameter). Because of their small size, microconidia are readily aerosolized and respirable and are the primary etiologic agents of disease. At 37° C, microconidia germinate and form mycelia that are transformed into small (2-5 μm in diameter), budding, oval yeasts. Budding occurs at the narrow end of the yeast cell, forming a narrow, often long and threadlike, distinctive neck.[1] Three to 6 weeks is required for the process of conversion to the mycelia and then to the yeast form of the organism in culture.[8]

Virulence

A variety of factors contribute to the virulence of *H. capsulatum*. The conidia of the filamentous fungus are infectious, but conversion to the yeast form is a requirement for virulence in the host. *H. capsulatum* is not an obligate intracellular parasite, but it lives within cells of the reticular endothelial system and is disseminated by them within the host.[58] The yeast is phagocytized by macrophages after opsonization with antibody or complement. The yeast binds to integrins on the surface of mononuclear cells through a recently discovered ligand (HSP60) on the yeast cell surface. *H. capsulatum* also binds to a specific receptor on the surface of dendritic cells. Dendritic cells have substantially greater anti–*H. capsulatum* activity than macrophages. The nature of these yeast/host phagocytic cell interactions, the subject of ongoing research, may influence the ability of the yeast to remain viable once engulfed by the phagocytic cell. Viable intracellular yeasts inhabit phagolysosomes with a higher pH than those containing dead *H. capsulatum* organisms. The yeast may be able to alter the intracellular environment to permit survival and growth. Production of calcium-binding protein by yeast cells is controlled by expression of the CBP1 gene. Expression of this gene during host cell infection is another requirement for virulence.[59]

Limiting availability of free iron is one mammalian host defense against invasion by bacterial and fungal pathogens, including *H. capsulatum*. The yeast has three mechanisms for acquiring iron that is essential for pathogenicity: (1) secretion of low-molecular-weight iron-chelating siderophores that scavenge ferric iron; (2) the ability to reduce ferric to ferrous iron and thereby utilize iron from ferric salts; and (3) acidification of transferrin-containing microenvironments in the host cell, releasing bound iron.[59]

Epidemiology

Histoplasmosis is the most common endemic mycosis of humans.[8] *Histoplasma* spp. are distributed worldwide. The fungus thrives in microclimates where the ambient temperature varies from 22° to 29° C (80°-90° F), the annual precipitation is 35 to 50 inches per year, and the relative humidity is 67% to 87%.[1] *H. capsulatum* is endemic in the Mississippi, Missouri, and Ohio River valleys, southwestern and eastern Ontario to Montreal, Ottawa, and the St. Lawrence River Valley, some regions of South America, and focal regions around the world where the climate is optimum for growth (Fig. 57-8). Within a favorable climatic zone, the fungi may be focally concentrated in locales where wild or domestic birds congregate. Infection in humans is associated with disturbance of soil that contains the fungus. Infection is not transmissible from host to host, but epidemics may occur after exposure to a common source (e.g., bird roosts, old houses or barns, contaminated soil disturbed during excavation or farming).[60] The organisms may be disseminated by prevailing winds and by migratory birds, particularly the starling.

Clinical disease is relatively uncommon in immunocompetent humans and very uncommon in horses; however, exposure to infectious propagules and asymptomatic infection are common. From 50% to 80% of healthy persons in endemic areas are reported to have positive delayed hypersensitivity reactions to intradermal *histoplasmin*, a filtrate of broth containing the fungal mycelia.[8,58,61] Of 467 healthy horses in central Kentucky, 50% reacted positively to histoplasmin in one survey,[62] whereas 8.7% of 51 horses in Uruguay were positive,[63] 7.9% of 2221 horses in Mexico were positive,[64] and 73% of 44 horses were positive in Missouri.[62,65]

Pathogenesis

Inhaled microconidia reach the small airways, where the spores germinate into the yeast form of the organism. Phagocytic cells of the reticuloendothelial system, particularly pulmonary macrophages and dendritic cells, engulf the yeast.

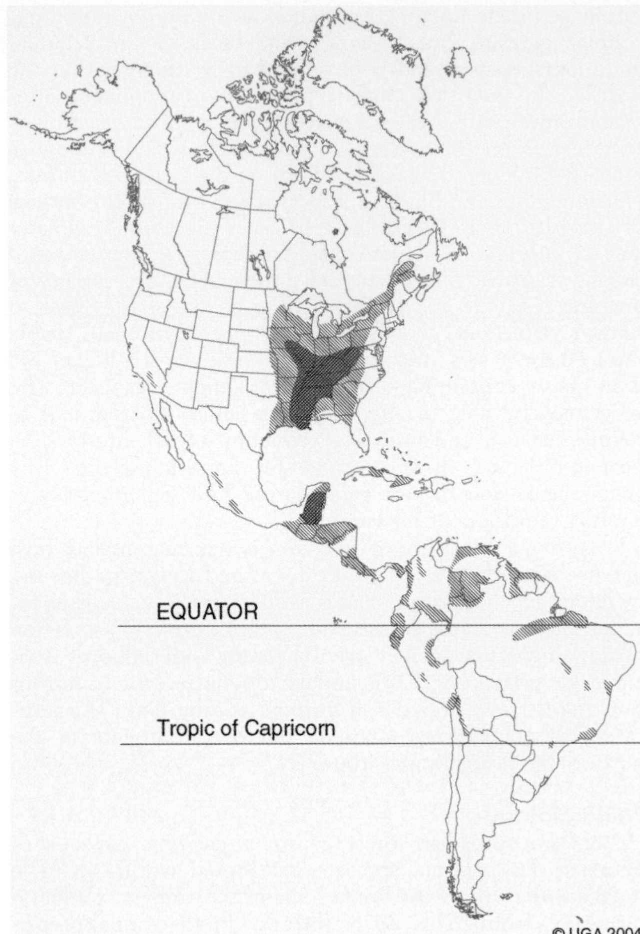

Fig. 57-8 Prevalence of histoplasmosis in North and South America based on seropositivity in people. Shading indicates areas of endemic histoplasmosis. Darker shading indicates areas of higher incidence. (From Greene C: *Infectious diseases of the dog and cat,* ed 3, Philadelphia, 2006, Saunders.)

Parasitized phagocytes efficiently disseminate the yeast to tissues rich in reticuloendothelial cells, such as lymph nodes, spleen, liver, and bone marrow. Occasionally the yeast may localize in the CNS. Reticuloendothelial cells throughout the body ingest and sequester the yeasts.[60] In immunocompetent hosts, a robust cell-mediated immune response occurs in 10 to 14 days. Antigen-specific T-lymphocyte–mediated immunity develops, and macrophages become fungicidal and kill the intracellular organisms.[58] Necrotic foci may develop at the site of infection. These foci become abscesses that are soon encased in a fibrous capsule. Calcification may occur over the ensuing several years.[60] Clinical signs of disease are often not observed when the fungal load is light and the invading yeasts are well controlled by the host's immune system. Viable yeast cells may be sequestered within granulomata and may subsequently be reactivated by the onset of another debilitating disease or by immunosuppression.

Exposure to a large inoculum may induce disease in immunocompetent hosts. Clinical signs in persons usually develop approximately 3 weeks after inhalation of the microconidia.[8] Recovery from natural infection confers some immunity. Persons may become hypersensitive to the yeast and may experience a severe or even fatal anaphylactic reaction on reexposure.[1] A poor cell-mediated immune response allows progressive dissemination of the yeast that may result in fatal disease.[60] Disseminated histoplasmosis usually occurs in persons with T-cell deficiencies.

Lymphatic tissue in the gastrointestinal (GI) tract may be a destination of disseminated yeasts. Additionally, the host may cough up and swallow infectious material from the lung. Resultant ulcerative enterocolitis and typhlitis in horses may be associated with protein-losing enteropathy, panhypoproteinemia, edema, diarrhea, or intestinal perforation.

Clinical Signs

Clinical manifestations of *H. capsulatum* infection in humans depend on inoculum size and the immune competence of the affected person. Immunocompetent patients may have asymptomatic infections or mild, flulike disease. In the latter case, thoracic radiographs may show a focal or miliary distribution of small, calcified nodules. Recovery may take weeks to months. Healthy or immunocompromised persons may develop chronic lung disease characterized by transient signs of pneumonia. This is followed by chronic indolent lung disease in immunocompetent persons or signs of progressive fibrosis, cavitation, necrosis, and death in patients who are or become immunocompromised.[8]

Surveys of the response to intradermal histoplasmin suggest that many horses residing in endemic areas have been exposed to the fungus, but disease is reported infrequently, suggesting that horses are relatively resistant to histoplasmosis. Among 22 cases of equine histoplasmosis reported in literature, 14 horses had pulmonary disease, eight had abdominal or GI disease, and one foal had CNS disease. Five mares aborted as result of *Histoplasma*-induced placentitis or histoplasmosis in the foal.[66-78] Some horses had more than one affected organ system, and one adult horse had disseminated histoplasmosis.[76] Clinical signs among infected horses include chronic weight loss, depression, fever, dyspnea, anorexia, edema, diarrhea, abortion, and neonatal death. *H. capsulatum* was isolated in cultures of the spleen from a clinically normal mare and from the fetal membranes of her foal.[74,79]

Gastrointestinal histoplasmosis is uncommon in humans and usually occurs in persons with mediastinal histoplasmosis or progressive disseminated disease.[80] Clinical signs in persons include hematochezia or melena, abdominal pain associated with peritonitis, toxemia caused by rupture of ulcerated bowel, or pain associated with colonic obstruction by a large inflammatory mass. Intestinal histoplasmosis has been described in two horses[69,74] and was found at necropsy in an additional five horses.[73] Both the reported horses had a history of chronic weight loss and progressive anorexia. Diarrhea, edema, and in one horse progressive toxemia resulted in the demise of these two horses.

Mycotic Keratitis

Keratitis caused by *Histoplasma* spp. was reported in a horse from Germany.[81] The horse displayed blepharospasm and endophthalmitis. A white opacity located ventrally and centrally in the cornea contained several subepithelial bullae and diffusely stained with fluorescein. The rest of the eye was not affected.

Diagnosis

Thoracic Radiography

Pulmonary disease is common in horses with histoplasmosis, and thoracic radiographs may demonstrate isolated, sometimes calcific nodules; multiple miliary nodules; diffuse interstitial densities; or focal cavitating lesions.

Cytology

Yeast cells may be identifiable in smears from transtracheal wash, BAL, peritoneal fluid, or blood specimens and in impression smears of tissues. Cytologic examination of bone marrow aspirates may also be helpful. The material should be fixed on a slide with methyl alcohol and stained with Wright's or Giemsa stain. The ovoid cells, 2 to 4 μm in diameter with a bud at the narrow end, are seen within macrophages or free in fluid or tissue. The yeast cell wall appears as an unstained halo around the cell.[1] Small, atypical *Blastomyces* or acapsular *Cryptococcus neoformans* (among other agents or artifacts) may be mistaken for *H. capsulatum*.[8] Cytology is an insensitive method of detecting *Histoplasma*, and confirmatory tests are required to establish the diagnosis.

Laboratory Tests

Assessment of a serum chemistry profile may be helpful, particularly in horses with GI histoplasmosis that are likely to have panhypoproteinemia associated with protein-losing enteropathy. Leukopenia and neutropenia may be evident if bowel wall integrity is lost. Other agents that could induce inflammatory bowel disease or diarrhea should be sought. One horse was reported to have concurrent salmonellosis with histoplasmosis.[74]

Culture

Culture of the organism remains the gold standard for diagnosis of histoplasmosis. The fungus will grow on Sabouraud dextrose agar or blood agar without antibiotics at 25° C under moist conditions to prevent the plates from drying out. Colonies that appear on blood agar are initially glabrous, pink to reddish brown, and develop into mycelia that are white to brownish. These colonies are very similar to those of *Blastomyces dermatitidis* and other fungi. Incubation at 37° C and demonstration of the characteristic yeast cell are required for identification of *H. capsulatum*. Cultures should be kept for 6 to 12 weeks.[1]

Limitations to the use of a positive culture as the basis for diagnosis and management of affected persons include (1) human patients with mild forms of histoplasmosis usually have negative cultures; (2) about 20% of patients with disseminated and 50% of those with chronic pulmonary histoplasmosis have false-negative cultures; (3) the slow growth of cultures precludes using culture results as a basis for therapy; (4) antibody production may be poor in immunocompromised hosts; and (5) invasive procedures may be required to obtain samples for culture.[61] An exoantigen test or molecular characterization may also be used for identification.

Histopathology

Tissue samples should be stained with GMS or PAS stains (Fig. 57-9). Experience is required to identify the yeast cells reliably in tissues and to distinguish them from other organisms. The sensitivity of histopathology for the diagnosis of human histoplasmosis is low (<50%).[61]

Serology

Immunodiffusion (ID) and complement fixation (CF) tests are standard for diagnosis of histoplasmosis in humans.[61] The ID test, which recognizes the H and M antigens of *H. capsulatum*, is less sensitive than CF. Host CF response is greater to the mycelial than to the yeast antigen. Positive CF titers are found in about 95% of persons with histoplasmosis, although only weakly positive titers (1:8 or 1:16) may be found in 25% to 33% of patients. Cross-reactions can occur in patients with blastomycosis, aspergillosis, coccidioidomycosis, or candidiasis.

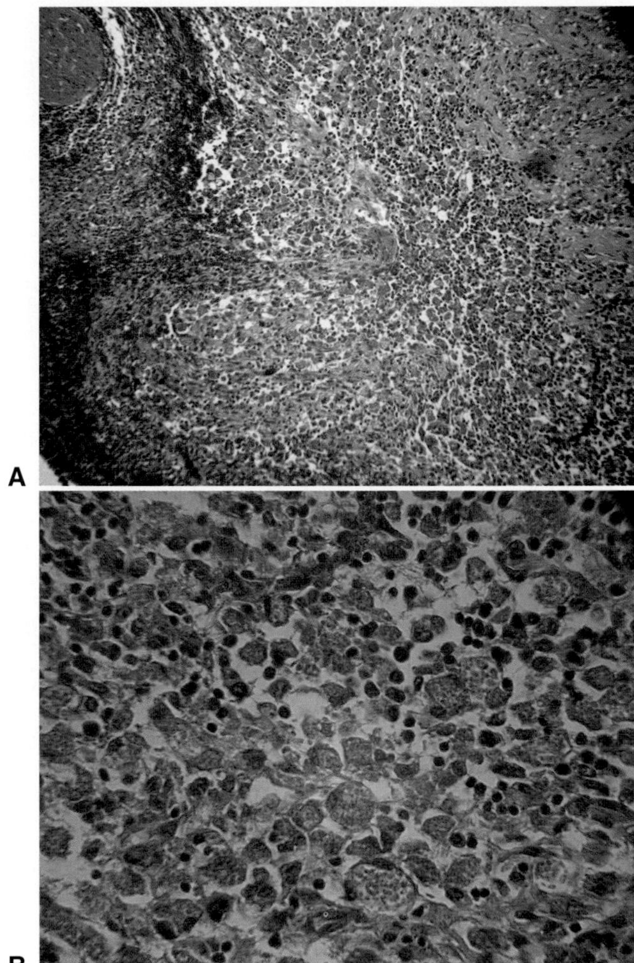

Fig. 57-9 A, Photomicrograph of *Histoplasma* yeast cells in spleen of weanling Standardbred filly with disseminated histoplasmosis. **B,** Photomicrograph of *Histoplasma* yeast cells in giant cells in spleen of weanling Standardbred filly with disseminated histoplasmosis.

Chronic histoplasmosis is associated with persistent antibodies, and prolonged exposure or latent infection may result in detection of antibodies for several years. Results of serologic testing do not provide a definitive diagnosis and should not be used as a basis for determining appropriate treatment. Antibodies to *H. capsulatum* were identified by AGID in one horse with pulmonary histoplasmosis.[72]

Antigen Detection. Antigens are released from yeast cells during active infection and may be detected in blood, urine, and other body fluids, particularly in human patients with disseminated or acute pulmonary histoplasmosis after inhalation of a large number of microconidia. For patients with acute pulmonary disease, BAL fluid antigen titers may be higher than serum or urine titers. In general, antigen detection is more sensitive in urine than in serum. False-negative tests may occur, probably because of low fungal burden. Serial determination of antigenemia or antigenuria is useful in monitoring response to therapy and in detecting relapse in human patients because reductions in antigenemia/uria are associated with successful treatment, whereas increasing values suggest recrudescence of disease. False-positive tests are rare in people, but cross-reactions may occur in patients with blastomycosis and other fungal diseases.[61]

Antigen detection would likely be useful in confirming a diagnosis of histoplasmosis in horses. To date, there are no reports of attempts at antigen detection in horses with histoplasmosis.[61]

Molecular Identification. Polymerase chain reaction (PCR) and DNA probe methods for detecting *H. capsulatum* in tissues have shown some promise and are currently under development. DNA probes are commercially available for identification of culture isolates.[61]

Intradermal Testing

Intradermal testing with histoplasmin is of no use diagnostically because of the large number of persons and horses in endemic areas with positive reactions to histoplasmin from exposure to *H. capsulatum*. False-positive results are observed in human patients with other fungal diseases. Exposure to histoplasmin increases serum antibody concentrations, further confounding the diagnosis.[61]

Pathology

Gross necropsy findings in affected horses include enlarged, firm lungs; swollen, mottled, yellow-tan liver; dilated, thickened, ulcerated or hemorrhagic intestine; enlarged tracheobronchial lymph nodes; and focal placental necrosis.[73] One horse with GI histoplasmosis had widespread, deeply ulcerated lesions in the cecum and colon.[74]

Histopathology of tissues from affected horses showed focal or coalescing pyogranulomatous inflammation with many macrophages and giant cells. In tissues from aborted fetuses and neonatal foals, focal infiltration with multinucleate giant cells containing yeast cells was seen in lung, liver, lymph nodes, and intestines.[73] In placental lesions the subchorionic stroma adjacent to blood vessels, the surface of the allantois, and chorionic villi were most prominently affected and were sites where organisms could be detected.[73] The submucosa of the cecum and colon was diffusely infiltrated with lymphocytes and macrophages laden with yeast cells (pyogranulomatous inflammation) in one horse with intestinal histoplasmosis.[74]

Tables 57-1 and 57-2 summarize the sensitivity of selected diagnostic tests for pulmonary and disseminated histoplasmosis, respectively, in human patients.

Table • 57-1

Sensitivity (% Positive) of Laboratory Tests for Diagnosis of Pulmonary Histoplasmosis in Humans

TEST	ACUTE OR SUBACUTE PULMONARY,* PERICARDITIS, RHEUMATOLOGIC	CHRONIC PULMONARY	MEDIASTINAL
Antigen	25-75	15	0
Fungal stain	10	40	<25
Culture	15	50-85	<25
Serology	95	100	67

From Wheat LJ: *Trends Microbiol* 11(10):488, 2003.

*In acute pulmonary, the sensitivity of antigen detection ranges from about 25% in patients with local manifestations to greater than 75% in those who present within the first month of exposure.

Table • 57-2

Sensitivity (% Positive) of Laboratory Tests for Diagnosis of Disseminated Histoplasmosis in Humans

TEST	NOT IMMUNE SUPPRESSED	IMMUNE SUPPRESSED
Histology	40-61	57-64
Serology	85-100	82
Immunodiffusion*	71-100	57-77
Complement fixation†	85-97	60-79
Culture	86-90	82-89
Antigen Detection		
Urine	80	82
Serum	67	60
Either	82	82

*For H and M bands.

†With yeast and mycelial antigens.

Mycotic Keratitis

In one horse with keratitis, a smear of a specimen obtained by corneal brushing and stained with Wright's stain showed intracellular and extracellular, spherical, globular structures up to 4 μm in size that were surrounded by an unstained halo. A presumptive diagnosis of histoplasmosis was made based on cytology. Fungal cultures were negative.[81]

Therapy

Histoplasmosis is a rare disease in horses, and data are insufficient to draw conclusions about equine treatment. Treatment of affected horses has been infrequently attempted because of the severity of clinical signs, failure to make the diagnosis, expense of treatment, and concerns of a poor prognosis for recovery from fungal disease.

One 2-year-old filly was successfully treated for *Histoplasma* pneumonia.[72] The horse was treated with AMB (Fungizone) using an escalating dosage regimen similar to that previously described for cryptococcal pneumonia in horses.[82] The filly was given AMB 0.3, 0.45, and 0.6 mg/kg IV in 1 L of D5W infused over 4 hours on days 1, 2, and 3 of treatment. After 4 days without treatment, 0.6 mg/kg AMB was administered every other day for approximately 4 weeks, to a cumulative dose of 6.75 mg/kg. The horse was lethargic for 18 to 24 hours after every treatment and became polyuric and polydipsic during the fourth week of therapy. The urine specific gravity remained at 1.024. The horse made a full recovery to athletic use.

Amphotericin B followed by itraconazole is the recommended therapeutic regimen for acute or chronic pulmonary or disseminated histoplasmosis in humans. Prolonged treatment is required. Recommendations include 6 to 12 weeks of treatment with itraconazole for immunocompetent persons with acute pulmonary histoplasmosis and 12 to 24 months of itraconazole (up to lifelong therapy) for immunocompromised patients with disseminated histoplasmosis.[60]

Mycotic Keratitis

One horse with an ulcer putatively caused by *Histoplasma* spp. was treated with topical fluconazole and 1% atropine for about 5 weeks.[81] To reduce the potential for developing iridocyclitis caused by rapid death of fungi in the stroma, treatments with fluconazole were introduced gradually and increased from twice daily to four times daily over a 4-day period. The cornea over the bullae was scarified to improve penetration of fluconazole. The horse recovered completely, except for a faint corneal scar.

HISTOPLASMA CAPSULATUM VAR. *FARCIMINOSUM*

Histoplasma capsulatum var. *farciminosum* (HCF) is the cause of epizootic lymphangitis of horses in the Middle East, Asia, and Africa. Infection results in ill thrift and decreased ability to work and is a source of major economic loss in countries where the horse is relied on for transport. HCF is not found in North America.

Etiology

As with *Histoplasma capsulatum* var. *capsulatum*, HCF is a thermally dimorphic organism. The saprophytic mycelia and the yeasts found in tissues can be cultivated on Sabouraud dextrose agar enriched with 2.5% glycerol, but PPLO dextrose glycerol agar may be the most useful medium.[83] At 25° C, mycelial colonies appear after 4 to 8 weeks of incubation. The mycelial colonies are yellow to light or deep brown, convoluted, waxy, and cauliflower-like.[83,84] Mycelia produce several types of conidia. Incubation of the mycelial colonies at 35° to 37° C on brain-heart infusion (BHI) agar with 5% blood results in transformation to the yeast form. In one study, transformation required four or five serial transfers to fresh media, performed at intervals of 8 days.[83] Transformation of the mycelial to the yeast phase was achieved within 3 to 4 weeks in another study.[85] The yeast cell closely resembles that of *Histoplasma capsulatum* var. *capsulatum*.

Epidemiology

Epizootic lymphangitis occurs in horses, mules, and donkeys, particularly in Egypt and India and in North Africa, the Middle East, southern Asia, southern Europe, and parts of Russia. It is endemic in countries that border the Mediterranean.[84] Of 2907 Ethiopian cart horses, 26% were infected with HCF based on clinical examination and culture.[86] In contrast, 83 (2.8%) of 3000 horses at a large racing facility in Iraq had enzootic lymphangitis during a 6-month period of observation.[85] Cases were more common in fall and early winter in Iran[85] and in January in Egypt.[1]

The disease is both contagious from equid to equid and zoonotic. Although the route of infection has not been definitively established, direct inoculation of infective propagules through abraded skin or mucous membranes is suspected to be common. Fomites, including harness, mangers, water buckets, and wound dressings, and flies also transmit the organism. Stallions may transmit HCF to mares during breeding. The less common respiratory manifestation of the disease may result from inhalation of HCF when dust is heavily contaminated.

Pathogenesis

After invading the skin, HCF disseminates through the lymphatics to regional lymph nodes or, in severe cases, to other organs.[84] Clinical signs are observed several weeks to 6 months after infection. Nodular lesions develop in the skin along the lymphatics and in the lymph nodes. These lesions eventually ulcerate and drain a thick, mucopurulent material containing yeast cells. Nodules occur wherever there is skin trauma (particularly under the harness and on the extremities). Horses that have a heavy systemic burden of fungi may succumb to pneumonia or failure of other affected organs. Some horses are asymptomatic carriers of HCF, based on the presence of calcified skin lesions, serologic evidence of antibodies, and positive reactions to intradermal tests. These methods do not distinguish exposure from chronic infection.

Clinical Signs

Affected horses display clinical signs referable to cutaneous (most common), ocular, or respiratory disease. In cutaneous disease, granulomatous, often ulcerated masses are seen in chains following lymphatic vessels[84] (Figs. 57-10 and 57-11). Draining ulcerated nodules eventually heal and scar, as others form. The forelimbs, neck, and head are common sites. After about 6 months, few new lesions develop. Mortality is not high (10%-15%), but inability to work because of these painful nodules results in significant economic hardship in countries where the horse is an important beast of burden. In the ocular manifestation of this disease, conjunctivitis, nodular enlargements over facial lymphatics, and nasolacrimal lesions are noted.[87] Serous ocular discharge and swelling of the eyelids are associated with the development of nodules on the conjunctiva or nictitans. Lacrimal and conjunctival lesions are reported to be the only clinical abnormalities noted in some horses in Egypt.[85,87] In the upper respiratory tract, usually near the external nares, HCF forms yellowish papules or nodules that ulcerate and bleed. Pulmonary granulomata may eventually cause fatal disease.[1,88] Disseminated disease has been infrequently reported.[1]

Diagnosis

Pattern recognition of clinical signs in horses in endemic regions is often the basis of diagnosis. Several confirmatory tests have been described. Culture of HCF from body fluids

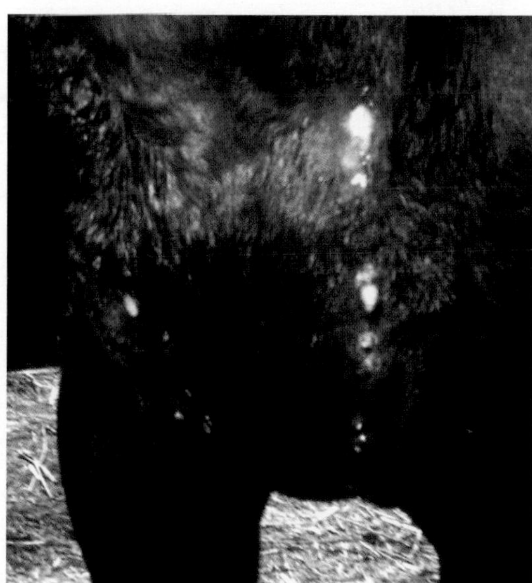

Fig. 57-10 *Histoplasma capsulatum* var. *farciminosum* in pectoral lymphatics of horse. (Courtesy Dr. John Barnes, North Carolina State University.)

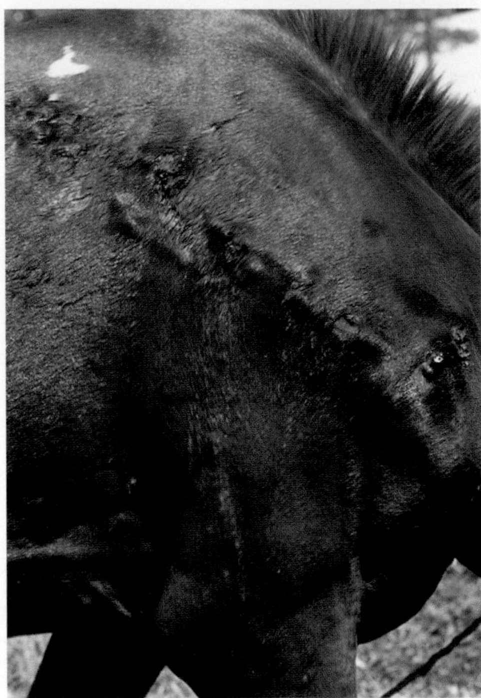

Fig. 57-11 *Histoplasma capsulatum* var. *farciminosum* in lymphatics of shoulder and neck of horse. (Courtesy Dr. John Barnes, North Carolina State University.)

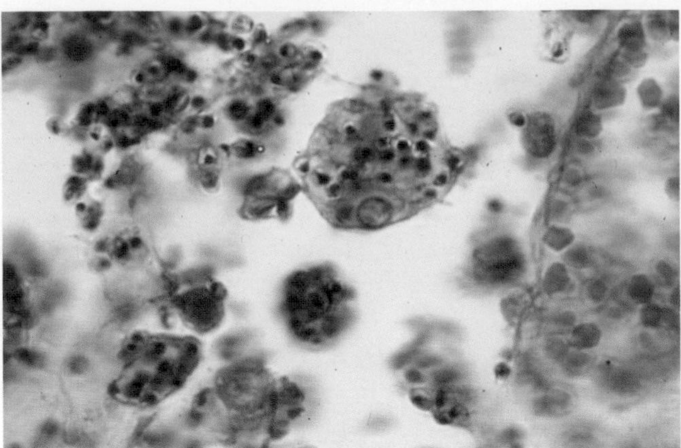

Fig. 57-12 Photomicrograph of *Histoplasma capsulatum* var. *farciminosum* in an infected nodule. (Periodic acid–Schiff stain; 400.) (Courtesy Dr. John Barnes, North Carolina State University.)

or tissues is the "gold standard" for confirming the diagnosis but may be impractical.

Cytology

Cytologic examination of material aspirated from a nodule that has not yet drained usually shows typical yeasts (Fig. 57-12). Giemsa or Gram staining demonstrates round cells 1 to 5 μm in diameter, usually within macrophages. In one study, direct microscopy yielded positive results in 79% of cases.[85]

Culture

The organism may be difficult and time-consuming to grow from body fluids and tissues, and false-negative results are likely. Samples can be cultured at 26° C to induce growth of the mycelial phase of the organism. Subsequent transformation to the yeast form is required to substantiate the diagnosis. In one study, HCF was isolated from 58% of infected horses.[85]

Pathology and Histology

Typical lesions are pyogranulomatous nodules that may be seen in lymphatic vessels, pleura, spleen, liver, bone marrow, and lung. Interstitial pneumonia may also be recognized. Lymphatic vessels may be thickened or fibrotic in chronic or locally resolved infections. Histologically, granulomas are characterized by the presence of many large macrophages, often containing yeast cells that are seen after staining with PAS or GMS stain.[84]

Serologic Tests

Tube agglutination and passive hemagglutination tests have been reported to identify increased titers in horses with epizootic lymphangitis,[89] and this assay can be used as a practical screening test. A serum agglutination titer of 1:80 or higher is reported to be positive.[84] Fluorescent antibody,[90] AGID, and ELISA[89] tests have also been described. Immunodiffusion and CF tests were positive in 26.5% of 200 horses from a farm where epizootic lymphangitis had previously been diagnosed, whereas 3% of horses on the farm were showing clinical signs of the disease when the blood samples were taken.[91] These findings suggest that serologic testing may not have a high degree of specificity for active disease, but it may reflect past exposure or asymptomatic infection.

Animal Inoculation

Immunosuppressed mice are susceptible to HCF and are suitable for diagnostic testing.[84]

Intradermal Testing

Intradermal histofarcin (a soluble antigen) induced a local reaction in all serologically positive horses in one study.[91] Intradermal testing may have low specificity for active disease.

Therapy

In many places, horses with epizootic lymphangitis must be reported to regulatory agencies, and a policy of slaughter and eradication is in effect. In endemic areas where treatment is allowed, oral and IV iodide or AMB have been administered. In conjunction with removal of crusts and exudates from cutaneous lesions, AMB treatment is reported to be successful.[84] In vitro tests have shown that nystatin is more effective than AMB and 5-fluorouracil in inhibiting growth of HCF,[92] and the author suggests using parenteral AMB and concurrent topical nystatin. In another in vitro study, clotrimazole was more effective than AMB at inhibiting the growth of four HCF isolates from sick horses. The MIC of clotrimazole for the mycelial and yeast forms of HCF was 1.25 μg/mL, whereas the MIC for AMB was 100 μg/mL.[93] There are no reports of clinical trials using either of these two therapeutic regimens.

Large lesions can be surgically debrided and packed with iodine.

Prevention

A killed vaccine prepared from the yeast and given subcutaneously to horses has been reported to provide protection. A modified live vaccine is reported to be in use for horses in China. Little information is in the accessible literature concerning these vaccines.

REFERENCES

See the CD-ROM for a list of references linked to the abstract in PubMed.

SUGGESTED READINGS

Gabal MA, Mohammed KA: Use of enzyme-linked immunosorbent assay for the diagnosis of equine histoplasmosis farciminosi (epizootic lymphangitis), *Mycopathologia* 91(1):35, 1985.

Saunders JR, Kaplan W, Matthiesen RJ: Abortion due to histoplasmosis in a mare, *J Am Vet Med Assoc* 183:1097, 1948.

Seslaw S, Maurice GE, Cole CR, et al: Experimental histoplasmosis in large domestic animals, *Proc Soc Exp Biol* 105:76, 1960

Timoney JF, Gillespie JH, Scott FW, et al: The opportunistic fungi. In *Hagan and Bruner's microbiology of infectious diseases of domestic animals*, ed 8, Ithaca, NY, 1988, Comstock Publishing Associates, Cornell University Press, p 407.

SECTION • V
Parasitic Diseases

CHAPTER • 58

Laboratory Diagnosis of Parasitic Diseases

Ellis C. Greiner

Parasites that are covered in this chapter include helminths and protozoans. Some parasites are easily diagnosed because the diagnostic stages passed in the feces are readily detected and identified. Other parasites require more effort to identify because the eggs are not distinguishable; larval fecal cultures are needed to determine the species or groups of nematodes present, and some require special procedures to enhance diagnosis. This chapter assists the equine clinician in sample selection and interpretation of results to facilitate rapid and accurate diagnosis of parasitic diseases of horses.

HELMINTH DIAGNOSIS

Some helminth parasites of horses have complex life cycles, and immature stages may go on circuitous journeys through viscera before attaining the site where the adult worms will develop and produce offspring. Sometimes these worms do not follow the correct route and migrate to the central nervous system, where they may cause severe damage. These conditions are usually confirmed at necropsy, when the parasites may be recovered and identified.

When larval stages of parasites migrate through tissues, normal parasite diagnosis by fecal examination is not possible because the mature adults have not developed and have not begun to produce and release the eggs or larvae. This interval is referred to as the *prepatent period*.

Diagnosis of helminth infection based on observation of eggs or larvae is facilitated by examination of fresh fecal samples. Some parasites are common in horses at any age, whereas others are restricted to the foals because the adult horses mount a sufficient immune response to prevent the adult worms from developing.

A large variety of nematode parasites infect horses. Most reside in the gastrointestinal tract and are detected by fecal examination; examples include the strongyles (Fig. 58-1), ascarids (Fig. 58-2), threadworms (Fig. 58-3), pinworms (Fig. 58-4), lungworms, and stomach worms. Some nematodes reside in solid tissues and do not pass any stages in the feces; these include the filarial worms, *Onchocerca cervicalis*, *O. reticulata*, and *Parafilaria multipapillosa*, which are detected by discovery of microfilariae, which are motile embryos (Fig. 58-5). Some worms cause problems as immature larval stages and do not produce any stages that leave the host. These are usually found by biopsy or are presumptive diagnoses, including summer sores caused by larval stomach worms, species of *Draschia*, and *Habronema*.

The diversity of flatworms is rather depauperate compared with the roundworms. Three species of tapeworms develop as adults in the small intestine, and the larval cyst (hydatid cyst of *Echinococcus*) of one tapeworm rarely develops in the liver. Two liver flukes infect horses in some parts of the world, but this is very uncommon. The latter flukes develop to adults that shed eggs into the feces, which can be detected by fecal examination.

PROTOZOAN DIAGNOSIS

Very few protozoal organisms infect the gastrointestinal tract of horses, and some are believed to be beneficial as the ciliate fauna of the large bowel. Others are pathogenic or potentially pathogenic, including flagellates such as *Giardia* (Fig. 58-6) and possibly *Leishmania* (Fig. 58-7) and coccidians such as *Eimeria* (Fig. 58-8) and *Cryptosporidium* (Fig. 58-9).

LABORATORY PROCEDURES

Procedures that are used to diagnose parasitic infections in horses include gross fecal examination, fecal flotation, fecal culture, fecal sedimentation, direct smear, Baermann procedure, cellophane (Scotch) tape test, McMaster's counts, stained fecal smears, impression smears, skin biopsy examination, and blood smears. It is highly desirable to have a compound microscope calibrated with an ocular micrometer to facilitate precise measurement of ova or other parasite structures.

Gross Fecal Examination

Before altering the feces for diagnostic purposes, examination without magnification for consistency, evidence of blood, and the macroscopic presence of worms should be performed. If the horse is impacted or there is delayed movement of ingesta, parasite ova may be more developed than normal. Conversely, if there is diarrhea, ova may not be as developed as expected. Blood might indicate high numbers of strongyles migrating within the intestinal mucosa, with resultant petechial hemorrhages and frank hemorrhage.

Fecal Flotation

Fecal flotation techniques use a variety of solutions, including sodium nitrate, zinc sulfate, sucrose, and sodium chloride, to identify parasite ova or larvae. The author prefers sodium nitrate as a fecal flotation solution because it will concentrate most nematode eggs and larvae, tapeworm eggs, flagellate cysts, and coccidian oocysts, as well as parasitic mites consumed when the host is trying to alleviate mite-associated pruritus. The goal is to establish a solution with a specific gravity that will allow the eggs to float to the top of a liquid column, effectively

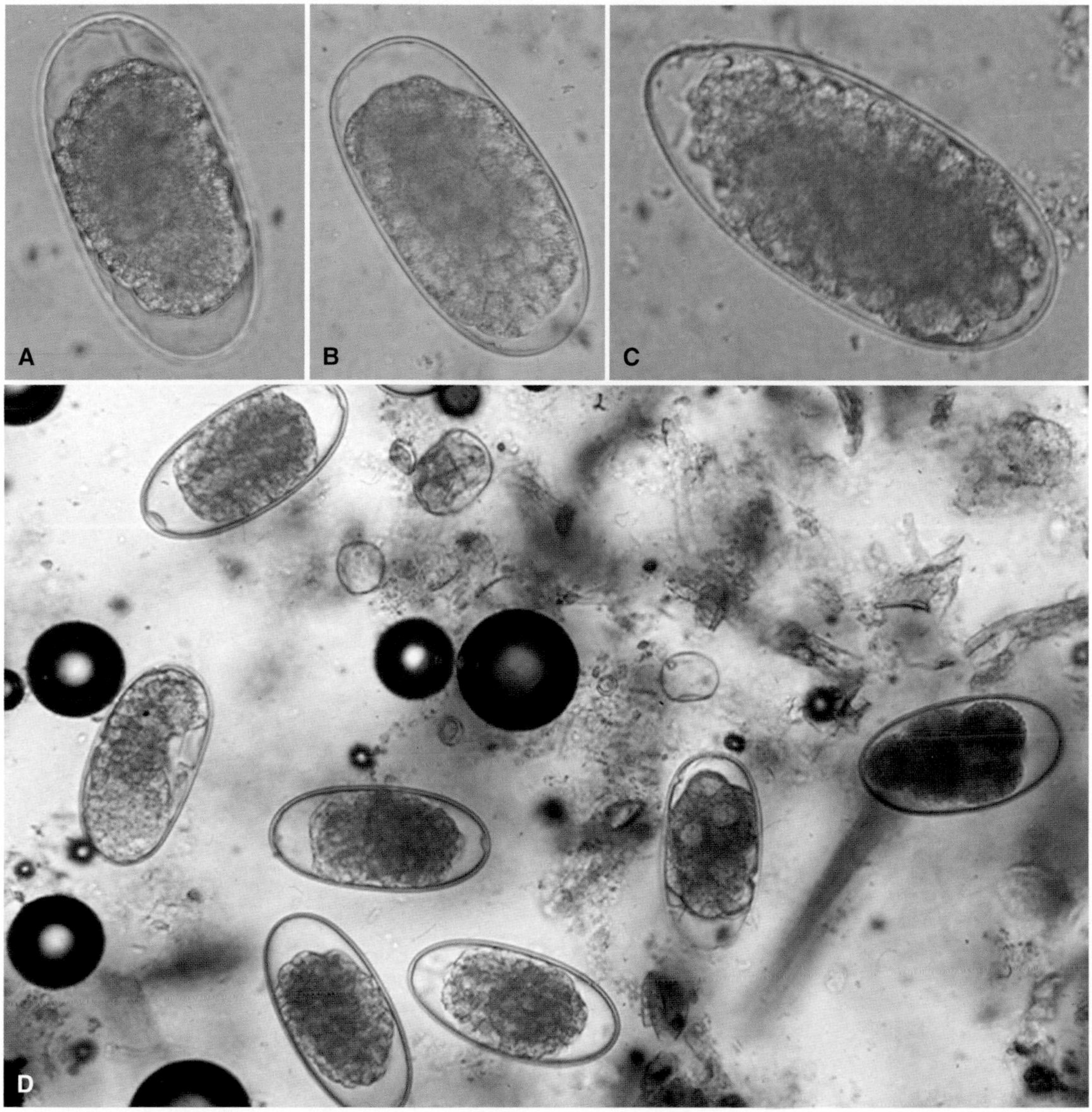

Fig. 58-1 **A,** Strongyle egg (112 × 54 μm). **B,** Strongyle egg (104 × 51 μm). **C,** Strongyle egg (90 × 69 μm). **D,** Strongyle eggs.

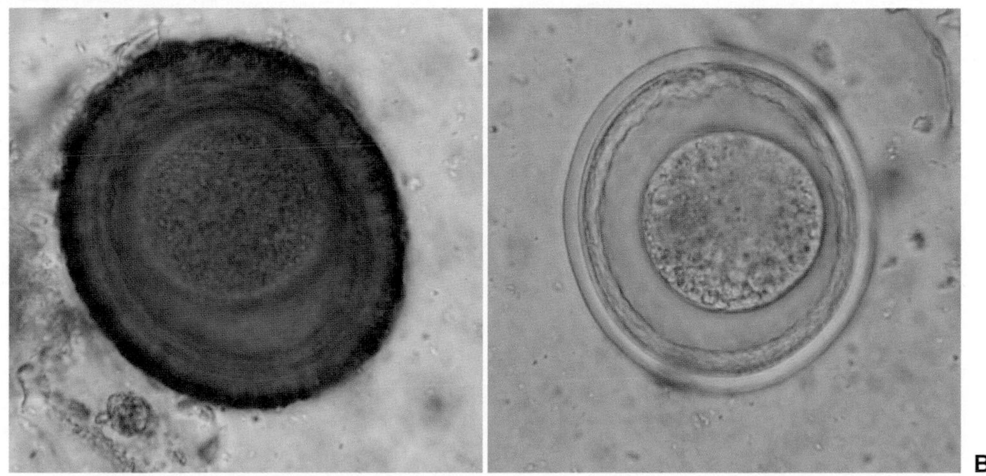

Fig. 58-2 **A,** *Parascaris equorum* egg (88 × 77 μm). **B,** *P. equorum* infertile and atypical egg (80 × 66 μm).

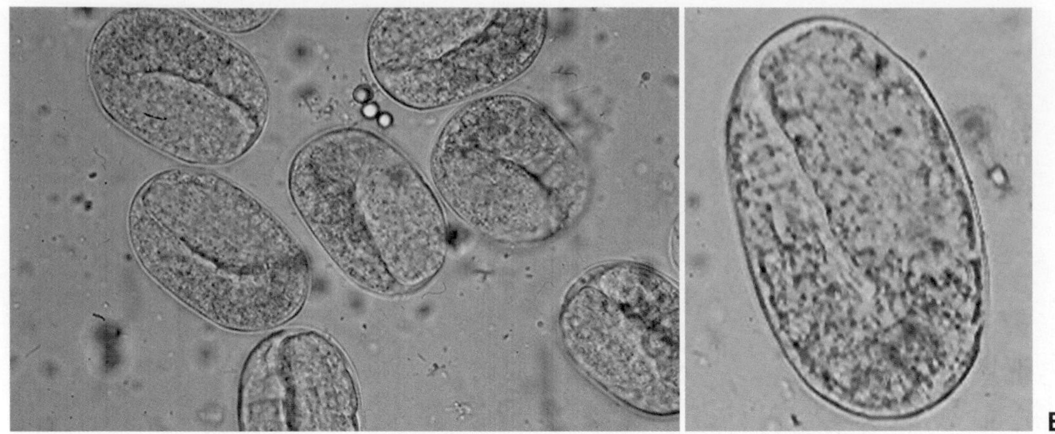

Fig. 58-3 A, *Strongyloides westeri* eggs. B, *S. westeri* egg (58 × 33 μm).

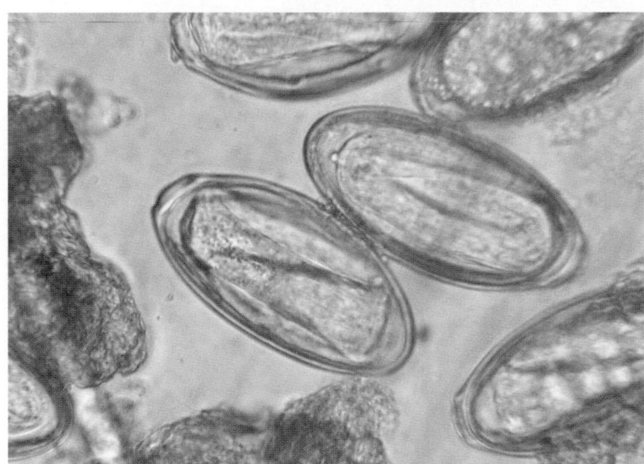

Fig. 58-4 *Oxyuris equi* eggs (88 × 42 μm).

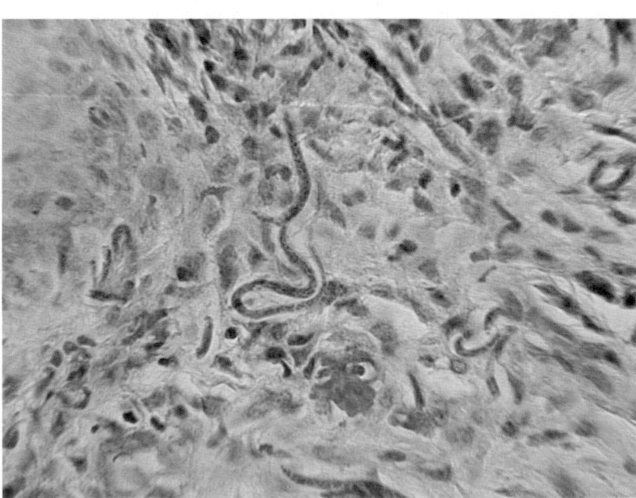

Fig. 58-5 *Onchocerca cervicalis* microfilariae in skin section (width, 3.5 μm).

concentrating and cleansing them in the process. The feces (preferably at least 2-4 g) should be homogenized thoroughly in the medium of choice in less volume than will fill the tube in which the flotation will be done. The fecal solution is then poured into the tube through a layer or two of gauze to eliminate large pieces of debris. The tube is topped off with more flotation medium until there is a slight positive meniscus in the tube opening. A 22 × 22–mm coverslip is placed on top of the tube, which is allowed to stand for at least 10 minutes. Alternatively, the tube may be centrifuged with the coverslip in place for 10 minutes. Most of the diagnostic stages will adhere to the surface film on the underside of the coverslip.

The coverslip is carefully removed and gently placed on a labeled microscope slide. The slide is first scanned systematically using the 10× objective using a high-quality microscope. High magnification may be used to clarify the identity of detected eggs. It is important to optimize light transmission through the slide by appropriately adjusting the substage iris diaphragm of the microscope.

Fecal Cultures

The largest and most diverse group of parasites in horses is the strongylate nematodes, referred to as "small" and "large" *strongyles* (or *strongyli*). Because more than 40 species of strongyles are found in horses and their ova have a similar microscopic appearance, specific species of strongyle ova cannot be identified by microscopy with any reliability. Fecal culture by an experienced parasitologist can facilitate species diagnosis if this speciation is considered necessary.

The feces are cultured for 10 to 12 days to obtain the infective third-stage (L_3) larvae to allow differentiation of some of the strongyles found from those of threadworms and stomach hair worms. A sample of 5 to 10 g of fresh feces is mixed with an equal quantity of vermiculate and formed into a ball in two layers of gauze. The top of the ball is tied closed with a piece of string, and the ball is moistened and placed into a jar with a lid that contains water about 5 to 10 mm deep. The string is held so the fecal ball is just above the surface of the water while the lid is screwed down to hold the string in place and secure the ball. The jar is labeled and placed into a dark chamber for 10 to 12 days at room temperature. When opened, the water at the bottom

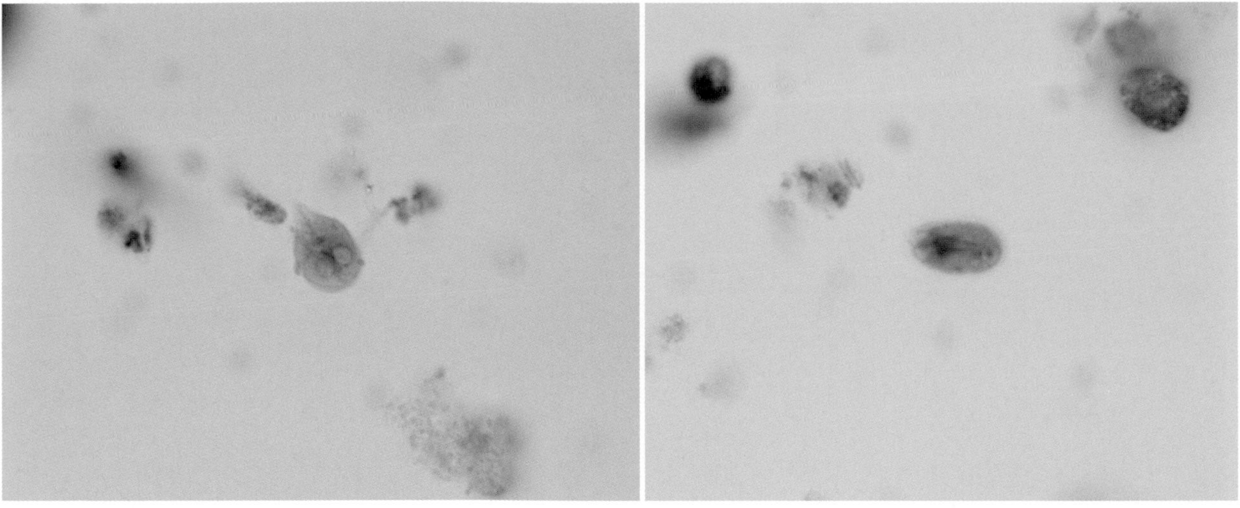

Fig. 58-6 **A,** *Giardia intestinalis* trophozoite (iron hematoxylin stain; 11 × 7 μm). **B,** *G. intestinalis* cyst (iron hematoxylin stain; 8 × 6 μm).

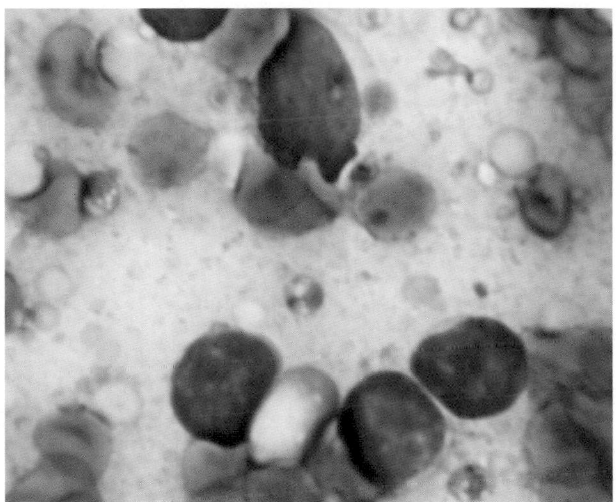

Fig. 58-7 *Leishmania* sp. amastigotes from skin lesion (3 × 3 μm).

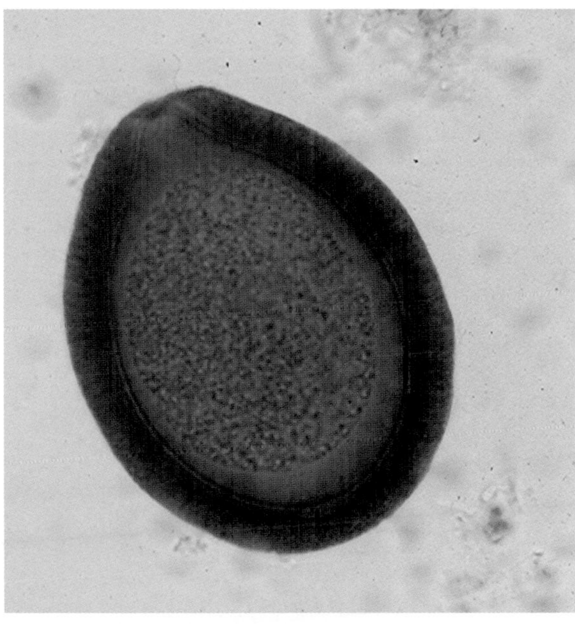

Fig. 58-8 *Eimeria leukarti* unsporulated oocyst (88 × 69 μm).

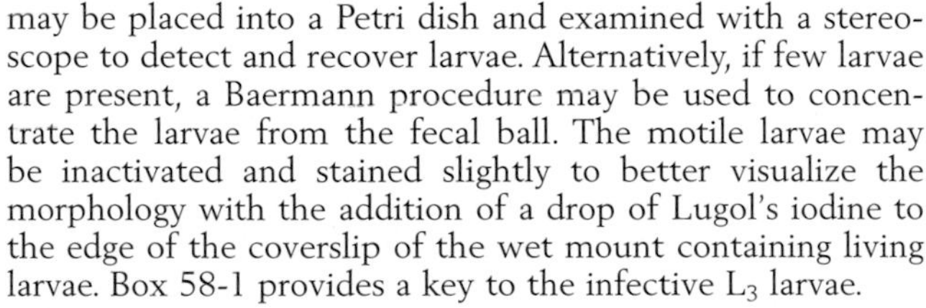

may be placed into a Petri dish and examined with a stereoscope to detect and recover larvae. Alternatively, if few larvae are present, a Baermann procedure may be used to concentrate the larvae from the fecal ball. The motile larvae may be inactivated and stained slightly to better visualize the morphology with the addition of a drop of Lugol's iodine to the edge of the coverslip of the wet mount containing living larvae. Box 58-1 provides a key to the infective L_3 larvae.

Fecal Sedimentation

Fluke eggs do not rise in normal flotation media, and thus the sedimentation procedure may be used to cleanse and concentrate such eggs. A simple procedure with soapy water (1 mL of inexpensive dish detergent in 500 mL of water loaded into a squeeze bottle) may be used. Two to 4 g of feces is placed into a sample cup and mixed thoroughly with approximately 40 mL of sedimentation solution. The solution is poured through a double layer of gauze into a vertical 50-mL centrifuge tube. After standing for 5 minutes, the solution is decanted or aspirated. The process is repeated with soap. The third sedimentation step uses fresh water. After the eggs have been cleaned and concentrated by these sedimentation steps, the sample of the sediment is placed on a glass slide and examined microscopically.

Direct Fecal Smear

A small amount of feces is placed on an applicator stick and mixed thoroughly in normal saline on a microscope slide. A coverslip is placed and the preparation examined using a compound microscope to identify flagellated and ciliated protozoa. This procedure is not as sensitive as fecal flotation or sedimentation because there is no cleansing or concentration of potential diagnostic stages present in the sample.

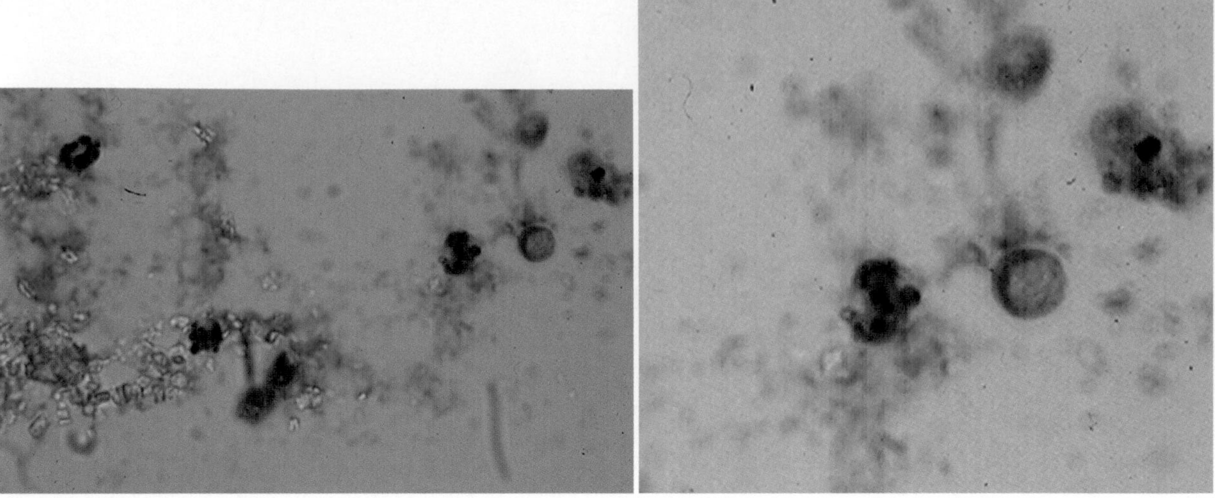

Fig. 58-9 A, *Cryptosporidium parvum* oocysts (Kinyoun acid-fast stain; 4.5 μm). **B,** *C. parvum* oocysts (Kinyoun acid-fast stain).

Box • 58-1

Key to Identification of Nematode Larvae from Equine Feces

1. Esophagus with obvious midlevel constriction (rhabditiform).	Free-living trematodes
Esophagus without such a constriction.	2
2. Body not enclosed in sheath; tip of tail has V notch.	*Strongyloides westeri*
Body not enclosed in sheath.	3
3. Containing fewer than 16 distinct cells.	Cyathostomes
Body with more than 16 gut cells.	4
4. Body with 16 gut cells.	5
Body with more than 16 gut cells.	7
5. Sheath tail is short and rounded.	*Trichostrongylus axei*
Sheath is long and whiplike.	6
6. Very large larvae with well-defined triangular cells.	*Oesophagodontus* spp.
Medium-sized larvae with rectangular gut cells.	*Posteriostomum* spp.
Long, thin, larvae; poorly defined gut cells; small trilobed process on posterior end.	*Strongylus equinus*
7. Larvae with 28 to 32 well-defined gut cells.	*Strongylus vulgaris*
Larvae with 18 to 20 gut cells.	8
8. Broad larvae, medium length, with well-defined gut cells.	*Triodontophorus* spp.
Small, slender larvae with blunt tail and poorly defined gut cells.	*Strongylus edentatus*

Baermann Procedure

The Baermann procedure is used to search for motile nematode larvae or tiny adult nematodes. It uses a simple device consisting of a funnel mounted vertically, a rubber tube that fits on the stem of the funnel, and a clamp to close off the tubing. The funnel is filled with warm water, and the clamp is shut to hold the water within the funnel. It is helpful to squeeze the tubing to express air trapped inside the tube or funnel stem. The feces or larval culture material is placed in a few layers of gauze, and the gauze is wrapped around the feces to make a ball. A hardware cloth support should be cut to fit in the funnel reservoir to act as a support for the ball of feces. The feces are added to the reservoir and allowed to stand from 2 hours to overnight. The fluid is then drawn into a small Petri dish, and the contents are examined under a stereomicroscope. If nematode larvae or tiny adults (e.g., *Probstmyaria*) are seen thrashing back and forth, some of these are placed onto a microscope slide with a drop of Lugol's iodine solution and a coverslip added. Nematodes lack circular muscles and thus cannot change the length of the body. They can only flex one way and then the other in a characteristic manner. The larvae may be examined and compared to standard larval diagrams to facilitate taxonomic identification (Fig. 58-10).

Cellophane (Scotch) Tape Test

The cellophane (Scotch) tape test is the preferred test for detection of pinworm *(Oxyuris equi)* ova (see Fig. 58-4).

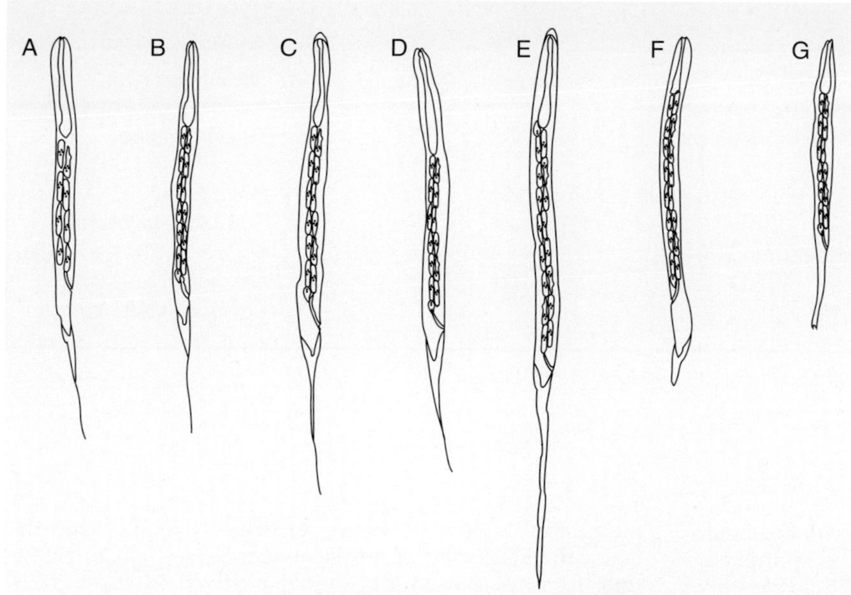

Fig. 58-10 Infective larvae of strongyles: A, Cyathostome; B, Posteriostomum; C, *Strongylus equinus;* D, *Strongylus edentatus;* E, *Strongylus vulgaris;* F, *Trichostrongylus axei;* G, *Strongyloides westeri.*

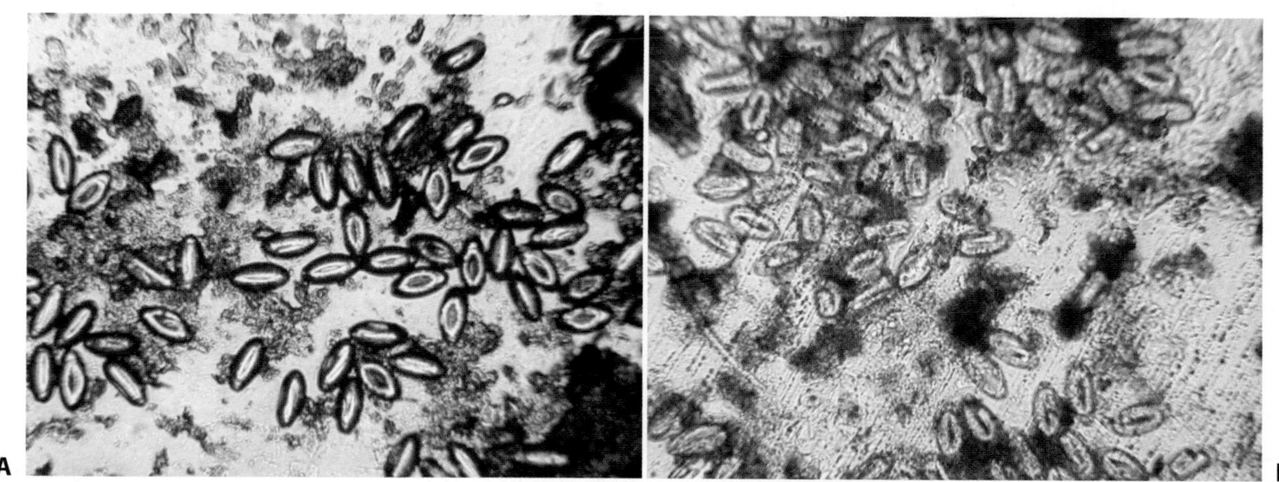

Fig. 58-11 A, *Oxyuris equi* eggs under tape without saline. B, *O. equi* eggs under tape with saline.

These ova adhere to the perineum and are rarely observed in routine fecal flotation or sedimentation samples. A length of clear cellophane tape is wrapped around three or four fingers with the sticky side out, and the tape is pressed against the perineum, then placed onto a glass slide. Saline or water may be placed over the tape and a long coverslip added to facilitate visualization of the ova (Fig. 58-11).

McMaster's Procedure

The McMaster's procedure is used to estimate the level of fecal contamination with parasite ova. Because it is a dilution technique, it may produce a false-negative result if low numbers of ova are present in a sample. Therefore, it is best used in combination with techniques that provide exact fecal egg counts. The McMaster's technique is often used to determine whether an anthelmintic treatment was effective. Pretreatment results are compared to results from samples collected 10 to 14 days after therapy.

A 4-g sample of fresh feces is added to a 120-mL screw-cap sample cup with sufficient sodium nitrate solution (fecal flotation medium) to bring the total volume to 30 mL and is mixed thoroughly. The solution is poured through one layer of gauze into another cup. After thorough mixing, the solution is used to fill the McMaster chamber. After standing for 10 minutes, the slide is placed on a compound microscope with the 10× objective in place. The width of each of the six lanes of the McMaster chamber is equal to the diameter of the field of view. The slide is systematically scanned to count the total number of each type of egg present on both sides of the chamber. If the counts between sides vary more than 20%, it is considered evidence of insufficient mixing of the sample, and the procedure should be repeated. The total count by parasite type present is multiplied by 25 to determine the eggs per gram of feces (EPG). (*Note:* The volume of fluid and the weight of feces used can vary and are based on the following: the volume under each grid is 0.15 mL, and thus the volume

Box • 58-2

Modified Key to Microfilariae of Horses

1. Microfilariae encased in membranous sheath; found in blood.	*Setaria equina*
Microfilariae not enclosed in sheath.	2
2. Microfilariae with round posterior ends, 200 μm long and present in hemorrhagic nodules in dermis.	*Parafilaria multipapillosa*
Microfilariae with pointed posterior ends, greater than 200 μm.	3
3. Tail is short.	*Onchocerca cervicalis*
Tail is long and whiplike.	*Onchocerca reticulata*

Modified from Soulsby EJ: *Textbook of veterinary clinical parasitology*, Philadelphia, 1965, Davis.

under both grids is 0.3 mL. This is $^1/_{100}$ the volume used (30 mL), and thus the number of eggs would be multiplied by 100; if 4 g of feces were used, this would be divided by 4 to obtain EPG. This is the same as multiplying by 25.)

Impression Smears

When horses are suspected of having cutaneous lesions attributable to *Leishmania*, a deep scraping that draws blood from the lesion is made. Smears of the exudate are stained with Wright's or Giemsa to reveal the presence of amastigotes. Impression smears of biopsies from spleen, liver, or bone marrow would reveal visceral amastigotes about 2 μm in length with recognizable nucleus and kinetoplast (see Fig. 58-9).

Skin Biopsy Examination

For diagnosis of microfilariae of *Onchocerca* spp., dermal biopsies are obtained from the unpigmented area of the ventral abdomen. These may be either fixed for histologic examination or teased apart in saline. If the latter approach is used, begin with warm saline and allow the teased preparation to stand for approximately 15 minutes before examining for motile microfilariae that have emerged from the tissue. Histologic sections will reveal the microfilariae in the superficial dermis (see Fig. 58-6). Box 58-2 provides a key to the microfilariae of the filarial nematodes of horses.

Blood Smears

Blood smears may be used to facilitate diagnosis of equine piroplasmosis and rarely microfilariae of *Setaria*. The microfilariae will be free in the blood, but the piroplasms of *Babesia equi* and *Babesia caballi* will be in erythrocytes (see Chapter 60).

Isolated Worms Recovered from Necropsy or Passed in Feces

Proper fixation of parasites will make identification easier for the parasitologist examining the specimens. Although most veterinary practices have formalin for fixing tissue, this is not the ideal solution to fix nematode, cestode, or trematode parasites. Nematodes should be fixed in stock glacial acetic acid if they are medium to small in size, then transferred and stored in 70% ethanol with glycerin (90 parts 70% ethanol, 10 parts glycerin). Flatworms should be relaxed about an hour in water, then fixed as flat as possible in AFA (85 parts 85% ethanol, 10 parts stock formalin, 5 parts glacial acetic acid). Some trematodes may need to be placed between two microscope slides and slight pressure applied, allowing AFA to diffuse around the specimens. Maintain pressure for a few minutes, then place the specimens into a vial with AFA. Maggots should be dropped into boiling water for a minute and then placed in 70% ethanol. Lice, ticks, and mites may be placed directly into 70% ethanol.

When shipping parasites to an identification service, provide appropriate contact information, including e-mail address, the host identity, the location from which the specimens originated (organ), and any other pertinent clinical information.

Suggested Readings

Bowman DD: *Parasitology for veterinarians*, Philadelphia, 1999, Saunders.

Jacobs DE: *A color atlas of equine parasites*, Philadelphia, 1986, Lea & Febiger.

Lichtenfels JR: Helminths of domestic equids, *Proc Helm Soc Wash* 42, Special Issue 92, 1975.

Manual of veterinary parasitological laboratory techniques, Technical Bulletin 18, London, 1979, Ministry of Agriculture, Fisheries and Food.

Soulsby EJ: *Textbook of veterinary clinical parasitology*, vol 1, Helminths, Philadelphia, 1965, Davis.

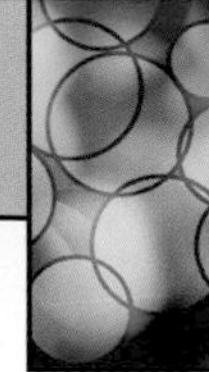

CHAPTER • 59

Equine Protozoal Myeloencephalitis

Debra C. Sellon and J. P. Dubey

In 1970, Rooney et al.[1] reported 52 cases of focal myelitis-encephalitis in horses from Kentucky and Pennsylvania, with the highest incidence in young Standardbreds. Horses were presented for evaluation of progressive spinal ataxia of one or more limbs. At necropsy, focal lesions of vascular damage, hemorrhage, mononuclear cuffing, gliosis, and neuronal and axonal degeneration were observed in one or more segments of the spinal cord. This report is now thought to be the first published description of *equine protozoal myeloencephalitis* (EPM).

In 1974, separate reports by Beech and Dodd,[2,3] Dubey et al.,[4] and Cusick et al.[5] described 14 horses in the United States with focal malacia and hemorrhage in the white and gray matter of the brain and spinal cord. Protozoal organisms observed in the central nervous system (CNS) tissues of each horse resembled *Toxoplasma gondii* but differed in several respects, including an absence of *T. gondii* antibody responses in affected horses. A subsequent serosurvey of horses revealed that 20% of 1294 serum samples tested by microtitration and indirect hemagglutinin test were positive for antibodies to *T. gondii*.[6] Attempts to induce disease in healthy ponies by oral administration of infective *T. gondii* oocysts with concomitant corticosteroid injections were unsuccessful,[7,8] and the etiologic agent of EPM remained a mystery for almost 20 years.

In 1991 a protozoan apicomplexan parasite was successfully cultured from the spinal cord of a horse with EPM,[9] and Dubey et al.[10] proposed the name *Sarcocystis neurona* for the parasite associated with encephalomyelitis in horses in North America. Subsequently, other investigators were able to isolate *S. neurona* from affected horses,[11] and the phylogenetic relationship of the organism to members of the family *Sarcocystidae* was confirmed based on small, ribosomal ribonucleic acid (rRNA) gene sequence.[12] Because of greater than 99.5% homology within a 742–base pair (bp) segment of the 18S rRNA gene, investigators mistakenly suggested that *S. neurona* was synonymous with *Sarcocystis falcatula*.[13] The opossum is the definitive host for *S. falcatula*, and birds are intermediate hosts. However, *S. neurona* is distinguishable from *S. falcatula* on the basis of its genetic composition, structure, biology, and ability to infect horses, and the two parasites are now recognized as separate species.[14-19]

In the past 15 years, numerous studies have advanced our understanding of the life cycle and epidemiology of *S. neurona* and enhanced our abilities to diagnose, treat, and prevent EPM. Despite these advances, however, EPM remains one of the most common infectious neurologic diseases of horses in North America.

ETIOLOGY

Sarcocystis neurona is the most common etiologic agent identified as a cause of EPM, but similar parasites, including *Neospora hughesi*, have been incriminated as etiologic agents in a few horses.[20-25] In this chapter, EPM refers to disease caused by infection of the equine CNS with *S. neurona* unless specified otherwise.

Sarcocystis neurona has a complex life cycle involving both sexual and asexual stages (Fig. 59-1). The definitive hosts for *S. neurona*, the opossums (*Didelphis virginiana* and *D. albiventris*),[26] become infected through ingestion of mature sarcocysts containing bradyzoites in tissues of intermediate hosts, such as the skunk,[27] raccoon,[28] nine-banded armadillo,[29,30] domestic cat,[31] and sea otter.[32] Bradyzoites are released from the sarcocysts in the gut lumen of opossums and transform directly in the small intestine into male and female *gamonts* without any replication.[33,34] The male gamonts divide into several *gametes*. An oocyst is produced after the fertilization of the female gamont by the male gamete; the entire process can be completed in the small intestine of the opossum within 24 hours of ingestion of sarcocysts. *Oocysts* sporulate in the lamina propria, producing two *sporocysts*, each containing four sporozoites. Fully sporulated oocysts or sporocysts are excreted in the feces of the opossum. *Sarcocystis neurona* sporocysts from opossum feces are approximately 10×8 μm in size.[35]

After ingestion of sporocysts by an intermediate host, sporozoites are released, invade the intestinal epithelium, and undergo asexual multiplication in many tissues. The number of asexual generations (schizogony) has not been determined. Studies in interferon-gamma (IFN-γ) knockout mice suggest that *S. neurona* multiplies in visceral tissues, lungs, and heart before invading the CNS. *Sarcocystis neurona* multiplies in the CNS and visceral tissues by a specialized form of schizogony, called *endopolygeny* (Fig. 59-2). In endopolygeny the nucleus becomes lobulated.[34] The lobes are connected by chromatin strands and may be arranged in groups. In early stages the uninucleate schizont sometimes resembles a macrophage or a degenerated host cell (Fig. 59-2, C). Finding multiple nucleoli in a nucleus helps to distinguish *S. neurona* from degenerating host cells. Several merozoites may develop within the same host cell[10,34] to become mature schizonts and produce merozoites without leaving the host cell; thus the developmental cycle may be asynchronous. *Merozoites* are formed centrally or peripherally in the schizont, often around a residual body (Fig. 59-3). Schizonts and merozoites are periodic acid–Schiff (PAS) reaction negative. Mature *schizonts* in the CNS are up to 30 μm long and may be oval, round, elongated, or irregular in shape.[34] The mechanism by which *S. neurona* is transported is unknown, but it has been proposed that it may reach CNS protected in mononuclear cells (Fig. 59-4).[36]

Both neural and inflammatory cells in the CNS may be parasitized. Several hundred merozoites may be present in a single neuron.[4] In histologic sections of CNS, individual merozoites are about 3 to 5 μm long and contain a single, centrally located, vesicular nucleus.[34]

Ultrastructurally, schizonts and merozoites are located in the host cell cytoplasm without a parasitophorous vacuole at

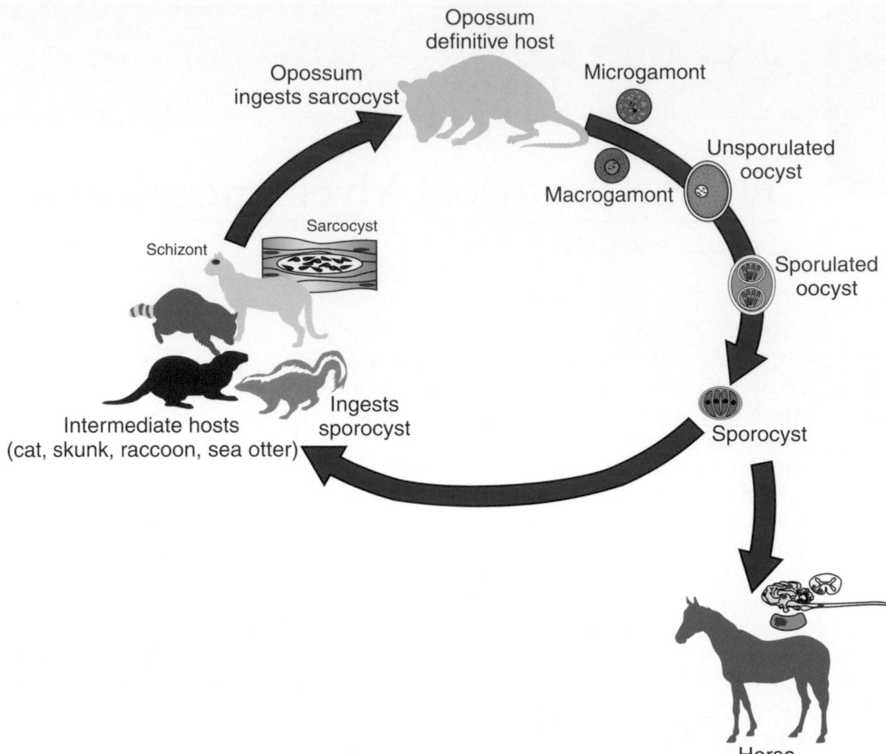

Fig. 59-1 Proposed life cycle of *Sacrocystis neurona.* (From Dubey JP: *J Vet Parasitol* 15:91-102, 2001).

any stage of development (see Figs. 59-2 and 59-3). Fully formed merozoites have the same organelles as found in most coccidians (except that rhoptries are absent in *Sarcocystis* merozoites).[37] Merozoites released from schizonts eventually give rise to encysted stages *(sarcocysts)*.[31] The earliest sarcocysts consist of a tissue cyst wall enclosing a few round forms, called *metrocytes*. Metrocytes divide into two organisms that eventually become *bradyzoites*. Unlike schizonts, sarcocysts are located in a parasitophorous vacuole inside host cytoplasm. It takes approximately 2 months or more for sarcocysts to mature in the intermediate hosts.[34] Sarcocysts observed in experimentally infected cats and raccoons were approximately 700 μm in length with a cyst wall 1 to 3 μm thick.[31,34,38] Bradyzoites are slender and approximately 5 μm in length. Intermediate hosts do not usually exhibit recognizable clinical signs as a result of *S. neurona* infection, but encephalomyelitis has been documented in the cat, raccoon, mink, skunk, sea otter, Pacific harbor seal, Canadian lynx, fischer, and dog.[39] Horses are considered aberrant intermediate hosts for *S. neurona* in which only schizonts have been identified with certainty. Raccoons, armadillos, sea otters, skunks, cats, and possibly other mammals are intermediate hosts of *S. neurona*.[27-31,39-41] In the intermediate hosts, sarcocysts are microscopic; bradyzoites are slender and tiny. The villar protrusions on the sarcocyst walls are up to 2.5 μm long and have microtubules that extend into the ground substance.[34]

There have been numerous reports of myeloencephalitis in horses associated with *Neospora* spp. infection.[20-23,25,42] A new species, *Neospora hughesi*, was isolated from infected horses and is considered distinct from *Neospora caninum* based mainly on genomic analysis of the first internal transcribed spacer (ITS-1) region of the rRNA gene[23] and amino acid differences in two immunodominant surface antigens.[24]

EPIDEMIOLOGY

In North America the opossum *(Didelphis virginiana)* is the only known definitive host for *S. neurona*.[26] Opossums in North America may be simultaneously infected with several *Sarcocystis* spp., including *S. neurona, S. falcatula, S. speeri,* and others.[34,43,44] Risk factors associated with the presence of *S. neurona* sporocysts in opossums include season and higher body condition score.[45] Approximately twice as many opossums trapped in spring were positive for sporocysts as opossums trapped in fall or winter. These investigators found no association between sporocyst presence in trapped opossums and age, gender, or the presence of young in the pouch of females.[45] A similar study of opossums in southern Michigan revealed that 31 of 206 opossums examined (15%) were infected with *S. neurona*.[46] This study confirmed that summer season was a risk factor for infection, but body condition score was not a factor. A higher frequency of *S. neurona* infection was observed in adult animals (12.6%) and females (9.2%) than in juveniles (2.4%) and males (5.8%). Multivariate analysis suggested that concomitant infection with other *Sarcocystis* spp. and presence of young in the pouch of females were risk factors for *S. neurona* infection in opossums.[46]

Armadillos,[29] raccoons,[28] skunks,[27] sea otters,[43] cats,[31,47] and possibly horses[48] have been identified as natural intermediate hosts for *S. neurona*. Sarcocysts isolated from the tongue of wild armadillos were identified as *S. neurona*, and all 19 armadillos were seropositive for *S. neurona* by immunoblot analysis.[30] Dubey et al.[28] demonstrated the presence of *S. neurona* sarcocysts in muscle of naturally infected raccoons. When these muscles were fed to opossums, *S. neurona* sporocysts were shed in the feces. Feeding sporocysts to IFN-γ knockout mice resulted in classic protozoal myeloencephalitis. After experimental

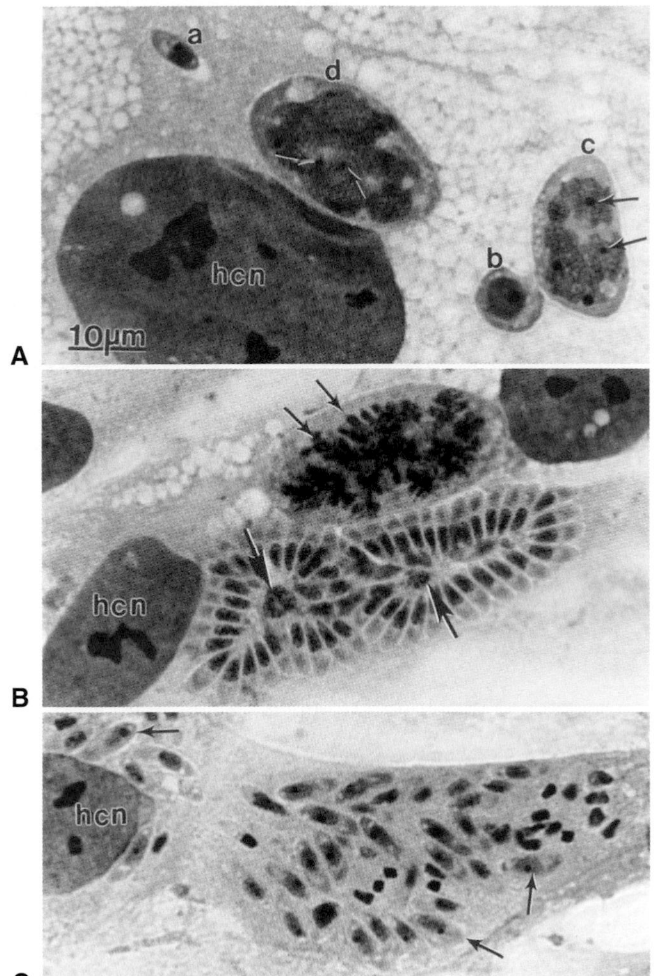

Fig. 59-2 Schizogonic stages of *Sarcocystis neurona* in bovine turbinate cells (Giemsa stain; *hcn*, host cell nucleus; bar applies to all figures). **A,** Differentiation of merozoite nucleus into schizont nucleus. Note a merozoite with enlarged nucleus *(a)*, globular schizont with nucleus containing one nucleolus *(b)*, lobulated nucleus *(c)* with five nucleoli *(arrows)*, and a schizont with large nucleus with two nucleoli *(arrows) (d)*. **B,** Three schizonts. Note merozoites budding at the surface *(small arrows)* and residual bodies *(large arrows)* in two mature schizonts. **C,** Development of second generation of schizonts without merozoites of the first generation leaving the host cell. Arrows indicate merozoites transforming to schizonts. (From Dubey JP: *J Vet Parasitol* 15:91-102, 2001.)

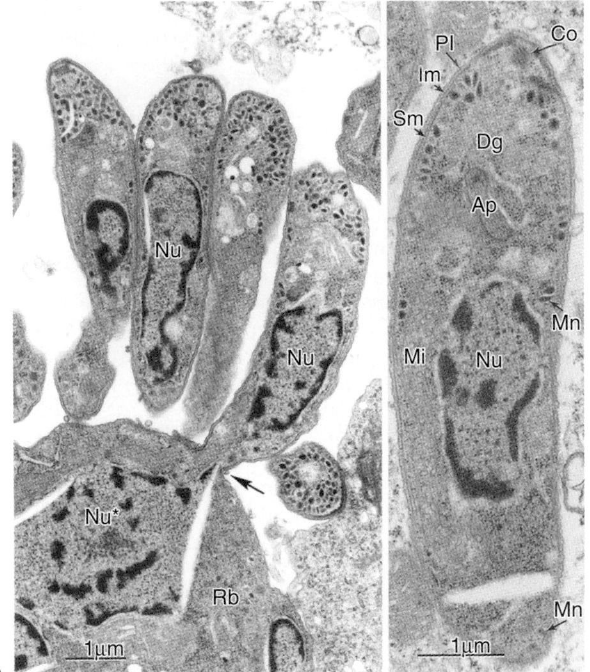

Fig. 59-3 Transmission electron micrographs of *Sarcocystis neurona* in brain of horse. *S. neurona* (isolate SN7) was obtained from this horse.[31] **A,** Portion of schizont showing several budding merozoites, one of which still attached *(arrow)* to the residual body *(Rb)*; *Nu*, nucleus of merozoite; *Nu**, nucleus of schizont still in residual body. **B,** Merozoite; *Ap*, putative apicoplast (Golgi adjunct); *Co*, conoid; *Dg*, dense granule; *Im*, inner membrane complex; *Mi*, mitochondrion; *Mn*, microneme; *Pl*, plasmalemma; *Sm*, subpellicular microtubule. (From Dubey JP: *J Vet Parasitol* 15:91-102, 2001.)

infection by feeding of *S. neurona* sporocysts, raccoons developed schizonts and merozoites in many tissues, including the brain, and sarcocysts in skeletal muscle, especially the tongue.[38]

The raccoon is probably the most important intermediate host for *S. neurona* in the United States because it is found throughout the country and is often infected with *S. neurona*. The role of the domestic cat and other intermediate hosts in the natural epidemiology of EPM is controversial, but most researchers consider it unlikely that the cat plays a major role. No *S. neurona* sarcocysts were observed in muscle sections from 50 free-roaming domestic cats, but *S. neurona* antibody was detected in 5 of 100 cats.[49] Only 5% of 196 feline serum

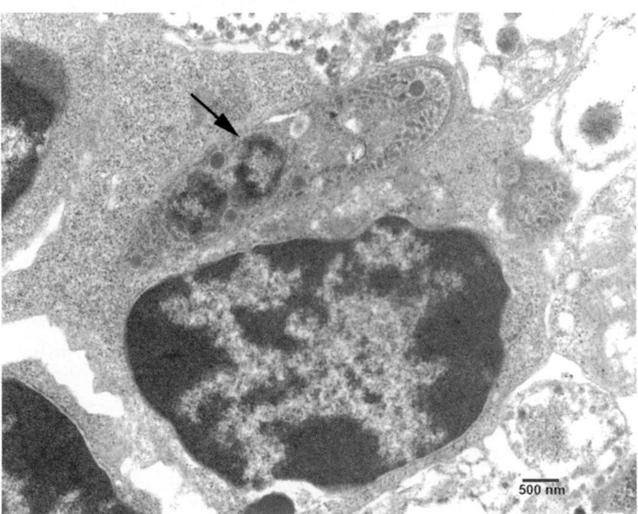

Fig. 59-4 Equine monocyte infected 24 hours previously with merozoites of SN-37R isolate of *Sarcocystis neurona*. Arrow indicates a single merozoite that is free in the cytoplasm of the monocyte.

samples submitted to the Michigan State University Animal Health Diagnostic Laboratory for *Toxoplasma gondii* testing were positive for antibodies to *S. neurona*. There was no correlation between *S. neurona* immunoblot results and *T. gondii* test results, age, gender, or the reason for *T. gondii* testing.[50] Fourteen of 35 cats (40%) from horse farms in southwestern Ohio with prior *S. neurona* infections in horses on the premises were seropositive for *S. neurona*. Horses from the same premises had a 93% seropositive rate. In contrast, only 27 of 275 cats (10%) from a spay/neuter clinic in Ohio were seropositive.[51]

The geographic range of clinical EPM in horses is defined by the range of the opossum, the definitive host of *S. neurona*. In areas where the opossum is common, approximately 50% of horses are seropositive, indicating exposure to *S. neurona*.[52-58] In central Wyoming and Montana, outside the natural range of opossums, only 6.5% and 0%, respectively, of wild horses are seropositive.[59-60] The South American opossum, *Didelphis albiventris*, is also a definitive host for *S. neurona*. Approximately 35% of horses in Brazil and Argentina are seropositive to *S. neurona* by immunoblot analysis.[61,62] *S. neurona* isolates from North America are genetically similar, regardless of the host, but are different from isolates from South America.[63]

The horse is the most common species in which myeloencephalitis caused by *S. neurona* infection is identified. In 1998 the U.S. Department of Agriculture (USDA) estimated the incidence of EPM to range from 0.06% in the southern states to 0.43% in the central United States, with a national average of 0.014%.[64] Clinical cases of EPM have been diagnosed in native horses of Panama[65] and Brazil,[66] but the incidence of EPM in seropositive horses in those countries is unknown. Horses in Europe, South Africa, and Asia diagnosed with EPM have invariably been imported from the Western Hemisphere.[67-71] Although serologic evidence indicates exposure of other equid species to *S. neurona*, the only reports of clinical disease in these species are in a single pony and a Grant's zebra.[72-74]

Most clinicians consider clinical EPM as a sporadic disease.[75] However, prior diagnosis on a premises is a risk factor for diagnosis of future cases of EPM,[76] and clusters of disease over a short period have been reported on single farms.[65,77] In 1990, Fayer et al.[78] reported on 364 histologically confirmed cases of EPM from many areas of the United States. Thoroughbreds, Standardbreds, and Quarter Horses were the breeds most often affected. There were no obvious patterns of infection based on geographic location, gender, or season. Also in 1990, Boy et al.[79] reported that the risk for EPM among 82 horses in Pennsylvania was higher in male and Standardbred horses. Neither study had control populations to confirm the significance of the demographic observations.

In 2000, Saville et al.[76] reported the results of a case control study of 251 horses diagnosed with EPM at Ohio State University on the basis of positive immunoblot or polymerase chain reaction (PCR) of cerebrospinal fluid (CSF). These horses were compared to a control group of 225 horses with neurologic diseases other than EPM and a control group of 251 horses admitted to the hospital for evaluation of nonneurologic disorders. In the final multivariable logistic regression analysis of EPM horses versus neurologic control horses, factors associated with increased risk of EPM included admission in the fall season, hay storage not secure from wildlife, wooded terrain around the premises, previous diagnosis of EPM on the premises, and a recent (<90 days) adverse health event for the horse.[76] Adverse health events included lameness, parturition, accident or injury, management changes, lacerations, surgical procedures, colic, and other medical problems. In the final multivariable logistic regression analysis of EPM horses versus nonneurologic control horses, factors associated with increased risk of EPM included admission to the hospital during the spring/summer/fall season, hay storage not secure from wildlife, use of the horse for racing or showing, age 1 to 5 years, previous diagnosis of EPM on the premises, and a recent adverse health event for the horse. Protective risk factors included age less than 1 year, use for breeding, and observation of birds, but not opossums, on the premises.[76]

In 2003, Rossano et al.[80] reported on a study of EPM in 1121 equids in 98 horse herds in Michigan. Serum samples were tested by immunoblot for presence of antibodies to *S. neurona*. Samples were stratified based on relative opossum abundance and herd size. Management factors such as age, fly control, wildlife control, and type of feed containment were examined. No single management factor was associated with herd seroprevalence. The authors speculate that it is difficult to restrict exposure of horses to *S. neurona* on farms located in areas with an abundance of opossums.[80]

Sarcocystis neurona has been associated with CNS infection and disease in many nonequid mammalian species, including southern sea otters,[81-83] Pacific harbor seals,[84,85] skunks,[72,86] mink,[72,87] raccoons,[88-90] dogs,[39,41] and cats.[72,91,92] An unconfirmed *S. neurona*–like infection has also been reported in a rhesus monkey[93] and Canadian lynx.[94] The presence of antibodies to *S. neurona* is a risk factor for myocarditis in southern sea otters.[95] Strains of *S. neurona* isolated from opossums and sea otters are morphologically and molecularly indistinguishable from equine isolates.* The role of *S. neurona* infection in these species in the natural history of EPM in horses is uncertain at this time.

PATHOGENESIS

The only known method of transmission of *S. neurona* to horses is through ingestion of sporocysts in opossum feces. Merozoites and schizonts may be observed in a variety of cell types in the CNS of horses with EPM, including neurons, mononuclear cells, and glial cells.[4] Only asexual stages of the parasite have been isolated from horses and, in the absence of evidence that sarcocysts form in the muscle of horses, equids are considered aberrant or "dead-end" hosts.

Several investigators have reported clinical signs of disease in one or more horses after experimental infection with *S. neurona* sporocysts or merozoites.[98-102] To date, however, none has successfully fulfilled all of Koch's postulates by isolating the organism from the experimentally infected horse and subsequently reproducing disease in another horse with that isolate.

In 1997, Fenger et al.[98] reported the results of feeding *S. neurona* sporocysts from opossums to five seronegative foals between 3 and 6 months of age. All foals developed an antibody response to *S. neurona* in both serum and CSF; four foals exhibited clinical signs of weakness, proprioceptive deficits, spasticity, hypermetria, or ataxia, first observed at 28 to 42 days after infection. Microscopic lesions consistent with EPM were found in three foals, but no protozoal organisms were observed. One foal in which no EPM-like lesions were observed had unilateral, noninflammatory lesions in the cervical and thoracic spinal cord that were consistent with cord compression. Attempts to culture *S. neurona* from spinal cord samples were unsuccessful.[98]

In 2001, Cutler et al.[102] infected eight seronegative yearling horses orally with sporocysts; concurrently, four of these horses

*References 14, 32, 63, 83, 85, 96, 97.

were treated with dexamethasone. All horses were seropositive for *S. neurona* within 32 days of challenge and were CSF antibody positive within 61 days. Signs of mild to equivocal neurologic disease were observed after 40 days. Mild to moderate multifocal gliosis and neurophagia were observed histologically in the spinal cords of seven horses. No protozoal organisms were identified in any section of the CNS of any of the infected horses. Immunosuppression with dexamethasone did not increase the severity of clinical signs or histologic changes observed in the CNS. Attempts to culture *S. neurona* from blood, CSF, and CNS tissues were unsuccessful.[102]

In 2001, Saville et al.[101] used a model of transport stress immediately before inoculation with *S. neurona* sporocysts. Twelve seronegative foals between 4 and 5 months of age were transported for 55 hours. Immediately after transport, three horses were inoculated with sporocysts. Three horses were infected after 2 weeks of acclimation; three horses were acclimatized for 2 weeks and treated with dexamethasone before infection; and three horses remained as untreated negative control horses. Horses infected with sporocysts immediately after transport seroconverted earlier than other horses (9-15 days after infection). All infected horses developed clinical signs of disease as early as 9 days after infection, with the most severe signs in horses infected immediately after transport. One negative control horse developed neurologic signs at 30 days after infection, seroconverted, and had minimal inflammatory CNS lesions at necropsy. One other control horse seroconverted. Histologic lesions observed in infected horses were minimal. All tissue sections from infected horses were negative for *S. neurona* by immunohistochemistry (IHC), tissue culture, and bioassay in IFN-γ knockout (GKO) mice.[101]

The experiment was repeated with 24 seronegative weanling horses.[103] Six groups of four horses each received varying numbers of sporocysts or placebo. Mild to moderate clinical neurologic signs were observed in challenged horses from all groups, with the most consistent signs observed in the group receiving the highest number of sporocysts. Histologic lesions suggestive of *S. neurona* infection were observed in 4 of 20 horses fed sporocysts, but parasites were not detected by light microscopy, IHC, or bioassay in GKO mice. Attempts to induce more severe clinical signs by transporting horses a second time 4 to 18 days after infection were unsuccessful.[100] All horses seroconverted, and clinical signs were observed as early as 5 days after infection. Parasites were not detected in CNS sections by light microscopy or IHC.[100]

Sarcocystis neurona has been isolated from the blood and tissues of immunodeficient and immunocompetent horses after experimental infection.[99,104,105] The parasite was isolated from the blood of an Arabian foal with severe combined immunodeficiency (SCID) at 21 days after oral infection with *S. neurona* sporocysts.[105] Parasitemia after infection was confirmed in a larger study in which six immunocompetent foals and three SCID Arabian foals were infected either orally with *S. neurona* sporocysts or intravenously with *S. neurona* merozoites.[99] Foals were stressed by weaning immediately before infection. Despite prolonged parasitemia and persistent infection of visceral tissues (skeletal muscle, cardiac muscle, lung, liver, and spleen), as demonstrated by PCR and culture, SCID horses did not develop neurologic signs after oral or intravenous infection.[99] In contrast, although parasitemia was undetectable, four of six orally infected immunocompetent foals developed neurologic signs consisting of ataxia and proprioceptive deficits. Parasites were detectable by PCR or culture in the CNS tissues of immunocompetent foals with neurologic signs. These studies demonstrate that specific immune responses (B and T cell mediated) are required to control parasitemia and infection of visceral tissues of horses, but these responses are often unable to control neuroinvasion and prevent development of clinical signs.[99] In 2005, Rossano et al.[104] confirmed the presence of parasitemia in immunocompetent horses after oral infection with *S. neurona* sporocysts by culturing the organism from blood of experimentally infected weanling horses.

Murine models of *S. neurona* infection provide additional clues to the pathogenesis and immune control of *S. neurona* in mammalian hosts. Infection of immunocompetent mice is not associated with disease; however, infection of GKO mice, incapable of producing IFN-γ, with either sporocysts or merozoites consistently results in fulminant neurologic disease and death, regardless of the genetic background of the mice.[18,106-108] Examination of the CNS of infected GKO mice that die after *S. neurona* infection reveals inflammatory infiltrates consisting mostly of neutrophils and macrophages, fewer eosinophils, rare multinucleated giant cells, scattered subacute perivascular cuffing, and intralesional protozoa.[109] Lesions and organisms are most common in the caudal brain, especially the cerebellum, and equally distributed in white and gray matter of the brain and spinal cord.[109]

In 2001, Dubey[110] described the pathogenesis of *S. neurona* infection in GKO mice fed sporocysts. Parasitemia was demonstrable by bioassay at 1 to 8 days after infection. Sporozoites were observed in histologic sections of all regions of the small intestine and in cells in Peyer's patches of a mouse killed 6 hours after ingesting sporocysts. At 1 day after infection, organisms were present in all regions of the small intestine and in mesenteric lymph nodes. Parasites were visible in extraintestinal tissues by 3 days after infection and in the brain within 2 weeks after infection.[110,111] Parasites could be found in the brain, liver, lung, heart, and eyes of mice examined at 20 to 62 days after infection.[111] Witonsky et al.[112] described splenomegaly, lymphadenopathy, mixed inflammatory infiltrate in the liver, perivascular infiltrate in the liver and lung, and interstitial pneumonia in GKO mice at 14 days after infection.

Although there is a paucity of specific information regarding the pathogenesis of *S. neurona* infection in horses, the information gleaned from pathologic and epidemiologic reports of natural infection, results of experimental equine infections, and extrapolation from murine models of disease suggest a likely theory for the pathogenesis of EPM.

After ingestion of sporocysts from opossum feces, *S. neurona* replicates to a limited extent in equine gastrointestinal epithelial cells.[113] Cell-associated parasitemia provides the parasites with access to visceral and CNS tissues, where subsequent rounds of asexual reproduction occur. After hematogenous spread to the CNS, *S. neurona* may localize in any area, from cerebrum to spinal cord, but is not found in peripheral nerves. Specific immune responses limit parasitemia and visceral organ infection, but do not always prevent CNS invasion and disease. The exact location of parasite replication in the CNS of an infected horse determines the type and severity of clinical signs that are observed. Some types of immune suppression and stress may increase the likelihood of neurologic disease after infection with *S. neurona*.

Most information regarding host immune response to *S. neurona* infection has been gained from murine models of infection. The consistent induction of disease in GKO mice clearly demonstrates the importance of IFN-γ in disease control.[18,106-108] IFN-γ is released in the mammalian brain in response to a variety of infectious agents and is considered an essential component of host immune response to CNS infection.[114] In C57Bl/6 mice, protection from neurologic disease is mediated by CD8+ T lymphocytes.[112,115,116] Mice lacking these cells develop clinical signs of meningoencephalomyelitis with typical histopathologic lesions.[115] The relevance of this observation to equine disease is uncertain because of reports that SCID foals (lacking B and T cells) do not develop neurologic disease after infection with *S. neurona* sporocysts or merozoites, despite persistent parasitemia and widespread replication of parasites in visceral tissues.[99]

Genetic background also influences development of clinical disease in mice.[106,117] Marsh et al.[117] reported that C57Bl/6 nude mice (lacking T cells) developed neurologic disease after experimental infection with *S. neurona,* but ICR SCID mice (lacking B and T cells) did not. This apparently contradictory observation remained unexplained until Ahlgrim et al.[106] demonstrated that nude and SCID mice with a C57Bl/6 genetic background develop severe neurologic disease and die after experimental infection with *S. neurona,* whereas nude and SCID mice on a BALB/c background consistently survive infection without clinical signs. Resistance to clinical disease in BALB/c mice appears to be related to a component of innate immunity other than natural killer (NK) cell function.[106,118] When BALB/c SCID mice were infected with *S. neurona* they failed to develop neurologic disease even when NK cells were depleted. However, these mice did develop fulminant neurologic disease when IFN-γ function was blocked.[118] These data suggest that BALB/c mice may have a cell type, other than B cells, T cells, or NK cells, that secretes more IFN-γ than secreted by similar cells in C57Bl/6 mice. The relevance of this observation to equine disease is uncertain, but it may indicate genetic differences in susceptibility to CNS infection and disease in horses.

Relatively little is known about immune responses to *S. neurona* infection in horses. Two surface proteins of *S. neurona,* Sn14 and Sn16, are expressed in vivo in the horse and are strong immunogens.[119] However, many horses readily develop clinical disease despite the presence of specific antibody, suggesting that humoral responses are not protective. Specific B-cell and T-cell responses limit and control parasitemia and replication of parasites in visceral tissues of horses, but these responses cannot prevent neuroinvasion and neurovirulence.[99] Parasites may be able to induce an immunosuppression toward parasite-derived antigens, including suppression of IFN-γ production, facilitating parasite survival in the horse.[120] The limited available data suggest that both innate and adaptive immune responses are important for control of infection of *S. neurona* in horses. Additional information is needed to determine better the nature of protective immune responses and guide production of better vaccines for prevention of disease.

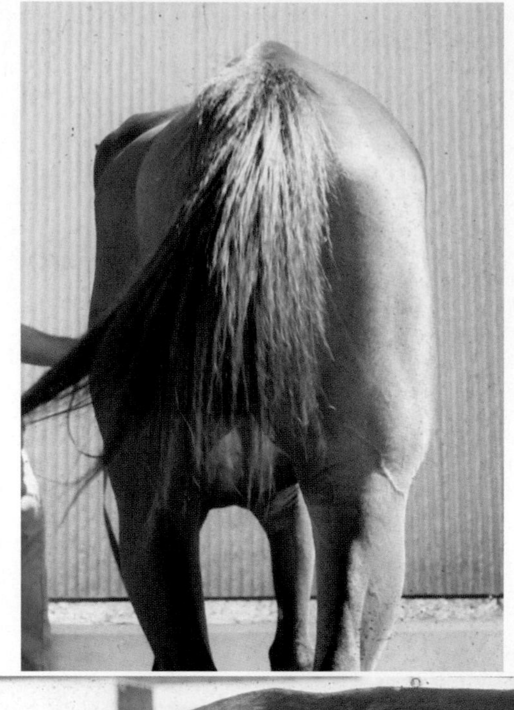

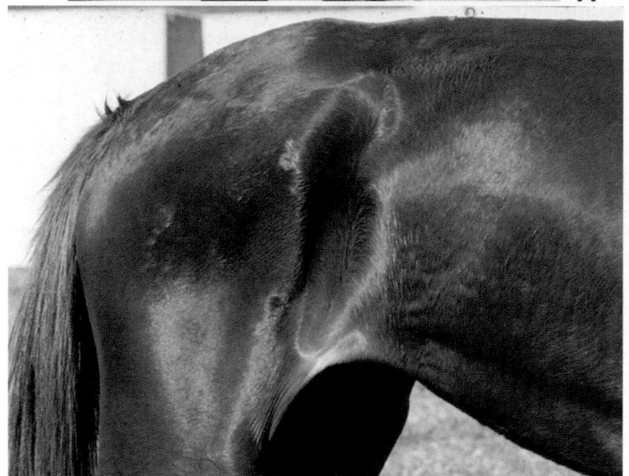

Fig. 59-5 Asymmetric muscle atrophy resulting from *S. neurona* infection. **A,** Atrophy of left gluteal muscles. **B,** Atrophy of right quadriceps, tensor fascia lata, and biceps femoris. (Courtesy Dr. Robert MacKay.)

CLINICAL FINDINGS

Clinical signs of EPM vary greatly because of the diffuse or multifocal localization of parasites and inflammatory lesions in gray or white matter of the brain, brain stem, or spinal cord.[75,121-123] Onset of disease may be acute or insidious, and signs may progress rapidly or remain stable for long periods. Most affected horses are bright and alert with normal vital signs, but focal asymmetric muscle atrophy may be obvious on initial examination (Fig. 59-5). Muscle atrophy is most common in the gluteal or quadriceps muscles but may also mimic sweeney, radial nerve paralysis, or polyneuritis equi.[123] Occasionally, affected horses exhibit more generalized, mild muscle atrophy. Complete blood count (CBC) and serum biochemical profile are usually unremarkable.

Initial reports of EPM described horses with progressive neurologic disease that might include ataxia and conscious proprioceptive deficits of one or more limbs, cranial nerve deficits, or cerebral signs.[1-5,124] In 1978, Mayhew et al.[125] reported that 8 of 32 horses (25%) with EPM had signs of brain disease. MacKay[126] reported in 1997 that a survey of 158 cases of EPM from Ohio State University revealed that 126 (80%) had spinal cord signs alone, 10 (6%) had only brain signs, and 22 (14%) had both brain and spinal cord signs. In 2000, Saville et al.[127] reported the frequency of specific clinical signs in 251 horses diagnosed with EPM. Spinal ataxia was observed in 88.8% of 251 horses with EPM, weakness in 80.5%, spasticity in 56.2%, muscle atrophy in 14.3%, cranial nerve dysfunction in 11.6%, and seizures in 6%. More than 74% of affected horses had clinical signs involving both front and rear limbs, 0.4% involved front limbs only, and 19.9% had signs only in the rear limbs. Severity of gait deficits ranged from mild (grade 1-2, 19.9%) to severe (grade 4-5, 22.2%). Clinical signs were asymmetric in 68.9% of horses.[127]

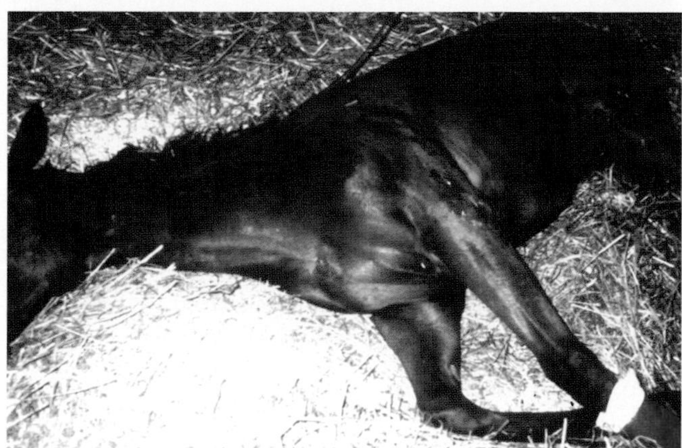

Fig. 59-6 Horse presenting with acute onset of recumbency and inability to rise caused by equine protozoal myeloencephalitis (EPM). Note the decubital ulcers after just 48 to 72 hours of recumbency.

Gait abnormalities are the most common presenting complaint for horses with EPM. Ataxia, spasticity, weakness, and conscious proprioceptive deficits of one or more limbs indicate spinal cord involvement. Mild conscious proprioceptive deficits and weakness resulting in an asymmetric gait are easily confused with lameness, occasionally resulting in misdiagnosis or delay in treatment. Some neurologic lesions may manifest as behavioral or training problems or injuries resulting from the abnormal gait. Examples of performance problems that have been attributed indirectly to EPM include frequent bucking, head tossing, excessively high head carriage, difficulty maintaining a specific lead, back pain, upward fixation of the patella, and difficulty negotiating turns.[121,126,128] Areas of hyporeflexia, hypalgesia, hyperhydrosis, or complete sensory loss may be identified.[122] Most horses with EPM exhibit gradual progression of the severity and range of clinical signs, but some horses may experience a sudden exacerbation in severity.[122] Occasionally, horses exhibit acute recumbency and inability to rise as the initial clinical sign recognized by owners (Fig. 59-6).

The most common signs of brain or brain stem involvement in horses with EPM are depression, head tilt, facial paralysis, and difficulty swallowing[122] (Fig. 59-7). Affected horses may also exhibit seizure activity, dementia, head shaking, amaurosis (central blindness), or narcolepsy-like activity.[75,121,123,129] Some horses with EPM have abnormalities of the upper airway, including laryngeal hemiplegia or dorsal displacement of the soft palate as a result of involvement of the nuclei of the vagus, glossopharyngeal, accessory, or hypoglossal nerve.[121] Difficulties with prehension, mastication, or deglutition of food may result from involvement of the nuclei of the facial, trigeminal, glossopharyngeal, hypoglossal, or vagus nerve. Head shaking, responsive to antiprotozoal therapy, has been reported in horses with EPM.[128] Urinary incontinence reported in horses with EPM presumably results from damage to sacral spinal cord segments.[130] Affected hoses had normal anal reflexes and normal anus and tail tone.

In a longitudinal retrospective study of 251 horses with EPM, Saville et al.[127] reported a 55.4% survival rate. Approximately 90% of horses in the study were treated for EPM, and 65% of treated horses showed some improvement in clinical signs. Of horses that improved after treatment, horses with mild neurologic deficits had a 92.3% survival rate, horses with moderate neurologic deficits had a 72.2% survival rate, and horses with severe neurologic deficits had a survival rate of 55.6%. The likelihood of improvement in clinical signs after diagnosis of EPM was lower in breeding and pleasure horses than in racing and show horses, possibly as a result of age or exercise factors.

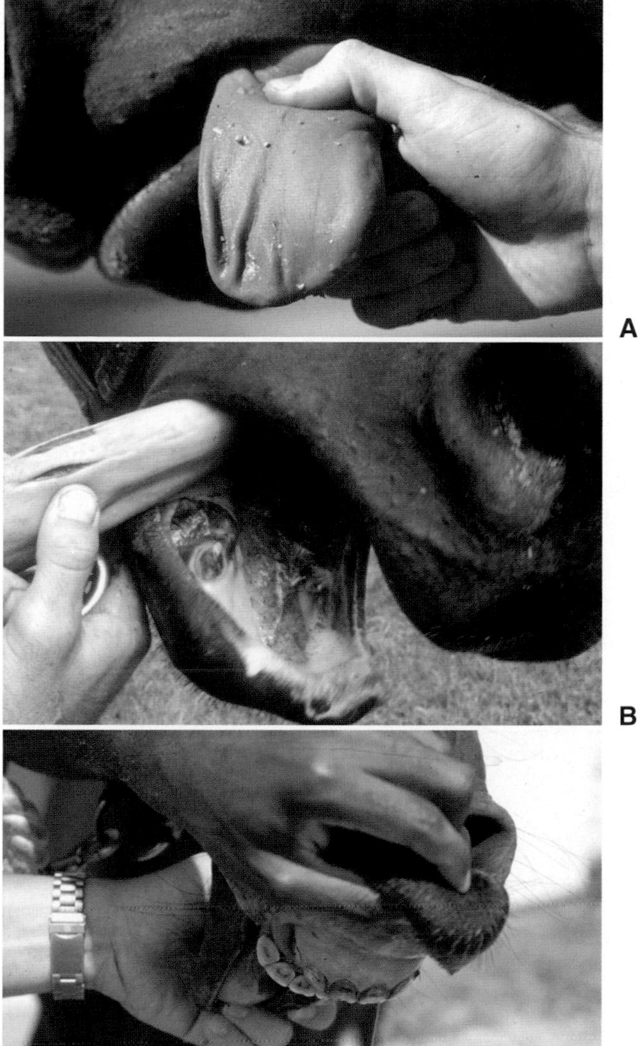

Fig. 59-7 Cranial nerve abnormalities in horses with EPM. **A,** Unilateral atrophy of tongue caused by impaired hypoglossal nerve (cranial nerve XII). **B,** Self-mutilation of tongue secondary to loss of trigeminal nerve (cranial nerve V) sensory function. **C,** Deviation of mandible to the right secondary to a loss of trigeminal nerve motor function. (Courtesy Dr. Robert MacKay.)

DIAGNOSIS

The considerable variability in presenting complaints and progression of neurologic disease in horses with EPM and the high prevalence of antibody to *S. neurona* in horses in North America make this disorder inherently difficult to diagnose definitively. A number of antemortem diagnostic tests for EPM, most of them based on detection of antibody to *S. neurona* in the serum or CSF, have been described. None of these tests is currently considered definitive when used alone, and the "gold standard" for diagnosis remains postmortem identification of characteristic lesions and parasites within the CNS.

In 2002 a consensus panel of experts was convened by the American College of Veterinary Internal Medicine to review available information related to diagnosis of EPM. The final published statement from this consensus panel recommends a systematic approach to diagnostic testing, beginning with a thorough physical and neurologic examination.[131] This examination should affirm the presence of neurologic abnormalities, and the absence of musculoskeletal disease, as the primary cause of the presenting complaint. The neurologic examination should localize probable neurologic lesion(s) and facilitate construction of an accurate list of differential diagnoses. The next step in the diagnostic process is to perform appropriate laboratory or other diagnostic tests to rule out as many differential diagnoses as possible, given limitations appropriate to the individual client and patient. In many cases the necessary diagnostic testing will require access to facilities, equipment, and laboratories capable of supplying specialty services. After exclusion of reasonable differential diagnoses, specific diagnostic tests for EPM may be considered. In some cases, response to antiprotozoal therapy is considered the diagnostic test of choice after excluding appropriate differential diagnoses.[131]

Routine laboratory testing, including CBC and serum biochemical profile, is within normal limits in most horses with EPM. CSF analysis may be helpful in ruling out other differential diagnoses. Horses with EPM do not consistently have changes in CSF color, clarity, cell counts, protein concentration or cytology. Iatrogenic contamination of CSF with even small quantities of peripheral blood can confound interpretation of immunoblot tests described below.[132]

The introduction of the Western immunoblot by Granstrom et al.[133] in 1993 offered a dramatic advance in antemortem diagnosis of EPM. Before that time, diagnosis was based solely on the presence of neurologic disease and exclusion of other differential diagnoses. In recent years, investigators have described modifications to the original procedure[134] as well as other serologic tests for immunoglobulin G (IgG) antibodies to *S. neurona*, including direct agglutination [135] and indirect fluorescent antibody[136] tests.

The Western immunoblot test (IBT) detects the presence of *S. neurona*–specific antibodies in the serum or CSF of horses. Proteins from cultured *S. neurona* merozoites are separated by polyacrylamide gel electrophoresis. Antibody responses to three proteins (14.5, 13, and <7 kDa) are specifically assessed in interpretation of IBTs (Fig. 59-8). A modification of IBT that eliminates cross-reactivity with *S. cruzi*, a parasite of cattle, and assesses reactivity to 30-kDa and 16-kDa bands as the criteria for a positive test is reported to have enhanced sensitivity and specificity.[134] However, technical differences in test conditions make it difficult to compare critically the diagnostic accuracy of different types of IBTs.[34]

Approximately 50% of clinically normal horses in many parts of the United States are seropositive for *S. neurona*, indicating exposure to the parasite. As a result, IBT of serum samples lacks specificity for diagnosis of clinical EPM. Granstrom[137] compared results of CSF IBTs from 254 horses with neurologic disease. A postmortem diagnosis of EPM was made in 124 horses. Sensitivity and specificity of immunoblot analysis of CSF samples were each reported to be approximately 89%. Positive and negative predictive values in this population were 85% and 92%, respectively. These results prompted the recommendation of IBT of CSF samples as a standard for antemortem diagnosis.[126]

Subsequent studies assessing the accuracy of IBT of CSF for diagnosis of EPM using postmortem evaluation as a "gold standard" concluded that IBT had a relatively low specificity with numerous false-positive results.[138-140] Daft et al.[140] compared CSF Western blot results to histopathologic evaluation of CNS tissues and reported that the IBT had a sensitivity of 87% and a specificity of 44% for diagnosis of EPM in 65 horses with neurologic disease. In horses without neurologic disease, sensitivity was 88% and specificity 60%. The high sensitivity in both groups of horses suggests that IBT of CSF is useful for ruling out EPM in horses when the prevalence of infection is low or moderate. However, IBT should not be used as the sole diagnostic criterion for confirmation of EPM and is inappropriate as a screening test for EPM in neurologically normal horses.[141]

False-positive immunoblot results may occur because of laboratory error, iatrogenic blood contamination of the CSF

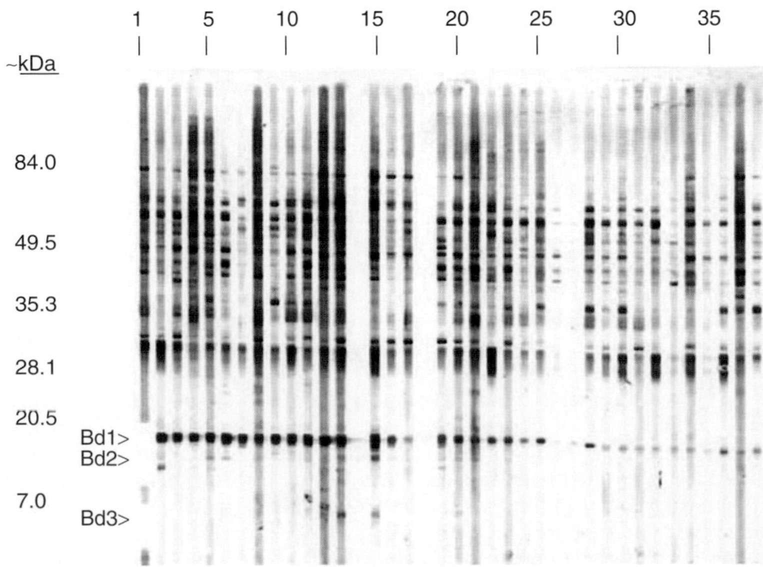

Fig. 59-8 Immunoblot of equine serum samples. The *Sarcocystis neurona*–specific bands are designated by the numbered arrows to the left of the first lane, and their approximate molecular weights are based on the migration of standards of known molecular weight *(far left)*. Band 1 = 14.5 kDa; band 2 = 12 kDa; and band 3 <7 kDa. Lanes 15, 16, and 17 contain positive, diluted positive (for assessing lower detection limit), and negative sera, respectively. Lanes 14 and 18 are blank. Lanes 1 through 13 contain sera that tested positive by immunoblot test (IBT). Lanes 19 through 23 contain sera with equivocal IBT reactivity. Lanes 24 through 38 contain sera that tested negative by IBT. (From Dubey JP, Mitchell SM, Morrow JK, et al: *J Parasitol* 89:716-720, 2003.)

at sampling, alterations in the permeability of the blood-brain barrier, normal presence of low levels of specific antibody in the CSF, or after passive transfer of colostral antibody to neonatal foals. Miller et al.[132] demonstrated in 1999 that false-positive immunoblot results may occur after introduction of microscopic quantities of seropositive blood into the sample.[132] Cytologic evaluation of CSF obtained for IBT analysis may aid in interpreting results by enabling the clinician to assess the degree of iatrogenic blood contamination at the time the sample was obtained. A total red blood cell count in the CSF of less than 50 cells/μL is recommended for accurate interpretation of immunoblot results.[132]

For several years the calculation of albumin quotient and IgG index was recommended to assist with interpretation of IBT for EPM.[142,143] However, the immunoblot can be falsely positive because of blood contamination despite a normal albumin quotient, and these indices are no longer widely used.[132]

Recent reports of *S. neurona*–specific antibody in the CSF of foals after ingestion of colostrum from seropositive mares suggest that antibody can cross the intact equine blood-brain barrier in sufficient quantities to result in a positive IBT.[144] This conclusion is supported by the observation that antigen-specific antibodies are detectable in the CSF of adult horses after vaccination with ovalbumin.[145] Most foals ingesting colostrum containing *S. neurona*–specific antibodies are seronegative by 9 months of age.[144]

False-negative serum or CSF immunoblot reactions are uncommon but may occur, especially if a horse is recently exposed to *S. neurona*. In a study by Rossano et al.[146] horses with a negative serum immunoblot result were highly likely to have a negative CSF immunoblot test as well. Approximately one third of seropositive horses in that study had negative CSF immunoblot results. The high negative predictive value of the IBT using either serum or CSF samples makes it a valuable tool for eliminating EPM as a differential diagnosis for horses with neurologic disease.

A direct agglutination test[135] and an indirect fluorescent antibody test (IFAT)[136,147] have been described for diagnosis of EPM in experimental and naturally infected animals. The direct agglutination test has been used primarily for detection of *S. neurona* antibodies in the serum of experimentally infected mice, with a reported sensitivity of 100% and specificity of 90%.[135] The accuracy of the IFAT using serum and CSF of horses naturally and experimentally infected with *S. neurona* was assessed by comparison to histopathologic diagnosis. Sensitivity and specificity of the IFAT using serum were 83.3% and 96.9%, respectively. Using CSF, the sensitivity and specificity were reported to be 100% and 99%, respectively.[136] A comparison of IFAT results with results from two types of immunoblot showed that the IFAT was more accurate for serologic diagnosis of EPM.[147]

Polymerase chain reaction testing of CSF to detect presence of *S. neurona* deoxyribonucleic acid (DNA) has a high specificity for EPM, but sensitivity is quite poor.[12,148] Merozoites rarely enter the CSF, and free parasite DNA is destroyed by enzymatic action, resulting in a very large number of false-negative results. Diagnosis of EPM in horses that have died may be facilitated by immunohistochemical studies to detect antigens in CNS tissue.[149,150]

PATHOLOGIC FINDINGS

At necropsy, gross lesions of the CNS may or may not be visible. The brain stem and spinal cord are more often affected than the cerebrum. When present, lesions usually consist of multifocal hemorrhagic foci varying from clearly demarcated areas of discoloration to larger lesions affecting the brain or multiple segments of the spinal cord[2,4,5,125,151] (Fig. 59-9). Microscopically, hemorrhage, nonsuppurative inflammation, and small areas of necrosis may be seen (Figs. 59-10 through 59-13).[34,122] Perivascular cuffing with mononuclear cells is common. Giant cells, gitter cells, and eosinophils are frequently observed in inflammatory foci and in the meninges overlying the lesion.[122] Organisms are seen in association with lesions in fewer than half of cases. Organisms are infrequently found in sections stained with hematoxylin and eosin. Prior administration of corticosteroids did not influence the likelihood of observing parasites in association with CNS lesions in a study by Boy et al.[79] but prior treatment with trimethoprim-sulfonamide alone or with pyrimethamine significantly decreased the likelihood of observing parasites. Merozoites may be

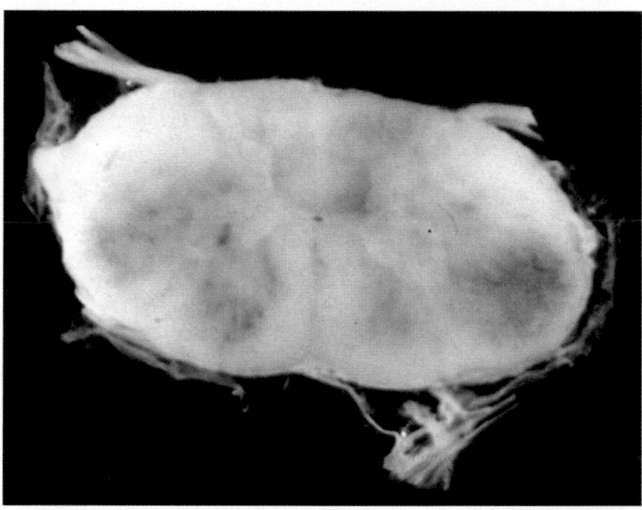

Fig. 59-9 Cross section of spinal cord of horse with EPM. Focal areas of discoloration indicative of necrosis. (Unstained.) (From Dubey JP: *J Vet Parasitol* 15:91-102, 2001.)

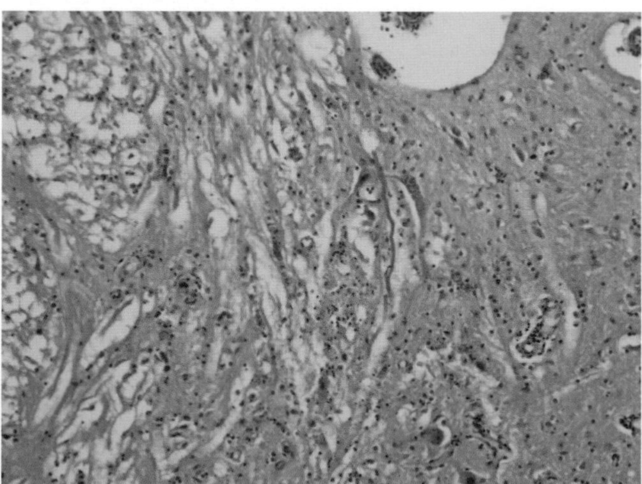

Fig. 59-10 Myelitis in spinal cord of naturally infected horse; *Sarcocystis neurona* was named based on the organism in this horse.[10] Focal necrosis with numerous basophilic merozoites scattered throughout the neural parenchyma.

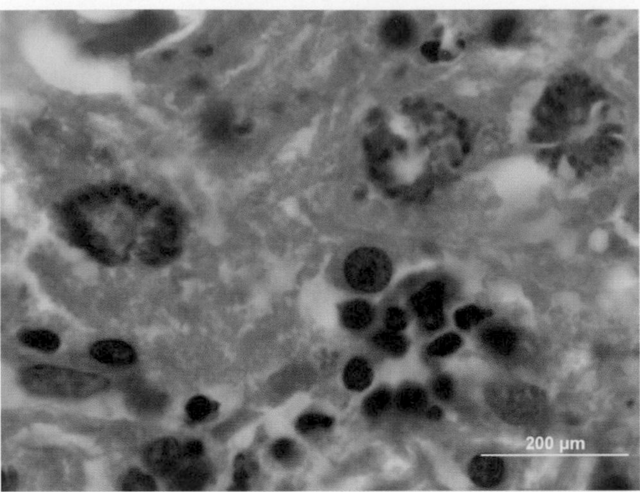

Fig. 59-11 Hematoxylin and eosin–stained section of neural tissue from the same horse as described in Figure 59-6. Higher-power magnification shows developing stages of the parasite.

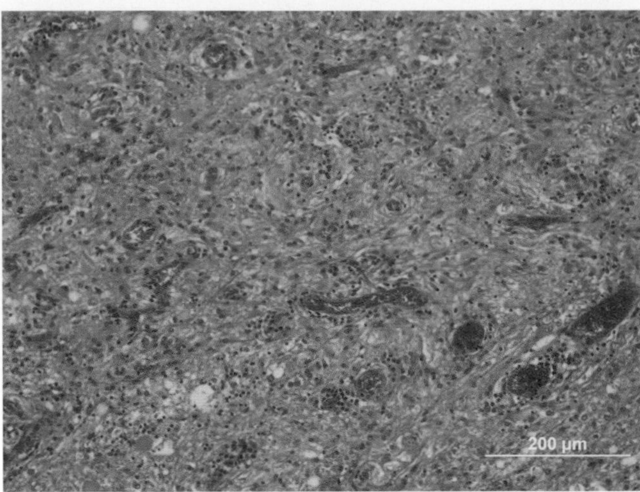

Fig. 59-13 Focus of mononuclear cell infiltration in spinal cord of another naturally infected horse.

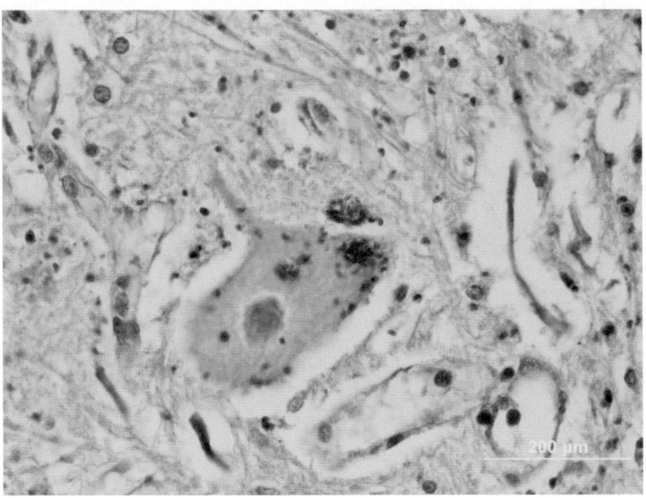

Fig. 59-12 Immunohistochemical staining of sections of neural tissue from the same horse as described in Figure 59-9. Numerous *S. neurona* organisms inside and outside neurons.

observed singly or in groups (schizonts) up to 20 µm in diameter. Parasites may be observed either free in tissues or within neurons, macrophages, glia, eosinophils, or vascular endothelium.[123] When observed, they are strongly basophilic, PAS negative, and agyrophobic.[122] Visualization of organisms may be improved with immunohistochemical staining using an *S. neurona*–specific antiserum (see Fig. 59-12) that does not cross-react with closely related species.[149,150]

In most naturally infected horses, macroscopic or microscopic lesions caused by *S. neurona* are not observed in any tissues other than the CNS. However, Mullaney et al.[48] identified mature sarcocysts in the tongue and skeletal muscle of a 4-month-old Shire filly with neurologic disease consistent with EPM. This horse also had schizonts in the brain and spinal cord.

THERAPY

Antiprotozoal Drugs

Three antiprotozoal drugs or drug combinations are approved for use in the treatment of EPM in horses: ponazuril, nitazoxanide, and a combination of pyrimethamine and sulfadiazine.

Ponazuril

Ponazuril (Marquis, Bayer Corporation, Kansas City, Missouri) is a primary metabolite of toltrazuril, a member of the triazine family of chemotherapeutic agents. Ponazuril has anticoccidial activity against a variety of parasites, including *S. neurona*, and was the first approved medication for treatment of EPM.[152] *Toltrazuril*, the parent drug, has activity on the mitochondria and respiratory chain of some avian coccidian parasites. Ponazuril may also have activity against the plastid body, an organelle of apicomplexan parasites that functions in amino acid synthesis, electron transport, and energy metabolism.[152] A chlorophyll complex of coccidian organisms, not found in mammals, appears to serve as the receptor for this drug.[153] Because ponazuril is a weak acid with high lipid solubility, it is able to cross the intact blood-brain barrier and enter the CSF, most likely by passive diffusion.

Ponazuril is absorbed well in horses after oral administration at 5 mg/kg body weight in a 15% paste formulation.[154] Concentrations of drug in the serum and CSF during a 28-day course of daily treatment were 4.33 ± 1.10 mg/L and 0.162 ± 0.05 mg/L, respectively. The terminal elimination half-life of ponazuril in serum was 4.3 ± 0.6 days.[154] At 1 µg/mL, ponazuril inhibits growth of *S. neurona* in vitro by 98.6%; at 0.1 µg/mL, growth is inhibited by 94.4%.[155]

Kennedy et al.[156] reported that administration of ponazuril 15% oral paste to 24 horses at 0, 10, or 30 mg/kg for either 28 or 56 days resulted in minimal changes in serum biochemical profiles, coagulation profiles, or hematology parameters. Uterine edema was observed at necropsy of three of four mares treated with ponazuril at 30 mg/kg. At 10 times the label dose (50 mg/kg) for 10 days, adverse effects included intermittent anorexia, weight loss, and mild colic.

In a field trial of ponazuril 15% oral paste, 101 horses with EPM were randomly allocated to treatment at either 5 or 10 mg/kg for 28 consecutive days.[157] Diagnosis of EPM was made based on a neurologic gait abnormality of grade 2 or greater, normal cervical radiographs, and the presence of *S. neurona*–specific antibodies in the CSF by immunoblot analysis. Treatment success was defined as conversion to a negative CSF immunoblot or demonstrated improvement of at least one neurologic grade on day 118 compared with findings on day 0. The outcome was considered successful for 63 horses (62%) and unsuccessful for 38 horses (38%). The majority of treatment successes (76%) demonstrated improvement by the end of the 28-day treatment period. Some horses (15 of 63) did not show improvement until after conclusion of therapy on day 28. Of the 38 horses with unsuccessful outcomes, eight showed noticeable improvement during the treatment period and then regressed during the 90-day follow-up period, suggesting that a longer period of treatment may have been needed. Possible adverse effects observed in a low number of horses during the field trial included blisters on the nose and mouth, skin rash or hives, loose feces, and mild colic. One horse, with a prior history of seizures, experienced a seizure while being treated. In experimentally infected horses, prophylaxis at 5 mg/kg starting 7 days before and continuing 28 days after inoculation with *S. neurona* sporocysts reduced clinical EPM in horses but did not eliminate infection.[158]

Furr et al.[159] assessed the ability of daily feeding of ponazuril to horses to prevent or limit clinical signs of EPM after experimental infection. A transport stress model of infection was used. All untreated horses developed signs of neurologic disease consistent with EPM; only 71% and 40% of horses in the 2.5 and 5.0 mg/kg ponazuril groups, respectively, developed neurologic abnormalities.

Nitazoxanide

Nitazoxanide is a thiazolide antiparasitic agent with in vitro activity against a wide variety of protozoa and helminths[160] that has been approved as a 32% paste formulation for treatment of EPM in horses (Navigator, Idexx Pharmaceuticals, Westbrook, Maine). It is rapidly metabolized in horses to the active metabolite, acetylnitazoxanide. Antiprotozoal activity is believed to result from interference with pyruvate:ferrredoxin oxidoreductase enzyme-dependent electron transfer reactions, essential to anaerobic energy metabolism. Nitazoxanide is approved for use in the treatment of diarrhea associated with *Giardia intestinalis* or *Cryptosporidium parvum* infection in some people.[160]

There is very little information in the peer-reviewed veterinary literature regarding the safety or efficacy of this drug in horses. With in vitro assays, 0.52-ppm nitazoxanide inhibited *S. neurona* merozoites by 50%. Two reports in 1999 describe a total of nine horses with suspected EPM that were treated with the drug.[161,162] Clinical signs were improved in eight of the nine horses; the only adverse effect reported was inappetence in three horses.

Nitazoxanide is sold with the recommendation to treat affected horses for 28 days. Because of the lack of peer-reviewed literature pertaining to the drug in horses, much of the available information relating to its performance is based on the manufacturer's package insert. The manufacturer's recommendation is to treat at 25 mg/kg for days 1 to 5 and 50 mg/kg on days 6 to 28. Administration of nitazoxanide can disrupt normal gastrointestinal flora of horses, leading to enterocolitis. Deaths caused by enterocolitis were observed in field studies. Other possible adverse effects include reduced appetite, lethargy, depression, scant feces, colic, laminitis, increased water consumption, discolored urine, fever, head and limb edema, and weight loss. Stallions may be more prone to develop laminitis while receiving nitazoxanide than are mares or geldings. If signs of high fever, scant or loose feces, diarrhea, colic, or laminitis are observed, treatment with nitazoxanide should be discontinued and appropriate veterinary care provided.

Field trials of nitazoxanide for treatment of horses with EPM were designed similar to those for ponazuril, as previously described. Based on improvement in neurologic examination scores and a negative result using CSF immunoblot, 28 of 49 horses (57%) were classified as treatment successes. In a second field study, 81% of 250 horses completing the study were classified as treatment successes. Success rate in horses that had been previously treated for EPM with other drugs was reported as 78%.

Folate Inhibitors

Folate inhibitors, the first drugs described for treatment of EPM in horses, are still widely used. The combination of sulfadiazine and pyrimethamine (ReBalance, Phoenix Scientific, St. Joseph, Missouri) blocks successive steps in protozoal folate synthesis. The recommended dosage is 20 mg/kg of sulfadiazine and 1 mg/kg of pyrimethamine once daily for at least 4 to 6 months.[122,126] This drug combination is now approved by the U.S. Food and Drug Administration (FDA) for treatment of horses with EPM.

In vitro studies demonstrate that pyrimethamine is coccidiocidal for *S. neurona* at 1.0 μg/mL and trimethoprim is coccidiocidal at 5.0 μg/mL.[163] None of the sulfonamides has activity against *S. neurona* in cell culture on its own at 50 or 100 μg/mL. However, combinations of sulfonamides (4 or 10 μg/mL) with 0.1 μg/mL of pyrimethamine had improved coccidiocidal activity.[163] Pharmacokinetic studies of pyrimethamine showed that repeated dosing at 1 mg/kg body weight is unlikely to produce sustained CSF drug levels greater than 0.1 μg/mL. Failures observed with sulfonamide/pyrimethamine treatment may be related to a failure to obtain sustained coccidiocidal concentrations of drugs in the equine CNS.[163,164] However, because pyrimethamine concentrates in the CNS tissue rather than plasma, the concentration at the desired site of action may be more than 0.1 μg/mL.[122,165]

The peer-reviewed veterinary literature contains very little information regarding the efficacy of folate inhibitors for treatment of EPM in field cases. A multicenter trial of 105 horses treated for 90 to 210 days reported that 66% of horses responded favorably to treatment. Treatment response was defined as improvement of two grades or more in evaluation of gait or reversion to negative immunoblot status.[122] Recommendations for duration of therapy are varied, and minimal data support them. Horses with a negative immunoblot when folate inhibitor therapy is discontinued are reportedly unlikely to relapse. Unfortunately, most horses do not obtain CSF immunoblot-negative status with treatment.[122]

Folate synthesis inhibitors are generally considered to be safe therapeutic options when administered for short periods. However, prolonged therapy, as is frequently needed for treatment of horses with EPM, has been associated with a variety of adverse effects in a few horses, including fever, depression, anemia, leukopenia, neutropenia, sexual dysfunction in stallions, abortion, and teratogenesis.[122,166-170]

In a report by Fenger[170] in 1998, 15.4% of 13 horses treated with standard doses and 50% of 12 horses treated with double doses of sulfadiazine/pyrimethamine developed anemia.[170] Neutropenia was reported in 7.7% of horses receiving standard-dose therapy and 50% of horses receiving double-dose therapy. An increase in mean corpuscular volume (MCV) of red blood cells was reported in 25% of standard-dose horses and 66.7% of double-dose horses. Hematologic abnormalities associated with prolonged sulfadiazine/pyrimethamine therapy in horses have been attributed to folate deficiency, and folic acid supplementation has been recommended.[121] However, subsequent reports suggest that folate supplementation paradoxically exacerbates folate deficiency in treated horses, and its use cannot be justified.[166,168]

Caution should be exercised in the treatment of pregnant mares with EPM because of the risk of teratogenic effects associated with folate synthesis inhibitor therapy. Foals born to mares treated with sulfonamides, trimethoprim, pyrimethamine, folic acid, and vitamin E orally during pregnancy have exhibited a fatal syndrome of myeloid, erythroid, and lymphoid aplasia and hypoplasia with epithelial dysplasia and renal nephrosis or hypoplasia.[122,168] Serum folate concentrations in affected mares and their foals were lower than those reported for normal broodmares.

Supportive Therapy

A variety of ancillary and supportive therapies may be indicated for the treatment of some horses with EPM. Short-term antiinflammatory therapy may be beneficial for treatment of moderate to severely affected horses during the first few days of antiprotozoal therapy or when the onset of signs is acute and rapidly progressive.[121,122] Nonsteroidal antiinflammatory drugs (NSAIDs) such as flunixin meglumine, 1.1 mg/kg intravenously (IV) twice daily, or phenylbutazone, 2.2-4.4 mg/kg IV or orally twice daily, are frequently used. For horses with moderate to severe clinical signs, dimethyl sulfoxide (DMSO) at 0.5 to 1 g/kg as a 10% solution IV or by nasogastric tube once or twice daily may be beneficial. Use of corticosteroids such as dexamethasone in horses with EPM is controversial because of the potential of these drugs to suppress immune responses to the parasite. However, judicious short-term use in horses with severe clinical signs may be beneficial in reducing CNS inflammation and associated clinical signs while waiting for antiprotozoal drugs to begin working.[122]

Many clinicians recommend supplementation of vitamin E, 6000 to 10,000 IU orally daily, as antioxidant therapy throughout the course of therapy and rehabilitation.[122] Biologic response modifiers have been recommended for treatment of horses with EPM because of the possibility that affected horses may be immunocompromised. Drugs that have been used include levamisole (1 mg/kg orally twice daily for 2 weeks), killed *Propionobacterium acnes* (Eqstim, Neogen, Lansing, Michigan), and mycobacterial cell wall extract (Equimune IV, Vetrepharm, London, Ontario, Canada).[122] No experimental or field trial data exist to support the efficacy of these drugs in the treatment of EPM.

General supportive care is indicated for horses with neurologic dysfunction that significantly impairs ability to stand and move, eat, drink, or perform other vital functions. This may include provision of appropriate fluid and nutritional support, deep bedding, sling support, and protective headgear.

PREVENTION

The only known route of transmission of *S. neurona* to horses is through ingestion of sporocysts shed in the feces of opossums. Therefore, prevention strategies are aimed at minimizing opossum access to horse feeds and pastures. Whenever possible, feed should be protected from wildlife access through use of enclosed facilities and containers with tight-fitting lids.[121,122] After feeding, scattered grain should be swept from aisle ways and other areas near horses. Cat, dog, and bird food should not be left out overnight in barns or near pastures. Insects, birds, and rodents may mechanically transfer sporocysts in barn areas, and control of these species may help reduce the incidence of EPM on a farm.[122] Risk factors associated with EPM include recent adverse health events.[76] Prompt treatment of illness and injury, close monitoring of pregnant mares, and minimizing stress associated with these events may be beneficial. Proximity of a creek or river to the premises where the horse resides is associated with a reduced risk of EPM. This may provide a preferred habitat for opossums, decreasing their presence near barns and equine feed supplies.[76]

The most effective means to kill *S. neurona* sporocysts in feed or in the environment is heat treatment. Heating to 55° C (131°F) for 15 minutes or 60° C (140° F) for 1 minute or more renders sporocysts noninfective to GKO mice.[171] Treatment with bleach (10%, 20%, and 100%), 2% chlorhexidine, 1% povidone-iodine, 5% *o*-benzyl-*p*-chlorophenol, 12.56% phenol, 6% benzyl ammonium chloride, or 10% formalin was not effective in killing sporocysts.[171]

Pyrantel tartrate kills merozoite and sporozoite stages of *S. neurona* in vitro.[172] However, the drug was ineffective in preventing infection in GKO mice.[173] In 2005, Rossano et al.[174] reported that daily feeding of pyrantel tartrate failed to prevent seroconversion associated with daily low-dose oral administration of *S. neurona* sporozoites to horses. Feeding *diclazuril* at 50 ppm was able to prevent infection in GKO mice fed sporocysts of *S. neurona*.[175] Similar studies have not been performed in horses.

A killed whole-parasite vaccine prepared from *S. neurona* merozoites is currently marketed in the United States under a conditional license for the prevention of EPM in horses (EPM Vaccine, Fort Dodge Animal Health, Fort Dodge, Kansas). To obtain conditional licensure in the United States, a vaccine manufacturer must show safety, purity, and a reasonable expectation of efficacy. Administration of this vaccine results in an antibody response that is purported to inhibit parasite replication in vitro. The antibody response induced by vaccination is indistinguishable by IBT of serum or CSF from the response to natural infection.[176] Intradermal skin testing of vaccinated horses suggests that some degree of cell-mediated immunity is also induced by vaccination.[177] Data demonstrating in vivo efficacy of the vaccine for prevention of EPM in horses are not currently available.

PUBLIC HEALTH CONSIDERATIONS

To the authors' knowledge, there are no reports of human disease caused by infection with *Sarcocystis neurona*.

REFERENCES

See the CD-ROM for a list of references linked to the abstract in PubMed.

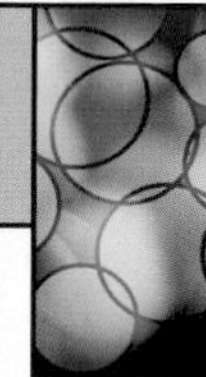

CHAPTER • 60

Equine Piroplasmosis

Chantal M. Rothschild and Donald P. Knowles

Equine piroplasmosis (EP) is a tick-borne protozoal disease of horses, mules, donkeys, and zebras that is characterized by acute hemolytic anemia.[1-6] The etiologic agents are two hemoprotozoan parasites, *Babesia equi* (Laveran, 1901)[7] and *Babesia caballi* (Nutall and Strickland, 1910),[8] that are transmitted primarily by ixodid ticks. Equine piroplasmosis is found globally where tick vectors are present and is endemic in tropical, subtropical, and some temperate regions.[1-3,5,9-11] Horses infected with *B. equi* remain seropositive for life; horses infected with *B. caballi* are seropositive for several years to life.[3,5,10-12]

Economic losses associated with EP are significant and include the cost of treatment, especially in acutely infected horses; abortions; loss of performance; death; and restrictions in meeting international requirements related to exportation or participation in equestrian sporting events.[13] Equine babesiosis–free countries, including the United States, limit the entrance of *Babesia*-seropositive horses into their countries. Equine piroplasmosis is synonymous with equine malaria,[14,15] equine biliary fever,[14-16] equine babesiasis,[15] Oyns,[16] horse tick fever,[15] equine babesiosis, and equine theileriosis.[17]

ETIOLOGY

The genera *Babesia* and *Theileria* belong to the family *Piroplasmidae.* The term *piroplasm* is derived from the pear-shaped appearance of intraerythrocytic replicative forms. The piroplasms are members of the phylum Apicomplexa, which also includes the genera *Plasmodium*, *Cryptosporidium*, and *Toxoplasma*. *B. caballi* is regarded as a true *Babesia* because it exclusively replicates within erythrocytes in the vertebrate host (Fig. 60-1). Currently, there is uncertainty as to the appropriate taxonomic classification for *B. equi*. Although considered a "small *Babesia*," *B. equi* has several characteristics that distinguish it from other species within the genus, including apparent initial development in lymphocytes before the erythrocytic stage[18,19] (as occurs with *Theileria* spp.), division into four merozoites within the erythrocytes (forming the "Maltese cross," Fig. 60-2), only transtadial transmission by ticks (not transovarial), and resistance to babesicidal drugs.[11,20,21] Phylogenetic studies using small-subunit ribosomal ribonucleic acid (rRNA) gene analysis suggest *B. equi* belongs to a distinct paraphyletic group, different from both the *Babesia* and the *Theileria* genus.[22] Currently, both nomenclatures may be found interchangeably in the literature. Because both *Babesia* and *Theileria* are piroplasms, the term *equine piroplasmosis* conforms with either classification.

Babesia caballi and *B. equi* share many of the same tick-vectors, are usually present in the same geographic regions, and frequently co-infect horses. *B. caballi* and *B. equi* are transmitted by more than 15 species of the tick genera *Dermacentor* (Fig. 60-3), *Hyalomma*, and *Rhipicephalus*.[2,23,24] *B. equi* can also be transmitted by *Boophilus microplus*.[25-27] Ticks serve as a reservoir for *B. caballi* because the organism persists in ticks throughout several generations, with transtadial and transovarial transmission (although not in all tick species). In contrast, horses are the only known reservoir for *B. equi*, and only transtadial (not transovarial) transmission occurs within the tick vector. Because of their longevity and mobility, male ticks can transmit *B. equi* to multiple horses.[5] Importantly, *Boophilus microplus* may acquire and transmit *B. equi* even when feeding on inapparent carrier horses with a low level of parasitemia.[28] Adult stages of *Hyalomma anatolicum* and *Rhipicephalus turanicus* transmit *B. equi* to horses after acquisition of the organism in nymph stages from infected horses under experimental conditions.[5]

Parasitemia (percentage of erythrocytes infected) typically does not exceed 1% in *B. caballi* infections and may be as low as 0.1% even in clinical cases.[3] Maximum reported parasitemia is 10%.[9] *B. equi* parasitemia usually ranges from 1% to 7%,[5] with a maximum of 95%.[9] Once infected with *B. equi*, horses remain carriers for life, regardless of whether clinical signs resolve naturally or with drug treatment.[10] Infection with *B. caballi* has been said to be self-limiting, lasting up to 4 years after infection.[9] However, many horses that recover from *B. caballi* infection later relapse, suggesting temporary nondetection of organisms with possible lifelong infection. Carrier horses represent a potential reservoir for maintenance and dissemination of parasites to ticks and horses.[23] Because new tick species capable of transmitting equine piroplasms are being recognized and reliable control methods do not currently exist, it is important to prevent the introduction of both infected horses and ticks into equine piroplasm-free areas.

No evidences exists for transmission of EP by hematophagous dipterans such as tabanids (horsefly) or *Stomoxys calcitrans* (stable fly).[23,29] *B. equi* can be transmitted iatrogenically by contaminated needles or surgical instruments, administration of

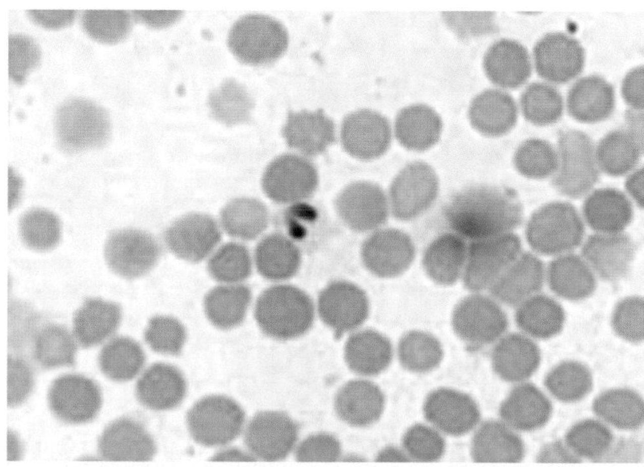

Fig. 60-1 *Babesia caballi* merozoites and trophozoites within erythrocytes.

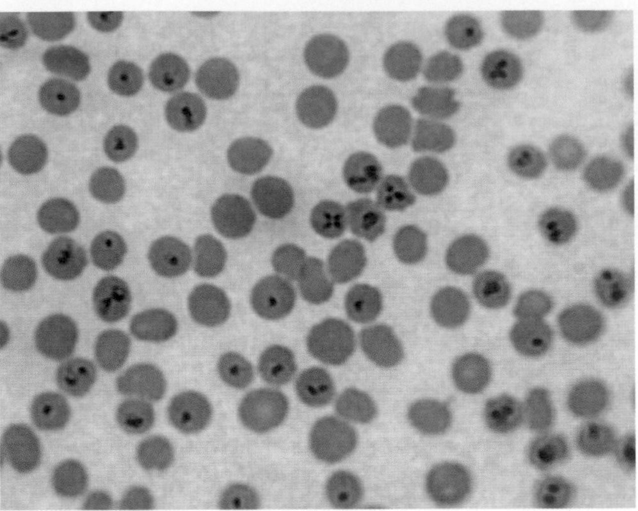

Fig. 60-2 *Babesia equi* merozoites in "Maltese cross" formation.

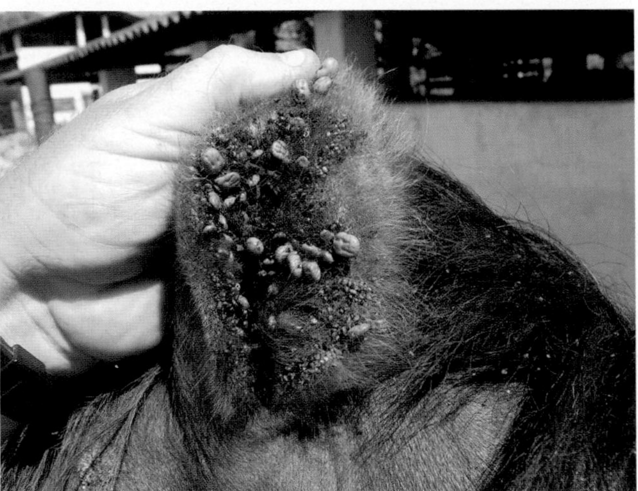

Fig. 60-3 Horse heavily infected with *Dermacentor (Anocentor) nitens*, one of the most common horse ticks capable of transmitting *Babesia caballi.*

contaminated blood transfusions, or failure to properly sterilize equipment that contacts equine blood (e.g., stomach tubes, dental instruments).[5,20] Chronically infected pregnant mares are at risk of transplacental transmission, resulting in abortion, stillbirth, or birth of a sick foal that typically succumbs to the disease. *B. equi* is most frequently involved in these cases.[3,30,31] Transmission of parasites in semen has not been documented; however, this may be possible if blood contamination of semen occurs.[32]

Life Cycle of *Babesia caballi*

The life cycle of *B. caballi* is typical of most *Babesia* species in that only erythrocytes are targeted in the mammalian host (Fig. 60-4). Infection is initiated by feeding of infected ticks, most often *Dermacentor nitens*, on a naive equine host. Sporozoites immediately invade erythrocytes. Within the erythrocyte, the parasite develops from a small anaplasmoid body (trophozoites), consisting predominantly of nuclear material, into a larger ameboid sphere that divides into two large pyriform bodies (merozoites) measuring approximately 2 to 5 µm long and 1.3 to 3 µm in diameter. When an uninfected tick subsequently feeds on the infected horse and ingests parasitized erythrocytes, most parasites are destroyed within the tick's midgut. However, some merozoites survive and form small, round bodies floating free within the gut contents of the tick. These spherical bodies give rise to large, clavate (club-shaped) bodies that penetrate the epithelial cells of the midgut and undergo multiple fissions. This is followed by infection of a variety of tick tissues, where a secondary cycle of multiple fissions occurs. Infected tissues in the female tick include all tissues and eggs except for the salivary glands. Small pyriform bodies produced in the salivary glands of the larvae, nymphs, and adults of the next tick generation are infective to the horse if these tick forms are feeding.[33] The large, paired merozoites joined at the posterior ends in the equine erythrocytes are a diagnostic feature of *B. caballi* infection[5] (see Fig. 60-1).

Life Cycle of *Babesia equi*

The details of the life cycle of *B. equi* may vary depending on the tick species involved.[34-37] Infected ticks feed on horses and inject *B. equi* sporozoites into the new mammalian host with their saliva. It has been reported that sporozoites initially are able to penetrate lymphocytes and form large *microschizonts* and *macroschizonts* (schizogony). These parasite forms ultimate give rise to approximately 200 merozoites per infected cell, each measuring approximately 1.5 to 2 µm in length. Merozoites invade erythrocytes and reproduce by binary fission (merogony), forming pyriform stages measuring approximately 2 to 3 µm. In erythrocytes, asexual division gives rise to four pear-shaped stages measuring approximately 2 µm and appearing as a "Maltese cross" form (see Fig. 60-2). After rupture of infected erythrocytes, merozoites enter new erythrocytes and continue to replicate. Some merozoites eventually become spherical in shape, forming ring forms, believed to be *gamonts*. When a tick ingests gamonts, gamonts grow in the tick's midgut, start nuclear reproduction, and initiate formation of "ray bodies" (protrusions). By 4 to 6 days after ingestion, ray bodies divide and form *microgamonts* and *macrogamonts*, which will fuse, forming zygotes (sexual replication). Inside the zygote a kinete is formed, which will later penetrate through the midgut of the tick into the hemolymph. *Kinetes* are observed 5 to 7 days after tick feeding and usually last 6 to 9 days. Kinetes penetrate into salivary gland type III cells 7 to 8 days after attachment. In these cells, sporonts, sporoblasts, and then sporozoites are formed (sporogony). Sporozoite development is typically complete between day 6 and 24 after completion of tick feeding.[17]

EPIDEMIOLOGY

Few countries in the world are free from autochthonus (native) infections with EP, and it is estimated that only 10% of horses globally inhabit regions that are free of EP. The countries currently recognized as nonendemic by the World Organization for Animal Health (OIE) include Australia, Canada, United States, England, Ireland, and Japan; the OIE website, http://www.oie.int, is available to confirm national information. Many areas currently free of EP are climatically suitable for appropriate tick vectors or already possess competent tick vectors.[3] Thus, there is the

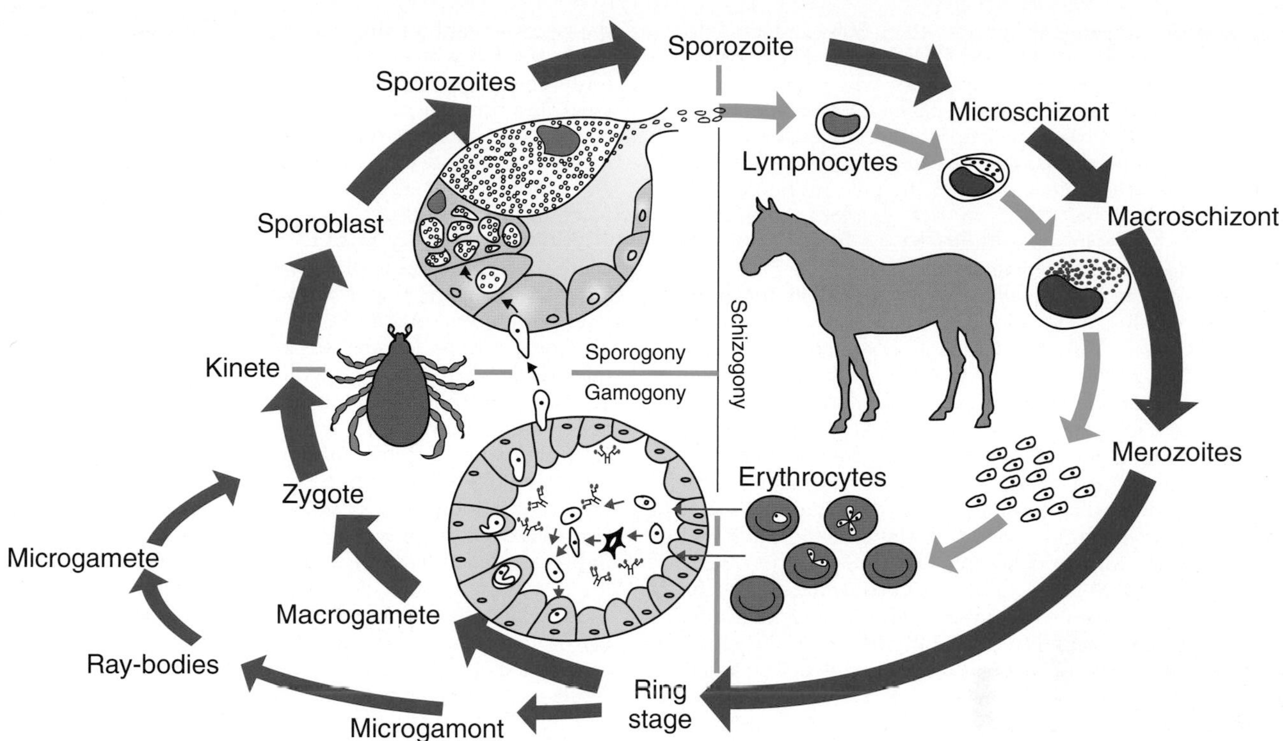

Fig. 60-4 Life cycle of *Babesia caballi*. *B. equi* life cycle is similar except for transovarial transmission within the tick and with the possible addition of a pre-erythrocytic stage within lymphocytes.

continual possibility of introducing *B. equi* and *B. caballi* into *Babesia*-free areas either by infected ticks or horses.

The worldwide prevalence of EP is consistent with worldwide distribution of competent tick vectors. Because *B. equi* and *B. caballi* share the same vectors in a given region, they are closely associated and are endemic in tropical and subtropical climates. In most regions, however, infections with *B. equi* are more common than infections with *B. caballi*.[2,3,20] Outbreaks of overt clinical disease are uncommon in endemic areas, with the exception of India, despite the endemic status of implicated parasites.[38] Outbreaks in Germany, Switzerland, and Australia in the past were attributed to the use of contaminated needles or instruments rather than tick transmission.[2] Acute clinical disease is most often observed when naive horses are moved into endemic areas.[39]

Babesia equi and *B. caballi* are endemic in almost all of Latin America, except for the southern parts of Chile and Argentina. Almost all horses in Brazil,[13,40-42] Colombia,[43] Puerto Rico, and Mexico[2,5] are seropositive for *B. equi* and *B. caballi*. Despite the widespread distribution of infection and the intense tick parasitism of the horse population in many parts of Latin America (see Fig. 60-3), data are limited regarding which ticks are responsible for transmission of EP in these countries. *B. caballi* is transmitted by *Dermacentor* (*Anocentor*) *nitens*, the "tropical horse tick."[40] *Boophilus microplus* is believed to be one of the ticks involved in the transmission of *B. equi*.[26,37] In a study in Brazil using nested polymerase chain reaction (PCR), both *B. equi* and *B. caballi* were identified in *B. microplus* ticks.[27] The significance of this finding is uncertain because these ticks are not generally considered to be a vector for *B. caballi*. *Boophilus microplus* primarily feeds on cattle, although it will occasionally feed on horses, especially if horses are kept in pasture with cattle. As a result, the seroprevalence of *B. equi* is higher in horses in close contact with cattle.[26,37,41] The most common species of tick found on horses in Brazil are *Dermacentor (Anocentor) nitens* (see Fig. 60-3) and *Amblyomma cajennense*.[26,40,41] Intense parasitism by these ticks is observed in horses at an early age in many regions of the country. In 1995, Barbosa et al.[40] found that 100% of foals in southeastern Brazil seroconvert to *B. equi* by 127 days of age and to *B. caballi* by 150 days. Yet, tick surveys using microscopy[40] or PCR[41] and experimental transmission studies fail to support *A. cajennense* as a natural tick vector for equine piroplasmosis.[2]

Babesia equi and *B. caballi* are widely present in Portugal, Spain, France, and Italy. Piroplasmosis is also endemic in the Balkan Peninsula, Hungary, Romania, several countries of the Commonwealth of Independent States (CIS, the southern parts of Russia), and the states of the Caucasus region. In central Russia, *B. caballi* infections have a common distribution with the tick vector *Dermacentor reticulatus*.[2,5] Most infections of horses in nonendemic European countries have been traced back to Spain, France, Italy, or the CIS. Belgium, Switzerland, Austria, the Czech Republic, and Poland are considered infection free, although autochthonous infections occasionally occur.[2,3,5] Potential vectors of the genus *Dermacentor* are present in most Northern European regions. *Hyalomma* and *Rhipicephalus* ticks predominate in southern Europe, the southern regions of Russia, and the CIS.[2]

Morocco,[45] Republic of South Africa, Madagascar, and nearly all other parts of the African continent are considered endemic for *B. equi* and *B. caballi*.[2,12,46-48] Virtually all horses and zebras are infected, except in a few regions. The seroprevalence in these countries is generally greater than 50% and 60% for *B. equi* and *B. caballi*, respectively. Ticks involved in transmission include *Rhipicephalus evertsi evertsi*, which can transmit both *B. equi* and *B. caballi*,[46] and *Hyalomma truncatum*, which transmits *B. caballi*.[49] An association between gender and the occurrence of antibodies against *B. caballi* has been observed in South Africa, with colts more likely to have antibodies than fillies.[50] This may be linked to tick gender predilection, because male horses in some studies have a higher burden of certain tick species than females.[50]

Babesia equi and *B. caballi* are widespread in the horse populations of Mongolia, China, and many parts of Southeast Asia and Asia.[27,51-53] In both China and Mongolia, *B. equi* is more prevalent and is primarily transmitted by *Dermacentor nuttallii*.[54,55] High infection rates are similarly reported in Korea.[5] Historically considered free of infection, recent reports demonstrate both *B. equi*–seropositive and *B. caballi*–seropositive horses in Japan.[56] The tick *Haemaphysalis longicornis* has been suggested as a potential vector for EP in Japan and was shown to acquire *B. caballi* from experimentally infected mice with severe combined immunodeficiency (SCID).[57] Further studies are necessary to verify if acquisition and transmission occurs in horses under natural conditions.[56] The "brown dog tick," *Rhipicephalus sanguineus*, listed as a potential *B. equi* vector, is also present in Japan. (This tick has been shown to transmit *B. caballi*, although it is not believed to be involved in the natural transmission of the disease because of its habit of feeding almost exclusively on dogs.[1,23])

High infection rates have also been reported in the Middle East, including Kuwait, Oman, and India, where *Babesia equi* is reported to have higher seroprevalence. Ticks involved are of the *Hyalomma* and *Rhipicephalus* species.[2,5,58,59] Jordan recently has reported fatalities in strenuously exercised horses with high-level *B. equi* parasitemia on blood smears and consistent necropsy findings.[60]

Although *B. equi* was introduced into Australia in the 1950s and 1960s with Quarter Horses imported from Texas and in 1976 with the importation of Andalusian horses from Spain, the organism did not become established in Australia. As in other nonendemic countries, transmission occurred by contaminated needles and instruments.[2,3,5,20] *Boophilus microplus* is present in parts of Australia, and other tick vectors capable of transmitting EP could potentially be introduced by horses or other hosts.[61,62]

Babesia caballi and *B. equi* were introduced into the United States (U.S.) in 1959 when Cuban horses were imported. Limited *B. caballi* infections became established in Florida, southern Georgia, Texas, and some adjacent states in which the tick vector *Dermacentor (Anocentor) nitens* was present.[9,15] Since then, a few new cases and epizootics have occurred in Florida, but with minor exceptions, further spread was prevented by intensive control measures.[15,29,63-65] Despite sporadic occurrence of EP in the U.S.,[66] it is considered free of EP. *Dermacentor nitens, D. albipictus*, and *D. variabilis* are potential tick vectors for *B. caballi* in the U.S. *Boophilus microplus* and *D. variabilis* are native to the U.S. and potential vectors of *B. equi*.[24] *B. microplus* has been eradicated from the U.S. but remains endemic in Mexico. The development of acaricide resistance in the U.S. at the border with Mexico increases the potential for reemergence of this tick in the U.S.[67]

PATHOGENESIS

In piroplasmosis-endemic areas, most horses become infected within the first year of life. Mortality in native horses may range from 5% to 10%, depending on the strain of protozoa, the general health of the animals, and the availability of treatment. Mortality rates exceeding 50% may occur when previously unexposed mature horses are introduced into endemic areas. Importation of infected animals into southern France resulted in 69% mortality among untreated horses.[1] The incubation period varies from 12 to 19 days for *B. equi* and 10 to 30 days for *B. caballi* and coincides with the peak in fever and erythrolysis.[3]

Alterations in erythrocyte membrane protein and lipid content and increases in plasma malondialdehyde during severe parasitemia suggest that accumulation of oxidative ions resulting from lipid peroxidation alters the erythrocytes' biochemical composition, leading to hemolysis.[68] These alterations may result in increased erythrocyte rigidity and decreased deformability, contributing to microvascular stasis.[68] The packed cell volume (PCV) typically decreases to 20% but may fall to 10% or lower. Extreme anemia is more common in *B. equi* infections.[29] Hemoglobinuria of varying severity, secondary to severe hemolysis, is observed in *B. equi* infection. Icterus, also caused by hemolysis, is the result of an increase in the indirect (unconjugated) bilirubin, which is deposited in mucosal surfaces and elsewhere, imparting a yellow color to those tissues. In the case of *B. caballi*, clumping of parasitized erythrocytes can lead to microvascular occlusion. Simultaneous thrombocytopenia and the systemic inflammatory response result in endothelial damage, increased vascular permeability, and in severe cases, disseminated intravascular coagulation (DIC). Severely affected horses experience edema, hemorrhage, ischemia, and anoxia, culminating in organ dysfunction.[1]

Thrombocytopenia has been described in association with EP and other protozoal infections. Although various theories as to its etiology have been proposed, the exact pathogenesis remains uncertain. Thrombocytopenia may be a result of low-grade DIC, as proposed in dogs with *Babesia canis* infections.[69]

Passage of infected erythrocytes across the placental barrier has been implicated as the probable mode of in utero transmission of disease and may result from damage to placental blood vessels, leading to mixing of maternal and fetal blood near or at the time of foaling.[16] Not all foals from an infected mare are born infected, and the factors that determine whether prenatal infection occurs have not been identified.[16]

Protective immunity is present as long as a horse harbors the *Babesia* organism, which in most cases is for life. There is no cross-immunity between *B. equi* and *B. caballi*.[1,29] The resistance to clinical disease acquired by horses after *Babesia* infection is a result of continued stimulation of immunity by the persisting parasite, but the exact mechanisms involved are unknown. Innate immunity likely plays a central role in control of *Babesia* parasites,[70,71] although the precise role of neutrophils, macrophages, and natural killer (NK) cells in parasite control is not defined.

The spleen is important in eliminating piroplasms. Horses with intact spleens often control infection and survive, whereas splenectomized horses develop severe parasitemia and succumb to the infection.[4,10,72,73] Despite its important role, the spleen and innate immunity are insufficient for protection against EP in the absence of adaptive immunity. In 1994, Knowles et al.[4] demonstrated that foals with SCID become severely anemic with a high level of parasitemia and die after experimental infection with *B. equi*. SCID foals lack mature T and B lymphocytes and are incapable of antigen-specific immune responses, but they have intact spleens and a competent innate immune system. This demonstrates that the spleen is unable to control *B. equi* infection in the absence of parasite-specific immune responses, and that erythrolysis caused by *B. equi* does not require a specific immune response.

High antibody titers correlate with parasite control in horses.[74,75] Immunoglobulin Ga (IgGa) and IgGb correlate with control of *B. equi* during the acute stage of infection, and IgG(T) increases during chronic infection.[76] Specific antibodies are first detected 7 to 11 days after experimental infection in ponies and reach a peak 30 to 45 days after infection.[77] *B. equi*–infected horses preferentially produce antibodies against highly conserved merozoite surface proteins, specifically *equi merozoite antigens* 1 and 2 (EMA-1 and EMA-2).[25,78] Passively transferred antibodies to *B. equi* and *B. caballi* may persist in the foal for 4 to 5 months.[79] However, foals born from *B. equi*–seropositive mares may be born infected without clinical disease and remain seropositive for life. Foals from endemic areas are particularly resistant to clinical disease.[41]

Despite the vigorous humoral immune response, in vivo and in vitro studies with serum of recovered animals failed to prove a full protective effect of antibodies,[80] suggesting that humoral antibodies are also insufficient for protection against EP.[75,80] Considering the importance of cell-mediated immune responses to other protozoan parasites, such as *Theileria parva* and *Babesia bovis*, it is expected that cell-mediated immunity plays a key role in immunity against *B. equi* and *B. caballi*.[4,81] The cell-mediated response to *Theileria* spp. schizont-infected cells is thought to be responsible for protective immunity.[81] Although this life-cycle stage may occur in *B. equi*, it does not seem to be as predominant as it is for *Theileria* species.

Mechanisms of protection against *Babesia* parasites in other species have been identified. Interferon-γ (IFN-γ), produced by CD4+ helper T lymphocytes, activates macrophages, enhancing phagocytosis and inducing production of antibodies.[82] Nevertheless, only superficial information is available demonstrating the contribution of cellular immunity to control of EP.[80,83] Donkeys immunized with *B. equi* immunogen, consisting of a lysate of parasitized erythrocytes combined with the adjuvant Quil A, developed a strong humoral and cell-mediated response and survived mortal challenge.[75]

CLINICAL FINDINGS

Horses infected with *B. caballi* and *B. equi* may present with similar clinical signs, although the signs associated with *B. caballi* infection tend to be milder or inapparent.[3] Clinical infections may be peracute, acute, subacute, or chronic.

Inapparent Carrier

The vast majority of *Babesia*-seropositive horses are inapparent carrier horses, with low levels of parasitemia and no obvious clinical signs. However, athletic or heavy working horses may have compromised athletic performance compared with uninfected horses. These horses are also at risk of developing overt infection with clinical illness.[45] Parasitemia levels are very low and may not be detectable with blood smears. These horses are reservoirs for the parasites and can potentially disseminate the organism in areas where vector ticks are present. Inapparent carrier mares may transmit *B. equi* by intrauterine infection throughout their breeding life, leading to abortion, stillbirth, or neonatal piroplasmosis.[3,30] A survey of Thoroughbred mares in South Africa reported that 11% of abortions in those herds were caused by *B. equi* infection.[12,30] Abortion usually occurs in the last trimester of gestation, and mares are usually clinical normal. However, *B. equi* has been identified in healthy fetuses at as early as 120 days of gestation, indicating that infection may actually occur early in gestation.[16,30] This form of transmission results in serious economic losses to horse breeders in EP-endemic areas.[3]

Peracute Equine Piroplasmosis

Peracute piroplasmosis occurs primarily in neonatal foals born infected in utero,[3,30,31] in adult horses suddenly introduced into areas with large numbers of infected ticks,[1] and in adult horses infected after strenuous exercise.[60] Neonatal piroplasmosis is characterized by weakness at birth or the rapid onset of listlessness, anemia, severe icterus, and malaise soon after birth. Affected foals become progressively lethargic and are ultimately unable to stand and suckle. Fever is usually present, and petechiae may be observed on the mucous membranes. Hemoglobinuria may also be evident.[16] Some foals are apparently normal at birth but develop clinical signs of EP 2 or 3 days later. Affected foals have a poor prognosis. Neonatal piroplasmosis may appear similar to equine neonatal isoerythrolysis, but differentiation is important so that adequate therapy can be implemented.[16,3]

Peracute infection with *B. caballi* results in organ damage and dysfunction caused by obstruction of capillaries or other small vessels with parasitized erythrocytes. Clinical signs in affected foals and adult horses therefore vary with the organ affected.[9] Central nervous system (CNS) involvement has been reported, with encephalitis, ataxia, and other signs, depending on the exact location of the lesions.[1,3]

During peracute *B. equi* infection, parasites replicate in erythrocytes, causing cell lysis and death from anemia.[9] Sudden death caused by piroplasmosis in adult horses is rare[5,84] but can occasionally occur when naive horses are introduced into *B. equi*–endemic areas.[1] *B. equi* has been implicated as the cause of death in two horses with high levels of parasitemia after strenuous exercise. Necropsy findings were also consistent with EP, and other horses on this property became severely sick with similar blood smear findings.[60]

Acute Equine Piroplasmosis

Acute cases of EP are characterized by pyrexia (typically exceeding 40° C [104° F]), moderate anorexia and malaise, frequent recumbency, dehydration, congested mucous membranes, tachypnea, tachycardia, sweating, limb edema, supraorbital edema and tearing, anemia and in severe cases icterus, hemoglobinuria/bilirubinuria (rare in *B. caballi* infections), and death.[1,3,5,29,63] Pneumonia may result as a complication of pulmonary edema and inflammation.[1] *B. equi* infection results in intermittent pyrexia; if untreated, mortality can be moderately high. Digestive tract involvement may occur terminally, with signs of colic, constipation, diarrhea, and catarrhal enteritis.[1,3,29,63] In severe cases, inflammation of mucous membranes and blood vessels occurs in various organs, and a variety of atypical presentations may result, including renal and liver failure.[1]

Subacute Equine Piroplasmosis

Horses with subacute EP exhibit varying degrees of anorexia, malaise, weight loss, intermittent pyrexia, normocytic normochromic anemia, limb edema, poor performance, tachycardia, and tachypnea. Mucous membranes vary from pale pink or pale yellow to bright yellow, with occasional petechiae and ecchymoses. Intermittent colic signs may occur. Constipation may be followed by diarrhea. Urine may be dark yellow to brown or reddish, depending on degree of hemoglobinuria. Horses with subacute EP typically have splenomegaly, which is palpable rectally.[3,5] If untreated, these horses may become severely anemic with marked general weakness.

Chronic Equine Piroplasmosis

Horses with chronic EP typically present with a history of nonspecific clinical signs, including mild inappetence, poor performance, weight loss, poor body condition, and malaise (Fig. 60-5). Anemia may be minimal. Clinical signs of chronic

EP may be similar to signs observed in horses with equine infectious anemia (EIA) or other chronic inflammatory conditions.

Clinicopathologic abnormalities in horses with *B. equi* or *B. caballi* infection may include reduced red blood cell count, platelet count, and hemoglobin concentration.[1,3,29] Acute infections are characterized by neutropenia and lymphopenia with occasional left shift.[14] Decreased plasma fibrinogen, serum iron, and phosphorus concentrations; increased serum bilirubin concentration; and prolonged clotting times[29] may also occur. Varying degrees of hemoglobinuria are observed in *B. equi*–infected horses. In experimentally infected horses, eosinopenia and monocytosis are observed during the initial stages of disease.[94] After approximately 10 days of infection, lymphocytosis develops, and PCV often decreases to approximately 20% but may fall to 10% or lower. Extreme anemia is more common with *B. equi* infection.[29] In chronic cases, serum bilirubin concentration is not usually increased, and only mild anemia may be observed.[29]

DIAGNOSIS

Clinical diagnosis of EP can be made based on clinical signs and examination of blood smears. Clinical signs may be nonspecific, and the disease may be confused with a variety of other conditions. Important differential diagnoses for EP include surra, equine infectious anemia, dourine, African horse sickness, purpura hemorrhagica, and toxicities, among others. Although it may be difficult to differentiate clinically between *B. equi* and *B. caballi*,[3] differentiation may be important for successful treatment. Serologic and PCR testing may be necessary in subclinical cases and for regulatory purposes. In a babesia-regulated country, the proper state and federal authorities should be contacted before collection or submission of samples from suspect animals. Careful and secure handling of samples is necessary, and samples should only be submitted to authorized laboratories. In the United States, the federal authorities (Area Veterinarian in Charge) can be found at http://www.aphis.usda.gov/vs/are_offices.html. For other countries, information can be found on the World Organization for Animal Health (OIE) website at http://www.oie.int.

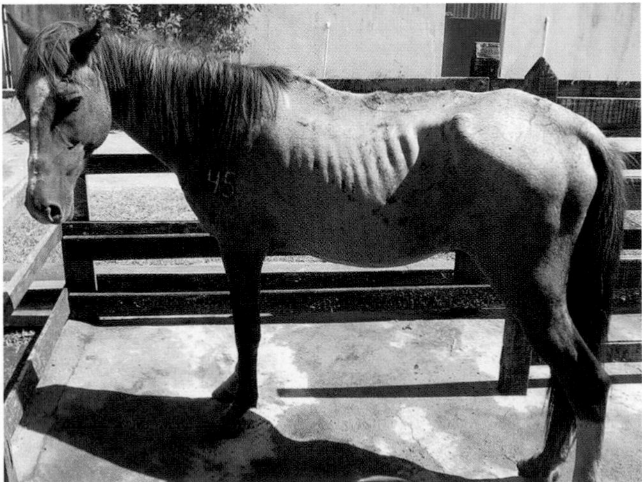

Fig. 60-5 Horse chronically infected with equine piroplasmosis.

Microscopy

If present, parasites can be observed in blood smears stained with a 10% Giemsa solution. In the acute phase of EP, diagnosis by microscopic examination of blood smears is possible. In inapparent carrier horses, however, the low number of piroplasms in circulation decreases the sensitivity of microscopy,[5,85] and serologic diagnosis is more reliable. Because parasitemia with *B. caballi* is very low, observation of parasites in thin blood smears is often difficult. The thick blood smear technique can be very useful.

The merozoites of *B. caballi* within erythrocytes are pyriform in shape and vary between 2 and 5 μm × 1 and 1.5 μm in size and often form pairs joined at their posterior ends[3] (see Fig. 60-1). Trophozoites may also be observed in erythrocytes and are polymorphic in shape, varying from round to oval or elliptic, measuring approximately 1.5 to 3 μm in diameter. *B. equi* merozoites in erythrocytes typically appear as four pyriform parasites, measuring approximately 1.5 μm long and arranged in a "Maltese cross" formation (see Fig. 60-2). The trophozoites can appear as oval, round, elliptic, or spindle in shape and can measure up to 3 μm in diameter within erythrocytes.[3]

Complement Fixation Test

The complement fixation test (CFT) was the previously officially standard test for equine piroplasmosis and has been used worldwide to test horses entering EP-free countries. Recently it has been determined that the regulatory assay for entrance of horses into the United States is the cELISA.

The underlying principle of the CFT is the fixation of complement during the reaction between specific antigen and antibody.[5,20] Horse sera that react positively at a dilution of 1:5 are considered positive. The CFT detects antibody titers from day 8 after infection, with titers declining at 2 to 3 months after infection. CFT reactions may become transiently negative within 3 to 15 months of treatment of *B. caballi*–infected horses and within 24 months for *B. equi*–infected horses.[20,86] For this reason, retesting of treated horses must be done 4 to 6 weeks after treatment.

Many disadvantages are associated with the use of CFT, including the need for production of large quantities of antigens, the occurrence of false-negative results,[87,88] and cross-reactivity between *B. caballi* and *B. equi* sera.[11,20] CFT is a very specific test; however, it has low sensitivity in chronic cases because of the presence of IgG(T) antibodies (noncomplement fixing).[87,88]

Indirect Immunofluorescent Antibody Test

The indirect immunofluorescent antibody test (IFAT) is more sensitive than the CFT and has been used as a supplementary test when CFT results are inconclusive.[5,20] In this assay, parasite antigens are bound to glass slides and allowed to react with test sera. Bound antibodies are visible under ultraviolet light after binding of a fluorescein-labeled antiequine serum. Sera are considered positive if they show strong fluorescence of the parasites at a dilution of 1:80 and higher. The earliest antibody responses in horses experimentally infected with *B. caballi* and *B. equi* in one study were at 3 to 20 days after infection, with titers still detectable during the latent period of infection. IFAT titers are detected more consistently than CFT titers, and sera remain positive by IFAT longer than by CFT. To increase specificity with IFAT, serum must be diluted, which concurrently results in loss of sensitivity.

The IFAT is time-consuming, requires large amounts of antigen, and because of subjectivity in interpreting fluorescence, is difficult to standardize.[5,20]

Enzyme-Linked Immunosorbent Assay

The enzyme-linked immunosorbent assay (ELISA) is used to detect dominant antibodies to both *B. equi* and *B. caballi*, although cross-reactivity may occur.[5,20] In 1991, Knowles et al.[78] using *B. equi* EMA-1 and specific monoclonal antibodies, developed a competitive inhibition ELISA (cELISA) for *B. equi* infection.[88] EMA-1 is a specific *B. equi* surface erythrocyte-stage protein that possesses an epitope shown to be both immunodominant and conserved worldwide.[25] This cELISA was later improved by the use of a recombinant protein instead of culture-derived whole parasites.[25] This test overcomes the problem of antigen purity because specificity depends only on the monoclonal antibody used. ELISA has improved performance compared with CFT and IFAT[5,89] and has detected latent infections of experimentally infected horses not detected by CFT.[20] The use of a recombinant protein facilitates standardization of the assay and overcomes the need for in vitro cultivation of the parasite or the artificial infection of horses for antigen production, making cELISA an ideal test for screening of *Babesia* infection.

In 1999 a cELISA using recombinant *B. caballi* rhoptry-associated protein-1 was developed by the same group.[90] In a field survey, this test identified 25% more sera as positive for *B. caballi* than the CFT.[90] In 2004, OIE (http://www.oie.int) approved the cELISA for both *B. equi* and *B. caballi* as the prescribed test for international horse trading.

A single-dilution ELISA using the whole-merozoite antigen was validated in the field in India by Kumar et al.[38] in 2003 to detect antibodies to *B. equi*. These authors reported the test to be economical and sensitive, with no cross-reaction with *B. caballi*, and suitable for large epidemiologic studies.

Polymerase Chain Reaction

Detection of parasite deoxyribonucleic acid (DNA) using polymerase chain reaction (PCR) is more sensitive than microscopic detection of parasites in blood smears and is ideal for the detection of carrier infections.[91] The PCR systems may be useful tools in the expeditious detection and identification of *B. equi* and *B. caballi* in blood, as supplements to microscopy and serology for augmenting diagnostic results; at this time, however, these systems are only used for research purposes. Surveys of horses in endemic areas are necessary for assessment of the diagnostic sensitivity and specificity of these assays.[85]

Primary PCR assays have been developed to detect both *B. equi* and *B. caballi* DNA in horses.[85] In one survey, PCR was able to detect calculated parasitemias as low as 0.0083% for *B. equi* and 0.017% for *B. caballi*. However, most horses with positive PCR results also had positive microscopic examination of blood smears. A nested PCR for *B. equi* based on the sequence of the EMA-1 gene has increased sensitivity and may be more reliable for the diagnosis of subclinical infection, detecting an equivalent calculated parasitemia of 0.000006%.[91] In a field study using the same nested PCR for *B. equi*, the test was able to detect 3.6 times more infections than microscopic analysis and 2.2 times more than with primary PCR. Many subclinical infections in apparently healthy horses that could not be detected with primary PCR were detected by nested PCR.[44] The same test has been successfully used to detect *B. caballi*–infected and *B. equi*–infected ticks in Mongolia[27,52]and to detect infected ticks and horses in Brazil.[27]

A PCR-based hybridization assay for *B. caballi* using a specific biotin-labeled DNA probe has been developed with good results but has not yet been tested in field conditions.[92] PCR testing is fairly straightforward and becoming more affordable and soon may become commercially available.

In Vitro Organism Cultivation

In vitro culture of blood samples from suspected animals for the identification of *B. caballi*[93] and *B. equi*[12,66] in carrier horses and zebras[6] has been described. This is an alternative to the traditional in vivo testing in which blood from a suspected infected horse is injected into a susceptible splenectomized horse, which is observed for development of typical clinical signs and clinicopathologic evidence of disease. Despite the considerable advantage of eliminating the need for use of live animals, in vitro culture methods are laborious, expensive, and inconsistent and therefore are not appropriate for commercial use.

PATHOLOGIC FINDINGS

Gross pathologic findings of EP include anemia, icterus, edema of subcutaneous and subserosal tissue, varying degrees of emaciation, hepatomegaly, splenomegaly, enlarged pale to red-brown kidneys, ascites, hydrothorax and hydropericardium with epicardial and endocardial hemorrhages, congestion and edema of the lungs, and enlargement of lymph nodes.[3,14,29,63,95] Catarrhal enteritis has been reported in some affected horses.[1,29]

Histopathologic examination reveals congestion and edema of the lungs and centrilobular necrosis of the liver with bile stasis. Renal changes consist of hydropic and fatty degeneration of the tubular epithelium and protein and hemoglobin casts in many tubules of the cortex and medulla. There is also a marked proliferation of the reticuloendothelial cell system in the liver, kidneys, lungs, and lymph nodes. Thrombi in the blood vessels of the liver and lungs have been reported. Many hemosiderin-containing macrophages may be present in pulmonary alveolar walls.[3,95] Lymph node sinuses are distended, with evidence of phagocytosis of parasitized erythrocytes. Syncytial accumulations of macrophages can be observed in the sinuses. Parasites within erythrocytes present in vessels can also be observed.[95] Hemosiderosis in the liver and spleen can be observed secondary to erythrolysis.[14]

THERAPY

The efficacy of drugs for treatment of EP is highly variable, and close monitoring of horses undergoing treatment is necessary to ensure success. Treatment strategies may aim at resolving the clinical signs during acute infection or at completely clearing the horse from the carrier state (sterilization). The latter is more difficult and possibly unattainable. Although it has been stated that horses with *B. caballi* infection may self-clear the infection,[2,3,5] it is important to remember that most reports of successful sterilization for both *B. caballi* and *B. equi* were before the development and availability of more sensitive tests such as nested PCR. Attempts to eliminate the carrier state of EP is not recommended in endemic areas, but may be desirable for movement of horses to areas that are considered EP free.[3]

Babesia caballi Infection in Adult Horses

For the treatment of adult horses with acute clinical signs of *B. caballi* infection, intramuscular (IM) administration of *imidocarb dipropionate* (Imizol, Schering-Plough Animal Health, USA) at 2.2 mg/kg body weight for two treatments with a 24-hour interval is considered most effective.[5,20,49,96] Although relatively safe, imidocarb can cause toxicity with fatal outcomes in some horses. Mild signs of toxicity include salivation, gastrointestinal (GI) hypermotility, and colic.[96] Donkeys can be particularly sensitive to imidocarb toxicity, with high mortality rates in treated animals.[97] The same imidocarb treatment regimen is recommended for sterilization, although this may actually result in temporary disappearance of the organisms, with later recrudescence. The time required for horses to become seronegative by CFT after imidocarb treatment varies substantially, with one study reporting an average of 39 days (maximum, 116 days) to "clearance."[96]

Diminazene (Berenil, Hoechst, Germany; Ganaseg, Squibb-Mathieson, Mexico) is effective for treatment of acute disease when administered intramuscularly (IM) at 11 mg/kg for two treatments 24 hours apart. This therapy may result in elimination of the organism.[3,5] Deep IM injections are recommended; swelling and necrosis at diminazene injection sites have been reported. The use of multiple injection sites for the administration of smaller volumes of drug per site helps obviate local reactions.[98] Respiratory distress and depression are primary signs of intoxication.

Amicarbalide (Diampron, May & Baker, England) administered at 9 to 10 mg/kg IM single dose is often sufficient for treatment of horses with acute signs of EP. When administered at 8.8 mg/kg for 2 consecutive days, amicarbalide therapy has been claimed to result in sterilization.[3] A delayed anaphylactic-type reaction, with respiratory and GI disturbances, periorbital and muzzle edema, and subcutaneous edema over the back and flank, has been reported in a few horses. A dosage of 2.2 mg/kg IM for 2 consecutive days may be used to treat clinical signs of *B. caballi* infection but does not result in clearance.[98]

Acridine dyes such as *euflavine* (Gonacrine, May & Baker, England), 4 to 8 mL/100 kg of a 5% solution with a maximum volume of 20 mL, and tetracyclines are reported to alleviate clinical signs but not clear infection.[3,20,98] It has been reported that it may take approximately 3 to 15 months for a horse to become seronegative by CFT after spontaneous or therapeutic clearance of *B. caballi*.[20]

Babesia equi Infection in Adult Horses

Babesia equi is resistant to most therapeutic agents, and sterilization or even temporary clearance may not be accomplished even with persistent and repeated efforts. Most horses that survive clinical infection remain lifelong carriers of the parasite. In some cases, treated horses become seronegative by CFT for a few weeks or months but remain positive by IFAT.[2] Additional supportive therapy is often necessary if severe hemolysis and enterocolitis are present. This may include intravenous (IV) fluid therapy and electrolyte replacement, glucose infusions, nonsteroidal antiinflammatory drugs (NSAIDs), and even blood transfusions.

Imidocarb dipropionate (Imizol) at a dosage of 4 mg/kg administered four times at 72-hour intervals is usually an effective treatment for clinical signs of *B. equi* infection.[3,5,99] This dose is near the 50% lethal dose (LD_{50}) for imidocarb and may cause moderate to severe signs of intoxication and even death.[3] Clinical signs of toxicity include salivation, restlessness, slight to moderate colic, and GI hypermotility. Local injection site reactions can also occur, although these generally resolve without complications.[97] Administration of half this dose initially, followed by the remainder of the dose, may decrease toxicity. The treatment should not be repeated before 30 days after the first treatment. Liver function should be monitored in treated horses. Increases in serum activities of aspartate aminotransferase (AST), alanine aminotransferase (ALT), alkaline phosphatase (AP), and sorbitol dehydrogenase (SDH) may be observed.[100] Necropsy findings in horses with imidocarb toxicity include acute periportal hepatic necrosis and renal cortical tubular necrosis.[101] It is unclear what factors predispose some donkeys to these adverse reactions, and care must be taken if treating these animals with imidocarb. High doses of imidocarb have been successfully used in zebras with no significant adverse reactions.[102] Administration of imidocarb at 6 to 8 mg/kg for 4 doses with a 72-hour interval between doses may induce clearance but has a very high risk of toxicity.[2,5] Some *B. equi* strains, such as those of European origin, may have differing susceptibility to treatments with imidocarb.[99,103]

Antitheilerial drugs have been used with variable success in the treatment of clinical signs of *B. equi* infection but cannot completely eliminate the parasite (parvaquone, Clexon, Coopers Animal Health, England).[99] *Buparvaquone* (Butalex, Coopers), 4 to 6 mg/kg given as a slow IV injection once a day for 3 consecutive days, successfully resolved clinical signs of *B. equi* infection in two experimentally infected splenectomized horses; however, these horses remained inapparent carriers. No toxicity was observed if treatment began before horses were severely ill and while PCV remained above 25%. IM administration of this drug resulted in severe local reaction and lameness that lasted 2 to 3 days.[103] The greatest activity of these drugs is against the schizont stages of the parasites. A combination of buparvaquone and imidocarb therapy may eliminate *B. equi* infection.[20] Experimental trials using this combination are necessary. The combination of IV buparvaquone with IM artheeter (E-Mal, Themis Laboratories, India), an antimalarial drug (each drug 5 mg/kg for 4 days), resulted in temporary clearance of infection in splenectomized donkeys.[100] This combination has not been administered to intact horses.

Other antiprotozoal drugs have had variable results against *Babesia* in vitro.[3,20,100,104,105] Imidocarb is recommended for treatment of mixed infections. It is believed to take approximately 24 months for a horse to become seronegative by CFT if complete elimination of *B. equi* occurs.[20]

Pregnant Carrier Mares (*B. equi* or *B. caballi*)

Effective measures to prevent abortion or stillbirth from EP have not been described.[30] It is unknown at what stage *B. equi* infects the fetus, and therefore the optimal time for treatment has not been determined. Abortions usually occur in the last trimester of gestation, but *B. equi* has been identified in healthy fetuses as early as 120 days of gestation.[16,30] Imidocarb is detectable in the fetal circulation at a similar concentration as found in the dam's blood, but correlation between treatment of mares with the birth of sick or healthy foals has not yet been described. Imidocarb is eliminated in the milk for approximately 2 hours after administration of a dose of 2.4 mg/kg in the dam.[106] It is uncertain if this can cause toxicity effects in nursing foals.

Neonatal Piroplasmosis

Even with appropriate intensive therapy, prognosis for most neonatal foals with EP is poor.[3,16] Infected foals frequently become severely anemic. Transfusion with a crossmatched noninfected blood donor should be performed. The PCV should be closely monitored for 2 weeks or longer for recrudescence of severe anemia. Other supportive therapy may include judicious fluid therapy, adequate nutrition (bottle, nasogastric tube, or parenteral), and broad-spectrum antibiotic therapy (if concomitant sepsis is a concern).

No data exist regarding the safety or efficacy of babesicidal drugs (e.g., imidocarb) in equine neonates. One brief report described the successful treatment of an infected equine neonate with one 0.5-mL dose of 12% imidocarb diproprionate IM combined with 3 mL of 10% oxytetracycline hydrochloride (Terramycin Q-100, Pfizer) intravenously. Twenty-four hours later the same dose of oxytetracycline was repeated. Three months later, this foal presented with the same clinical signs, and treatment was repeated for 2 consecutive days. Recovery was uneventful.[107]

PREVENTION

Several experimental immunization strategies have been tested for EP. At present, however, there are no effective, commercially available vaccines for *B. equi* or *B. caballi*.[75] Control of EP largely relies on drug therapy, tick-vector control, and restrictions in the movement of infected horses. Control measures vary depending on the piroplasmosis status of the location. In disease-free areas, tick-borne infections typically do not occur, and the entrance of infected horses and ticks is closely monitored. Currently, the countries that restrict the movement of serologically positive horses include the U.S., Canada, Australia, Japan, Mexico, and Brazil.[71] For import into the U.S., a horse testing positive for *B. caballi* is quarantined. The horse may be allowed entry after appropriate drug treatment and subsequent serologic testing demonstrate lack of *B. caballi* antibody. Horses that test positive for *B. equi* are denied entrance. If a domestic horse is found to be seropositive for *B. equi*, it must be quarantined, exported, or euthanized. Implementation of compliance is through the respective state and federal authorities.* If a domestic horse is seropositive for *B. caballi*, the horse may be allowed to remain in the country under quarantine and treated until the infection is cleared. Under all these circumstances, immediate notification of appropriate state or federal authorities is required, and compliance is usually monitored by these authorities.

Preventing the introduction of infected ticks can be difficult or impossible, especially if neighboring countries have high tick infestations. Strict quarantine and treatment of horses with acaricides at the time of import are usually performed to minimize the risk of introducing ticks. Introduction of infected ticks by domestic, wild, and zoo or other exotic animals is also a threat.[2]

In endemic areas, premunition strategies may be an important method to control outbreaks of disease caused by EP. *Premunition* is a state of prior infection and obtainment of carrier status for maintenance of protective immunity. Attempts to chemosterilize horses should be avoided in endemic areas, and only moderately to severely sick horses should be treated with babesicidal drugs. Under highly intensive management systems, it may be feasible to control EP by eliminating tick infestation on horses with regular application of acaricides.[2,20] In these endemic areas, strategic tick control should agree with seasonality of tick infestation, when animals are not being moved.[20] Exposure of foals to ticks and natural infection may result in immunity without overt signs of disease.[3,20] Development of acaricide resistance is a serious problem in many heavily tick-infested areas and is a consideration for limited use.[67]

*http://www.aphis.usda.gov/vs/sregs/official.html, http://www.aphis.usda.gov/vs/area_offices.htm.

PUBLIC HEALTH CONSIDERATIONS

Although a strain of *B. equi* has been implicated in rare human cases, there have been no confirmed reports of human infection with either *B. caballi* or *B. equi*. The *Babesia* species known to be transmitted to humans are the bovine pathogens *B. bovis* and *B. divergens* (the most virulent causing fulminant disease), the canine pathogen *B. canis*, and the white-footed mouse and white-tailed deer pathogen *B. microti*. Infection with *B. divergens* is most virulent and likely to cause fulminant disease. Transmission can occur through infected ixodid ticks or as a result of contaminated blood transfusions.[108]

REFERENCES

See the CD-ROM for a list of references linked to the abstract in PubMed.

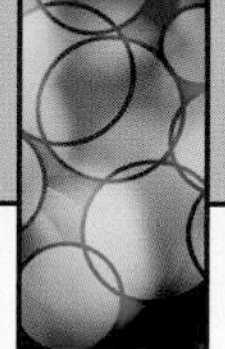

CHAPTER • 61

Miscellaneous Parasitic Diseases

Debra C. Sellon

TRYPANOSOMIASIS

The trypanosomes are spindle-shaped protozoal parasites, most of which propel themselves with a flagellum and undulating membrane. Infection of horses with *Trypanosoma equiperdum*, *Trypanosoma evansi*, and *Trypanosoma brucei brucei* has traditionally been associated with the diseases dourine, surra, and African animal trypanosomiasis (AAT), respectively. These species make up the subgenus *Trypanozoon* (Protozoa: Sarcomastigophora: Kinetoplastida: *Trypanosomatidae*).[1] Differentiation of the parasite species in this subgenus on a morphologic, serologic, and molecular basis is unclear, and recent reports suggest that current species designations may ultimately prove to be incorrect.[1-5]

The other trypanosomes that infect horses, *Trypanosoma congolense* (subgenus *Nannomonas*) and *Trypanosoma vivax* (subgenus *Duttonella*), with *T. brucei brucei*, are etiologic agents of AAT. Because of the considerable confusion in nomenclature for specific trypanosomes that infect horses and the considerable overlap in clinical disease that may result from infection with these parasites, this chapter discusses the trypanosomal infections of horses as clinical syndromes (dourine, surra, and AAT) rather than individual etiologic agents.

Dourine

Etiology

Dourine is a chronic trypanosomal disease of horses that is transmitted predominantly by coitus and is characterized by genital edema, neurologic dysfunction, and death. A disease similar to dourine was described in early Arab texts[4]; the first mention of this disease in European literature was in 1796.[6] In 1894, Rouget[7] isolated *T. equiperdum* from the blood of an Algerian horse. Disease was later reproduced by subcutaneous inoculation of a horse with another isolate of the parasite, and the name *Trypanosoma equiperdum* was proposed by Doflein in 1901.[8-10]

Epidemiology and Pathogenesis

Historically, dourine has been present in Europe, North America, Asia, and Africa.[4] After World War I, the disease was eradicated from Western Europe by serologic screening, strict sanitation, and treatment of some horses with trypanosides.[4] Currently, dourine is considered a reportable disease by the World Organization for Animal Health (OIE) and is present in most of Asia, southeastern Europe, South America, and Africa. Dourine has been reported recently in Kyrgyzstan, Botswana, Lesotho, Namibia, and South Africa.[2]

Equids are considered the only natural host for *T. equiperdum*. Clinical signs are less obvious in donkeys than in horses, and these animals may be a reservoir for infection.[2] Disease is not observed in zebras, although they may be seropositive by complement fixation test (CFT).[2] A variety of animal species, including dogs and rabbits, may show clinical signs of disease after experimental infection with *T. equiperdum*. The organism is present in the urethra of infected stallions and in vaginal discharges of infected mares. Transmission in horses primarily occurs by coitus, although mechanical transmission by arthropod vectors is also possible.[11,12] *T. equiperdum* can pass through intact mucous membranes. Transmission is considered most likely during the early stages of disease. The incubation period between exposure and initial clinical signs is highly variable; it may be as short as 1 to 2 weeks or as long as several years.[11]

Foals born to mares infected with *T. equiperdum* may be infected in utero or may become infected during parturition. Transmission to foals by ingestion of infected colostrum or milk is considered rare. Foals that ingest colostrum from infected mares will become seropositive due to passive transfer of antibodies; these foals are usually seronegative by 4 to 7 months of age.

Clinical Findings

In endemic regions, clinical signs of dourine are milder in native equids than in recently introduced breeds. The strain prevalent in southern Africa may be less virulent than the European, Asian, or North African strains, producing a very chronic, insidious disease with a long incubation period. Clinical signs may be precipitated by stress.[13] The observations of geographic differences in disease severity are supported by a recent report of genetic differences between African *T. equiperdum* isolates and isolates from China and South America.[1]

The first signs of dourine in mares are vaginal discharge with edema of the vulva, perineum, mammary gland, and ventral abdomen. Some mares exhibit signs of vulvitis and vaginitis with polyuria or other signs of perineal discomfort. Abortion may occur if mares are infected with virulent strains. In stallions, initial clinical signs include edema of the external genitalia and perineum. Paraphimosis may occur.[13] Cutaneous plaques, when they occur, are considered pathognomonic for dourine ("silver dollar plaques"); however, these plaques do not occur with all strains of the parasite.[4] Conjunctivitis and keratitis may occur in some infected horses. Chronically infected horses develop signs of neurologic dysfunction with progressive weakness and ataxia, leading ultimately to recumbency and death. These horses usually exhibit wasting despite a good appetite and frequently have anemia. Clinical signs may wax and wane for many months or years before death, depending on the strain of infecting parasite and the host immune response.[13]

Diagnosis

In endemic regions, the diagnosis of dourine is usually made on the basis of characteristic clinical signs. Serum, whole blood in ethylenediaminetetraacetic acid (EDTA) and blood smears from affected horses may be submitted for identification of the parasite (Fig. 61-1); however, these attempts are not often successful. The OIE-prescribed test for diagnosis of dourine is the CFT; this test does not distinguish between infection with *T. equiperdum* and infection with the closely related *T. evansi*, *T. gambiense*, or *T. brucei*.[14,15] Despite this cross-reactivity, the CFT has been used effectively for the eradication of dourine in many countries, including Canada,[16] Ethiopia,[17] Italy,[12] Morocco,[18] South Africa,[11,19] and Russia.[20-22] Alternative serologic tests include indirect fluorescent antibody (IFA), card agglutination, agar-gel immunodiffusion (AGID), arrayed immunodiffusion, and enzyme-linked immunosorbent assays (ELISA).[19,23-25]

Therapy

In most situations, treatment of horses with dourine is not recommended because it may result in an inapparent carrier state.[13] There are reports of treatment of affected horses with neoarsphenamine,[26] suramin,[27] and quinapyramine dimethylsulfate.[28] Of these, neoarsphenamine and suramin have been used in large dourine eradication programs.[18,21,22,29] In vitro testing suggests that *T. equiperdum* is also susceptible to diminazene, melarsomine, and isometamidium.[30-32]

Prevention and Public Health Considerations

Dourine has been successfully eradicated from many parts of the world using programs based on CFT testing. The Terrestrial Code of the OIE contains recommendations for testing and quarantine of horses imported from an endemic

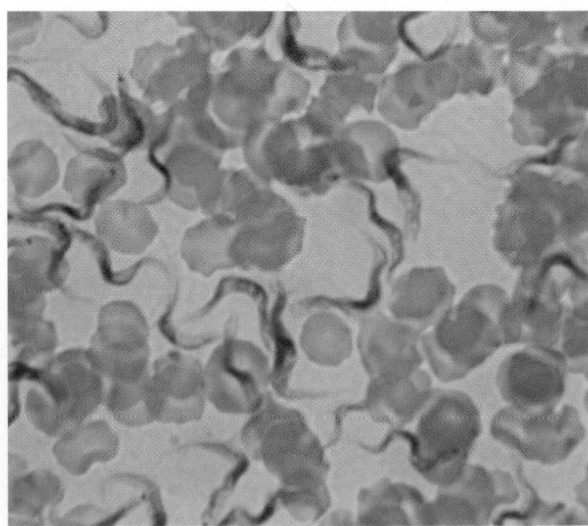

Fig. 61-1 *Trypanosoma equiperdum* in blood smear from infected mouse. (Courtesy Dr. Ellis Greiner.)

area into a dourine-free country. Two conditions should be met before importation of semen from a stallion that resides in a country that is not considered free of dourine: (1) the stallion should be housed for 6 months before semen collection in an establishment or artificial insemination center where no case of dourine was reported during that period, and (2) the stallion should be seronegative for *T. equiperdum*.

Surra

Etiology

Surra is caused by infection with the hemoparasite *Trypanosoma evansi*. The name is a Hindi word meaning "rotten."[33] Surra, the first pathogenic trypanosome to be discovered, was originally described by Griffith Evans, a British veterinarian, who described the condition in horses and camels in India in 1880.[33] Surra is characterized by anemia, weight loss, recurrent fever, and death in a wide variety of domestic animals, including horses, cattle, buffalo, and camels, in Asia, Africa, and South America.

Epidemiology and Pathogenesis

Surra is most severe and most frequently diagnosed in horses and camels. It may also affect cattle, buffalo, llamas, dogs, cats, sheep, goats, pigs, and elephants. In some species, only occasional mild or inapparent infections are seen. The disease is seen in South America, northern Africa, the Middle East, Asia, Indonesia, and the Philippines.[34,35] The etiologic agent, *T. evansi*, is transmitted mechanically by hematophagous biting flies of the species *Tabanus* and *Stomoxys*. Transmission by vampire bats is also possible.[35] Mortality rate in horses can be quite high in areas where the disease has been newly introduced. Outbreaks of surra tend to occur in areas where there are large numbers of commingled horses, large numbers of appropriate vectors, and reservoir hosts. The incubation period after infection is approximately 1 to 2 weeks. There is no known age, breed, or gender predilection.

Clinical Findings

Horses with surra present with fever, progressive anemia, weight loss despite a good appetite, and neurologic abnormalities.[36] Disease is usually acute, although some horses will experience chronic manifestations. Intermittent fever correlates with intermittent episodes of parasitemia. Urticarial lesions and edematous plaques may appear on the ventral abdomen; distal limb edema and petechial hemorrhages are common. Horses with severe anemia have pale mucous membranes. Neurologic signs, when they occur, lead to progressive weakness and ataxia, most apparent in the hindlimbs.[35] Experimentally, acute infection is associated with monocytosis (up to 35%) followed by lymphocytosis.[36] In an outbreak of surra on a breeding farm in Thailand, 42% of pregnant mares aborted or gave birth to stillborn foals. On this farm, 40% (19/47) of affected horses and 10% (1/10) of affected mules died.[37]

Diagnosis

A diagnosis of surra is suspected on the basis of compatible clinical signs in a horse residing in an area endemic for this disease. In the early stages of disease, this diagnosis is confirmed by observation of typical trypanosomes in blood or tissue fluids. This approach to diagnosis is more difficult in equids with chronic disease.[38,39] Centrifugation of a blood sample and examination of the buffy coat layer may increase the sensitivity of this technique.[35] Available serologic assays include ELISA, card agglutination test, and latex agglutination test. Data on their sensitivity and specificity for the field diagnosis of equine surra are largely lacking. The mouse inoculation test[40] is considered the most accurate diagnostic test for surra but takes up to 6 weeks to complete and is therefore not practical for routine screening.[36] The mouse inoculation test and direct review of wet blood films or buffy coat preparations are accurate for diagnosis early in disease (48 and 96 hours of infection, respectively).[41,42] The reported sensitivity and specificity of other antigen detection (antigen-ELISA,[39] latex agglutination[43,44]) and antibody detection (antibody-ELISA,[39] card agglutination,[45,46] IFA[47]) methods have varied depending on methodology and investigator.[36,41,42]

Therapy

Suramin is the drug that has most frequently been used for treatment of surra in horses. The recommended dose is 10 mg/kg body weight intravenously (IV), repeated 1 week later.[35] Quinapyramine sulfate at 3 mg/kg has a risk of adverse local reactions, and the dose should be divided between two or more sites.[35] Isometamidium chloride at 0.25 to 2 mg/kg imtramuscularly (IM)[35] and melarsen oxide[33] have also been suggested as treatments for surra. On a breeding farm in Thailand treatment of affected horses with diminazene aceturate at 3.5 mg/kg was initially effective in clearing *T. evansi* from the peripheral blood but was less effective with a second treatment. Approximately 50% of treated horses and mules showed moderate to severe signs of adverse reaction to the drug, including lip edema, salivation, recumbency, restlessness, and dyspnea.[37]

Prevention and Public Health Considerations

There are no vaccines for prevention of surra in horses. Prevention relies on identification and treatment of infected horses, appropriate vector control, and hygiene. Repeated treatment with antitrypanosomal medications such as suramin, quinapyramine, or isometamidium chloride has been suggested.[34]

There is a single report of human *T. evansi* infection in an Indian farmer with fluctuating parasitemia and fever who was successfully treated with suramin.[48]

African Animal Trypanosomiasis

Etiology

African animal trypanosomiasis (tsetse disease, tsetse fly disease, African animal nagana) is a disease complex caused by infection with *Trypanosoma congolense*, *T. vivax*, or *T. brucei brucei*, either singly or in combination.[49-52] In East Africa, *T. congolense* is the most important cause of AAT. Cattle, sheep, goats, horses, and pigs develop significant clinical disease if infected. In West Africa, *T. vivax* is the most important cause of AAT in cattle. The polymorphic trypanosome *T. brucei brucei* causes significant disease in horses, dogs, cats, camels, and pigs.

Epidemiology and Pathogenesis

Infection of cattle, sheep, goats, pigs, horses, camels, dogs, cats, and monkeys with the etiologic agents of AAT results in disease that ranges from subclinical to mild to chronic to fatal.[49] Numerous laboratory and wild animal species may also be infected. Wild ruminants are considered reservoirs of infection.[49] In Africa, the most important biologic vectors for transmission of AAT are three species of tsetse flies: *Glossina morsitans*, *G. palpalis*, and *G. fusca*. Large hematophagous flies *(Tabanus, Haematopa, Liperosia, Stomoxys, Chrysops)* may act as mechanical vectors in some situations.[49] The natural range of AAT infection is largely defined by the range of the principal vector, the tsetse fly, and includes the area from the southern edge of the Sahara desert to Angola, Zimbabwe, and Mozambique.[49] Only *T. vivax* occurs in the Western Hemisphere (Caribbean and South and Central America), where tabanid and hippoboscid flies probably transmit the parasite mechanically.[49]

Trypanosomes that cause AAT replicate in the skin at the site of initial inoculation, causing a sore or chancre, and then spread to draining lymph nodes and blood. Parasitemia is detectable within a few days of experimental infection. *T. congolense* localizes in endothelial cells, whereas *T. vivax* and *T. brucei brucei* localize in tissues. Antibodies to the glycoprotein coat of the parasite are produced, killing the parasite and forming immune complexes with released coat protein. Parasites are not eliminated because antigenic changes in the surface coat proteins of the trypanosome occur. The result is cycles of parasitemia, antibody production, death of parasites, immune complex formation, and glycoprotein coat antigenic changes. Many of the lesions observed in animals with AAT are probably the result of immune complex disease (e.g., anemia, glomerulonephritis).[49,53] Marked immunosuppression predisposes to secondary infections.

Clinical Findings

Clinical signs of AAT, regardless of the specific trypanosome involved, include anemia, intermittent fever, edema, and weight loss.[49,54] Abortion and infertility may be observed. Stressors such as malnutrition or concurrent disease increase the likelihood and severity of disease. Infection with *T. congolense* has an incubation period that varies from 4 to 24 days; it causes severe disease in horses, cattle, sheep, goats, and camels, with milder disease in pigs. In donkeys, it may cause chronic infection with longer persistence in the blood.[55] In contrast, *T. vivax* has an incubation period of 4 to 40 days and causes relatively mild disease in horses. Infection of horses with *T. brucei brucei* has a comparatively short incubation period (5-10 days) and causes severe, frequently fatal, infection of horses, camels, dogs, and cats, with mild, chronic or subclinical disease in cattle, sheep, goats, and pigs.[49] Clinical signs of trypanosomiasis may be complicated by clinical signs of secondary diseases that develop as a result of immunosuppression.

Diagnosis

A diagnosis of AAT should be suspected in horses in endemic areas with anemia and poor body condition. The diagnosis is usually confirmed by demonstration of the organism in blood or lymph node smears. Parasites, especially *T. vivax* and *T. congolense*, are readily observed in whole-blood or buffy coat smears early in infection. Stained lymph node smears are most useful for diagnosis of early infection with *T. vivax* and *T. brucei brucei* or chronic *T. congolense* infection.[49] An ELISA for detection of antigen-specific, species-specific deoxyribonucleic acid (DNA) probes for trypanosomes and polymerase chain reaction (PCR) assays to identify specific trypanosome species have been described for diagnosis of AAT in ruminants and horses.[51,52,56-61]

Therapy

A variety of antitrypanosomal medications have been used for the treatment and prevention of AAT; however, the development of drug resistance has complicated this approach to disease control.[49,62] Quinapyramine derivatives provide effective protection against *T. brucei brucei* in horses for up to 3 months. Other drugs suggested for control of AAT include isometamidium chloride,[62,63] homidium bromide,[63] diminazene aceturate,[63] and melarsen oxide; however, potential adverse effects may limit the usefulness of some of these drugs in horses.

Prevention and Public Health Considerations

The most effective way to control AAT is to control vector populations. This may include habitat manipulation (discriminative brush clearing), sterile male eradication techniques similar to those used for eradication of screwworm in the United States, ground and aerial spraying, use of synthetic pyrethroids, and odor-baited targets impregnated with insecticides.[49]

The trypanosomes associated with AAT are considered nonpathogenic for people.

ENTERIC COCCIDIOSIS

Etiology and Epidemiology

Horses may be infected by three species of coccidia: *Eimeria leuckarti*, *E. solipedum*, and *E. uniungulsti*.[64-66] Infection with *Cryptosporidium parvum*, another coccidial parasite of horses, is discussed later. The most common coccidial oocyst identified in equine feces is that of *Eimeria leuckarti*. It is a rare parasite of the small intestine of horses and donkeys worldwide.[64,65,67-72] Oocysts are most frequently observed in the feces of foals and yearlings but may occasionally be detected in older horses.[65,67,69,73] Studies of oocyst shedding on Kentucky horse farms in 1986 and 2003 revealed shedding in approximately 40% of foals on more than 80% of farms.[74,75] The mean age for the first appearance of oocysts in the feces was 70 days; the age of the oldest foal shedding oocysts was 185 days. The longest oocyst shedding period was about 4 months.

Pathogenesis and Clinical Signs

The prepatent period for experimentally induced *E. leuckarti* infection in horses is approximately 35 days.[64,69] Early gametocytes of *E. leuckarti* are found in cells of the lamina propria of villi in the equine small intestine.[64] Microgametes and microgametocytes are visible by 23 days after infection; at 28 days, macrogametes have begun formation of an oocyst wall in the cytoplasm of host cells. These findings suggest that the life span of parasitized host cells is up to 28 days, much longer than the expected life span for normal intestinal epithelial cells (approximately 2-3 days). The host cells parasitized by *Eimeria* species appear to be epithelial cells that have been displaced to the lamina propria.[66] Most horses shedding oocysts of *E. leuckarti* show no clinical signs of gastrointestinal (GI) disease, and it is largely regarded as nonpathogenic in horses.[65,73,76] It has been recorded as an incidental finding in horses with diarrhea,[77,78] intestinal hemorrhage,[71] and catarrhal inflammation of the jejunum.[79] Experimental infections of ponies and foals have not been associated with any clinical signs attributable to coccidiosis.[69,80]

Diagnosis and Therapy

Oocysts can be detected in the feces of horses by standard fecal flotation with saturated sugar or sodium nitrate solution (see Fig. 58-8).[67,69,72,74,81] They are dark brown, thick walled, and ovoid and contain a prominent micropyle on the narrower end.[76] The oocysts of *E. leuckarti* are larger than those of most *Eimeria* spp. (80-90 μm × 49-69 μm).[76] Because infection with *E. leuckarti* is generally considered to be nonpathogenic, no therapeutic regimens have been reported.

CRYPTOSPORIDIOSIS

Etiology, Epidemiology, and Pathogenesis

Cryptosporidium parvum is a coccidian parasite in the suborder Eimeriorina that infects the microvilli of intestinal epithelial cells in many domestic and wild animal species, including horses and humans. Strains that infect calves, horses, and humans are cross-transmissible, and cryptosporidiosis is considered a zoonotic disease.[82,83]

Horses become infected with *C. parvum* by ingestion of oocysts. Oocysts are approximately 4 to 5 μm in diameter, smaller than those of most coccidia (see Fig. 58-9). Cryptosporidia develop in the apical surfaces of parasitized GI epithelial cells, beneath the limiting cell membrane, but separate from the host cell cytoplasm.[84] In contrast to other coccidia, *Cryptosporidium* oocysts are sporulated and infectious at the time they are excreted into the feces. Some oocysts have a thick wall that enhances survival outside the host. Other oocysts have thinner walls and the potential to release sporozoites during passage through the lower gut with immediate infection of host cells and propagation of clinical disease.[76,82] Damage to intestinal microvilli results in malabsorption, maldigestion, and diarrhea.

There are relatively few studies of the prevalence of cryptosporidiosis in horses,[85-90] and the prevalence of fecal shedding of oocysts is low.[85,86,88-90] In contrast, a serosurvey of horses in England demonstrated that 91% of 22 horses were seropositive, suggesting that subclinical infection is common.[87]

A cross-sectional study of 152 horses at a large horse show, admitted to a veterinary teaching hospital, and on a breeding farm examined the prevalence and risk factors for shedding of *C. parvum* oocysts.[85] Fecal samples from only 13 horses were positive. Risk factors for fecal shedding included residence on specific breeding farms, age less than 6 months, and history of diarrhea during the preceding 30 days. Exposure to mature horses and cattle were not identified as risk factors for cryptosporidial infection of foals, suggesting that these are not important sources of infection for foals.[85]

Clinical Findings

The incubation period for *C. parvum* infection is approximately 3 to 7 days. The primary clinical sign associated with cryptosporidiosis in animals is severe, persistent diarrhea leading to dehydration, weakness, and death if untreated.[91] In immunocompetent animals, clinical signs usually last for 5 to 14 days.[76] Infection is common in foals with severe combined immunodeficiency (SCID).[92-94] *C. parvum* has also been isolated from foals that develop diarrhea while hospitalized for other problems, suggesting that the stress of hospitalization and disease may predispose to clinical cryptosporidiosis. Most reports of equine cryptosporidiosis describe the disease in foals; however, there is one report of cryptosporidial oocyst shedding in an adult Quarter Horse stallion with diarrhea.[95] The large number of seropositive horses in one serosurvey and documented shedding of oocysts in foals and horses with no clinical signs suggest that subclinical infection is common.

Diagnosis

Cryptosporidial oocysts are very small and difficult to identify by light microscopy on a routine fecal flotation. Visualization of oocysts in fecal samples can be enhanced by acid-fast or acridine orange staining. Alternatively, immunofluorescent staining or flow cytometry may be used to identify oocysts in fecal samples.[96]

Therapy

There is no known specific therapy for treatment of cryptosporidiosis. Affected animals should receive appropriate supportive care for dehydration and acid-base and electrolyte imbalances associated with severe diarrhea.

Public Health Considerations

Cryptosporidiosis is considered a zoonotic disease.[82,83,88,97-99] The strains of *C. parvum* that predominate in calves and humans are cross-transmissible.[82] Because cryptosporidiosis is transmitted by a fecal-oral route, disease can be prevented by using good sanitation and hygiene practices, including appropriate handwashing. Oocysts are highly resistant to most chemical disinfectants.[100] Therefore, emphasis should be placed on effective removal of all fecal material rather than use of a chemical disinfectant to kill oocysts.[82] Moist heat (pasteurization to >55° C [131° F] or live steam), freezing, or thorough drying may be the most effective means of killing oocysts.[101] Exposure to 5% ammonia solution or 10% formalin for 18 hours will also kill oocysts.[100]

Concerns have been raised regarding the potential contamination of the environment with *Cryptosporidium* oocysts shed by inapparent carrier horses. However, a study of 91 horses used for backcountry riding in California revealed that none of the horses was shedding *Cryptosporidium* oocysts.[102]

GIARDIASIS

Giardia intestinalis (previously known as *Giardia lamblia*) is a protozoan parasite of the GI tract of many domestic and wild animals and humans. The parasite has a characteristic teardrop shape with twin nuclei and four pairs of flagella (see Fig. 58-6). It has a two-stage life cycle consisting of trophozoite and cyst. Cysts are ingested by the host and release trophozoites that reproduce by binary fission after attachment to the intestinal epithelium in the duodenum. Ultimately, trophozoites develop into inactive, environmentally resistant cysts that are excreted in feces.

There are infrequent reports of *Giardia* infection in horses; some of these reports indicate that infected horses had compatible clinical signs of diarrhea or colic.[103-110] Shedding of cysts in the feces of normal foals may be common.[111] In a survey of breeding farms in Ohio and Kentucky, shedding of *Giardia* appeared to be common in apparently healthy nursing mares, the presumed source of infection for foals, leading to speculation that there may be a periparturient relaxation of immunity.[111] In one report, a 4-year-old Thoroughbred gelding with a 6-month history of intermittent diarrhea, weight loss, poor hair coat, lethargy, inappetence, and exudative dermatitis was shedding *Giardia* cysts that were detected by zinc sulfate fecal flotation.[104] Diarrhea ceased on the second day of treatment with metronidazole at 5 mg/kg three times a day for 10 days. Subsequent fecal samples obtained over a 6-week period after treatment were negative for *Giardia* cysts.

Giardia intestinalis is an important GI zoonosis. Symptoms in affected people vary from inapparent to severe, chronic diarrhea. Symptoms begin approximately 7 days after exposure to the parasite and continue for 2 to 6 weeks or longer. Concerns have been raised regarding the potential contamination of the environment with *Giardia* cysts shed by inapparent carrier horses. However, a study of 91 horses used for backcountry riding in California revealed that none of the horses was shedding *Giardia* oocysts.[102]

BESNOITIOSIS

Besnoitia spp. are tissue, cyst-forming protozoa that cause a serious systemic disease in cattle (*Besnoitia besnoiti*) and have been occasionally implicated as agents of disease in horses (*Besnoitia bennetti*).[76] The natural definitive hosts for most *Besnoitia* spp. are domestic cats; however, this is considered unlikely for *B. bennetti*, and the definitive host remains unknown.[112] *Besnoitia bennetti* was first reported by Bennett in four horses from Sudan.[113,114]

Equine besnoitiosis has been described in horses, donkeys, and burros in Africa, Central America, and North America.[115-118] Infective oocysts are ingested and develop into large, thick-walled cysts in connective tissue. Horses are presumed to be an intermediate host in the life cycle of this parasite. Cysts are usually located in the skin, which becomes quite thickened (Fig. 61-2). In addition to alopecic dermatitis of the legs, ears,

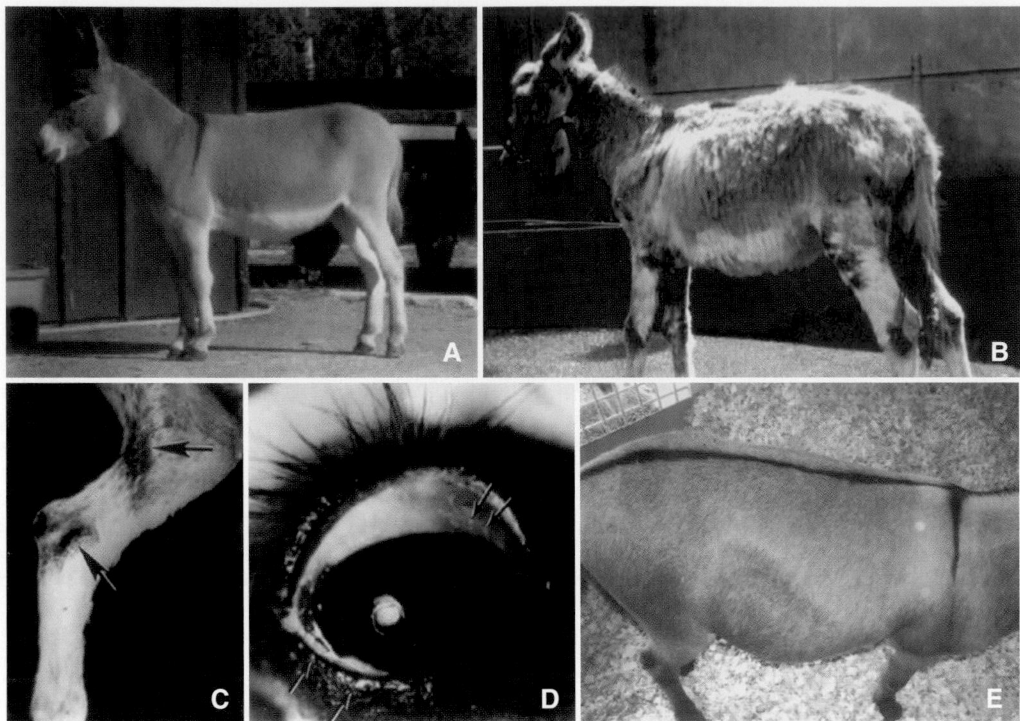

Fig. 61-2 Lesions of *Besnoitia bennetti* in donkey. **A,** Before onset of clinical signs at approximately 1 year of age. **B,** Eight months after onset of clinical signs. Note marked cachexia, poor hair coat, and skin lesions (alopecia, hypotrichosis, hyperpigmentation, thickening, and crusting) over lateral neck, shoulders, carpi, stifle, hock, periocular region, around ears, and muzzle. **C,** Lateral aspect of hindlimb. Note alopecia and hypotrichosis, with thickened, irregular, crusty hyperpigmented skin over caudal aspect of stifle and lateral hock *(arrows)*. **D,** Multifocal white pinpoint granular structures (*Besnoitia bennetti* tissue cysts) within sclera and conjunctiva *(arrows)* of eye. **E,** Dorsolateral view of donkey after treatment with trimethoprim-sulfa. (Courtesy Dr. J.P. Dubey; from *J Parasitol* 35:659-672, 2005.)

eyelids, and scrotum, affected horses may exhibit signs of depression, weakness, and fever.[76,119] Diagnosis of besnoitiosis is made by identification of the pathognomonic cysts in biopsied skin or conjunctiva.[76,115]

Administration of pyrimethamine and sulfamethoxazole for 7 months was effective for treatment of a donkey infected with *B. bennetti*.[112]

SARCOCYSTOSIS

Sarcocystis spp. are coccidian parasites with an obligate, two-host life cycle. Intermediate hosts ingest sporulated oocysts that are shed in the feces of definitive hosts. Mature tissue cysts develop in the muscles of the intermediate host. When that host dies, ingestion of infected muscle by the definitive host completes the life cycle. The most common *Sarcocystis* infection of horses is equine protozoal myeloencephalitis (EPM) caused by *Sarcocystis neurona* (see Chapter 59).

Horses act as intermediate hosts for at least two species of *Sarcocystis: S. equicanis* and *S. fayeri*. Dogs are the definitive host for both species. Experimental infection of horses results in formation of sarcocysts in muscle, especially in the esophagus and diaphragm.[120-125] Surveys of horses at slaughter in Germany and the United States reveal that 13% to 23% of horses had sarcocysts in the muscle of the esophagus and diaphragm.[76,122,123] Fever, mild anemia, anorexia, and depression may be seen in some horses after experimental infection. In most horses, the presence of sporocysts in muscles is not

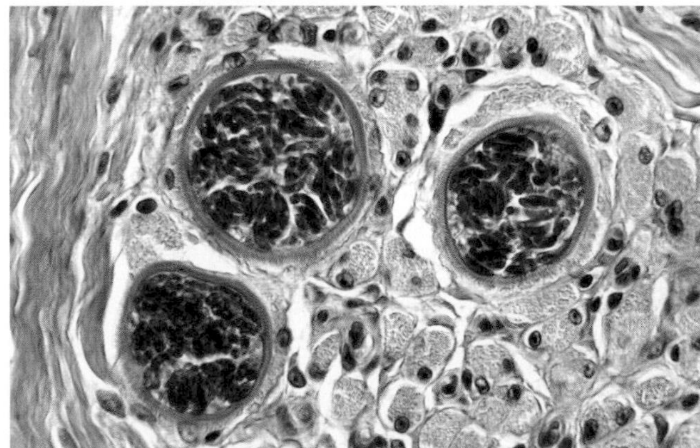

Fig. 61-3 Photomicrograph of biopsy specimen from tongue of 10-year-old Thoroughbred gelding with 2-week history of extensive swelling of anterior portion of tongue. Note the large sarcocyst in the muscle and associated severe eosinophilic glossitis/myositis. (Courtesy Dr. Kevin Snekvik.)

accompanied by an inflammatory response. However, multifocal granulomatous myositis has been occasionally described[121,126] (Fig. 61-3). The possibility of a *Sarcocystis*-related toxin was suggested in one 3-year-old Quarter Horse mare with weight, loss, weakness, depression, and dysphagia and large numbers of intramuscular cysts, presumed to be *S. fayeri*.[127]

A 7-year-old Quarter Horse gelding with multifocal myositis and probable *S. fayeri* cysts in the muscles was successfully treated with trimethoprim-sulfamethoxazole, pyrimethamine, and phenylbutazone. Therapeutic regimens described for treatment of EPM in horses would be reasonable for treatment of horses with myositis caused by sarcocystosis (see Chapter 59).

ABERRANT PARASITES

A variety of parasites that primarily infect other species have been described as causing sporadic disease in horses resulting from aberrant migration through numerous organs and tissues. This is most often described in relation to central nervous system (CNS) disease. One of the most common of these aberrant CNS parasites, *Halicephalobus gingivalis*, is discussed in Chapter 4.

In addition to *H. gingivalis*, several helminth and dipteran parasites have been described as etiologic agents of CNS disease in horses. These include *Strongylus vulgaris* larvae (Chapter 62),[128-130] the filarial nematode *Setaria* spp.,[131,132] the spirurid stomach worm *Draschia megastoma* (Chapter 62),[133] hydatid cysts of *Echinococcus* spp.,[134] and dipteran larvae belonging to the genus *Hypoderma* (Chapter 7).[130,135-137] Clinical signs vary depending on the affected area of the CNS and may be either acute or chronic. The diagnosis is usually made by histopathologic examination of tissues obtained at necropsy.

Adult canine heartworms were recovered from the heart and pulmonary vessels of one horse.[138] The ruminant liver fluke *Fasciola hepatica* has been implicated as a cause of liver disease in horses.[139-149]

ECHINOCOCCOSIS

Etiology and Epidemiology

Echinococcosis, or hydatid disease, is a zoonotic disease caused by infection with a metacestode of the genus *Echinococcus*. Hydatid cysts of *Echinococcus granulosus* have been reported in the liver and lungs of horses after natural or experimental infection.[150-155] The life cycle of *Echinococcus* spp. begins with passage of eggs containing a six-hooked larva (hexacanth or oncosphere) in the feces of carnivore definitive hosts. Eggs are ingested by the intermediate host. Humans may serve as accidental intermediate hosts. The larvae penetrate the intestinal mucosa and migrate via lymphatic and blood vessels to other sites, where they develop into a metacestode, forming a hydatid cyst containing numerous protoscolices. Affected tissues are ingested by a carnivore, and protoscolices develop into adult tapeworms in the carnivore's intestines to complete the life cycle.

The taxonomy of the genus *Echinococcus* is presently undergoing changes.[156-158] Currently, four species are recognized in Europe, one of which, *E. equinus*, uses equids (horses, donkeys, mules, zebras) as an intermediate host.[159] In Europe, equine echinococcosis has been described in Great Britain, Ireland, Belgium, Switzerland, Italy, and Spain.[160] The disease is also prevalent in equids in the Middle East and Africa.[161] There have been at least four reports of hydatid disease in horses in the United States.[153,155,162,163] All the horses in these reports originated from the United Kingdom and Ireland, where hydatid disease is endemic. The prevalence of disease in horses in the United Kingdom is higher in horses used for hunting. In Ireland the prevalence in horses at slaughterhouses varies between 10% and 62%.[153,164] Disease has been correlated with the feeding of raw or improperly cooked offal from horses to dogs.[164,165]

Clinical Findings and Diagnosis

The most common site of hydatid cyst formation in horses is the liver, followed by the lung. Involvement of other organs is rare.[153] The parasite may persist for many years in some equids with no obvious clinical signs.[153,166] When clinical signs do occur, they are often related to pressure of the enlarging cyst on adjacent organs and tissues. Most cysts range in diameter from 1 to 7 cm, but they may occasionally be up to 20 cm in diameter.

There are no definitive antemortem tests for echinococcosis in equids, and the diagnosis is usually made at necropsy. However, ultrasonography of the liver of affected horses might provide evidence of cystic lesions in affected horses.

Public Health Considerations

Although humans are at risk for development of echinococcosis, the level of risk posed by equine strains of the parasite is unclear. Epidemiologic data from Europe suggest that *E. equinus* may not be infective to humans.[159] Regardless, the infective stage of *Echinococcus* is shed in the feces of the definitive host, usually a canid species, and the life cycle stages present in horses would not be directly infectious to people.

BOTS

Larvae of horse botflies are internal parasites of horses worldwide. The two species that most often infect horses are *Gasterophilus intestinalis* (horse botfly) and *Gasterophilus nasalis*. Occasional infections with *Gasterophilus haemorrhoidalis* (nose botfly) and *Gasterophilus pecorum* are reported.[167-169] Second-stage and third-stage larvae of these flies typically attach to the mucosa of the equine stomach or intestine, where they cause focal mucosal ulceration.[170]

Adult botflies are hairy and similar in size and appearance to honeybees. The common horse botfly usually lays its yellow to gray eggs on the hairs of the forelegs, mane, and flanks (Fig. 61-4). Throat botfly eggs are attached to the long hairs beneath the mandible and chin. Nose botfly eggs are deposited most often on the hairs around the muzzle of the horse. The hatching of botfly eggs is stimulated by warmth and moisture when the horse licks eggs off the hair during grooming. Larvae spend about 3 weeks migrating in the soft tissue of the

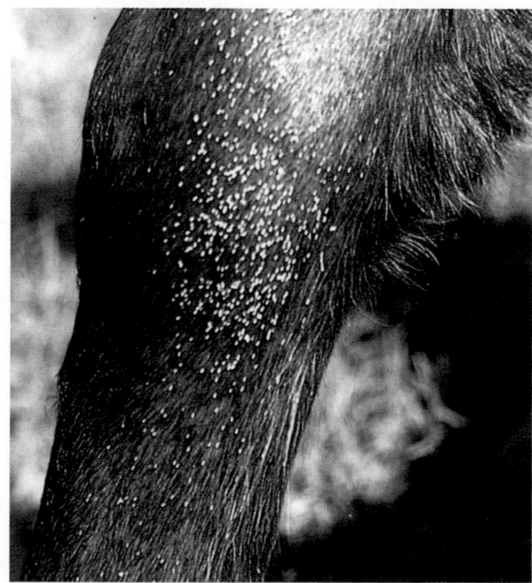

Fig. 61-4 Botfly eggs on leg of horse. (Courtesy Dr. Wendy Duckett.)

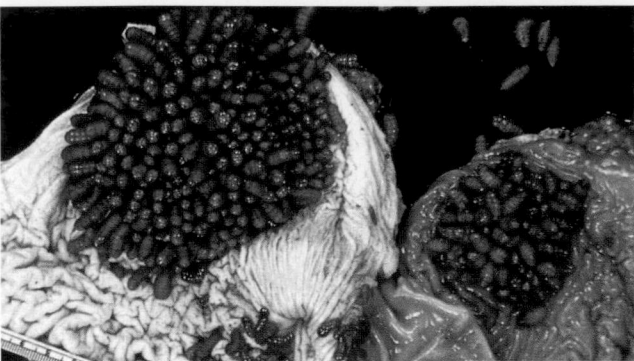

Fig. 61-5 Botfly larvae attached to gastric mucosa of horse. (Courtesy Dr. Wendy Duckett.)

oral cavity, then migrate to the stomach or small intestine, where they attach to the mucosa (Fig. 61-5). They remain in the stomach until spring or early summer, when they detach, are passed in the feces, enter the soil below the manure pile, and pupate. In weeks to months, they emerge as adult flies. Nonfeeding adult flies mate, and females lay their eggs during fall until the first hard frost. Adult *G. pecorum* bots lay eggs in batches on grass, and eggs are ingested when horses graze.

Bot larvae cause minimal pathology in most horses. The egg-laying activity of female flies can irritate horses and lead to abnormal behavior in an attempt at fly evasion. Larvae of *G. nasalis* burrow into the spaces around the teeth and can cause gingival irritation and necrosis. Minor irritation may be associated with attachment of larvae in the stomach or intestine. High numbers of parasites have been implicated as causes of gastric ulceration and rupture, intramural gastric suppuration, peritonitis secondary to gastroduodenal perforation, and gastroesophageal reflux.[171-175] In a recent report, septic peritonitis in an adult mare was caused by colonic perforation associated with aberrant migration of a *G. intestinalis* larvae.[176] In Asia, *G. pecorum* has been associated with esophageal constriction and hypertrophy of the musculature of the oropharynx and esophagus with resultant dysphagia and death.[177] This species has also been associated with epidemic deaths of horses resulting from attachment of large numbers of bots to the soft palate.[167,178]

Bots can be controlled by (1) applying insecticides to prevent adult flies from laying eggs on the horse, (2) clipping hairs or removing eggs from hairs before they can be ingested by the horse, and (3) administering appropriate anthelmintic agents. Avermectin anthelmintics are highly effective for the control of bots. The most effective time to administer boticides is in the late fall after the first hard frost, when adult fly activity has ceased.

There are occasional reports of infection of humans with horse botfly larvae.[178-185] Several of these reports involved patients with known exposure to horses.[178,180,184,185] Burrowing of larvae behind the lips or inner cheek is said to elicit discomfort. Migration of first-stage larvae is associated with cutaneous and ocular myiasis in people. The burrowing of larvae beneath the skin may produce a visible tortuous path with severe pruritus.

REFERENCES

See the CD-ROM for a list of references linked to the abstract in PubMed.

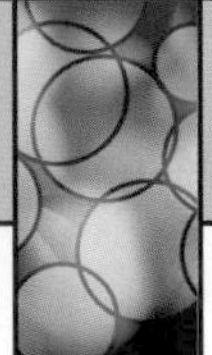

CHAPTER • 62

Nematodes

Numerous nematode parasites infest and infect horses. The first section of this chapter describes the important nematodes of the gastrointestinal tract of horses. Nematode infections with clinical manifestations affecting the skin (onchocerciasis, habronemiasis) and the respiratory tract (lungworm infection) are discussed later in this chapter. Chapter 4 discusses nematode infection of neural and somatic tissues (*Halicephalobus* spp.); Chapter 10 discusses infection of ocular tissues (*Thelazia* spp.).

GASTROINTESTINAL NEMATODES

Craig Reinemeyer and Martin Krarup Nielsen

Strongylosis

The term *strongylosis* refers to infection with any of dozens of species of similar nematodes that reside as adults within the large intestine of equids. These parasites are classified in the family *Strongylidae* and are commonly known as "strongylid nematodes" or "strongyles." Differences in morphology, biology, pathogenicity, anthelmintic susceptibility, and management strategies support the practicality of discussing the strongyles as two major groups: the subfamily *Strongylinae* ("large strongyles," strongylins) and the subfamily *Cyathostominae* ("small strongyles," cyathostomins, cyathostomes).[1]

Strongylinae (Large Strongyles, Strongylins)

Etiology. The *Strongylinae* occurring in North America belong to four genera: *Strongylus, Triodontophorus, Craterostomum,* and *Oesophagodontus*. Compared with small strongyles, the large strongyles possess substantial, globular, buccal capsules (oral cavities) by which they can attach firmly to the mucosa of the cecum or colon. Specimens of the genus *Strongylus* are large, stout nematodes (~1.5-4.5 cm × 2 mm), whereas *Triodontophorus, Oesophagodontus,* and *Craterostomum* are smaller and resemble the cyathostomins in size.

All strongyles invade gut tissues after initial infection, but only larval stages of the genus *Strongylus* migrate to organs beyond the alimentary tract. Larvae of *Strongylus vulgaris* wander within the vascular system; those of *Strongylus edentatus* invade the liver and retroperitoneum; and *Strongylus equinus* larvae migrate within the liver and pancreas[2] (see Pathogenesis). Because of their protracted migration, members of the genus *Strongylus* have long prepatent periods ranging from 5.5 to 12 months, depending on the species.

Epidemiology. The role of the environment in the transmission of strongylosis is virtually identical for large and small strongyles. The cycle of transmission begins when strongylid eggs are passed in the feces of an infected host. Strongylid eggs are homogenous, and large strongyle eggs cannot be differentiated from those of cyathostomins. Equine feces usually contain adequate levels of moisture (>24%)[3] and oxygen to support hatching and development of larval stages, and eggs are able to hatch when environmental temperatures exceed 8° C (46° F).[4,5] The first larval stage (L_1) hatches from an egg, feeds on organic material in the manure, molts to the second larval stage (L_2), and eventually develops into an infective, third-stage larva (L_3). Rates of egg hatching and larval development increase in direct proportion to environmental temperatures. Under field conditions, the minimum interval between egg passage and development to the infective stage is approximately 1 week.

After larvae reach the infective, third stage, prolonged survival is fostered by a different set of environmental conditions, and larvae persist better at low temperatures. Third-stage strongylid larvae are surrounded by a durable sheath that protects them from desiccation but does not allow them to feed. Accordingly, infective larvae survive by metabolizing energy reserves that are stored within intestinal epithelial cells. These limited energy stores are depleted more rapidly at higher temperatures, so infective larvae can survive only briefly in hot weather. Because larvae persist well in cold conditions, the concept of a "killing frost" does not exist. Horses can acquire strongyle infections while grazing pastures during winter and through the subsequent spring.

Environmental conditions during spring and autumn are ideal for strongyle transmission in all regions. However, geoclimatic variations result in seasonal differences in strongyle transmission patterns during winter and summer. In northern temperate climates (above ~40 degrees north latitude), summer is a favorable season for hatching of strongyle eggs and development into infective larvae.[6] Northern winters are too cold for eggs to hatch, but larval survival is excellent. In contrast, southern temperate summers are too hot and dry for sustained larval persistence, but winter conditions are mild enough to allow some egg hatching as well as excellent survival of existing larvae.[3,7] In terms of transmission potential, horses in southern temperate regions experience substantial risk during autumn through spring, whereas transmission in pastured, northern horses is virtually perennial.

In northern temperate climates, migrating *Strongylus* larvae return to the gut and begin egg production during spring.[8] Third-stage larvae develop during spring and summer, and ingestion by grazing horses completes transmission. Adult large strongyles survive in the host through summer and autumn, become senescent during winter, and are replaced in the following spring by a new population.[8] The annual epidemiology of *Strongylus* infection has not been studied in southern temperate regions.

Pathogenesis. Large strongyles damage the host as both larval and adult stages. Within days of infection, L_3 *Strongylus vulgaris* larvae invade the submucosa of the small intestine and molt to the L_4 stage.[9] These larvae enter local arterioles, burrow beneath the intima, and migrate proximally to the root of the anterior mesenteric artery (AMA).[10] A proportion of *S. vulgaris* larvae continue to wander past this site, and migratory lesions have been observed in the root of the aorta and in other arterial branches.[11] Larvae within the intima of the proximal AMA cause severe local arteritis, accompanied by focal enlargement, thrombi within the vessel lumen, and hypertrophy of the medial layer (Fig. 62-1). This lesion is classically described as a "verminous aneurysm," although the arterial walls are neither thin nor dilated. Verminous arteritis is associated with an increased incidence of colic, although the pathophysiologic mechanisms are unknown. The simplest hypothesis is that emboli from the thrombus are carried distally and occlude the arterial supply of the gut. However, a necropsy survey of ischemic bowel lesions of horses failed to demonstrate emboli in the majority of cases.[12] Other hypotheses for inducing colic include primary changes in gut motility[13] and interference with local neurologic control.[14]

Migrating larvae of *Strongylus edentatus* and *S. equinus* have been associated with hemorrhagic and inflammatory lesions in the liver, pancreas, and retroperitoneal tissues. These lesions do not cause distinct clinical signs but may contribute to the general inflammatory component of strongylosis. In the final stage of migration, all *Strongylus* larvae return to the large intestine and form nodules within the gut wall.[15] Adult large strongyles emerge from these nodules to take up residence within the gut. The parasitic nodules can be greater than 1 cm in diameter and often are filled with purulent material whether occupied or vacant.

Adult large strongyles can use their buccal capsules to attach firmly to the mucosa of the cecum or ventral colon. These worms are said to "plug feed," drawing small amounts of gut mucosa into the oral cavity and presumably ingesting tissue proteins. Rupture of local vessels may cause focal hemorrhage, but the consequences of adult feeding activities are only a minor component of strongylosis. One noteworthy species of large strongyle, *Triodontophorus tenuicollis*, feeds in colonies of 20 or more adults and causes large (1-3 cm), deep ulcers in the dorsal colon.[2]

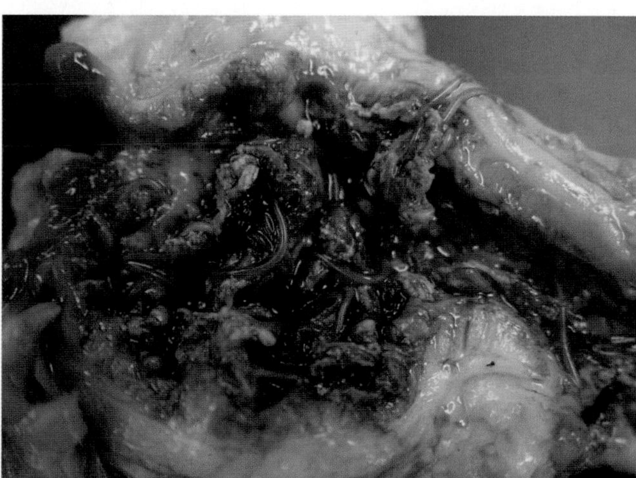

Fig. 62-1 Verminous arteritis caused by migrating larvae of *Strongylus vulgaris*. (Courtesy Dr. Charles Faulkner, Department of Comparative Medicine, University of Tennessee College of Veterinary Medicine, Knoxville.)

Clinical Findings. Strongylosis is characterized by nonspecific signs of weight loss and poor growth, rough hair coat, and compromised performance.[16] Experimental infections caused pyrexia, tachycardia, anorexia, diarrhea, and listlessness.[17] Larval *S. vulgaris* infections do not cause distinct clinical signs but are associated with an increased incidence of colic.

Diagnosis. Infection with adult strongyles is easily demonstrated by using a variety of concentration techniques to detect strongylid eggs in the feces (see Chapter 58). Concentration techniques include simple fecal flotation using saturated salt or sugar solutions, as well as quantitative procedures such as the McMaster's, modified Wisconsin, or modified Stoll technique.[18] Regardless of methodology, the presence of strongyle eggs in the feces of grazing horses is ubiquitous, so the diagnostic value of fecal examination is not robust. Even quantitative techniques that calculate the numbers of eggs per gram of feces have limited interpretive value because strongylid egg counts are not correlated to the numbers of parasites that produced them, and they are not predictive of the severity of clinical parasitism.[19,20]

Strongylid eggs are homogenous, and those of cyathostomins cannot be differentiated from large strongyle eggs (Fig. 62-2). In mixed infections, more than 95% of strongyle eggs passed in the feces are produced by cyathostomins. Proportional contributions of various strongylid genera or subfamilies to the total egg count can be determined by fecal culture, which requires that feces containing strongyle eggs be kept moist, aerated, and incubated at room temperature for 10 to 14 days. The L_3 larvae that develop in these conditions are collected and examined, and the proportional contributions by cyathostomins (Fig. 62-3) and the various genera of large strongyles (Fig. 62-4) can be calculated.[18]

In the 1990s, the ribosomal deoxyribonucleic acid (rDNA) from several species of large and small strongyles was sequenced and cloned.[21] This allowed the first and second internal transcribed spacers (ITS-1 and ITS-2) to be used for species-specific amplification in polymerase chain reactions (PCR).[22] This technology holds potential for the development of PCR-based diagnostic assays to detect and quantify the presence of large strongyle eggs in fecal samples. Such assays are currently under development, but no commercial tests are available at present.

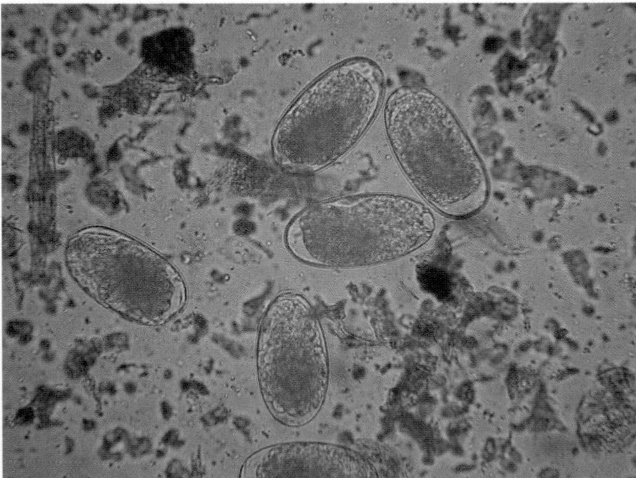

Fig. 62-2 Photomicrograph of typical strongylid eggs passed by large strongyles and cyathostomins. (Courtesy Dr. Charles Faulkner, Department of Comparative Medicine, University of Tennessee College of Veterinary Medicine, Knoxville.)

Hematology and serum chemistry of horses with strongylosis often indicate mild anemia, leukocytosis with eosinophilia, hypoalbuminemia, beta-globulinemia, and elevations of IgG(T).[15,23] Essentially all abnormalities are consequences of inflammation and protein-losing enteropathy.

Pathologic Findings. Discrete hemorrhages, approximately 1 cm in diameter and occurring beneath the serosa

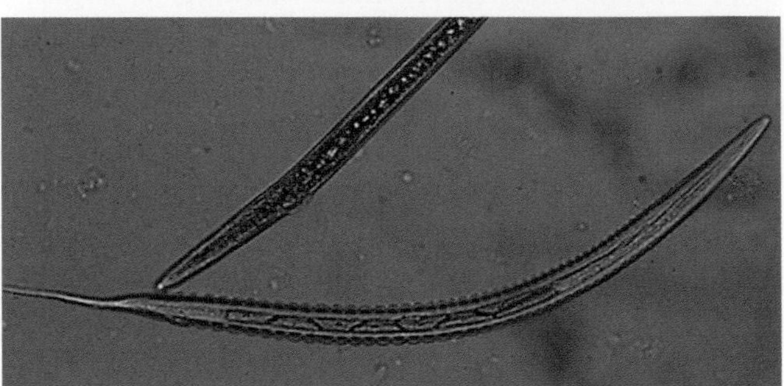

Fig. 62-3 Third-stage larva (L_3) of cyathostomin nematodes. (Courtesy Dr. Martin Krarup Nielsen, Department of Large Animal Sciences, Royal Veterinary and Agricultural University, Frederiksberg, Denmark.)

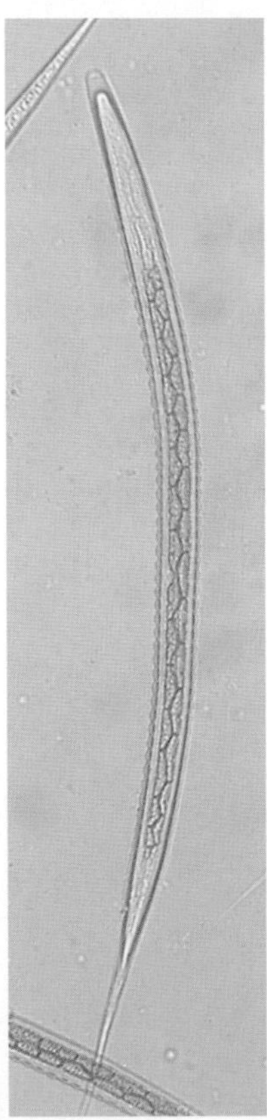

Fig. 62-4 Third-stage larva (L_3) of *Strongylus vulgaris*, a large strongyle. (Courtesy Dr. Martin Krarup Nielsen, Department of Large Animal Sciences, Royal Veterinary and Agricultural University, Frederiksberg, Denmark.)

of the ileum, have been termed *hemomelasma ilei* and are considered to be pathognomonic for recent *S. vulgaris* infection.[11] The pathologic lesions caused by fourth-stage and fifth-stage *S. vulgaris* larvae within blood vessels have been characterized by scanning electron microscopy.[24] Typical lesions consist of large thrombi surrounding larvae located within vessels with dilated lumens and thickened walls. Active coagulation is evident on the surfaces of larvae, thrombi, and vascular endothelium, where aggregations of red blood cells, platelets, and fibrin can be observed. The concurrent existence of a mature thrombus with additional, active thrombi indicates cumulative formation over time. The arterial walls become thickened by fibrosis and occasionally by dystrophic calcification.[15] After thrombotic lesions are fully developed, the artery may never return to normal.[25]

On rare occasions, migrating *Strongylus* larvae have been associated with cerebrospinal disorders.[15] More common are eosinophilic lesions in the pancreas[26] or eosinophilic granulomas in the liver and epicardium.[27]

Therapy. Several anthelmintics belonging to three chemical families are effective for treatment of adult large strongyles, but migrating larvae are susceptible to only three anthelmintic regimens (Table 62-1). Because of the inflammatory nature of lesions associated with migrating larvae, specific chemotherapy cannot be expected to result in immediate alleviation of clinical signs of strongylosis.

Prevention. General approaches to strongyle control are discussed in greater detail in the following section on *Cyathostominae.* Chemotherapeutic approaches to control large strongyles include daily administration of *pyrantel tartrate* (2.64 mg/kg), which kills ingested strongylid larvae before they can invade gut tissues and establish infection.[28] Unlike some populations of cyathostomins, resistance to pyrantel tartrate has not been demonstrated in large strongyles to date.

Eradication of large strongyles from a herd not only is feasible, but has been accomplished at a majority of well-managed horse farms in North America.[29] Because larvicidal anthelmintics (see Table 62-1) can kill all stages of *Strongylus* larvae within the host, at least 6 months would be required after treatment before another adult population could develop and begin to contaminate pasture with eggs. By repeating larvicidal treatments at intervals of no greater than 6 months, new infections could not arise on a farm where all animals had been maintained on this program. Also, because the maximum duration of survival of free-living stages in the environment is approximately 1 year, no infective large-strongyle larvae could remain on pastures where this program had been maintained for 18 months or longer.[30]

Public Health Considerations. The large strongyles have no zoonotic potential and cannot infect any domestic animals other than equids.

Cyathostominae (Cyathostomes, Cyathostomins, Small Strongyles, Trichonemes)

Etiology. The *Cyathostominae* found in North America belong to eight genera: *Cyathostomum, Cylicocyclus, Cylicodontophorus, Cylicostephanus, Coronocyclus, Parapoteriostomum, Poteriostomum,* and *Petrovinema.*[31] Another genus, *Gyalocephalus,* has been assigned to a different taxonomic group, but it behaves biologically as a cyathostomin. In contrast to large strongyles, cyathostomins have shallow or cylindrical buccal capsules with which they attach weakly to the mucosa of the large intestine. Most small strongyle species are moderately sized nematodes, less than 1.5 cm in length by about 1 mm in diameter.

After ingestion by a grazing horse, L_3 cyathostomins invade the mucosa of the cecum, ventral colon, or to a minor extent, the dorsal colon.[32] Within 1 to 2 weeks after infection, a fibrous capsule develops around the larva,[33] which is now said to be "encysted." Small-strongyle larvae develop through multiple, sequential stages. The invading stage (early third-stage larva, or EL_3) grows into a late third-stage larva (LL_3), then molts into an early fourth-stage larva (EL_4) and ultimately a late fourth-stage larva (LL_4). All larval growth and maturation occur within the confines of a mucosal or submucosal cyst. The LL_4 stage emerges from the cyst into the lumen of the large intestine and develops into a reproductive, adult nematode. Larval development may be progressive, producing an adult worm in as quickly as 5 to 6 weeks, or larvae may arrest

Table • 62-1

Spectra of Various Anthelmintics Labeled for Efficacy against Strongylid Nematode Parasites of Horses

			LARGE STRONGYLES		CYATHOSTOMINS	
CHEMICAL CLASS	**COMPOUND**	**DOSAGE**	**ADULTS**	**MIGRATING LARVAE**	**ADULTS AND LUMINAL LARVAE**	**ENCYSTED LARVAE**
Benzimidazoles	Fenbendazole	5 mg/kg	Yes	Yes*	Yes	Yes *†
	Oxfendazole	10 mg/kg	Yes	No	Yes	No
	Oxibendazole	10 mg/kg	Yes	No	Yes	No
Heterocyclic compounds	Piperazine	88 mg/kg	No	No	Yes	No
Macrocyclic lactones	Ivermectin	0.2 mg/kg	Yes	Yes	Yes	No
	Moxidectin	0.4 mg/kg	Yes	Yes	Yes	Yes‡
Tetrahydropyrimidines	Pyrantel pamaote	6.6 mg/kg	Yes§	No	Yes	No
	Pyrantel tartrate¶	2.64 mg/kg/day	Yes	No	Yes	No

*Requires a regimen of 10 mg/kg daily for 5 consecutive days.
†Label claims for efficacy against early third-stage (EL_3), late third-stage (LL_3), and fourth-stage (L_4) cyathostomin larvae.
‡Label claims for efficacy against late third-stage (LL_3) and fourth-stage (L_4) cyathostomin larvae.
§Efficacy against *Strongylus edentatus* is less than 90%.
¶When fed daily, aids in the control of certain nematode parasites.

development in the EL_3 stage,[34] and not undergo further maturation for up to 2.5 years.[35]

Epidemiology. The bionomics of cyathostomin development and persistence in the environment are virtually identical to those of large strongyles, discussed previously. An annual cycle has been hypothesized for cyathostomin populations within the host.[23] A large proportion of encysted larvae emerge from gut tissues during late winter or early spring and mature into adult cyathostomins. The reproductive activity of this new population is manifested by the spring increase in fecal egg counts.[36] This population continues to reproduce through the summer months, when conditions are favorable for egg hatching and larval development. In northern climates, a second generation of adult cyathostomins may arise in late summer as a direct product of infection earlier in the grazing season. The majority of larvae ingested during autumn are destined to undergo arrested development within the host. This population overwinters within host tissues and emerges in the following spring to initiate another annual cycle.

Arrested development is a strategy employed by many nematode species to avoid unfavorable environmental conditions. Cyathostomin larvae specifically interrupt their development at the EL_3 stage and can remain encysted in tissues for 2 years or longer.[34,35] Small strongyle populations in northern climates undergo arrested development during winter, presumably to avoid environmental conditions that are unfavorable for egg hatching. Similarly, cyathostomin populations in the south would arrest during summer to evade hot, dry weather, which favors neither larval development nor persistence.

Pathogenesis. Cyathostomin third-stage larvae cause mucosal inflammation of the cecum and ventral colon when they first invade the gut after ingestion.[37] Within a few weeks, these larvae become surrounded by a fibrous capsule within the mucosa or submucosa of the host organ.[33] The capsule protects the horse from the parasitic products inside the cyst, but it also shields the nematode from inflammatory and immune responses of the host. Minimal inflammation is observed around encysted larvae as long as the capsule remains intact (Fig. 62-5). Rupture of the cysts during larval emergence releases excretory and secretory products that have accumulated over time. Larval excystment results in lesions of focal edema, congestion, and hemorrhage, with accompanying leakage of tissue fluids into the bowel lumen. The cumulative severity of the lesions and their effect on the host are correlated to the numbers of larvae emerging. Adult small strongyles are ineffective plug feeders and cause minimal damage as mature parasites.[38]

Clinical Findings. Strongylosis is characterized by weight loss and poor growth, rough hair coat, and compromised performance.[16] Cyathostomins can cause these general clinical signs in the absence of a large-strongyle component. One specific syndrome, *larval cyathostominosis*, is a seasonal condition caused by synchronous emergence of large numbers of encysted cyathostomins.[23] This syndrome is characterized by severe diarrhea, rapid weight loss, marked hypoproteinemia, and passage of numerous larval cyathostomins in the feces. In northern climates, larval cyathostominosis occurs most frequently in late winter, when encysted larvae are expected to emerge from arrested development. In southern regions, larval cyathostominosis is most common in late summer and autumn for the same reasons.[39]

Diagnosis. Diagnosis of the nonspecific aspects of strongylosis is discussed in the section on *Strongylinae.*

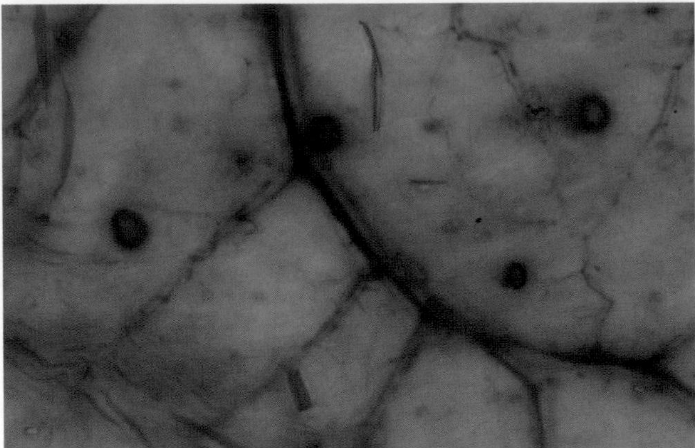

Fig. 62-5 Cyathostomin larvae encysted in mucosa of cecum. (Courtesy Dr. Andrew Peregrine, Department of Pathobiology, Ontario Veterinary College, University of Guelph, Ontario, Canada.)

Strongylid eggs are homogenous, and those of cyathostomins cannot be differentiated from large-strongyle eggs. In mixed infections, more than 95% of strongyle eggs passed in the feces would be produced by cyathostomins, and this proportion can be confirmed by coproculture, as discussed previously.

Recent attempts to develop serologic assays to detect infection with encysted larval cyathostomins have shown great promise.[40,41,42] Such assays would be of great value in equine practice because these stages cannot be detected by fecal examination, yet clearly are the most pathogenic. In addition, a PCR-ELISA (enzyme-linked immunosorbent assay) has been validated that can identify six different species of cyathostomins by fecal analysis.[43,44] This technology allows parasitologists to study the relative impact of specific species in natural infections, as well as to identify species with higher levels of anthelmintic resistance.

Pathologic Findings. Soon after larval ingestion, L_3 cyathostomins penetrate the basement membrane of the epithelial cells of the tubular glands in the large intestine, where they provoke a fibroblastic reaction. This increases as the larvae grow, eventually leading to goblet cell hyperplasia and hypertrophy and distortion of the glands. Modest infiltration with lymphocytes and (in some cases) eosinophils occurs below and around the encapsulated larvae.[37]

The major lesions of cyathostomin infection occur during larval emergence and include typhlitis and colitis, which contribute to protein-losing enteropathy.[45] Intense, focal eosinophilia may develop when the cyst wall is breached by an emerging larva.[37]

Therapy. Adult cyathostomins are susceptible to several anthelmintics belonging to four chemical families, and two anthelmintic regimens demonstrate activity against encysted larvae (see Table 62-1). The efficacy of a dewormer against adult cyathostomins can be evaluated simply with a *fecal egg count reduction* (FECR) test (Box 62-1).

Most equine anthelmintics are labeled only for removal of adult and larval cyathostomins from the lumen of the gut; larvae encysted in the gut wall may not be affected. When mature worms are killed by deworming, larval stages emerge from tissues at varying intervals thereafter, apparently to reestablish reproducing populations. Anthelmintic treatment

Box • 62-1

Fecal Egg Count Reduction (FECR) Test

Fecal samples are collected from individual horses before treatment and examined by a quantitative egg-counting technique. The results are reported as strongyle eggs per gram (EPG). An accurate dose of the product to be tested is administered, based on a current body weight and consistent with label recommendations. Ten to 14 days after treatment, another fecal sample is examined from the same animal, and the percentage reduction of egg counts is calculated, using the following formula:

$$\frac{\text{EPG (pretreatment)} - \text{(posttreatment)}}{\text{EPG (pretreatment)}} \times 100 = \text{FECR}$$

The FECR proportion is synonymous with percentage efficacy. Effective anthelmintics should decrease strongylid egg counts by greater than 90%, whereas reductions less than 80% indicate resistance to the class of anthelmintic being evaluated. Reductions between 80% and 90% are equivocal and the efficacy of that drug class should be reevaluated in the future.

purportedly can even induce parasitic disease by promoting the emergence of arrested cyathostomin larvae from tissue cysts.[47] In addition to the endogenous supplementation of adult populations, horses grazing on infective pastures rapidly acquire a new generation of larvae to maintain the cycle.

Prevention. Strongyle infection is ubiquitous in grazing venues, so the major objective of control is to limit pasture contamination with feces containing strongylid eggs. This can be accomplished by targeting the general fecal component. In fact, the use of commercial vacuum units to remove manure from pastures at biweekly intervals was very effective for controlling the transmission of strongyles in the United Kingdom.[48] However, pasture hygiene is labor intensive and requires expensive machinery and relatively flat paddocks for effective implementation. For grazing horses, pasture rotation has not been a successful control strategy because it is extremely complicated and requires extensive monitoring beyond the capacity of laypersons.

Rather than limiting fecal contamination, most strongyle control programs attempt to reduce the numbers of parasite eggs contained in the feces. This requires chemical intervention, so anthelmintics are the keystone of almost all strongyle control programs for horses. Administering *pyrantel tartrate* (2.64 mg/kg) daily in the feed is a preventive, chemical approach because it kills ingested strongylid larvae before they can invade gut tissues and establish infection. One concern about this program is that perennial use could interfere with the development of acquired immunity, especially by younger horses. In addition, populations of cyathostomins can develop resistance to pyrantel tartrate, rendering its daily use ineffective.[49]

A common strategy is to administer anthelmintics at a frequency that removes reproducing adults but also limits cumulative egg production by the herd over the course of a grazing season. Egg counts should decrease by more than 90% after the successful removal of a small-strongyle population. Ultimately, however, adult populations are replaced, reproduction resumes, and egg counts return to previous levels. The interval between effective treatment and resumption of significant egg production is known as the *egg reappearance period* (ERP).[50] ERPs are quite predictable for various classes of equine anthelmintics. *Benzimidazole* or *pyrantel pamoate* treatments typically provide an ERP of 4 weeks, *ivermectin* prevents contamination for 6 to 8 weeks after treatment, and the ERP of *moxidectin* is approximately 12 weeks. By administering subsequent anthelmintic treatments at an interval determined by the ERP of the previous drug class, replacement worm populations are killed before they achieve full reproductive potential. Thus the quantities of eggs produced are limited, and pasture contamination is minimized. Fewer eggs yield fewer larvae, with a lowered risk of future infection for horses grazing that pasture.

Unfortunately, suppressive treatment tends to select for anthelmintic resistance, or at least for populations that reproduce faster and have shorter ERPs. Cyathostomin populations that are resistant to benzimidazole anthelmintics were first identified in the 1960s and are now widespread in most countries. Resistance to pyrantel salts is found primarily in North America, where it was documented on approximately 40% of horse farms in one survey.[49] The lower prevalence of pyrantel resistance in the rest of the world is possibly explained by the exclusive availability of daily pyrantel tartrate in North America. The *macrocyclic lactones* ivermectin and moxidectin remain the only anthelmintics that are fully effective against equine strongyles. Consequently, these drugs are the most widely used in equine establishments. The potential evolution of macrocyclic lactone resistance by cyathostomins has been discussed extensively.[51,52,53] Because no new classes of equine anthelmintics are anticipated in the near future, current control strategies must be revised to preserve the efficacy of available drugs for as long as possible.

Biologic control with nematode-trapping fungi has potential as a nonchemical approach to equine parasite control.[54] These fungi are natural predators of nematodes and kill free-living larvae by trapping them in a network of hyphae. Fungal spores can be fed to animals so that they pass though the alimentary tract and inoculate the feces. Fungi trap nematode larvae as they develop in the feces and significantly reduce the numbers of larvae on pasture. At present, fungal products are not commercially available.

Modern approaches to cyathostomin control emphasize the use of effective drugs, high levels of parasite surveillance, and decreased intensity of treatment within the herd. These approaches can maintain health, limit pasture contamination, and decrease selection pressures for anthelmintic resistance. One such approach, termed *selective treatment*, is based on characterizing the contaminative potential of each horse in a herd, then designing control programs based on individual characteristics.[55-58] The magnitude of strongylid egg counts of horses after a long sojourn from deworming can be used to classify individual animals as low, moderate, or high contaminators. Horses that are "low contaminators" apparently control parasitism on their own and do not contribute significantly to overall contamination of the premises. Such animals do not need to be dewormed at all if only cyathostomins are present on the premises. If large strongyles are a potential threat, low contaminators only need to be dewormed twice annually with a larvicide, at the beginning and end of a grazing season, to maintain eradication of large strongyles. Horses that are "high contaminators" should be the major focus of control and probably need repeated anthelmintic treatment throughout the grazing season. Finally, those horses that are "moderate contaminators" can be dewormed on a schedule that is intermediate between the two extremes. Eradication of cyathostomins is not a realistic goal for any control program.

Public Health Considerations. The cyathostomin nematodes that infect horses have no zoonotic potential and cannot infect any domestic animals other than equids.

Parascarosis

Etiology and Epidemiology

Parascaris equorum (ascarids, roundworms), as with other members of the superfamily *Ascaridoidea*, resides as an adult in the small intestine of its host. *P. equorum* is the largest nematode that infects horses, growing to approximately the size of a pencil when mature (Fig. 62-6). Thick-walled eggs are passed in the feces 10 to 15 weeks after infection[59-61] (Fig. 62-7). Development of eggs to the infective stage in the environment requires about 10 days at optimal temperatures (25°-35° C [77°-95° F])[62] and probably several weeks in cool conditions. The infective stage is an egg containing a second-stage larva (L_2).[2] Larvated eggs are ingested from the environment, hatch in the small intestine, and the liberated L_2 ascarids enter the portal circulation and are carried to the liver. Larvae are migrating through the liver within 24 hours of infection.[60] After approximately 1 week, larvae are carried to the lungs, where they break out of the vasculature and enter alveoli. These larvae migrate up the airways or are coughed up into the pharynx, where they are swallowed and return to the small intestine to complete maturation.

The major features of the epidemiology of parascarosis are the extreme persistence of the infective stage in the environment and the predominance of infection in juvenile horses. Larvated *Parascaris* eggs remain viable for 10 years or more, so one patent infection on a premise can affect several future generations of foals. Susceptible animals acquire infection by ingesting larvated eggs from the environment. Unlike strongylids, ascarid infections can be transmitted in confinement venues as well as on pasture. *Parascaris* eggs possess a sticky, protein coating[63] that allows them to adhere to a variety of surfaces, including vertical walls and the hair coat or udder of a mare. *Parascaris* infection is found almost exclusively in juvenile horses less than 18 months of age.[64] Horses develop extremely effective acquired immunity against *Parascaris*, and it is unusual to see patent infections in mature horses. Infections in juvenile horses often involve hundreds of worms, comprising a liter or more of parasites. Weanlings and yearlings ultimately lose their ascarid infections, probably through a combination of acquired immunity and senescence of the adult worm population. *Parascaris* is transmitted solely by equids; no alternate definitive hosts exist.

Pathogenesis

The pathogenesis of adult ascarid infections is poorly understood, but parasitized foals exhibit reduced weight gain and inferior body composition, with elevated total body water and decreased total body solids. The simplest explanation for their impact is that the large mass of worms in the small intestine competes with the host for digested nutrients, especially amino acids. This hypothesis was supported by an experiment showing that ascarids absorbed radiolabeled methionine after oral administration to foals.[65] In addition to competition for amino acids, reduced dietary intake by infected foals can result in hypoproteinemia.

Clinical Findings

Hepatic migration (1 week after infection) is not accompanied by apparent clinical signs. Invasion of the lungs (2-4 weeks after infection), however, can cause frequent coughing and a grayish white, purulent nasal discharge.[64,66] This exudate may also be visualized within the trachea by endoscopic examination. Affected foals often experience secondary bacterial infection, especially with *Streptococcus equi* subsp. *zooepidemicus*. Weanlings or yearlings infected with adult ascarids may exhibit poor growth, ill thrift, rough hair coats, and a pot-bellied appearance, but juveniles with modest worm burdens often appear normal. A large mass of ascarids can cause impaction of the small intestine, with accompanying colic and eventual intestinal rupture if not relieved. The likelihood of intestinal rupture is not directly correlated to worm numbers. In addition to signs of abdominal pain, foals with ascarid impaction may have gastric reflux (containing intact worms)

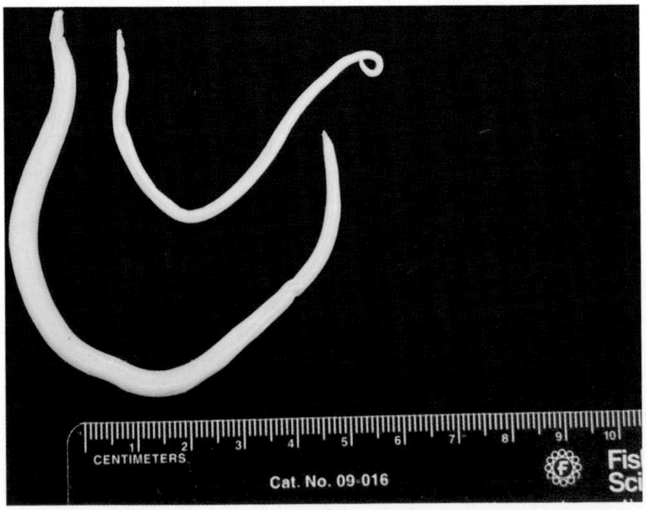

Fig. 62-6 *Parascaris equorum* adults; male *(top)* and female *(bottom)*. (Courtesy Dr. Charles Faulkner, Department of Comparative Medicine, University of Tennessee College of Veterinary Medicine, Knoxville.)

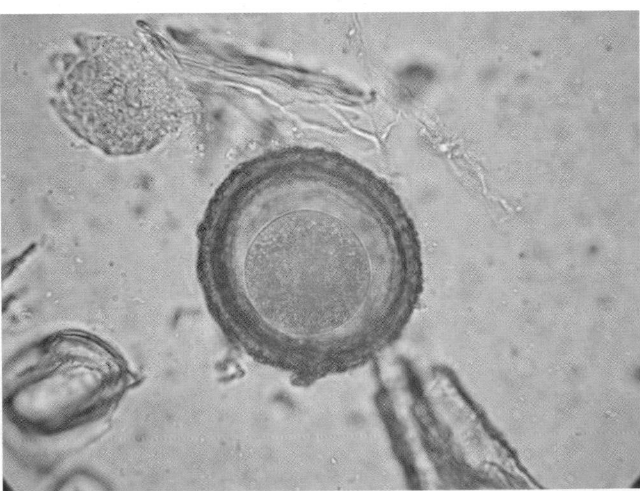

Fig. 62-7 Egg of *Parascaris equorum*. (Courtesy Dr. Charles Faulkner, Department of Comparative Medicine, University of Tennessee College of Veterinary Medicine, Knoxville.)

and shock secondary to possible toxic or hypersensitivity reactions to parasite antigens.

In a retrospective study of foals with ascarid impaction that were treated surgically, the median age at presentation was 5 months (range, 4-24 months).[85] Males were affected more often than females (67% and 33%, respectively). Approximately 75% of cases occurred during the fall season (late August to early November). At presentation, foals tended to be tachycardic and febrile, with injected and toxic mucous membranes and a prolonged capillary refill time. Gastrointestinal tract sounds were often reduced or absent.

Diagnosis

Patent ascarid infections are easily detected by fecal examination using one of the qualitative or quantitative concentration techniques discussed previously. Infections involving immature (i.e., nonreproducing) worms in the intestine, lungs, or liver, however, cannot be detected by this method. Infected horses often pass intact ascarids in the feces, especially within 1 to 2 days after anthelmintic treatment. Endoscopic and radiographic findings for the pulmonary stage of infection have been described.[66,67]

Foals with ascarid impactions often have abnormal abdominal fluid ranging from serosanguineous to purulent in nature.[85] Definitive diagnosis before surgery or necropsy may be difficult. However, presence of intact parasites in feces or gastric reflux of a foal or horse 4 to 24 months of age with acute colic suggests the diagnosis. A history of recent anthelmintic treatment also supports a diagnosis of ascarid impaction in foals. In a retrospective study of 11 foals treated surgically for ascarid impaction, three were dewormed less than 24 hours before the onset of colic signs and three were dewormed 2 to 5 days before the onset of signs (54% dewormed <6 days before onset of colic). In eight cases in which the type of anthelmintic was reported, three foals were treated with ivermectin, three with pyrantel pamoate, one with fenbendazole, and one with trichlorfon.[85] Ultrasound examination of the abdomen may facilitate presurgical or antemortem diagnosis by visualization of worms within the small intestine (Fig. 62-8).

Pathologic Findings

Hepatic migration during the first week after infection is accompanied by focal hemorrhage beneath the hepatic capsule and eosinophilic tracts within the parenchyma.[69] The hemorrhages heal by fibrosis, leaving depressed, white areas under the hepatic capsule. Pulmonary migration initially causes petechial hemorrhages and inflammatory changes. Four to six weeks after infection, lymphocytic nodules develop beneath the pleura.[70] These gray-green nodules may contain remnants of dead larvae and are more numerous after reinfection than after primary exposure.

Therapy

Parascaris is the dose-determining parasite for some equine dewormers, especially the benzimidazoles. This means that a higher dosage of a given anthelmintic is required to kill ascarids than other internal parasites, and this parameter often determines the approved label dosage of an equine parasiticide. Adult and juvenile ascarids in the lumen of the small intestine are susceptible to numerous anthelmintic products (Table 62-2). The ascaricidal efficacy of an anthelmintic can be evaluated by FECR testing (see Box 62-1) based on pretreatment and posttreatment counts of *Parascaris* eggs. Interpretation of FECR for ascarids, however, has not been characterized as well as for strongyles. In recent years, ascarid populations at some breeding farms in Canada,[71] The Netherlands,[72] and Denmark[73] have developed apparent resistance to the macrocyclic lactone anthelmintics moxidectin and ivermectin, as indicated by poor FECR. In 2005, Kaplan et al. reported that ivermectin failed to reduce egg counts or worm counts in foals that had been inoculated with a purportedly resistant strain of *Parascaris* from Canada.[73a] Anecdotal reports of ascarid resistance are common in the United States, but no data have been gathered to document the validity or extent of this phenomenon.

Foals that are suspected to have heavy ascarid burden should not be immediately treated with highly efficacious antihelminthics. Initial administration of a drug with lesser efficacy, specifically fenbendazole (5 mg/kg), may lessen the risk of posttreatment ascarid impaction. If ascarid impaction is suspected, treatment should include administration of mineral oil by nasogastric tube, appropriate supportive care to maintain hydration and treat shock, and analgesic therapy.

If medical therapy fails to relieve the impaction, surgical exploration with small intestinal enterotomy to remove worms may be attempted. In a retrospective study of 11 horses presented for surgical treatment of ascarid impaction, only one horse survived.[85] Impactions in these horses were usually at multiple sites, and postoperative complications leading to death included colic, endotoxemia, fever, adhesions, severe peritonitis, focal necrotizing enteritis, intestinal perforation, and abdominal incision infections.[85]

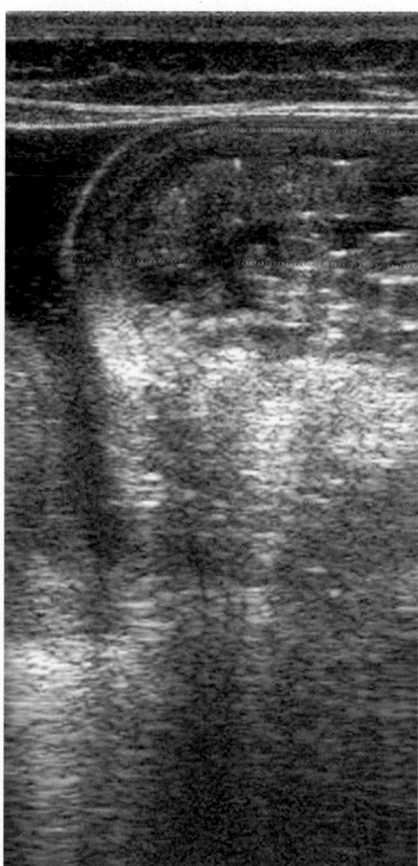

Fig. 62-8 Ultrasound image of ascarids within lumen of small intestine of foal with signs of colic. (Courtesy Dr. Maureen T. Long.)

Table • 62-2

Spectra of Various Anthelmintics Labeled for Efficacy against Nonstrongylid Nematode Parasites of Horses

CHEMICAL CLASS	COMPOUND	DOSAGE	*PARASCARIS EQUORUM*	*STRONGYLOIDES WESTERI*	*OXYURIS EQUI*
Benzimidazoles	Fenbendazole	5 mg/kg	Yes*	No	Yes
	Oxfendazole	10 mg/kg	Yes	No	Yes
	Oxibendazole	10 mg/kg	Yes	Yes†	Yes
Heterocyclic compounds	Piperazine	88 mg/kg	Yes	No	Yes
Macrocyclic lactones	Ivermectin	0.2 mg/kg	Yes	Yes	Yes
	Moxidectin	0.4 mg/kg	Yes	N/A‡	Yes
Tetrahydropyrimidines	Pyrantel pamaote	6.6 mg/kg	Yes	No	Yes
	Pyrantel tartrate§	2.64 mg/kg/day	Yes	No	Yes

*Requires a dosage of 10 mg/kg.
†Requires a dosage of 15 mg/kg.
‡Moxidectin may not be used in foals less than 5 months of age.
§Aids in the control of certain nematode parasites when added to the feed daily.

Prevention

The objective of an ascarid control program is to limit environmental contamination with reproductive products (i.e., passage of eggs in feces). Contamination can have far-reaching effects because of the extreme persistence of the infective stage in the environment. In contrast to strongylids, ascarid control efforts must be applied to the entire farm premises, not only pasture venues.

If administered daily in the feed, *pyrantel tartrate* (2.64 mg/kg) kills ingested ascarid larvae after they hatch from the egg but before they can invade the tissues of the small intestine. This approach is limited to horses that reliably ingest the pelleted product but can be very effective. Ascarid resistance to pyrantel tartrate has not been reported.

Control recommendations for breeding farms are based on a prepatent period of approximately 70 days or longer. It is recommended that treatments for ascarid infection begin when foals are 45 to 60 days old, and that subsequent treatments thereafter be repeated at 2-month intervals until the horse is at least 15 months of age. The ERP of effective anthelmintics does not differ as widely for ascarids as it does for cyathostomins. Acquired immunity usually develops well before a horse's second birthday, and ascarid control efforts are not required for mature equids.

Because resistance to at least one drug class (macrocyclic lactones) has been reported, it is an excellent recommendation to monitor fecal samples of foals for ascarid eggs during the intervals between regularly scheduled treatments. The presence of large numbers of eggs 2 to 4 weeks after treatment suggests that the previous deworming was ineffective, and anthelmintic resistance could be confirmed with a standard FECR test.

Because ivermectin has some activity against larval ascarids migrating in the liver or lungs,[74] many breeding operations use it at monthly intervals in foals. This frequency is excessive, and all premises with documented *Parascaris* resistance to macrocyclic lactone anthelmintics had a history of using ivermectin or moxidectin at monthly intervals.

Ancillary ascarid control efforts are directed at reducing exposure to infective stages from the environment. These measures include rigorous hygiene of foaling stalls or other housing areas to be occupied by suckling foals. Numerous disinfectants, including Lysol, phenol, chlorine bleach, and even live steam, have been evaluated in the field.[62] None has been entirely successful in eliminating infective eggs. Because ascarid eggs can adhere to the hair coat of a horse, a standard practice at many breeding farms is to bathe mares thoroughly before introducing them to foaling stalls, with particular efforts to clean the udder.

Public Health Considerations

Parascaris equorum has no zoonotic potential and does not infect other domestic animals in the adult stage.

Strongyloidosis

Etiology and Epidemiology

Strongyloides westeri is a small, thin nematode (<1 cm × 1 mm) that resides in the proximal small intestine of foals. Only females are parasitic, and they reproduce by parthenogenesis. Thin-walled, oval eggs containing a coiled larva (Fig. 62-9) are passed in the feces. In the environment, *Strongyloides* undergoes a complex life cycle with alternating free-living and parasitic generations.[2] Eggs hatch and larvae develop to become either free-living males and females or infective third-stage larvae. Sexual reproduction by free-living stages produces only larvae that are destined for a parasitic existence. Environmental development requires moist conditions and warm temperatures. Horses are infected when third-stage larvae penetrate the skin or mucous membranes. In immune adult horses the infective larvae migrate to somatic tissues and suspend further development. In mares the hormones of pregnancy and lactation apparently stimulate the arrested larvae to mobilize and migrate to the mammary gland. Third-stage larvae are passed in the milk of mares within a few days after foaling, and foals ingest infective larvae while they suckle.[75] Within the foal, larvae undergo pulmonary migration and return to the small intestine. Egg production by adult females usually begins in foals at 10 to 14 days of age,[2] but patent infections have been observed in foals as young as 5 days.[76]

Most foals develop permanent immunity against reinfection with *Strongyloides* by 5 or 6 months of age. However, foals

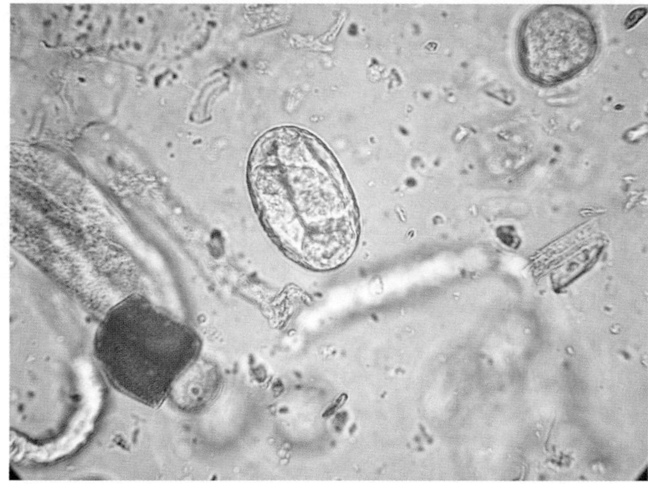

Fig. 62-9 Egg of *Strongyloides westeri*. (Courtesy Dr. Charles Faulkner, Department of Comparative Medicine, University of Tennessee College of Veterinary Medicine, Knoxville.)

with no prior exposure to *Strongyloides* may be susceptible to primary challenge.[77] A recent, coprologic survey of foals from central Kentucky revealed a prevalence of *Strongyloides* infection (1.5%) that was much lower than historical observations in a similar population.[78]

Pathogenesis

Strongyloides westeri occasionally causes diarrhea in infected foals,[77] but mechanisms other than simple enteritis have not been described. Although *S. westeri* patency and foal heat diarrhea both occur contemporaneously during the second week of life, no causal relationship has been established. Foal heat diarrhea continues to be common despite the declining prevalence of *Strongyloides* infections.

Clinical Findings

The most common clinical sign of strongyloidosis is diarrhea during the first month or two of life. Heavily infected foals may become emaciated, listless, and dehydrated from enteritis. This clinical syndrome must be differentiated from other causes of diarrhea in foals.

A syndrome of "frenzy" (hyperactivity and extreme discomfort) has been reported in foals that were confined on moist soil, sand, or sawdust with an acid pH.[76,79] Affected animals exhibited swelling of the lower legs within 2 days of an attack, and some developed skin lesions. This clinical manifestation was attributed to percutaneous invasion by third-stage *S. westeri* larvae. Exposed foals developed patent infections within 1 week after a frenzied episode, and *Rhodococcus equi* was recovered from regional lymph nodes.[76]

Diagnosis

Infection is confirmed by demonstrating small, thin-shelled, oval eggs containing a coiled larva in the feces of foals from 1 week to about 5 months of age (see Fig. 62-9). The observation of *Strongyloides* eggs in the feces of a diarrheic foal, however, does not necessarily implicate the nematode as the cause of the diarrhea. In a case-control study of foal diarrhea in the United Kingdom, the presence of *Strongyloides* eggs was significantly correlated to clinical diarrhea only when egg counts were very high (>2000 EPG), suggesting the presence of large numbers of adult parasites.

Pathologic Findings

Little is known about the pathologic lesions associated with *Strongyloides* infection in foals. Enteritis in the proximal small intestine is the most common lesion, but edema of the entire alimentary tract was described in one severe case.[77] Systemic migration during the prepatent period may be accompanied by petechial hemorrhages and inflammatory foci in pulmonary tissues.

Therapy

Only two currently marketed equine anthelmintics have label claims for efficacy against *S. westeri*. Oxibendazole (15 mg/kg) and ivermectin (0.2 mg/kg) are both effective after oral administration (see Table 62-2). Another macrocyclic lactone, moxidectin, is also effective, but this compound is not labeled in the United States for use in foals less than 5 months of age.

Prevention

Attempts to minimize lactogenic transmission by deworming the mare with ivermectin during the last weeks of gestation have not been completely effective.[80] Environmental hygiene to remove foal feces and application of basic chemicals to adjust the pH of moist confinement areas may reduce percutaneous transmission. Many breeding farms routinely deworm foals at about 2 weeks of age with one of the products listed previously to reduce transmission and obviate clinical disease. However, the incidence of *S. westeri* infection has declined so dramatically in recent years that many breeding operations would be justified in deleting specific *Strongyloides* control measures from the facility herd health program.

Public Health Considerations

Although human lesions of cutaneous larva migrans resulted from an accidental laboratory exposure to infective larvae of *S. westeri*,[81] this parasite is generally considered to have little zoonotic potential. Humans and all domestic mammals serve as definitive hosts of various *Strongyloides* species other than *S. westeri*.

Oxyurosis

Etiology and Epidemiology

Oxyuris equi is a fairly large nematode (~1-6 cm in length) that resides as an adult in the small colon and dorsal colon of equids.[2] *Oxyuris* is known as a *pinworm* because the tail end of the female is sharply pointed. Pinworm eggs are rarely passed in feces because gravid females protrude from the anus and deposit eggs in a sticky film directly onto the anus and perianal tissues. Development is facilitated by proximity to a warm host, and eggs become infective in about 5 days. The masses of infective eggs flake off into the environment, and transmission to other horses is accomplished by ingestion. As with ascarids, pinworms can be transmitted in confinement venues as well as on pastures. When an infective egg is ingested, a third-stage larva hatches out and invades the mucosa of the large intestine. These molt to fourth-stage larvae, which are small, wedge-shaped worms that attach to the mucosa of the proximal large intestine. Larvae ultimately molt into adults, which live in the distal colon to reduce the commuting distance for nocturnal oviposition by females. The prepatent period of *O. equi* is approximately 5 months. Equine pinworms apparently invoke acquired immunity because the prevalence of patent infections is much lower in mature horses. Adult horses can develop oxyurosis, however, if never previously infected.

Pathogenesis

Larval pinworms attach to the mucosa of the cecum and ventral colon, where their plug-feeding activities may cause superficial typhlitis or colitis. Adult pinworms apparently do not have any primary pathologic impact.

Clinical Findings

As a consequence of anal pruritus associated with the egg-laying activity of female worms, affected horses rub their rumps against stall fixtures, trees, and fence posts, causing hair loss of the tail and abrasions to the perianal region.[2] Adult pinworms occasionally are observed in freshly passed feces or adhering to a rectal palpation sleeve, and adult females may be observed protruding from the anus. Fresh or dried egg masses can be observed on the anus. The fresh material is greenish yellow and pasty, and the dried masses are gray, yellow, or green.

Diagnosis

Diagnosis is confirmed by recovery of *Oxyuris* eggs in samples collected from around the anus of a suspected host. Typical *Oxyuris* eggs are oval, flattened on one side, have a single operculum, and contain a coiled larva (Fig. 62-10). Various techniques can be used to collect perianal samples. In the cellophane (Scotch) tape technique, the sticky side of a small piece of adhesive tape is applied to the perianal area and then attached directly to a glass slide for microscopic examination. Diagnostic material can also be collected by scraping the perianal region with a tongue depressor dipped in mineral oil or lubricant and transferring the scrapings to a microscope slide for examination.

Pathologic Findings

Mild, superficial colitis has been attributed to attachment of fourth-stage larvae on the mucosa of the proximal large intestine. In one case, lesions of hemomelasma ilei on the serosa of the ileum were found to contain eggs of *O. equi*.[82]

Therapy

Virtually all broad-spectrum equine anthelmintics are effective against adult and larval *O. equi*. These include drugs of the benzimidazole, tetrahydropyrimidine, and macrocyclic lactone classes. Any of these products could be used as a specific therapy when the objective is to alleviate clinical signs caused by adult pinworm infection.

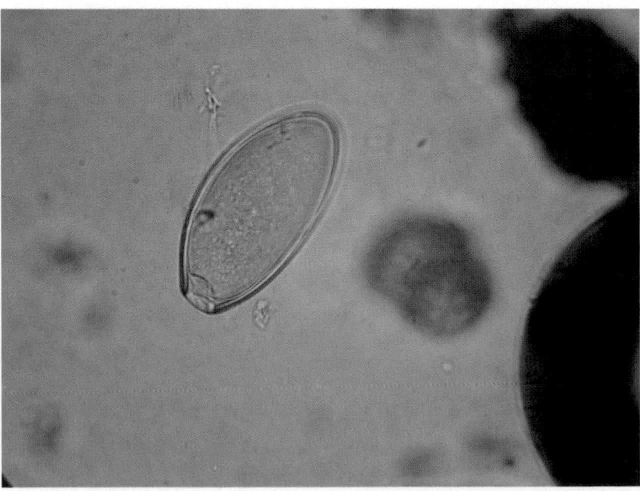

Fig. 62-10 Egg of *Oxyuris equi*.

Prevention

Environmental hygiene would be beneficial for pinworm control but would not be expected to eliminate infective stages completely. The routine use of anthelmintics in horses less than 2 years of age should provide adequate control of pinworm infections. Because of the long prepatent period of *Oxyuris*, routine strategies for strongylid control are sufficient against pinworms as well. Since 2004, numerous reports have circulated of adult horses with pinworm infections that were refractory to treatment with macrocyclic lactone anthelmintics, even with frequent treatments and increased dosages. Macrocyclic lactones are not 100% effective against adult *Oxyuris*,[83,84] so these observations should not be construed as unequivocal evidence of resistance.

Public Health Considerations

Oxyuris equi has no zoonotic potential and does not infect other domestic animals. Humans serve as definitive hosts of *Enterobius vermicularis*, a pinworm that is unique to primates.

NONENTERIC NEMATODES

Debra C. Sellon

The adult stages of most nematode parasites that affect horses reside within the gastrointestinal tract. However, a few parasites cause significant disease within other body systems, including the skin (*Onchocerca, Habronema/Draschia*), respiratory tract (*Dictyocaulus*), eye (*Thelazia;* discussed in Chapter 10), and central nervous system *(Halicephalobus;* discussed in Chapter 4).

Onchocerciasis

Etiology and Epidemiology

At least three species of nematode parasites from the genus *Onchocerca* are associated with cutaneous and ocular lesions in horses. *Onchocerca gutturosa* affects cattle and horses in North America, Africa, Australia, and Europe.[86] Adult worms are up to 60 cm in length and live in connective ligamentum nuchae of horses. Adult parasites produce microfilariae (200-230 μm in length) that are most numerous in the dermis of the face, neck, back, and ventral midline.[87] A number of *Simulium* spp. and *Culicoides* spp. may serve as intermediate hosts.[88-90]

Onchocerca reticulata infects horses in Europe and Asia. Adult worms may be up to 50 cm in length and live in the connective tissue of the flexor tendons and the suspensory ligament of the fetlock, especially in the front legs. Microfilariae are 310 to 395 μm in length and are most numerous in the dermis of the legs and ventral midline. *Culicoides* spp. act as intermediate hosts.[86]

Onchocerca cervicalis causes a nonseasonal dermatitis in horses worldwide.[86,91-93] Clinical disease occurs year-round but may be worse in the spring and summer. The small, threadlike adult nematode is approximately 30 cm in length and resides in the ligamentum nuchae. Microfilariae migrate to the dermis of the ventral midline, pectoral area, withers, inguinal region, and eyelids,[94] with highest numbers in the spring, when *Culicoides* spp., the predominant intermediate host, are most active.[95] Mosquitoes may also serve as vectors in some geographic areas. Microfilariae undergo development to infective larval stages over a 25-day period within the *Culicoides* vector. The estimated prevalence of *O. cervicalis* infestation in clinically normal horse populations in the United States varies from 25% to 100%.[86,96] There are no apparent breed or gender predilections for onchocerciasis, but affected horses are usually older than 4 years.[86] Because O. *cervicalis* is the most common member of the *Onchocerca* genus to affect horses, the remainder of this discussion focuses on this parasite unless otherwise indicated.

Pathogenesis

Cutaneous lesions related to O. *cervicalis* are thought to result from type I and type III hypersensitivity reactions to microfilariae.[86,91,93,97] The severity of the reaction varies between horses, and many horses have dermal microfilariae without any evidence of reaction. Ocular lesions are the result of microfilariae in the eyelids, conjunctiva, cornea, anterior chamber, uvea, and fundus. Concurrent uveitis, presumably an immune-mediated event, may be observed. In either cutaneous or ocular lesions, sudden death of parasites with chemotherapy may produce a severe exacerbation of disease, presumably as a reaction to antigens released by dead and dying microfilariae.

Clinical Findings

Lesions of cutaneous onchocerciasis secondary to O. *cervicalis* microfilariae begin as areas of thinning hair, with or without mild scaling or crusting. These areas are observed most often on the face, neck, chest, withers, and ventral midline and usually are accompanied by mild to moderate pruritus[86,91,93,97] (Fig. 62-11). Over time, lesions progress to areas of alopecia with scaling, crusting, and plaques. Chronic lesions become ulcerated and excoriated with crusts and lichenification. Depigmentation eventually occurs and is irreversible.[86,92,93] Affected horses may exhibit extreme pruritus and attempt to rub lesions on the face and ventral abdomen. However, tail rubbing is seldom seen with onchocerciasis, helping to differentiate this disorder from *Culicoides* hypersensitivity reactions.[93]

The most common clinical abnormality associated with ocular onchocerciasis is depigmentation (vitiligo) of the bulbar conjunctiva at the temporal limbus.[93] Sclerosing keratitis originating at the temporal limbus and extending toward the center of the eye may be observed.[86] Other clinical signs and lesions may include conjunctivitis, chemosis, blepharospasm, lacrimation, corneal edema, and faint multifocal corneal deposits. Signs of concurrent uveitis may be observed in some horses. Chronic infection may result in formation of nodules 0.5 to 1 mm in diameter in the pigmented conjunctiva of the temporal limbus. Peripapillary choroidal sclerosis (round or crescent-shaped area of depigmentation bordering the optic disc) has been described in some affected horses.[86,93]

Clinical signs of O. *reticulata* infestation of horses include subcutaneous nodules overlying or within the flexor tendons and suspensory ligaments around the fetlock, especially in the front legs. Severely affected horses may have associated swelling and lameness.[86]

Diagnosis and Pathologic Findings

Differential diagnoses for cutaneous onchocerciasis include dermatophytosis, fly-bite dermatoses, mite infestations, and food hypersensitivity. Skin scrapings and direct smears of blood or cutaneous lesions are unreliable for diagnosis. Diagnosis is most easily confirmed by identification of microfilariae in minced skin biopsy preparations from horses with compatible history and clinical signs (Fig. 62-12). A standard 4- or 6-mm skin punch biopsy specimen is minced with a sharp blade and mixed with physiologic saline in a Petri dish. After incubation at room temperature for 30 minutes, the specimen is examined under a microscope for identification of rapidly moving microfilariae.[86,93] Routine skin biopsies reveal superficial perivascular eosinophilic dermatitis, often with visible microfilariae in the superficial dermis surrounded by degranulating eosinophils.[86,98] Chronic lesions may have evidence of fibrosis. Occasionally, necrosis of hair follicle epithelium, focal areas of collagenolysis in the superficial dermis, or lymphoid nodules in the deep dermis or subcutis may be observed.[86] Because microfilariae may be observed in the skin of normal horses, diagnosis cannot be made solely on the basis of observation of these parasites in a biopsy specimen. The final diagnosis can only be made after consideration of biopsy results, history, and clinical signs and observation of a positive response to appropriate therapy.

Therapy

Ivermectin at a dose of 200 μg/kg orally is the treatment of choice for elimination of microfilariae in the skin or ocular tissues.[99,100] A single dose may result in improvement in clinical signs within 2 to 3 weeks, with complete resolution in 2 months.[99] One study suggested that some horses may remain free of cutaneous microfilariae for 4 to 5 months or longer

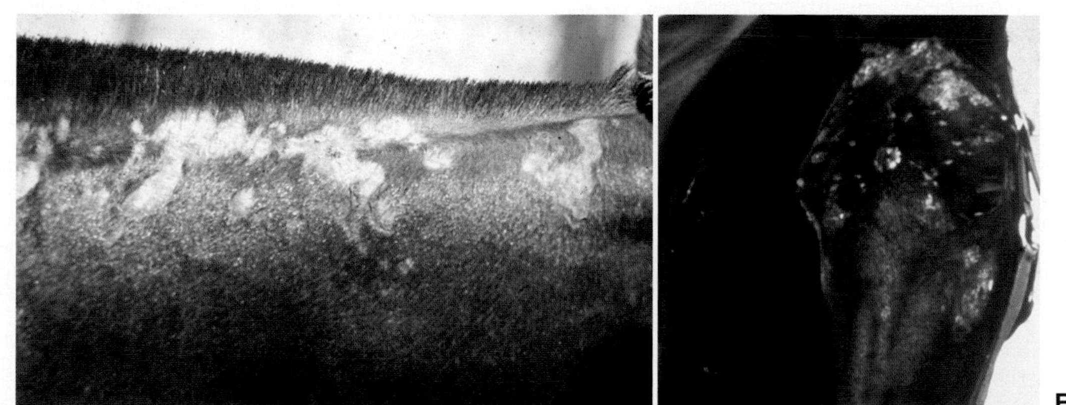

Fig. 62-11 Thinning of hair and hair loss caused by *Onchocerca cervicalis* microfilariae in neck (A) and head (B) of horse. Note the inflammation and ulceration secondary to pruritus. (Courtesy Dr. Melissa T. Hines.)

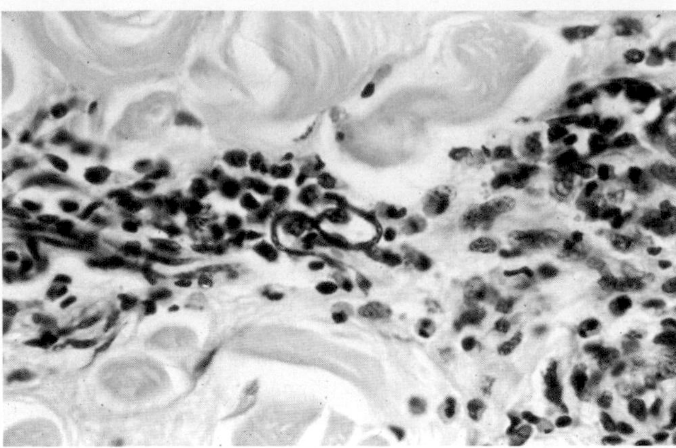

Fig. 62-12 Photomicrograph of skin biopsy specimen from horse with *Onchocerca cervicalis*. Note the numerous eosinophils and presence of microfilariae. (Courtesy Dr. Melissa T. Hines.)

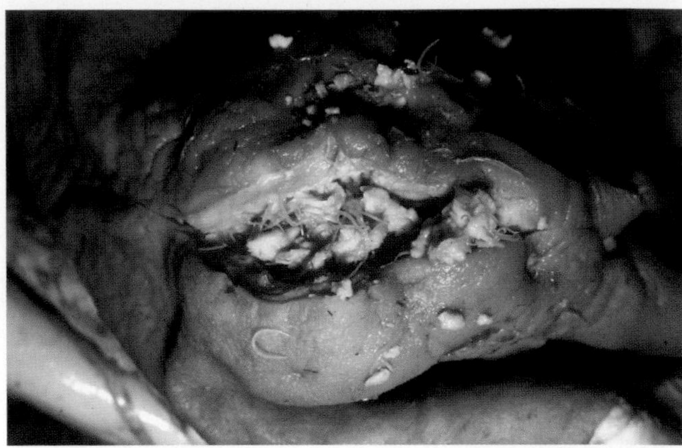

Fig. 62-13 Large granuloma containing *Draschia megastoma* parasites in stomach of horse. (Courtesy Dr. John Barnes.)

after treatment with injectable ivermectin. Some horses may require two or three monthly treatments before clinical signs resolve. Approximately 10% to 25% of horses with onchocerciasis have an adverse reaction (e.g., ventral midline edema or pruritus) to ivermectin treatment within 7 to 10 days. In rare cases, severe ventral midline or eyelid edema and fever may develop. Anecdotal reports suggest that treatment may precipitate uveitis in horses with ocular microfilariae.[92] These horses should be treated with corticosteroids before or during ivermectin therapy to decrease the likelihood or severity of adverse reactions. There is no known therapy to eliminate adult O. *cervicalis* from the ligamentum nuchae of horses. Therefore, affected horses will need periodic re-treatment with ivermectin to prevent or control recurrence of clinical signs.[92-94]

Alternative drugs that have been recommended for treatment of equine onchocerciasis include diethylcarbamazine at 5 mg/kg orally (PO) for a minimum of 5 consecutive days or levamisole at 10 mg/kg PO daily for 7 to 10 days. However, with the widespread availability of ivermectin, these drugs are now rarely used.

Habronemiasis

Etiology and Epidemiology

Habronemiasis, also known as "summer sores," bursatti, "swamp cancer," and granular dermatitis, is caused by a reaction to larvae of the equine stomach worms *Habronema muscae, Habronema majus (Habronema microstoma)*, and *Draschia megastoma*.[101] Adult *H. muscae* and *H. majus* are 1 to 2.5 cm in length and can be found free in the mucus covering the glandular area of the stomach.[101] They are rarely pathogenic, although large numbers may cause nonspecific gastritis or ulceration of the gastric mucosa.[102] In contrast, adult *D. megastoma* worms are 0.5 to 1.25 cm in length, invade the gastric mucosa, and cause granulomatous masses up to 10 cm in diameter. Large *D. megastoma* granulomas within the stomach contain colonies of adult parasites and have a central opening through which larvae pass into the lumen of the stomach (Fig. 62-13). Occasionally, these lesions may be large enough to obstruct the flow of ingesta or may perforate the stomach wall, resulting in diffuse or localized peritonitis, occasionally fatal.[101]

Regardless of species, adult worms produce first-stage larvae (L_1) that are passed in feces. The L_1 stages are ingested by fly maggots. The housefly *(Musca domestica)* is an intermediate host for *H. muscae* and *D. megastoma*; the stable fly *(Stomoxys calcitrans)* is the intermediate host for *H. majus*.[86] After maturation, infective third-stage larvae (L_3) on the mouthparts of adult flies are deposited around a horse's mouth or in horse feed; the larvae are ingested; and the life cycle is complete. Cutaneous habronemiasis occurs when infective L_3 parasites are deposited on wounds or other moist areas of the body, such as the penis, prepuce, or periocular tissues. Occasionally, the parasite may penetrate unbroken skin to cause lesions.

Cutaneous habronemiasis has been reported in horses from most parts of the world as a seasonal, sporadic, recurrent disease.[101-115] Lesions are most frequently observed in the spring and summer and may regress in the winter. Larvae do not appear to overwinter in the skin.[86] No breed, gender, or age predilection exists. Some horses appear to have particular susceptibility to disease and have recurrent lesions each year, whereas other horses on the same premises never exhibit lesions.

Pathogenesis

The characteristic ulcerative granulomatous lesions of cutaneous habronemiasis are probably the result of a hypersensitivity reaction to parasite larvae. Evidence for the role of hypersensitivity reactions in the pathogenesis include the seasonal recurrent nature of lesions, predilection of some horses for lesions, and response to systemic glucocorticoids as a sole treatment.[86,101] The reaction of specific immunoglobulin E (IgE) with larvae is speculated to result in mobilization of eosinophils; peripheral eosinophilia may reach 15% to 20%.[101]

Clinical Findings

Cutaneous habronemiasis is characterized by large, granulomatous, ulcerative lesions most often observed in areas of wounds or on moist areas of the body, such as the penis, prepuce, periocular tissues, or distal limbs (Figs. 62-14 and 62-15). Early lesions often appear as slow-healing wounds that gradually enlarge and develop the typical appearance of exuberant granulation tissue.[116] They may be solitary or multiple and can affect more than one part of the body in a single horse. The ulcerated granulomatous tissue frequently exudes a serosanguineous exudate. Pruritus varies from mild to severe. Small (1-mm) yellow granules consisting of caseation, calcification, fibrosis, and necrosis surrounding dead larvae may be observed. As lesions enlarge, they frequently take on a circular shape. These granules must be differentiated from the

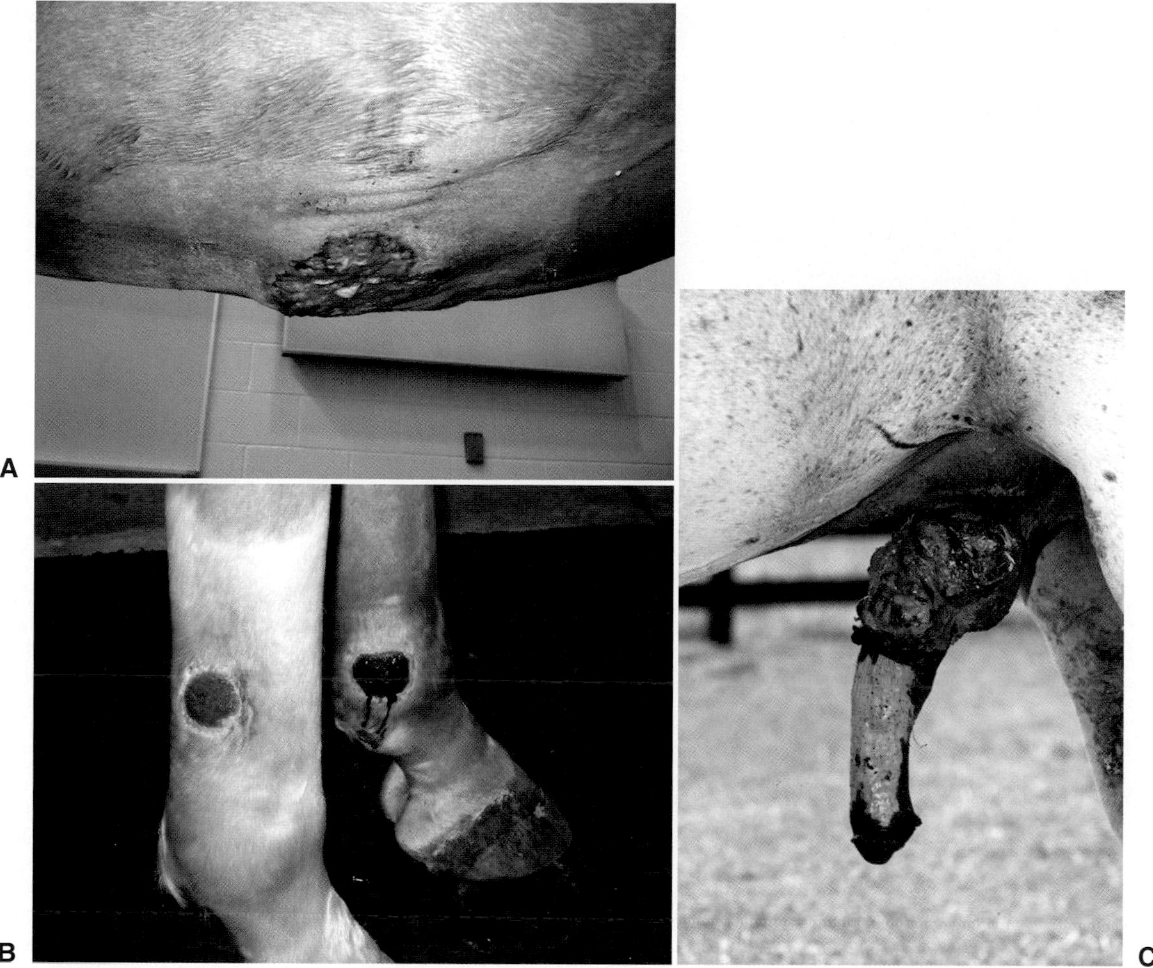

Fig. 62-14 Equine habronemiasis of **A,** ventral abdomen; **B,** distal limbs; and **C,** penis. (*A* courtesy Dr. Steeve Giguere; *B* courtesy Dr. Robert MacKay; C courtesy Dr. Margo Macpherson.)

"leeches" observed in lesions of phycomycosis and zygomycosis (see Chapter 55). Lesions of the urethral process may obstruct urine flow, with resultant dysuria and pollakiuria.[117]

Ocular lesions are most frequently observed as yellowish, gritty plaques in the conjunctiva of the medial canthus. Lesions may also involve the conjunctival sac, the lacrimal duct, or the third eyelid (see Fig. 62-15). Lesions of the nictitans may be more proliferative. Lacrimal duct lesions typically result in a circular lesion from a few millimeters up to 2 cm in diameter, approximately 2 to 3 cm below the medial canthus.[86,101,116,118]

Pulmonary habronemiasis is uncommon and rarely associated with clinical respiratory disease. Nodular granulomas with central necrosis are present in the interstitial and peribronchial areas of the lung.[86,120-122] One foal had a *Rhodococcus equi* pulmonary abscess from which *D. megastoma* larvae were recovered.[119] Another report described small, white, necrotic foci containing *D. megastoma* in the liver of a horse.[115] It has been proposed that these types of lesions represent aberrant dissemination of larvae through the blood or lymphatic circulation; however, the horses in these reports did not have concurrent cutaneous lesions.[101]

Diagnosis and Pathologic Findings

A presumptive diagnosis of habronemiasis can often be made on the gross appearance of the lesions. Differential diagnoses should include bacterial granulomas, phycomycosis, zygomycosis, other fungal granulomas, exuberant granulation tissue, squamous cell carcinoma, sarcoid, and other neoplastic lesions. Definitive diagnosis is confirmed by direct smears or biopsy. Deep scrapings or smears of lesions, especially from lesion granules, may reveal nematode larvae.[86] These larvae are typically large (2-3 mm wide and 60 mm long) with a large, spiny process on their tails.[116] Caution should be exercised in interpreting these types of smears because they may be negative despite the presence of the parasite, and larvae may be present in other ulcerative lesions of equine skin, including those differential diagnoses previously listed. Biopsy usually reveals varying degrees of nodular to diffuse dermatitis, numerous eosinophils and mast cells, areas of coagulative necrosis that may contain nematode larvae, and palisading granuloma formation around necrotic foci.[86]

Therapy

A wide variety of therapeutic strategies have been described for treatment of habronemiasis in horses. An individual therapeutic plan should be developed for each horse, taking into consideration the site of the lesion, size of the lesion, number of lesions, financial concerns, and practical considerations. Medical therapy alone may be efficacious for many horses; however, horses with large or refractory lesions may

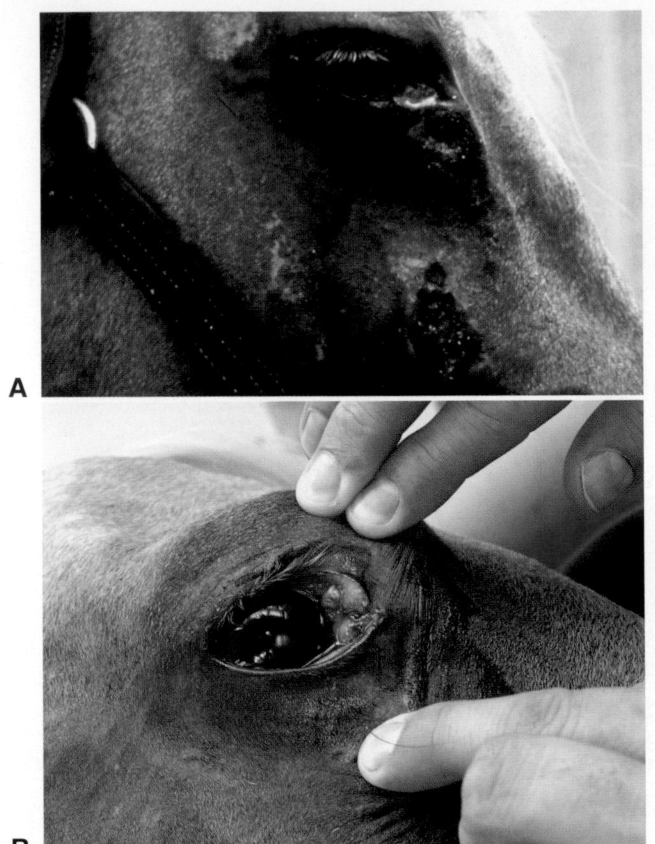

Fig. 62-15 A, Typical lesions of ocular habronemiasis involving lacrimal gland at medial canthus of eye. B, Ocular habronemiasis involving nictitans. (*A* courtesy Dr. Melissa T. Hines; *B* courtesy Dr. Alison Morton.)

benefit from surgery to debulk the lesion before initiating medical therapy. Cryosurgery may also be performed with a double freeze-thaw cycle.[123]

A variety of topical preparations for treatment of habronemiasis have been described. Most of these contain some combination of organophosphates plus corticosteroids and/or dimethyl sulfoxide (DMSO). Also, antimicrobial drugs are often included. These preparations are usually applied daily and covered with a bandage. Injectable or oral ivermectin therapy is also indicated for its larvacidal effects. Organophosphates have been used orally or intravenously (IV) for treatment of equine habronemiasis. Trichlorfon is the most commonly used agent and is administered IV at 25 mg/kg in 1 L of 5% dextrose or physiologic saline.[124] The solution is autoclaved before use and should be repeated at 1- to 2-week intervals if necessary.[116] Adverse effects may occur, including restlessness, pawing, and colic.

Systemic corticosteroids are indicated for primary treatment of many horses with habronemiasis and to minimize hypersensitivity reactions to dead or dying parasites. These drugs have been used successfully as sole therapy for some horses with habronemiasis, supporting the theory that lesions are the result of a hypersensitivity reaction.[116] Prednisolone at 1 mg/kg PO once daily for 7 to 14 days is reported to be effective for treatment of many horses.[86,116]

Conjunctival habronemiasis may be treated topically with 0.03% echothiophate drops twice daily in combination with an antimicrobial/dexamethasone ophthalmic ointment.[86] Occasionally, conjunctival granulomas require excision or curettage.[116]

Prevention

Regular deworming of horses with ivermectin will kill adult stomach worms and minimize larval contamination of manure. Regular removal of manure, prompt treatment of wounds, and appropriate use of insecticides will also aid in the control and prevention of cutaneous habronemiasis in susceptible horses.[116]

Lungworm Infection

Etiology, Epidemiology, and Pathogenesis

Donkeys and mules are the reservoir hosts for *Dictyocaulus arnfieldi*, the equine lungworm.[125] Infestations in the reservoir hosts do not cause clinical signs even when large worm burdens are present.[126] Prevalence of lungworm infection is estimated to be approximately 68% to 80% in donkeys, 29% in mules, and 2% to 11% in horses.[127,128]

Infection is initiated by ingestion of second-stage larvae (L_2), which migrate through the gut wall and are carried to the lungs through the lymphatics. After 13 weeks of maturation in the peripheral bronchioles, parasites begin to shed ova that are transported by mucociliary clearance to the pharynx, swallowed, and passed out in feces to become infective within 4 days. First-stage larvae (L_1) can survive up to 7 weeks in warm soil but do not tolerate cold weather well.[129] In most horses and ponies, infection is arrested at the L_5 stage and are usually nonpatent, although ova may be passed in the feces of some horses.[126] Because lungworms have been identified in horses with no known contact with donkeys or mules, it is assumed that direct horse-to-horse spread is possible.[127,130]

Experimental studies suggest that *Pilobolus* fungi may facilitate the spread of lungworm infection in a manner similar to that which occurs in cattle lungworm infections.[131] Infective larvae invade the sporangia of the fungi as they grow on manure and are dispersed in the environment when sporangia rupture.[130]

Clinical Findings

Horses with lungworm infections frequently present with signs of coughing and increased expiratory effort that may mimic the signs of reactive airway obstruction (chronic pulmonary obstruction).[129,132] Auscultation frequently reveals crackles and wheezes, most often over the dorsocaudal lung fields.[132] Infected donkeys rarely show clinical signs of respiratory disease.

Diagnosis and Pathologic Findings

Diagnosis should be suspected in horses with typical clinical signs and history of exposure to donkeys or mules. Endoscopic examination usually reveals large quantities of exudate in the large airways,[130] with a preponderance of eosinophils. Diagnosis can be confirmed by visualization of the parasite, identification of ova on fecal examination with the Baermann technique, or response to appropriate therapy. Occasionally, larval stages of the parasite may be observed in tracheal wash or bronchoalveolar lavage samples or in centrifuged mucus.[129,133] Iodine may be useful to stain larvae and facilitate their visualization. On rare occasions, adult lungworms may be visualized endoscopically in the bronchi. These parasites may be up to 16 cm in length.[130] The Baermann fecal flotation technique should be performed on the patient and any potential reservoir hosts. However, infections in horses are usually not patent, and a negative Baermann procedure does not rule out the possibility of lungworms. At necropsy, adult lungworms are most often found in the peripheral bronchi. Circumscribed, pale, overinflated areas may be observed in lung parenchyma, especially in caudal lung regions.[126]

Therapy and Prevention

Ivermectin at 200 μg/kg PO is effective for treatment of *D. arnfieldi* and is not associated with significant adverse effects.[134,135] Moxidectin was 99.9% effective for treatment of lungworm infections in donkeys.[136] Thiabendazole, mebendazole, and fenbendazole may also be effective for treatment of lungworms. In donkeys, however, fenbendazole only transiently suppressed fecal larval counts.[137]

Lungworm infections may be prevented by housing horses in areas where no donkeys or mules are present. It is advisable to avoid areas where donkeys and mules have previously been housed, unless a freeze has occurred since last habitation.

REFERENCES

See the CD-ROM for a list of references linked to the abstract in PubMed.

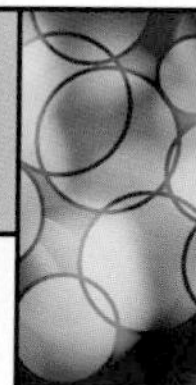

CHAPTER • 63

Cestodes

Merijo Eileen Jordan and Joseph A. DiPietro

ETIOLOGY

Three species within the family *Anoplocephalidae* (Kholodkovskii, 1902) infect the gastrointestinal (GI) tract of horses and donkeys: *Anoplocephala perfoliata* (Goeze, 1782; Blanchard, 1848), *Anoplocephala magna* (Abildgaard, 1789; Sprengel, 1905), and *Anoplocephaloides mamillana* (Mehlis, 1831; Rausch, 1976; Schmidt, 1986). All members of the family *Anoplocephalidae* are similar in that the scolex is devoid of rostellum, hooks, or hooklets during all stages of development, and the suckers are unarmed.[1,2] Within this family, four subfamilies have been described based on type of uterine development.[2] All members of the subfamily *Anoplocephalinae* (Blanchard, 1891), including the three equine tapeworm species, can be defined by the following characteristics: morphologically, the uterus persists in gravid proglottids, and biologically, members have a cysticercoid larval type that occurs within the hemocele of oribatid mites.[2,3]

Of the three tapeworm species infecting horses, *A. perfoliata* is the most prevalent and the most frequently associated with clinical disease. Therefore, this chapter focuses primarily on *Anoplocephala perfoliata*.

Morphology

Distinguishing characteristics of adult *Anoplocephala perfoliata* (Fig. 63-1, *A*) include the following: (1) the length of gravid adult specimens is usually 25 to 40 mm but may reach 80 mm; (2) the width of the body is generally between 8 and 14 mm; and (3) the scolex or holdfast organ is distinct and much smaller than the body, measuring only 2 to 3 mm.[1]

The scolex of *A. perfoliata* has four ear-shaped lappets measuring 0.5 to 1.0 mm that are situated posterior to the four apical muscular suckers.[4] In contrast, *Anoplocephala magna* is generally larger, measuring up to 80 cm in length and 2.5 cm in width, with a scolex 4 to 6 mm wide (Fig. 63-1, *B*), and *Anoplocephaloides mamillana* is smaller, measuring 6 to 50 mm in length and 4 to 6 mm in width.[3] The scolices of the latter two species do not have lappets as does *A. perfoliata*.

The morphology of proglottids of *A. perfoliata* has been described extensively.[1] Individual proglottids are always much wider than long. Each proglottid is hermaphroditic, containing a single set of both male and female reproductive organs. Each proglottid has a single genital apparatus; the apertures are unilateral and are found in the cranial half of the lateral margin. The gravid uterus is transverse, large, saclike, and lobed.[3] The female reproductive system also consists of a poral ovary, a vagina posterior to the cirrus sac, and a seminal receptacle. Both internal and external seminal vesicles are present as part of the male reproductive system, and the testes are scattered throughout the medulla.[2] Each proglottid also contains a muscular system, a tegument, and an excretory system.

The morphology of mature eggs of *A. perfoliata* is unique (Fig. 63-2). The eggs are 65 to 80 μm in diameter, whereas eggs of *A. magna* measure 50 to 60 μm in diameter and *Anoplocephaloides mamillana* about 51 by 37 μm.[3] *A. perfoliata* eggs are round to D shaped, with an outer vitelline membrane and a thick (8-10 μm), dark, albuminous middle shell. The innermost membrane is flame or pear shaped and consists of a chitinous pyriform apparatus. The length of the pyriform apparatus is approximately equal to the radius of the egg, measuring about 48 μm. This pyriform apparatus in turn contains the hexacanth embryo characteristic of cyclophyllidean cestode eggs.[1,5] The diameter of the embryo measures approximately 16 μm. Eggs seen on fecal flotation often have an amber cast resulting from contact with excreta; however, eggs dissected from gravid proglottids of the adult tapeworm are colorless.[1]

The morphology of anoplocephalid larval development is very similar among many species. In fact, it is difficult to impossible to determine the genus from studying the cysticercoid.[1] The morphology of the larval stages of *Anoplocephala perfoliata* within the intermediate host has been described.[6] However, literature generally presents a detailed ontogenesis of the tapeworm of sheep and goats, *Moniezia expansa* rather than this parasite.[1,7] Briefly, the stages of ontogenesis of *A. perfoliata* begin after the tapeworm egg has been ingested.

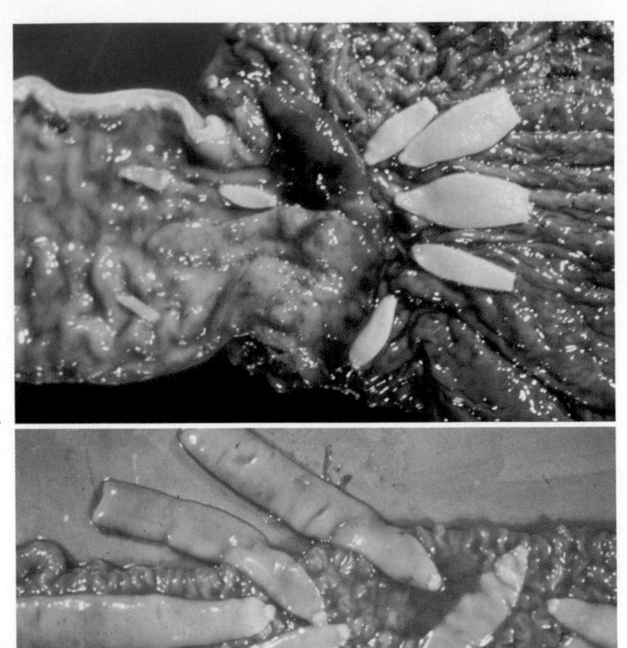

Fig. 63-1 A, Mature *Anoplocephala perfoliata* attached to gastrointestinal mucosa of horse at level of ileocecal valve. B, Mature *Anoplocephala magna.* (Courtesy Dr. William Foreyt.)

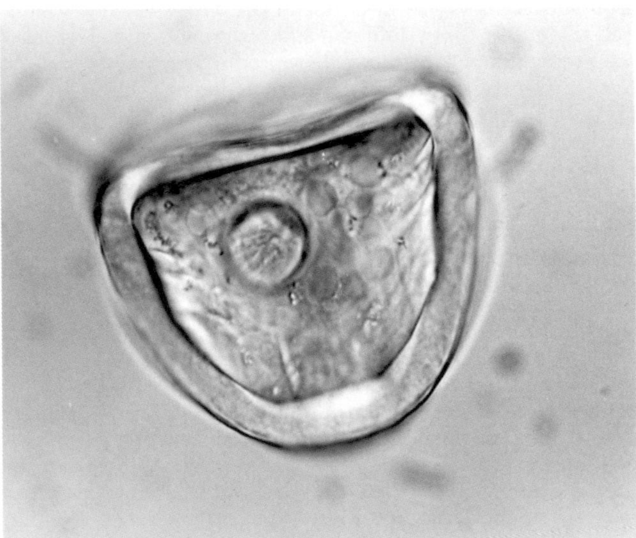

Fig. 63-2 Photomicrograph of ova of *Anoplocephala perfoliata.* (Courtesy Dr. William Foreyt.)

The oncosphere emerges and penetrates the intestinal wall of the oribatid mite. The oncosphere appears in the mite's body cavity within 48 hours and is very motile and active for several days to weeks. The second stage of development is the "large sphere" stage, in which the oncosphere form is lost and the larva becomes immobile. During this period, the oncosphere increases in size and undergoes internal reorganization of the organs. The six hooks lose positioning and move to the tail of the larva while the body of the larva fills with round cells. The third stage of growth within the mite's hemocoele is the "extended larva" stage, in which the body lengthens. The fourth stage is called the "segmented larva" stage. In this phase of development, the body continues to elongate but also divides into two parts that are separated by a constriction. The portion anterior to the constriction has four suckers, which will become the scolex of the tapeworm, and the portion posterior to the constriction is a spherical capsule. Embryonic hooks are positioned caudal to the capsule. During the fifth stage of larval development, the anterior portion of the larva invaginates into the posterior capsule portion. The "cysticercoid stage" is the final stage of larval development. Morphologically, the body is spherical with a dense cuticle. Within the cuticle is the scolex, with four suckers. The wall of the cyst is stratified. At this phase of development, the larva is infective for the final host. In six experimentally infected *Scheloribates* spp. the average size of the *A. perfoliata* cysticercoids was 141 by 119 μm.[8]

Life Cycle

The life cycle of the three tapeworm species that infect the GI tract of horses and donkey are *indirect* because they require an intermediate host as well as a definitive host. Stunkard[9] completed the developmental cycle of Anoplocephaline cestodes in 1937 when he discovered that certain members of one genus of oribatid mites (Acari: Oribatida), *Galumna* spp., could serve as the intermediate hosts of the sheep tapeworm, *Moniezia expansa,* a closely related cyclophyllidean that infects ruminants. A few years later, Bashkirova[6] determined the complete developmental cycle of *Anoplocephala perfoliata.* With an indirect life cycle, the prevalence of cestode infection in the intermediate host is low, whereas it is high in the definitive host.[10] Intermediate host specificity is low in the various anoplocephaline cestode species, and many species of oribatid mites may become infected.[11]

Adult *A. perfoliata* parasites attach near the ileocecal valve of horses, whereas *A. magna* and *Anoplocephaloides mamillana* attach in the small intestines of the horse's digestive tract. Horses with patent infections shed tapeworm eggs in their feces. The proglottids of *A. perfoliata* are broken up by digestion during transit through the large intestines, and thus only eggs are passed in the feces.[12,13] After a gravid proglottid is shed, more than 48 hours may elapse before its ova are passed in the feces.[13]

Survival time of an infective egg on pasture is important because it potentially allows for an improved chance of exposure to the intermediate host. Little is known about the longevity of *A. perfoliata* eggs in the environment. It has been hypothesized that cestode egg survival may be shortened in tropical climates.[14] However, the infectivity of cestode eggs over time in natural conditions has not been determined. Stunkard[15] believed that the redistribution of the anoplocephaline tapeworm eggs by rain into the upper layers of the soil would allow the eggs to remain viable for a longer period and enable the intermediate hosts in the soil to encounter the eggs, pick them up, and feed on them.

The life cycle continues when oribatid mites ingest viable eggs of *A. perfoliata* on the pasture. Oribatid mites are free-living mites found on herbage and in the soil of pastures. Because the cestode eggs are presumably too large to be accidentally eaten, the intermediate host may interpret them as prospective or preferred food.[16] Mackiewicz[10] hypothesized that Anoplocephaline tapeworm eggs may use chemoattraction to increase the likelihood of being eaten by the oribatid mites.

This would especially hold true if the tapeworm eggs were eaten as a food item rather than as a food contaminant. On the other hand, the oribatid intermediate hosts and *A. perfoliata* eggs may be so abundant that chance encounters between the egg and mite may be the sole strategy of transmission.[10,11]

Whatever the transmission strategy, once ingested by the intermediate host, the larva or oncosphere is freed from within the tapeworm eggshell or embryophore, presumably through digestion. Activation factors that stimulate the oncosphere to tear through the intestinal wall using its hooks are unknown.[17] Once in the mite's body cavity, the development time to an infective cysticercoid within the invertebrate intermediate host is variable. Growth of the cysticercoid within the mite's hemocele depends on environmental conditions, especially temperature. The infective cysticercoid stage is formed within 8 to 20 weeks under natural conditions. Once the cysticercoid is fully developed and infective within the oribatid mite, it is ingested by a grazing horse.

The infective cysticercoid has a scolex with four fully developed suckers. It is assumed that the excysted larvae of *A. perfoliata* move along the GI tract with ingesta until reaching the ileocecal valve area, at which point the larvae attach to the GI mucosa. Behind the scolex of the larvae, germinal cells will multiply through proglottid development or asexual reproduction to produce the proglottids of the adult tapeworm.[15,18,19] The caudal end of the larvae contains the excretory pore that becomes the terminal segment of the adult tapeworm.[15] The prepatent period following ingestion of an infected oribatid mite is 6 to 16 weeks.[5,20,21,22]

No actual data are available on the life span of adult *A. perfoliata*, but the life span of an adult cestode may vary from a few months to several years.[18,23] A basic cestode life cycle strategy, based on repeated production of egg-laden proglottids, infers a long adult cyclophyllidean life span that often lasts for years or as long as the definitive host lives.[10,18,24] Furthermore, there is selection for repeated production of proglottids and eggs and high fecundity when the pre-reproductive life span is long.[18] In the case of *A. perfoliata*, this pre-reproductive life span may be 1 to $1^1/_2$ years while the cysticercoid is in the oribatid mite.[25,26]

EPIDEMIOLOGY

The distribution and prevalence of *A. perfoliata* are high enough to cause concern among both horse owners and veterinarians. *A. perfoliata* is found worldwide and is currently accepted as the most common and the most pathogenic of the equine tapeworm species.[3,22,27-31]

The prevalence of *A. perfoliata* in North America has been reported extensively. Many epidemiologic studies report prevalence of infection at necropsy. In 1979, necropsy data collected from eight states, including Kentucky, found that 18% of foals and 26% of adult horses were infected with tapeworms.[32] The most common tapeworm identified was *Anoplocephala magna*. Other studies reported prevalences of *A. perfoliata* in the United States that vary from 13% to 54% and worldwide from 14% to 81.5%* (Box 63-1). Why different regions have such varying prevalence rates for these parasites is not known. The differing rates could be caused by differences in pasture type (thus creating a better or worse environment for the intermediate hosts), pasture stocking rates, climate, or other management or environmental factors. Even with the variation in prevalence, there seems to be a trend toward higher prevalence of infection in countries with temperate climates.[13]

Box • 63-1

Prevalence (%) of* Anoplocephala perfoliata *in United States (US) and Other Countries

North Carolina (US)	13%
Kentucky (US)	52%-54%
Louisiana (US)	47%
New England (US)	53%
Ohio (US)	18%
Canada	14%
New Zealand	81.5%
England	31%-69%
The Netherlands	21%
Sweden	65%

Many parasitologists have speculated about the factors that may have caused an increase in reports of *A. perfoliata* infection. Edwards[44] and Geering and Johnson[45] proposed that extensive use of *ivermectin*, which was new to the market, removed the nematode parasites with greater efficacy than drugs previously available. This selective removal of other intestinal parasites allowed tapeworms to flourish because of lack of competition, thus the increase in prevalence of *A. perfoliata* in recent decades. This hypothesis was refuted by French et al.,[46] who reported that the use of ivermectin for 5 years did not promote increase of *A. perfoliata*. Others propose that antiparasitic drugs, such as pyrantel pamoate and fenbendazole, used before ivermectin was available may have had some cestocidal activity.[39,47,48] Other hypotheses include changes in climactic factors, which may in turn have a positive influence on intermediate host numbers, and changes in stocking rates and other pasture management practices.[45] However, no unequivocal data suggest that a true increase in the prevalence of *A. perfoliata* over time has occurred. Lyons et al.[29] reported that the prevalence of tapeworm remained essentially unchanged in necropsies of Thoroughbred horses conducted from 1951 to 1990.

Equids of all ages can be infected with tapeworms, and unlike cattle and small ruminants, there is no acquired or age resistance.[22,29,31] Living in the lumen of the gut usually does not trigger pronounced immune responses. This allows the same host to be repeatedly infected over the course of its life.[10]

Horses of all ages, and as young as weanlings, can have patent infections with tapeworm species. The prepatent period is between 6 and 16 weeks. Adult horses as old as 40 years reportedly have been infected with *A. perfoliata*.[31] Prevalence is lower in foals less than 1 year (30%-31%) than in animals that are yearlings or older (52%-60%).[31,49] No gender difference in the prevalence of *A. perfoliata* has been reported. In foals, prevalence was similar for colts and fillies, at 33% and 24%, respectively. In adult horses, prevalence between genders also was similar, at 59% to 61% in mares, 43% to 57% in geldings, and 41% to 57% in stallions.[31,49]

PATHOGENESIS

Much has been published regarding the pathology associated with *A. perfoliata* infection. Although the mechanisms are not completely understood, presumably both mechanical

*References 20, 21, 27, 33-40, 42, 43.

damage and parasite antigens play a role in the process.[13] The four unarmed suckers on the scolex of *A. perfoliata* cause pathologic changes at the attachment site. The anatomy of the scolex can be directly related to the features of the lesion when viewed with a scanning electron microscope, in that pegs of mucosa are pulled up into the four suckers.[50] The distance between the tissue pegs corresponds to the distance between the suckers. Long before scanning electron microscopy was available, Skrjabin and Spasskii[1] described ulceration caused by the scolex of *A. perfoliata* embedded in the intestinal wall. These ulcers were inflamed and contaminated with food and intestinal microflora. Perforation, peritonitis, and death resulting from infection with *A. perfoliata* have been reported.[1]

Adult *A. perfoliata* cestodes inhabit the intestinal tract, attaching in clusters primarily at the ileocecal junction, in the cecum near the ileocecal junction, and less often in the terminal ileum and ventral colon[41,50] (see Fig. 63-1, *A*). This clustering of the adult tapeworms can greatly exacerbate the lesions associated with tapeworm attachment. In areas of tapeworm clustering, lesions were found to extend into the submucosa and therefore were more likely to disrupt intestinal blood supply and the nervous regulation.[41] There is no scientific explanation for the clustering of the tapeworms at or near the ileocecal junction, but it may be caused by the production of an aggregation pheromone. There has been documentation and study of an aggregation pheromone, nippolure, secreted by the female of the nematode *Nippostrongylus brasiliensis*.[51,52]

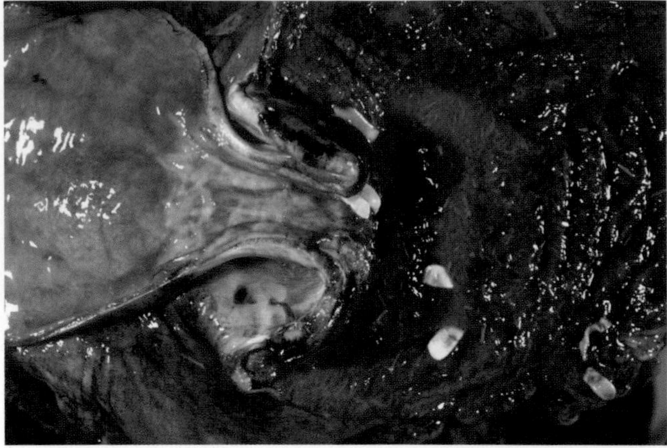

Fig. 63-3 Ileocecal intussusception in horse with adult *A. perfoliata* attached to mucosa at ileocecal junction. (Courtesy Dr. William Foreyt.)

CLINICAL FINDINGS

Clinical signs such as poor body condition,[41] poor growth or chronic ill thrift, recurring diarrhea, progressive weight loss, and anemia have been associated with infections by *A. perfoliata*.[5] These parasites do not appear to cause blood loss that would result in anemia. The anemia could be an anemia of chronic or inflammatory disease.[53]

The literature throughout the 1980s contains many clinical reports of intestinal crises in horses, such as intussusception, cecal perforation, and cecal torsion, that were circumstantially related to concurrent infection by *A. perfoliata*.[44,54,55] Barclay et al.[54] associated intussusception with *A. perfoliata* in five cases admitted to the Illinois Equine Hospital, which accounted for 55% of the intussusceptions seen during a 1-year period at that clinic (Fig. 63-3). The intussusceptions all involved the ileum or the cecum (ileoileal, ileocecal, or cecocecal). The association between *A. perfoliata* and acute GI crisis was described in three reported cases of peritonitis. The peritonitis was attributed to perforation of the cecum, which in all cases was associated with infection by *A. perfoliata*.[55] Horses described in these three cases of peritonitis harbored high numbers of the parasite, up to 300 worms. In contrast, as few as two adult tapeworms were observed during laparotomy or necropsy of horses with intussusception.[54]

Even after an extensive review of the literature, Owen et al.[56] could make no direct conclusions as to the role of tapeworms in association with equine intestinal disease. This interpretation began to change in the early 1990s when Proudman and Edwards[57] demonstrated an association between the presence of equine tapeworms and ileocecal colic. Although the association was not very strong, they found that the risk of ileocecal colic was increased by the presence of tapeworms. More recently, *A. perfoliata* was determined to be a significant risk factor for spasmodic colic and ileal impaction, with the risk of spasmodic colic increasing with the numbers of parasites.[58] Twenty-two percent of the spasmodic colic cases and 81% of ileal impactions were tapeworm associated based on serologic and coprologic diagnoses. Their matched case-control studies suggested a dose-response link between infection intensity (as revealed by ELISA) and risk of clinical disease.[13,58]

It is possible to relate the gross and microscopic pathology caused by *A. perfoliata* to factors predisposing horses to intussusceptions involving the ileocecal area of the GI tract, the most common site of intussusception in horses.[59] Two factors, segmental atony and hyperperistalsis, are thought to be necessary for intussusception to occur.[60] Lesions associated with tapeworm attachment may alter the pattern of intestinal motility and thus may be a potential cause of intussusception.[44] Other tapeworm-associated changes that may predispose to intussusception include local inflammatory changes at the site of parasite attachment and changes in bowel wall diameter at the ileocecal junction.[61]

DIAGNOSIS

Diagnosis of infection by *A. perfoliata* can be made at necropsy. Location and appearance best identify adults of *A. perfoliata* (see Fig. 63-1). The tapeworms are found in clusters at or near the ileocecal junction. Finding eggs on fecal examination (see Fig. 63-2) or using serologic antibody tests can facilitate an antemortem diagnosis of *A. perfoliata infection*. Additionally, an indirect enzyme-linked immunosorbent assay (ELISA) that detects coproantigen is being developed.[62] Once validated, this test may offer early detection of *A. perfoliata* infection, may provide information about the current status of the animal, and may be used to monitor response to therapy.

Coprologic examination for parasite eggs is the most common diagnostic technique to detect any GI parasite. Infection with equine cestodiasis is likely underestimated because veterinary practitioners use a standard flotation solution for microscopic fecal examination.[28] One study proposed that diagnosis has proved difficult because eggs levitate poorly with common fecal flotation solutions.[34] Another study found that 3% of horses were positive for eggs of *A. perfoliata* using flotation with sodium chloride solution (specific gravity of 1.18)[27] and 7% of horses were positive using zinc sulfate solution.[35] At necropsy, 54% of these same horses were infected with *A. perfoliata* adult worms. Another study found that the eggs, when present, appear to float with all the standard flotation solutions.[46] Although saturated sugar solution is the most sensitive of the standard flotation media,[21] this levitation medium is not typically used by veterinary practitioners. Zinc sulfate solution can be prepared more quickly and easily than the saturated sugar solution.

Most flotation techniques are inconsistent primarily because of sporadic shedding of egg-laden proglottids.[28] When proglottids are shed, the structure (and eggs) may disintegrate before the feces pass from the horse's GI tract.[22,41] An alternative hypothesis is that tapeworm eggs are retained in the small, easily overlooked proglottids, making few eggs available in the feces for diagnosis.[5,63] Treating suspect animals with ivermectin is reported to increase the visualization of *A. perfoliata* eggs.[46]

Alternatives to simple flotation for fecal diagnosis of equine tapeworms are double-centrifugation techniques that use sedimentation followed by flotation. Although more time-consuming, these techniques improve diagnostic accuracy. Beroza et al.[28] found that the use of double centrifugation first in water and then in sucrose solution improved the recovery of known numbers of formalin-fixed equine tapeworm eggs by 10 times over a technique using only gravitational flotation in sucrose solution. Centrifugal techniques improve accuracy, but as with other fecal diagnostic techniques, they often lack sensitivity because of the sporadic-shedding egg that is an inherent feature of equine tapeworms. Regardless of the fecal diagnostic method used, no correlation has been recognized between numbers of adult tapeworms and egg detection using these techniques.[43,64,65]

Serologic testing that measures serum antibodies specific for antigens of *A. perfoliata* have been developed. The first group to develop an ELISA used a scolex antigen of *A. perfoliata*.[66] This test did not show cross-reactivity to concurrent nematode infection. However, the specificity of the test is low.

Proudman and Trees[67] developed and validated an ELISA using excretory and secretory antigens of *A. perfoliata*. The diagnostic sensitivity of this test was 68% (n = 38). The specificity was 95% (n = 20) when helminth-naive horses were used, but fell to 71% with horses that were *A. perfoliata* negative at necropsy. These horses may have had prior exposure to the parasite, and thus residual circulating antibodies were present. Antibody concentrations correlate with tapeworm infection intensity.[13] This immunodiagnostic test may improve the ability to diagnose and treat horses that have high numbers of *A. perfoliata*, allow monitoring of herd levels of infection, and may be used as a tool for epidemiologic studies.[13,66]

PATHOLOGIC FINDINGS

Lesions caused by *A. perfoliata* account in part for the parasite's association with colic. Mild prolapse of the terminal ileum into the lumen of the ileocecal junction was observed in 5 of 50 horses examined at necropsy that had adult tapeworms attached to the mucosal surface of this area.[50] Extensive mucosal ulcerations near the ileocecal valve were found at necropsy in 63.1% of horses in a highly endemic area.[20]

Damage to the intestinal lining varies with the intensity of *A. perfoliata* infection.[30,41,50] The primary feature of the gross pathologic lesions found at the site of tapeworm attachment, either at the ileocecal junction or on the cecal wall, is *mucosal ulceration*.[50] The depth and severity of the ulceration increase as the numbers of tapeworms attached to the surrounding area increase. Pearson et al.[30] associated numbers of tapeworms with severity of damage. Superficial congestion with slightly raised focal ulceration is seen in horses infected with up to 20 tapeworms, whereas the mucosa is raised, thickened, and ulcerated, with nodular swellings at the area of worm attachment, in horses infected with more than 100 tapeworms. Other significant gross pathologic changes associated with attachment of *A. perfoliata* include a yellow diphtheritic membrane and gross edema of the mucosa.[20,41,50] A verrucose granulomatous lesion projecting from the mucosa of the ileocecal junction was described in 2 of 20 horses examined by Pearson et al.[30] and in 7.8% of the 65 horses examined by Bain and Kelly.[20]

Histopathologic sections from the areas of tapeworm attachment reveal ulcerations of various depths from the superficial mucosa to the muscularis mucosa and submucosa.[30] In severe cases the mucosal damage may be so extensive that the glandular anatomy is distorted by fibrosis and infiltration of eosinophils into the lamina propria.[50] Inflammatory cells, eosinophils, and lymphocytes infiltrate the areas of damage, and in one case a submucosal abscess was reported.[30] Verrucose granulomatous lesions are composed of granulation tissue, primarily lymphocytes, and associated fibrinoid necrosis, primarily neutrophils.[20]

THERAPY

In the United States, paste dewormers containing *ivermectin* or *moxidectin* in combination with *praziquantel* are marketed for treatment of the equine tapeworm, *A. perfoliata*. In these products the cestocidal activity of praziquantel is combined with a broad-spectrum anthelmintic (e.g., ivermectin or moxidectin) effective against nematodes and *Gasterophilus* larvae. A high degree of efficacy was demonstrated for these products when administered at the label dose of ivermectin (0.2 mg/kg) and praziquantel (1.0 mg/kg) orally.[68] Cestode egg counts were reduced by 98%, and more than 96% of the horses positive for cestode eggs before treatment were negative on posttreatment fecal tests.

Historically, there is disagreement regarding cestocidal activity of *pyrantel pamoate*. Early studies indicate partial efficacy against cestodes, but a more recent study only demonstrated dislodgement of gravid segments, with retention of the scolex. At the double dose of 13.2 mg/kg, greater than 96% efficacy was achieved. A recent study examining a paste dewormer at the 13.2-mg/kg dose in five different U.S. locations demonstrated significant reductions in fecal egg counts 7 to 16 days after pyrantel pamoate treatment.[69] This study demonstrated greater than 95% efficacy overall.

PREVENTION

Good management will help prevent and control tapeworm infection by reducing both the numbers of eggs passed into the environment in equine feces and the exposure of horses to cysticercoid-containing mites. Reasonable stocking rates should be maintained on pastures. Overcrowding of pastures with infected animals in the cool, dry season, when oribatid mites may have peak populations, would likely produce heavy parasite burdens in the definitive host.[14] Rotation of pastures also has been recommended as a means of prevention. Although this could reduce egg numbers on the pasture, given the longevity of the adult mites on pastures (1-1$^1/_2$ years), transmission probably would not cease unless the horses were kept off of the pasture for at least that time.[25,26]

One of the most important control methods is to isolate new animals on arrival at the farm. Because fecal testing may produce false-negative results, all new horses should be treated with an appropriate cestocidal drug before entering the grazing area.[68] If this recommendation is not followed, the potential for initiating the life cycle in a previously uninfested pasture is great. Resident horses should be routinely tested and dewormed as well.[20] Plowing and reseeding pastures have been suggested to reduce the number of oribatid mites.[5,20]

In reality, control of *A. perfoliata* infection by reduction of mite numbers is impractical for most horse owners because of the ubiquitous nature of these mites; thus the only viable alternative is prophylactic cestocidal treatment. Many parasites of livestock can be controlled by a limited number of strategically timed treatments,[71,72] but at present, not enough is known about the transmission of tapeworms to allow complete recommendations. If there were a seasonal fluctuation in mite numbers on pastures, strategically timed treatment of horses to reduce shedding of tapeworm eggs in feces just before the seasonal increase in mite populations would be advantageous.[14]

REFERENCES

See the CD-ROM for a list of references linked to the abstract in PubMed.

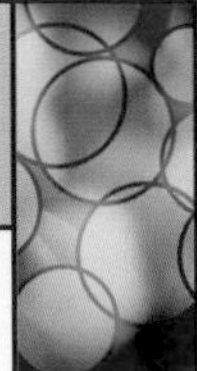

CHAPTER • 64

Ectoparasites of Horses

Joy L. Barbet

Equidae around the world are afflicted by ectoparasites. In addition to annoyance from these parasites, some are capable of transmitting infectious agents and inducing hypersensitivity reactions, toxic reactions, and even death, if exposure is overwhelming. Some of these ectoparasites are ubiquitous and found in most locations where horses and other livestock live; some are reportable in certain countries; and some are highly contagious, spreading easily from animal to animal. Increasing international movement of horses as well as other livestock makes it important for the veterinarian to be able to anticipate, recognize, and treat ectoparasitic conditions early, preventing spread of equine and livestock diseases.

This chapter discusses the major crawling and flying ectoparasites that afflict horses and the pertinent etiologic, epidemiologic, pathogenic, clinical, treatment, and control factors for the particular arthropod.

TICKS

Etiology

Horses are susceptible to tick infestations by many species of ticks that feed on wild or domestic ungulates in different regions. Soft ticks (Argasidae) and hard ticks (Ixodidae) may be involved. *Ixodes* spp., *Dermacentor* spp., *Boophilus* spp., *Amblyomma* spp., and *Otobius megnini* (spinose ear tick) are most often involved. Exotic ticks, such as *Anocentor nitens* (tropical horse tick), if found on horses in the United States, are reportable.

Epidemiology

Life cycles among tick species may require one, two, or three hosts and a few weeks to 2 years to complete, depending on environmental conditions. Details of life cycles and hosts can be found elsewhere.[1] With multihost ticks, the larvae and nymphs usually require small vertebrate hosts, while the adults feed on larger animals. Tick infestations occur in spring or summer months (the exception being the winter tick, *Dermacentor albipictus*) or nonseasonally in the tropics. In warm climates, if rainy and dry seasons are distinct, ticks will be more active during the rainy season. Most ticks live in forests, grasslands, and scrub, infesting passing animals. Some live in the burrows or nesting areas of the host, enabling them to reach the host easily whenever conditions are favorable.

Pathogenesis

Clinical manifestations of tick infestation result from tick feeding. Local reactions result in papules, nodules, wheals, and sometimes pustules around the feeding site. Highly pruritic reactions with papular to urticarial lesions have been attributed to hypersensitivity to *Boophilus* spp. Other species of ticks, including *Otobius megnini* nymphs, *Anocentor nitens* (an important vector of equine babesiosis), and *Amblyomma maculatum*, feed in the ear canals of horses. The resulting irritation results in head shaking, ear rubbing, head tilt, or a lop-eared appearance and creates conditions conducive to the development of secondary bacterial otitis externa.

Infectious agents are readily transmitted by ticks for several reasons: (1) ticks feed multiple times throughout their life cycle; (2) many infectious agents are transmitted during tick maturation to the next stage in the life cycle; (3) ticks take relatively large blood meals, which are concentrated by secreting the host's own fluids back into the host directly or as coxal secretions; and (4) immunosuppressive substances are present in the tick saliva that reduce host defenses, allowing the microbe to become established.[1] Heavy tick infestations can result in poor nutritional and immunologic condition and even anemia from blood loss. Tick paralysis results from salivary proteins found in females of some tick species, which secrete the neurotoxic proteins during feeding. Just one tick may cause partial paralysis, but a more severe or extensive paralysis may result from larger numbers of ticks feeding. Foals and ponies are more likely to be affected.[1,2]

Clinical Findings

Clinical syndromes resulting from tick infestation include (1) mild to severe papulonodular dermatitis, with or without pruritus; (2) otitis externa; (3) systemic infection with tick-borne agents such as *Babesia caballi* or *B. equi* (Chapter 59), *Anaplasma phagocytophilum* (previously *E. equi*, Chapter 42), *Borrelia burgdorferi* (Chapter 35), *Francisella tularensis*, and *Theileria annulata;* (4) anemia and poor condition; and (5) flaccid, ascending motor paralysis, particularly in foals or ponies.[1,3,4]

Diagnosis

Finding ticks on the horse is diagnostic. Identification of ticks is useful in determining which control measures will be most effective. Keys to aid identification can be found in parasitology texts and elsewhere.[5,6,7] When exotic ticks are suspected or tick management problems arise, consultation with governmental authorities or a parasitologist for proper identification is strongly recommended.

Pathologic Findings

Histopathologic findings for tick-induced papules and nodules range from eosinophilic and neutrophilic perivascular dermatitis with dermal edema to intraepidermal vesiculopustular dermatitis. Chronic, nodular lesions often contain large numbers of lymphohistiocytic cells forming lymphoid nodule or follicles.[8,9]

Therapy and Prevention

Control measures for tick infestations depend on the species involved. Topical or systemic acaricidal treatments are normally combined with management changes such as clearing brush, keeping pastures mowed, and avoiding tick habitat during the season of greatest tick activity. With multihost ticks, control of other tick hosts in the environment (rodents, mice, deer) may prove helpful when possible. Acaricides normally used include synthetic pyrethroids, organophosphates, and avermectins. Chlorinated hydrocarbons and formamidines (amitraz) are contraindicated because of environmental danger and toxicity to horses, respectively. Products are usually applied as sprays or dips, or administered systemically. Resistance to acaricides varies regionally.

Public Health Considerations

Infestation of horses with ticks should alert their human owners that they too are at risk of tick exposure and thus potential exposure to tick-borne diseases. Humans in contact with tick-infested animals should inspect themselves for similar infestation and remove ticks as soon as possible before engorgement occurs. The longer a tick remains attached, the greater the likelihood for transmission of infectious agents to the host.

MITES

Sarcoptic Mange

Etiology

Sarcoptic mange, caused by the mite *Sarcoptes scabei* var. *equi*, is very uncommon in horses in Western Europe, North America, and Australia. It is a reportable disease in some countries, and regulatory authorities should be contacted for advice when it is strongly suspected.

Epidemiology

Sarcoptes scabei var. *equi* is a host-specific mite that completes its lifecycle on members of the family Equidae, but it may survive long enough on humans and other species to induce an allergic dermatitis. The female mite lays eggs in epidermal burrows in the skin. They hatch and pass through larval and nymphal stages, reaching maturity in 2 to 3 weeks. Transmission is by direct contact between animals but may also occur by fomites (e.g., riders' clothing, stable blankets, harness). Mites can live off the host for only a few days, dying of desiccation, but survival could be prolonged in conditions of warmth, darkness, and humidity.

Pathogenesis and Clinical Findings

Irritant and hypersensitivity reactions to the burrowing mites and their excrement are thought to be the cause of the intense pruritus associated with sarcoptic mange. Clinical lesions consist of crusted papules, scaling, and alopecia beginning on the head, ears, and neck and progressing caudally to involve the rest of the body. Over time, excoriations, lichenification, and secondary infections result. Untreated, sarcoptic mange can lead to serious generalized debility, weight loss, and even death.

Diagnosis

Infestation is suspected in animals with a typical history and clinical signs. Diagnosis may be confirmed by microscopic examination of scale and debris obtained by deep and superficial scrapings of multiple affected areas. However, as in other species, negative scrapings do not completely rule out sarcoptic mange, and response to therapy is often used for diagnosis in highly suspicious cases.

Therapy

All infested animals and those suspected of infestation must be isolated; their blankets, harness, grooming equipment, and stables should be treated or disinfected. Handlers must change clothing and wash thoroughly before tending unaffected animals. Affected animals and in-contact animals may be treated topically using organophosphate, synthetic pyrethroid preparations, or 2% lime sulfur applied as a dip, spray, or wash at 7- to 10-day intervals for three or more treatments. These preparations may also be used when necessary for treatment of infested buildings, vehicles, and equipment after thorough cleaning. In chronic cases or when lichenification is excessive, it may be necessary to treat over a longer period. Although not licensed for this condition in horses, ivermectin, given orally at 200 μg/kg body weight every 2 weeks for three treatments, is effective in the treatment of sarcoptic mange in other species. Its use, however, does not eliminate the need for strict isolation of animals and environmental cleaning and treatment.

Public Health Considerations

As with all sarcoptic mange mites, transient infestation of humans may occur. The mites do not reproduce on humans, but reinfestation may continue as long as contact with infested animals continues.

Psoroptic Mange

Etiology

Psoroptic mange in horses has been attributed to several species of psoroptic mites that may or may not be truly distinct species. *Psoroptes equi*, *P. ovis*, *P. natalensis*, and *P. cuniculi* have been implicated in equine infestations. Because *P. ovis* is reportable in cattle and sheep and because these mites are very similar to one another (possibly one species), appropriate authorities should be contacted for advice, especially if infested horses have had exposure to sheep or cattle or have been acquired recently.

Epidemiology

Mites are readily transmitted by direct contact or contact with fomites. Psoroptic mange mites live on the skin surface and feed by puncturing the epidermis, causing serous exudation, erythema, crusting, and pruritus. The female mite lays eggs in the surface debris. Eggs hatch within 2 to 3 days and develop to maturity within 11 to 14 days. Off-host survival of adult mites is shortest during periods of high temperature and low humidity. On average, survival on premises is 2 to 3 weeks but may be longer depending on conditions.[10]

Pathogenesis and Clinical Findings

As with sarcoptic mange, pruritus from psoroptic mange is thought to be caused by irritant and hypersensitivity reactions to the presence and secretions of the mites. Papules, crusts, scaling, alopecia, and lichenification are the initial lesions. Lesions tend to be distributed around the outer ear, forelock, mane, tail, ear canal, and inguinal and axillary areas, with less involvement of the trunk and legs. Secondary bacterial infections may result.

Diagnosis

Diagnosis requires microscopic identification of *Psoroptes* spp. mites from multiple superficial scrapings and crusts obtained from lesions. Unlike sarcoptic mange, mites are found more readily with psoroptic mange.

Therapy

Treatment is similar to that for sarcoptic mange. The long potential environmental survival time for psoroptic mites makes vacating premises for a minimum of 3 to 4 weeks advisable. Thorough cleaning of the premises should be carried out with complete removal of bedding and debris. Insecticidal premise treatment is recommended.

Prevention

Thorough physical examination and isolation of newly introduced horses should prevent introduction of *Psoroptes* mites into the herd. Fomites that could potentially transmit the infestation indirectly (e.g., buckets, tack, blankets, grooming equipment) should not be shared between new horses and other horses on the farm.

Chorioptic Mange

Etiology

The most frequently diagnosed mange in horses, chorioptic mange is caused by the surface-living mange mite *Chorioptes bovis* (Fig. 64-1). As with the previously discussed mange mites, there is likely only one species of *Chorioptes* mites that infests several hosts.

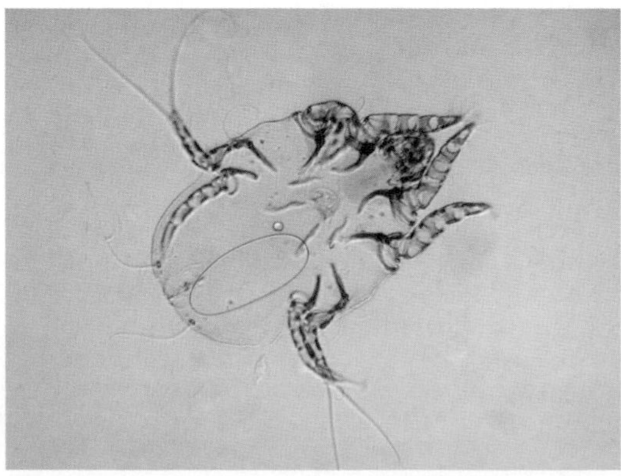

Fig. 64-1 Female *Chorioptes bovis* mite. (Courtesy Ellis Greiner.)

Epidemiology

Transmission occurs by direct and indirect contact. The mite feeds on cutaneous scale and debris without burrowing or puncturing the epidermis. Mite eggs are laid and subsequently develop in skin debris, completing the life cycle in 2 to 3 weeks. Mites and mite eggs can survive on debris within buildings, bedding, and on grooming equipment for extended periods, depending on temperature, humidity, and conditions of hygiene. Asymptomatic carriage of mites is common in sheep and cattle and may occur in horses. Mite populations and subsequently clinical signs appear to increase in the winter and decrease in the drier summer months.

Pathogenesis and Clinical Findings

Because pruritus can range from severe to nonexistent in chorioptic mange, it is presumed that, as with other mite infestations, hypersensitivity plays a role in the pathogenesis of lesions. Chorioptic mites have a predilection to infest the skin of the legs from below the carpus and the hock. Chronic lesions may spread to the ventral thorax and abdomen and occasionally extend up to the tail base. Initial lesions include erythema, papules, and crusts arising on the lower limbs. With time these may progress to more extensive crusting, ulceration, lichenification, and secondary infection. A difficult-to-treat, chronic, pastern dermatitis may result. Draft breeds with feathered (long-haired) fetlocks seem especially suited to maintaining infestations. Foot stamping, biting at the lower limbs, and rubbing of the lower limbs are symptoms usually noted by the owner.

Diagnosis

Diagnosis, by demonstrating the mite in superficial skin scrapings taken from multiple sites, can be difficult. Recommended techniques for catching these fast-moving mites include (1) using clear cellophane tape to pick up mites and crusts from the skin surface (although mites can be difficult to remove or position for identification, and parasitologists find such preparations frustrating); (2) adding insecticide to the oil used for the scrapings; and (3) vigorous brushing into a pan of soapy water. With the third technique, allow the mixture to settle out in a deep, narrow container. Decant and then centrifuge the settled material for microscopic examination of the pellet, or process the settled material as for fecal flotation.[9,11] Field collections of crusts and debris can be placed in a blood sample tube for transportation to the laboratory for examination. In warmer weather the mites may only be obtained from scrapings of the coronary band.[9]

Therapy

Chorioptic mange can be difficult to treat because of its superficial location on the skin and mites' ability to survive in the environment. Oral ivermectin is effective at reducing mite populations but cannot eliminate them.[12] Effective topical treatments include a series of three whole-body baths, 5 days apart, using 1% selenium sulfide shampoo, and two treatments, 2 to 3 weeks apart, with 0.25% fipronil spray.[13,14] Fipronil spray should be applied to all affected areas, including both the forelimbs and the hindlimbs from above the carpus and stifles, respectively, distally to the hoof and in sufficient quantity to dampen the hair and wet the skin. Other topical products that should be effective include 2% lime sulfur, organophosphate products, and synthetic pyrethroids. Ideally, the legs of heavily feathered animals should be clipped (owners often resist this for cosmetic reasons) and the legs thoroughly washed and skin debris removed before each parasiticidal application. Dips or washes may need to be repeated at 5- to 7-day intervals for 3 to 4 weeks. Care should be taken to apply these products to all areas vulnerable to infestation, including rear quarters, tail base, ventral abdomen and thorax, and even the head, if the horse is biting at or rubbing infected forelimbs with its head. One author suggests a combined approach using ivermectin systemically in combination with topical treatment.[15] A key component to treatment is isolation of infested horses and treatment of the environment and fomites. All bedding should be removed from the stables, followed by thorough cleaning and treatment of premises with insecticide. If stalls or paddocks can be vacated for 3 or more weeks, there is less likelihood mites will survive in the environment. All bedding for infested horses should be replaced with fresh product daily, if possible, or on treatment days, at a minimum. Grooming and feeding equipment should be segregated, cleaned, and treated.

Prevention

Prevention of chorioptic mite infestation includes examination of newly introduced horses for clinical lesions, followed by scrapings and cytologic preparations of any suspect lesions, such as crusted papules or scaling of coronary bands. Isolation from other horses for 2 to 3 weeks to observe for suggestive clinical signs is also helpful. Good stabling hygiene with frequent bedding changes and keeping horses in their own stalls help reduce spread. These procedures are most important in the management of breeds with heavy feathering of the lower limbs because these horses are most frequently infested.

Demodectic Mange

Etiology

Clinical demodectic mange in the horse is extremely rare. Two species, *Demodex caballi* (eyelids and muzzle) and *Demodex equi* (body), have been described in the horse. Disease caused by *D. caballi* has not been reported.

Epidemiology

Demodex mites are host specific and considered as normal fauna. They complete their life cycle within the pilosebaceous apparatus of the skin. Most animals harbor a few mites without evidence of skin disease. It is thought that mites are transmitted shortly after birth by contact between the dam and foal.

Pathogenesis and Clinical Findings

Poor immune status, local changes in skin chemistry, and other unknown factors may allow mite proliferation and the development of clinical lesions. Lesions may take two forms: (1) patchy, nonpruritic alopecia and scaling of the head, neck, shoulders, and forelimbs, which may resolve spontaneously, or (2) a papulonodular form with many mites found within follicular cysts.

Diagnosis

Microscopic examination of multiple deep skin scrapings or nodular contents should be sufficient to confirm diagnosis. Efforts should be made to detect underlying conditions making the animal susceptible to demodectic mange. Systemic glucocorticoid treatment is the most frequently implicated cause.[9] However, endocrine diseases, other systemic diseases, nutritional factors, and immunosuppressed states should be considered.

Therapy

Some cases of demodectic mange in horses resolve spontaneously. Any underlying conditions that may weaken immune status or alter skin chemistry should be corrected when possible. Resolution of lesions may follow. Topical therapy to aid self-clearing includes benzoyl peroxide shampoos followed by application of 2% lime sulfur dip every 5 to 7 days and/or daily application of antibacterial ointment such as mupiricin or fusidic acid. If significant secondary bacterial dermatitis is present, a 3-week course of trimethoprim-sulfonamide or fluoroquinolone antibiotics is indicated. Most authors do not advocate attempts to treat equine demodicosis systemically. Amitraz is contraindicated in horses. Nodular lesions are refractory to treatments and may persist for years.

Trombiculid and Other Mite Infestations

Etiology

Mites inhabiting vegetation, vegetable matter, hay, straw, cereals and other stored foods, and bedding may cause dermatitis in animals contacting the infested environment or feed. These mites belong to the suborders Sarcoptiformes (Astigmata), Trombidiformes (Prostigmata), and Parasitiformes (Mesostigmata). Forage mites include mites in the genera *Acarus, Tyrophagus, Tyrolichus, Glycyphagus, Pyemotes, Neoschoengastia, Euschoengastia, Caloglyphus, Lepidoglyphus, Cheyletus,* and *Suidasia*. Many species of larval *Trombiculidae* (harvest mites, red bugs, or chiggers) are capable of producing skin lesions and irritation in the horse. Genera represented include *Eutrombicula, Neotrombicula,* and *Leptotrombium*.

Epidemiology

Forage mites can induce dermatitis in either stabled animals or those on pasture at any time of the year, depending on their source. The source may be pasture, hay, bedding, or grain products. Trombiculid mites cause seasonal dermatitis in horses on pasture or those being housed or ridden in natural areas. The larvae range from red to orange or yellow in color and are active in late summer and early autumn. In tropical areas, they may be present almost year-round. After feeding on lymph and disintegrated skin cells, they drop off the host and progress to free-living nymph and adult stages.

Pathogenesis and Clinical Findings

Lesions associated with these mite infestations may result from irritant, pharmacologic, or hypersensitivity reactions to the salivary secretions of the mite. Lesions caused by forage mite infestation arise in areas of primary contact: face and head for feeds and lower limbs or entire body for bedding products. Forage mite and trombiculid mite infestations contracted by horses at pasture most frequently involve the lower limbs, ventral and lateral trunk, face, and lips. Depending on the host response, a range of lesions may be observed, including a fine papulocrustous dermatitis; patches of erythema, exudation, and scaling; papular urticaria; or urticarial plaques. Pruritus may vary from absent to severe.

Diagnosis

In forage mite infestations, demonstration of the mite in the feed, in the environment, or from the lesions is diagnostic. One author suggests that using a flea comb is more successful than skin scrapings for finding forage mites on the skin.[9] More frequently, the mites will be found in the feed or bedding rather than on the animal. The collected material can be placed into Berlese funnels and left overnight to facilitate collection of insects and arthropods. This method was effective for retrieving *Pyomotes tritici* from hay samples in one outbreak of forage mite–induced dermatitis in horses.[16] In early cases of trombiculid infestations, it may be relatively easy to find the distinctly colored larvae attached in the center of a typical papule. Skin scrapings of lesions may dislodge enough mites for diagnosis. Later, the mites may have already detached, and the diagnosis must be based on seasonality, contact with an infested environment, and response to treatment.

Therapy

Animals infested with forage or trombiculid mites at pasture should be removed immediately from the infested environment. Although forage mites may have dropped off already, topical insecticides should be applied to kill remaining mites. Relief from pruritus may be required, using topical steroids or a brief course of short-acting systemic corticosteroids. It may require up to 8 weeks before the trombiculid mite season is finished. During this time, further contact with the infested environment should be avoided. Because infestation is likely to recur from year to year, infested pastures should be vacated at the same time in following years. Forage mite populations in the environment fluctuate significantly year to year and cannot be reliably predicted; however, it is usually safe to return animals to the same fields after 8 weeks. Forage mites are capable of massive proliferation in stored feeds and bedding when humidity and temperature are favorable. These increases in number often may be confined to one small portion of the stored product. Infested materials must be completely removed and replaced by product from a different source.

Public Health Considerations

People are also susceptible to forage and trombiculid mite infestations and may have lesions in areas of contact with infested vegetation or feed products at the same time animals are affected.

PEDICULOSIS

Etiology

Horses and other *Equidae* are hosts for two species of lice: the sucking louse, *Haematopinus asini*, and the biting louse, *Bovicola (Damalinia) equi* (Fig. 64-2), which is more common.

Epidemiology

Lice are host specific and survive for just a few days off the host, even under optimal conditions of high humidity and cool temperatures. The life cycle is completed on the host. Female lice produce eggs that are cemented firmly onto hair shafts. After hatching, nymphs undergo three molts, reaching maturity in 3 weeks. In temperate climates, louse activity is greatest during the autumn, winter, and early spring, coinciding with increased crowding of animals (facilitating transmission), reduced use of topical insecticides, and ideal living conditions in the host's dense winter coat. Transmission is by direct contact with the infested animals or fomites, such as brushes that contain nymphs, adults, or hair with viable louse eggs attached. Crowded, unsanitary conditions promote transmission. The sucking louse, *Haematopinus asini*, literally sucks blood from superficial vessels through a hollow tube, or stylet. Preferred feeding areas are the mane, tail, and fetlocks. Survival time off-host is shorter than that for biting lice. The biting louse, *Bovicola equi*, feeds on superficial skin debris, hair, and secretions, using the mandibles to bite and scrape. Although preferring areas on the trunk, especially the neck, flanks, and tail base, biting lice may be found in the mane and tail as well. No known equine pathogens are transmitted by lice.

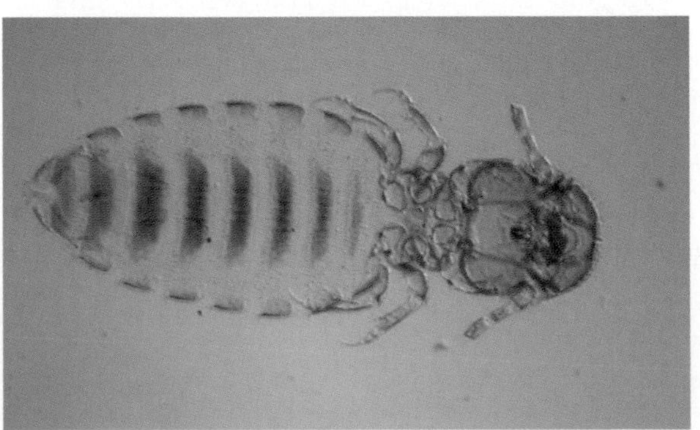

Fig. 64-2 *Bovicola equi*. (Courtesy Ellis C. Greiner.)

Clinical Findings

The main clinical sign of louse infestation is pruritus, manifested by biting at the flanks, kicking and stamping, restlessness and irritability, and rubbing against objects. This results in an unkempt appearance, alopecia, scaling, abrasion, and even secondary infection, if pruritus is severe. Rarely, louse infestation may be severe enough to result in poor condition or debility.

Diagnosis

Louse infestation is common in the horse and should always be a differential diagnosis for pruritus. Demonstration of fast-moving, biting lice can be difficult when numbers are low. Nits, cemented to the hair shafts, are more easily found. Under good lighting, a careful search, parting the hair coat in many places, is necessary to find adults and identify hairs bearing nits. In addition, a stiff brush may be used to collect lice by brushing hair downward, collecting hair and debris into a pan held close beneath. Lice may be observed moving among the collected debris.[11]

Therapy

Louse infestation is usually treated with applications of insecticidal shampoos, sprays, or dips applied at 10- to 14-day intervals for at least 3 to 4 weeks to eliminate newly hatching nits. Pyrethrins or synthetic pyrethroids are most often used, but organophosphate compounds and 1% selenium sulfide shampoo (left on 5-10 minutes, once lathered) are also effective.[17] Label directions for insecticides should be followed carefully. Although not always completely effective for treating biting lice infestations, sucking lice are susceptible to oral ivermectin, 200 μg/kg, two doses administered 2 weeks apart. Tack, blankets, and grooming equipment and even the environment may harbor infective hairs. Such items should be cleaned and treated with insecticides. Particularly valuable items that may not withstand harsh treatments might be salvaged by thorough cleaning followed by placement in a sealed garbage bag and storage in a warm, preferably sunny, place for 3 to 4 weeks, allowing time for any nits present to hatch and die before the equipment is used again. All infested and in-contact horses should be treated.

Prevention

Newly acquired animals should be inspected carefully for louse infestation, treated with appropriate insecticidal products, and held in quarantine until they are ascertained to be disease free before commingling with other horses.

BITING FLIES

One of the most common pests of horses and other animals, biting flies are numerous in species and found throughout the world. Lesions resulting from the bites of tabanids (*Tabanus, Haematopota*, and *Chrysops* spp.), stable flies *(Stomoxys calcitrans)*, and black flies (*Simulium* spp.) are crusted papules that fade within a few days. Mosquito bites result in papules without crusts and also fade in a few hours to days. Hypersensitivity reactions ranging from urticaria to eosinophilic (collagenolytic) granulomas or pruritic dermatoses have been associated with the bites of these insects.[18] "Fly worry," characterized by incessant hoof stamping, tail switching, bunching, and running, can result from large numbers of biting insects. This section discusses the major types of dipterans that harass horses, with reference to epidemiology, specific clinical syndromes, and control measures.

Tabanids

Epidemiology

Tabanid flies (*Tabanus, Chrysops,* and *Hybomitra* spp.), commonly known as horseflies and deerflies, serve as mechanical vectors of several livestock diseases, including *Microsporum gypseum* (Chapter 54), equine infectious anemia (Chapter 23), and *Trypanosoma evansi* (Chapter 61; the causative agent of surra). Mostly daytime feeders, their bites are painful, and thus these flies cause considerable annoyance to many species of large animals. They are not host specific, feeding on other animals and humans. The breeding grounds for these pests are aquatic and semiaquatic habitats, including mud and wet vegetation near bodies of water. Terrestrial species lay eggs on vegetation or in forest litter.

Therapy and Prevention

Control of tabanid flies is difficult. Frequent applications of insecticides and repellents provide only short-term protection. Vegetation barriers more than 2 meters ($6^1/_2$ feet) in height may deter flies from entering pastures.[19] Avoiding forested pastures and daytime stabling can help reduce tabanid access to animals. Anecdotally, horse farms in Florida have relocated because of intractable tabanid activity.[11] Excessive nighttime lighting may extend tabanid feeding into the nighttime hours as well.

Stable Flies

Epidemiology

Another daytime feeder, the stable fly *(Stomoxys calcitrans)*, feeds mostly on the lower limbs, ventrum, chest, and back. A pattern of three or four bites grouped or in a chain suggests stable flies.[20] The bite is painful, and feeding is not host specific. They can cause considerable annoyance to humans. Stable flies have been implicated in the transmission of dermatophilosis (Chapter 31) and dermatophytosis (Chapter 54).[19] Additionally, they are a primary transmitter of the stomach worm *(Habronema microstoma)*. Stable flies breed in decaying vegetable matter, bedding, and feces, where the stomach worm larvae is ingested by the larval fly. Stomach worm larvae are deposited on the skin when the adult stable fly bites the horse. To continue the life cycle, the *Habronema* larvae must be ingested as the horse bites at the flies or at the itchy papules that result from the fly bite. These larvae also may be deposited at mucocutaneous junctions or in superficial wounds, where they migrate into the tissues and, in sensitized horses, incite the hypersensitivity reaction, resulting in proliferative lesions of cutaneous habronemiasis. Only 12 days, but usually 15 to 30 days, are required to complete maturation from egg to adult stable fly.[21] Breeding season is year-round in the tropics and the subtropics, whereas immature forms are suspected to overwinter in northern climates.

Therapy and Prevention

Control of stable flies is best accomplished by eliminating breeding grounds. Strict attention to proper removal and disposal of manure and decaying vegetation is essential. Composted manure needs to be kept hot for effective killing of eggs and larvae. Manure piles that are too large to turn regularly may be covered with weighted, black, plastic sheets to keep them hot. To prevent breeding in manure in pastures and paddocks, breaking up and scattering of the piles should be done every 1 to 2 weeks. Topical insecticides applied to the animal are not highly effective because the stable fly spends very little time on the host, and efficacy of repellents is short lived.[21] Insecticides applied to favorite resting places of the flies (sunny walls, tree foliage), insecticide misters, and fly traps may help. Screening to exclude flies can be effective, and daytime stabling may be useful.

Horn Flies

Epidemiology

Horn flies *(Haematobia irritans)* are primary pests of cattle, bison, and water buffalo but will feed on other large animals housed in proximity to these species. Infection with *Corynebacterium pseudotuberculosis*, the cause of ulcerative lymphangitis, subcutaneous abscesses, and folliculitis, is thought to be spread by biting flies, especially horn flies[21] (Chapter 30). The eggs develop in the fresh feces of the bovine species and not in feces of other large mammals. Maturation from egg to adult may take only 9 days.[21] Adults feed on the dorsal back withers, shoulders, flank, and neck, often facing downward, or on the ventral midline of horses.

Clinical Findings

Horn flies are a common cause of ventral midline dermatitis, which often occurs in horses kept in proximity to cattle. This dermatitis is characterized by focal to multifocal areas of alopecia, crusting, depigmentation, and ulceration, usually starting at or involving the umbilical area. Because this is not considered a hypersensitivity disease, most horses on the premises will be affected. Treatment of the lesions involves cleansing and using topical antibacterial products with or without corticosteroids.

Therapy and Prevention

Control of the problem requires daily application of topical insecticides and repellents. In some areas, horn flies may be resistant to pyrethroids, and alternative products may be required. For best results, appropriate horn fly control measures (sanitation, insecticide applications) applied to cattle housed in proximity to horses are recommended to reduce numbers of flies.

Black Flies

Epidemiology and Public Health Considerations

Running water is required for black fly (*Simulium* spp.) egg deposition and larval/pupal development. More than 1000 species, with differing abilities to overwinter and survive drought, are found worldwide. Equine encephalitis viruses have been found in black flies, but transmission has not yet been demonstrated. Adult flies are active in the late spring and early summer and can travel many miles from their breeding grounds. These flies inflict painful bites around the face, ears, neck, ventrum, and legs. Evidence suggests that some species of black fly are natural transmitters of vesicular stomatitis virus (Chapter 24) and possibly other viruses.

Black flies have significant public health importance in transmitting human pathogens, causing considerable annoyance, and inducing "black fly fever," a flulike syndrome in persons with multiple bites.[22]

Clinical Findings

A crusting dermatitis on the concave surface of the ear pinnae is often attributed to bites of black flies. Also found on the concave surface of the pinna, aural plaques or aural flat warts (raised, depigmented, wartlike lesions) are likely to be caused by infection with papillomavirus, for which the black fly is the suspected vector (Chapter 25).[23] *Simuliotoxicosis* is a syndrome resulting from massive attacks of black flies, which occur most often in large river basins, especially after breeding grounds are expanded by flooding.[22] Cardiotoxic or allergenic components in the saliva trigger cardiopulmonary dysfunction, possibly resulting in death of the animal. Alternatively, animals may die of blood loss from massive attacks.

Therapy and Prevention

Because black flies generally do not enter enclosed spaces, provision of shelters for animals is important. Application of permethrin insecticides to the affected horses may offer some protection. White petroleum jelly applied to the insides of horses' ears may reduce black fly feeding in that location. In some regions, environmental control of black flies has been attempted by governmental agencies.[22]

MOSQUITOES

Epidemiology and Public Health Considerations

The most important species of mosquito in equine medicine are included in the genera *Culex, Aedes,* and *Anopheles.* Mosquitoes breed in standing water almost anywhere. Depending on the species, a film of water on leaf litter, maintained for the duration of larval and pupal periods, is sufficient.[24] They feed predominantly around dusk and dawn and continue at lower levels throughout the night. Daytime feeding may be a problem in heavily shaded, damp areas. They serve as vectors of several viruses causing equine encephalitis, including Venezuelan (VEE), eastern (EEE), and western (WEE) equine encephalitis (Chapter 20) and Japanese encephalitis (JE) and West Nile virus (WNV) (Chapter 21). Mosquitoes are unlikely to transmit equine infectious anemia virus because large amounts of blood are usually necessary for efficient transmission (Chapter 23). In addition to their role as disease vectors, mosquitoes can cause considerable annoyance when their numbers are high, and rarely, potentially fatal anemia may result. They have been implicated in some cases of equine insect hypersensitivity.

The public health significance of mosquitoes is great because they transmit several human pathogens, including some of the same encephalitis viruses that infect horses.

Therapy and Prevention

Because the larvae develop in standing water, drainage or treatment of standing water is essential to mosquito control. If such areas cannot be eliminated, treatments to kill larvae in the water include (1) *Bacillus thuringiensis israelensis,* (2) light mineral oils, (3) organophosphate insecticides, (4) insect growth regulators such as methoprene, and (5) mosquito fish *(Gambusia)* that feed on mosquito larvae.[24,25] Environmental offices of the local government should be contacted for advice. Because of their limited duration of efficacy, repellents or insecticides should be applied to affected horses twice daily. Stabling at night in screened stalls and use of fly sheets will limit mosquito access. Propane-powered mosquito traps that produce carbon dioxide (CO_2) may be useful in limited areas of 1 acre or less.[9]

BITING MIDGES

Epidemiology and Public Health Considerations

Species in the genera *Culicoides* and *Leptoconops* are tiny flies also known as "midges," "no-see-ums," "punkies," "sandflies" (erroneously), and other names, depending on geographic location. Despite its diminutive size, this insect inflicts a painful bite by lacerating the skin and capillaries with its mandibles. In most geographic locations, *Culicoides* spp. feed primarily at dusk and dawn, less so during the night, and sometimes during the day. However, *Leptoconops* spp., which breed in sandy or arid, alkaline soils (deserts, beaches, tidal marshes), may be active during the day as well as dusk and dawn. Most midges breed in areas of moist, muddy ground around ponds, marshes, ditches and tidal flats, standing water in tree holes, in decaying vegetation, in rotting wood, and in manure. Because they are weak fliers, windless conditions with temperatures above 10° C (50° F) are ideal for their activity, but some species tolerate cooler temperatures and winds up to 18 kph (11 mph) or higher.[26] Females of many species are able to travel an average of 2 km (1.2 miles) from their breeding grounds.[26] Midges transmit the virus causing African horse sickness (Chapter 15), the filarial worms *Onchocerca cervicalis* and *Onchocerca reticulata* (Chapter 62), and other diseases of importance in other animal species.

In addition to annoyance from being bitten, humans may develop hypersensitivity to the bites, and several human pathogens are transmitted by midges.

Clinical Findings and Diagnosis

Biting midges are the most common cause of equine insect hypersensitivity, also known as "sweet itch," "kasen," "Queensland itch," "muck itch," "dhobie itch," and "Sommerekzem." Types I and IV hypersensitivity reactions are implicated in the pathogenesis, and a genetic predisposition is suspected because certain major histocompatibility types are highly represented in affected horses of susceptible breeds.[27] It is not unusual to see the condition in related horses. Affected animals should be removed from breeding programs.

Clinical signs arise between 1 and 4 years of age or 1 to 4 years after first exposure to the insects. In temperate climates a seasonal onset is characteristic, occurring in the summer and early autumn. Horses in tropical and subtropical locations may be exposed for 9 or 10 months of the year, possibly from successive species emerging throughout the season.[27] During the first season the condition tends to be mild, worsening each year as long as exposure to the insects continues. Pruritus is the major symptom, resulting in self-inflicted lesions. Classically, the head, ears (Fig. 64-3), mane, withers (Fig. 64-4), rump, and tail (Fig. 64-5) are affected. However, some species of *Culicoides* feed in other areas on the animal, resulting in lesions with a different distribution. A ventrally distributed form, described in the southeastern United States, involves the head and ears, the intermandibular space, chest (Fig. 64-6), upper forelegs, ventral abdomen, inguinal region, and usually the tail.[28] Rubbing and self-trauma result in alopecia, lichenification, crusting, erosions, ulcerations, and eventual wrinkling or corrugation of the skin. Secondary infections of the traumatized skin often follow.

Tentative diagnosis should be possible based on history and clinical signs. Response to appropriate insect control measures is diagnostic. Intradermal skin testing can be a useful method for confirming the clinical diagnosis. Biopsy findings of perivascular cuffs of mononuclear cells and eosinophils suggest allergic dermatitis but are not diagnostic for an etiologic agent because similar results can be seen with many ectoparasitic conditions.[18] The parasitic manges, louse infestation, other causes of allergies, and cutaneous onchocerciasis should be ruled out.

Therapy and Prevention

The only effective treatment is to prevent further exposure to the insects. Housing in insect-proof stables from late afternoon until well after dawn and daily to twice-daily application of insect repellents containing at least 2% permethrin are the minimum efforts required. Nightly stabling of affected animals should begin before the onset of the insect season and continue until the insects subside in the fall. In the author's experience, one night's exposure during the insect season can result in itching that may last as long as 2 to 4 weeks. Additionally, fine-mesh screening (32 × 32 or 2 mm × 2 mm) or netting, ceiling fans or strategically placed box fans, and automated insecticide misters may aid in situations where the stables cannot be fully enclosed or midge populations are particularly overwhelming. Screening can be treated with insecticide to kill midges trying to pass through. Fly sheets and insect masks may be of some use if started early in the season before the horse starts to itch. After pruritus has ensued, such items will not remain on the horse for long. In selected situations where exposure is not overwhelming, CO_2 traps stationed near barn or stable areas may attract insects away from animals housed inside. One author suggests adding octenol strips to the traps to make them more attractive to midges and mosquitoes.[9] The source of these insects is usually nearby; however, because some species are able to travel more than 2 km from breeding grounds, distant sources may not be immediately obvious. Drainage of ponds, ditches, marshes, or other wet areas in the horse's immediate surroundings reduces breeding grounds, but environmental regulations may prohibit such efforts. Transfer of affected animals to higher, drier, open, and breezy pastures or to drier geographic locations often results in complete or near-complete resolution of signs.

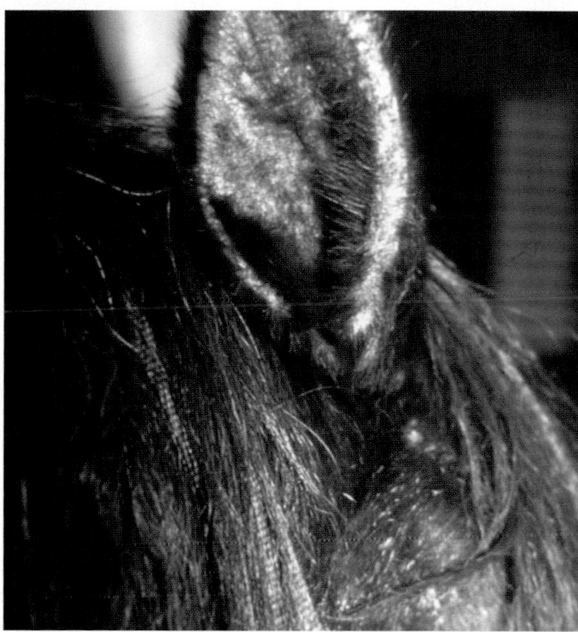

Fig. 64-3 Alopecia, lichenification, and crusting of pinna typical of that seen in chronic *Culicoides* hypersensitivity. (Courtesy Gail Kunkle.)

Immediate relief from pruritus is achieved using systemic glucocorticoids. Initial doses of *prednisolone* required to control severe itch may be as high as 1.5 mg/kg daily, tapering to the lowest possible dose on alternating days. If insect exposure is not controlled, it is usually difficult to reduce this induction dose significantly without relapse. Should prednisolone be ineffective, oral *dexamethasone*, starting at 0.02 to 0.1 mg/kg every 48 hours (q48h), tapering the dose after the first week of treatment, may provide better results.[29] Additional relief of pruritus can be achieved by treating secondary bacterial infections using appropriate systemic antibiotics and weekly topical therapy with antibacterial (benzoyl peroxide or ethyl lactate) or antiseborrheic (tar and sulfur, sulfur and salicylic acid) shampoos and rinses (2% lime sulfur).

One controlled study of immunotherapy (hyposensitization) using whole-body extracts of these midges was unsuccessful.[30] In an uncontrolled study using a *Culicoides* extract with adjuvant, reduced clinical signs were reported in 9 of 10 horses.[31] Some authors report better success with immunotherapy in horses that have pollen allergies concurrent with their insect allergies, questioning the clinical relevance of positive

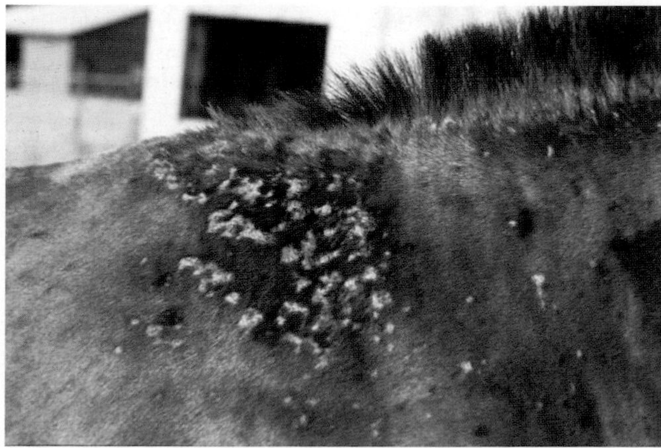

Fig. 64-4 Patchy alopecia and crusting on withers, resulting from severe pruritus seen in *Culicoides* hypersensitivity.

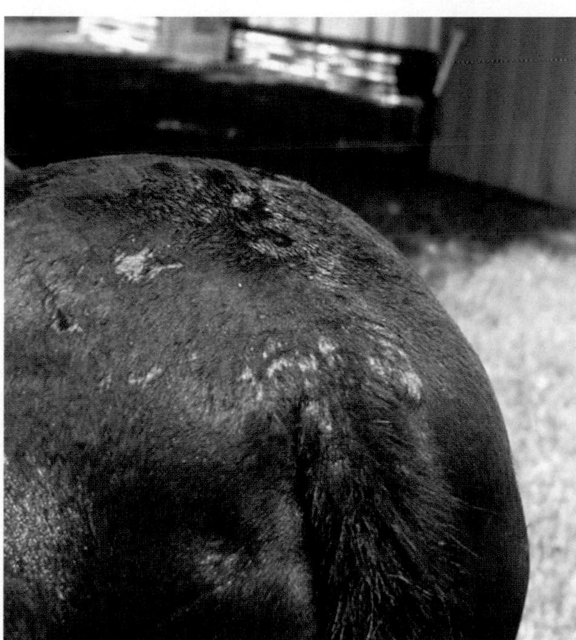

Fig. 64-4 Alopecia, ulcerations, and crusts on rump with severe hair breakage and alopecia of base of tail in horse with *Culicoides* hypersensitivity.

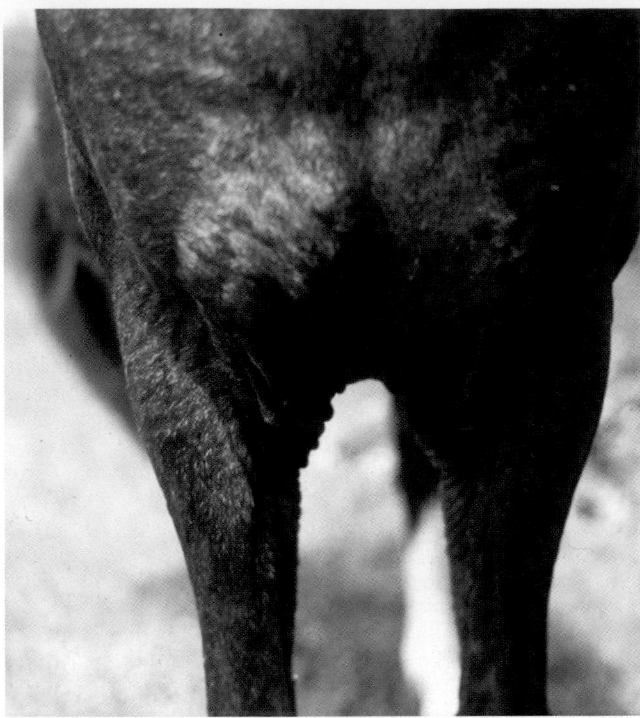

Fig. 64-5 Chronic lesions of lichenification and alopecia on chest of pony with *Culicoides* hypersensitivity.

reactions to the *Culicoides* allergen in such horses.[29,32] As possible explanations, successful immunotherapy to the relevant pollen allergens may raise the pruritic threshold in the affected horses to a level such that the insect allergy is not clinically manifested, or some positive insect allergen reactions may not be clinically relevant in some horses and may reflect insect exposure. Adjunctive treatments used by some authors include antihistamines (hydroxyzine at 400 mg orally twice daily) and fatty acid supplements.[29,33,34] Results with fatty acid supplements have been inconsistent.

NONBITING FLIES

Flies in the genera *Musca* and *Hydrotea* deposit eggs in fecal material, garbage, and decomposing organic matter. They feed on moist secretions in wounds or near mucocutaneous junctions. The housefly *(Musca domestica)*, the bush fly *(Musca vetustissima)*, and the bazaar fly *(Musca sorbens)* serve as developmental hosts for the horse stomach worms, *Habronema muscae* and *Draschia megastoma*, the larvae of which may induce the hypersensitivity syndrome of cutaneous habronemiasis in susceptible horses (Chapter 62). Rarely, myiasis can result from oviposition in wounds.[35] The face fly is a developmental host for *Thelazia lacrimalis*, the eyeworm of horses (Chapter 10). Similar to stable flies, removal and appropriate disposal of garbage, dung, and other decomposing organic material is essential to control fly populations. Topical insecticides and repellents reduce feeding on the animal. Good wound care and bandaging prevents secondary myiasis and cutaneous habronemiasis. Because the flies alight on sunny walls to rest, insecticidal applications to such areas are helpful. As mechanical transmitters of enteric infections in humans, these flies represent a significant public health problem.

WOUND MYIASIS

Etiology and Epidemiology

In *obligatory myiasis*, a reportable disease, the infestation of living host tissues is required for completion of the fly life cycle.[35] Species involved are the New World and Old World screwworms of the genera *Cochliomyia* and *Chrysomyia*, respectively. Screwworm infestation of healthy tissue of wounds, fly bite lesions and dermatitis, ulcerated masses, and mucocutaneous junctions occurs in the Americas (primarily Central and South America), Africa, and Asia. The adult fly deposits eggs in the exudative lesions or moist areas. When the larvae hatch, they burrow into the healthy subcutaneous tissue, causing liquefaction and enlargement of the lesion. After 3 to 6 days, they drop out to pupate.

Myiasis caused by blowflies and fleshflies is facultative (not requiring a living host).[35] It is uncommon in horses. Genera involved are *Lucilia*, *Calliphora*, *Phormia*, *Chrysomyia*, and *Sarcophagus*. These flies lay their eggs in decomposing tissue of wounds, macerated skin lesions, and areas of fecal soiling or accumulation, as well as in carcasses of dead animals. Larvae feed on the decomposing matter and secrete enzymes that cause wound enlargement.

Accidental myiasis, a rare finding, occurs when species of the family *Muscidae* deposit eggs in decomposing tissue of wounds while feeding on exudates.[35] It is termed "accidental" because living or decaying tissues are not the normal breeding ground for these flies.

Clinical Findings

Lesions of myiasis are painful and malodorous with exudation. Exploration of the wound under sedation will reveal maggots within the necrotic tissue. Larger lesions may result in septicemia resulting from secondary bacterial infection. If untreated, screwworm myiasis almost always results in the death of the host.

Diagnosis

Diagnosis is by larval identification. If screwworm is suspected, larvae should be dropped into boiling water for 30 to 60 seconds and then preserved in 70% alcohol for official identification.[11] Appropriate authorities should be notified. In cases where tumors or granulomas are secondarily invaded, biopsy to determine the underlying pathology is recommended. For best results, this should be done in an unaffected area of the mass or after the infestation and infection has been cleared.

Therapy and Prevention

Treatment includes removal of maggots, debridement and cleansing of lesions, application of topical insecticides, and administration of systemic antibiotics and other supportive therapy if septicemia is present. Avoiding surgical procedures during the fly season, prompt wound care with bandaging and application of thick topical insecticidal preparations, and keeping skin and hair free of manure deposits and soiling will prevent myiasis.

Widespread control of screwworms using sterile-male release programs and complementary insecticidal pelleted baits that attract female flies have been very successful in eliminating the problem in North America and much of Central America.[35] Similar attempts to control *Lucilia cuprina*, an Australian blowfly, have met with some success.[35] Control of other blowflies can be aided by deep burial or cremation of carcasses and placental materials. Good sanitation practices, such as composting or spreading manure and other decaying vegetable matter and strategic use of insecticides on premises and animals, will help control flies causing accidental myiasis.

Public Health Considerations

People are susceptible to wound myiasis, especially those who are very young, very old, infirm, or working in or near livestock operations. Prompt and appropriate wound care and good fly control practices should minimize the risk. Blowfly maggots, particularly *Phaenicia sericata*, have been used clinically in people to clean wounds and promote formation of granulation tissue.[35]

HYPODERMIASIS (WARBLES)

Etiology

Warbles are caused by the larval stages of the heel flies *Hypoderma bovis* and *H. lineatum*. These are primary parasites of ruminants, and horses, a dead-end host, are only sporadically affected.

Epidemiology

Warbles flies are similar in appearance to bumblebees and fasten their eggs to hairs on the legs and ventrum. After a few days, the larvae hatch and burrow through the skin, migrating through the body via the connective tissues. *Hypoderma lineatum* migrates through the submucosa of the esophagus, and *H. bovis* migrates in the epidural fat of the spinal canal. In the spring the larvae migrate to the subcutaneous tissues of the dorsal back, where they cut an air hole and become stationary, forming a nodule. After about 2 months, they emerge through the hole and fall to the ground to pupate. The larvae fail to develop normally in the horse and are unable to complete their life cycle. Horses housed near infested cattle are at the greatest risk of developing these nodules.

Clinical Findings and Diagnosis

Although cattle can have large numbers of nodules, the horse, as an aberrant host, seldom has more than one or two nodules, usually located on the dorsal back or withers. Warbles are easily distinguished from other nodules (dermoid cysts, eosinophilic granulomas, neoplasms) by the presence of the breathing pore. Identification of the larvae removed from the cyst is confirmatory.

Therapy

The best treatment for horses is careful surgical removal of the intact larva. Care must be taken to avoid crushing the larva during surgery because leakage of its internal contents can cause an anaphylactic reaction in the host.

Prevention

Control of the warble in the primary host is important. Avermectins are effective larvicides for the control of warbles in cattle, and their use in horses for regular intestinal parasite control probably prevents many cases from developing. Before the availability of avermectins, organophosphate insecticides were used to control cattle warbles. Preventing adult flies from laying eggs on animals requires use of topical insecticides and repellents.

MISCELLANEOUS FLIES

The horse botfly (*Gasterophilus* spp.) may cause restlessness and stamping as the flies hover and lay eggs on the hair of the horse's lower limbs and head. *Dermatobia hominis*, the human botfly, may infest horses in Central and South America. The resulting nodules have breathing pores, similar to warbles.[35] Louse flies of the genus *Hippobosca* are reported in Europe, North Africa, Western Asia, and South America. Preferring perineal and inguinal regions, these flies have painful bites, causing considerable annoyance. They may be vectors of equine babesiosis, Q fever, and other rickettsial organisms.[36] In Africa, multiple species of tsetse flies *(Glossinia)* bite horses, other domestic livestock, and many wild animals. They transmit *nagana* to livestock and horses, a chronic disease of anemia and weakness caused by protozoans in the genus *Trypanosoma*. The method of choice for control of tsetse flies is using traps baited with attractants.[37] Occasional reports of *Leishmania* in horses suggest that some species of sandflies (*Phlebotomus* and *Lutzomyia*) feed on horses as well as humans and other animals.[38,39]

ACCIDENTAL ECTOPARASITES

Horses can be affected by *Dermanyssus gallinae*, a mite of poultry, if housed close to poultry. Clinical signs include nocturnal pruritus, papules, erythema, and crusts on the feet and legs.[20] One author reported finding poultry lice on horses.[40] Rarely, cat fleas *(Ctenocephalides felis)* and poultry fleas or "stick-tights" (*Echidnophaga gallinacea*) have been reported on horses.[41,42] Control measures are similar to those for pets and poultry, respectively. In addition, the source of fleas, pets or poultry, should be treated.

ANTS, BEES, AND SPIDERS

In the southern United States, fire ants (*Solenopsis* spp.) are common. Horses tend to be stung by these insects on the legs, nose, or ventrum. Lesions are painful and rapidly develop a pustule, followed by crusting. Severe exposure may occur if the animal rolls on an anthill. Anaphylaxis may result, and sloughing of the epidermis may occur in the severely stung skin.[43] Bee and wasp stings result in edematous wheals or plaques at the sites of envenomation. If there has been previous sensitizing exposure, angioedema or anaphylaxis can result from stings. Spider bites, depending on the spider species involved, result in hot, painful, edematous lesions at the site of the bite, vesicular lesions, or necrotic lesions. Some spider bites progress from acute edematous lesions to necrosis and sloughing.[44] In cases of fire ant, bee, wasp, or spider envenomation, unless witnessed, it is difficult to tell, after the fact, which species is responsible for the lesions unless good circumstantial evidence implicates a certain species. Treatment is symptomatic and palliative.

REFERENCES

See the CD-ROM for a list of references linked to the abstract in PubMed.

SECTION • VI
Prevention and Control of Infectious Diseases

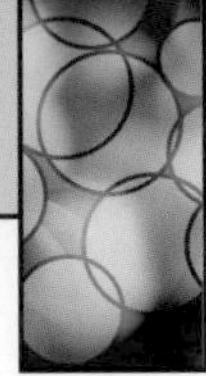

CHAPTER • 65

Epidemiology of Equine Infectious Disease

Paul S. Morley, Ashley E. Hill, and Paulo C. Duarte

BASICS

Definition

Epidemiology is the study of the occurrence of disease in populations[1] and the application of this knowledge to control or prevent disease. The underlying tenet of epidemiology is that *disease does not occur randomly in a population.* This means that there are always reasons why some horses become sick and others stay healthy, even if we do not always understand those reasons. This has tremendous implications for veterinarians: they can identify causes and risk factors for disease and take actions to prevent or decrease the impact of a disease. In this sense, it is critical to consider more than just disease agents and hosts; it is also critical to consider the environment and management factors that impact interactions among agents and hosts. Because of this broader implication, epidemiology is also sometimes defined as "medical ecology," as discussed below.

The mare reproductive loss syndrome outbreak in Kentucky in 2001 was an excellent example of epidemiology in action.[2] Even before veterinarians and producers understood the etiology of this disease, veterinarians were able to use epidemiology to identify risk factors for disease (exposure to eastern tent caterpillars[2] or pasture[3]), which allowed farm managers to implement control measures and prevent some abortions that would have otherwise occurred.

Epidemiologic Approach

A key epidemiologic approach to understanding and controlling disease involves looking for patterns of disease in the population of interest. Which horses are sick, and what do they have in common? Which horses are healthy, and what do they have in common? Which groups have been most affected? Great insight can be gained into causal mechanisms and control points that can be exploited in disease prevention efforts by (1) describing a population and identifying patterns, (2) making comparisons among different groups within a population, (3) comparing different populations, and (4) comparing the same population at different time points.

It is useful to consider the "five Ws" when trying to understand disease occurrence in a population: who, what, where, when, and why. **Who** is affected (and unaffected)? Include age, breed, gender, housing, water source, and vaccination status, as well as any other variables that may be relevant. **What** are the circumstances related to disease occurrence, and has anything changed? **Where** are the affected and unaffected animals located? Use a map of the barn or farm with food, water, and ventilation sources marked, and spatially locate the ill animals. **When** did each ill animal develop disease? Use this information to identify groups most affected (e.g., age groups, barns, breeds) using the tools described later in this chapter. All this should be interpreted with a focus on ultimately identifying "why." **Why** did these animals develop disease, and **why** were others not affected? Understanding why disease occurs allows identification of ways that disease can be prevented.

Disease Ecology

When trying to understand reasons why particular animals become diseased, it is clearly important to consider more than just an individual host and a particular agent as causes for a specific occurrence. The population to which an individual belongs must also be considered, in addition to the patterns of interactions and the environment that influences these interactions and impacts the likelihood of contagious transmission. Because of the importance of these broader considerations, epidemiology is sometimes referred to as *medical ecology*, or the interactions of all organisms and their environment as these pertain to health.

Mare reproductive loss syndrome (MRLS), which was initially reported among broodmares in central Kentucky in 2001, is one example of disease arising from a combination of host, agent, and environmental factors. An epidemic of equine abortion, endophthalmitis, and pericarditis began in late April 2001 and lasted until June 2001;[4-6] fetal losses occurred both early and late in pregnancy[3,7] and affected more than 60% of mares on some farms.[7] Multiple bacterial species were identified[8] in tissue of aborted fetuses. The syndrome was subsequently found to be associated with ingestion of the eastern tent caterpillar,[4] and it has been proposed that bacterially contaminated barbed caterpillar hairs migrated out of the alimentary tract, spread hematogenously, and were directly responsible for the observable signs of MRLS.[9] Eastern tent caterpillars are ubiquitous in the eastern United States but were particularly abundant in Kentucky that spring because a rapid temperature increase in early spring was superimposed on an unusually dry winter and spring.[10] These climatic conditions caused an explosion of biologic activity, including growth of black cherry trees on which eastern tent caterpillar eggs are laid and larvae develop.[11] During that spring with its unusual climactic conditions, grazing on pasture[4] with black cherry trees[12] exposed horses to disease; fetuses were particularly vulnerable. The sensitivity of the fetus to disease, the environmental conditions that led to the overgrowth of caterpillars, the bacteria themselves, and the management of the broodmares all contributed to the occurrence of MRLS.

Disease Agent

Characteristics of the disease agent, including infectivity, contagiousness, pathogenicity and virulence, immunogenicity, host range, life cycle, and antimicrobial susceptibility, influence the speed and scope of disease spread. *Infectiousness* (infectivity) refers to the ease with which an agent infects susceptible hosts, which is sometimes quantified in relation to the amount of agent required to reliably infect an individual. *Contagiousness* relates to the likelihood that an agent will move between infected and susceptible hosts; it is sometimes quantified by the number of new infections that will likely result from exposure to an infected animal or as the speed with which a disease agent is transmitted through a susceptible population. Equine influenza virus and equine herpesvirus are both highly infectious, but influenza virus is more contagious. Although equine protozoal myeloencephalitis (EPM) is an infectious disease, it is not a contagious disease because the etiologic agent is not transmitted directly between horses. *Pathogenicity* describes the likelihood that an infected horse will develop clinical disease, and *virulence* describes the likelihood that disease will be severe. West Nile virus (WNV) is highly virulent in horses; more than 30% of horses with clinical disease die.[13] In contrast, EPM is not highly pathogenic; most equids exposed to the disease agent do not develop clinical disease.[14-16]

Characteristics of the disease agent that enable it to survive and spread without detection are particularly important to consider when instituting preventive or control measures. Agents that can persist in the environment, such as *Clostridium difficile*[17] or *Streptococcus equi* subsp. *equi*, require different control measures than does equine influenza, which does not persist well outside the host. Some diseases spread undetected through infected horses without clinical signs of illness. Subclinically, persistently, and latently infected animals are often important reservoirs and sources of exposure for susceptible animals in a population because they go unnoticed or undiagnosed. Animals often are infected with a potentially pathogenic organism without showing clinical signs, and this can even be the predominant presentation depending on the pathogenicity of the agent. The term *subclinical* is also used to describe animals during the induction or incubation period for infectious diseases. Animals that remain infected for extended periods are sometimes described as being "persistently infected," especially if infections continue after clinical signs of disease resolve. Persistent infection and long-term shedding of *S. equi* subsp. *equi* are common[18-20] and important to the spread of disease among populations.[20,21] In contrast, *latency* describes a state of dormant viral infection in which shedding stops and the virus cannot be detected until later, when the infection reactivates or recrudesces. This is a common feature among alpha herpesviruses, such as equine herpesvirus (EHV) types 1 and 4.[22-29]

Host

Many host characteristics are intrinsic to the horse and relatively unchangeable, such as age, gender, and breed. Other host characteristics are highly variable among individuals and can change over time, perhaps most notably, inherent susceptibility to infectious agents or immunity. Characteristics of the host can affect both its exposure to disease and its likelihood of becoming infected if exposed. For example, geldings or spayed mares are less likely to be exposed to *Taylorella equigenitalis*, the agent that causes contagious equine metritis, and foals can be more vulnerable to disease than adults, as with *Rhodococcus equi* pneumonia.

Environment

A horse's environment includes its location, climate, and the local surroundings and interactions created by its management.[30] Characteristics of a horse's environment affect which diseases and vectors a horse is exposed to, the magnitude of that exposure, and the likelihood of developing disease if exposed. Horses that have been vaccinated with efficacious vaccines or immunized by natural exposure are more resistant to a particular disease than naive horses. Horses that are stressed for any reason, including poor diet, concurrent disease, weaning, transport, or mixing, are more likely to develop a disease than their unstressed counterparts. The risk of disease is not equal for similar horses when managed differently or housed in different environments.

Individual. Environmental characteristics that affect risk of disease in individual horses include climate, landscape, flora and fauna, cleanliness, air quality, housing, diet, and events that affect stress levels. Some of these factors (e.g., cleanliness, ventilation, housing, diet, stress level) are directly related to management practices and may be changeable, thus affecting risk of disease. Some management strategies (e.g., housing in open pastures, using outdoor drinking-water sources) increase potential exposure to insect vectors and also increase the risk of other diseases, such as Potomac horse fever (*Neorickettsia risticii* infection) and vesicular stomatitis. On the other hand, indoor housing, especially if it is high density or poorly ventilated, can increase exposure to diseases transmitted by aerosol or oral-fecal routes, such as influenza virus and *Salmonella*. Some environments and climates support larger vector populations than others, thus increasing potential risks for diseases, such as equine infectious anemia (EIA) or the equine encephalitides, including western equine encephalitis (WEE), eastern equine encephalitis (EEE), and WNV encephalitis. Although the climate itself cannot be changed, management practices, such as using animal-safe insect repellents, treating open-water sources with larvicides, and housing horses indoors at dusk and dawn, can be used to reduce disease risk.

Population. In addition to characteristics of individuals that affect their disease risk, the aggregate characteristics of the population to which the individual belongs affects the disease risk for that individual. This aggregate of the population's susceptibility to disease is often called *herd immunity*, described as immunity of an individual that is conferred by the population to which it belongs, or the ability of a population of animals to withstand exposure without succumbing to disease because the immunity of a population is more than the sum of its parts.[31] Herd immunity is created when the likelihood is small that an infected horse shedding a disease agent will encounter a susceptible horse (Fig. 65-1). If most horses are immune or if contact among horses is heavily restricted, it is unlikely that the few susceptible horses will have contact with the infected horse sufficient to allow transmission. For example, consider a barn in which 90% of horses are immune to influenza virus, and each horse in the barn contacts four other horses per day. If a newly introduced horse happens to be infected with influenza virus, and conditions are adequate for transmission of virus to in-contact horses, the probability that any other horse in the barn will become infected is about 35%, and the probability that more than one horse will become infected is about 12% (Fig. 65-1). For herd immunity to be effective, the disease agent (e.g., influenza) must only reside in horses, must not have an environmental reservoir, must be transmitted directly from horse to horse, and must have a short infectious period.[32]

Disease Causation

Many veterinarians are accustomed to thinking that infectious diseases have a single cause: the disease agent. Epidemiologists think of cause in a more general sense. Any "exposure" that leads to new cases of disease can be considered a "cause" of

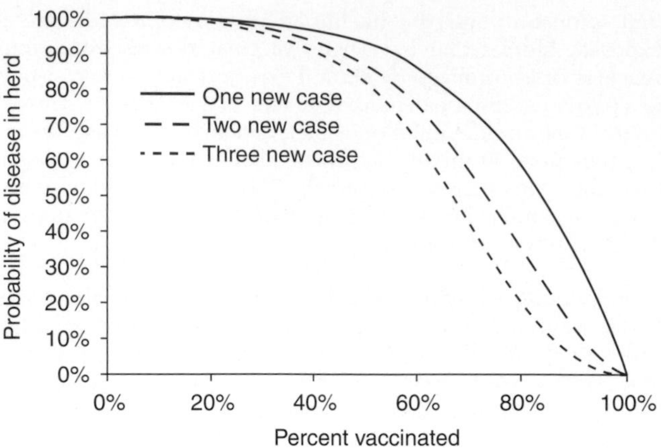

Fig. 65-1 Probability of new cases of disease with 1-day infectious period as a function of percentage vaccinated in a herd of horses where each horse contacts four other horses per day.

that disease. By removing that exposure, therefore, some cases of disease can be prevented. Causation has multiple levels. Again, consider MRLS. What "exposures" are associated with MRLS? The bacteria on the caterpillar hairs,[8] the caterpillars themselves,[33] exposure to cherry trees,[2] pasture grazing,[3,7] and the convergence of climatic factors resulting in caterpillar overgrowth have all been implicated in the epidemic occurrence of MRLS. Epidemiologically, all these factors are causes. Cases of disease can be reduced by removing bacteria from the caterpillars (an obviously impractical approach), minimizing exposure to caterpillars, reducing exposure to environments shared with the caterpillars (cherry trees or pasture), or returning to a more typical climate, as happened in subsequent years.

Likewise, consider encephalitis associated with WNV infection. This agent is propagated in a mosquito-bird-mosquito life cycle.[34] West Nile virus can replicate in multiple mosquito species,[35] although its primary vectors are *Culex* mosquitoes[36] The primary hosts are birds,[37] which develop transient viremia followed by long-term (lifelong) immunity. Ticks may also play a role in maintenance of WNV.[35,38,39] New cases of equine disease can therefore be reduced by minimizing exposure to mosquitoes and ticks (e.g., controlling vector populations, using animal-safe repellents, housing horses inside at dusk and dawn) or by increasing immunity to the virus, either in birds or in horses. In birds the natural immunity that develops after initial exposure reduces the total amount of virus circulating in the mosquito population, which in turn reduces equine exposures. The increase in WNV immunity among birds is one likely reason that the number of reported equine cases of WNV-associated disease in Colorado was 378 and 426 in 2002 and 2003, respectively, and then decreased to 33 in 2004.[40]

One useful model used to understand complex causal relationships is to classify causes as component causes, necessary causes, or sufficient causes.[31] In this model, a *component cause* is anything that contributes to new cases of disease. Component causes can be characteristics of the host (e.g., age, vaccination status), the agent (e.g., subtype), or the environment (e.g., presence or absence of caterpillars). A *sufficient cause* is any set of components that, when present together, is capable of causing disease; once a sufficient cause is present or complete, disease will occur. A *necessary cause* is a component cause that must be present for disease to occur; without the necessary cause, disease cannot occur. For infectious diseases, exposure or infection with the infectious agent is never sufficient by itself, but it is necessary for disease to occur.

Using this model, we can see that there may be multiple sufficient causes, and that disease can "flow" through any of these paths. Thus, removing exposure to one component cause will only mitigate disease through the sufficient causal paths that include that particular component cause. When a particular component cause is part of a high proportion of sufficient pathways, then exposure to this particular component cause will be strongly associated with disease occurrence. The extreme of this example is when a component cause is included in all sufficient causes, in which case the component cause can also be called a "necessary cause." Necessary causes are rare among all component causes, and there are always multiple sufficient causal sets. Thus, by removing exposure to some of the component causes, we only expect to prevent some disease occurrence and not all occurrences. The objective is to maximize efficiency of disease prevention efforts by targeting component causes that are strongly associated with disease occurrence.

IDENTIFYING CAUSAL FACTORS

In epidemiologic studies the main objective is to determine the factors (risk factors) associated with occurrence of disease so that they can be targeted in control and prevention programs. In general, we identify risk factors for a disease by comparing measures of disease frequency between different populations or groups. More specifically, this is accomplished by summarizing the occurrence of disease in the population, measuring disease frequency, and then comparing the risk of disease among horses with different exposures. By identifying differences in disease risk for groups with different exposures, we determine which exposures are associated with disease. Multiple studies are required to label exposures confidently as risk factors that are truly causal, which can then be targeted for minimizing exposure and thereby reducing the occurrence of new cases.

For example, in a study to identify the risk factors associated with equine protozoal myeloencephalitis (EPM), horses affected with EPM and nonaffected horses were compared using a case-control study design.[41] In that study, presence of opossums on the premises, lack of feed security, and recent occurrences of major health events, among other factors, were associated with an increased likelihood of disease and thus were identified as potential risk factors for the disease.[41]

Measuring Disease

The *frequency* of disease occurrence is measured for different purposes, including determining and comparing the health status of populations, monitoring changes in disease occurrence over time, and establishing the risks associated with certain events in the population. For example, the practitioner might be interested in the number or proportion of diseased horses in a herd, the increase or decrease in the number of disease cases over time, or the risk of disease introduction associated with new horses introduced to the herd. Common measures of disease frequency include prevalence and incidence, as well as related measures such as attack, case-fatality, and mortality risks.

Disease can be measured in whole populations or in specific subgroups. Measuring disease in the whole population (sometimes called a "crude" measure) tells you about the overall scope of the problem. Measuring disease in subgroups (called "specific" measures) enables you to compare those groups, which is essential when attempting to identify factors affecting the occurrence of disease. For example, if you had 10 cases of neurologic disease on a farm of 100 horses, you could report that 10% of horses on the farm are affected, as a crude prevalence estimate. In contrast, you could also report that 8 of 25 (32%) horses grazing in Pasture A were affected and 2 of 75 (3%) horses in Pasture B were affected. These pasture-specific attack rates suggest that something associated with housing in Pasture A may be the problem.

Population-at-Risk

The term *population-at-risk* (PAR) refers to the group of individuals susceptible to the event of interest (e.g., infection, disease, death) at or during the time period of interest. The PAR is used as the denominator in calculations of measures of disease frequency and can include the entire population or only a population subset, depending on susceptibility or specific interest in certain subgroups. For example, in describing the frequency of pneumonia caused by *Rhodococcus equi* infections, only foals would likely be included in the PAR because adult horses are not considered susceptible to this disease.[42]

Types of Data

The types of data available largely determine which methods will be most appropriate for measuring disease frequency or comparing disease risk. Most data can be described as interval (measurement) or categorical data. *Interval data* quantify a characteristic such as temperature, age, or weight, which can be measured as an infinite number of possible values. For example, in a group of five horses, you might take temperature measurements of 100°, 100°, 101°, 101.5°, and 102° F. Average or median values are often used to summarize interval data, and for this example the average temperature for these five horses is 100.9° F. Interval data are often compared by subtracting one average or median from another, and differences in interval measurements among groups are often statistically tested using z-tests, t-tests, and analyses of variance (ANOVA).

Categorical data divide groups into mutually exclusive categories (e.g., young horses vs. older horses, Quarter Horses vs. Thoroughbreds), and counts are used to characterize horses fitting into each category. Categorical data can be further characterized as "ordinal" if categories have an inherent order to them (e.g., young or old, light or heavy) or "nominal" if categories cannot be numerically ordered (e.g., categories for gender or breed). Interval measurements can be converted to ordinal measurements by dividing your range of values into categories. For example, if you wanted to describe temperature ordinally, as <101.5° F vs. temperature ≥101.5° F for these five horses, you would report that three horses had temperatures <101.5° F, and two had temperatures ≥101.5° F. Categories for nominal or ordinal data can be *dichotomous* (only two values are possible; e.g., live/dead, yes/no, sick/well) or can have more than two possible values (e.g., breed, age group). Ordinal and nominal data are summarized using ratios, proportions, and rates. These summary measurements can then be compared using relative risks, odds ratios, and attributable risks. These comparisons are often tested statistically using different types of chi-square tests.

Generally, all characterizations of disease occurrence in populations include some type of categorical assessment of presence or absence of disease signs using a specific case definition. In summarizing these measurements, the data are standardized to account for population sizes using the number of affected animals as a numerator, and some context measurement of the "opportunity" for disease to have occurred in the population (e.g., the population at risk). The denominator that we choose greatly affects the conclusions we can draw from these measurements of disease frequency. In general, these measures of disease frequency take the form of ratios, proportions, or rates.

Using Interval Data

Interval data are usually summarized using a measure that describes *central tendency* (e.g., means, medians, or modes) and some measure of the *variability* in data, such as the range of observed values, percentile rankings (e.g., values corresponding with the 25th and 75th percentiles), or the standard deviation or standard error of the mean. A simple arithmetic average summarizes the data well if the distribution of values looks like the well-recognized "normal" or "bell-shaped" curve. However, in distributions that do not have this balanced shape or in situations in which there are relatively few observations, averages can be strongly influenced by extreme values and may not represent the "center" of the data very well. In these situations the median or mode will likely provide better measures of centrality in the data.

Using Categorical Data

Ratios, Proportions, and Rates. When using ratios, proportions, and rates to summarize disease occurrence, a count of affected animals meeting a specific case definition is used as the numerator. Do 10 affected horses represent a significant number of cases? The answer depends on the type of disease and the size of the population in which these observations were made. Are we referring to 10 sick horses in a barn of 15 horses, or 10 sick horses at an entire racetrack facility with 3500 horses? The denominator provides context (e.g., is the PAR 15 or 3500 horses) and improves standardization and the ability to extrapolate or make comparisons. The type of denominator we choose affects the conclusions we can draw. The ratios, proportions, and rates used as epidemiologic measures principally differ in how the denominator is calculated (e.g., which animals are included, is time considered).

Ratios. Ratios are used to express the magnitude of two events in relation to each other. Ratios vary between 0 and infinity and can also be expressed as the number of events in one group per number of events in another group. In a ratio, the numerator is not part of the denominator. For example, in a population of horses a ratio of *infectious upper respiratory tract disease* (IURD) of 0.25, or 1:4, indicates that there is one diseased for every four nondiseased horses. In this case we can also say that the odds of IURD in the population is 1:4. Ratios are also used to compare measures of disease frequency between groups.

Proportions. A proportion is a special type of ratio in which the numerator is included as part of the denominator. For disease measurement, this fraction is calculated as the number of events over the total number of possible events. A proportion varies between 0 and 1 and is usually expressed as percentage. For example, during a regular clinical examination, 10 of 100 horses examined were identified with IURD. The proportion of IURD among these 100 horses at the time of examination was 10/100, or 10%. In another situation, 100 horses were followed for 1 year. During that year, 20 new cases of IURD were identified. The proportion of new IURD cases during that 1-year period was 20/100, or 20%.

Rates. A rate is another special type of ratio. In epidemiologic terms, rate represents the average "speed" that health events will occur in a population over a specific or standardized amount of time. A rate is calculated as the number of events over the product between the total number of possible events and the time period during which each event could have occurred. A rate varies between 0 and infinity, and the units of the denominator are expressed in *event-time* (e.g., horse-years, horse-months). For example, 100 horses were followed for 1 year. Assume that 10 horses developed IURD in the middle of the year (0.5 year) and after this point were no longer at risk of IURD because of acquired immunity. The rate of IURD would be calculated as 10 cases/90 horses × 1 year + 10 horses × 0.5 year and expressed as 0.11 cases per horse-year, or 11 cases per 100 horse-years. Notice that the time units of the denominator can be changed as desired, and 11 cases per 100 horse-years is the same as 11 cases per 1200 (100 × 12) horse-months, which means that you expect approximately 11 cases of IURD if you follow 100 horses for 1 year or 1200 horses for 1 month. Similarly, 33 cases of IURD would be expected to occur if 100 horses were followed for 3 years. The word "rate" is commonly used to refer to a proportion; however, rates and proportions are different quantities and are calculated differently, even though they are sometimes used as approximations of each other.

Epidemiologic Measures of Disease Frequency

Prevalence. Prevalence (P) is the proportion of cases of disease in a population at a specific point in time[43] and is calculated as follows (*PAR*, population-at-risk):

$$\text{Prevalence} = \frac{\text{Number of affected animals at a specific point in time}}{\text{PAR of being affected at that specific point in time}}$$

Prevalence is used to assess the health status of the population at a single point in time. Therefore it is a static measure of disease frequency and does not allow strong inferences about previous or future occurrences of disease or how fast these occurrences accumulate over time. Prevalence measures are also used to describe the risk or probability of a condition being present in a population (Box 65-1). Note that in prevalence estimates the numerator includes all cases of disease present at the specific point in time (recent and chronic).

Cumulative Incidence. The cumulative incidence (CI) is the proportion of new cases of disease occurring in a population during a specific time period[43] and is calculated as follows:

$$\text{Cumulative incidence} = \frac{\text{Number of new cases of disease during a specific time period}}{\text{PAR of becoming a case at the beginning of that time period}}$$

Cumulative incidence is used to assess the progression of disease in the population during a specific time period and can be used to predict disease occurrence. The cumulative incidence measures the risk or probability of becoming diseased in a population during a defined time period (Box 65-2).

The cumulative incidence is an appropriate measure of disease incidence when the population is relatively "closed" (i.e., minimal movement of animals in and out of the population). When there is substantial movement of animals ("open" population), the cumulative incidence might underestimate or overestimate (bias) disease incidence,[43] and the *incidence rate*, also called *incidence density*, is a more appropriate measure of disease incidence.

Other common measures that could be described as specific types of cumulative incidence include the attack rate, mortality rate, and the case-fatality rate. The *attack rate* is simply a different name attributed to the cumulative incidence in an outbreak situation and is calculated exactly as the cumulative incidence. The *mortality rate* is the proportion of all deaths ("crude" mortality rate) or deaths attributable to a specific disease ("cause-specific" mortality rate) over the total PAR of death at the beginning of the time period (Box 65-3). Note that these measures are called "rates," but in reality they are *proportions* because they do not include time measurements in their denominator.

Mortality can be calculated as a proportion, as just noted, or as an incidence using one of the methods described next. The term "mortality rate" is commonly used to describe mortality in the population whether it is a proportion or an

Box • 65-1

Prevalence

A population of 100 horses was examined for presence of infectious upper respiratory tract disease (IURD). At the time of examination, a total of 30 horses were diagnosed as having IURD. The prevalence of IURD in this population can be calculated as follows:

$$\text{Prevalence} = \frac{30}{100} = 0.3 = 30\%$$

In this population, at the time of examination, 30% of the horses had IURD; therefore the risk or the probability of having IURD in this population was 30%. If, for instance, someone were to buy a horse from this population without any information, the risk of buying one with IURD would be 30%.

Box • 65-2

Cumulative Incidence

A population of 100 horses was followed for 1 year to detect new cases of IURD; 20 new cases were observed during the year. The cumulative incidence of IURD in this population during that year was:

$$\text{Cumulative incidence} = \frac{20}{100} = 0.2 = 20\% \text{ in 1 year}$$

In this population, during a 1-year period, 20% of the horses developed IURD. If the conditions remain the same, we can expect 20% of the susceptible, healthy horses in that population to develop IURD in the following year. Thus the risk or probability of developing or becoming affected with IURD in that population is 20%.

actual rate.

The *case-fatality rate* is the proportion of deaths attributable to the disease of interest during a specific period of time (Box 65-4).[43] The case-fatality rate is calculated as follows:

$$\text{Case-Fatality Rate} = \frac{\text{Number of deaths attributable to the disease during a specific time period}}{\text{Total number of cases of disease in that time period}}$$

This measure of disease occurrence is often used to characterize the severity of disease and the effectiveness of treatment. Therefore the specific case-fatality rates for treated and untreated animals are often cited and compared.

Mortality rates and case-fatality rates are two of the most frequently confused epidemiologic measures, and they actually describe very different disease characteristics. Mortality rates are used to describe the risk or probability of death in a population (whether estimated by prevalence, cumulative incidence, or incidence density). This can be death attributable to all causes or death associated with a specific condition. In contrast, the case-fatality rate characterizes the likelihood of death once a condition is present. As such, the cause-specific mortality rate can be very low for a given disease, whereas the treated or untreated case-fatality rate for the same disease can be very high. For example, the mortality rate for rabies is very, very low among horses in most parts of the world. This means that very few deaths are associated with this disease in most equine populations. However, both the treated and untreated case-fatality rate is essentially 100% for rabies. This means that on the rare occasions that horses develop rabies, all affected horses can be expected to die.

Incidence Rate. The incidence rate (IR) is the number of new cases of disease per unit of animal-time. There are different ways to calculate incidence rate depending on the information available. The most accurate is as follows:

$$\text{Incidence Rate} = \frac{\text{Number of new cases of disease in a specific time period}}{\text{Sum of each individual's disease free time in the PAR in the specific time period}}$$

The incidence rate, as the cumulative incidence, is used to assess the progression of disease in the population and can be used to predict disease occurrence. It is calculated for a specific time period, but it represents a measure of the "speed" of the disease in the population over time. In practice, incidence rate and cumulative incidence are used as an approximation of each other and are given the same interpretation. The type of the population (open or closed) and the data available are what drives the calculation of one versus the other. The incidence rate is not a true measure of risk but can be and is used as such (Box 65-5).

In the example in Box 65-5, we can say that, if everything remains constant, the disease is "moving" through the population at an average "speed" of 26 cases per 100 horses per year. For practical purposes, we might also say that there is a 26% risk of developing IURD in this population in 1 year, although this is a less precise interpretation.

Two other approximations can be used to estimate the denominator incidence rates when information on disease-free time for each individual horse is not available: (1) average the PAR at the beginning and at the end of the time period of interest, or (2) use an estimate of the total population at a certain point in time during the period of interest (usually the middle of the time period) as the average PAR. In both cases, we assume that the average population represents the average number of horses at risk for a period of time equivalent to the follow-up period, and we calculate the incidence rate denominator as the product between the average PAR and the follow-up period.

In these examples, we assumed that once a horse developed IURD, it also developed immunity to the disease, and thus there

Box • 65-3

Mortality Rate

In a population of 100 foals followed for 1 year, eight deaths were attributable to *Rhodococcus equi* pneumonia, one to neonatal septicemia, and one foal was euthanized because of an intestinal torsion. The crude mortality rate for this population during that year was:

$$\text{Crude mortality rate} = \frac{10}{100} = 0.1 = 10\% \text{ in 1 year}$$

The cause-specific mortality rate for deaths attributable to *R. equi* pneumonia was:

$$\text{Cause-specific mortality rate} = \frac{8}{100} = 0.08 = 8\% \text{ in 1 year}$$

In this population the risk or probability of a foal dying from any cause during that year was 10%, and the risk or probability of a foal dying from *R. equi* pneumonia was 8%.

Box • 65-4

Case-Fatality Rate

A population of foals was followed for 1 year. During that period, there were 20 new cases of *R. equi* pneumonia identified. Ten of the 20 affected foals died as consequence of the disease during the year. The case-fatality rate for *R. equi* pneumonia in that population of foals during that year was:

$$\text{Case-fatality rate} = \frac{10}{20} = 0.5 = 50\% \text{ in 1 year}$$

In this population, once a foal is affected by *R. equi* pneumonia, the risk or probability of dying from the disease is 50%.

Box • 65-5

Incidence Rate

A total of 100 horses were followed for 1 year. During the year, there were 20 new cases of IURD, all of which occurred in the third month of the year (0.25 year). In addition, 10 horses were sold and left the population at 6 months (0.5 year) into the year, and another five horses died of other causes. Among these five horses, one died at 2 months (0.2 year) into the year, two at 4 months (0.3 year), and the other two at 9 months (0.75 year) into the year. The incidence rate was:

$$\text{Incidence rate} = \frac{20}{(65\times 1)+(10\times 0.5)+(1\times 0.2)+(2\times 0.3)+(2\times 0.75)+(20\times 0.25)} = \frac{20}{77.3}$$

Incidence Rate ≅ 0.26 cases/horse-years or 26 cases/100 horse-year

Explanation of the calculations in the denominator:

65 × 01 = Time-at-risk accumulated by horses that never developed IURD and were at risk for the disease for the entire 1 year (disease-free time).

10 × 0.5 = Time-at-risk accumulated by horses that left the population in the middle of the year and thus were at risk for IURD for 0.5 year each.

(1 × 0.2), (2 × 0.3), and (2 × 0.75) = Time-at-risk accumulated by horses that died of other causes and were at risk of IURD during the time they were alive: 0.2 year for 1 horse, 0.3 year for two horses, and 0.75 year for two horses.

20 × 0.25 = Time-at-risk accumulated by horses that developed IURD at 3 months into the year and were at risk for the disease for 0.25 year each.

Box • 65-6

Prevalence and Incidence

In Box 65-2 the cumulative incidence of IURD was 20%. Assume average disease duration of 7 days (or 0.02 year). The prevalence of IURD at any given day of the year is approximately:

$$\text{Prevalence} \cong \frac{\text{Cumulative incidence} \times \text{Duration}}{(\text{Cumulative incidence} \times \text{Duration})+1} = \frac{0.20\times 0.02}{(0.20\times 0.02)+1} = 0.4\%$$

were no recurrences during that year. To account for recurrences, the total number of occurrences per horse would be included in the numerator, with the total disease-free time between occurrences for each horse included in the denominator.

Relationship between Prevalence and Incidence. Prevalence of disease is a function of disease incidence and duration.[43] In general, prevalence increases as the incidence and duration of disease increase, and vice versa (Box 65-6). This relationship can be used for approximation of incidence or prevalence if one measure or the other is available.

Temporal Patterns of Disease

Characterizing and understanding the occurrence of disease over time in populations are very useful and can provide great insight into the infectivity and contagiousness of disease. One standard method of graphically summarizing disease temporally is to generate an epidemic curve by plotting the number of new occurrences that develop per units of time (time is traditionally graphed on the x axis in whatever intervals make sense; case frequency is plotted on the y axis; Fig. 65-2). In general, the occurrence of disease over time can be grouped into four categories: endemic, epidemic, pandemic, and sporadic.[30]

A disease is *endemic* (Fig. 65-2, *A*) if it occurs at some predictable rate regardless of whether that rate is high, low, or varies during a given year or other specific time period. For example, in some regions of the United States (U.S.), Potomac horse fever (PHF) is endemic because the number of new cases is relatively constant from year to year. Salmonellosis is also endemic throughout the U.S., although the rates predictably increase in the summer and early fall.

A disease is *epidemic* (Fig. 65-2, *B*) when it occurs at a level beyond that which is typical or expected in the population.[30] For example, introduction of WNV into the U.S. created epidemics in horse populations throughout North America.[13,44-50] Strangles is endemic in the U.S. as a whole but often occurs as outbreaks at the local level. When epidemics affect populations across multiple continents, then disease is sometimes considered pandemic (e.g., H5N1 avian influenza in 2004–2005,[51] "type 2" (H3N8) equine influenza in 1963[52-55]) (Fig. 65-2, C). Epidemics and pandemics occur when a highly contagious disease is introduced into a susceptible population.

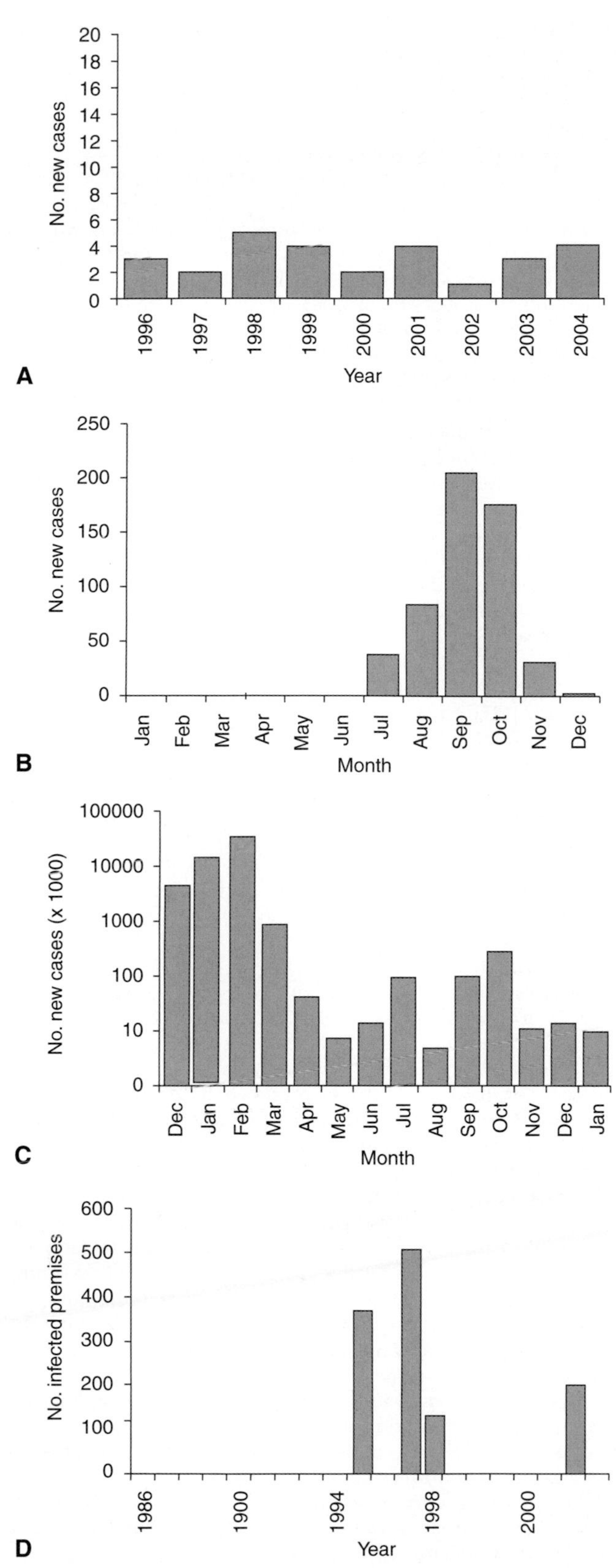

Fig. 65-2 Epidemic curves associated with **A**, endemic disease (Potomac horse fever); **B**, epidemic disease (equine West Nile encephalitis cases in California[70]); **C**, pandemic disease (H5N1 avian influenza in Asia 2003–2005[51]); and **D**, sporadic disease (vesicular stomatitis in western United States[57,58,71-73]).

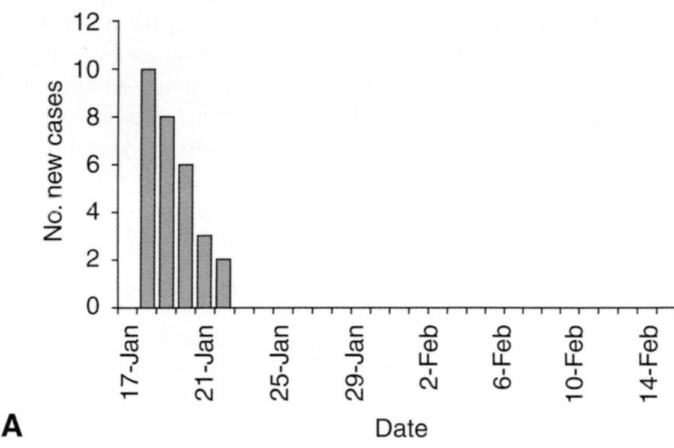

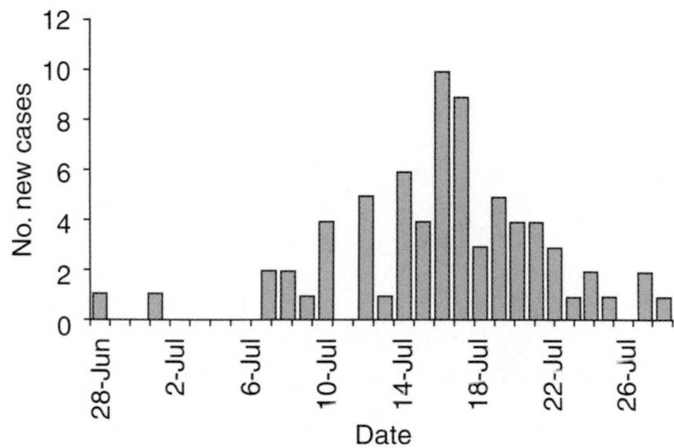

Fig. 65-3 Epidemic curves from point-source outbreak of neurologic signs associated with **A,** consumption of mycotoxin-contaminated ryegrass,[59] and **B,** propagated outbreak of infectious upper respiratory disease.[60]

A disease is considered *sporadic* (Fig. 65-2, *D*) if it occurs irregularly and haphazardly; sporadic disease can occur as a single case or as a cluster of cases. Vesicular stomatitis occurs sporadically in horses in the western U.S.[56-58] Sporadic disease can be the result of infrequent contact between a susceptible animal and a reservoir of disease.

From a conceptual perspective, epidemics can be further separated into two general patterns: point-source and propagated (Fig. 65-3). A *point-source epidemic* occurs when many horses in a population are exposed at the same time to a specific disease agent. For example, a point-source epidemic might occur if a group of horses are all exposed at the same time to a toxin in the feed, such as mycotoxin-contaminated ryegrass hay.[59] An epidemic curve of a point-source outbreak (Fig. 65-3, *A*) shows a high number of initial cases, but the number of new cases often taper off quickly when the exposure to the agent is removed or disappears. *Propagated epidemics* occur when an infectious agent, equine influenza virus,[60] is spread from one or a few initially infected horses ("primary" cases) to other susceptible horses ("secondary" cases) that spread disease themselves (Fig. 65-3, *B*). For propagated epidemics of contagious disease, the number of new cases classically increases exponentially over days to weeks as susceptible horses become infected, then tapers off gradually as the number of susceptible horses in the population decreases and concomitantly exposures decreases.

This conceptual model of different epidemics is very useful, but differentiating between point-source and propagated outbreaks is not always easy based on the shape of their epidemic curves. For example, a group of horses could all develop salmonellosis after consuming contaminated feed; the horses may then shed *Salmonella* in their feces, thus infecting other horses in their paddocks. Although the disease outbreak originated from a single source, it was then propagated through fecal-oral transmission. The shape and time scale of a propagated epidemic curve are affected by the disease incubation period, how contagious the disease is, what proportion of horses in the herd are susceptible, and how densely the horses are housed.[30]

Comparing Groups

There are two important questions to answer when comparing data from two or more groups. First, how "big" is the difference between groups? One way of evaluating how "big" is "big" is to consider whether the difference seems biologically or economically meaningful. The second question that must be considered is whether the observed difference is "real," or could it be caused more by chance variation than by a systematic difference? To quantify the size of differences between groups, typically a *summary measure*, such as averages or proportions, is compared or a measure of association such as an odds ratio or relative risk is calculated. Using this comparative information, it is necessary to evaluate whether the observed differences are meaningful or trivial. For example, in a study evaluating *Salmonella* shedding among colic patients, the association between having a fever and shedding *Salmonella* was reported[61] as an odds ratio of 9.0 with a *P* value of <0.01, indicating that horses shedding *Salmonella* were about nine times more likely to have a fever than horses not shedding *Salmonella*. That seems like a meaningful difference (i.e., 9 times more likely is biologically meaningful), and the *P* value suggests that this difference is unlikely to have occurred from chance alone.

To evaluate whether there is a "real" difference versus a difference that occurred from chance variation, we typically use some type of *statistical evaluation* (e.g., chi-square test, z-test) and consider the *P* value. The *P* value indicates the *statistical significance* of the association, or how likely we are to see results this extreme if no association existed between the factor and the disease.[62] A *P* value of <0.01 suggests that if there truly were no causal association between fever and *Salmonella* shedding, we would still see an odds ratio of 9.0 in a similar study less than 1% of the time. In other words, it is likely that the association is real, not just coincidence. The *P* value is greatly affected by the number of horses in the study (i.e., study power), the magnitude of the difference being measured (i.e., strength of association), and the degree of variation in the groups being compared (did *all* febrile horses and *none* of the afebrile horses shed *Salmonella*, or was there more variation in shedding within febrile and afebrile groups?). In general, the *P* value decreases as the number of animals being studied increases, as the magnitude of difference increases, and as the variation within each group decreases. The *P* value does *not* provide any information about whether the difference between groups is meaningful.

Using Measurement Data

Is the Difference Real? If data follow a bell-shaped curve, the z-test can be used to determine how likely it is that the difference is real and not caused by chance variation. To use the z-test, the standard deviation (SD) of each group's data (a $20 calculator can do this for you), the number (count) of horses in each group, and the z-score values (95% = 1.96; 90% = 1.64; 80% = 1.28) must be known. The following formula is used to calculate a confidence interval, using the 95% z-score of 1.96:

$$\text{average1} - \text{average2} \pm \text{z-score} \times \sqrt{\frac{\text{SD1}^2}{\text{count1}} + \frac{\text{SD2}^2}{\text{count2}}}$$

If the range does not include zero, there is 95% confidence that the observed difference is real and not caused by chance. If the range does include zero, the equation is recalculated using the 90% z-score of 1.64. If the new range does not include zero, there is 90% confidence that the difference is real. If the 90% range includes zero, the equation is recalculated using the 80% z-score. If the range does not include zero, there is 80% confidence that the difference is real; if the range does include zero, there is less than 80% confidence that the difference is real.

For example, if there was a concern that poor ventilation in Barn A was affecting the horses, temperature data on 10 horses in Barn A and 15 horses in Barn B could be collected. If the average temperature of horses in Barn A was 102.0° F with SD of 0.56, compared with 100.6° F with SD of 0.71 for horses in Barn B, this would yield the following equation with a 95% z-score of 1.96:

$$102.0 - 100.6 \pm 1.96 \times \sqrt{\frac{0.56^2}{10} + \frac{0.71^2}{15}} = 1.4 \pm 0.50 = 0.9, 1.9$$

The range 0.9 to 1.9 does not include zero, so there is 95% confidence that the difference is real and not caused by chance variation. Is an average body temperature difference of 1.4° F biologically meaningful? That cannot be determined by a statistical test and is better determined using clinical experience and judgment.

Using Categorical Data

In epidemiology, it is common to use the term *exposure* to refer to an individual's experience with a risk factor. In a study of EPM occurrence, lack of feed security was identified as a potential risk factor for the disease.[41] Horses "exposed" to "lack of feed security" were more likely to have EPM than horses "not exposed" to "lack of feed security" (i.e., horses that had their feed safely stored). Thus it is important to notice that "exposure" is used broadly in epidemiology and does not necessarily refer to the physical contact between the risk factor and the individual, as it might initially suggest.

Various measures of association can be used to characterize relationships between risk factors and disease. The timing of data collection relative to disease occurrence dictates to a great extent which measures of association are appropriate. If horses exposed and not exposed to a potential risk factor are followed over time to determine occurrence of disease (*cohort* studies), measures of incidence are obtained, and measures of association (e.g., attributable risk, attributable fraction, relative risk, odds ratio) can all be estimated. If diseased and nondiseased horses are compared in relation to their past or current exposure to a potential risk factor (*case-control* and *cross-sectional* studies), the odds ratio is the measure of association estimated.

Comparing Cumulative Incidence: Attributable Risk and Attributable Fraction. The attributable risk (AR) measures the absolute amount of risk attributable to exposure in the group of individuals exposed to the risk factor. The attributable risk is calculated as the difference between the cumulative incidence in horses exposed and not exposed to the risk factor. The attributable fraction (AF) is the proportion of risk attributable to exposure to the risk factor and is calculated as the attributable risk divided by the cumulative incidence in the exposed group (Box 65-7).

In Box 65-7, 50% (10% of 20%) of the risk of IURD in horses housed in poor bedding conditions is attributable to the actual exposure to poor bedding conditions. In other words, if you could transfer all horses in poor bedding conditions to good bedding conditions, you would prevent 50% of disease in that group. In the population there is a mixture of horses exposed and not exposed to poor bedding conditions. Therefore the reduction in disease occurrence in the population as a whole (not only in the exposed group) will depend on the proportion or prevalence of exposure in that population.

To determine the impact of control and preventive measures in the population, two other measures can be calculated: the population attributable risk and the population attributable fraction. The *population attributable risk* measures the amount of risk attributable to exposure in the population and is calculated as the product of the attributable risk and the prevalence of exposure in the population.[43] The *population attributable fraction* is the proportion of risk attributable to exposure in the population and is calculated as the population attributable risk divided by the cumulative incidence of the disease in the entire population (CI_{TP}) (Box 65-8).[43]

Comparing Cumulative Incidence: Relative Risk. The relative risk (RR) is the ratio between the cumulative incidence in the exposed and nonexposed groups. It measures how large the cumulative incidence is in the exposed group compared with the nonexposed group (Box 65-9).

Comparing Prevalences: Odds ratio. The odds ratio (OR) is the ratio between the odds of disease in the exposed group and the odds of disease in the nonexposed group. It measures how large the odds of disease are in the exposed group compared with the nonexposed group. Frequently, diseased and nondiseased horses are the groups selected in epidemiologic studies, and differences in exposure between groups are determined. In these cases, strictly speaking, the odds ratio is the ratio between the odds of exposure in the diseased group over the odds of exposure in the nondiseased group. However, mathematically, the odds ratio calculated as the odds of exposure in the diseased and nondiseased groups and the odds of disease in the exposed and nonexposed groups are the same (Box 65-10).

The relative risk and odds ratio are also called "measures of strength of association." They indicate not only the

Box • 65-7

Attributable Risk

Assume that veterinarians at a racetrack believe that housing conditions contribute to the risk of IURD occurrence, and that exposure to dusty environments with high levels of ammonia increase likelihood of IURD occurrence. In other words, they believe that poor bedding conditions serve as a risk factor for IURD. A cohort study was designed to determine whether there was an association between poor bedding conditions and occurrence of IURD. A sample of 100 horses housed in poor bedding conditions and another sample of 100 horses housed in good bedding conditions were followed for 1 year. The cumulative incidence (CI) was calculated for both groups and compared. The data are presented below:

	Poor Bedding	Good Bedding	
IURD+	20	10	30
IURD–	80	90	170
	100	100	

$$\text{Cumulative incidence}_{PB} = \frac{20}{100} = 20\% \quad \text{Cumulative incidence}_{GB} = \frac{10}{100} = 10\%$$

$$\text{Attributable risk} = CI_{PB} - CI_{GB} = 20\% - 10\% = 10\%$$

$$\text{Attributable fraction} = \frac{CI_{PB} - CI_{GB}}{CI_{PB}} = \frac{20\% - 10\%}{20\%} 50\%$$

In this example, the attributable risk indicates that 10% of the 20% total risk of IURD in horses exposed to poor bedding conditions was actually attributable to the horses being housed in poor bedding conditions. The attributable fraction indicates that this 10% of the risk represented 50% of the total risk of IURD in the horses exposed to poor bedding conditions. Note that IURD also occurred in horses housed in good bedding conditions. Therefore, poor bedding conditions contribute to an increase in IURD but are not the only factor associated with its occurrence.

Box • 65-8

Attributable Fraction

Based on the information obtained in the study described in the Box 65-7, the veterinarians at the racetrack decided to implement a program to improve bedding conditions in the entire racetrack (the population). They want to know the impact such a program will have in reducing IURD in the population. According to a previous survey conducted at the racetrack, approximately 30% of the horses were housed in poor bedding conditions (exposure prevalence). Using the data from Box 65-7, the population attributable risk (PAR) and the population attributable fraction (PAF) were:

$$\text{Population attributable risk} = AR \times \text{Exposure prevalence} = 10\% \times 30\% = 3\%$$

$$\text{Population attributable fraction} = \frac{\text{PAR}}{\text{CI}_{\text{TP}}} = \frac{3\%}{13\%} = 23\%$$

Where:

CI_{TP} = Cumulative incidence of IURD in the entire population

$$\text{CI}_{\text{TP}} = (\text{CI}_{\text{PB}} \times \text{exposure prevalence}) + \{\text{CI}_{\text{GB}} \times (1 - \text{exposure prevalence})\}$$

$$\text{CI}_{\text{TP}} = (20\% \times 30\%) + (10\% \times 70\%) = 13\%$$

By implementing a program to improve bedding conditions at the racetrack, practitioners may expect an absolute reduction of 3% in the total IURD incidence. This reduction represents approximately 23% of the total current incidence of IURD (13%) at the racetrack. In other words, the veterinarians might expect to reduce the total incidence of IURD at the racetrack from 13% to 10%. The PAR and the PAF can also be calculated as:

$$\text{Population attributable risk} = \text{CI}_{\text{TP}} - \text{CI}_{\text{GB}}$$

$$\text{Population attributable fraction} = \frac{\text{CI}_{\text{TP}} - \text{CI}_{\text{GB}}}{\text{CI}_{\text{TP}}}$$

Where:

CI_{TP} = Cumulative incidence of IURD in the entire population

CI_{GB} = Cumulative incidence of IURD in the nonexposed (good bedding) horses

existence of an association but also the strength of the association. An RR or OR of 5 indicates a much stronger association between the risk factor and the disease than an RR or OR of 1.5. An RR or OR equal to 1 indicates no association between the risk factor and the disease. In other words, it indicates that disease is as likely to occur in the exposed as the nonexposed group. An RR or OR less than 1 indicates that the risk factor is actually protective for the disease and technically is not a risk but a protective factor. A common example is vaccination. An RR or OR of 0.5 obtained when comparing occurrence of disease in vaccinated (exposed) and nonvaccinated (nonexposed) horses indicates that disease occurrence in vaccinated horses is about half of that in nonvaccinated horses.

Outbreak Investigations: Attack Risk Table. An attack risk table is a quick and simple way to summarize exposures and disease occurrence and also to look for factors strongly associated with disease. It is often used to analyze data quickly during an outbreak. Consider a farm on which 10 cases of strangles are diagnosed in a population of 100 horses. Several potential disease sources exist on the farm: a newly arrived horse, a used feed trough recently purchased from a neighbor, and participation in a recent horse show. Exposure data are collected on all horses; all horses are categorized as sick/well using a standardized case definition and as exposed or not exposed to each potential risk factor; and the attack risk table is constructed (Table 65-1).

For each potential disease source, the total number of horses exposed and unexposed should equal the number of horses on the farm. The attack risk for horses exposed to a factor is calculated by dividing the number of horses exposed and ill by the total number exposed. Likewise, the attack risk for horses not exposed to the factor is calculated by dividing the number of horses unexposed and ill by the total number unexposed. The risk ratio is calculated by dividing the attack risk for exposed horses by the attack risk for unexposed horses. The higher the risk ratio, the stronger is the association between factor and disease. In this example, it appears the horse show was the source of the strangles outbreak. Horses that went to the show were six times more likely to have strangles than those that did not go.

Box • 65-9

Relative Risk

As in Box 65-7, a cohort study was designed to determine whether there was an association between poor bedding conditions and occurrence of IURD. A sample of 100 horses housed in poor bedding conditions and another sample of 100 housed in good bedding conditions were followed for 1 year. The cumulative incidence (CI) was calculated and compared between groups. The data are presented below:

	Poor bedding	**Good bedding**	
IURD+	**20**	**10**	**30**
IURD–	**80**	**90**	**170**
	100	**100**	**200**

$$CI_{PB} = \frac{20}{100} = 20\% \qquad CI_{GB} = \frac{10}{100} = 10\%$$

$$RR = \frac{CI_{PB}}{CI_{GB}} = \frac{20\%}{10\%} = 2$$

A relative risk (RR) of 2 indicates that the cumulative incidence of IURD in horses exposed to poor bedding conditions is twice the cumulative incidence of IURD in horses in good bedding conditions. Horses in poor bedding conditions are twice as likely to develop IURD as horses in good bedding conditions.

Box • 65-10

Odds Ratio

A study was conducted to evaluate risk factors associated with development of equine protozoal myeloencephalitis (EPM). Using a case-control study design, horses with EPM were identified for enrollment. "Security" of the hay fed to the horses from wildlife was evaluated as one of the potential risk factors.[41] Horses fed hay from "nonsecure" sources were considered "exposed," whereas horses fed hay that was protected from exposure to definitive hoses (secure hay) were considered "nonexposed."

	EPM+	**EPM–**	
Hay Not Secured	**86**	**51**	**137**
Secured Hay	**43**	**48**	**91**
	129	**99**	**228**

Calculations for the odds ratio for EPM occurrence in the exposed and nonexposed groups is shown below:

$$\text{Odds Ratio} = \frac{86 \times 48}{51 \times 43} \cong 2$$

An odds ratio of 2 indicates that horses exposed to nonsecure hay were approximately two times more likely to develop EPM than horses fed secure hay. Note that the interpretation of the odds ratio is similar to the interpretation of the relative risk (see Box 65-9), even though measures of disease incidence were not calculated. In epidemiologic studies the odds ratio is used as an approximation of the relative risk when the study design does not allow the calculation of measures of incidence. This approximation is more precise when the disease is rare in the population.[30]

Table • 65-1

Attack Risk Table (Constructed as Described in Text)

FACTOR	EXPOSED	ILL AND EXPOSED	ATTACK RISK FOR EXPOSED	NOT EXPOSED	ILL AND UNEXPOSED	ATTACK RISK FOR UNEXPOSED	RISK RATIO
New horse	14	3	$\frac{3}{14}=0.21$	86	7	$\frac{7}{86}=0.08$	$\frac{0.21}{0.08}=2.6$
New trough	25	3	$\frac{3}{25}=0.12$	75	7	$\frac{7}{75}=0.09$	$\frac{0.12}{0.09}=1.3$
Horse show	20	6	$\frac{6}{20}=0.30$	80	4	$\frac{4}{80}=0.05$	$\frac{0.30}{0.05}=6.0$

Table • 65-2

A 2 × 2 Table Constructed for Chi-Square Test (as Described in Text)

	SICK	WELL	TOTAL
Exposed	A	B	C
Unexposed	D	E	F
Total	G	H	I

Table • 65-3

Example of Chi-Square Table (as Described in Text)

	STRANGLES	HEALTHY	TOTAL
Attended horse show	6	14	20
Did not attend horse show	4	76	80
Total	10	90	100

Is the difference real? If data can be summarized in a 2 × 2 table, a chi-square test can help determine how likely it is that an observed difference is real and not just caused by chance variation. To use the chi-square test, data must be organized in a 2 × 2 table, and the following chi-square values are used: 95% = 3.84; 90% = 2.70; and 80% = 1.64. The 2 × 2 table is constructed as shown in Table 65-2.

Sick/well categories are placed in columns and exposed/unexposed in rows. Sickness goes to the left of health, and exposure (in this case, attending the horse show) goes on top of nonexposure. An example using data from the attack rate table on horses with and without strangles that did and did not attend a recent horse show (see Table 65-1) is shown in Table 65-3.

The chi-square value is calculated by using the following formula:

$$\frac{[(A\times E)-(B\times D)]^2\times I}{C\times F\times G\times H}$$

$$\frac{[(6\times 76)-(14\times 4)]^2\times 100}{20\times 80\times 10\times 90}=\frac{[400]^2\times 100}{1,440,000}=11.11$$

This value is compared to the value obtained with the 80%, 90%, and 95% chi-square values. If the chi-square value is greater than the 95% chi-square value (3.84), there is 95% confidence that the difference is real. If the chi-square value is less than the 95% value but greater than the 90% value (2.70), there is 90% confidence that the difference is real. Similarly, if the chi-square value is less than the 90% value but greater than the 80% value (1.64), there is 80% confidence that the difference is real. In this example, the chi-square value of 11.11 is greater than the 95% value of 3.84, so there is 95% confidence that the difference in strangles occurrence between horses that did and did not attend a recent horse show is real and not caused by chance variation.

PROPERTIES OF DIAGNOSTIC TESTS

In a medical context, a *diagnostic test* can be defined as any process or device designed to detect or quantify a sign, substance, tissue change, or body response[43] and used to gain additional information regarding the health or exposure status of an individual or population. Laboratory tests (e.g., antibody detection, cultures, PCR, histology) and imaging procedures (e.g., plain radiographs, ultrasonography, endoscopy, MRI) are some of the most obvious diagnostic tests used. However, a clinical examination and a questionnaire designed to obtain information about the health status of an individual can also be considered a test. This section focuses on diagnostic tests as they apply to the diagnosis of infectious disease in horses; however, the principles presented here are valid for any other type of test.

Box • 65-11

Sensitivity and Specificity

A study was conducted to estimate the sensitivity and specificity of the Western blot (WB) test for the diagnosis of equine protozoal myeloencephalitis (EPM) caused by *Sarcocystis neurona*.[63] This study included serum samples from 63 neurologic horses necropsied at the California State Laboratory. All horses were evaluated using the "gold standard" method and classified as having or not having *S. neurona* parasites or lesions characteristic of EPM in their central nervous system. Serum samples were tested by the Western blot for detection of antibodies against *S. neurona*. The data are presented below.

Western Blot	Gold Standard Test: Positive	Gold Standard Test: Negative	
Positive	12	30	42
Negative	3	18	21
	15	48	63

$$\text{Sensitivity (Se)} = \frac{12}{15} = 80\% \qquad \text{Specificity (Sp)} = \frac{18}{48} = 38\%$$

$$\text{False-negative (1} - \text{Se)} = \frac{3}{15} = 20\% \qquad \text{False-positive (1} - \text{Sp)} = \frac{30}{48} = 62\%$$

Types of Measurement

Test results can be broadly divided into qualitative and quantitative. *Qualitative* test results are reported in a nominal (positive or negative) or ordinal (positive, weak positive, or negative) scale and most often represent the presence or absence of antibodies or antigens in body fluids or tissues. Examples of qualitative test results in horses include the Western blot test for detection of serum antibodies against *Sarcocystis neurona*[63] and the reverse transcriptase–polymerase chain reaction (RT-PCR) test on nasal swabs for detection of ribonucleic acid (RNA) from equine influenza virus.[60]

Quantitative test results are reported in an interval scale (titers) or continuous scale (e.g., ELISA optical densities, mg/dL) and usually represent direct or indirect measures of antibody, antigen, or enzyme concentrations. Examples include the indirect fluorescent antibody test (IFAT) for detection of serum antibody titers against *S. neurona*,[64] the enzyme-linked immunosorbent assay (ELISA) used to detect antibody concentrations (based on optical densities) against WNV,[65] and liver function tests to detect enzyme concentrations in blood.[66] Quantitative test results are often categorized (dichotomized) into positive or negative to facilitate interpretation of test results and estimate certain test characteristics.

Test Accuracy

Test accuracy is the ability of a test to determine correctly the true status of an individual. In the context of infectious diseases of horses, test accuracy is the ability of the test to differentiate correctly between infected and noninfected horses. Test accuracy is basically determined by two characteristics: sensitivity and specificity. Test *sensitivity* is the proportion of infected horses correctly identified by the test as infected. Test *specificity* is the proportion of noninfected horses correctly identified by the test as noninfected. When sensitivity and specificity are less then 100%, their complement (1 – sensitivity and 1 – specificity) represent the proportion of false-negative and false-positive results, respectively.

Estimation of Sensitivity and Specificity

Diagnostic test sensitivity and specificity should ideally be characterized using appropriately designed, population-based studies (test validation studies).[67] There are several variations in study designs, but in general, these studies should include a representative (e.g., various ages, gender, breeds) random sample of the population of horses in which the test will ultimately be applied.[67] Typically, horses enrolled in validation studies are identified as infected or noninfected based on another diagnostic test that is considered the definitive, "gold standard" test. Traditionally, sensitivity and specificity have often been estimated by comparing test results from the test of interest (often a newly developed test) with the results from the gold standard test in the infected and noninfected groups, respectively (Box 65-11).

Estimation of sensitivity and specificity in Box 65-11 is straightforward because the test results are inherently dichotomous. In such cases the data can be simply cross-tabulated into a 2 × 2 table and the values for sensitivity and specificity calculated. However, when test results are quantitative (e.g., titers, white blood cell counts, optical densities), it is necessary to determine a *cutoff value* for a positive test result in order to estimate test sensitivity and specificity. The choice of a cutoff value is somewhat arbitrary and is affected by the purpose of the testing.[68] For example, in a screening program to detect exposure to some infectious agent, the purpose is to detect all horses possibly exposed to that agent. In such cases, choosing a lower cutoff value will maximize test sensitivity and minimize the number of false-negative results. On the other hand, an equine clinician may want to determine whether a horse is infected with a certain agent, with minimal chances of misclassification. In such cases the cutoff of choice will be the one that maximizes

Box • 65-12

Sensitivity and Specificity: Indirect Fluorescent Antibody Test

A study was designed to evaluate the indirect fluorescent antibody test (IFAT) for the diagnosis of EPM caused by *S. neurona*.[64] The study included serum samples from 109 horses necropsied at the California State Laboratory. All horses were identified as having or not having *S. neurona* parasites in their central nervous system (gold standard test). Serum samples were tested by IFAT for detection of antibody titers against *S. neurona*. The data are presented in Tables A and B below.

Table A. Frequency of IFAT serum titers for horses having or not having *S. neurona* parasites in their central nervous system

IFAT Titer	Gold Standard Positive	Gold Standard Negative
0	0	85
10	0	6
20	2	2
40	0	1
80	4	0
160	3	2
320	2	1
640	1	0
Total	12	97

Table B. Sensitivity and specificity of IFAT using each titer as a potential cutoff value for a positive test result

Cutoff Value for a Positive Result	Sensitivity	Specificity
0	12/12 = 100%	0/97 = 0%
10	12/12 = 100%	85/97 = 88%
20	12/12 = 100%	91/97 = 94%
40	10/12 = 83%	93/97 = 96%
80	9/12 = 75%	93/97 = 96%
160	6/12 = 50%	94/97 = 97%
320	3/12 = 25%	96/97 = 99%
640	1/12 = 8%	97/97 = 100%

In this example, an IFAT titer of 20 was the test result that yielded the lowest combined proportion of false-negative (0%) and false-positive (6%) results and is one potential choice for a cutoff value. Notice that there is a decrease in sensitivity and an increase in specificity as the cutoff value increases. The opposite occurs as the cutoff value decreases.

sensitivity and specificity and minimizes the number of both false-negative and false-positive results. This cutoff value that yields the highest sensitivity and specificity is frequently the choice. To determine that cutoff value, values of sensitivity and specificity are calculated using all test results as possible cutoff values (Box 65-12).

Another option to measure accuracy of a quantitative test is the use of likelihood ratios for specific test results. *Likelihood ratios* measure how likely a specific test result will occur in an infected horse compared with a noninfected horse. Likelihood ratios for specific test results are calculated as the proportion of infected horses that have a certain test result over the proportion of noninfected horses that have that same test result. The advantages of likelihood ratios are that each test result has its own interpretation, and there is no need to choose a cutoff value for a positive test result. Thus there is more flexibility in test interpretation[64] (Box 65-13).

INTERPRETATION OF TEST RESULTS: PREDICTIVE VALUES

The ultimate question to answer after testing a horse for an infectious agent is whether or not that horse is really infected and has a particular disease. If a test could be found that was 100% sensitive and 100% specific, the answer to this question would be straightforward; a positive test result would indicate that a horse is infected, and a negative test result would indicate that a horse is not infected. Unfortunately, although some tests are more accurate than others, probably no tests truly have either 100% sensitivity or 100% specificity. In addition, regardless of how accurate a test is thought to be, the probability that tests will correctly predict disease or infection status is not the same for all populations.

Therefore, we need to understand and use the predictive values to help us correctly interpret test results. Predictive values refer to the probability of being affected/infected given the test result (positive or negative). As such, the *positive predictive value* is the probability that a horse is infected given a positive test result. The *negative predictive value* is the probability that a horse is not infected given a negative test result. Predictive values are calculated as the proportion of truly infected horses among the test-positive horses (positive predictive value) and the proportion of truly noninfected horses among test-negative horses (negative predictive value) (Box 65-14).

At this point, it is important to distinguish between true prevalence (TP) and apparent prevalence (AP). *True prevalence*

Box • 65-13

Likelihood Ratio: Indirect Fluorescent Antibody Test

In the study evaluating the IFAT for the diagnosis of EPM, titer-specific likelihood ratios were calculated.[64] Frequency of IFAT titers in *S. neurona*–infected and noninfected ("gold standard") horses and titer-specific likelihood ratios are presented below.

IFAT Titer	Gold Standard Positive	Gold Standard Negative	Likelihood Ratio
0	0	85	0.03
10	0	6	0.7
20	2	2	1.7
40	0	1	4.4
80	4	0	11.2
160	3	2	28.7
320	2	1	73.4
640	1	0	187.8
Total	12	97	

A likelihood ratio (LR) of 0.7 for an IFAT titer of 10 indicates that a titer 10 is 1.4 (1/0.7) times more likely in noninfected horses than in infected horses. On the other hand, a LR of 4.4 for a titer of 40 indicates that a titer 40 is 4.4 times more likely in infected horses than in noninfected horses. In this study, because of zero counts for some titers in both groups, a more sophisticated modeling technique was used to calculate the likelihood ratios and "smooth out" the data.[64] However, the basic principle of LR calculations can be illustrated using the non-zero cells as an example. For example, the LR for a titer of 20 would be calculated as the proportion of infected horses with a titer 20 (2/12) over the proportion of noninfected horses with that same titer (2/97).

Box • 65-14

Predictive Value: Western Blot

From Box 65-11, data on serum Western blot test results for 63 neurologic horses identified as having ("gold standard" positive) or not having ("gold standard" negative) *S. neurona* in the central nervous system are presented below.[63] Positive and negative predictive values were calculated.

Western Blot	Gold Standard Positive	Gold Standard Negative	
Positive	12	30	42
Negative	3	18	21
	15	48	63

$$\text{Positive predictive value} = \frac{12}{42} = 29\% \quad \text{Negative predictive value} = \frac{18}{21} = 86\%$$

In this example, only 29% of the test-positive horses were actually infected with *S. neurona*, whereas 86% of the test-negative horses were truly noninfected.

is the proportion of horses that actually have the infection or disease in the population, whereas *apparent prevalence* is the proportion of horses that test positive for the infection or disease.[43] True prevalence is the prevalence value used in calculating predictive values. In Box 65-14, TP was 24% (15/63), whereas AP was 67% (42/63). The true prevalence and apparent prevalence relate to each other as follows:

$$\text{True Prevalence} = \frac{\text{Apparent Prevalence} + \text{Specificity} - 1}{\text{Sensitivity} + \text{Specificity} - 1}$$

Notice that if the sensitivity and specificity are 100%, the true prevalence and apparent prevalence are equal.

Predictive values can be directly calculated only from 2 × 2 tables when the study is conducted using a representative sample of the population, because in such cases the prevalence of the disease in the study group is an unbiased estimate of the prevalence of disease in the population. When this is not the case, the predictive values from 2 × 2 tables will be biased and should be calculated using an independent prevalence estimate by the following formulas:

$$\text{Positive predictive value} = \frac{\text{Prevalence} \times \text{Sensitivity}}{(\text{Prevalence} \times \text{Sensitivity}) + (1\text{-Prevalence}) \times (1\text{-Specificity})}$$

$$\text{Negative predictive value} = \frac{(1\text{-Prevalence}) \times (\text{Specificity})}{[(1\text{-Prevalence}) \times (\text{Specificity})] + [(\text{Prevalence}) \times (1\text{-Sensitvity})]}$$

Predictive values are greatly affected by differences in test sensitivity, test specificity, and prevalence of disease in the population. For fixed values of sensitivity and specificity, the positive predictive value increases and the predictive value negative decreases as the prevalence increases (Fig. 65-4). This means that even when sensitivity and specificity are high, the probability of infection given a positive test result is low when the prevalence is low, and probability of infection is high when the prevalence is high. Similarly, the probability of no infection given a negative test result is high when the prevalence is low and low when prevalence is high (Box 65-15).

When likelihood ratios for specific test results are used instead of sensitivity and specificity, the probability of disease for each specific test result can be calculated using the following formula:

$$\text{Probability of disease given a specific test result} = \frac{\left(\dfrac{\text{Prevalence}}{1-P}\right) \times \text{Likelihood ratio}}{\left(\dfrac{\text{Prevalence}}{1-\text{Prevalence}} \times \text{Likelihood ratio}\right) + 1}$$

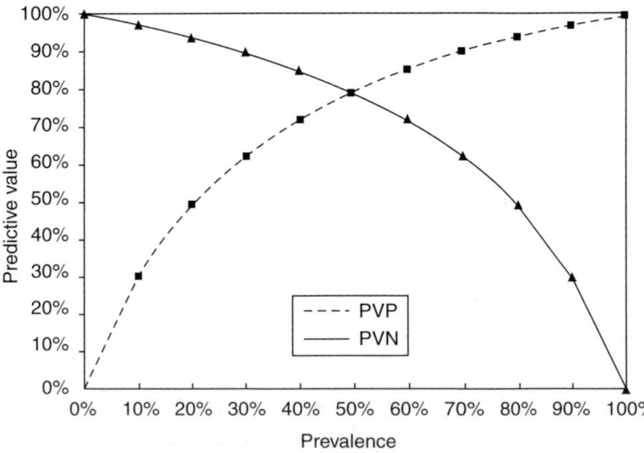

Fig. 65-4 Relationship among positive predictive value *(PVP)*, negative predictive value *(PVN)*, and prevalence.

Using Tests in Combination

Frequently, two or more tests are used in the diagnosis of disease or infection. The tests can be used simultaneously or in sequence, and the results can be interpreted in parallel or in series. In *parallel* interpretation, horses testing positive in one or more tests are considered positive.[43] For example, horses might be considered infected with *Salmonella enteritidis* after testing positive in at least one of several fecal cultures performed in sequence. In *series* interpretation, horses are considered positive only if they test positive in all tests.[43] For example, horses tested for EPM might be considered infected only if they test positive for *S. neurona* antibodies in serum and in cerebrospinal fluid (CSF). Note that the serum and CSF tests can be run simultaneously or in sequence when a CSF test is run only in seropositive horses. When multiple tests are used, the sensitivity and specificity of the combination of tests are different than the sensitivity and specificity of each test separately. In parallel interpretation the combination of tests has higher sensitivity but lower specificity than each individual test. In series interpretation the combination of tests has lower sensitivity and higher specificity than each individual test.

Other Diagnostic Test Characteristics

Other characteristics of diagnostic tests that should be evaluated before or concomitantly with population-based accuracy studies include analytical sensitivity and specificity and reliability. *Analytical sensitivity* indicates the minimum detectable amount of the material (e.g., antibodies, antigens) being measured by the test. *Analytical specificity* indicates the potential for cross-reactivity with materials of no interest. Analytical sensitivity and specificity are assessed in laboratory conditions and affect the population estimates of sensitivity and specificity; however, they are different quantities. For example, information on the minimum amount of serum antibodies detected by an ELISA test for the diagnosis of a certain disease might be important to establish the optimum serum dilution to be used in the plaques when testing field samples. Similarly, samples from animals infected with various potential cross-reacting agents should be tested to assess occurrence of false-positive results.

Reliability is the ability of the test to produce the same results when samples are tested multiple times in the same laboratory (repeatability) or in different laboratories (reproducibility).[43] There are various measures of reliability, including the coefficient of variation and the correlation coefficient for quantitative tests and the kappa measure of agreement for qualitative tests.[43]

Overall, these measures assess how concordant test results are in multiple testing.

STRATEGIES FOR PREVENTION OF INFECTIOUS DISEASE

In general, prevention of infectious disease involves altering the host, agent, or environment to make it more difficult for disease to occur or spread. We usually have little control over the disease agent, so we focus on the disease host (the horse) and its environment. A herd is best able to resist infection if the horses in it are immunized, properly nourished, and minimally stressed. An environment in which new equine arrivals are quarantined, tested for disease, and immunized before mixing with the herd minimizes the likelihood of introduction of a new disease, as does an environment where contact between disease vectors (e.g., mosquitoes, ticks) and horses is minimized. Disease spread is more easily controlled in

Box • 65-15

Predictive Value: Enzyme-Linked Immunosorbent Assay

Assume a hypothetical scenario where two populations of neurologic horses (i.e., from two veterinary hospitals in different parts of the country) were serologically tested for diagnosis of West Nile virus (WNV) infection. In Population 1, independent virus isolation studies have shown that the true prevalence of WNV is 1%, and in Population 2 the same studies have shown that WNV true prevalence is 90%. Both populations were tested with the same test, an enzyme-linked immunosorbent assay (ELISA), for detection of antibodies against WNV and determination of the infection status. Assume that the test has been shown to be 90% sensitive and 90% specific and that 1000 horses from each population were tested. The 2 × 2 tables below show the data for each population. The data in each cell of these 2 × 2 tables were distributed based on the prevalence and test characteristic information.

Population 1

		Infected		
		Yes	**No**	
ELISA	**Positive**	**9**	**99**	**108**
	Negative	**1**	**891**	**892**
		10	**900**	**1000**

$$\text{Positive predictive value} = \frac{9}{108} \cong 8\% \qquad \text{Negative predictive value} = \frac{891}{892} \cong 99\%$$

Population 2

		Infected		
		Yes	**No**	
ELISA	**Positive**	**810**	**10**	**820**
	Negative	**90**	**90**	**180**
		900	**100**	**1000**

$$\text{Positive predictive value} = \frac{810}{820} \cong 99\%$$

$$\text{Negative predictive value} = \frac{90}{180} = 50\%$$

Despite the use of the same test, the probability that a test-positive horse is infected in Population 1 is only 8%, compared with the 99% in Population 2. This means that the majority (99/108) of the test-positive horses in Population 1 were actually false-positive results. Similarly, the probability that a test-negative horse is actually not infected in Population 1 is 99% versus 50% in Population 2. Therefore, 50% of the test-negative horses in Population 2 were actually infected and were false-negative results.

a well-ventilated environment with easily cleanable, nonporous surfaces. Standing water in which mosquitoes breed should be minimized. Water and feed troughs should be cleaned regularly; a contaminated trough can quickly amplify an outbreak of salmonellosis or strangles.

To prevent the arrival or spread of a specific infectious disease, an understanding of the disease's life cycle and risk factors is important. How do horses become infected? Through a vector, as with WNV encephalitis? By direct contact, as with equine influenza? By indirect contact, as with salmonellosis? Through aerosol spread, as with equine influenza? Minimize horses' exposure to the source of infection. How pathogenic or virulent is the disease? Does it have a lengthy incubation period, or a carrier or persistently infected state (e.g., strangles)? Identify and isolate or treat asymptomatic horses that may be sources of infection. Does the disease agent survive in the environment (e.g., *Salmonella*)? If so, institute biosecurity measures such as foot baths to minimize environmental contamination. What are known risk factors for the disease? Is it associated with pasture grazing, as with MRLS or strongyles? Change management as necessary to minimize known risk factors for the disease.

MANAGING AN OUTBREAK OF INFECTIOUS DISEASE

An outbreak investigation is a systematic approach to identifying the cause(s) and source(s) of an epidemic (see Chapter 67). The goals of an outbreak investigation are to identify the problem, identify steps that can be taken immediately to deal with the problem, and identify means by which future outbreaks can be prevented. The standard steps in an outbreak investigation are described next.

Make a diagnosis. After initial contact with the client, review relevant diagnoses before a farm visit. For each potential diagnosis, review the biology, epidemiology, diagnostic method, and treatment. At the farm, listen carefully and say nothing that might influence your client's perception of events. Take samples as needed, look for patterns that may be relevant, and define natural groups (housing, use, age, gender, or breed) that should be compared. Use clinical observations and test results to make a tentative diagnosis. If the initial diagnosis is a zoonotic or reportable disease, take appropriate action.

Verify the diagnosis. When a tentative or final diagnosis of disease has been made, ensure that it is medically sound. Use medical records, laboratory test results, and clinical examinations to confirm that the diagnosis is consistent with the information available. If the data are not consistent with the diagnosis, seek a better diagnosis.

Define a "case." To facilitate identification of cases associated with the outbreak, specify the clinical signs and test results that define a case of disease. Some illness in the population may be unrelated to the outbreak. By defining an outbreak-associated "case" of disease, unrelated illnesses may be excluded from analysis.

Determine the magnitude of the problem. Is there an epidemic? Are more horses affected by this disease than typically seen? Compute an attack rate, as described earlier, and compare it to the normal or expected occurrence of disease, if known.

Describe the outbreak temporally, spatially, and by animal characteristics. Examine the temporal characteristics of the outbreak by creating an epidemic curve (see Temporal Patterns of Disease). Use the client's calendar to obtain the most accurate information on disease onset. Does it appear to be a point-source or a propagated epidemic? Does disease onset coincide with any management changes or recent additions to the farm? Describe disease spatially by making a map recording the total number of horses in each region (e.g., field, pasture, barn, farm) and the number of ill horses in each region. Be sure to record the location of feed and water sources on the map, as well as locations where horses might come in contact with wildlife or other livestock species. Record age, gender, breed, vaccination status, use, housing type, location, and feed and water sources of all animals in the population—those unaffected as well as those affected.

Analyze data. For each factor of interest (age, gender, breed, vaccination status, use, housing type, location, feed and water sources), construct an attack risk table, as described earlier. Look for differences among groups. Which factor has the strongest association?

Working hypothesis. Based on data analyses, develop hypotheses regarding the type of epidemic that is occurring (point-source vs. propagated), the source of the epidemic, and possible modes of spread (e.g., direct contact, vector, fomites).

Implement disease controls. Standard disease control measures include mass treatment, quarantine, environmental hygiene, mass immunization, and applied ecology.[69] *Mass treatment*, such as administration of antimicrobials during a *Salmonella* outbreak, is intended to reduce transmission of disease by decreasing the amount and duration of shedding by infectious individuals and decreasing the likelihood of infection in susceptible animals. *Quarantine* restricts movement of horses suspected of being infectious; it is intended to reduce the likelihood that infected horses will come in contact with susceptible horses. *Environmental hygiene* incorporates actions that remove or prevent environmental contamination, reducing the likelihood of disease exposure for horses in that environment; use appropriate cleaning agents, and rinse thoroughly. *Mass immunization* (vaccination) acts to decrease the susceptibility of both the individual horse and the herd (through herd immunity). *Applied ecology* refers to disease control methods that target some factor other than the disease agent, such as the vector or the disease reservoir; the goal is to reduce the likelihood that horses will be exposed to disease. To apply these methods, an understanding of the disease's life cycle is important.

Intensive follow-up. Intensive follow-up includes confirmation of the diagnosis (clinical, pathologic, or microbiologic data) and confirmation of the disease source (microbiologic or toxicologic examination of feeds, fomites, or suspect carrier horses) if possible. Detailed diagrams or flowcharts of animal movements or feed preparation and distribution may be helpful in identifying points where preventive measures could be implemented.

Report. Summarize findings, and present them to the client. Colleagues and local veterinary associations may also be interested in the investigation and its results.

REFERENCES

See the CD-ROM for a list of references linked to the abstract in PubMed.

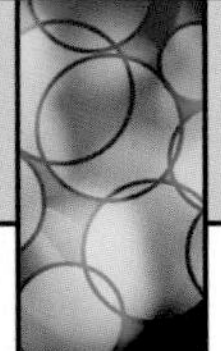

CHAPTER • 66

Biosecurity

Magdalena Dunowska, Paul S. Morley, Josie L. Traub-Dargatz, and David C. VanMetre

OVERVIEW AND VETERINARIAN'S ROLE

The importance of control measures for prevention of infectious diseases in individuals and populations has been realized for centuries, long before the modern microbiologic era. Throughout this chapter, we use the term "biosecurity" interchangeably with "infection control" to encompass all practices intended to prevent introduction and spread of infectious diseases within a group of equine patients and their human caregivers. Although used frequently by a variety of groups, the term *biosecurity* is not defined in any of the commonly used English dictionaries. Traditionally, biosecurity focused on prevention of the introduction of a disease agent into a population, whereas *biocontainment* focused on control of spread of the agent once introduced. Although this distinction is reasonably straightforward with relation to a unit such as a farm, a breeding station, or even a country, it is more difficult to separate "biosecurity" from "biocontainment" in the environment of an equine veterinary clinic, where disease agents are introduced and dealt with on a daily basis. Recently, the word "biosecurity" has been defined in a broader term as "work of strategy, efforts, and planning to protect human, animal, and environmental health against biological threats."[1]

The need for infection control in human medical settings first became broadly recognized during the nineteenth century.[2] Hospital-acquired or community-acquired infections have long been perceived as important problems for hospitals, day care centers, hospice or geriatric care centers, and similar institutions.[3-5] In the United States, national surveillance for human hospital-associated infections using standardized methods was first implemented in 1970. Such surveillance provided a basis for development of control strategies, which ultimately resulted in improved quality of patient care, as measured by reduced infection rates, reduced morbidity and mortality, improved patient and hospital personnel safety, and reduced costs of hospitalization.[6-8]

Protecting the public health and promoting animal well-being are part of the veterinarians' oath[9] and have always been taken very seriously. Veterinarians have been recognized for their leadership role in control of zoonoses and food-borne diseases. However, concerns regarding nosocomial infections in veterinary hospitals have lagged behind those for human health care settings, despite veterinarians facing similar challenges associated with nosocomial infections in their patients, in addition to risk of zoonotic disease in caregivers and clients. As awareness increases among veterinary clinicians and their clients, infection control strategies at veterinary care facilities for horses and other animal species will develop in a manner similar to the advancement seen in human health care settings. A survey conducted in 2004 among equine veterinary hospitals indicated that all veterinary teaching hospitals in North America and many in other regions have implemented some type of infection control program, as have some of the more progressive private veterinary hospitals.[2] As an indication of the rising prominence of this aspect of veterinary medicine, the Dorothy Russell Havermeyer Foundation sponsored a workshop dedicated solely to the topic of biosecurity and infection control in equine hospitals. This workshop resulted in the creation of the Veterinary Infection Control Society and publication of an issue of *Veterinary Clinics of North America: Equine Practice* dedicated to this topic[10] (P.S. Morley, personal communication, 2005).

IMPORTANCE OF BIOSECURITY

Quality of Care and Liability

Application of the concepts of biosecurity and biocontainment is important not only in veterinary hospitals, but also for ambulatory practices, equine breeding facilities, training facilities, and any other facilities that house horse populations. Contagious diseases can significantly endanger the well-being of horses in addition to having potentially devastating financial and emotional effects. As such, a high standard of care cannot be attained without addressing strategies to control selected infectious diseases.

There is an inherent risk of nosocomial infection for any hospitalized patient, and therefore it is the hospital's obligation to implement practices that will minimize those risks. According to a survey conducted among veterinary teaching hospitals in 1997, 12 of 18 responders reported 18 outbreaks of nosocomial disease between 1985 and 1996. Six of these outbreaks resulted in hospital closure, with conservative estimates of cost ranging from $10,000 to $550,000.[11] These estimates did not include indirect costs related to loss of client-provider relationships, emotional stress inflicted on horse owners, loss of learning opportunity for students and residents, diminished morale of hospital staff and clinicians, and "bad" publicity. At the same time, even with well-developed infection control programs, it may not be possible to eliminate all nosocomial infections. Therefore, it is important to recognize that occasional nosocomial infections will occur even in hospitals that provide excellent quality care for their patients.

Nosocomial infections and iatrogenic injury (e.g., fractures) have been listed as one of the top 10 reasons for malpractice claims against human hospitals, and these cases were more likely to be adjudicated in favor of the patients than were all other types of cases.[12] In the past, veterinary clients seemed to be more "forgiving" and willing to accept some risk of nosocomial infections as being normal. This attitude is changing, however, and it is increasingly likely that equine hospitals will face legal claims associated with nosocomial infection, and that these claims will inevitably lead to significant costs in both monetary and professional terms. It will therefore become increasingly necessary to develop comprehensive infection control plans to manage this risk.

Zoonotic Infections

Another important aspect of biosecurity is prevention of zoonotic infections. People working with animals have inherently increased risks of infection with zoonotic agents compared to the general public.[13] Considering the wide variety of microbial agents that may infect horses, a relatively small number can be transmitted from horses to people, but these zoonotic infections may be devastating for affected individuals.[14] This creates the potential for liability among veterinarians when people interact with animals in the hospital environment or because of the instructions or recommendations made by the veterinarians. This aspect of liability becomes particularly important as the percentage of the general public at increased risk, or those with some degree of immunocompromise, increases for a variety of reasons, including steroid treatment, cancer treatment, and chronic illness (e.g., infection with HIV or other agents); very young and elderly persons are also at increased risk.

Although the risks of acquiring a zoonotic infection from horses are generally low, a number of known and emerging pathogens can affect both horses and humans.[15] In the United States the three agents most likely to pose a threat of zoonotic transmission (particularly to immunocompromised individuals) include *Salmonella enterica*, *Rhodococcus equi*, and methicillin-resistant *Staphylococcus aureus* (MRSA).[14] *R. equi* was regarded as an equine-specific pathogen until recent reports of *R. equi* infections in immunocompromised people; contact with horses is not a clear risk factor for this infection in humans.[16-18] Similarly, MRSA infection in horses and potential transmission between horses and people have been described only recently.[19,20] Several equine viruses that cause encephalitis can affect both people and horses. Horses are usually "dead-end" hosts, with the exception of Venezuelan equine encephalitis, which can be transmitted from equids to humans.[21] Although rabies is relatively infrequent among horses, it should be considered as one of the differential diagnoses in all cases of progressive neurologic disease.[31,32] Reports have also described possible zoonotic transmission from a horse of *Trichophyton equinum*,[22,23] *Cryptosporidium parvum*,[24-26] *Microsporum equinum*,[27] *Streptococcus equi* subsp. *zooepidemicus*,[28] and *Pasteurella caballi*.[29] In one study, isolation of *Clostridium difficile* from an equine hospital environment suggested that there was a potential risk of zoonotic infection.[30]

The emergence of Hendra virus in Australia dramatically demonstrates the importance of maintaining standard infection control precautions.[33-35] One of the human patients who died from Hendra virus infection assisted in necropsies of affected horses without using barrier precautions, such as gloves, masks, and protective eyewear.[14] This incident emphasizes the importance of maintaining high levels of infection control as standard practice, because it is likely that new infectious agents will be encountered in the future.

Similarly, pathogens of historical significance may reemerge as threats to human health. The extreme example of this is the emergence of biologic materials as potential bioterrorism agents, most of which are zooneses.[36] The organism *Burkholderia mallei*, the equine pathogen that causes glanders, is listed as a select agent for potential as a biologic weapon.[14] The ability to recognize animals with clinical signs consistent with diseases such as glanders and to stop spread of a bioterrorism agent among animals or between animals and humans may be very important in a potential outbreak situation.

Antimicrobial Resistance

Antimicrobial resistance is an emerging problem that affects our ability to treat individual patients (whether animals or humans), affects the control of disease in animal populations, and has significant public health implications. Antimicrobial resistance arises from interaction between bacteria and antimicrobial agents. Theoretically, all uses of antimicrobial drugs have the potential to promote the evolution of resistance in bacterial populations. Antimicrobial drugs provide a survival advantage for bacteria that are resistant to the drug used for treatment, which in turn promotes propagation of the genetic traits conferring this resistance. Drug resistance can develop stepwise by the accumulation of chromosomal mutations, or resistance genes can be transferred between bacteria from different taxonomic and ecologic groups by means of mobile genetic elements such as plasmids, transposons, or bacteriophages. Resistance genes acquired through these mobile elements are often linked together, so selection for resistance to one antimicrobial can promote resistance to a number of other antimicrobial drugs, with development of multidrug-resistant strains.[37] In addition, genes rendering bacteria resistant to disinfectants (e.g., quaternary ammonium products) can be located on the same plasmid as antimicrobial drug resistance genes, therefore providing a survival advantage in the hospital environment to resistant bacteria.[38]

As noted in human hospitals, many of the nosocomial pathogens associated with equine hospitals also are multidrug resistant. This may be caused by high selection pressures applied through common use of antimicrobial drugs and disinfectants in hospital environments.[20,39] In addition, many bacteria are very efficient at forming biofilms in the environment. These *biofilms* consist of an extracellular matrix that is produced by organized bacterial communities attached to a surface. Organization of bacteria in biofilms enhances their survival from a variety of environmental insults, including disinfectants and other antimicrobial treatments.[40-47a] Because bacteria in biofilms survive well in the environment, they may provide a continuous source of infectious pathogens that can cause nosocomial infections.

Several actions can be taken to minimize the impact of antimicrobial use. On one level, although antimicrobial drugs should be used when needed to aid the health of animals, they also should be used as conservatively as possible in accordance with published guidelines.[48,49] Inevitably, however, bacteria will be exposed to antimicrobial drugs and disinfectants in hospitals, so patients will be exposed to resistant microorganisms in the hospital environment. Therefore it is essential that appropriate infection control precautions be used to help prevent spread of such agents from patient to patient and between patients and caregivers, as well as to help prevent resistant bacteria from establishing themselves in the environment.

METHODS FOR DESIGN OF AN EFFECTIVE BIOSECURITY PROGRAM

In designing a biosecurity program for an equine facility, it may be useful to apply a systematic approach, such as the Hazard Analysis and Critical Control Point (HACCP) system. The application of HACCP principles to biosecurity programs in veterinary hospitals and clinics has been described in detail.[11] Most of the examples in this section address veterinary clinics. However, infection control programs must be tailored to each individual operation, and the same general principles guiding design of a hospital infection control program can be applied to any facility with a number of horses on the operation, whether an adjustment facility, a riding or boarding facility, or a breeding farm. Although the choice of rules governing infection control will vary between facilities, it is important that the rules are designed with all animals in mind, not only those suspected of having an infectious disease. For example, implementation of hand hygiene protocols and use of clean clothing and equipment should be encouraged as a part of basic standard care. Good biosecurity practices may prevent the spread of infectious agents from subclinical shedders of infectious agents that do not show overt clinical signs of disease.

Risks and Hazards

The first step in any control efforts should be to identify risks and hazards specific for a given facility. The pathogens and diseases considered for control should include those that are zoonotic, those foreign to a given region, diseases with a high risk of nosocomial transmission between patients, and those likely to have an impact on patient welfare and management. The contagious pathogens likely to be of importance for equine facilities in North America include *Salmonella enterica*, equine influenza virus, equine herpesviruses, *Streptococcus equi* subsp. *equi*, *Clostridium difficile*, multidrug-resistant enteric bacteria that can cause incisional or wound infections, rabies virus, rotavirus, and MRSA. Veterinarians are legally and ethically obliged to make reasonable attempts to protect themselves, their families, clients, and employees from the potentially serious consequences of acquiring a zoonotic infection.

In addition, several diseases foreign to a given region should be considered in a control program. The most important diseases will vary with the geographic location of an equine establishment. For example, at the Colorado State University Veterinary Teaching Hospital (CSU-VTH), these include foot-and-mouth disease (FMD) and vesicular stomatitis (VS). As such, appropriate precautions are instituted during periodic outbreaks of VS in the region. Also, all visitors to CSU-VTH are asked to disclose recent foreign travel in an effort to exclude the possibility of FMD virus exposure.[11]

Control Points

The next step in designing a biosecurity protocol for an equine establishment is to identify the areas or processes where transmission of pathogens is likely to occur (control points) and implement measures aimed at minimizing the possibility of such transmission. Despite the existence of a large number of agents that pose a potential threat to the well-being of horses and their human care providers, there are some common features in the way these pathogens are spread and transmitted. The three main types of infection important from a biosecurity point of view are gastrointestinal (GI), respiratory, and surgical infections. Thus, efforts designed to minimize the spread of GI pathogens will likely be similar for all potential agents that have similar routes of transmission. Similarly, efforts designed to minimize nosocomial respiratory or surgical infections will likely be applicable to a variety of agents spread via these routes. The physical areas that should be targeted in a biosecurity program will vary between establishments, but usually these will include areas where the most susceptible animals (e.g., severely ill, immunocompromised, young, surgical patients) and animals most likely to be shedding contagious pathogens are housed (e.g., critical care or isolation units), away from high-traffic areas such as waiting rooms, examination rooms, and surgery. For an ambulatory practice, the focus should be prevention of spread of infectious agents from sick to healthy horses on a given equine facility and, as ambulatory practitioners, between facilities (see later discussion).

Preventive Measures

Several preventive measures can be implemented to minimize risks of nosocomial spread of infectious diseases between animals and from animals to humans.

Hand Hygiene

Hand hygiene is a proven aid to preventing transmission of infectious agents.[50] Personnel in contact with horses should maintain short fingernails to minimize accumulation of contaminants underneath fingernails and to facilitate effective hand hygiene. Hands should be washed before and after attending each individual animal. Gloves should be used in addition to, rather than instead of, good hand hygiene practices. Clean areas (e.g., doorknobs, drawer or cabinet handles or contents, equipment, medical records) should not be touched with soiled hands or gloves. Although handwashing is an effective way to control spread of infectious agents, frequent handwashing can also lead to skin damage and increased risks of colonization of hands with bacteria.[51] Therefore it is important to provide not only soap and water to all employees of any equine establishment, but also lotions and moisturizers to promote frequent hand hygiene and maintenance of healthy skin.

In addition to soap and water, alcohol-based hand sanitizers can be a useful adjunct to handwashing in veterinary hospitals and can provide a practical option for improving hand hygiene for ambulatory clinicians (Fig. 66-1). Alcohol rubs are as effective as or more effective than handwashing in reducing bacterial contamination on hands when evaluated after study subjects performed physical examinations on horses.[52] Alcohol can also be used in situations where fresh water is not easily available, such as at the stall side during a sporting event or in transit. Dispensers for hand-sanitizing solutions can be easily installed in any equine barn, and their frequent use should be encouraged to minimize potential spread of infectious agents. In particular, they should be used after handling any sick horses or quarantined horses. The cost associated with the use of alcohol hand rubs is less than that associated with products needed for handwashing.[53]

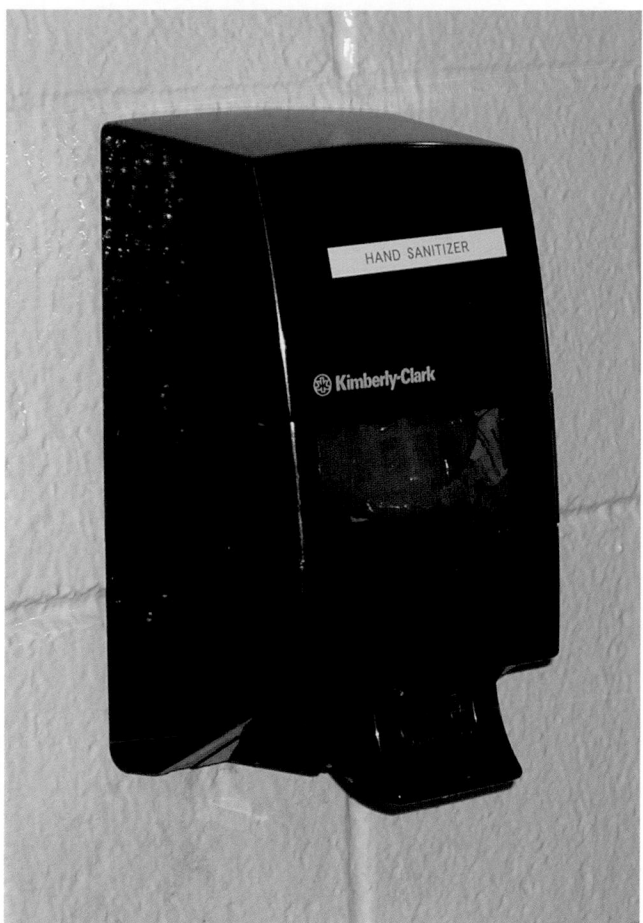

Fig. 66-1 Hand sanitizer on wall at Colorado State University Veterinary Teaching Hospital (CSU-VTH).

Protective Clothing

Daily attire for hospital personnel should be neat, clean, and professional. Footwear must be safe, protective, and cleanable. Footwear should not be constructed of a porous or absorbent material. Closed-toe footwear is strongly recommended for all hospital personnel. Standard outerwear should be clean and should be changed if contamination occurs. It should be a standard recommendation that personnel wear dedicated clothing and footwear in high-risk areas, such as isolation, intensive care, or foaling facilities. Designated surgical scrub clothes and dedicated shoes or protective shoe covers should be worn while working in surgery areas.

Barrier Nursing

Barrier nursing is another proven step in preventing the transmission of infectious agents[54] (Fig. 66-2). In veterinary settings, this usually includes the use of disposable gowns, gloves, masks, and footbaths to prevent movement of organisms from one patient to another. This technique should be used in all isolation areas and for patients with special needs (e.g. foals, immunocompromised patients). Different practices have preferences as to how barrier nursing is accomplished. For example, opinions vary regarding the use of disposable plastic boots versus reusable rubber overboots. Similarly, opinions regarding efficacy of disinfectant footmats or footbaths vary among practitioners. In most situations, barrier precautions are effective if they are implemented in a knowledgeable way and all personnel understand the rationale behind their use. For example, disposable gloves will be ineffective as barrier precautions if the same pair is used on a number of animals. Gloves will serve their purpose only if they are used when working with one patient and then disposed of immediately when such contact is finished. Specifically, gloves

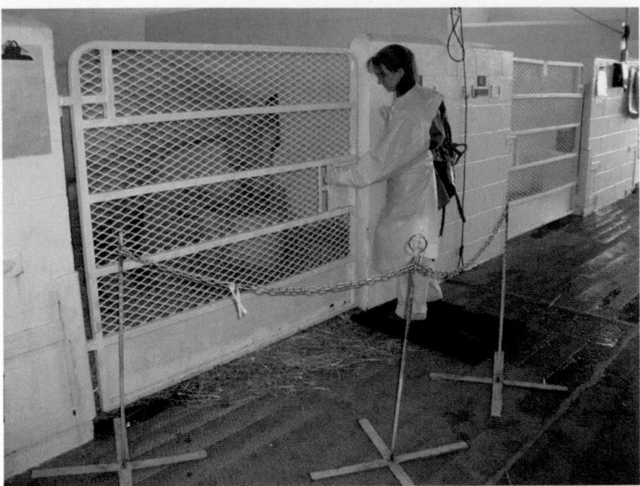

Fig. 66-2 Student working with horse under barrier precautions in main hospital at CSU-VTH. The student is wearing disposable gloves and a disposable gown. The chain barricade is placed around the stall to limit traffic, and a disinfectant foot mat is placed at the entry to the stall.

that have been used to examine or treat a patient should be taken off before reaching for any supplies from a common shelf or drawer, before answering a phone, or before entering data on a computer.

Care should be taken not to contaminate one's hands or clothing while taking off protective garments. It is easy for such a contamination to occur, for example, when taking off either reusable or disposable shoe covers. All personnel must be aware of which areas or materials are thought to have different likelihood of contamination (i.e., the distinction between "clean" and "dirty") and make every effort to keep "clean" areas (including clothing, equipment, and supplies) free of contamination. It is equally important for all personnel to be able to recognize when contamination might have occurred so that appropriate actions can be taken to avoid transmission of the contaminants to another area (e.g., change of clothing, disinfection of contaminated supplies, disinfection of hands).

Area Separation

Establishment of separate areas within a veterinary hospital with different levels of biosecurity precautions for patients in these areas is a useful strategy. The number of areas and level of separation that could be achieved will be dictated by the physical and operational limitations of any given facility. The most common separated areas include large and small animal facilities (in a mixed-animal practice), critical care units, and isolation units. Personnel and equipment movement between different biosecurity areas should be limited or prohibited. Similarly, separated areas for the purpose of division of the animals can be established on any equine facility. For example, on a breeding farm, such areas may include those that house pregnant mares, foaling mares, mares and foals, weanlings, and yearlings. The movement of personnel and equipment between these areas should be minimized or, at the minimum, governed by clearly defined procedural protocols (e.g., use of protective clothing and gloves for patient contact, hand-washing, disinfection of equipment between patients).

Cleaning and Disinfection

Effective cleaning and disinfection are critical for breaking transmission cycles for contagious agents.[55] With this in mind, it is critical that cleanable surfaces be maintained throughout any equine facility, particularly equine hospitals. Use of dirt floors or porous surfaces (e.g., untreated wood) should be avoided because these cannot be effectively disinfected. If porous surfaces are present, they can be rendered less porous by certain treatments, such as painting or sealing the surface.[56,57] Care should be taken to ensure that proper dilutions of disinfectants are used and that the disinfectant used is effective against the pathogens in question. The latter becomes particularly important with difficult-to-kill pathogens such as parvovirus or rotavirus. Also, it is important to make sure that the product used is registered with the U.S. Environmental Protection Agency (EPA) and that all safety precautions recommended by the manufacturer are followed. All disinfectants should be stored in a safe place, particularly when access by children or domestic pets is a possibility.

A number of commercial products are available for environmental disinfection. It is beyond the scope of this chapter to review all available products, but it is important for personnel responsible for choosing these products to be familiar with major groups of disinfectants, their efficacy against different classes of pathogens, and conditions that limit their effectiveness[56,58] (Table 66-1). For example, temperature can greatly affect the efficacy of some products, which is an important consideration when disinfectants are applied in areas that are not climate controlled. It is imperative that all surfaces are thoroughly cleaned before any disinfectant is applied. Applying disinfectant to soiled surfaces, such as those grossly contaminated with feces or nasal exudates, will likely be ineffective because most disinfectants have diminished or reduced efficacy in the presence of organic matter.[55]

Proper cleaning and disinfection should be employed regularly for areas used to house and manage *all* patients, not only those known to be or suspected of being infected with contagious agents. For example, all stalls should be routinely cleaned and disinfected between patients. Proper disinfection helps to minimize bacterial environmental burden and accumulation of resistant flora that may serve as a source of antimicrobial resistance genes to pathogenic organisms (see Antimicrobial Resistance). Proper cleaning and disinfection are of primary importance when dealing with patients that may be shedding infectious agents. All areas that these patients contact (e.g., examination rooms, surgery suites) should be cleaned and disinfected immediately after use to minimize inadvertent tracking of the infectious agent from contaminated to clean areas. It is critical that any equipment in contact with animals having an infectious disease be cleaned and disinfected before reuse and that these items be handled so as to prevent contamination of the hospital surfaces. For example, a rectal thermometer used to check the temperature of a horse with salmonellosis can contaminate the hands of personnel as well as any surface where it is laid if not promptly cleaned and disinfected or discarded.[59]

In addition to traditional surface disinfection, aerosol application or "fogging" with a disinfectant may be considered for control of airborne infections or difficult-to-reach areas such as ceiling areas or overhead beams[60,61] (Fig. 66-3). This approach is not a panacea and does not negate the importance of appropriate cleaning, but it may be a useful adjunct to cleaning and more traditional methods of disinfection. The use of aerosolized compounds should be performed with appropriate respiratory protection for personnel.

Use of Pasture

Although pasture or open paddocks in many ways may be optimal housing environments for horses, they are impossible to disinfect. Therefore the use of pasture for horses with

Table • 66-1

Common Disinfectants Used in Veterinary Medicine

CLASS	DISINFECTANT	APPLICATION IN VETERINARY MEDICINE	ACTIVITY IN ORGANIC MATERIAL	COMMENTS
Acids	Acetic acid, citric acid	Disinfectants for foot-and-mouth disease virus	Poor	Nontoxic and nonirritating at typical dilutions.
	Lactic acid	Carcass decontamination	Poor	Nontoxic and nonirritating at typical dilutions. Immediate bactericidal effect and delayed bacteriostatic effect result in extended shelf life of meat and decreased risk of food-borne pathogen transmission.
Alcohols	Ethanol, methanol, isopropanol	Surface disinfectants, topical antiseptics, hand-sanitizing lotions	Very poor	High concentrations for effective use in most situations as a germicide. Commercially available hand-sanitizing lotions have been shown to greatly reduce bacterial counts on skin; also effective against many viruses. Highly flammable. Irritating to injured skin, but low toxicity.
Aldehydes	Formaldehyde	Surface disinfectant, fumigant	High	Highly irritating and toxic, both through contact and fumes. Exposure to formaldehyde vapor has associated carcinogenic risk. Contact sensitization can develop rapidly. Active against nonenveloped viruses, and glutaraldehyde is an effective sporicide with sufficient contact. Noncorrosive on metals, rubber, plastics, lenses, and cements. Activity of aldehydes is significantly compromised at lower temperatures. Glutaraldehyde is most active at alkaline pH.
	Glutaraldehyde	Surface disinfection and sterilization	High	
Alkalis	Sodium hydroxide (lye, soda lye)	Environmental disinfection, surface disinfectant	High	Highly caustic. Strong concentrations can be used for prion disinfection.
	Calcium hydroxide (slaked lime)	Environmental disinfection	Moderate	Sometimes used as a whitewash that kills or inhibits growth of non–spore-forming bacteria.
	Sodium carbonate	Cleansing agent	Moderate	Used extensively in foot-and-mouth disease (FMD) outbreaks.
Biguanides	Chlorhexidine	Surface disinfectant, topical antiseptic	Very poor	Very low toxicity potential. Typical dilutions are nonirritating even when contacting mucosa. Inactivated by anionic detergents and other anionic substances (e.g., phosphate, citrate, carbonate, bicarbonate, chloride salts). Bactericidal activity on skin is more rapid than many other compounds, including iodophors. Activity in aqueous alcohol solutions is superior to activity in strictly aqueous solutions. Residual effect on skin diminishes regrowth. Variable activity against fungi. Not active against nonenveloped viruses, mycobacteria, or spores.

Continued

Table • **66-1**

Common Disinfectants Used in Veterinary Medicine—cont'd

CLASS	DISINFECTANT	APPLICATION IN VETERINARY MEDICINE	ACTIVITY IN ORGANIC MATERIAL	COMMENTS
Chlorine-releasing agents	Sodium hypochlorite (bleach)	Surface disinfectant	Very poor	Bactericidal activity is reduced with increasing pH, lower temperatures, and in presence of ammonia and nitrogen compounds, which can be important when urine is present. Not affected by water hardness. Considered to have relatively low toxic potential with standard dilutions. Chlorine gas can be produced when mixed with other chemicals. Strong oxidizing (bleaching) activity that can damage fabric and is corrosive on metals (silver and aluminum, not stainless steel) and concrete. Strong solutions can deactivate prion material. Chlorine dioxide is irritating and toxic.
	Calcium hypochlorite	Surface disinfectant	Very poor	
	Chlorine dioxide	Fumigant, gas sterilization	Moderate	
Iodine-releasing agents	Iodine solutions	Surface disinfectants, topical antiseptics	Very poor	Absorption of iodine and associated toxicity are greatest with tinctures and solutions and reduced with iodophores. People can become sensitized to skin contact. Generally less active than chlorine-releasing agents. Bactericidal activity is slowed at lower temperatures and alkaline pH, but affected less by organic material than chlorine-releasing agents. Dilution of iodophors increases free iodine concentration and antimicrobial activity. Metal surfaces can be oxidized. Staining of tissues and plastics also occurs.
	Iodophors	Surface disinfectants, topical antiseptics	Very poor	
Peroxygens	Peroxymonosulfate (PMS) and "accelerated" hydrogen peroxide compounds	Surface disinfectants, aerosol fumigants	High	Wide spectrum of activity, including nonenveloped viruses and mycobacteria. PMS and HP have low toxicity potential and do not form harmful decomposition products. PMS and HP act as drying agents on skin but generally are nonirritating at appropriate dilutions. Safety of animal exposure to dilute aerosol solutions has been described. PAA may be a weak carcinogen. PMS is labeled for use against FMD virus and can be used in the presence of animals. HP has brief germicidal activity when applied to tissues, but poor lipid solubility. Less active at low temperatures. Excellent against spores. PAA is germicidal at much lower concentrations than HP. Corrosive to plain steel, iron, copper, brass, bronze, and vinyl, rubber, and concrete.
	Hydrogen peroxide (HP)	Surface disinfectant, topical antiseptic, gas sterilization	Low	
	Peracetic acid (PAA)	Surface disinfectant, fumigant	High	

Table • 66-1

Common Disinfectants Used in Veterinary Medicine—cont'd

CLASS	DISINFECTANT	APPLICATION IN VETERINARY MEDICINE	ACTIVITY IN ORGANIC MATERIAL	COMMENTS
Phenols	Various phenols (2-phenylphenol, benzylphenol, 4-chloro-3,5-dimethylphenol, etc.)	Surface disinfectants	High	Irritation is variable among products, but these compounds in general are highly irritating and should not be used on surfaces that contact skin or mucosa. Environmental safety is also variable. Not affected by hardness of water. Extended residual activity after drying. Activity variable against nonenveloped viruses and spores. Some residual activity after drying.
Quaternary ammonium compounds	Various ammonium salts (mono-alkyltrimethyl ammonium salts, etc.)	Surface disinfectants	Moderate	Irritation and toxicity are variable among products, but these compounds in general are nonirritating and have low toxicity at typical dilutions. Not effective against nonenveloped viruses. Inactivated by anionic detergents. Some residual activity after drying. Good hard water tolerance; more effective at neutral or slightly alkaline pH.

Modified from Morley PS: *Vet Clin North Am Food Anim Pract* 18:133, 2002.
Data from Block SS, editor: *Disinfection, sterilization, and preservation*, ed 5, Philadelphia, 2001, Lippincott, Williams & Wilkins; and Linton AH, Hugo WB, Russell AD, editors: *Disinfection in veterinary and farm animal practice*, Oxford, 1987, Blackwell Scientific Publications.

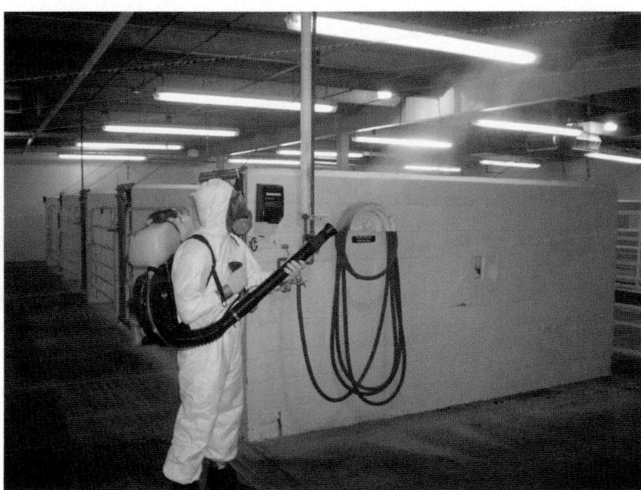

Fig. 66-3 Misting with Virkon using solo backpack mister during annual "bug out" at CSU large animal hospital.

infectious disease should be carefully considered. In a situation where only a small area of pasture is available, its use for any horses infected with contagious disease agents should probably be avoided to prevent establishing a source of infection for other animals. Alternatively, the best method for cleaning and "resting" the pasture is to allow sufficient time for die-off of the agent before other horses are introduced to such a pasture. The amount of time needed will vary depending on several factors, including the agent in question, type of pasture, and climate.

The survival time of *Streptococcus equi* subsp. *equi* on wood under laboratory conditions was reported to be 63 days at 2° C (35.6° F) and 48 days at 20° C (68° F) in one study. Measurable decline in the viable count did not occur until at least 7 days had elapsed.[62] In another study, *Salmonella* survived on apical parts of plants for up to 5 days, whereas it survived near the base of the plant or in the topical part of the soil for as long as 77 days.[63] A minimum waiting period before reintroduction of animals to a pasture treated with *Salmonella*-contaminated slurry is 3 to 6 weeks.[63-65] It is worth noting that these studies emphasize cattle. The susceptibility to *Salmonella* infection of horses, particularly compromised hospitalized patients, may be different.

Waste Disposal

Infectious waste, including any material contaminated with bodily excretions (e.g., needles, bandages, bedding), can be a source of infection for other horses. Transmission can occur either through mechanical transfer by shoes, hands, or shared equipment (e.g., stall-cleaning equipment) or through biologic vectors such as rodents or flies. In addition, waste contaminated with zoonotic agents such as *Salmonella* can pose a human health hazard. Therefore, management of infectious waste is an important part of biosecurity.

All sharps should be discarded in designated sharps containers and disposed of according to local laws. Similarly, any material that may be contaminated with an infectious agent(s) should be rendered noninfectious by autoclaving or incineration before disposal (e.g., bandages contaminated by discharge from infected wound). Alternatives to this approach would include contractual arrangement with a biomedical waste company. Because of large volumes, proper disinfection of equine bedding often becomes problematic. Acceptable ways of dealing with infectious bedding include autoclaving, composting, disposal at the designated landfill, or steaming. The latter involves attaching a source of steam (e.g., from building's heating system) to a covered Dumpster filled with contaminated bedding so that high temperature is achieved inside. It is a relatively inexpensive and very effective way of rendering any infectious bedding noninfectious and is used by several North American veterinary teaching hospitals (VTHs) as a standard treatment of bedding before disposal (B.P. Smith and A. Nguyen, Dorothy Havermyer Symposium, personal communications, 2004).

Footbaths and Footwear

In a recent survey, the practice of using disinfectant footbaths as part of infection control was reported by 30 of 31 of the VTHs in the United States and Canada.[66] Among those that used disinfectant footbaths, 73% used a single type of disinfectant solution, and 27% reported using more than one type of disinfectant solution (in different footbaths, not mixed). The disinfectants most often used were quaternary ammonium compounds (45%) and phenolics (39%), followed by hypochlorite solutions (19%) and peroxygens (16%). Other disinfectants used in footbaths were povidone-iodine, chlorhexidine, and ammonia-based products (each was used at 1 of 31 VTHs). In addition to footbaths, seven (23%) hospitals reported also using disinfectant foot mats in some locations.

Footbaths should be considered for use in traffic areas where personnel will be moving between groups of animals of different status, such as between colic patients and the remainder of an equine population. All personnel should be instructed to use footbaths when present. The use of rubber boots that can readily be worn into footbaths may be considered when fecal soiling of footwear is likely. These boots should be kept clean at all times when moving between patients. The efficacy of a footbath depends on a number of factors, including type of disinfectant used, frequency of changing disinfectant, amount of organic debris on boots, and environmental temperature. In one study, a 1% Virkon footbath used under conditions typically encountered in the large animal veterinary hospital reduced bacterial load on rubber boots by 0.48 to 0.66 $\log_{10}$.[66]

Disinfectant foot mats are another option for use in equine facilities (Fig. 66-4). Although more expensive than traditional footbaths, increased compliance is likely because mats can be used without the requirement for rubber overboots. In the authors' experience, Virkon-filled foot mats were as effective as Virkon-filled footbaths and resulted in 1.3 to 1.4 $\log_{10}$ reduction in bacterial load on rubber boots in one set of experiments (unpublished data). Use of dedicated hospital footwear should be encouraged to minimize the possibility of trafficking infectious agents from or to the outside of the hospital. Also, use of hospital dedicated footwear would increase the compliance in using foot mats, because people may be less inclined to step onto a disinfectant mat when wearing expensive footwear.

Some practitioners prefer to use disposable plastic overboots instead of footbaths or footmats to minimize risk of spreading disease agents on footwear.

The relative efficacy of one method over another has not been documented. Most likely, any method will be effective at minimizing bacterial load in the environment and trafficking of infectious agents provided it is properly implemented and consistently used by all personnel. Factors such as cost-effectiveness and convenience are likely to influence preference. However, environmental consideration related to disposal of used plastic boots should also be considered.

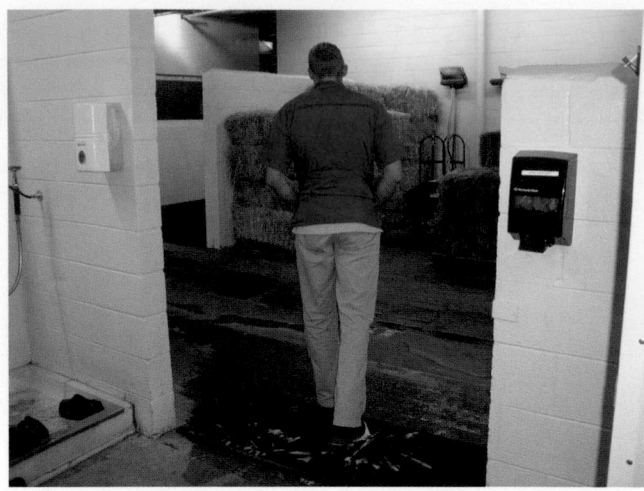

Fig. 66-4 Student walking through disinfectant foot mats at entry to equine barn at CSU large animal hospital.

Visitors and Foot Traffic

The presence of visitors in any equine facility should be assessed with regard to the risk they pose to the facility and the need for such visitation. In some areas (e.g., isolation area) it may be better to forbid visitation. In a situation where some traffic is unavoidable, it can be minimized and more closely monitored by establishing visiting hours. Consideration should be given to the rules governing visitation by small children. The actions of young children can be more difficult to predict and control, and therefore they can pose more biosecurity risk than adult visitors. Similarly, clients' dogs or other pets should not be allowed in the hospital. The CSU-VTH has a policy of inquiring if visitors have been in foreign countries in the previous 72 hours, and if so, special policies apply to their visit.

Impact of Insects, Rodents, and Other Animals

Control of insect, rodent, and other wildlife is an important part of biosecurity efforts at equine establishments. Both insects (e.g., flies, mosquitoes) and rodents (e.g., mice, rats) can serve as biologic or mechanical vectors for dissemination of infectious agents.[67] However, this is based mostly on logical assumption; minimal scientific data are available to further prove or disprove these statements. Similarly, pets such as barn cats or dogs can serve as biologic or mechanical vectors for infectious agents, and this possibility should be considered when designing a hospital biosecurity program. Cats have been epidemiologically linked to *Salmonella* outbreaks in several investigations.[68-72] In one study, cats were found on 65% of *Salmonella*-positive dairy farms versus 85% of *Salmonella*-negative farms and were therefore regarded as a protective factor.[73] In addition, pets can serve as reservoirs of antimicrobial-resistant bacteria.[74] Wildlife can also serve as a source of infectious agents for domestic animals; for example, feces of the opossum may contain the infective form of *Sarcocystis neurona*, which is the causative agent for equine protozoal encephalomyelitis.[75] West Nile virus is spread by mosquito bites,[76-79] and insects are proposed vectors for the spread of VS virus.[80;81]

Protocol for Dealing with Patients with Suspected Infectious Disease

Every effort should be made to minimize contact between patients with a history or clinical signs suggestive of infectious disease and the remainder of patients. Therefore, patients with clinical signs suggestive of GI or respiratory infection should be taken to an examination room or isolation facility as soon as possible to minimize the time they spend in common areas. Acquiring a thorough history before admission can often help avoid contamination because the astute clinician will recognize that the patient poses a risk to other patients and the facility. At CSU-VTH the clinical signs considered suggestive of GI infectious disease for large animal patients include diarrhea plus fever and/or leukopenia.

The index of suspicion for infectious respiratory disease should be increased for patients with recent onset of fever, ocular or nasal discharge, or frequent coughing, particularly if the animal is from a facility with a mobile equine population, such as a training, breeding, or boarding facility. It is important to be alert to such patients and to realize they may not be admitted for an infectious disease problem but may still pose a risk. For example, a foal admitted for correction of an angular limb deformity may arrive with a fever and purulent nasal discharge. All equine patients with signs of respiratory disease, particularly if there is a history of other animals being ill on the same farm, should be regarded as potentially infectious. It would be optimal if patients referred from another veterinarian were examined for potential infectious disease. If any suspicion exists regarding a referred patient, the receptionists at the referral hospital should be informed of the potential infection status of the animal, and diseases of concern should be clearly indicated on the hospital record.

Patients with clinical signs suggestive of GI or respiratory infection should be housed in an isolation area. If treatment or diagnosis of animals with infectious disease requires use of the main hospital's equipment or facilities, such as radiology, surgery, or endoscopy, these procedures should be performed at the end of the day and all areas thoroughly cleaned and disinfected immediately after use. It may be helpful to establish a policy of mandatory testing of all hospitalized animals that develop specified clinical signs, such as *Salmonella* culture of animals with fever, diarrhea, or leukopenia; rapid influenza testing of animals with fever and cough; and bacterial cultures for *Streptococcus equi* subsp. *equi* of animals with clinical signs of respiratory disease that come from farms with a history of *S. equi* strangles infections.

Monitoring

It is important that protocols are designed to maintain a maximum attainable biosecurity level within limitations dictated by available resources. Introduction of biosecurity protocols that are too strict to be practically implemented in a given practice would result in a failure of any biosecurity efforts due to lack of compliance. In addition, education of all employees regarding biosecurity practices is an essential part of a successful program. Personnel should know what is expected from them and why these procedures are important. Availability of written protocols would greatly assist in these efforts. The principles of surveillance and monitoring for control of nosocomial infections in veterinary hospitals have been detailed.[7,11,82]

In a successful biosecurity program, it is important to establish a way of monitoring the effectiveness of implemented protocols. Monitoring is important for several reasons. First, the challenges identified during the establishment of biosecurity protocols might have changed, and current protocols may no longer be adequate. An example is emergence of VS in the southwestern United States every few years. Once VS is identified in the region, then-current biosecurity protocols need to be changed to reflect this new challenge of reducing the risk of introducing VS-infected animals into the general patient population. Second, monitoring is important to maintain compliance. A successful biosecurity program should minimize occurrence of nosocomial infections. It is natural for people to revert to the most convenient practices (but not necessarily the safest for biosecurity) when little or no nosocomial infections are detected over time. As such, monitoring and reporting of bacterial contamination detected as part of a surveillance program can help to keep hospital personnel aware of the potential hazards of reduced biosecurity efforts. Early detection of increased environmental contamination may allow correction of any problems before they lead to an increased number of nosocomial infections.

Patient Monitoring

The optimal goal of a comprehensive surveillance system is to detect all occurrences of nosocomial infection and disease. However, achieving such a goal may not be possible because of limited resources available for this purpose in veterinary health care settings or because of limitations of diagnostic modalities. Further, experiences with infection control in human health care settings have suggested that it is possible to be more efficient and just as effective if special high-risk or high-cost problems are targeted. Therefore, *targeted surveillance* is more often used in veterinary hospitals. In focused efforts the population of patients that is monitored may be targeted (e.g., all patients vs. inpatients vs. critical care patients or colic patients only), specific pathogens may be targeted for surveillance (e.g., *Salmonella*, MRSA), and the methods of identifying patients may be varied (e.g., active vs. passive surveillance, bacteriologic cultures vs. syndromic surveillance). The specific focus and methods for surveillance need to be matched to the needs and resources of each establishment. The major benefit of targeted surveillance is that it decreases the cost and effort of data collection, but the trade-off is the inability to detect potential problems in the patients that are not being monitored. At the same time, increasing awareness about infection control methods for common or high-risk diseases will increase general awareness and compliance with control measures that relate to other potential hazards.

A number of methods can be employed to monitor for nosocomial infections among hospitalized patients. These could include weekly rounds of all clinicians to exchange and discuss any possible problems, regular analysis of computerized clinical data to look for predefined clinical signs, and full microbiologic monitoring for specific agents. Common clinical presentations of potential nosocomial infections include fevers of unknown origin, diarrhea, catheter-associated infections, postoperative infections, and multidrug-resistant wound infections. A combination of different monitoring methods may be used for surveillance. For example, at the CSU-VTH, all large animal patients are monitored for *Salmonella* shedding based on fecal cultures performed twice weekly throughout the period of hospitalization. However, other potential nosocomial infections are passively monitored based on syndromic surveillance, which may or may not be followed by bacteriologic cultures. The principles behind *syndromic surveillance* include monitoring of clinical signs suggestive of nosocomial infection without specific microbiologic diagnosis. Typically, the clinical signs that syndromic surveillance focuses on include fever of unknown origin, diarrhea, surgical wound infections, intravenous (IV) catheter–associated infections, urinary catheter–associated infections, and signs of respiratory infection (e.g., cough, nasal discharge). Syndromic surveillance can be incorporated into a computerized medical record system so that any trends (e.g., increased frequency of catheter-associated infections) can be quickly recognized. This would allow the clinician to investigate suspicious episodes further and potentially implement corrective actions before the situation escalates.

Environmental Monitoring

Environmental monitoring can be used as an adjunct to patient monitoring in a comprehensive biosecurity program.[7,83] It can be more efficient than monitoring every patient and can identify important reservoirs for nosocomial exposure. It is the authors' experience that in a veterinary hospital, environmental contamination with *Salmonella* is common in the vicinity of where infected horses are housed or managed. Therefore, if individual patient monitoring based on fecal cultures for *Salmonella* is not a feasible option, periodic monitoring of the environment can provide a less expensive alternative, assuming that culture or other detection methods have been appropriately optimized. Typically, high-traffic areas such as treatment rooms, examination areas, or aisles in the housing areas are targeted. In addition, environmental monitoring for one agent that survives in the environment reasonably well (e.g. *Salmonella*) gives a good indication of the overall quality of cleaning and disinfection and therefore can provide useful feedback for the cleaning personnel. It can also indicate the source of problems with infection related to other agents.

Important factors to consider when introducing environmental surveillance include sample collection, shipping conditions, and culture methods. In one study, for example, approximately 12% of environmental samples collected from CSU-VTH using electrostatic household wipes were positive for *Salmonella enterica*.[83] As an alternative to culturing environmental samples for the specific agent (e.g., *Salmonella*), the clinician can perform a nonspecific bacterial count. Contact plates (e.g., RODAC) are one convenient way of estimating general bacterial counts on various surfaces.[84-87] This technique involves pressing an agar contact plate against a tested surface, followed by an overnight incubation and enumeration of bacterial colonies without further identification of specific agents. As such, it requires minimal investment of labor and, when used on regular basis, can provide valuable information regarding cleanliness of hospital surfaces. Such data can be used as feedback for the cleaning personnel, for monitoring of quality of cleaning, or for pinpointing problem areas. To gain meaningful information, contact plate cultures should be performed regularly so that the normal baseline level of microbial contamination of various surfaces is known and any unexpected increases from that baseline can be detected.

SPECIFIC ASPECTS OF BIOSECURITY

Equine Veterinary Hospital

In a veterinary clinic, large numbers of animals are concentrated in a small area, thus increasing the risk of transmission of infectious disease from one animal to another, particularly if animals with infectious disease are housed in proximity to animals with increased susceptibility to infection, such as immunocompromised patients or neonatal foals. In addition, intensive management or care of patients increases the possibility of exposure to infectious agents because of frequent contact between medical personnel and a number of sick equine patients. Design of the facility can impact the ability to control spread of infectious agents. Specifically, factors such as area separation, type of surfaces, airflow, and air-exchange rate can influence the success of implemented infection control measures.[82] Therefore, these factors should be taken into consideration when designing equine hospital facilities.

It is important to recognize that nosocomial infections are an inherent risk of hospitalization. This fact should be communicated clearly to clients. The amount of effort aimed at preventing nosocomial disease in an equine clinic depends on specific circumstances, such as size of the operation, type of clientele, financial resources available for this purpose, and risk aversion as perceived by clients. For example, a two-veterinarian clinic may not need and probably will not be able to justify as extensive a biosecurity program as would be appropriate for a large referral hospital. Many factors can be influenced by education and communication. In general, clients who are highly educated about their horses and willing to pay for advanced medical care are likely to expect high-quality care, and for the long term they would choose a provider who fulfills these criteria. This includes more comprehensive infection control efforts. As mentioned earlier, because nosocomial infections are an inherent risk of hospitalization, good-quality care cannot be achieved without efforts to prevent these infections. A summary of two comprehensive biosecurity programs for VTHs at CSU University of California–Davis have recently been published.[11,82]

Equine Ambulatory Practice

The proximity of animals with different disease status is not usually a concern for an ambulatory practice, where a veterinarian treats patients in their home environment. However, diseases can still be transmitted from one client's premises to another's through movement of veterinary personnel or their equipment, if appropriate biosecurity precautions are not observed. The greatest risk for transmission between clients' premises is posed by pathogens that survive well in the environment or that are difficult to disinfect. Examples include canine parvovirus, rotaviruses, FMD virus, *Salmonella enterica*, *Streptococcus equi* (strangles), *Corynebacterium pseudotuberculosis* (pigeon fever), and external parasites. The authors investigated an outbreak of salmonellosis on a ranch where *Salmonella* was cultured from the attending veterinarian's truck. Important potential sources for transmission of infectious agents include the veterinarian's hands, clothing, footwear, equipment, and vehicle. Although transmission of infectious agents on wheels of vehicles is possible, this is likely not as important as other sources of contamination. Thus, attention to personal hygiene (frequent handwashing, use of alcohol-based waterless hand rubs, prompt changing of contaminated clothing, use of disposable gloves and gowns, prompt cleaning and disinfection of footwear) as well as proper cleaning and disinfection of medical equipment between patients are essential. Thorough cleaning and disinfection of reusable equipment (e.g., rectal thermometers, endoscopes, nasogastric tubes) between patients is particularly important.[55,58,88,89] The use of waterless surgical hand scrub (e.g., Avagard) is as effective as a traditional 10-minute surgical scrub with chlorhexidine and water, and it can be easily used in any field situation to minimize the risk of nosocomial infection associated with invasive procedures.[90-92]

Equine Owner

Protection of Resident Horses

Unlike the situation in the equine veterinary hospital, where biosecurity efforts are focused on controlling spread of pathogens from one animal to another, biosecurity at horse farms, stables, stud farms, and similar facilities should focus primarily on preventing entry of an infectious agent onto the premises and secondly on controlling the spread of an infectious agent, should it enter the establishment. To some degree, all the control measures previously discussed can be implemented on any equine facility. The general equine population will likely be less susceptible to common infectious agents because they are not exposed to the stresses of hospitalization and illness. Therefore, use of fewer biosecurity precautions will likely be effective at keeping this population healthy. Nonetheless, lack of minimum biosecurity practices can lead to the introduction of a new disease agent to a naive population, sometimes with serious emotional and financial consequences.

All resident horses should be vaccinated on a regular basis. The type of vaccines and frequency of administration should be determined by an attending veterinarian based on published evidence of efficacy, knowledge of local disease risks, and consideration of factors such as geographic region, size of the facility, extent of movement of people and horses onto and off the operation, and the age of the resident equine population.[93]

All new arrivals, including resident horses returning from competitions, breeding facilities, or sales, should be quarantined for a period that exceeds the maximum incubation period for a disease of concern. According to a survey conducted by U.S. Department of Agriculture in 1997 among representative samples of equine operations in 28 states, only approximately one third of equine operations that added resident equids routinely isolated new arrivals. The majority of those that isolated newly arrived horses used a separation period of more than 2 weeks, with an average length of quarantine of 28.5 days.[94]

Any traffic to and from equine facilities should be minimized or controlled. For example, any commercial vehicles that are likely to have visited other farms may be restricted from entering horse stabling areas. Visitors can be asked to wear clean clothing, wash their hands before touching horses, or step on a disinfectant foot mat before entering the stabling area. It may be advisable to ask the medical history of all horses coming onto the operation and specifically inquire about recent episodes of respiratory infection or diarrhea. Similarly, all visiting horses on arrival should be inspected for clinical signs of infectious disease, such as diarrhea or nasal discharge, and access may be denied to animals showing such signs. It may also be helpful to require all visiting horses to be dewormed and vaccinated against specified pathogens.

Protection of Traveling Horses

An equine owner should be concerned with the possible exposure of horses to pathogens at sales, competitions, training stables, breeding facilities, or anywhere horses congregate from multiple different sources. In addition to difficulties in controlling exposure to possible pathogens in these situations, traveling horses may have a compromised immune system and therefore may be more likely to develop clinical disease when exposed to common pathogens.[95,96] The principles of biosecurity for these horses are similar to those discussed for resident horses, with day-to-day hygiene and use of efficacious vaccines playing major roles in maintaining health.

Although it is often difficult to restrict traffic around traveling horses (e.g., at sale barns or competitions), it is possible to limit direct contact to only essential people. It is also possible to provide stall-side hand sanitizers and disinfectant mats to further minimize trafficking of pathogens. Stalls at equine events can be thoroughly cleaned and disinfected between uses either by the event coordinators or by the participants, although the efficacy of these actions may be hindered by porous construction materials (e.g., wood) and dirt stall floors. In addition, good ventilation and temperature control can help to reduce stress on the respiratory tract of horses and reduce circulation of pathogens.

CONCLUSIONS

Biosecurity and infection control are important aspects of day-to-day operation of any equine facility and are especially important for equine hospitals. A successful infection control program requires the commitment and participation of all personnel. It is essential that the people in charge, such as clinicians (in the hospital) and owners or trainers (in an equine facility), observe the implemented infection control measures. Leadership by example is the best way to ensure compliance of all personnel. In addition, educational efforts should be undertaken to make sure all workers understand the importance of biosecurity and their role in maintaining the facility as a safe place for horses and their human caregivers.

REFERENCES

See the CD-ROM for a list of references linked to the abstract in PubMed.

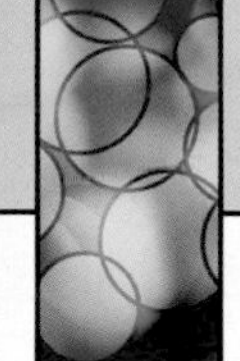

CHAPTER • 67

Control of Infectious Disease Outbreaks

Roberta M. Dwyer

Owners rely on veterinarians for advice on containment of infectious disease outbreaks on farms. Some of the most important pathogenic diseases of concern include salmonellosis, herpesvirus abortions, rotaviral diarrhea, and strangles. This service is most effective if offered before the outbreak of disease because appropriate preventive measures facilitate and enhance responses in the face of an outbreak.

Many recommended control measures are based on anecdotal information. First, although veterinarians are formally trained in disease prevention, especially vaccination and deworming, the typical veterinary school curriculum spends comparatively little time on instruction specifically related to equine biosecurity compared to time spent on this topic with other species. Second, because of the heterogenous nature of equine facilities, few scientific studies have evaluated the efficacy of biosecurity measures on one farm compared with other farms. As a result, recommendations for disease control on horse farms are made based on the personal experiences of the attending veterinarian, descriptions of disease control and prevention in veterinary hospitals, scientific studies in other species, and colleagues' observations. The author has used the following methods successfully to facilitate the integration of preventive medicine and biosecurity education in equine veterinary practice

PATHOGENS

The pathogens in North America most frequently associated with disease outbreaks on equine farms are listed in Table 67-1. Method of spread, transmission, and degree of environmental contamination all contribute to the overall biocontainment plan. For example, rotavirus is the most difficult to kill with disinfectants because it is a nonenveloped virus, and thus the type of disinfection is critical to control. Salmonellosis is one of the most challenging to control environmentally because it can be highly contagious and is readily spread by fomites, avian species, and insects. Airborne viral pathogens such as influenza and herpesvirus are aerosolized, contaminating an entire barn and seeding the environment before institution of control measures is possible.

In the event of a suspected infectious disease outbreak, affected horses should be isolated immediately, pending diagnostic test results. If subsequent diagnostic testing eliminates the possibility of contagious disease and no further horses develop clinical signs, the affected animals may be released from isolation. If a highly contagious disease is diagnosed, however, the client will have been correctly advised, and the rapid quarantine may dramatically reduce potential spread through a barn or herd and diminish related morbidity and mortality.

Diseases of Unknown Etiology

Veterinarians are often faced with outbreaks of disease of unknown etiology because of limited client resources or diagnostic tools. If multiple horses are exhibiting clinical signs, which should signal the high probability of infectious disease, a response level equal to that for an outbreak of the worst possible scenario (e.g., salmonellosis for fecal-oral or strangles for respiratory outbreak) is appropriate. A response of this level immediately imposes strict limitations on the traffic of animals and human caregivers to limit spread of disease.

If a foreign animal disease (FAD) is suspected, the farm should immediately (1) restrict all animal movement and (2) contact the state's U.S. Department of Agriculture (USDA) veterinary office. A USDA veterinary medical officer (VMO) or a specialist trained in FAD detection will inspect the farm, collect data, and obtain appropriate diagnostic samples. At the time of VMO involvement, the USDA recommends and enforces quarantine measures and makes further recommendations for disease control, usually in coordination with the respective state department of health (see Chapter 68.)

FARM FACILITIES

Stalls

Equine farms that experience frequent infectious disease outbreaks are often overcrowded and have poor sanitation. A limit of one acre per horse is appropriate for farms with well-tended pastures, and horses supplemented with hay when necessary. Organic debris is a major contributory factor to environmental contamination by pathogens. Management practices that may predispose to this debris include inadequate cleaning and sanitation of buckets and waterers, feces in hay mangers or feed buckets, manure buildup in stalls and run-in sheds, and on-site long-term storage of animal waste. The veterinarian should emphasize in client education that these conditions predispose to disease outbreaks and to increased expense in the form of labor, medications, veterinary visits, loss of use of animals (especially pertinent to performance horses and breeding stock), and potential mortality.

Where possible, stalls should ideally be constructed of nonporous materials such as painted concrete block (Fig. 67-1) or varnished or polyurethane-treated wood. Raw wood stalls cannot be thoroughly disinfected. Type of flooring is also critical for pathogen control; there is no reliable methodology for decontamination of dirt floors. Removable rubber mats can harbor infectious organisms beneath them and are difficult to remove, disinfect, and replace routinely because of their weight and size. Regardless of materials present at

Table • 67-1

Common Causes of Equine Disease Outbreaks

PATHOGEN	DISEASE
Salmonella spp.	Acute and chronic diarrhea, septicemia, localized infections, abortion
Rotavirus	Diarrhea in foals
Influenza virus	Respiratory disease, high fever
Equine herpesvirus	Abortions, respiratory disease, neurologic disease
Equine viral arteritis	Abortions, respiratory disease
Streptococcus equi subsp. *equi*	Strangles, bastard strangles, and potentially, purpura hemorrhagica
Leptospira spp.	Abortions
Trichophyton and other fungi	Skin lesions

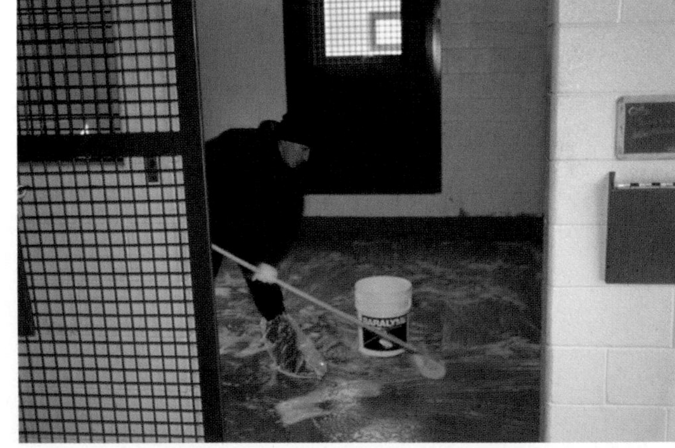

Fig. 67-1 Nonporous concrete-block stalls with concrete floors provide surfaces that can be completely cleaned, the most labor-intensive part of cleaning and disinfecting stalls.

the time of an outbreak, a routine cleaning and disinfection plan should be prepared (Box 67-1). Raw wood stalls can be thoroughly swept, removing as much organic matter as possible. Dirt, clay, sand, and porous stall floors should be completely mucked out and wet areas sprinkled with barn lime and allowed to dry. Fans may be necessary to facilitate drying. Aisleways and tack rooms should not be neglected in yearly cleaning.

Pest Control Plan

Farms should implement plans for year-round rodent control to prevent transmission and buildup of potential pathogens in the environment. Mice can ingest very small amounts of *Salmonella* that exponentially grow in their gut and are excreted in fecal pellets, seeding the equine environment with high concentrations of bacteria. Vermin may also act as mechanical fomites and physically carry pathogens around the barn and farm. Proper storage of feed and use of approved baits and humane traps may help in control, although a professional exterminator may need to be consulted in many cases. The use of rodenticides must be carefully monitored because horses are susceptible to most of these poisons.

Birds may also harbor pathogenic organisms and participate in the mechanical spread of infectious materials after an outbreak begins. Unfortunately, the movements of birds can be extremely difficult to control. Netting to prevent birds from nesting in rafters may be effective but is not foolproof and comes at significant cost in materials and labor. An alternative is to close off barn rafters and remove nesting sites that routinely appear in equine housing.

Bat nests should always be removed by a professional because of the risk of inhalation of rabies virus from dried saliva in these areas. Bat houses should never be built around barns to reduce insect populations because of the risk of rabies to humans, horses, and other mammals.

Insects may serve as biologic or mechanical vectors for the transmission of pathogens from one horse to another or from one area of the farm to another. Information regarding barn insect sprays, fans, and management techniques for removing standing water has been widely disseminated since the emergence of West Nile virus into North America.[1]

Box • 67-1

Routine Stall Disinfection Procedures for Nonporous Surfaces

1. Remove all buckets, feed tubs, and bedding from the stall.
2. Sweep the walls and floor of the stall to remove as much organic matter as possible.
3. Using a hose and garden nozzle sprayer (or pressure sprayer at <120 psi), wash down all stall surfaces using a detergent or a disinfectant that also has detergent capabilities. For stubborn stains, keep the surface wet for 10 to 20 minutes, then scrub by hand. Rinse by starting at the top of the stall, then working from the edges of the stall toward the drain area, or exit of stall. Remaining dirty areas, especially corners and drains, might need a second cleaning and rinsing.
4. After all surfaces are cleaned and rinsed, remove as much excess water as possible, especially from floors, by using a broom or rubber squeegee. Because the disinfectant will be diluted according to label instructions, it should not be further diluted by standing water.
5. Put on protective clothing, gloves, and goggles before working with the disinfectant. Follow label instructions and dilute the disinfectant into an applicator (e.g., garden sprayer). Spray the disinfectant on the walls (begin at the top) and floors and allow to dry. *Do not rinse.*
6. If an outbreak of infectious disease is ongoing, repeat the spraying and drying of the disinfectant.
7. Scrub all buckets, feed tubs, and other feeding equipment with a detergent. Spray on the diluted disinfectant, allow to soak for 10 minutes, then completely rinse with potable (drinkable) water. Anything that the horse will eat from needs to be completely rinsed of disinfectant. Dry these containers and return them to the disinfected stall.
8. All equipment (e.g., pitchforks, shovels, grooming tools) also should be cleaned, rinsed, then soaked in disinfectant solution for 10 minutes. Natural bristle brushes should be rinsed, and other equipment can be allowed to dry. Keep in mind that any disinfectant will be tough on leather handles of brushes, so these should be protected.
9. Towels, contaminated clothing, and other machine-washable materials should be rinsed of gross filth, soaked for 10 minutes in a disinfectant solution, then washed with laundry detergent.

Modified from Dwyer RM: *Horse* 16:67-80, 1999.

Traffic Control

Horses should be housed in groups that are matched according to age and use. Whenever possible, groups should not be commingled. Figure 67-2 provides a general overview of appropriate and practical equine groupings. This organization places animals of similar disease risk together to minimize the potential for pathogen transmission between horses by commingling or inadvertent transfer of pathogens by humans. People (hands, shoes, and clothing) and vehicle tires can be efficient fomites for transfer of pathogens between groups of horses. Therefore, human traffic (veterinarians, farriers, farm deliveries) between groups of horses should follow the order indicated in Figure 67-2. These traffic patterns result in people working first with animals at high risk of morbidity or mortality from disease (e.g., pregnant mares, foals) before going to areas of the farm where there are horses at high risk of harboring and shedding pathogens (e.g., show horses, 2-year-olds in training).

Horse groupings should be maintained in pasture assignments as well. Random rotation of horses between pastures increases the likelihood of transmission of disease. Whenever possible, one horse should be housed in one stall. If there are more horses than stalls, pairs or small groups of horses should always enter the same stall. Preplanning for this type of traffic takes logistical effort but reduces the amount of cross-contamination between horses.

An isolation area for horses that will ultimately join the resident herd should be established. This area is used for newly acquired horses, resident horses returning from travel (especially horses returning from a veterinary hospital), and any horse that will be entering the resident herd from high-risk groups. Horses should be maintained in this isolation area for a minimum of 2 weeks (3-4 weeks if they come from a farm with a history of strangles). While in isolation, horses should have their temperatures recorded daily, receive appropriate vaccinations and anthelmintic treatments, and be monitored for signs of disease.

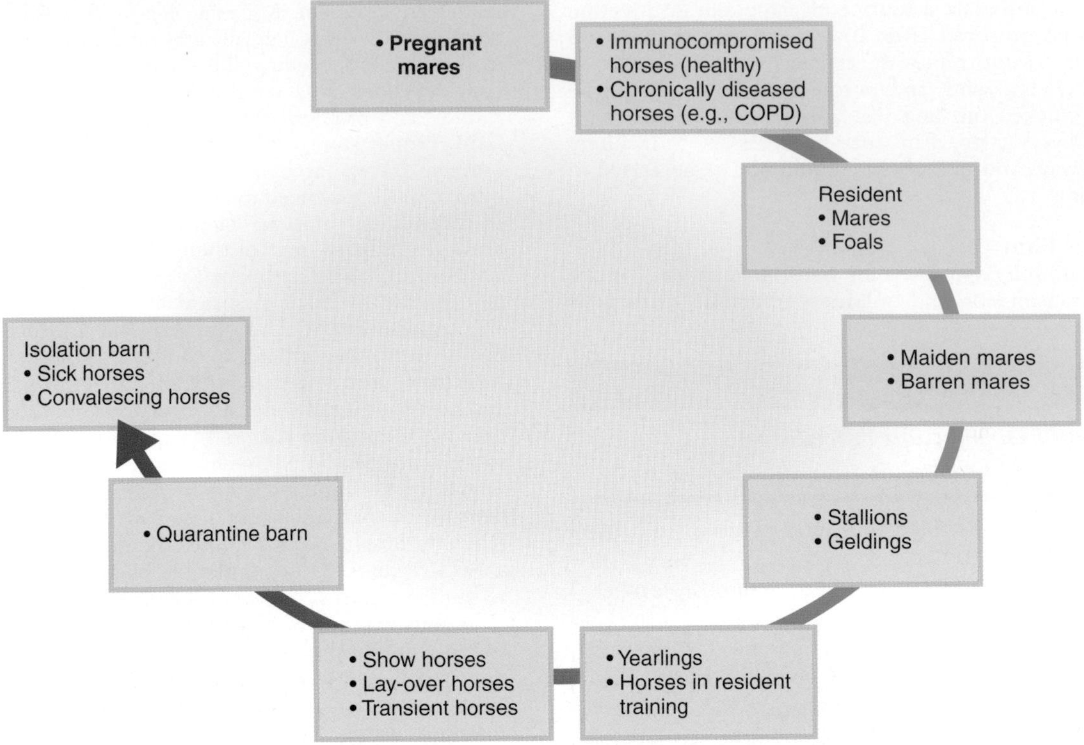

Fig. 67-2 Overview of appropriate and practical equine groupings.

Handwashing Facilities

All employees should have access to handwashing facilities. Ideally, this is a water basin with hot and cold running water, liquid hand soap, and disposable paper towels (Fig. 67-3). Bar soaps should be discarded because they may harbor pathogens. To be effective in killing pathogens, hands should be washed with soap for 15 to 30 seconds. In less-than-ideal conditions, a garden hose or other source of potable water, liquid hand soap, and paper towels will suffice.

During an outbreak, or when running water is not available, waterless hand disinfectants containing at least 62% ethyl alcohol are effective solutions. Commercially available at grocery stores and medical supply houses, these foams and gels are rubbed on the hands and dissipate within 10 to 15 seconds. Organic matter significantly interferes with the disinfectant activity, so these should be used on hands without gross evidence of dirt and organic matter. Frequently used products include Alcare (STERIS, St. Louis, Missouri) and Purell (GoJo Industries, Alton, Ohio). Owners should be specifically instructed that such products are highly flammable because of their alcohol base. In human hospitals, compliance with use of alcohol foams was superior to handwashing[2,3] and resulted in reduced transmission of pathogens.[4,5] These products are increasingly being used in veterinary hospitals and are effective in reducing bacterial load on hands of veterinary staff performing physical examinations on horses.[6]

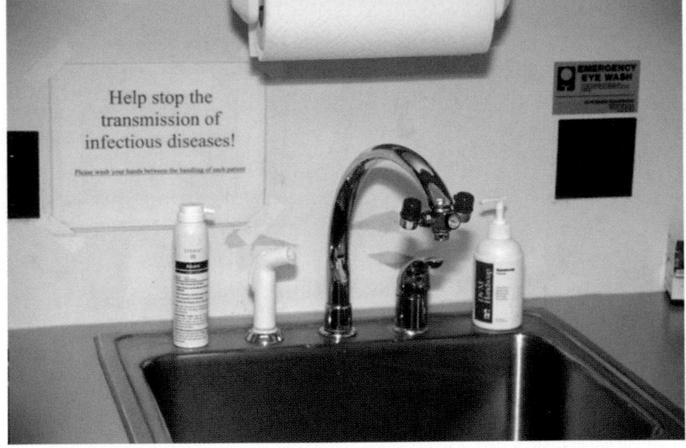

Fig. 67-3 Handwashing facilities, including liquid hand soap (right of faucet), paper towels, and 62% alcohol hand disinfectant (left of faucet), complete with a visible reminder during outbreak situations.

EMPLOYEE EDUCATION

Owners must not only "buy into" preventive medicine but also educate their employees for outbreak prevention and control to succeed. A lay article on outbreak control on horse farms is available.[7] In many cases, information must be communicated verbally and in writing in the native language of farm employees. Everyone working with the animals must understand the importance of disinfection, traffic control, and other measures, or the entire plan will fail or be seriously compromised.

The previous prevention techniques set the stage for effectively dealing with an outbreak. Knowing which pathogens are likely to cause outbreaks of disease, having a disinfection and traffic program in place, controlling vermin and pests, and understanding isolation methods are the first steps in outbreak control.

OUTBREAK PROCEDURES

Isolation and Traffic Control

Sick Horse Population

As soon as a horse is suspected of having a contagious disease, it should be quarantined to its stall and the owner advised that this horse is to be considered contagious until proved otherwise, including the time it takes to obtain confirmatory diagnostic laboratory results. Especially in cases of suspected salmonellosis and rotavirus, multiple daily diagnostic samples may need to be obtained before a veterinarian can reasonably conclude that a horse does or does not have the disease.

If a veterinarian is called to a farm where multiple horses have developed similar clinical signs and an infectious disease outbreak is highly suspect, sick horses should be immediately quarantined to their stalls or pastures, unless there is an empty barn or pasture geographically separate from where other horses are housed. Few horse farm owners have this luxury, but in the face of an outbreak, taking all potentially contagious animals to a separate facility will reduce the contamination in the barn where in-contact horses still reside. The factors of animal stress in a new location and the availability of personnel to care for sick animals need to be considered in this decision.

Exposed or In-Contact Horses

In-contact horses (same barn or pasture with sick animals) should *not* be moved to other areas of the farm. These animals need to be considered as horses that are potentially incubating the disease. If conditions permit, keep healthy, unexposed horses out of the barn to lessen the opportunity for cross-contamination with material from sick horses and their stalls.

Often an owner's first inclination is to move apparently healthy in-contact horses to other barns on the farm, or to different pastures than those that house sick horses. This practice spreads the contagion to as-yet-unaffected barns. The best way to deal with the situation is to "divide and conquer" by keeping in-contact horses in their same pastures. Horses can be further subdivided with portable fencing; separate water troughs must be accessible in each area. Exposed horses should have their temperature recorded daily, and if they develop a fever, they should be removed to the barn with other sick animals and treated as contagious.

Barns are excellent concentration areas for pathogens, with mice, cats, people, water hoses, and other equipment carrying organisms from one area of the barn to another. This is a primary reason to keep healthy horses out of barns housing sick horses whenever possible.

The barns and pastures where sick horses are housed should be off-limits to casual visitors and people unaware of biosecurity procedures. Clients should be advised that farriers and other necessary visitors (including the veterinarian) should wear rubber boots or disposable plastic booties while in the barn. These can be effectively scrubbed and disinfected (or discarded) before leaving the barn housing sick horses.

Access to Sick Horses' Stalls

Horses with clinical signs of infectious disease should be isolated in their stalls, and personnel entering the stall should wear disposable gloves, footwear, and separate coveralls or protective clothing (Fig. 67-4). The objective is to minimize contamination from entering and leaving the stalls, especially on hands and feet. After disposable gloves are removed, hands should be thoroughly washed or a hand disinfectant (>62% ethyl alcohol) used.

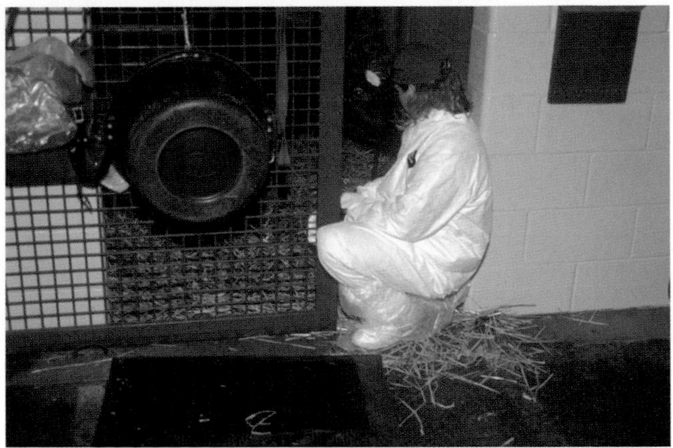

Fig. 67-4 Animal caregiver during an outbreak wearing disposable gloves, plastic booties, and coveralls. The coveralls can be reused only with the patient in that stall until they are soiled.

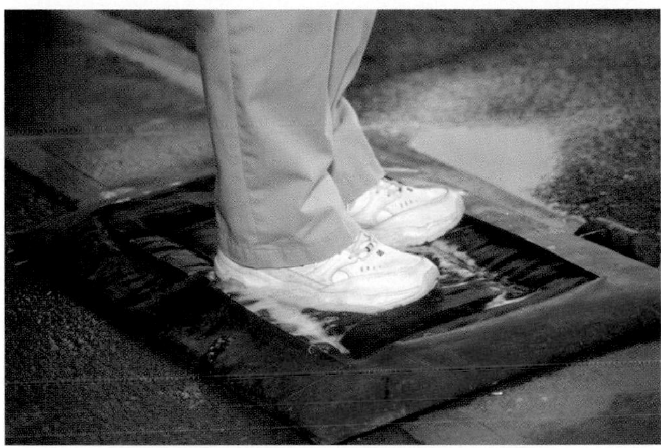

Fig. 67-5 Biosecurity foot mats are user-friendly. Visitors and employees stand on the mats with both feet and press their feet several times. Notice foaming action of disinfectant. Disposable plastic boots are not being worn because this is a high-risk but disease-free barn.

Footbaths

The effectiveness of footbaths depends on the disinfectant, the cleanliness of the footwear being disinfected, and the regularity with which the disinfectant solution is changed. Not even the best disinfectant will work effectively in the presence of manure-encrusted shoes. In a recent study, a quaternary ammonium compound used in a footbath was ineffective in reducing bacterial counts from boots, whereas a peroxygen disinfectant (Virkon S, Antec International, Sudbury, Suffolk, United Kingdom) reduced bacterial load on boots by more than 70%. Virus loads were not analyzed.[8]

An effective alternative to footbaths are foot mats (Biosecurity Mats, FarmTek, South Windsor, Connecticut). These contain disinfectant and can be placed in front of stalls and at the entrances and exits to affected barns (Fig. 67-5). Foot mats must be routinely cleaned and replenished with fresh disinfectant but are more user-friendly than foot baths, where people sometimes tend to "dip their toe" instead of sinking their entire shoe into the disinfectant solution.

Because some equine pathogens have considerable zoonotic potential, employees should be advised always to disinfect their hands with alcohol gel or foam before leaving the farm. Separate shoes may also be recommended, especially in *Salmonella* outbreaks. Questions regarding the implications of human exposure to potential zoonotic pathogens should be referred to a physician. This is especially important if immunocompromised individuals or young children have been exposed or possibly exposed to a zoonotic pathogen.

Equipment

Separate equipment (e.g., brushes, lead shanks, pitchforks) is needed for sick animals (Fig. 67-6). Alternatively, equipment can first be used on unaffected horses and their stalls, then on sick animals and thoroughly disinfected.

Tractors, Hay Wagons, and Other Vehicles

Tires of any farm implement or vehicle can easily carry infective material to other barns. The horse-grouping diagram is a template for traffic between barns (see Fig. 67-2). Within a barn with sick animals, implements should travel in a direction from healthy animals' stalls toward the sick animal stalls if possible. Muck from these barns should be handled separately, as described later. Tires on vehicles can be washed between barns to limit the amount of organic debris carried between areas.

Disinfection of Stalls

The area immediately outside the stall must be considered contaminated by personnel entering and leaving the stall, even when using protective footwear. This area should be kept as clean as possible; nonporous aisleways should be cleaned and disinfected daily until the outbreak is over.

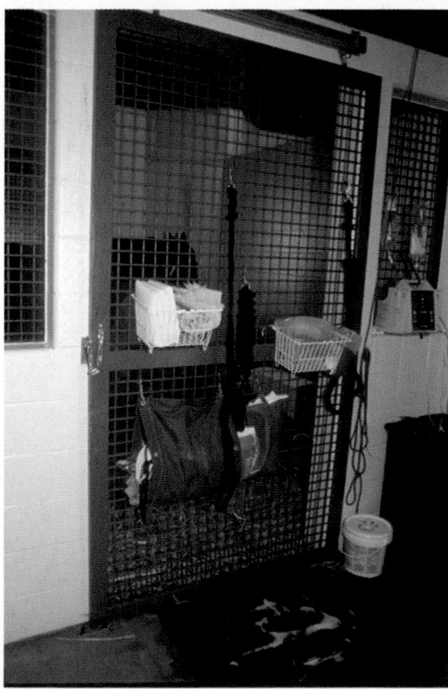

Fig. 67-6 During an outbreak situation, or with contagious cases in hospitals, separate equipment is used for each patient, including brushes, lead ropes, towels, and plastic booties. This prevents cross-contamination to other horses.

A general outline of a stall disinfection protocol is shown in Box 67-1. The cleaning step is the most important because approximately 90% of bacteria are removed from concrete surfaces with appropriate cleansing.[9] Another 6% to 7% of bacteria may be removed by disinfectants,[10] but the choice of disinfectant is critical to success. General classes of disinfectants used on equine facilities are presented in Chapter 66 (see Table 66-1);[10,11] however, phenols are one of the few types of disinfectants effective against rotavirus, even in the presence of feces.[12] Hypochlorites and many quaternary ammonium compounds are readily inactivated in the presence of organic matter.[13] Some modern quaternary ammonium compounds have been successfully used on thoroughly cleaned, nonporous stalls.

Pressure washing should not be used in a barn or stable housing horses with potentially contagious pathogens, especially in salmonellosis outbreaks, because of the risk of aerosolization of pathogens to rafters, where the material dries and may ultimately be re-aerosolized into stalls. Steam cleaning does not sterilize surfaces because steam rapidly cools between the end of the spray nozzle and the surface.[14]

If a stall with an organic or dirt floor is found to be harboring a pathogen (e.g., *Salmonella*) after an outbreak, the optimal way to rid the premises of the pathogen and render the stall safe to house horses or other livestock is to remove 6 to 12 inches (15-30 cm) of flooring and replace it with new materials.

Pasture Management

Pastures and fields where diarrheic animals have been housed cannot be disinfected without killing healthy soil and plant microorganisms. If feasible, remove surface manure from pastures or paddocks, and chain-harrow the area to break up remaining manure and allow exposure to the sun and drying. The duration of survival of *Streptococcus equi* subsp. *equi* in the environment is unknown;[15] however, fence posts, gates, and other materials should be cleaned and disinfected of obvious discharges and watering containers routinely cleaned and disinfected.

Hospital Visits

Clients should be provided with or should bring their own protective clothing when visiting any horse that is hospitalized. This will help prevent clients from introducing new pathogens into the clinic and from taking any hospital pathogens (from their own horse or others) back to their farm. This protective clothing should include disposable booties and gloves and protective coveralls (see Fig. 67-4).

SPECIAL CIRCUMSTANCES

Horse Trailers

Often the weakest link in infection control is the one behind the barn. Any horse trailer or van transporting a sick, potentially infectious horse should be thoroughly cleaned and disinfected, as done for a stall, before its next use. Use of a dirty trailer after hauling an animal shedding a pathogen is equivalent to placing a healthy animal in the stall of a sick horse with double the environmental contamination, because the horse van is at least 50% smaller than the size of a horse's stall.

Likewise, trailers that are used for transient horses (e.g., show, racing, trail riding) should be thoroughly cleaned and disinfected before being used by a resident animal (e.g., transport of a broodmare to the breeding shed). Transient horses may be shedding viruses and bacteria to which they are immune but a resident broodmare is not immune.

Horse Show and Horse Sales Stalls

Substantial commingling of horses from unknown backgrounds and with uncertain vaccination status, combined with transportation stress, is a recipe for infectious disease disaster, with outbreaks of strangles, herpesvirus, and other pathogens frequently traced back to such events.

On reaching the show or sales barns, stalls should be inspected before unloading and all muck and bedding removed. Any remaining wet spots should be sprinkled with barn lime. Clients should use their own buckets, hay nets, and mucking equipment. It is ideal if an owner has the opportunity to scrub fecally contaminated walls and completely disinfect a stall, but this is not possible at many events. However, if a stall is totally unacceptable (e.g., unsafe, inches of manure on floor), the owner should request to be reassigned to another stall if possible.

Owners should be cautioned to avoid nose-to-nose contact between horses and to graze and exercise their horses in areas away from other animals, if possible. Routine quarantine precautions should be taken when horses are returned to the farm of origin and before reintroduction to the resident herd.

Box • 67-2

Basic Principles of Outbreak Control

Prevention of Outbreaks

- Vaccinate and deworm horses regularly.
- Evaluate the ability to disinfect facilities adequately, and recommend nonporous surfaces in stalls whenever possible.
- Implement pest control measures as needed.
- Organize horses into groups based on age and use.
- Organize traffic of vehicles and human caregivers from healthy animals most at risk to sick animals (except in an emergency).
- Update handwashing facilities and keep them properly maintained.
- Quarantine all new horses and animals returning from an extended absence for at least 14 days; for a horse from a farm with a recent history of strangles, quarantine for 21 to 28 days.
- Routinely disinfect horse vans or trailers.
- Educate employees; advise owners to write a short summary of procedures for farm biosecurity.

Responses to Outbreaks

- Immediately quarantine sick horses, and attempt to confirm a diagnosis.
- Do not move in-contact horses on or off the farm.
- Implement measures to decrease pathogen contamination and cross-contamination through disinfection, protective clothing, and traffic control.
- Emphasize biosecurity to owners when visiting horses in hospitals; visitors should always use protective clothing, which is disposed of on leaving the clinic.

Manure Disposal

Manure and bedding from the stalls of sick horses should not be spread on pastures or fields. Each jurisdiction, county, or city of the United States has rules and regulations regarding manure disposal. Some areas will allow bedding and manure to be disposed of in garbage Dumpsters, whereas others allow composting (as long as other horses and animals do not have access to the area). *Rhodococcus equi, Salmonella* spp., *Clostridium* spp., rotavirus, and other equine pathogens can have a long life span in the environment. Horse owners should not seed their pastures with pathogens; waste should be disposed of properly.

WORDS OF CAUTION

Veterinary professionals making recommendations regarding hand and surface disinfectants should understand the label information, advise clients of potential hazards, and strongly urge use of protective clothing and eye protection when working with these chemicals. Owners, even those of commercial operations, know little about safety data. Websites that contain the appropriate documentation and material safety data sheets can be accessed.

The potential zoonotic nature of diseases should be emphasized by the veterinarian and communicated by the owner to all farm personnel. Immunocompromised individuals and people with young children or immunocompromised family members at home also need to be alerted that a potential zoonotic disease is on the farm. Thorough handwashing and a change of footwear and even clothing may be required at the end of each workday during an outbreak.

CONCLUSIONS

Horses may be housed in a wide variety of facilities, from open ranges to concentrated breeding and boarding operations. However, the basic principles of outbreak control can be custom-fit to any horse operation (Box 67-2).

The veterinarian's expertise in outbreak prevention and control is crucial at the farm level. Owners appreciate the necessity of disease prevention when the costs associated with an infectious disease outbreak (e.g., additional labor, veterinary services, loss of animal use, risk of asymptomatic carriers) are considered. Commercial operations have the added risk of loss of clientele and community trust. Preventing infectious disease outbreaks is much more cost-effective than dealing with such outbreaks without a plan. An effective outbreak control plan can halt or slow an outbreak simply by the initial isolation of a suspected contagious animal.

REFERENCES

See the CD-ROM for a list of references linked to the abstract in PubMed.

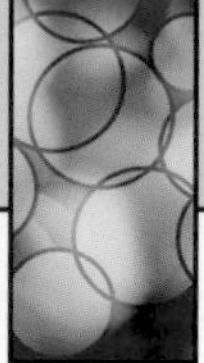

CHAPTER • 68

Recognition of Foreign Animal Diseases

Corrie C. Brown

Globalization has created a new landscape for animal health and disease recognition. Decades ago, foreign disease incursions were an extremely rare event, and primarily only regulatory veterinarians and those working at the ports or in overseas positions were concerned about international disease issues and threats. Currently, the term *foreign animal diseases* is rapidly becoming both more meaningful and less meaningful. The term may be less meaningful because of the rapid movement of diseases around the world, so that fewer diseases are now considered "foreign" (e.g., monkeypox, bovine spongiform encephalopathy). At the same time, "foreign animal diseases" is more meaningful for exactly the same reason; that is, more pathogenic microbial agents are entering new territories than ever before.

The initiation of the World Trade Organization (WTO), fueled by the combined forces of information flow and fluidity of markets, has created a new set of rules for those involved in transnational commerce. Designed to "level the playing field" and allow all countries access to global markets, the result has been not only a new game plan for international marketers, but also a revolution in expectations for the entire animal health community. At present, with the increasing traffic of people, animals, and animal products, the chances of a foreign animal disease (FAD when referring to its investigation) entering the United States are very high. U.S. borders are porous, and a foreign animal disease could just as easily appear in the middle of the country as at one of the border ports of inspection. A private practitioner who may never venture more than a hundred miles from home needs to be aware that the world is at his or her doorstep. A hitchhiking vector or a fomite on someone's clothing could bring a disease to any of the 50 states.

Horses are a unique species, treading the line between companion animals and livestock. Historically based in agriculture, horses now serve more as pleasure animals or as athletic performance animals. Because many equids have significant commercial value, regulatory issues and international commerce are closely monitored to ensure health of the populations and preservation of industry value. Oversight is supplied in most cases by federal agricultural agencies, and overall global coordination is through the multilateral animal health regulatory body known as the World Organization for Animal Health (formerly the Office International des Epizooties and still referred to by the abbreviated designation of OIE).

EQUINE DISEASES AS LISTED BY OIE

The OIE maintains lists of diseases of animals that must be monitored in order to participate in international trading. Before January 2005, there were two "lists": List A and List B. There were 15 List A diseases, of which only two affected horses: African horse sickness and vesicular stomatitis. The defining characteristic of a List A disease was its ability to spread rapidly and have serious socioeconomic impact. Member countries were bound to report the occurrence in their country of a List A disease to the Central OIE Bureau in Paris within 24 hours of diagnosis. List B diseases were defined as diseases of potential socioeconomic impact, and these 94 diseases had to be reported to the OIE Central Bureau on an annual or semiannual basis. Over time, the assignment of specific diseases to these lists was questioned. For example, bovine spongiform encephalopathy was a List B disease, so immediate reporting was not necessary, and Hendra was not on either list, so it never would be reported.

The OIE convened an ad hoc group that spent 2 years developing a new list and a new set of criteria for inclusion. The overriding criterion for inclusion on the list is a disease's *potential for international spread*. Other qualifications include a capacity for significant spread within naive populations or potential for zoonotic infection. The list is now fairly lengthy, including a total of 130 pathogens (for a complete listing, see http://www.oie.int/eng/maladies/en_classification.htm). Box 68-1 lists the pathogens that impact horses, and Table 68-1 provides the preferred diagnostic tests for these diseases.

Reporting requirements to the OIE Central Bureau have also changed. Now, if one of these diseases is diagnosed, immediate reporting is not necessary unless one of the following epidemiologic events is applicable: it is the first occurrence within a country; it is a recurrence after the country was declared free of the disease; it is a new strain of a known pathogen; or there is a sudden or unexpected increase in morbidity or mortality. In addition, countries are now bound to report any emerging disease with significant morbidity or mortality; therefore, even a new disease that is not yet listed must be reported if it is causing notable illness or death.

Of the listed equine diseases, the following are considered foreign to the United States: screwworm (see Chapter 64), dourine (see Chapters 8 and 61), epizootic lymphangitis (see Chapter 57), equine piroplasmosis (see Chapter 60), glanders (see Chapter 39), horse pox (see Chapter 7), Japanese encephalitis (see Chapter 21), surra (*Trypanosoma evansi;* see Chapter 61), Venezuelan equine encephalomyelitis (see Chapter 20), and African horse sickness (see Chapter 15).

FIELD RECOGNITION

Glancing through the listed diseases, particularly those specifically foreign to the United States that would require immediate reporting, it is apparent that none comes with a unique signature or "red flag." Any of these diseases could conceivably be confused with domestic diseases and probably will be when first encountered. The clinicopathologic features, epidemiology, and diagnostics for each of these diseases are discussed in detail in other chapters. However, it is important to remember that definitive diagnosis of a foreign animal disease is made only at the level of the laboratory. For the government to initiate the cascade of regulatory events that would contain the disease, the etiologic agent must be confirmed through an internationally approved laboratory test. Laboratory diagnosis can be made only if samples are submitted with initial reporting of suspicious clinical signs to the respective state or federal veterinarian.

Box • 68-1

Diseases Notifiable to the OIE

Multiple-Species Diseases
- Anthrax
- Aujeszky's disease
- Bluetongue
- Brucellosis (*Brucella abortus*)
- Brucellosis (*Brucella melitensis*)
- Brucellosis (*Brucella suis*)
- Crimean Congo hemorrhagic fever
- Echinococcosis/hydatidosis
- Foot-and-mouth disease
- Heartwater
- Japanese encephalitis
- Leptospirosis
- New World screwworm (*Cochliomyia hominivorax*)
- Old World screwworm (*Chrysomya bezziana*)
- Paratuberculosis
- Q fever
- Rabies
- Rift Valley fever
- Rinderpest
- Trichinellosis
- Tularemia
- Vesicular stomatitis
- West Nile fever

Equine Diseases
- African horse sickness
- Contagious equine metritis
- Dourine
- Equine encephalomyelitis (eastern)
- Equine encephalomyelitis (western)
- Equine infectious anemia
- Equine influenza
- Equine piroplasmosis
- Equine rhinopneumonitis
- Equine viral arteritis
- Glanders
- Surra (*Trypanosoma evansi*)
- Venezuelan equine encephalomyelitis

Table • 68-1

Prescribed and Alternative Diagnostic Tests for OIE-Listed Equine Diseases

DISEASE NAME	PRESCRIBED TESTS*	ALTERNATIVE TESTS
Diseases That May Affect Multiple Species		
Aujeszky's disease	ELISA, VN	
Leptospirosis		MAT
Rabies	VN	ELISA
New World screwworm		Agent identification
Old World screwworm		Agent identification
Vesicular stomatitis	CF, ELISA, VN	
Diseases That Affect Only Horses		
African horse sickness	CF, ELISA	
Contagious equine metritis	Agent identification	
Dourine	CF	IFA, ELISA
Equine encephalomyelitis (eastern and western)		HI, CF, PRN
Equine infectious anemia	AGID	ELISA
Equine influenza		HI
Equine piroplasmosis	IFA, ELISA	CF
Equine rhinopneumonitis		VN
Glanders	Mallein test, CF	
Equine viral arteritis	VN, agent identification (semen only)	
Venezuelan equine encephalomyelitis		HI, CF, PRN

AGID, Agar-gel immunodiffusion; *CF*, complement fixation test; *ELISA*, enzyme-linked immunosorbent assay; *HI*, hemagglutination inhibition; *IFA*, indirect fluorescent antibody test; *MAT*, microscopic agglutination test; *PRN*, plaque reduction neutralization; *VN*, virus neutralization.
*"Prescribed tests" are those considered optimal for determining the health status of animals before shipment. "Alternative tests" do not demonstrate the absence of infection in the tested animals with the same level of confidence as the prescribed tests. However, the OIE Terrestrial Animal Health Standards Commission considers that an alternative test chosen by mutual agreement between the importing and exporting countries can provide valuable information for evaluating the risks of any proposed trade in animals or animal products.

Therefore, although the most astute clinician or the most diligent pathologist might have strong suspicions based on disease presentation and gross or histopathologic lesions, it is still imperative that appropriate samples be submitted for confirmation. The first case of a foreign animal disease to enter the United States might be presented as a complete mystery or might appear similar to any of a number of domestic diseases. Also, if samples were not submitted to the laboratory, the chances of ever discovering that a foreign animal disease had just entered would slip away, perhaps allowing for significant amplification of the problem before the realization that a foreign animal disease was at hand.

RESPONSE PLAN FOR FOREIGN ANIMAL DISEASES

Incursion of any of the foreign animal diseases will initiate a response plan, activated at the moment the diagnosis is rendered.[1] Depending on the urgency of containment and eradication, the extent of the response will vary. However, all responses will involve the participation of a number of entities, including local, state, and federal agencies, as well as private practitioners and volunteer organizations.

As a result of Homeland Security Presidential Directive 5, issued in February 2003, and its mandated development of the National Response Plan, which went into effect in March 2004, all emergencies will be administered under a system known as the National Incident Management System (NIMS), which uses a structure known as the Incident Command System (ICS).[2] Originally developed by the U.S. Forest Service to combat forest fires, ICS is now in routine use for disasters and incidents throughout the United States. The ICS would become the structure in which veterinarians and animal health professionals would be working in the event of an eradication campaign. The ICS is composed of five major sections and is highly flexible, with sections growing or shrinking depending on the extent of the outbreak and its complexity. It is designed to streamline activities, maximize resources, and clarify chains of command. For an FAD outbreak, the ICS would include veterinarians, technicians, disease specialists, and many support personnel, drawn from the military, universities, industry, and private practice, as well as federal and state governments.

The five major sections of incident management are command, finance, logistics, operations, and planning (Figs. 68-1 and 68-2). The Command Section is led by one

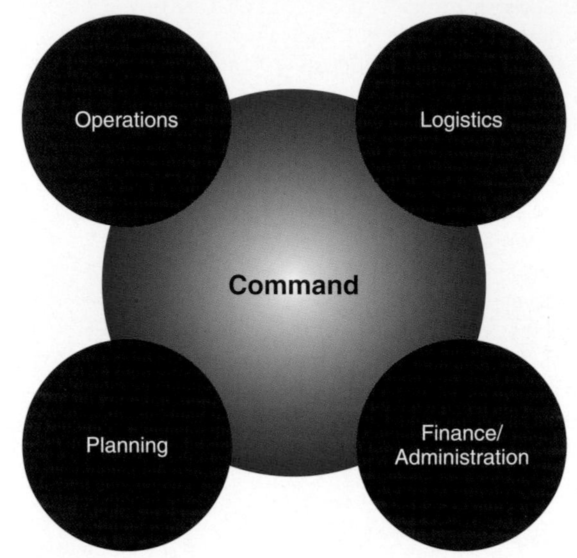

Fig. 68-1 Schematic of Incident Command System (ICS) structure.

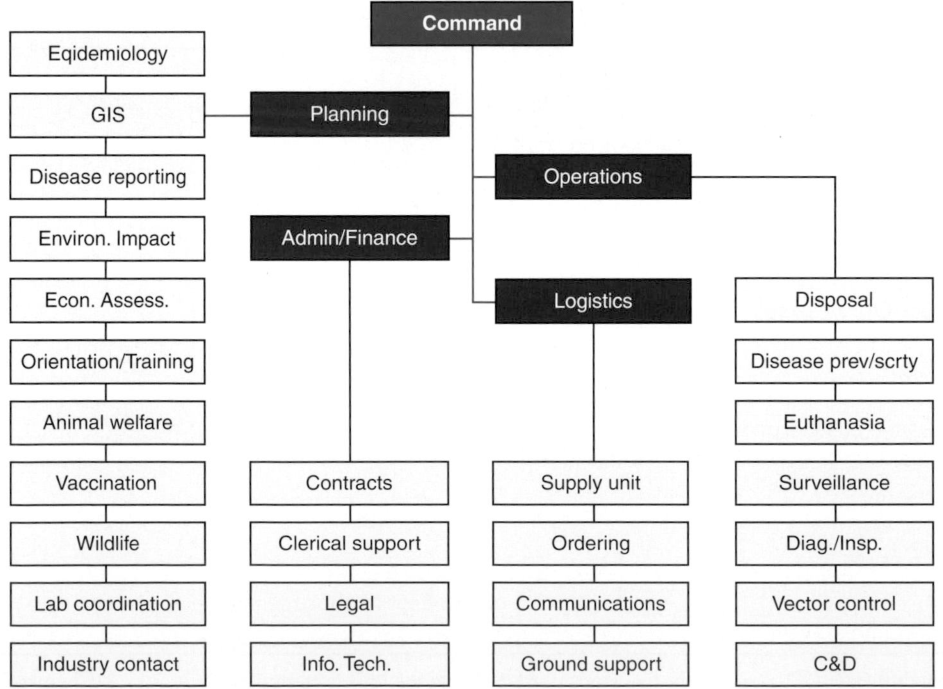

Fig. 68-2 Organizational chart depicting functions of various sections in Incident Command System (ICS). *GIS*, Geographic Information System; *Prev/Scrty*, Prevention/Security; *Diag./Insp.*, Diagnosis/Inspection; *C&D*, Cleaning and Disinfection.

incident commander and controls all personnel and equipment, maintains accountability for task accomplishment, and serves as a liaison with outside agencies. In a foreign animal disease ICS, the incident commander would be a veterinarian. The Planning Section must create the Incident Action Plan, which defines the response activities and use of all resources. During an FAD outbreak response, the Planning Section will be concerned with animal welfare, vaccinations, epidemiology, wildlife, laboratory coordination, the Geographic Information System (GIS), and disease reporting. The Operations Section carries out the response plan; activities and duties include quarantine, vector control, slaughter, and disposal of carcasses. The Logistics Section functions in long-term or extended operations and deals with a number of personnel and equipment issues. The Finance Section manages the expenditures required by all sections and participants to respond to a disaster. In the event of an FAD response, veterinarians, whether from government, industry, or private practice, would be primarily involved in the Planning Section or Operations Section.

The ICS has now been used successfully in combating FAD outbreaks, most notably during the California Exotic Newcastle disease problem in 2002–2003. It provides a structure whereby efforts from multiple organizations can be unified into a functional whole. The ICS replaces the former Regional Animal Disease Eradication Organization (READEO).

CONCLUSIONS

The likelihood of having to respond to a foreign animal disease incursion is very high. Recent experiences involving outbreaks of exotic Newcastle disease virus, highly pathogenic avian influenza virus, bovine spongiform encephalopathy, monkeypox virus, spring viremia of carp, and West Nile virus have highlighted the United States' heightened vulnerability to disease incursions. These diseases have also underscored that our best preparation is to recognize the disease as soon as possible and mount an effective and coordinated response. The value of U.S. animal industries depends on their awareness and capacity to control and contain any diseases that threaten the health of animal or human populations.

It is important to note that the amount of damage that a foreign animal disease will cause is directly proportional to the time between introduction and accurate diagnosis. In other words, we must accurately recognize a foreign animal disease at first contact if we are to implement effective control measures. It is imperative that practitioners consider foreign animal diseases in their diagnostic rule-outs.

Two main adages convey the "gestalt" regarding recognition of foreign animal diseases. The first is a new follow-up to the age-old admonition, "When you hear hoofbeats on the covered bridge ...." Historically, the standard response was, "... don't think about the zebra." Presently, in our new climate of globalization, the admonition needs to be adjusted to, "When you hear hoofbeats on the covered bridge... please think about the possibility of a zebra!" The second adage that is relevant to the recognition of foreign animal diseases is that a veterinarian can become "famous" in two ways when a foreign animal disease enters the neighborhood. One way is to diagnose it; the other is to miss it.

REFERENCES

See the CD-ROM for a list of references linked to the abstract in PubMed.

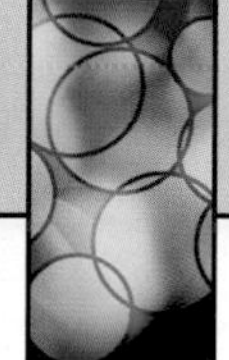

CHAPTER • 69

Infectious Diseases and the International Movement of Horses

Peter J. Timoney

We are living in an era in which the world could be said to have become a "global village," with "shrinking" national borders. No longer can countries consider themselves remote from the risk of incursion of a wide variety of infectious diseases of public health or veterinary significance.[1,2] Globalization of trade and the ever-increasing volume of international movement, primarily of humans, have given rise to a major paradigm shift in the geographic distribution of many diseases. The frequency with which diseases are transferred from country to country and within countries continues to escalate. Fewer and fewer diseases can now be regarded as "geographically restricted" or "compartmentalized" to certain areas of the world.

The list of human and animal pathogens that have been accidentally introduced or reintroduced into regions or countries where they were never previously known to occur or from which they were eradicated in the past continues to grow.[3] Examples of the more important human diseases and disease agents spread through international travel include tuberculosis, severe acute respiratory syndrome (SARS virus), influenza, malaria, cholera, Lassa fever, and Ebola virus. The roster of animal diseases with convincing evidence of spread through international trade is also extensive. Foot-and-mouth disease, hog cholera, exotic Newcastle disease, equine influenza, canine parvovirus, West Nile virus (WNV), and more recently, highly pathogenic avian influenza (H5N1 virus), well illustrate the point. Some animal disease pathogens (e.g., WNV) are important zoonoses and can give rise to significant morbidity and mortality in humans as well as in various animal species.

Many transboundary animal disease incursions are relatively transient in duration; the diseases are effectively controlled and eradicated within a limited time after their introduction. However, this is not always the case. Some disease pathogens are highly adaptable and very successful in establishing themselves in a new geographic environment. This is well illustrated by the behavior of West Nile virus subsequent to its first discovery in the northeastern United States in 1999.[4] Over the span of relatively few years after its initial detection, WNV adapted itself remarkably well to the diversity of physical and climatic environments found not only in the continental United States, but also in Canada and numerous other countries in the Western Hemisphere. In only 5 years, WNV is considered to have become endemic in 48 of the 50 states in the United States.

ROLE OF HORSES AND THE EQUINE INDUSTRY

Besides humans, equids best exemplify the ease with which infectious diseases can be spread through international movement. The horse is unique not only because of the longevity of the species and significant financial value of individual animals, but more importantly, because of the frequency with which horses are shipped between countries and between continents for various commercial purposes. In today's world, the horse can truly be considered no less an "international jet-setter" than its human counterpart. Changing trends in the equine industry worldwide have contributed significantly to the evolving nature of the international trade in equids, semen, and embryos and in the process have inevitably increased the risk of spread of various equine diseases. However, before elaborating on specific factors involved in the international dissemination of equine diseases in detail, it is important to appreciate the transformation that the equine industry in different countries has undergone over the past 40 to 50 years.

Since the 1960s, there has been an unprecedented upsurge in the growth of the horse industry in many countries, both for commercial and recreational purposes. The most significant factor in this development has been the favorable economic climate enjoyed by these countries over this period. National economics flourished from changes in the global market structure under various multinational trade agreements.[5] Among the industries to benefit from the economic upswing has been the horse industry, with a resultant increase in the volume of international trade in equids and semen. The trend toward globalization of the horse industry received further impetus after establishment of the World Trade Organization (WTO) in January 1995.[6] The primary goal of the WTO is to promote freer economic exchange between member countries through reduction or elimination of protectionist barriers to trade.[7]

Any consideration of the increased prominence of the equine industry in many countries must include the resurgence of interest in the horse as a leisure animal. The 2005 Economic Impact Study carried out in the United States identified recreation as the single largest equine-related activity, involving 3.9 million horses of an estimated national equid population of 9.2 million animals.[8]

INTERNATIONAL TRADE IN EQUIDS, SEMEN, AND EMBRYOS

An appreciation of the nature of international movement of equids is fundamental to understanding how trade in horses, apart from semen or embryos, contributes to the spread of equine diseases.[9] Horses are shipped internationally for various reasons. Some are intended for permanent entry and others for temporary entry into the importing country. Most frequently, horse travel between countries is for the purpose of competing in a particular performance event. Among the more prominent and better known performance activities are racing, show jumping, dressage, eventing, driving, polo, vaulting, reining, and endurance riding.

Shipment of stallions and mares for breeding purposes is another important facet of the international movement of equids. This is especially significant in the case of the Thoroughbred industry worldwide, which bans the use of artificial insemination or embryo transfer in the breed. In the last 10 to 20 years, significant growth has occurred in the practice of "shuttling" stallions, the majority Thoroughbreds, between countries in the Northern and Southern Hemispheres.[10] Financially, there is much to be gained from breeding a stallion in both northern and southern breeding seasons in the same calendar year. Horses are also shipped internationally to be sold at a commercial sale or in the case of a change in ownership.

A final category of horse movement that applies primarily to countries other than the United States is the shipment of horses for slaughter and the provision of meat, primarily for human consumption. Several hundred-thousand horses are shipped annually from eastern Europe and northern Africa to various countries in western Europe, including (but not only) Italy, Germany, France, and Belgium, for this purpose.[3]

As with live animal movements, the international trade in equine semen and embryos has expanded significantly in recent years.[9] This is largely the result of acceptance of artificial insemination in all the major horse breeds except Thoroughbreds.[11,12] Another contributing factor has been the technical advances in successfully cryopreserving equine sperm and embryos, enabling them to be shipped to countries worldwide.[12]

Air Transportation

Frequently taken for granted, the advent of commercial jet aircraft transportation has been the single most important factor in helping to bring about the unparalleled growth in international trade in equids, semen, and embryos that has taken place over the past 40 years.[9] It revolutionized the speed and ease with which horses could be shipped between or within countries and largely replaced other means of transporting horses over considerable distances by land or by sea.

Economic Significance

A second major contributory factor to the importance of international trade in equids, semen, and embryos has been the increased economic significance of the equine industry in a growing number of countries worldwide. The horse has joined the list of animal and plant commodities that are traded globally.[3]

To date, relatively few countries have attempted to assess the impact of their respective industries on their national economies. Limited studies have been done in the United Kingdom, Ireland, and Mexico, all of which underscore the important cultural and economic value of the horse in these countries. [13] Australia and the United States have carried out comprehensive studies of their respective equine industries.[8,14-16] The American Horse Council Foundation commissioned an economic impact study of the horse industry in the United States in the mid-1990s and again 10 years later.[8,15] Comparison of the findings of the two studies revealed that the U.S. equid population had increased considerably over the intervening period, from an estimated 6.9 million in

consideration was given to the need to prevent and respond to a bioterrorist attack against the U.S. agricultural industry and equine population in particular.[36] Regretfully, past events serve to underscore the reality of the threat posed to agricultural industries. Whereas the transfer of diseases between countries occurs most often accidentally or inadvertently, such incursions could also be deliberate, the consequence of an act of bioterrorism.

In view of the major economic importance of the U.S. equine industry, certain transboundary diseases could have a huge financial impact if deliberately introduced into the unprotected equine population. Of the entire array of equine infectious diseases, AHS and VEE have the potential to cause the most serious and devastating epidemics of disease among all categories of horses. Such an occurrence would also cripple the ability of the United States to export equids or semen throughout the world.

Clearly, the potential threat of agroterrorism should neither be underappreciated nor oversensationalized. Widespread acceptance of the reality of the threat is the important issue, as well as the awareness that a national emerging response plan has been developed to deal with any bioterrorist-related health emergency involving the horse or other livestock industries.

REDUCING THE RISK OF INTERNATIONAL SPREAD OF EQUINE DISEASES

Historically, veterinary regulatory authorities worldwide have responded to the threat of infectious disease spread inherent in international trade by formulating import policies that maximize disease preventive safeguards but minimize facilitation of trade. It has become increasingly difficult, however, for countries to uphold policies based on overly restrictive import controls in today's global economic climate. They are perceived in conflict with the overall goal of the WTO, which is to eliminate or reduce unjustified protectionist barriers to trade among member countries.[7]

It is freely accepted that the economic viability and success of the horse industry worldwide is critically dependent on the ability to ship horses within a state, a country, or internationally, without excessive restrictions on movement. With the aim of reducing the level of risk of disease spread from such movements, regulatory authorities have developed specific control measures to prevent the introduction and potential dissemination of a range of equine diseases into the importing country. To assist in formulation of their animal health import policies, the Office International des Epizooties (OIE), now the World Organization for Animal Health as recognized by the WTO, has developed a Terrestrial Animal Health Code that provides countries worldwide with principal control standards for preventing the spread of specific diseases listed by the OIE, including those of equids.[37] Regardless of country of origin or destination, horses are shipped internationally under license/permit issued by the appropriate regulatory agent in the exporting country. This documentation serves as a means of individual animal identification, certification of health and freedom from contact with various equine diseases, and a declaration that the exporting country or its region/zone has been confirmed free of evidence of certain diseases within a particular time frame.

Preexport Measures

In addition to certification of freedom of the exporting country or region/zone from specified equine diseases (e.g., AHS, VEE, glanders), current regulations governing the import of equids into the United States and most other countries require similar certification with respect to the premises of origin of the horse(s) being exported, other premises within a stated radius of that location, and most importantly, the individual animal(s) being exported. Horses must be held in preexport quarantine for a specified period, during which they are subjected to the necessary clinical examination and laboratory tests prescribed by the importing country. Of critical importance to ensuring the integrity of sampling and testing of horses for export is the need for some form of permanent individual identification, such as a unique animal identification number. Poor or inferior systems of animal identification increase the potential for willful substitution of horses before shipment and enhance the disease risks involved.

Postimport Measures

Assuming all the preexport certification and testing meet the requirements of the importing country, the horse(s) being shipped are approved for temporary or permanent entry into the United States. Immediately after arrival, the U.S. Department of Agriculture (USDA) requires that all horses imported from non–AHS-affected countries are transported in a federally sealed conveyance to a USDA-approved quarantine station closest to the port of entry. The animals are held in isolation for at least 48 hours and no longer than 72 hours, during which they are clinically monitored and serologically tested for evidence of dourine, glanders, equine infectious anemia, and equine piroplasmosis. Subject to a satisfactory health report and negative serologic findings for these diseases, horses are released from quarantine and shipped to their state of destination.

Intact male or female horses over 730 days of age originating in a CEM-affected country and approved for permanent entry into the United States are required to undergo additional testing to confirm their freedom from *Taylorella equigenitalis*, the causal agent of CEM. To accomplish this, such individuals are shipped in a sealed conveyance to a state that is federally approved to accept and quarantine stallions and mares from CEM-affected countries. There they are quarantined on a premises approved for that purpose in accordance with federal and state guidelines and subjected to the necessary testing for CEM. They are released from quarantine once they have been confirmed not to be carriers of *T. equigenitalis*.

Clearly, a balance must be struck between allowing movement of equids and providing the necessary safeguards to prevent the spread of various equine diseases. In light of the risks associated with international trade in horses and semen, countries need to have in place adequate postentry risk management strategies. Countries can no longer be passive to the health risks involved.

Some in the international community espouse the concept of "equivalency" and advocate that the importing country accept the reliability of preembarkation laboratory testing conducted in the exporting country, thereby obviating the need for a period of postentry quarantine and repeat laboratory testing in the country of destination. However, experience has shown that failure to provide adequate postentry screening of equids for specific infections can pose an unacceptable disease risk for the horse industry in the United States or other importing countries. For example, over the past 10 years alone, a total of 23 horses, comprising 16 stallions and 7 mares imported into the United States from Europe, were confirmed carriers of *T. equigenitalis*, on postentry quarantine and testing. All the animals involved were tested in the countries of origin and certified free of evidence of this bacterium. If this transboundary disease had been reintroduced into the United States breeding population through any of these importations, it would have had major economic repercussions on the horse industry. Another example of the existing federal postimport inspection and testing program successfully preventing the introduction of a transboundary disease is screwworm myiasis. In repeated but infrequent cases, horses imported from certain South American countries and certified free from this parasite were confirmed infested with the larvae of *Cochliomyia hominivorax* in postentry quarantine.

In addition, horses shipped from various European countries have occasionally been found to be clinically affected with diseases such as strangles or equine rhinopneumonitis on arrival in the United States. Collectively, these incidents bring into question the reliability of preimport laboratory testing and clinical veterinary inspection conducted by the exporting country. Also, they reaffirm the importance of maintaining the current system of postentry safeguards that has served the horse industry well over the years and protected it from the introduction of various transboundary diseases.

Disease Surveillance and Reporting

Surveillance of equine diseases at a national level and prompt reporting to the relevant authorities and industry organizations are critical to the effectiveness of national and international equine health control programs. Essential to any disease or early-warning monitoring program is the availability of adequate diagnostic capability for the disease(s) under surveillance. Accuracy and timeliness of a laboratory diagnosis of the suspected disease are of paramount importance.

In any national reporting system, primary consideration should be given to the equine diseases listed by the OIE. In addition to OIE notification of occurrences of listed diseases and any newly emergent disease problem, an informal disease-reporting system is supported by a number of countries worldwide. It involves each participating country providing a quarterly report of any confirmed occurrences of a range of equine diseases, many but not all listed by the OIE, to the International Collating Center at the Animal Health Trust in the United Kingdom.

The value of timely exchange of accurate, up-to-date information on occurrences of specific equine diseases at an international level cannot be overemphasized. Such sharing of information facilitates the process of risk assessment analysis between countries and enhances opportunities for a reduction or elimination of unjustified restrictions on international trade in equids, semen, and embryos.

Industry Initiatives

No program for the national or international control of equine infectious diseases can expect to be successful if it lacks the participation and support of the horse industry. With this in mind, several international groups have been formed over the years that represent the racing, equestrian sports, and breeding sectors of the industry. They include the Federation of Horseracing Authorities Permanent Liaison Committee on the International Movement of Horses, the Federation Equestre Internationale (FEI), and an international grouping of national Thoroughbred breeders' associations. These respective organizations or groups are broadly representative of the international community of countries with significant horse-breeding/performance industries. Their overall goal is to enlist industry involvement in identifying specific equine health issues that adversely affect international movement of horses and to seek ways to resolve them. Greater control over the international spread of equine diseases can be maximally effective only if horse industries and regulatory authorities worldwide work cooperatively toward this end.

REFERENCES

See the CD-ROM for a list of references linked to the abstract in PubMed.

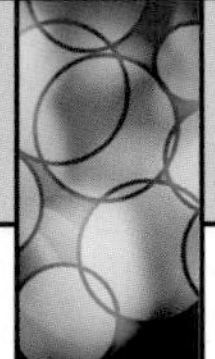

CHAPTER • 70

Immunoprophylaxis

W. David Wilson and Nicola Pusterla

Immunoprophylaxis is the prevention of infectious disease through induction or enhancement of specific protective immune responses. Immunity can be passively acquired by natural transfer or by exogenous administration of humoral or cellular factors from animals previously immunized through natural exposure or vaccination. However, the preferred approach is to induce protective responses actively through administration of vaccines containing (1) inactivated or live pathogens modified to attenuate their pathogenicity, (2) microbial components, (3) inactivated microbial products such as toxoids, or (4) genetic material encoding for expression of protective antigens. Of the infectious agents, viruses typically have the least complex set of antigenic determinants involved in protective immune responses; therefore, viral diseases are generally more amenable to control through active immunization than diseases caused by bacteria and, to an even greater extent, by fungal, protozoal, and metazoal agents.

ACTIVE IMMUNIZATION

Basic Principles

Active immunization typically involves administration of a primary series comprising one or more doses of vaccine to "prime" the immune system and generate *effector proteins* (antibodies) as well as clones of *memory cells* (lymphocytes and plasma cells) that are the basis for immunologic memory and "recall." Typically, "booster" doses of vaccine are administered periodically to enhance the level of specific antibody and memory. On subsequent exposure to the specific pathogen, memory cells can be recruited to quickly generate specific antibodies and effector cells such as cytotoxic T lymphocytes (CTLs) to neutralize the pathogen before it causes disease. Some vaccines are capable of inducing sterile immunity, in which case infection and replication of the pathogen are completely blocked, whereas many vaccines induce clinical protection without completely blocking infection or replication of the organism, although the latter is typically at a much reduced level.

Types of Vaccines

Vaccines currently licensed for use in horses in North America include traditional inactivated vaccines (bacterins, toxoids, and inactivated viral vaccines) and inactivated subunit vaccines containing bacterial cell wall components or toxoid for intramuscular (IM) administration; modified live viral and bacterial spore vaccines for parenteral administration; modified live viral and bacterial vaccines for intranasal administration; and recombinant vectored vaccines and deoxyribonucleic acid (DNA) vaccines for parenteral administration.

Dead Vaccines

Inactivated Pathogen Vaccines. Inactivated pathogen vaccines are the most common form of equine vaccine in current use and comprise microorganisms that have been treated with heat or chemicals to inactivate them while preserving their immunogenicity (Table 70-1). Phenol, formaldehyde, and β-propiolactone are among the inactivating agents used most frequently in the preparation of inactivated bacterial and viral vaccines.[1] Inactivated vaccines are inherently biologically safe because they have, in theory, no residual virulence and have a high stability in storage. They are typically suitable and safe for use in pregnant mares, debilitated or immunocompromised animals, geriatric horses, and colostrum-deprived foals. However, such vaccines typically require multiple doses and regular boosters, and efficacy frequently depends on use of potent adjuvants and high antigenic mass. Compared with vaccines of other types, disadvantages often associated with inactivated vaccines include slow onset of immunity, increased risk of local and allergic complications (high antigenic mass and inclusion of adjuvants are two factors that increase the likelihood of reactions), need for multiple doses in the primary series, need for parenteral (typically IM) administration, need for regular boosters at frequent intervals to maintain reasonable immunity, and shorter duration of immunity than achieved with modified live vaccines. Further, because inactivated vaccines are known to be weak inducers of cell-mediated immunity, they are not very efficient in eliminating virus-infected cells.[2]

Protein or Subunit Vaccines. Extracted and purified proteins naturally produced by pathogens can be used to formulate inactivated vaccines. Such vaccines can be developed only if the immunogens responsible for inducing the protective immune response are known. These vaccines often need high antigenic mass and strong adjuvants to stimulate the immune system. The major advantage of subunit vaccines is their inherent biologic safety because there is no risk of residual virulence. These vaccines have been associated with fewer injection site reactions than vaccines containing whole bacterial products. The best known examples of equine subunit vaccines are vaccines against tetanus containing tetanus toxoid and vaccines against strangles based on the M protein of *Streptococcus equi* subsp. *equi* (SeM).

Recombinant DNA technology permits synthesis of specific antigens that are important for immunity to pathogens. Such subunit immunogens can be produced only if the genetic

Table • 70-1

Types of Equine Vaccines Commercially Available

	DEAD VACCINES		LIVE VACCINES		
DISEASE/VIRUS	INACTIVATED	SUBUNIT	MODIFIED LIVE	RECOMBINANT	DNA VACCINE
Tetanus		X			
Equine western	X				
encephalitis					
Equine eastern	X				
encephalitis				X	X
Equine Venezuelan	X		X	X	
encephalitis			X		
West Nile	X	X		X	X
Equine influenza	X		X	X	
Equine herpesvirus 1	X		X		
Equine herpesvirus 4	X				
Strangles	X	X	X		
Equine viral arteritis			X		
Rabies	X				
Potomac horse fever	X				
Botulism	X				
Equine protozoal	X				
myeloencephalitis					
Rotavirus	X				

sequence encoding for expression of the specific protective protein antigens, as well as the immunogenic characteristics of these proteins, are known. Recombinant subunit equine herpesvirus type (EHV) 1 and equine influenza vaccines have been produced experimentally but, as yet, have shown poor protection, probably because of the poor immunogenicity of the recombinant proteins.[3,4]

Live Vaccines

Modified Live Vaccines. Modified live vaccines (MLVs) consist of attenuated microorganisms that replicate in vivo, thereby eliciting an immune response similar to that induced by natural infection, but without the associated symptomatology typically seen with natural exposure to the specific pathogen. MLVs typically induce rapid onset of immunity that includes both humoral and cell-mediated responses, produce a long-lasting duration of immunity, and require fewer doses to immunize the host. Depending on the route of administration, some MLVs are capable of inducing local mucosal responses. Compared with killed vaccines, MLVs generally contain a lower antigenic mass and usually do not require inclusion of an adjuvant; therefore they are less likely to induce adverse local reactions. Because the mutations responsible for attenuation of virulence in MLVs often are poorly defined, one of the major concerns is the possibility that the vaccine organism regains its virulence or combines with a wild strain to generate a more pathogenic reassortant that could induce clinical disease, death, and possibly outbreaks. Therefore, modified pathogens with multiple mutations on different genes are more suitable candidates for MLVs because they are less likely to revert to virulence than pathogens with single mutations. Further, lack of safety data in immunocompromised or pregnant horses compromises the appropriateness and, in some instances, precludes the use of such vaccines in these animals.

Attenuation usually is achieved by in vitro passage through one or more cell types, selection of spontaneous or induced temperature sensitive mutants, use of reassortants obtained by co-infection of the same cell with two different viruses with segmented genomes, or use of chemicals that induce mutations.[5-7] Several modified live vaccines are currently marketed for use in horses, including vaccines for prevention of equine influenza, strangles, EHV-1, and equine viral arteritis (EVA).

Recombinant Vectored Vaccines. Viruses and bacteria can be genetically engineered to serve as carriers or vectors for the expression of foreign DNA through the use of recombinant technology. A prerequisite to using this technology is thorough definition of the protective antigens of the specific pathogen of interest. Such vectors allow the introduction of the transgene into host cells, leading to production of protein antigens and stimulation of both B-cell and T-cell responses.[8] Adenoviruses and herpesviruses are being considered and evaluated as potential vaccine vectors, and a recombinant modified vaccinia Ankara virus (rMVA) vaccine for equine influenza has already shown efficacy in challenge studies in horses.[9,10] In addition, a variety of recombinant poxviruses are currently commercially available. In contrast to many poxviruses, which have a very broad vertebrate host range, the canarypox and fowlpox viruses are host restricted to certain avian species and produce an abortive infection in mammals. Canarypox and fowlpox are therefore ideal candidate vectors for mammalian vaccines because they express the inserted foreign genes in the absence of productive replication. Avian poxvirus–vectored vaccines have the potential to induce a broad array of immune responses in the absence of an adjuvant, although the canarypox-vectored West Nile virus (WNV) and influenza vaccines currently marketed for use in horses do contain a polymer adjuvant.[11-13] Further, it appears that canarypox virus recombinants do not trigger a neutralizing response against the vector, which would preclude an immune response against the transgene when subsequent booster doses of vaccine are administered.

Chimera Vaccines. Chimera vaccines are similar to live vectored vaccines in that they use components of one viral agent to transport genes encoding for expression of important protective antigens of the pathogen of interest. In the case of chimera vaccines, the vector and the pathogen of interest are typically in the same family. To date, this technology has been applied most extensively to immunize against dengue, Japanese encephalitis (JE), and WNV, all of which are flaviviruses, using the highly attenuated 17D vaccine strain of the related flavivirus, yellow fever virus (YF), as the vector. The premembrane (prM) and envelope (E) structural proteins of the pathogen of dengue, JE, or WNV are exchanged for the homolog proteins of YF 17D using complementary DNA (cDNA) templates encoding for these proteins.[14] A single dose of the nonadjuvanted YF-WNV chimeric vaccine generated using this technology has been shown to induce solid protection in horses subjected to intrathecal challenge with virulent WNV as a part of USDA immunogenicity studies as required for licensing. In addition, this vector, while affording high levels of protein expression, does not replicate to detectable levels in the horse, thereby further enhancing its safety.[15]

DNA Vaccines

Another novel vaccination technology currently under investigation, and recently licensed for use in an equine WNV vaccine, is DNA vaccination. The basis for DNA immunization is that host cells take up naked DNA, and these in vivo transfected cells express the foreign genes that signal in vivo synthesis of antigenic proteins in a manner identical to that occurring in natural infection.[6,16] Consequently, DNA vaccines appear to stimulate both humoral and cellular immunity. DNA vaccines offer many of the potential benefits of live vaccines without the same inherent risks, such as reversion to virulence. Because the vaccine consists of a single gene, it will not induce infection or disease. In addition, DNA vaccines typically induce expression of only one or a few of the many protein antigens present in the parent microorganism, thereby raising the possibility of developing companion diagnostic tests to differentiate vaccinated animals from animals that are carriers of the disease. Another advantage of having the host respond to a single protein rather than the myriad of proteins present in a pathogen is that many pathogens have proteins that can downregulate the immune response to the desired protein. Further, DNA vaccines are typically able to overcome maternally derived immunity in neonates or in very young animals.[6]

To date, no adverse effects have been associated with the use of DNA vaccines; however, safety concerns, including the potential integration of plasmid DNA into the host genome or the generation of anti-DNA antibodies, have been determined to be of remote risk. DNA vaccines stimulate a relatively weak serologic response. This response can be improved by the co-expression of the antigen along with cytokines, the administration of the DNA-containing plasmid through needleless devices, and the use of adjuvants. Investigations of the use of equine DNA vaccines are at an early stage, but already it has been demonstrated that they are effective at protecting horses from influenza virus and WNV infection.[17,18] Recently, an adjuvanted DNA WNV vaccine was licensed by the U.S. Department of Agriculture (USDA) for use in horses and represents the first DNA vaccine licensed for use in any species.[19] As of August 2006, this vaccine has not been marketed for use in the horse.

Marker Vaccines

Marker (or DIVA) vaccines are needed in situations where the differentiation between a naturally infected and a vaccinated animal is important. Such vaccines can be subunit, gene-deleted, vectored, or DNA vaccines and are always used in conjunction with a diagnostic test. The basis of marker vaccines is that vaccinated animals do not induce antibodies to a marker protein that is absent from the vaccine, but included in a diagnostic test. No marker vaccines are yet available for use in equids, but such vaccines are being developed against equine arteritis virus.[20] This approach will permit control by serologic testing and exclusion to continue in parallel with vaccination to prevent acquisition of infection, and it may greatly facilitate international movement of horses as well as ultimate eradication of this disease from horse populations in individual countries, should industry and regulatory authorities deem this approach to be desirable.

Adjuvants

Definition

Vaccine adjuvants are chemicals, microbial components, or mammalian proteins that enhance the immune response to a vaccine. When developing a vaccine, it is essential to know what type of immune response will provide optimal protection and then select an adjuvant that will help induce that type of immune response without unacceptable adverse effects. Adjuvants in development or already incorporated in animal vaccines include aluminum salts, oil emulsions, liposomes, microparticles, saponins, immune-stimulating complexes (ISCOMs), nonionic block co-polymers, cytokines and a wide variety of bacterial derivatives. Adjuvants can be broadly divided into two classes, based on their principal mechanisms of action: vaccine delivery systems and immunostimulatory adjuvants. Some vaccines contain proprietary adjuvants, the composition of which has not been made public.

Mechanisms of Action

The mechanisms of action of most adjuvants remain poorly understood because immunization often activates a complex cascade of responses, and the primary effect of the adjuvant is difficult to discern clearly. In general, adjuvants appear to exert their effect by enhancing antigen presentation, improving antigen stability, or acting as immunomodulators.[21,22] A single adjuvant may have more than one mechanism of action. Adjuvants that influence antigen presentation can affect this complex process by improving antigen uptake by *antigen-presenting cells* (APCs), the cells that process antigens and present epitopes to T cells in association with major histocompatibility complex (MHC) molecules. Some adjuvants appear to trap the antigen at the injection site and provide a continuing supply to local APCs, whereas others may work by saturating Kupffer cells in the liver and subsequently may increase the amount of antigen reaching the APCs. Most adjuvants can effectively stimulate T-helper (Th) cells and humoral immunity (Table 70-2). Some, such as liposomes, also appear to deliver antigens to pathways that lead to the presentation of MHC class I molecules and the induction of a CTL response. Immunomodulation is another mechanism of action of adjuvants and is achieved by altering the cytokine network. Adjuvants can influence the type of immunity by enhancing some cytokines and reducing the concentration of others, which may shift the immune response toward a T-helper cell type 1 (Th1, cell-mediated) or T-helper cell type 2 (Th2, humoral) response. By shifting the balance of cytokines, adjuvants such as saponins may stimulate cell-mediated immunity to an antigen that would normally induce only antibodies.

Table • 70-2

Adjuvants Used in Veterinary Medicine with Induced Immune Responses

	IMMUNE RESPONSE		
ADJUVANT	**CELL MEDIATED (Th1)**	**ANTIBODY MEDIATED (Th2)**	**CTL**
Aluminum salts (alum)	X	X	
Oil emulsion		X	
Liposomes		X	X
Nanoparticles	X	X	X
Saponins	X	X	X
ISCOMs	X	X	X
Nonionic block co-polymers		X	X
Cytokines	X	X	
Bacterial products		X	X

Th1, Th2, T-helper type 1 and type 2 cells; *CTL,* cytotoxic T lymphocyte; *ISCOMS,* immune-stimulated complexes.

One particular type of adjuvant deserving special mention is the mucosal adjuvant. Mucosal immunity has a critical role in resistance to a wide variety of pathogens, such as equine influenza and *Streptococcus equi* subsp. *equi*. Generating mucosal immunoglobulin A (IgA) responses with killed vaccines is challenging, and the only effective mucosal adjuvants defined to date are the bacterial exotoxins of enteric bacterial pathogens, such as cholera toxin or the labile toxin of *Escherichia coli*.

Adverse Effects

In addition to enhancing the immune response, adjuvants can also increase the adverse effects of the vaccine. Adverse effects are influenced by the interactions of the specific adjuvant and antigen.[23] Systemic, nonspecific adverse effects can include lethargy, anorexia, fever, arthritis, uveitis, and soreness. More often, however, adjuvants cause local reactions, including inflammation and, more rarely, granulomatous or sterile abscesses. Although most of these reactions are minor and transient, severe inflammation can trap antigens at the injection site and prevent them from being recognized by the immune system. Further, local inflammation and granulomas after vaccination have been linked to the development of vaccine-associated tumors in small animals. Such association has not been reported for horses. Adverse reactions should be reported to the vaccine's manufacturer or the USDA (1-800-752-6255).

Licensing and Safety of Vaccines

The USDA Animal and Plant Health Inspection Service (APHIS) is the federal agency charged with licensing and overseeing the production and use of veterinary vaccines and other biologic products marketed in the United States. The Canadian Department of Agriculture has similar authority in Canada. These agencies license the facilities in which vaccines are produced and regularly inspect them to ensure that facilities and production methods meet established standards. All vaccines are checked for potency, stability, and safety before licensing and at regular intervals thereafter. Safety is established by testing for sterility, toxicity, freedom from extraneous organisms and other material (i.e., purity), and confirmation of the identity of the antigens or organism(s) included in the vaccine. Both "in-house" and field safety studies involving several hundred animals (typically >500 in the case of horses) are also completed before final licensing to confirm that the risk of inducing local or systemic adverse reactions is at an acceptably low level.

The starting point in potency tests is to determine the immunogenicity of a vaccine or the *minimum dose* of antigen that induces a defined immune response, either determined serologically or in challenge studies. Because organisms included in live attenuated or vectored vaccines inevitably die over time, a substantial excess of the organism above the minimum immunizing dose is included in the marketed product to ensure that at least this minimal amount of antigen is present in the vaccine up to the expiration date, assuming appropriate storage and handling of the product. Potency of each batch (serial) of vaccine is therefore tested before and after accelerated aging. Similarly, excess antigen is also in inactivated vaccines, even though they are considerably more stable than live vaccines. Vaccines must not be used after the stated expiration date, even though most will retain potency beyond that date if stored properly. Because live vectored vaccines are governed by the same regulations as MLVs, they typically contain substantially higher amounts of the live vector than the minimum dose needed to immunize horses. This not only adds to the expense of vaccine production, but also may be responsible for some to the systemic reactions observed occasionally in horses after administration of recently released serials of the canarypox-vectored WNV vaccine that presumably contain higher titers of the vector as a result of minimal "die-off" after release. These systemic adverse effects may include fever, lethargy, inappetence, tachycardia, abdominal discomfort, hyperemic mucous membranes, and mildly delayed capillary refill time.

The USDA has traditionally placed more emphasis on documentation of the purity, stability, and safety of veterinary vaccines than on their efficacy.[24,25] Consequently, vaccines for use in horses are typically safe when stored, handled, and administered according to label directions. Many vaccines, however, particularly those directed at pathogens of the respiratory and gastrointestinal tracts, have been found to be of questionable efficacy in the field. Furthermore, published data documenting the efficacy of equine vaccines in well-controlled blinded challenge or field studies have been sparse until recently. For those vaccines for which challenge data were available, duration of immunity (DOI) was rarely established because challenge was typically performed a few weeks after completion of the primary series, when immunity would be expected to be maximal. Without data to define DOI, label directions for revaccination were often arbitrary or ambiguous. Similarly, efficacy studies were not typically performed on foals; therefore the potential inhibitory effects of maternally derived antibodies and the age at which to commence primary immunization were typically not established. Fortunately, "the bar has been raised" considerably during recent years, to the extent that solid challenge data, including information on DOI, are available for virtually all new equine vaccines granted full licenses during the last decade. It is hoped that this type of information will be generated in the future for vaccines that were first licensed many years ago.

In addition to full licenses, USDA has the prerogative to grant conditional licenses to vaccines or antibody products that have met requirements for purity, safety, and stability but have not had efficacy documented in either experimental challenge or field studies. Other criteria used in the granting of a conditional license include a determination that the disease is an imminent and significant threat, that currently available measures for prevention and treatment are inadequate, and that the vaccine or plasma product has a reasonable expectation of efficacy. For vaccines, this expectation of efficacy is typically based on documentation of a detectable serologic response in vaccinated animals and a reasonable likelihood that this serologic response will be protective. Conditional licenses are issued for a limited period and are renewable while the manufacturer works toward documentation of efficacy to support granting of a full license. Each respective state department of agriculture decides whether to allow marketing of a particular conditionally licensed product in that state. The benefit of the conditional licensing procedure was clearly evident when Fort Dodge Animal Health (Fort Dodge, Iowa) was granted a conditional license to market an inactivated WNV vaccine (West Nile-Innovator) in 2001, before the disease had spread beyond eastern and southern states. Widespread use of this vaccine undoubtedly saved the lives of thousands of horses during the interval leading up to granting of a full license supported by challenge data in early 2003. In contrast, inactivated rotavirus and equine protozoal myeloencephalitis (EPM) vaccines have been marketed under conditional licenses for many years without apparent progress in documenting efficacy to support granting of a full license.

Although uncommon, the possibility always exists for adverse reactions (including anaphylaxis) associated with administration of a vaccine; therefore, vaccines should be administered by, or under the direct supervision of, a veterinarian. Adverse reactions should be reported to the vaccine's manufacturer and to the USDA (1-800-752-6255) or the USP Veterinary Practitioners Reporting Program (Forms may be obtained or reports submitted by calling USP at 1-800-487-7776). Anaphylaxis constitutes a life-threatening emergency requiring prompt treatment with epinephrine, 5 mL of a 1:10,000 dilution intravenously (IV) or, in less acute situations, 1 to 2 mL of a 1:1000 dilution intramuscularly (IM) or subcutaneously (SC). Local irritant tissue reactions occur more frequently, particularly when polyvalent combination vaccines are used. These reactions are usually self-limiting, but resolution can be promoted by parenteral or oral administration of nonsteroidal antiinflammatory drugs (NSAIDs), topical application of warm compresses or the cutaneously absorbed NSAID, diclofenac (Surpass, Idexx Pharmaceuticals, Greensboro, North Carolina), and gentle exercise. Significant reactions in the neck muscles may make the horse reluctant to lower or raise its head; therefore, feed and water buckets should be positioned accordingly. The incidence of local reactions can be reduced by administration of the vaccine deep in the semimembranosus and semitendinosus muscles of the hindleg rather than in the neck, and by allowing the horse to exercise after vaccination. In addition, horses that repeatedly react to polyvalent vaccines may benefit from administration of an NSAID before administration of the vaccine, administration of the individual antigenic components separately in different sites, or use of a different brand of vaccine containing a different adjuvant or administered by a different route, such as intranasal rather than intramuscular.

If unacceptable reactions occur repeatedly, the need for continued annual or more frequent revaccination against individual antigens should be carefully reevaluated, taking into account risk of disease, balanced against the risk of an adverse reaction. Many of the horses that experience adverse reactions have received many doses of many vaccine antigens, repeated over many years. In these horses the vaccination protocol should be "pared down" so that only the most essential antigens are administered and the maximum possible interval between boosters is employed. For diseases such as rabies and tetanus for which resistance can reasonably be correlated with circulating antibody titer, one possible approach to define the maximum or optimal interval between booster doses would be to measure the antibody titer to define the need for revaccination. Unfortunately, this approach is currently limited by a paucity of laboratories that offer this type of testing on a routine basis, inexpensively, and with a short turnaround time. The introduction in recent years of commercially available enzyme-linked immunosorbent assay (ELISA) testing for antibodies to the SeM protein (Equine Biodiagnostics-Idexx, Lexington, Kentucky) and neutralizing antibody testing for WNV (Cornell University, Ithaca, New York, and EDART Laboratory, University of Florida, Gainesville, Fla) has made it possible to refine vaccination protocols for these diseases in horses that experience adverse reactions to vaccination. In addition, testing for antibodies to other pathogens may be available through state diagnostic laboratories.

Safety of Vaccines in Broodmares

Consideration of vaccine safety in broodmares must take into account risks to the pregnancy and safety to the fetus. Potential adverse effects of vaccines on pregnancy are difficult to document, even when large numbers of mares are used, unless obvious problems occur. Because fetal organogenesis occurs early in gestation and this period is also characterized by substantial embryonic loss, even in normal mares, it is sound practice to avoid administering vaccines to mares during the first 60 days of gestation unless conditions of imminent risk prevail.

Few vaccines carry specific label recommendations for use in pregnant mares, and little published data exist to document the safety of equine vaccines during pregnancy. Of the available fully licensed vaccines, the two EHV-1 vaccines (Pneumabort-K + 1b, Fort Dodge, and Prodigy, Intervet) marketed for use in pregnant mares as an aid to prevention of EHV-1 abortion, the vaccine marketed for prevention of type B botulism in foals (BotVax-B, Neogen), and the Calvenza line of influenza and EHV vaccines (Boehringer Ingelheim, St. Joseph, Missouri) include directions for use in pregnant mares. In addition, the conditionally licensed vaccine for prevention of rotavirus infection in foals (Equine Rotavirus Vaccine, Fort Dodge) is similarly labeled for use in pregnant mares. Although not specifically labeled for administration during pregnancy, widespread use in practice over many years has failed to document that any of the inactivated vaccines currently marketed for use in horses poses an unacceptable risk to pregnant mares. Therefore, pregnant mares are routinely vaccinated with inactivated vaccines directed against tetanus, eastern equine encephalomyelitis (EEE), western equine encephalomyelitis (WEE), WNV, influenza, EHV-4, strangles and to a lesser extent Potomac horse fever (PHF), rabies, and Venezuelan equine encephalomyelitis (VEE). Similarly, adverse impacts on pregnancy have not been documented for intranasally administered strangles and influenza MLVs or the parenteral EHV-1 MLV (Rhinomune, Pfizer). In addition, safety of the recombinant WNV vaccine (Recombitek, Merial) should not be a significant concern because the modified live canarypox vector lacks the ability to infect mammalian cells. In contrast, modified live-virus EVA and VEE vaccines and live–anthrax spore vaccines should not be used in pregnant mares. Protection of mares against the potential abortigenic effects of EVA infection is therefore best accomplished by completing the primary immunization series before the mare enters the broodmare band and by administering subsequent boosters during the open period before rebreeding.[26]

The practice of booster-vaccinating mares against multiple diseases to maximize colostral transfer of antibodies to the foal, and because mares in broodmare bands are generally middle aged or older, results in the typical broodmare receiving multiple doses of many vaccine antigens and adjuvants during her lifetime. In addition to stimulating high levels of antibody against a range of antigens for the benefit of the foal, this practice may also predispose these mares to a higher rate of local and systemic adverse reactions, an issue that not only warrants further investigation but also may force horse owners and veterinarians to consider strategies for revaccination carefully.

PASSIVE IMMUNIZATION

Use of Exogenous Antibodies

Passive immunization through administration of exogenous plasma or serum products from immune donors is commonly practiced as a means of providing temporary protection from infection during a defined period of risk. Plasma and serum products from hyperimmunized donors are also used as an adjunct to the treatment of specific disease conditions such as tetanus, botulism, WNV infection, endotoxemia, neonatal septicemia, and hypoalbuminemia secondary to other diseases (see appropriate chapters covering these diseases for further information). The degree and duration of protection depend on the amount of total and specific immunoglobulin administered, but the rapid decay of exogenous antibodies inevitably provides only temporary protection.

By far the major indication for passive immunization through the use of plasma products is the treatment of partial or complete *failure of passive transfer* (FPT) of maternal antibodies in neonatal foals. Although the definitions of "complete" and "partial" FPT remain the subject of debate, most veterinarians agree that a plasma transfusion using 1 to 2 liters (20-40 mL/kg) of high–immunoglobulin G (IgG) plasma is indicated for foals with postnursing total serum IgG concentrations of less than 400 mg/dL. Some veterinarians also recommend transfusing foals with serum IgG concentrations between 400 and 800 mg/dL, particularly if other risk factors or signs suggestive of sepsis are present. All plasma products that make specific label claims must be licensed by the USDA to ensure purity, potency, sterility, stability, safety, and efficacy in treating the label indication. The sole indication for products marketed as immunoglobulin supplements is the treatment of FPT. USDA licensing requires documentation that at the recommended dose, these products increase the total IgG concentration by 400 mg/dL. USDA-licensed plasma products for intravenous (IV) administration and containing at least 2500 mg/dL of IgG include Polymune-Plus (Plasvacc USA, Templeton, California), HiGamm Equi (Lake Immunogenics, Ontario, New York), and High-Glo (Mg Biologics, Ames, Iowa). These products should be used to treat foals with complete FPT. Licensed products containing at least 1750 mg/dL of IgG (Foalimmune, Lake Immunogenics) and at least 1500 mg/dL of IgG (Polymune, Plasvacc USA) are also available and may be indicated for treating foals with partial FPT. In addition, a serum-derived concentrated IgG product containing at least 30 g of IgG per 250-mL bottle (I.V. Seramune Equine IgG, Sera, Shawnee Mission, Kansas) is available for IV administration. The same company markets a similar serum product containing at least 30 g of IgG per 300-mL bottle (Oral Seramune Equine IgG) for oral administration (20-40 mL/kg) to foals less than 24 hours of age to prevent FPT.

Several USDA-licensed tetanus antitoxin products have been available in North America for many years as adjuncts to the prevention of tetanus (see later section on tetanus) In recent years, two plasma products (Polymune R and

Polymune REA, Plasvacc USA) have been granted full USDA licenses for prevention of *Rhodococcus equi* pneumonia. A third product (*Rhodococcus equi* Antibody, Lake Immunogenics) has been granted a conditional license pending acceptance by USDA of results of a published study documenting a high level of efficacy in preventing *R. equi* pneumonia on farms where the disease is endemic. Efficacy of these products is optimized if one dose is administered during the first week of life and a second dose is administered 3 to 6 weeks later.[27] Other USDA-licensed plasma products include Polymune-J (Plasvacc USA) harvested from donors immunized against the J5 core antigen of *E. coli*. This product has documented efficacy as an adjunct to treatment of horses with endotoxemia and colitis and is also indicated for the treatment of foals with gram-negative sepsis.[28] Polymune-B (Plasvacc USA) is a *Clostridium botulinum* type B antitoxin licensed by the USDA for prophylactic administration to horses experiencing likely exposure to *C. botulinum* type B toxin or spores. This product has also been used in treatment protocols to neutralize type B toxin in foals with shaker foal syndrome and horses of all ages suspected of experiencing exposure. This univalent type B antitoxin will not neutralize other toxin types. One conditionally licensed plasma product, *Streptococcus equi* Antibody, Equine Origin (Mg Biologics), is marketed for use in horses that are clinically ill from infection with *S. equi* subsp. *equi* and claims to reduce duration of signs, severity of disease, and mortality. Another potential indication would be prevention of disease in horses exposed to *S. equi* subsp. *equi*, although published data regarding efficacy of this product are not available at this time. Similarly, one conditionally licensed plasma product, West Nile Virus Antibody, Equine Origin (Lake Immunogenics), is currently marketed as an aid in the treatment and control of WNV infection. Efficacy is supported by data showing reduction in the level of viremia experienced by hamsters challenged either 1 day before or 1 day after administration of plasma. Evidence of efficacy of this product, and two similar products manufactured by Plasvacc USA and Mg Biologics, in horses has not yet been documented in either experimental or field studies.

Manufacturers of plasma products often infer efficacy for prevention or treatment of specific diseases by stating that the donors were hyperimmunized against specific infectious agents. This practice, although commonplace, does not indicate that efficacy in preventing or treating the specific disease has been proved in controlled studies; therefore, practitioners should view these implied efficacy claims with caution.

Passive Transfer of Maternal Immunity

Passive transfer of maternal antibodies from the mare to the foal through colostrum constitutes by far the most important form of passive immunization in horses. The epitheliochorial placentation present in the mare prevents transfer of maternal immunoglobulins to the fetus during gestation, rendering the foal essentially agammaglobulinemic at birth. Therefore, protection of the foal against specific infectious diseases that it is likely to encounter during the first few months of life, as its own immune system matures, relies heavily on postnatal absorption of specific antibodies and perhaps other factors that the dam has concentrated in colostrum during late gestation. The duration of protection afforded by maternally derived antibodies (MDAs) depends on many factors, the most important of which are the characteristics of the specific infectious agent, the challenge dose, and the magnitude of the postnursing titer of specific antibody. The latter is influenced by the dam's history of disease exposure and vaccination, age, parity, normalcy of gestation, and prepartum leakage of colostrum (i.e., factors that influence concentration of specific antibody in colostrum). Above all, interval between foaling and nursing, the volume of colostrum ingested, and ingestion of macromolecules other than colostrum before ingesting colostrum play major roles in determining passive transfer of specific MDAs. Although several immunoglobulin isotypes are present in colostrum, the subisotypes of IgG are absorbed into the systemic circulation of the foal in much higher concentration than either IgM or IgA.[29] Specific IgA, however, is secreted continuously in milk and may provide passive protection against pathogens such as *S. equi* and enteric organisms by helping coat the pharyngeal and intestinal mucosa, thereby neutralizing pathogens.[29,30] When foals ingest adequate amounts of high-quality colostrum during the first 12 to 24 hours after birth, titers of specific antibody in the serum of the foal are typically very similar to the serum titer in the dam at the time of foaling. Whereas the rate of decay of specific subisotypes of IgG varies to some extent, the overall half-life of decline of maternal IgG antibodies is typically between 25 and 40 days.[31-37] Thus the magnitude of the postnursing antibody titer and the sensitivity of the assay used to detect passively transferred antibodies will determine persistence of these antibodies at measurable levels in the serum of foals. Use of ELISA and other sensitive assays has made it possible to detect persistence of MDAs at detectable levels for 6 months or longer in some cases.[32,37]

Whereas passively acquired MDAs are important for protecting the foal against infection with many pathogens, they play a particularly critical role in prevention of infection with enteric pathogens such as rotavirus, *E. coli*, and other Enterobacteriaceae to which neonates are particularly susceptible. Passive transfer of immunity to these and other agents (e.g., botulism) that affect foals can be enhanced by stimulating either a primary or an anamnestic response in the mare during late gestation. This is typically an important focus of immunization programs for mares and can be accomplished through planned exposure, if the infectious agent does not pose a threat to the mare, as is the case with rotavirus, or more appropriately through administration of booster doses of vaccines to mares, 30 to 60 days before foaling. Maintaining consistent vaccination protocols for mares will maximize the likelihood that a uniformly high level of colostral antibody transfer and passive protection will be achieved within the foal crop. Whereas intranasally administered vaccines may afford good protection to the mare, they are typically less effective than parenterally administered inactivated vaccines in stimulating high levels of circulating IgG, the isotype that is passively transferred to the foal in highest concentration. Parenteral vaccines are therefore preferred over intranasal vaccines for vaccination of mares during late gestation.

It is widely assumed that pregnant mares are fully capable of mounting appropriate cellular and humoral immune responses to vaccines; however, this issue has received little research attention. Whereas mares that have been primed before breeding appear to mount appropriate anamnestic responses to vaccines administered during late gestation, it appears that the humoral response to primary vaccination with at least the inactivated WNV vaccine is downregulated during gestation. In one study, more than 75% of naive mares, vaccinated for the first time against WNV while pregnant, failed to mount a detectable serologic response to two doses of an inactivated WNV vaccine administered 4 weeks apart.[38] Consequently, their foals failed to acquire any WNV antibodies through colostrum and were rendered potentially susceptible to infection. At this time it is not known whether this apparent pregnancy-associated suppression of serologic responses to primary immunization applies to vaccines other than the inactivated WNV vaccine. Nevertheless, it is wise to complete primary immunization before breeding and administer booster doses of selected antigens late in gestation rather than attempting to complete the primary series during gestation, regardless of the vaccine. The common practice of administering booster doses of multiple antigens to mares during late gestation raises the possibility that "competition" between multiple antigens will compromise the response to some or all of them and increase the risk of an adverse local or systemic reaction. Although these issues have not been addressed in controlled research studies, it is nevertheless good practice to administer no more than four antigens at one time and to allow an interval of 3 to 4 weeks between administration of vaccines containing additional antigens.

VACCINATION OF FOALS AND INFLUENCE OF MATERNAL ANTIBODIES ON VACCINE RESPONSES

Whereas foals are considered to be immune competent at birth and are capable of mounting both humoral and cellular immune responses to a range of antigens, continued maturation of the immune system after birth is believed to be necessary to achieve optimal immune function. However, few studies have been done to determine the age at which various elements of the innate and adaptive immune system become fully competent and optimal responses to vaccines can be achieved. Maternal antibodies, and perhaps other important immune effectors (e.g., lymphocytes) that are concentrated in colostrum and are passively transferred to the foal, play a crucial role in defense against pathogens encountered during the first few months of life while endogenous immune function continues to mature.

In addition to passively protecting the foal, maternal antibodies have been shown to exert a profound inhibitory effect on the immune response of foals to antigens, including those contained in vaccines. Several studies reported by groups in Holland, Ireland, and the United States during the 1990s brought this issue into focus by demonstrating that foals less than 6 months of age consistently failed to mount serologic responses to inactivated influenza vaccines.[33,35,37,39-42] Of potentially greater concern was the finding that not only a high proportion of foals vaccinated under the cover of MDAs failed to seroconvert in response to the recommended primary series of two or three doses of influenza vaccine, but also many failed to respond to multiple additional doses administered during the next year, suggesting induction of a potentially detrimental "immunotolerance-like" phenomenon.[39,40,43] Our studies confirmed an apparent lack of response of foals to multiple doses of inactivated influenza vaccines when the hemagglutination inhibition (HI) test was used to detect serologic responses. When the same samples were retested using sensitive isotype-specific ELISA tests, it was found that 6-month-old foals did mount a response that included all IgG subisotypes but that was less vigorous for the more important virus neutralizing IgGa and IgGb subisotypes than for the less effective IgG(T) subisotype.[37] Whereas there appeared to be some differences in responses to different vaccines containing different adjuvants, this "misdirection" of isotype responses in favor of IgG(T), likely influenced by MDAs, was consistently observed.[37] Subsequent studies, in which titers of total, rather than antigen-specific, IgG subisotypes were determined, documented that the age-related increase in concentrations of IgGb lagged significantly behind increases in concentrations of other isotypes and remained below adult levels beyond 6 months of age.[44]

Maternal antibody interference has now been documented as a significant issue for many other antigens, including tetanus, EEE, WEE, EHV-1, and EHV-4, contained in vaccines administered to foals.[36,37,45-48] Even low levels of antibody, below those detectable by many routine serologic tests and below those thought to be protective, can completely block the serologic response to some vaccines, resulting in a potentially prolonged period of susceptibility before the foal is capable of responding appropriately to vaccines.[47] These findings also indicate that it is not typically feasible to test samples from foals serologically to predict whether they will respond to particular vaccines. We now recommend that primary immunization with most vaccines containing inactivated antigens should be delayed until foals are 6 months of age or older and, with the exception of rabies vaccine, three doses of vaccine should be included in the primary series rather the two doses routinely recommended by vaccine manufacturers. Typically, the third dose stimulates a serologic response of greater magnitude and durability than two doses and may also contribute to a higher "set point" for the response to subsequent booster doses.[37,38,47,49] In contrast to the results previously cited, MDAs do not appear to exert a marked inhibitory effect on the response of foals to either the inactivated or recombinant live WNV vaccines (West Nile-Innovator, Recombitek), thus permitting antibody-positive foals as young as 3 months of age to be immunized successfully.[38]

Results of studies investigating MDA interference with responses to vaccines should be interpreted with caution because only humoral responses are typically assessed. In these studies, infectious challenge may not be performed to confirm that lack of serologic response equates to lack of protection. Lack of a serologic response may correlate well with lack of protection for some diseases and some vaccines, whereas for others this may not be the case. In contrast, the presence of a serologic response may not correlate well with protection, as is frequently the case for respiratory tract pathogens. Except for the intranasally administered strangles and influenza vaccines (Pinnacle I.N., Fort Dodge, and Flu-Avert I.N., Intervert), the EHV-1 MLV (Rhinomune), the EVA MLV (Arvac, Fort Dodge), and the canarypox-vectored WNV vaccine (Recombitek), most commercially available vaccines are inactivated, adjuvanted, and administered by IM injection. Because inactivated vaccines administered by injection have limited potential to stimulate cellular and mucosal responses, serologic responses to these vaccines likely correlate well with their potential to induce protection. In turn, MDA interference with serologic responses to inactivated vaccines likely equates to failure to induce protection. In contrast, failure to detect a serologic response to a modified live, vectored, DNA, or mucosally administered vaccine may not equate to lack of protection because vaccines of these types induce a broader array of systemic and local responses that may not be affected by MDAs.

If maternal antibody interference were not an issue, the approach to vaccination of foals would be greatly simplified because primary vaccination against all important diseases could be completed before MDAs had declined to nonprotective levels. In effect, the "window of susceptibility" would be eliminated. In reality, a realistic goal is to maximize the beneficial effects of MDAs while minimizing their negative impact on primary immunization. To best meet this goal, it is necessary to decide which one (or both) of the following is the primary focus:

1. To protect the foal and weanling against specific high-risk infectious diseases that affect this age group and have the potential to cause significant disease, either directly or by predisposing to other secondary infections.
2. To initiate primary immunization to protect against disease later in life.

Assessing risk takes into account both the incidence of disease (i.e. the likelihood that the foal will become infected) and the risk of serious sequelae or death if the horse does become infected. If the disease affects the foal early in life, as with rotavirus infection, there is usually insufficient time to induce a protective immune response by actively immunizing the foal. Under these circumstances, the approach should be to maximize the degree of protection passively transferred from the dam through colostrum. Other diseases, such as rabies, affect horses of all ages, but the risk of acquiring infection is generally low.

Diseases of moderate to high risk to young foals but low risk to adults include rotavirus infection (on certain breeding farms in certain years) and, in geographic areas such as Kentucky and some other eastern states, type B botulism. For these diseases, the following approach is appropriate:

- Booster-vaccinate the dam before foaling to maximize uniformity of passive transfer.
- Ensure good passive transfer of maternal antibodies.
- Introduce management practices to reduce exposure to the infectious agent.
- Vaccinate the foal if risk continues beyond the first few months of life.

Diseases of moderate to high risk for weanlings and older horses but lower risk to young foals born to vaccinated mares include EHV-4, EHV-1, strangles, influenza, tetanus, EEE, WEE, and WNV. For these diseases, the following approach is appropriate:

- Vaccinate the dam before foaling to maximize uniformity of passive transfer.
- Ensure good passive transfer of maternal antibodies.
- Start foal vaccination after the risk of MDA interference is no longer present in *most* foals. When several vaccine types are available for a particular disease, the vaccine that is least subject to MDA interference should be used. Introduce management practices to reduce exposure to the infectious agent while primary vaccination is being completed.
- If a two-dose primary series is recommended for adult horses, use three or more doses of vaccine in the primary series to improve the chances that foals that do not respond to earlier doses will respond to additional doses administered later.

Diseases of low risk to foals in most circumstances include rabies, PHF, WEE, and EVA. For these diseases, the following approach is appropriate:

- Vaccinate the dam before foaling if the disease is a significant risk to adult horses and a vaccine shown to be safe for use in pregnant mares is available. If the available vaccines are not considered safe for use in pregnant mares, administer boosters before breeding.
- Ensure good passive transfer of maternal antibodies.
- Start foal vaccination after the risk of MDA interference is no longer present in *any* foal (typically 9 months to 1 year of age).

AVAILABLE VACCINES AND CONCEPT OF CORE AND NONCORE VACCINES

Fully licensed vaccines are now available in North America as aids to the prevention of tetanus, viral encephalomyelitis (EEE, WEE, VEE), West Nile virus (WNV) infection, influenza, equine herpesvirus type 1 (EHV-1) and EHV-4 infection, strangles, rabies, equine viral arteritis (EVA), Potomac horse fever (PHF), and type B botulism. In addition, conditionally licensed vaccines are available to immunize horses against rotavirus infection and equine protozoal myeloencephalitis (EPM). Tetanus and viral encephalomyelitis caused by EEE, WEE, and WNV pose a threat to horses in all geographic areas and are therefore considered to be "core" diseases against which all horses in North America should be vaccinated. In addition, the public health consequences of infection and the 100% mortality rate warrant inclusion of rabies as a core disease for horses residing in, or being transported to, those many areas of North America where rabies is endemic in the wildlife population. The abortogenic potential of EHV-1 warrants inclusion of this disease in the core for all pregnant broodmares. Although influenza is not routinely included as a core disease, vaccination against this highly contagious respiratory tract infection is strongly recommended for all horses that are likely to be co-located with horses from other facilities during transportation or at sales, shows, trail rides, races, or other events. The remaining diseases for which vaccines are available are considered "noncore." Indications for use of vaccines against these diseases are discussed in the relevant sections that follow.

VACCINATION RECOMMENDATIONS FOR SPECIFIC DISEASES

Tetanus

All horses are at risk for developing tetanus, an often-fatal disease caused by a potent neurotoxin elaborated by the anaerobic, spore-forming bacterium *Clostridium tetani*. These organisms are present in the intestinal tract and feces of horses, other animals, and humans and are ubiquitous in soil. Tetanus is expensive to treat and has a high mortality rate; therefore all horses should be actively immunized using tetanus toxoid as part of the core vaccination program. Active immunization reduces the need to administer tetanus antitoxin, the use of which is associated with risk of inducing potentially fatal serum hepatitis. Protection against tetanus appears to be mediated by circulating antibodies, and these antibodies are transferred efficiently through colostrum. The many available vaccines are typically formalin-inactivated, adjuvanted toxoids that are inexpensive and safe and that induce an excellent serologic response and solid, long-lasting immunity. Manufacturers recommend administration of a primary series of two doses of toxoid at 3- to 6-week intervals, followed by annual boosters. Titers of specific antibody increase within 14 days after administration of the second dose in the primary series and, in adult horses, persist at detectable levels for 12 months or longer, depending on the adjuvant system used in the vaccine.[50,51]

No published challenge studies are available to document the speed of onset or duration of protection induced by tetanus toxoid preparations currently licensed in North America; conclusions regarding their efficacy are therefore based on the serologic response obtained in laboratory animals. However, a challenge study conducted in Europe more than 40 years ago found that horses were resistant to challenge 8 days after receiving a single injection of tetanus toxoid, before antibody could be detected in their serum.[52] A second study demonstrated that a series of three doses of tetanus toxoid induced protection lasting for at least 8 years, and perhaps for life, even when antibodies could no longer be detected.[53] In contrast, tetanus has been documented in vaccinated horses in North America,[54] although survival was strongly associated with previous vaccination. Thus it would not be prudent to recommend extension of the annual interval for revaccination with tetanus toxoid, pending publication of data documenting duration of immunity. Vaccinated horses that sustain a wound or have surgery more than 6 months after receiving their previous tetanus booster should be revaccinated with tetanus toxoid.

The annual booster for pregnant mares should be administered 4 to 8 weeks before foaling to protect the mare if she sustains foaling-induced trauma and to enhance concentrations of specific immunoglobulins in colostrum. Colostrum-derived antibodies significantly interfere with the immune response of foals vaccinated with tetanus toxoid until they are about 6 months of age.[37,51] If a foal received appropriate transfer of colostral antibodies from a vaccinated mare, that foal should receive its primary series of three doses of tetanus toxoid beginning at age 6 months or older. Foals born to nonvaccinated mares should receive this initial three-dose series starting at 1 to 4 months of age. The three-dose primary series is recommended for foals because a high proportion of foals fail to seroconvert in response to two doses of tetanus toxoid, regardless of whether maternal antibodies are detectable at administration of the first dose.[37,51] Optimally, the third dose in the primary series should be administered 2 to 3 months after the second dose.

Tetanus antitoxin is produced by hyperimmunization of donor horses with tetanus toxoid. Administration of one vial of antitoxin (1500 IU) to nonvaccinated horses induces immediate passive protection that lasts no longer than 3 weeks.[51] More prolonged protection may be accomplished with higher doses. In addition to the use of high doses of tetanus antitoxin to treat tetanus, indications frequently cited include administration to newborn foals born to nonvaccinated mares and to nonvaccinated horses that sustain an injury. In these cases the concurrent administration of tetanus antitoxin and tetanus toxoid at different sites using separate syringes has been advocated, followed by administration of additional doses of toxoid at 4- to 6-week intervals to complete the primary series.[55] Because a small but significant number of horses experience serum sickness and fatal hepatic failure (serum hepatitis) several weeks after receiving tetanus antitoxin,[56,57] a preferred approach to the nonvaccinated horse that sustains a puncture or deep laceration is to thoroughly clean and debride the wound, initiate active immunization by administering tetanus toxoid, and institute a course of antimicrobial treatment with penicillin or an alternate antimicrobial that is active against *C. tetani.*

Equine Encephalomyelitis (Sleeping Sickness)

The encephalomyelitis viruses (EEE, WEE, VEE) are transmitted by mosquitoes, and infrequently by other bloodsucking insects, to horses from wild birds or rodents, which serve as natural reservoirs for these viruses. Risk of exposure and geographic distribution of the encephalomyelitis viruses vary by season and from year to year with changes in distribution of insect vectors and wildlife reservoirs. The distribution of EEE has historically been restricted to the eastern, southeastern, and some southern states, whereas outbreaks of WEE have been recorded in the western and midwestern states, with sporadic cases in the Northeast and Southeast United States. Because EEE or WEE (or both) is endemic in most areas of North America, vaccination against these diseases should be part of the core vaccination program for all horses. Venezuelan equine encephalomyelitis occurs in South and Central America but has not been diagnosed in the United States or Mexico for many years; therefore, routine vaccination of horses in these regions against VEE is not recommended at this time, unless transportation to endemic areas is planned.

Although correlates for protection against EEE, WEE, and VEE are not well established, circulating antibodies are assumed to be important because infection is acquired by vascular injection (mosquito bites), and current inactivated vaccines are protective.[58,59] However, despite that virtually every manufacturer of equine vaccines in North America produces one or more equine encephalomyelitis vaccines, no randomized, double-blind challenge trials using these vaccines have been published. Available vaccines are inactivated, adjuvanted, bivalent whole-virus products containing EEE and WEE (Encevac with Havlogen, Intervet; Encephaloid Innovator, Fort Dodge; Cephalovac EW, Boehringer Ingelheim) or trivalent products that also contain VEE (Cephalovac VEW, Boehringer Ingelheim). Veterinarians and horse owners often use combination products containing other antigens, such as tetanus, influenza, WNV, or equine herpesviruses for primary or booster immunization of horses against encephalomyelitis viruses.

Primary immunization of nonvaccinated adult horses is accomplished by administration of two doses of inactivated vaccine 3 to 6 weeks apart. In areas where EEE is not a threat and mosquito vectors are active for less than 6 months of the year, annual revaccination in the spring, before the peak insect vector season, is recommended. In areas such as the Gulf States where EEE is endemic and mosquitoes are active virtually year-round, most veterinarians prefer to revaccinate horses semiannually to ensure more uniform protection throughout the year. Inactivated encephalomyelitis vaccines are considered to be safe for use in pregnant mares; therefore, booster vaccination 4 to 8 weeks before foaling is routinely recommended to enhance colostral concentrations of specific immunoglobulins. Neutralizing antibodies to WEE and EEE are transferred passively to foals through colostrum and decline with an estimated half-life of 33 and 20 days, respectively. Maternally derived antibodies (MDAs) appear to confer protection and are detectable in the serum of many foals from vaccinated mares for at least 3 months and up to 7 months, depending on the postnursing titer.[31,36,60,61]

Several studies have shown that MDAs exert a profound inhibitory effect on the ability of foals to mount serologic responses to inactivated bivalent WEE/EEE vaccines, which likely accounts for some of the reported cases of vaccine failure and resultant clinical EEE in vaccinated horses, particularly those less than 2 years of age.[31,36,43,47,60] Studies have shown that 3-month-old foals born to immune mares consistently failed to mount a serologic response to two doses of inactivated bivalent WEE/EEE vaccine, and the majority had not responded even after administration of a third dose.[38,47] Whereas many 6-month-old foals failed to seroconvert after administration of two doses of vaccine, most responded following administration of a third dose.[47] Based on these data, inclusion of a third dose in the primary series, 8 to 12 weeks after administration of the second dose, is strongly recommended for foals and yearlings.

Western equine encephalomyelitis has a lower mortality rate than EEE, and prevalence of WEE in many western states is sufficiently low that the risk of foals acquiring infection during their first year of life is also low. Therefore, primary vaccination of foals in areas where mosquitoes die off in the winter and the risk of infection is low is best completed when foals are 6 month of age or older, to minimize the potential for maternal antibody interference. Because foals born in the late spring and summer months are still less than 6 months of age by the time the mosquito season comes to an end in many regions, primary vaccination of these foals can be delayed until the spring of the yearling year. In contrast, EEE is a highly fatal disease that poses a significant risk to foals during their first year of life, particularly in the Gulf States, where competent vectors are present year-round.[31,43,62] Therefore, most veterinarians in these regions recommend commencing primary vaccination of foals at 3 to 4 months of age using a three-dose primary series followed by a fourth dose at 1 year of age and semiannual boosters thereafter, to maximize the chances of overcoming the inhibitory effects of maternal antibody and inducing protection.[31]

West Nile Virus

In the few years since WNV infection was first diagnosed in horses in the northeastern United States in 1999, it has spread across the entire North American continent and is now considered to be endemic in all mainland areas of North America and Mexico, where it has become an important consideration in the differential diagnosis of horses presenting with signs of neurologic disease. As of late 2005, the disease had been confirmed in more than 23,000 horses in the United States, approximately 35% of which had died or been euthanized. West Nile virus, as with the other encephalomyelitis viruses, is transmitted by mosquitoes, and infrequently by other bloodsucking insects, to horses, humans, and a number of other mammals from avian hosts, which serve as natural reservoirs for these viruses. Horses and humans are considered to be "dead-end" hosts of WNV and therefore do not contribute to the transmission cycle. The virus is not directly contagious from horse to horse or from horse to human. Similarly, indirect transmission by mosquitoes from infected horses is highly unlikely because horses do not experience a significant level of viremia.[63] Risk of infection and death appears to increase with increasing age; however, the disease has been confirmed in foals as young as 3 weeks of age. Although cases have been seen virtually year-round in the southeastern United States, the risk of acquiring infection is highest during those months in which mosquito activity peaks, typically July, August, September, and October in most areas of North America. WNV infection is a core disease against which all horses residing in the continental United States and Canada should be vaccinated.

As of late 2005, two fully licensed vaccines (West Nile-Innovator, Recombitek) are marketed for use in horses in North America. West Nile-Innovator is an inactivated whole-virus vaccine that contains a metabolizable oil adjuvant.[64] This vaccine is available as either a monovalent (single component) or a multivalent vaccine containing other encephalitis virus antigens (EEE and WEE). Recombitek is a canarypox-vectored recombinant MLV.[13,65] Both vaccines have met USDA requirements for safety in tests involving more than 600 horses. Needle and mosquito challenge models have shown that both significantly reduce the magnitude of viremia in experimentally infected, vaccinated horses compared with nonvaccinated control horses for as long as 12 months after primary vaccination with two doses of vaccine.[13,64] There is clear evidence that vaccination reduces the risk of infection and death after natural challenge in the field setting, although clinical disease may not be fully prevented.[66,67]

Directions for use include administration of two doses of vaccine 3 to 6 weeks apart (consult the specific label). Optimal protection cannot be expected until 2 weeks after administration of the second dose, although Recombitek is capable of inducing significant protection as early as 26 days after administration of the first dose.[65] The vaccine manufacturers recommend revaccination of previously vaccinated horses on an annual basis, or more frequently when local conditions are conducive to a prolonged period of potential exposure to infected mosquito vectors. Annual revaccination is best completed in the spring (late February through early April), before the onset of the insect vector season. In areas where the mosquito season is prolonged, revaccination twice annually, once in the spring and again in the late summer or early fall (late July through early September), may be necessary to maximize protection.

Neither of the licensed vaccines currently marketed in the United States carry label recommendations for administration to pregnant mares; therefore it is recommended that mares be vaccinated before breeding whenever possible. It is well recognized, however, that pregnant mares are at risk of acquiring infection from infected mosquitoes. Consequently, it has become accepted practice by many veterinarians to administer vaccines to pregnant mares on the reasonable assumption that the risk of adverse consequences of WNV infection greatly exceeds the reported adverse effects of use of vaccines in pregnant mares. Thousands of doses of West Nile-Innovator vaccine have been administered safely to pregnant mares, and a recent study failed to document vaccine-associated adverse effects in a large population of pregnant mares.[68] Although the Recombitek vaccine is a live vectored vaccine, the canarypox vector is incapable of replication in mammals and does not induce a viremia that could infect a fetus. In addition, a canarypox-vectored influenza vaccine available in Europe is licensed for use in horses during pregnancy; thus the vectored WNV vaccine is unlikely to induce adverse effects in pregnant mares. As with other vaccines, it is sound practice to avoid administering WNV vaccines to mares during the first 60 days of gestation unless conditions of imminent risk prevail.

Booster vaccination of previously primed pregnant mares, 4 to 6 weeks before foaling, using either WNV-Innovator or Recombitek vaccine, appears to induce a strong anamnestic serologic response that provides their foals with passive colostral protection lasting 3 to 4 months.[38] In contrast, preliminary data suggest that a significant proportion of naive pregnant mares failed to seroconvert when the primary series of West Nile-Innovator vaccine was administered during the second half of gestation, perhaps reflecting pregnancy-associated downregulation of Th2 responses. If subsequently proven, this preliminary observation adds further justification to the recommendation that the primary series is best completed before breeding.

In contrast to findings with many other vaccines in the foals of immune mares, MDAs do not block the response of foals as young 3 months of age to vaccination with either the inactivated or the recombinant vaccine.[38] Although this finding is somewhat surprising for the inactivated vaccine, it might reasonably have been expected for the recombinant vaccine because the canarypox vector system accomplishes transfection of cells and expression of the major E-peptide and M-peptide antigens of WNV on the surface of APCs in association with MHC class I and class II antigens. These peptide antigens are therefore not free in the tissues and circulation to be neutralized by MDAs.

Primary vaccination of foals from properly vaccinated mares should be started by administration of the first dose of vaccine at 3 to 4 months of age, followed by a second dose approximately 1 month later, then a third dose 8 to 12 weeks after the second dose. This third dose increases the likelihood that foals with high MDA levels, which may have attenuated the response to the first dose of vaccine, will become primed and protected. Even in foals that have no maternally derived WNV antibodies after nursing, the third dose of inactivated vaccine in the primary series induces significantly higher and more persistent levels of antibody than two doses. A booster should be administered during the spring of the yearling year, after which the recommendations for vaccination of adult horses should be followed. Primary vaccination of foals from nonvaccinated, nonexposed mares should commence at 3 to 4 months of age or younger (as early as 1 month of age), depending on month of birth and seasonal level of activity of mosquito vectors in the area. The three-dose primary vaccination protocol previously outlined should be followed. The duration of protection from reinfection in horses that have recovered from natural infection is unknown, but likely extends to more than 1 year. It is good practice, however, to include recovered horses in the routine vaccination program used for herdmates, in the year following recovery from natural infection.

In 2005, Fort Dodge Animal Health was granted a license to market a plasmid DNA vaccine to protect horses against WNV infection. However, this vaccine has not been marketed as of August 2006. Protection against viremia has been documented in mosquito challenge studies similar to those performed for licensing of the inactivated West Nile-Innovator vaccine.[18,69] Two doses of vaccine administered 3 to 4 weeks apart induced significant protection in horses challenged 1 year later. A fourth WNV vaccine, a chimeric yellow fever–vectored vaccine produced by Intervet, should receive final licensing and be marketed by the fall of 2006. A single dose of this vaccine has been shown to prevent clinical disease in 4- to 6-month-old horses as well as viremia in a rigorous intrathecal challenge model that, unlike models used previously, reliably induces severe clinical disease.[15] This vaccine will be labeled for protection against viremia and as an aid in the prevention of disease and encephalitis caused by WNV. It is remarkable that in little more than 6 years after WNV disease was first encountered in the Americas, four vaccines with documented efficacy based on challenge studies will be marketed for the benefit of horses, including three that apply the most modern technologies available for either animals or humans at this time.

Equine Influenza

Infection of the respiratory tract of horses with the orthomyxovirus, influenza A/equine/2 (H3N8), remains one of the most common causes of rapidly spreading outbreaks of respiratory disease, despite the widespread practice of frequently revaccinating horses with inactivated vaccines by IM injection. The influenza A/equine/1 subtype (H7N7) has not been recognized as a cause of clinical disease for many years and is likely extinct in nature. Influenza is endemic in the equine populations of the United States and much of the world, with the notable exceptions of Iceland, Australia, and New Zealand. Rapid national and international transportation of horses facilitates spread of the virus. Concentrating young horses at racetracks, training facilities, boarding stables, breeding farms, shows, or similar athletic events increases the risk of infection, as does a low serum concentration of specific antibody.[70] Older horses are generally less susceptible to infection but may become ill when partial protection is overwhelmed by exposure to horses excreting large amounts of virus. Although the disease is endemic in many countries and infection cycles continuously, explosive outbreaks occur at intervals of several years when the immunity of the equine population wanes and sufficient antigenic drift has occurred to generate a new viral strain. In contrast to herpesviruses, equine influenza virus is not maintained in asymptomatic carrier horses and does not circulate constantly, even in large groups of horses. Rather, the disease is introduced sporadically by a symptomatic or asymptomatic infected horse. This epidemiologic finding and the rapid elimination of the virus by the equine immune response suggest that infection can be avoided by preventing entry of the virus into an equine population (e.g., by quarantine of newly arriving horses for at least 14 days) and by appropriate vaccination.[71]

Equine influenza virus is highly contagious and spreads rapidly through groups of horses in aerosolized droplets dispersed by coughing. Contaminated buckets, grooming or feeding equipment, tack, and transport vehicles may serve as fomites because the virus can survive for hours on such objects. Severity of clinical signs of influenza, which include nasal discharge, fever, lethargy, anorexia, cough, and myalgia, depends on the degree of existing immunity and other factors. Infected horses shed virus for up to 10 days in their nasal secretions. Inactivated vaccines do not induce sterile immunity; therefore, recently vaccinated horses can become infected, shed virus, and contribute to interepidemic persistence of infection within the equine population and propagation of infection during outbreaks.[72]

Immunity to the same (homologous) strain of virus following natural infection persists for more than a year and involves both local and systemic humoral and cellular mechanisms. These include induction of large amounts of virus-specific neutralizing IgG and secretory IgA antibody in nasal secretions, high levels of circulating IgG antibodies, and genetically restricted antigen-specific cytotoxic T lymphocytes (CTLs) that kill infected cells.[73-77] Memory CTLs can be detected in peripheral blood for at least 6 months after infection, and solid immunity persists even when circulating antibody titers have declined to low or nondetectable levels.[74,75,78,79] Similarly, protection induced by the licensed modified live intranasal influenza vaccine (Flu-Avert I.N., Intervet) is presumably mediated through induction of local immune responses in the respiratory tract because this vaccine does not typically induce high levels of circulating antibody.[80,81] Except possibly for ISCOM vaccines, inactivated vaccines administered by IM injection have limited potential to induce CTL or nasal secretory IgA responses and induce only low levels of neutralizing antibody in nasal secretions.[73,79,82] The degree of protection induced by inactivated influenza vaccines is highly correlated with postvaccination titers of circulating antibody, predominantly of the IgGa and IgGb subisotypes, as measured by HI or single radial hemolysis (SRH) tests.[70,83-86] SRH levels of 100 mm^2 or greater are considered to be at least partially protective; however, levels greater than 140 mm^2 are required for successful prevention of disease.[85] The partial protection induced by inactivated vaccines is of limited duration (a few weeks up to about 7 months, depending on the vaccine) and is manifested as a reduction in clinical signs and attenuation of viral shedding in horses exposed to infection.[71,73]

The magnitude of the serologic response to inactivated influenza vaccines depends on many factors, including the preparation of antigen contained in the vaccine, antigenic mass, the nature of the adjuvant, history of previous vaccination or infection, interval since the last dose of vaccine, antibody titer at the time of vaccination, age, and maternal antibody status. Relatedness of the vaccine strain to circulating field strains of influenza virus is another important determinant of efficacy, at least for inactivated influenza vaccines.[83,87,88] Antigenic drift of the A/equine/2 subtype has resulted from point mutations in the genes encoding the amino acid sequences of the hemagglutinin (H) and neuraminidase (N) glycoprotein antigens on the surface of the virus. The result is emergence of viral strains representing two antigenic lineages, American and Eurasian, of the H3N8 virus. Further antigenic drift within each lineage has generated variants that, as with the prototypic strain A/equine 2/Miami 63, are named according to the location and year that they were first isolated. Antigenic drift, by generating antigenically heterologous viruses, reduces the degree and duration of protection conferred by previous infection or vaccination because of the specificity of immunoglobulins, and it allows horses with high titers to become infected and develop clinical signs of disease if the vaccine strain is not closely related to the drifted infectious field strain.[89] Although antigenic drift of equine influenza virus is slower than that of human influenza viruses, it is recommended that inactivated equine influenza vaccines include viral antigens from isolates obtained within the most recent 5 years, and ideally, representatives of each (American and Eurasian) lineage should be included. An expert surveillance panel meets annually to recommend strains that should be included in influenza vaccines in subsequent years (www.equiflunet.org.uk). To comply with federal regulations for licensing and marketing of vaccines, any change of a vaccine, such as including the most recently isolated influenza virus, usually leads to costly and time-consuming evaluation of the revised product. Consequently, viral antigens contained in inactivated vaccines typically lag more than the recommended 5 years behind the antigenic drift of field viruses, resulting in suboptimal protection. Even though Flu-Avert I.N. contains only a 1991 H3N8 strain of North American lineage, it has been shown to protect against challenge with Eurasian strains and recently isolated North American strains.

The short-lived immunity after vaccination with inactivated equine influenza vaccines was the impetus for past recommendations for frequent revaccination, at intervals as short as 2 months. However, too short an interval between revaccination may compromise efficacy because influenza vaccination in the horse with a high titer inhibits development of an optimal anamnestic response.[90] An additional consideration that potentially limits the efficacy of influenza vaccines is the phenomenon termed "original antigenic sin," whereby horses exposed to a drifted field A/equine/2 virus will mount an anamnestic immune response directed more strongly against the strain with which they were vaccinated initially than against the drifted field virus.[91]

A considerable amount of published efficacy data, based both on challenge studies and on field epidemiology studies, has been available for many years in Europe to support the use of influenza vaccines. In contrast, information regarding the efficacy of influenza vaccines marketed in North America has remained sparse until recently. Large, cross-sectional and longitudinal, prospective epidemiologic studies conducted during 3 consecutive years in the early 1990s at a Thoroughbred racetrack in Saskatchewan failed to document any reduction in risk of influenza in recently vaccinated horses.[70] Furthermore, a double-masked, randomized field trial conducted by the same researchers showed that vaccination of horses with the then-leading influenza vaccine marketed for use before an anticipated influenza epidemic did not significantly reduce the risk of developing respiratory tract disease or reduce the severity of disease, although the duration of clinical disease was shortened in vaccinates.[72] Serologic testing performed during these studies indicated that vaccine failure was caused by failure of the influenza vaccines in use at the time to induce protective antibody titers. Indeed, many horses failed to mount a detectable serologic response, a finding that was subsequently confirmed in a field study involving 173 horses on six premises in northern Colorado during 1997 and 1998 using aluminum hydroxide–adjuvanted vaccines (Flumune and Rhino-Flu, Smith Kline Beecham Animal Health, now Pfizer) containing an inactivated Miami/63 H3N8 strain.[92] In contrast, Newton and Lakhani et al.[93] found that 73% of previously vaccinated 2-year-old Thoroughbreds in England achieved a protective SRH antibody titer of 140 mm^2 2 weeks after administration of a booster dose of a European licensed inactivated aluminum hydroxide–adjuvanted influenza vaccine containing a more recent H3N8 isolate and likely also a higher antigenic mass.

Fortunately, vaccine manufacturers in North America have responded to the challenge of producing more efficacious equine influenza vaccines during the last few years by incorporating more relevant recent viral strains, by increasing antigenic mass of relevant strains, by eliminating the seemingly irrelevant H7N7 strain, by modifying adjuvant systems, and by introducing novel technologies. An important advance occurred in 1999 when Heska Corporation marketed an attenuated live, cold-adapted influenza vaccine (Flu-Avert I.N., Intervet, Millsboro, Delaware) for intranasal administration. This vaccine, which contains a Kentucky/1991 strain of North American lineage, was found to be highly efficacious in blinded, controlled challenge studies conducted 5 weeks, 6 months, and 1 year after administration of a single dose to naive horses.[81] Subsequently, Flu-Avert I.N. was shown to cross-protect against European H3N8 strains, as well as against North American strains isolated during the late 1990s and early 2000s, and to induce a rapid onset of protection within 7 days of administration of a single dose to naive horses.[80,94] Although horses challenged 1 year after administration of a single dose showed a significant but only partial reduction in severity of clinical signs and virus shedding, a more marked reduction in clinical signs and viral shedding was found when the challenge was performed 6 months after vaccination.[81] Based on these results, revaccination at 6-month intervals is recommended. Field experience indicates that this regimen induces solid clinical protection after natural challenge. Currently, Flu-Avert I.N. is licensed for use in nonpregnant horses 11 months of age or older, primarily because this was the youngest age of the horses used in the challenge studies for licensing. Horses may shed small amounts of vaccinal virus for several days after vaccination with Flu-Avert I.N., but the amount of virus shed is so low that in-contact horses will not generally become infected or immunized with vaccinal virus shed by recently vaccinated horses, and the likelihood of reversion to virulence is extremely low.[95]

In the years since Flu-Avert I.N. was licensed in North America as the first equine influenza vaccine with documented efficacy based on independent published challenge studies, several manufacturers have updated their inactivated vaccines and demonstrated efficacy in challenge studies. Inactivated influenza vaccines containing one or more relevant H3N8 strains are currently marketed by Boehringer Ingelheim (Calvenza EIV), Fort Dodge Animal Health (Fluvac Innovator), and Intervet (Equicine II). Calvenza EIV and Equicine II also contain an H7N7 strain. These companies also market a large number of multicomponent combination vaccines that contain the same inactivated influenza antigens as in their single-component products, but also contain tetanus, WEE and EEE virus, EHV, or WNV antigens.

A study in which naive 9-month-old horses were challenged by aerosol with a recent influenza H3N8 strain (KY/99), 16 weeks after the last dose of a three-dose vaccination series (0, 4, and 16 weeks), documented that Calvenza EIV and two EIV/EHV combination vaccines [Prestige II (Intervet) and Fluvac EHV-4/1 (Fort Dodge), containing the same influenza antigens as contained in Equicine II and Fluvac Plus, respectively] reduced clinical signs and viral shedding in vaccinated horses compared with nonvaccinated control horses.[96] The group vaccinated with Calvenza EIV developed significantly higher serum antibody titers after vaccination and experienced less fever, nasal discharge, and viral shedding than horses vaccinated with either Prestige II or Fluvac EHV-4/1. Based on these findings, the authors concluded that Calvenza EIV, a vaccine developed, formulated, and efficacy-tested according to European Union guidelines, was the most effective inactivated influenza vaccine available in North America at that time. This vaccine is adjuvanted with Carbopol and is the only vaccine licensed in North America to contain antigens from H3N8 viruses of both the American and the European lineages (Kentucky/95 and Newmarket/2/93). This vaccine also contains an H7H7 virus (Newmarket/77). The initial two doses of this vaccine are administered IM; subsequent doses may be administered IM or intranasally. It is proposed, but not proved, that administration of booster doses by the intranasal route may provide a stronger local mucosal immune response. This vaccine is licensed for use in horses older than 6 months of age, including pregnant mares. The metabolizable oil (MetaStim), adjuvanted Fluvac Plus vaccine evaluated in the previous challenge study contained the KY/92 strain of H3N8 virus. Fort Dodge Animal Health has since replaced this strain with a KY/97 strain in their Fluvac product line, now named Fluvac Innovator. Equicine II (Intervet) currently contains a Kentucky/93 H3N8 and a Pennsylvania/63 H7N7 strain along with a polymer adjuvant (Havlogen). An updated version of this vaccine containing the KY/93 and KY/2002 North American strains and the Newmarket/93 Eurasian H3N8 strains, but no H7N7 strain, will likely be licensed in 2006. The recent updates to these vaccines will further improve their efficacy, but published challenge data confirming this assumption are not yet available.

In 2006 it is anticipated that Merial will be granted a North American license to market an injectable canarypox-vectored recombinant equine influenza vaccine that has been used with success in Europe for several years. This vaccine, named ProteqFlu in Europe, has been shown to induce strong protection in challenge studies and shows great potential to have a positive impact on influenza prevention in North America.[12] The vaccine incorporates the HA gene from the Kentucky/94 and Newmarket/2/93 H3N8 strains into the same vector delivery platform as the efficacious recombinant WNV vaccine (Recombitek) and contains a carbomer polymer adjuvant in the diluent. Consequently, this vaccine invokes a broad array of humoral and cellular immune responses. It is likely that the vectored influenza vaccine will be able to circumvent the inhibitory effect of maternal antibodies, an issue that significantly impacts primary immunization of foals using inactivated influenza vaccines.

Vaccination Protocols for Influenza

Influenza should be considered a core vaccine on all facilities that are not totally closed so as to preclude contact with "outside" horses from other locations. Pending availability of published efficacy data for other equine influenza vaccines, we advocate use of the intranasal MLV (Flu-Avert) as a central component of control programs for equine influenza in North America. Incorporation of the MLV into a program that has relied on inactivated vaccines can occur when routine administration of inactivated vaccines would otherwise be scheduled.

As with other diseases, the full benefit of vaccination against influenza can be realized only if the primary vaccination series is completed, or booster doses of vaccine administered, several weeks before anticipated exposure. The following five issues should be considered when planning an influenza vaccination program: (1) primary vaccination of adult horses, (2) routine revaccination, (3) vaccination of pregnant mares, (4) primary vaccination of foals, and (5) vaccination in an outbreak.

Primary Vaccination of Adult Horses. The following administration of the primary series is for adult horses that have not previously been vaccinated:

1. Flu-Avert: administer a single dose intranasally. A second dose administered 3 months later may be beneficial, particularly for horses vaccinated at less than 11 months of age.
2. Inactivated IM-administered vaccines: administer two doses, 3 to 6 weeks apart according to label directions. Although not specifically recommended by some manufacturers, administration of a third dose of vaccine, 8 to 12 weeks after the second dose, is indicated because it significantly enhances the magnitude of the primary response and duration of persistence of antibodies at protective levels.
3. Canarypox-vectored vaccine: administer two doses, 4 to 6 weeks apart, and revaccinate again 5 months later.

Routine Revaccination. The poor efficacy of inactivated influenza vaccines marketed in the past contributed to development of recommendations for revaccination of horses at 2- to 4-month intervals, with the goal of maintaining a consistently high level of immune protection. Improvements in injectable vaccines and introduction of new vaccine types has extended the duration of clinical protection achievable through vaccination; therefore, a routine revaccination interval of 6 months appears to be appropriate for most of the influenza vaccines currently marketed in North America. This "routine" protocol should be customized, by adjusting timing of boosters or inclusion of an additional booster, to achieve maximum protection during periods when the risk of exposure is high. For example, strategic revacccination 1 month before being placed at high risk of exposure, such as at a show or sale, or being transferred to a training or boarding facility, is justified to maximize protection.

Vaccination of Pregnant Mares. For the mare to produce colostrum that contains a high level of antibodies against equine influenza, she should be revaccinated 4 to 8 weeks before foaling with a vaccine that stimulates a robust serologic response. Although the intranasally administered Flu-Avert I.N. vaccine induces good protection, it does not routinely stimulate high levels of circulating antibody, at least when used for primary immunization. An inactivated injectable vaccine is therefore recommended for prefoaling booster vaccination of pregnant mares at this time.[38] The canarypox-vectored recombinant vaccine (ProteqFlu) will likely also prove suitable for booster vaccination of pregnant mares.

Vaccination of Foals. The antibody status of a mare at the time of foaling is the main determinant of the postnursing circulating antibody titer in her foal and therefore has a profound impact on the ability of the foal or weanling to respond to influenza vaccines administered during the first year of life. Foals born to seronegative, nonvaccinated mares respond appropriately to influenza vaccines; therefore, primary vaccination can commence at 3 months of age, or younger if significant risk of exposure to influenza exists. In contrast, maternal antibodies have been shown to completely block the serologic response of foals to a primary immunization series comprising two or more doses of inactivated influenza vaccines when the first dose is administered at 6 months of age or younger.[33,35,37,39-42,47] Interference from MDAs may persist until 9 months of age or beyond for foals with high antibody titers after nursing.[38]

In a study to investigate the finding that many yearling horses had low or undetectable levels of HI antibody despite having received multiple doses of inactivated influenza vaccine during the first year of life, Cullinane et al.[40] found that a substantial number of foals vaccinated at 3 months of age not only failed to respond serologically to the subunit vaccine used in the primary series, but also failed to respond to four or more additional doses of either an inactivated subunit or a whole-virus vaccine administered over the next year. This result suggested that early vaccination in the presence of maternal antibody had induced immunotolerance to influenza vaccines, at least as defined by lack of serologic responses. Similar results were obtained in our laboratory when the responses of 3-month-old antibody-positive foals to inactivated whole-virus influenza vaccines were assessed using the HI test.

However, when the same samples were retested using a sensitive ELISA assay that detects subisotypes of IgG, evidence of induction of tolerance was not found. Instead, misdirection of the immune response in favor of IgG(T), rather than the IgGa and IgGb subisotypes believed to be important for protection, was documented.[37] In the same study we found that whereas the response of 6-month-old foals from seropositive mares was superior to that of 3-month-old foals, both in terms of the percentage of foals seroconverting and the magnitude of the resulting antibody titers, the response of yearlings was clearly superior to that of 6-month-old foals.[47] Whereas 60% of the yearlings seroconverted to influenza A/equine/2 after two doses of vaccine, all seroconverted after three doses, and more than 50% developed HI titers of more than 1:1000. Based on these data, it was concluded that titers will likely persist at a protective level for a much longer duration after a three-dose primary series than after a two-dose series. This conclusion is also supported by results of studies in Europe, to the extent that administration of a third dose, 2 to 4 months after the second dose, is now strongly recommended.* Because the inhibitory effects of MDAs on responses to inactivated influenza vaccines may persist up to 9 months of age in foals born to mares with high titers, primary vaccination of foals from immune mares should be delayed as long as possible, and preventive measures should focus on preventing introduction of infected horses.† Studies in Newmarket, United Kingdom, have shown that influenza virus infection is rare in Thoroughbred yearlings before they enter training, suggesting that the risk of influenza is low in horses less than 1 year of age born to mares in herds that are well vaccinated.[88,98,99] Therefore, little justification appears to exist for vaccinating young foals from vaccinated mares against influenza, as recommended in the past.[61,100,101]

The intranasal MLV (Flu-Avert I.N.) is licensed for vaccination of horses 11 months of age or older. Whereas this vaccine has been shown to be safe in foals as young as 2 months of age,[102] published data regarding the potential for MDAs to interfere with the response are lacking. Unpublished observations suggest that MDAs interfere with the response of foals age 3 to 6 months, whereas foals with MDA vaccinated at 7 months of age were protected against virulent challenge (Holland and Chambers, personal communication). Pending publication of well-controlled studies, it is recommended that if the first dose of Flu-Avert I.N. vaccine is administered before 11 months of age, a second dose should be administered at 11 months of age or older.[103] The live canarypox-vectored recombinant influenza vaccine is licensed in Europe for use in pregnant mares and foals as young as 4 months of age.[79] Although there are no published reports regarding the influence of MDAs on responses to this vaccine, the recommended minimum age for vaccination of foals from immunized dams is 5 months. If the foal experiences failure of passive transfer of maternal antibodies, or if the mare is seronegative for influenza, the manufacturer recommends commencing vaccination at 4 months of age and including an additional dose in the primary series.

Vaccination in an Outbreak. Definitive diagnosis of equine influenza infection should be pursued during outbreaks of suspected viral respiratory disease because specific measures can then be initiated to contain spread of the disease. Rapid (same-day) diagnosis of influenza can be accomplished using the highly sensitive and specific polymerase chain reaction (PCR) or antigen-capture ELISA tests. In addition, virus isolation should be pursued during outbreaks to characterize new isolates and assess efficacy of current vaccines.

The decision whether to vaccinate in an outbreak depends on many factors, most importantly the age, vaccination status, and size of the population of horses at risk; the elapsed time since onset of the outbreak; the rapidity with which a diagnosis can be confirmed; the layout of the physical facilities; and availability of personnel. Outbreaks of influenza at racetracks and similar facilities typically take 1 month or more to spread through the entire population; therefore, sufficient time exists to enhance immune protection of many at-risk horses while implementing other management strategies to minimize disease spread.[94] It is prudent to booster-vaccinate those horses that have been on a regular influenza vaccination program but have not been revaccinated within the previous 3 months. It is also important to induce protection as quickly as possible in horses that have not previously been vaccinated. Of the vaccines currently available, Flu-Avert I.N. induces protection most rapidly, within 7 days of administration of a single intranasal dose; therefore, this is currently the product of choice for vaccination of naive horses and those of unknown vaccination status during an outbreak. No evidence suggests that adverse effects will occur when Flu Avert I.N. is administered to horses that are incubating infection, although vaccination of horses that are already clinically ill is not recommended.

*References 33, 35, 37, 40, 47, 79.
†References 33, 35, 37, 40-42, 47, 97.

Future Influenza Vaccines

In addition to the modified–canarypox virus vector described earlier,[12] a recombinant modified vaccinia Ankara (rMVA) vector that delivers genetic material encoding for relevant HA antigens of an H3N8 influenza virus has been developed.[9,10] The rMVA system is designed to focus the CTL response on the recombinant antigen and was initially tested in a prime-boost strategy in which the priming dose consisted of a DNA plasmid encoding for expression of the HA antigen. The intent of this DNA prime-rMVA boost regimen was to invoke both cellular and humoral immune responses involved in protection.[9] A subsequent study showed that the rMVA system was capable of inducing virus-specific lymphoproliferative and interferon gamma (IFN-γ) messenger ribonucleic acid (mRNA) responses; antigen-specific IgGa, IgGb, and IgA antibodies; and protection from challenge, both with and without a priming dose of the DNA vaccine. These data indicate that vaccination of horses with rMVA alone, or as part of a prime-boost regimen, is an effective means of inducing protective immunity to influenza virus infection.[10] Considerable research has been performed to document the efficacy of the DNA vaccine used in these studies against equine influenza. However, the delivery system used (multiple sublingual, conjunctival, and subcutaneous injections delivered with a gene gun under general anesthesia) is impractical for use in the field.[10,17] Recent licensing of a naked plasmid DNA vaccine that can be conveniently administered to horses by IM injection to prevent WNV infection clearly documents the potential for development of a DNA vaccine to prevent influenza in horses in the future.

Equine Herpesvirus (Rhinopneumonitis)

The respiratory tract is the primary route of infection for both equine herpesvirus type 1 (EHV-1) and equine herpesvirus type 4 (EHV-4), agents that are often cited as important causes of primary and secondary respiratory tract disease. Seroepidemiologic studies indicate that the vast majority of foals become infected with EHV-1 and EHV-4 during the first few months of life, but the clinical disease syndrome resulting from these infections is not well defined. Similarly, surveillance studies involving racehorses document that seroconversion to both EHV-1 and EHV-4 occurs sporadically during the course of a racing season but is not clearly associated with outbreaks of respiratory disease that follow an epidemiologic pattern consistent with an infectious agent. EHV-1 and EHV-4 are spread by aerosolized secretions from infected horses, by direct and indirect (fomite) contact with nasal secretions, and in the case of EHV-1, by aborted fetuses, fetal fluids, and placentae associated with abortions. Management practices are therefore of primary importance for control of clinical disease caused by equine herpesviruses.

Viremia occurs frequently after infection with EHV-1, potentially leading to paralytic neurologic disease (myeloencephalopathy) secondary to vasculitis of the spinal cord and brain, abortion of virus-infected fetuses, or birth of infected nonviable foals. In contrast, manifestations of infection with EHV-4 (rhinopneumonitis) are generally confined to the respiratory tract because EHV-4 does not typically infect endothelial cells or produce a cell-associated viremia.[104] As with herpesvirus infections in other species, horses typically fail to clear primary infections with either EHV-1 or EHV-4, the result being that most horses in the population remain latently infected with both viruses.[105,106] Latently infected horses do not show clinical signs but may experience recrudescence of infection, with or without clinical signs, an increase in antibody titer, and shedding of the virus when stressed. Consequently, many horses have detectable levels of SN antibody to both EHV-1 and EHV-4 in their serum.[105,107] These features of the epidemiology of herpesvirus infections seriously compromise efforts to control these diseases and explain why outbreaks of EHV-1 or EHV-4 can occur in closed populations of horses. Whereas most mature horses have antibodies to EHV-1 and EHV-4 and do not show respiratory signs when they become infected, horses do not appear to become resistant to the abortogenic or neurologic forms of infection with EHV-1, even after repeated exposure.[108]

Correlates for protection against EHV-1 and EHV-4 infection have been investigated extensively but are not yet clearly defined. Infection with EHV-1 induces a strong humoral response, but protection from reinfection is short lived and is not achieved until the horse has experienced multiple infections with homotypic virus. No clear relationship exists between protection from EHV-1 infection and concentrations of circulating antibody induced by vaccination or infection, but the duration and amount of virus shedding from the nasopharynx are reduced in animals with high levels of circulating neutralizing antibody.[104] Mucosal immunity and cell-mediated responses likely play a role at least as important as circulating neutralizing antibodies in protection against EHV-1 infection,[109] since the presence of MHC class I–restricted CTL precursors in peripheral blood is correlated with protection. Because EHV-4 replication is largely confined to epithelial cells of the upper respiratory tract, it is likely that mucosal immunity is important in protection. Whereas circulating antibodies alone do not prevent EHV-4 infection, high levels of vaccine-induced circulating VN antibody greatly reduce virus shedding and clinical signs after challenge infection.[104]

The principal indication for use of equine herpesvirus vaccines is prevention of EHV-1–induced abortion in pregnant mares. Consistent vaccination appears to reduce the frequency and severity of herpesvirus-induced disease. Although convincing evidence is lacking, field experience suggests that, whereas the incidence of sporadic EHV-1–induced abortions in individual mares has not changed, the incidence of abortion storms caused by EHV-1 has declined significantly since the introduction and widespread use of EHV-1 vaccines in the United States.[105,108] Outbreaks of abortion and associated perinatal foal death, however, do continue to occur on occasion in herds of vaccinated mares. Of the vaccines currently licensed for use in pregnant mares in North America, only inactivated monovalent EHV-1 vaccines (Pneumabort-K + 1b, Fort Dodge Animal Health, and Prodigy, Intervet) containing abortogenic strains of EHV-1 carry a label claim for preventing abortion, whereas at least one bivalent EHV-1/4 vaccine is licensed for prevention of abortion in Europe (Duvaxyn EHV-1/4, Intervet). One of the vaccines available in North America (Pneumabort-K + 1b) incorporates both the 1p and 1b subtypes of EHV-1 to reflect the documented increase in the proportion of EHV-1 abortions caused by the 1b subtype that occurred during the 1980s as compared to earlier years.[110] Pregnant mares should be vaccinated during the fifth, seventh, and ninth months of gestation. Many veterinarians also recommend a dose during the third month of gestation. Similarly, vaccination of mares with an inactivated EHV-1/EHV-4 vaccine at the time of breeding and again 4 to 6 weeks before foaling is commonly practiced to enhance concentrations of colostral immunoglobulin for transfer to the foal. However, no published reports document the effectiveness of this approach in raising titers of specific antibody in mares that have already been vaccinated against EHV-1 three times during the previous 5 months. Vaccination of barren mares and stallions with either a bivalent EHV-1/4 vaccine or a monovalent EHV-1 vaccine before the start of the breeding season, and thereafter at 6-month intervals, is recommended, with the goal of increasing herd immunity in an attempt to reduce viral shedding and challenge to pregnant mares on breeding farms.[105]

A modified live-virus EHV-1 vaccine (Rhinomune, Pfizer) has been used as an aid to prevention of EHV-1 abortion by some practitioners for many years, even though this vaccine is not currently labeled for this use. However, several recent developments have created a renewed interest in the potential for use of modified live vaccines (MLVs) for protecting horses against manifestations of EHV-1 and EHV-4 infection. Sequencing of the EHV-1 genome has made it possible to document the nature of the mutation encoding for attenuation, mediated through truncation of the gp2 glycoprotein, of the KyA strain.[111] Similar studies may soon yield information regarding the mutation underlying attenuation of the RAC-H strain from which Rhinomune was derived. In addition, studies in Europe have documented the efficacy of an intranasally administered, temperature-sensitive, live EHV-1 vaccine in preventing abortion, neurologic disease, and respiratory disease after experimental challenge with virulent EHV-1.[109,112] This renewed interest in MLVs, as well as ongoing investigation of recombinant vaccines expressing the major EHV glycoprotein antigens, will likely lead to improved approaches to immunoprophylaxis in the near future.

Because currently available inactivated vaccines do not block infection with equine herpesviruses, the most we can hope for when using inactivated vaccines is reduction of severity of clinical signs and attenuation of virus shedding to help protect herd mates. Challenge studies in weanlings age 5 to 8 months have clearly demonstrated the efficacy of an inactivated whole-virus EHV-1/4 vaccine in reducing clinical manifestations and virus shedding induced by virulent EHV-1 challenge administered 2 weeks after completion of the two-dose primary series.[113] Efficacy was clearly correlated with vaccine-induced antibody levels at the time of challenge in this study. Studies investigating the serologic response of 3-month-old and 5-month-old foals to this same vaccine documented failure of a high proportion of foals to seroconvert, suggesting that this vaccine is likely to be less effective in protecting younger foals than in protecting the foals age 5 to 8 months cited in the previous challenge study.[48]

Specific antibodies against both EHV-1 and EHV-4 are passed in colostrum.[34,45,46,48,114] Field studies with EHV-1 MLVs indicate that colostral antibodies exert a profound inhibitory effect on serologic responses to vaccination up to at least 5 months of age.[45,115,116] However, a cytotoxic cellular immune response to both EHV-1 and EHV-4 was induced in a substantial percentage of foals vaccinated with an EHV-1 MLV in the presence of maternal antibody, even though humoral responses were often absent.[117] It is uncertain whether these responses would provide protection against natural challenge. Recent studies with two commercially available, inactivated bivalent EHV-1/4 vaccines, and one inactivated EHV-4/influenza vaccine, have shown that the majority of foals from EHV-vaccinated mares do not mount a detectable neutralizing antibody response to vaccines administered at 3 and 4 months of age, even when three doses are administered in the primary series.[46-48] An increased proportion of foals responded when vaccinated with a three-dose series starting at 5 or 6 months of age, but a substantial number still failed to seroconvert.[47,48] Some foals with low or undetectable levels of SN antibody at the time of vaccination failed to mount a serologic response, suggesting that low levels of antibody, below the lower limit of detection of the SN test based on EHV-1 antigen, are capable of inhibiting the serologic response to inactivated EHV-1/4 vaccines.[48] The failure of a large proportion of foals less than 6 months of age to mount serologic responses to inactivated EHV-1/4 vaccines and the influence of antibody titer at the time of vaccination on failure to respond has been confirmed using sensitive gD and gG ELISAs in studies on commercial stud farms in Australia.[118] In parallel studies, these researchers concluded that mares were the source of infection for foals, and that intensive use of inactivated EHV-1/4 vaccines on breeding farms in Australia had minimally impacted the infection rate of young foals and weanlings with EHV-1 and EHV-4.[106,107,119]

Considering the uncertainty regarding the role of EHV-1 and EHV-4 as causes of clinically important respiratory disease, the lack of published data regarding the efficacy of available vaccines in preventing infection and establishment of latency, and results of a recent study documenting the poor serologic responses of naive horses to a number of killed-EHV respiratory vaccines currently marketed in North America,[120] there appears to be little rationale to support the common practice of frequent revaccination of foals, weanlings, yearlings, and young performance horses against EHV-1 and EHV-4.[121] Furthermore, an obvious dilemma in designing a vaccination strategy to prevent EHV-1 and EHV-4 infection in foals and weanlings is that if primary immunization is delayed until 6 months of age or older to reduce the likelihood of maternal antibody interference, foals are likely to encounter field infection before completion of the three-dose primary series. Thus it is unreasonable to expect a high degree of efficacy for vaccination programs designed to protect foals and weanlings against EHV infection using available vaccines. Despite these uncertainties, many practitioners elect to vaccinate against both EHV-1 and EHV-4. Under these circumstances, a reasonable compromise would be to start foal vaccination at 4 to 6 months of age using two doses of an inactivated bivalent vaccine or an EHV-1 MLV administered 3 to 4 weeks apart, followed by administration of a third dose 8 to 12 weeks later. Revaccination at 4 to 6 month intervals thereafter using either an inactivated bivalent vaccine or an EHV-1 MLV appears appropriate for yearlings and young performance or show horses that experience contact with other horses. Frequent vaccination of nonpregnant mature horses, except those on breeding farms, with EHV vaccines is generally not indicated. Available vaccines make no labeled claim to prevent the myeloencephalitic form of EHV-1 infection.

Future Vaccination Strategies to Prevent Herpesvirus Infection

To be completely effective in blocking primary infection and establishing a lifelong carrier state with EHV-1 and EHV-4, future vaccination strategies should be directed at inducing a strong mucosal immune response in the upper respiratory tract during the first few weeks of life, at a time when high levels of maternal antibodies are present. Promising progress toward this goal was reported recently by Patel et al.,[122] who documented that intranasal administration of a single dose of temperature-sensitive EHV-1 MLV to MDA-positive foals aged 1.4 to 3.5 months afforded partial but significant protection against febrile respiratory disease, viremia, and virus shedding after intranasal challenge with virulent EHV-1 performed 8 weeks after vaccination.

Streptococcus equi subsp. *equi* Infection (Strangles)

Strangles is a highly contagious disease caused by the bacterium *Streptococcus equi* subsp. *equi (S. equi)*. Strangles primarily affects young horses (weanlings and yearlings), although horses of any age can become infected if not protected by previous exposure to the organism or by vaccination. The organism is transmitted by direct contact with infected horses or subclinical carriers, or indirectly by contact with water troughs, feed bunks, pastures, stalls, trailers, tack, or grooming equipment contaminated with nasal discharge or pus draining from lymph nodes of infected horses. The organism survives for only a few weeks in the environment. Because *S. equi* is a clonal organism, there is minimal antigenic variation between different isolates, even though isolates vary in their pathogenicity. Most horses develop a solid immunity during recovery from strangles, which persists in more than 75% of animals for 5 years or longer.[122a] The acquired immune response is directed predominantly at the cell wall M protein of *S. equi* (SeM) and involves a combination of circulating opsonophagocytic antibodies and local antibodies produced in the nasopharynx.[123-125] The predominant opsonophagocytic antibodies are of the IgGb subisotype but also include IgGa and IgA, whereas IgGb and later mucosal IgA predominate in nasopharyngeal secretions.[29,123]

Licensed strangles vaccines include two inactivated, adjuvanted cell wall SeM extracts (Strepvax II, Boehringer Ingelheim, and Strepguard with Havlogen, Intervet) and one attenuated live vaccine (Pinnacle I.N., Fort Dodge) derived from a nonencapsulated mutant of *S. equi* for intranasal administration.[126] Infection of horses with *S. equi* continues to cause troublesome outbreaks of strangles throughout North America, despite the availability and widespread use of these vaccines, indicating that their efficacy is suboptimal.[127] M-protein vaccines induce a good opsonophagocytic antibody response in serum but a minimal mucosal IgA response, which likely accounts for the incomplete protection observed when they are used in the field.[123,128] However, data do exist to document that vaccination using injectable SeM vaccines significantly reduces the attack rate and severity of strangles in herds with endemic infection.[128-130] The live intranasal vaccine has been shown to induce a relevant mucosal immune response and partial or complete protection, but may do so without inducing a strong serologic response.[127,131]

Vaccination against *S. equi* is not routinely recommended for pleasure or performance horses kept in low-risk situations, but it is a consideration for horses that are resident on, or being transported to, premises such as breeding farms where strangles is a persistent endemic problem or where a high risk of exposure is anticipated. The bacterial MLV is generally preferred over inactivated injectable vaccines for primary vaccination of foals and weanlings and for routine use in older horses that are at high risk for infection. On breeding farms, efforts should be concentrated on preventing infection of foals and weanlings by booster-vaccinating broodmares 4 to 6 weeks before foaling to maximize colostral content of antibodies. Whereas the intranasal vaccine has been shown to be safe for use in mares at all stages of pregnancy and can be used in mares during an outbreak, it does not reliably stimulate high levels of circulating antibody. For this reason, IM-administered inactivated SeM products are preferred for prefoaling booster immunization of mares. Antibodies of the IgG and IgA class recognizing the SeM are passively transferred to the foal through colostrum and are also present in the milk of immune mares.[30] Antibodies of predominantly the IgGb isotype are absorbed from colostrum and redistribute to the nasopharyngeal mucosa.[29] These IgGb antibodies, along with the SeM-specific IgA antibodies that are present in milk and passively coat the pharyngeal mucosa of nursing foals, provide protection to most nursing foals up to the time of weaning.[29,30,125] Resistance of nursing foals to strangles during the first few months of life appears to be mediated by IgGb antibodies in nasal secretions and milk and not by IgA.[30] Serologic (ELISA) responses to M-protein vaccines are poor in foals, most likely because of the inhibitory effect of maternal antibodies.

Whereas the intranasal MLV may be less susceptible than the inactivated extract vaccines to MDA interference, this issue has not been investigated, and the manufacturer does not recommend administration of this vaccine to horses less than 9 months of age. Considering that on farms where strangles is endemic, foals often become infected around the time of weaning, at 4 to 8 months of age, it is difficult to protect them if vaccination is delayed until 9 months of age. Therefore a reasonable compromise on breeding farms where the risk of strangles infection is high and mares are on a regular vaccination program would be to begin foal vaccination using the intranasal live vaccine as early as 4 months of age. The recommended two-dose primary series administered 2 to 3 weeks apart should be followed by a third dose 3 months later and boosters at 6- to 12-month intervals thereafter, depending on risk of infection. The intranasal vaccine has been administered to foals as young as 5 or 6 weeks of age during outbreaks. If used in this manner, a third dose of the vaccine should be administered 2 to 4 weeks before the foal is weaned to optimize protection during this high-risk period. Although there are few reports of adverse effects attributable to use of the intranasal strangles vaccine in young foals, the inability of foals to mount an adequate mucosal IgA response during the first month of life and the potential for interference by maternal antibodies suggest that foals are unlikely to benefit fully from intranasal strangles vaccine administered before 4 months of age. When an inactivated M-protein vaccine is used for primary vaccination of foals, it is recommended that the initial series begin at 4 to 6 months of age, using three doses administered at 3- to 6-week intervals, followed by semiannual boosters for as long as high-risk conditions prevail.

Outbreaks of strangles generally persist for several months to more than 1 year, particularly on breeding farms, where each foal crop adds new susceptible animals to the population. Thus, strangles vaccines are frequently administered during an outbreak in an attempt to bring outbreaks under control, as an adjunct to management practices designed to reduce spread of infection. Whereas all horses, except those that are clinically ill or incubating infection, can be vaccinated under these circumstances, the likelihood of preventing strangles is greatest for horses that have not yet been exposed and can be kept isolated from infected horses until the vaccination protocol can be completed. Horses that have been vaccinated previously will generate a response more rapidly than naive horses. Similarly, the attenuated live intranasal vaccine is preferred over inactivated vaccines for immunization of naive horses in an outbreak because it is likely to generate a protective immune response more rapidly.

Injectable strangles vaccines tend to cause local reactions at the site of injection more often than do other equine vaccines, particularly when administered in the muscles of the neck. In addition, *purpura hemorrhagica*, a serious and sometimes life-threatening systemic immune complex (Arthus-type) vasculitis manifested as edema with or without petechial hemorrhages on mucosal surfaces, has been observed with low frequency in the weeks after administration of strangles vaccines. Inactivated extract vaccines are implicated more often than the intranasal live vaccine, but all strangles vaccines have the potential to induce purpura. The antigen present in immune complexes is SeM, along with antibodies of the IgA class. Because a high serum IgG titer against *S. equi* appears to be associated with an increased risk of developing purpura, routine testing for specific IgG antibodies using a commercially available ELISA test has been recommended as a means of preventing vaccine-associated purpura. Horses with titers of 1:1600 or greater in the SeM ELISA should not be vaccinated.[127]

The bacterial MLV for intranasal administration will cause injection site abscesses if inadvertently injected IM. To avoid inadvertent contamination of other vaccines, syringes, and needles, it is advisable and considered good practice to administer all parenteral vaccines before handling and administering the intranasal strangles MLV. Other reported adverse responses after administration of the intranasal MLV include nasal discharge, submandibular or retropharyngeal lymphadenopathy with or without abscessation, limb edema, internal abscesses (bastard strangles), and purpura hemorrhagica. The overall frequency of adverse events is low but appears to be higher than reported to the manufacturer (4.8 per 10,000 doses). On the other hand, the majority of reported adverse events, including the development of nasal discharge, lymph node abscesses, and purpura hemorrhagica, occur in horses on farms with endemic or epidemic strangles. Thus it is often uncertain whether the adverse event was caused by the vaccine or by a wild strain of *S. equi*.

Rabies

Rabies is an infrequently encountered neurologic disease of horses that results when horses are inoculated with the rabies virus through the bite of infected (rabid) wildlife. Even though the incidence of rabies in horses is low, the disease is invariably fatal and has considerable public health significance. Wildlife species that serve as the natural reservoirs for infection with this rhabdovirus differ among regions of North America. All horses kept in areas where rabies is endemic in the wildlife population are at risk and should be vaccinated. Therefore, vaccination of horses against rabies is recommended using one of the three inactivated, tissue culture–derived products currently licensed for use in horses (Rabvac3, Fort Dodge; RM Imrab3, Merial; and Rabguard TC, Pfizer). These vaccines induce strong serologic responses after a single dose. Although correlates for protection against infection with rabies virus in horses are not well defined, it is logical to assume that protection correlates with titers of circulating antibody because infection is usually acquired by systemic injection through bites by rabid animals, In humans, postvaccination antibody titers are used to predict protection and to assess the need for postexposure vaccination or administration of immune serum. In dogs, however, postvaccination serologic test results were not found to be completely predictive of resistance to challenge exposure during tests performed with certain inactivated vaccines.[132] Published results of challenge studies to assess efficacy of rabies vaccines licensed for use in horses in North America are not available.

Label directions on inactivated rabies vaccines licensed for use in horses suggest administration to foals age 3 months or older using one dose of vaccine in the primary series, followed by a second dose at 1 year of age. Thereafter, annual revaccination is recommended. None of the licensed vaccines carries a specific label approval for use in pregnant mares; therefore it is recommended that mares be revaccinated before breeding whenever possible. However, it should be recognized that some veterinarians administer the killed-virus vaccine to pregnant mares and do not encounter adverse consequences. Because rabies antibodies persist in serum for a prolonged period, foals born to mares that are revaccinated while open acquire substantial titers of rabies antibody after ingesting colostrum. It should be recognized that some veterinarians administer the killed-virus vaccine to pregnant mares and do not encounter adverse consequences.

Documentation of rabies in reportedly vaccinated horses, most of which were less than 2 years old, has brought into question the efficacy of label recommendations for primary vaccination of foals against rabies.[133] Recent studies in our laboratory have shown that the serologic response of most 3-month-old foals from antibody-positive mares is completely blocked, even when a two-dose primary vaccination series is used. Although the response to the first dose of vaccine is typically blocked in 6-month-old foals from antibody-positive mares, these foals appear to seroconvert after administration of a second dose administered 4 weeks later. Primary vaccination of foals from vaccinated mares should therefore be delayed until they are 6 months of age or older and should include two doses of inactivated vaccine administered approximately 4 weeks apart, followed by a third dose at 1 year of age. For foals from nonvaccinated mares, the primary vaccination series can be started as early as 3 months of age and may comprise only one dose, although a two-dose series will likely induce more durable protection.

Equine Monocytic Ehrlichiosis (Potomac Horse Fever)

Equine monocytic ehrlichiosis, also known as Potomac horse fever (PHF), is caused by *Neorickettsia risticii* (formerly *Ehrlichia risticii*) and was originally described in 1979 as a sporadic disease affecting horses residing in the northeastern United States near the Potomac River. PHF is known to occur in 43 states, three provinces in Canada (Nova Scotia, Ontario, Alberta), South America (Uruguay, Brazil), Europe (The Netherlands, France), and India. The disease does not appear to be directly contagious, and it now appears that accidental ingestion of aquatic insects harboring metarcercariae infected with *N. risticii* is at least one mode of transmission.[134] PHF is seasonal, occurring between late spring and early fall in temperate areas, with most cases in July, August, and September at the onset of hot weather. The disease may affect individual horses sporadically or cause outbreaks involving multiple horses. Foals appear to be at low risk for the disease. If PHF has been confirmed on a farm or in a particular geographic area, it is likely that cases will occur in future years. Documentation of the involvement of operculate freshwater snails and aquatic insects such as caddisflies and mayflies in the life cycle of *N. risticii* has permitted formulation of focused control measures directed at minimizing exposure of horses to the habitats occupied by these species during the summer and fall months, when disease risk is highest in endemic areas.[134] Risk reduction is best accomplished by denying horses access to river banks, creek beds, and irrigation ditches, as well as pastures that have recently been flooded or flood-irrigated.

Recovery after natural infection with *N. risticii* induces a strong antibody response and durable protection from reinfection lasting 20 months or longer. However, the presence of antibodies does not necessarily correlate with protection, and cell-mediated responses likely play a crucial role.[135] A β-propiolactone inactivated host cell-free *N. risticii* vaccine protects mice against homologous challenge.[136] Several inactivated PHF vaccines for IM administration (Mystique, Intervet; Potomavac, Merial; PotomacGuard, Fort Dodge; PHF-Gard, Pfizer; Equovum PHF, Boehringer Ingelheim) are licensed for use in horses with the label claim that they aid in prevention of equine monocytic ehrlichiosis. The high rate of serious complications and mortality associated with this disease has been considered adequate justification for vaccinating horses residing in or traveling to endemic areas. In a series of studies in which ponies were challenged IV with *N. risticii* approximately 4 weeks after completion of the two-dose primary vaccination series using a formalin-inactivated, aluminum hydroxide–adjuvanted vaccine (PHF-Vax, Schering-Plough), Ristic et al.[137] reported that 78% of experimentally infected ponies were protected against all clinical manifestations of disease except fever, and 33% were protected against all signs, including fever. A published noncontrolled field study involving the same vaccine documented induction of serologic responses in most vaccinated horses and a substantial reduction in disease prevalence, morbidity, and mortality compared with data collected in a previous year when horses were not vaccinated.[135,138]

In contrast to the results of the previous studies, an epidemiologic investigation involving a large number of horses failed to demonstrate any clinical or economic benefit from annual vaccination with currently available vaccines in New York State.[139,140] Failure of a substantial number of individual horses to mount an immune response to inactivated PHF vaccines, heterogeneity of *N. risticii* isolates, the presence of only one *N. risticii* strain in vaccines, and much more rapid waning of immunity after vaccination than after natural infection likely account for the observed failure of vaccines to provide protection against field infection.[135,141] Despite the lack of documented efficacy of approved vaccines to prevent infection in the field setting, many practitioners who work in endemic areas believe that severity of disease is attenuated and mortality is reduced in vaccinated horses when vaccines are administered at 4- to 6-month intervals, with administration of one booster timed to precede the anticipated period of peak challenge.

If vaccination is elected, a primary series of two doses should be administered 3 to 4 weeks apart. Manufacturers recommend revaccination at 6- to 12-month intervals, although a 4-month revaccination interval appears to be necessary to achieve a reasonable likelihood of protection of horses in endemic areas because protection after vaccination is incomplete and short lived. Because the disease has a distinct seasonal pattern, revaccination in the late spring, about 1 month before the first cases are expected, followed by a second dose 4 months later, appears to be a reasonable approach for strategic immunization to maximize the chances of protection during the period of peak challenge. Available vaccines are licensed for use in stallions and pregnant mares and can be administered to gestating mares 4 to 6 weeks before foaling to maximize passive transfer of specific antibodies to foals through colostrum.

Whereas approximately 67% of foals from antibody-positive mares were antibody negative by 12 weeks of age, antibody was detectable in 33% of foals up to 5 months of age. On the basis of these findings, the low risk of clinical disease in young foals, and the apparent susceptibility to infection of two foals vaccinated earlier than 12 weeks of age, Sessions and Dawson[138] recommended that vaccination of foals from antibody-positive dams should begin with a two-dose primary series starting at 3 to 5 months of age, followed by administration of one subsequent booster dose 8 to 12 weeks later. However, the efficacy of this recommendation requires further study. Vaccination of foals in endemic areas is further complicated by the distinct seasonal incidence of disease in July, August, and September, when the majority of foals are 2 to 6 months of age and may be subject to maternal antibody interference with vaccination.

Botulism

Three forms of botulism—toxicoinfectious botulism (shaker foal syndrome), forage poisoning, and wound botulism—have been observed in horses as a result of the action of the potent toxins produced by the soil-borne, spore-forming bacteria of *Clostridium botulinum*. "Wound botulism" results from vegetation of spores of *Cl. botulinum* and subsequent production of toxin in contaminated wounds. "Shaker foal syndrome" results from toxin produced by vegetation of ingested spores in the intestinal tract. "Forage poisoning" results from ingestion of preformed toxin produced by decaying plant material or animal carcasses present in feed. Currently, toxicoinfection with *Cl. botulinum* type C is being investigated as a cause of "equine grass sickness," a largely fatal, pasture-associated dysautonomia affecting horses mainly in Great Britain, continental Europe, and Australia.

Botulinum toxin is the most potent biologic toxin known and acts by blocking transmission of impulses at motor end plates, resulting in weakness progressing to paralysis, inability to swallow, and frequently death. Of the eight distinct toxins produced by subtypes of *Cl. botulinum*, types B and C are associated with most outbreaks of botulism in horses. Almost all cases of shaker foal syndrome are caused by type B. Shaker foal syndrome is a significant problem in foals age 2 weeks to 8 months in Kentucky and in the mid-Atlantic seaboard states and occurs sporadically in other areas.[142-144] A toxoid vaccine (BotVax-B, Neogen Corporation, Tampa, Florida) directed against *Cl. botulinum* type B is licensed for use in horses in the United States, with its primary indication being the prevention of shaker foal syndrome. A similar toxoid is available to protect foals in endemic areas in Australia.[145] For primary vaccination, mares should be vaccinated during gestation with a series of three doses administered 4 weeks apart, scheduled so that the last dose will be administered 4 to 6 weeks before foaling to enhance concentrations of specific immunoglobulin in colostrum. Subsequently, mares should be revaccinated annually with a single dose 4 to 6 weeks before foaling.

Passively derived colostral antibodies appear to protect the foal for 8 to 12 weeks.[143,145] Maternal antibodies do not appear to interfere with the response of foals to primary immunization against botulism;[146] therefore a primary series of three doses of vaccine, administered 4 weeks apart, can be started when foals in endemic areas are 2 to 3 months of age or older. Reliance on MDAs directed against *Cl. botulinum* type B does not confer 100% protection, and the clinician must be aware of the status of transfer of passive immunity of each foal. Failure of transfer of specific immunity to botulinum toxin, insufficient specific antibody production by the dam in response to the vaccination, overwhelming toxin production, and loss of passive immunity by the time of exposure to the toxin may be reasons for vaccine failure. Other horses can be immunized using a primary series of three doses of vaccine administered at 4-week intervals, followed by annual revaccination. Currently, no licensed vaccines are available for preventing botulism caused by *Cl. botulinum* type C or other subtypes of toxins, and cross-protection between the B and C subtypes does not occur; thus routine vaccination against *Cl. botulinum* type C is not currently practiced. A type C toxoid approved for use in mink was used successfully in horses under special license to protect them during an outbreak of forage poisoning caused by contaminated alfalfa cubes in southern California.

Horses and foals with clinical botulism may be treated with botulinum antitoxin administered IV. Antitoxin is not effective against toxin that has been translocated to motor end plates. Therefore, clinical sings may progress for 12 to 24 hours after administration of the antitoxin or until all internalized toxin has attached to motor end plates. The dose of botulinum type B antitoxin recommended for treating a foal is 30,000 IU and for an adult is 70,000 IU.

Equine Viral Arteritis

Equine viral arteritis (EVA) is a contagious disease of equids caused by equine arteritis virus (EAV) and is found throughout the world. All breeds appear to be susceptible to the virus, but the prevalence of infection, as determined by seroconversion, is much higher in some breeds, notably Standardbreds, than in others. Despite the high seroprevalence of infection in Standardbreds, clinical disease is rarely observed in this breed, indicating that subclinical infection is common.[26,147] Conversely, Thoroughbreds and most other breeds have a low seroprevalence of infection but are likely to show fulminant clinical signs when they become infected. EVA is of special concern because the virus can cause abortion in pregnant mares, result in death of young foals, and establish a long-term carrier state in stallions.[26,148] Outbreaks of EVA are infrequent and sometimes difficult to diagnose because of clinical similarity to several other diseases (e.g., equine rhinopneumonitis, influenza, equine infectious anemia, purpura hemorrhagica). Clinical signs vary in severity and may include fever; anorexia; depression; edematous swelling of the eyelids, face, limbs, trunk, mammary glands, and genitalia; lacrimation and conjunctivitis; rhinitis and nasal discharge; skin rash; and infrequently, pneumonia and death of young foals. Aerosolized droplets of respiratory secretions containing virus can transmit the virus from horses with acute clinical disease. Of perhaps greater concern is transmission of the virus from subclinically infected carrier stallions to mares through semen during natural breeding or artificial insemination with fresh, chilled, or frozen semen. Carrier stallions are primarily responsible for maintenance of EAV in populations of horses. Identification of these individuals through serologic testing, followed by PCR testing or virus isolation from semen, forms the cornerstone of eradication measures.

A modified live vaccine (MLV) based on an attenuated strain of EAV was developed by researchers in Kentucky in 1969.[149] This vaccine (Arvac, Fort Dodge) was first used extensively in the field during the 1984 outbreak of EVA in Kentucky and proved to be safe and very helpful in bringing the outbreak under control.[26] Subsequently, this vaccine was developed further and licensed for commercial use, with the primary indications being (1) to prevent infection and establishment of the carrier state in previously unexposed stallions and (2) to protect nonpregnant mares being bred to carrier stallions. The vaccine has also been shown to be effective in controlling outbreaks of the disease in concentrated populations of performance horses at racetracks. Primary immunization involves administration of a single dose of vaccine, with boosters administered annually thereafter.

Vaccination of stallions, nonpregnant mares, and prepubertal colts has been shown to be a safe and effective means of controlling EVA. Strategic use of the MLV has formed the cornerstone of a highly successful program to control EVA in the Kentucky Thoroughbred breeding population during the past 15 years. Annual revaccination of breeding stallions, 28 days before the start of breeding season, is highly recommended as a means of preventing establishment of the carrier state. Mares being bred to carrier stallions should be revaccinated annually at least 21 days before breeding. Vaccinated mares may shed virus transiently after being bred to carrier stallions; therefore, isolation of these individuals for 21 days after breeding is recommended.[26] The vaccine is not recommended for use in pregnant mares, especially during the last 2 months of gestation, or in foals less than 6 weeks of age, except in emergency situations when there is a high risk of exposure. Mares should therefore be vaccinated after foaling before being rebred. Foals born to seropositive mares become seropositive after ingesting colostrum. The MDAs decay with a mean half-life of approximately 32 days, with the result that foals are generally seronegative by 7 months of age. Maternal antibodies are unlikely to interfere with the response to vaccine administered at 8 months of age or older.[32] Establishment of the carrier state appears to depend on the high levels of androgens circulating in intact stallions and can be prevented by vaccinating colts, preferably prior to puberty, before they are used for breeding.[26] In breeds or in areas where EAV is prevalent, vaccination of intact males between 8 and 12 months of age should therefore be strongly encouraged to prevent them from becoming carriers when exposed to EAV later in life through breeding or aerosol contact. Routine vaccination of Standardbred colts would be a logical approach to reducing the number of stallions that later become chronic carriers and would likely result in a substantial reduction in the incidence of infection in this breed.

Horses vaccinated with the MLV can be expected to become seropositive for life. Titers resulting from vaccination with the MLV currently licensed in North America or the inactivated vaccines licensed in Europe and in Japan cannot be distinguished from titers resulting from natural infection. Therefore, vaccination may complicate testing of horses for export. Although only a few countries currently restrict the importation of horses that test positive for neutralizing antibodies against EAV, several countries restrict entry of seropositive stallions because of the likelihood that they are chronically infected and may shed the virus in semen. It is advisable to collect a blood sample for serologic testing before administering the first dose of vaccine. Coordination of vaccination with state and federal regulatory officials, along with results of serologic tests that provide evidence the horse was seronegative before vaccination, may be helpful in resolving disputes but do not guarantee that entry will be granted into foreign countries or onto breeding farms. Development and marketing of a marker vaccine that allows vaccinated horses to be distinguished from inapparent infected carriers would greatly facilitate control, and even eradication, of EAV from horse populations.

Rotaviral Diarrhea

Equine rotavirus is one of the most important causes of infectious diarrhea in foals during the first few weeks of life and often causes outbreaks involving the majority of the foal crop on individual farms.[150-152] Older foals and adult horses are more resistant to infection. Equine rotavirus is transmitted via fecal-oral contamination and causes diarrhea by damaging the tips of villi in the small intestine, resulting in cellular destruction, maldigestion, and malabsorption. Rotaviruses are classified into seven serogroups (A through E) based on common antigens in each group.[152] Until recently, all equine rotavirus isolates were classified as belonging to serogroup A, which includes 14 serotypes (G1 through G14), of which five (G3, G5, G10, G13, and G14) representing four genotypes (P1, P7, P12, and P18) have been identified and characterized in horses.[153,154] Most equine rotavirus isolates are of the P12 genotype and G3 serotype (previously referred to as H-2) and include two subtypes (1 and 2).[155] A number of rotavirus isolates remain untyped, so it is possible that other equine rotavirus serotypes, and perhaps other serogroups, are active in the equine population.

An inactivated rotavirus A vaccine (Equine Rotavirus Vaccine, Fort Dodge) containing the G3 (H-2) serotype in a metabolizable oil-in-water emulsion is conditionally licensed in the United States and is indicated for administration to pregnant mares in endemic areas as an aid to prevention of diarrhea in their foals caused by infection with rotaviruses of serogroup A. Foal vaccination is not indicated. Label recommendations call for a three-dose series of the vaccine to be administered during each pregnancy at 8, 9, and 10 months of gestation. This protocol has been shown to induce significant increases in serum concentrations of neutralizing antibody in vaccinated mares and in concentrations of antibodies of the IgG, but not IgA, subclass in the colostrum and milk of vaccinated mares.[156,157] After nursing, the concentration of passively derived rotavirus-specific antibody of the IgG subclass in the serum of foals up to 90 days of age from vaccinated mares is significantly higher than that measured in serum of foals born to nonvaccinated mares. A field study showed this vaccine to be safe and provided circumstantial evidence of at least partial efficacy. An approximately twofold higher incidence of rotaviral diarrhea was found in foals from nonvaccinated mares compared with those from vaccinated mares, although this difference did not prove to be statistically significant.[156] Similarly, a controlled field study in Argentina, in which an inactivated aluminum hydroxide–adjuvanted vaccine containing the SA11 (G3P2), H2 (G3P12), and Lincoln (G6P1) strains was administered to 100 mares at 60 days and again at 30 days before foaling, demonstrated a substantial reduction in the incidence and severity of rotaviral disease in foals from vaccinated mares compared with foals from nonvaccinated mares.[158]

Challenge studies involving two inactivated rotavirus vaccines administered in a similar manner to pregnant mares in Japan showed that their foals were not completely protected against infection but had a substantial reduction in severity of clinical signs after challenge.[153] The major correlate for protection against rotaviral infection appears to be mucosal immunity, predominantly mucosal IgA, in the gastrointestinal tract. Studies of the immunoglobulin isotype responses of mares and of antibodies passively transferred to their foals after parenteral vaccination of their dams with inactivated rotavirus vaccines indicate that this approach is unlikely to provide foals with intestinal mucosal protection in the form of IgA.[157] Consequently, it is not surprising that current protocols do not provide complete protection. In addition, because the conditionally licensed vaccine available in the United States contains only the G3 serotype of the A serogroup, it cannot be expected to protect against infection with all field strains.

Equine Protozoal Myeloencephalitis

Equine protozoal myeloencephalitis (EPM) is a multifocal neurologic disease caused by the apicomplexan parasites

Sarcocystis neurona and, less often, *Neospora hughesi*. Serologic studies indicate that exposure to *S. neurona* occurs in most regions of North America, and in some areas, seroprevalence exceeds 50%. Prevalence of clinically apparent neurologic disease caused by *S. neurona* and *N. hughesi* is much lower than the prevalence of antibodies, indicating that many horses become infected and mount an immune response that is effective in clearing infection before substantial damage occurs in the central nervous system. It is not known whether all seropositive horses have experienced neural infection or whether the immune response in these individuals is successful in clearing parasites before neural invasion occurs. The life cycles of *S. neurona* and *N. hughesi* have not been determined definitively, although opossums are a definitive host for *S. neurona* and horses are likely dead-end hosts that inadvertently become involved in the life cycle.[159]

There is widespread exposure of horses in North America to *S. neurona* and a high level of owner concern (in some cases, hysteria) within the equine industry, leading to the perception that EPM is of economic importance. This, coupled with inadequate diagnostic techniques for antemortem confirmation of a disease and the suboptimal effectiveness of current treatment and control protocols, led the USDA to grant a conditional vaccine license to Fort Dodge Laboratories in 2000. This vaccine is an inactivated whole-parasite *S. neurona* vaccine with a metabolizable oil adjuvant (EPM Vaccine, Fort Dodge Animal Health) in which the USDA requirements for quality assurance and purity in the manufacturing process were met. The criteria for safety were also met by performance of a field study involving vaccination of more than 700 horses. The manufacturer met the requirement for documenting "a reasonable expectation of efficacy" by demonstrating seroconversion in vaccinated horses using a plaque reduction assay to measure neutralizing antibodies.

Development of a clinically relevant experimental model for *S. neurona* infection has proved to be difficult; therefore the efficacy of this vaccine has not been determined in experimental challenge studies or in prospective, controlled, double-blind field studies. Because antibody to *S. neurona* is detectable in the cerebrospinal fluid (CSF) as well as blood of some horses after vaccination,[160] prospective field-efficacy studies will be difficult to complete because one of the criteria now used to confirm a diagnosis—the presence of antibodies detectable by immunoblotting (IB) or immunofluorescent antibody test (IFAT) in CSF not contaminated with blood—will be rendered invalid in vaccinated horses. This vaccine has not gained widespread use, even though it may ultimately prove to be effective in preventing EPM. However, such use has inevitably generated controversy within the veterinary and scientific communities. Many veterinarians have expressed concern regarding widespread use of a vaccine of unknown efficacy, particularly with regard to potential adverse effects in horses already infected with the parasite. In addition, one of the most useful aspects of currently available serologic tests, the finding of a negative IB test result to rule out a diagnosis of EPM, will be invalidated in vaccinated horses. Critics also note that although an inactivated whole-parasite vaccine may induce a detectable serologic response, it is unlikely to induce a cellular Th1 response, which is probably important in preventing and clearing infection with an intracellular protozoan parasite such as *S. neurona*. Proponents of the vaccine note that many other vaccines currently licensed for use in animals and people lack data to support efficacy. In addition, the vaccine manufacturer has indicated that a modified IB procedure currently being tested may be effective in differentiating vaccinated horses from those that have experienced natural exposure. It is hoped that answers to these questions and concerns will be revealed in the future.

Anthrax

Anthrax is a serious and rapidly fatal septicemic disease caused by proliferation and spread of the vegetative form of *Bacillus anthracis* in the body. *B. anthracis* is acquired through ingestion or contamination of wounds by soil-borne spores of the organism and is encountered only in limited geographic areas where alkaline soil conditions favor survival of the organism. A Sterne's strain, nonencapsulated, live-spore vaccine (Anthrax Spore Vaccine, Colorado Serum Company, Denver) has been used to vaccinate horses. A primary series consisting of two doses of that vaccine should be administered subcutaneously 2 to 3 weeks apart, followed by annual revaccination. Adverse systemic or local effects may occasionally occur. Little objective information is available regarding use of this vaccine in horses, but clinical evidence suggests that it provides protection; however, vaccination of pregnant mares is not recommended.[161] Because it is a live bacterial product, appropriate caution should be used during storage, handling, and administration of the vaccine. Concurrent administration of antimicrobial drugs that are effective against *B. anthracis* is contraindicated if the vaccine is to function as intended.

REFERENCES

See the CD-ROM for a list of references linked to the abstract in PubMed.

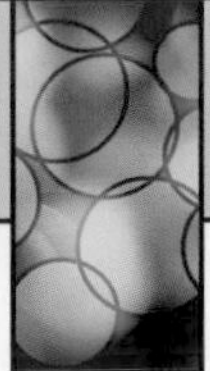

CHAPTER • 71

Antimicrobial Therapy

Mark G. Papich and Jennifer L. Davis

PRINCIPLES OF THERAPY

Antibiotic therapy for horses has always been challenging because of their poor oral absorption, the large volumes required for administration, and the high cost of some drugs. The risk of some adverse drug reactions that affect the gastrointestinal tract is a greater concern in horses than in other animals. Despite these drawbacks, it is essential that horses with serious infections receive appropriate therapy to prevent a chronic or life-threatening condition. Drug-resistant bacterial infections are an emerging problem, and the use of highly active drugs has become more important than ever before. Foals, in particular, need highly active drugs because they may be immunocompromised at the time of treatment. Drug treatment for foals has additional challenges because of differences in drug disposition in foals versus adults. Differences in oral absorption, volumes of distribution, metabolism, and clearance between foals and adults must be considered when selecting their antibacterial dosage regimens.

To assist veterinarians in prescribing effective antibiotics for their equine patients, pharmacokinetic-pharmacodynamic relationships have been used to provide guidelines for effective use. The selection of the most appropriate drug has been facilitated by new approaches to bacterial identification and susceptibility testing. This chapter reviews some of these concepts that guide antibiotic therapy for equine patients and provide important strategies for effective dosing.

MICROBIAL SUSCEPTIBILITY

Many microbes have predictable susceptibility patterns. Therefore, if the infectious agent can be accurately identified, rational antimicrobial therapy can be selected. For those bacteria and fungi that are usually highly susceptible, empiric-therapy antimicrobial agents may be chosen initially before susceptibility results are available.

Streptococcus and Pasteurella

These bacteria are consistently susceptible to β-lactam antibiotics such as the penicillins and cephalosporins. Resistance among *Streptococcus* spp. to trimethoprim-sulfonamide (TMS) combinations and chloramphenicol appears to be increasing. Trimethoprim-sulfonamide combinations for the horse may include either trimethoprim-sulfadiazine or trimethoprim-sulfamethoxazole; these drugs are also referred to as "potentiated sulfonamides". (See Appendix C for dosing information.) Many of the fluoroquinolones (e.g., enrofloxacin, orbifloxacin, marbofloxacin) used in veterinary medicine have low activity which is reflected in high minimum inhibitory (MIC) values against *Streptococcus* spp., whereas *Pasteurella* organisms are frequently susceptible to fluoroquinolones as well as other drugs. Aminoglycosides have good activity against *Pasteurella* spp., but against streptococci, they should be combined with a penicillin.

Actinobacillus

Actinobacillus spp. have historically been susceptible to many of the β-lactam antibiotics and the potentiated sulfonamides, although resistance has been documented in the last several years. One report of postoperative wound infection showed that 100% and 60% of the isolates were resistant to penicillin and TMS, respectively.[1] This resistance to penicillin may be caused by the production of β-lactamases by some strains.[2] Susceptibility to the cephalosporins and aminoglycoside antibiotics is usually anticipated.

Staphylococcus

Staphylococcus spp. that do not produce β-lactamase have a predictable susceptibility pattern to many of the penicillins and cephalosporins. *Staphylococcus* spp. are usually susceptible to oxacillin and dicloxacillin, but these are not typically administered to horses. Most staphylococci are sensitive to the fluoroquinolones and aminoglycosides. The majority of strains are also sensitive to chloramphenicol, TMS, or erythromycin, but resistance is possible. Susceptibility of β-lactamase–positive staphylococci is less predictable. The β-lactamase will inactivate penicillins, aminopenicillins (e.g., ampicillin, amoxicillin), and some of the extended-spectrum penicillins (e.g., ticarcillin). The addition of a β-lactamase inhibitor (clavulanate or sulbactam) or the use of β-lactamase–resistant β-lactam antibiotics such as cephalosporins (e.g., cefadroxil, cefpodoxime, cefazolin) will increase activity to include β-lactamase–producing strains of staphylococci.

Recent reports have raised concerns of staphylococcal resistance in horses.[3-5] The isolated methicillin-resistant *Staphylococcus aureus* (MRSA) strains colonized both horses and people who were in contact with the horses (see Chapter 44). Evidence for human-to-animal transmission was reported. These strains were resistant to other antibiotics, in addition to β-lactams. MRSA has been reported more often in some referral centers. These MRSA strains present an important problem for veterinarians because they are resistant to all β-lactam antibiotics, regardless of whether they are combined with a β-lactamase inhibitor. Some of these strains remain sensitive to fluoroquinolones and TMS, but there may be cases for which the only active drugs are the glycopeptide vancomycin or the oxyzolidinone linezolid (Zyvox). Vancomycin has been used sporadically in the treatment of equine MRSA as an intravenous (IV) infusion at doses of 4.3 to 7.5 mg/kg body weight every 8 hours (q8h).[6,7] There are no reports of clinical use of linezolid in horses, and at the time of this writing, its use is considered to be cost prohibitive. (Linezolid is a human drug, and current retail costs exceed $55 per tablet.)

Anaerobic Bacteria

If the bacteria are anaerobic, predictable susceptibility patterns also are available. In horses, anaerobic bacteria causing infection include *Clostridium*, *Fusobacterium*, *Peptostreptococcus*, and *Bacteroides* spp.[8] These bacteria are usually sensitive to penicillin, chloramphenicol, metronidazole, or one of the second-generation cephalosporins, such as cefotetan or cefoxitin. If the anaerobe is from the *Bacteroides fragilis* group, resistance may be more of a problem because these organisms can produce a β-lactamase that inactivates first-generation cephalosporins, penicillins, and ampicillin/amoxicillin. The incidence of resistant strains of *Bacteroides* has increased in recent years.[9] Because many anaerobic infections in horses may be caused by *B. fragilis*,[10] metronidazole is a logical choice for treatment. This drug is consistently active against anaerobes, including *B. fragilis*, and doses have been established from pharmacokinetic studies. Chloramphenicol also has consistent activity against many anaerobic bacteria. Clindamycin frequently has good activity against anaerobic bacteria, although resistance has increased over the last several years. However, clindamycin should never be used in the horse because of the likely development of a severe, often fatal, diarrhea. The activity of first-generation cephalosporins, TMS, or fluoroquinolones against anaerobic bacteria is unpredictable. None of the aminoglycosides is active against anaerobic bacteria.

Pseudomonas, Enterobacter, Klebsiella, and E. coli

If the organism is *Pseudomonas aeruginosa*, *Enterobacter*, *Klebsiella*, *Escherichia coli*, or *Proteus*, resistance to many common antibiotics is possible, and a susceptibility test is advised. Many *E. coli* isolates are resistant to common antibiotics such as penicillins, aminopenicillins, first-generation cephalosporins, and tetracyclines. Based on susceptibility data, gram-negative enteric bacteria are usually expected to be susceptible to fluoroquinolones and aminoglycosides. However, some reports suggest that resistance to fluoroquinolones may be increasing in small animals.[11,12] Such resistance trends have not been reported for isolates from horses. Resistance to gentamicin among equine pathogens is increasing and has been documented in veterinary teaching hospitals for more than 15 years.[13] Amikacin is the most active of the aminoglycosides against gram-negative bacteria in horses, including *P. aeruginosa*, and may be more suitable for the treatment of resistant gram-negative infections. *P. aeruginosa* is inherently resistant to many drugs, but it may be susceptible to fluoroquinolones, aminoglycosides, or extended-spectrum penicillins (e.g., ticarcillin, piperacillin). If a fluoroquinolone is used to treat *P. aeruginosa*, a large dose is necessary because the MICs of *Pseudomonas* spp. are higher than for other gram-negative organisms. Although pharmacokinetic studies have documented effective plasma concentrations for most gram-negative bacteria from typical doses of fluoroquinolones, no studies have used high enough doses to produce plasma concentrations considered to be effective against *Pseudomonas* spp. Moreover, the high doses recommended for treating *Pseudomonas* in dogs have not been tested for safety in clinical studies in horses. Of the currently available fluoroquinolones (human or veterinary drugs), ciprofloxacin is the most active against *P. aeruginosa*, but it is not absorbed well orally in horses.[14]

The extended-spectrum cephalosporins (second-, third-, and fourth-generation cephalosporins) have been used in horses for some of the refractory gram-negative infections. They have greater activity against gram-negative bacteria than first-generation cephalosporins such as cefazolin. Only ceftazidime has consistent activity against *P. aeruginosa*. Because the extended-spectrum cephalosporins are expensive, use of drugs such as cefotaxime and ceftazidime has been limited in horses. However, one of the veterinary drugs, ceftiofur (Naxcel, Pfizer; 50 mg/mL), has been frequently used in horses, and some dosing regimens may be effective (see later discussion under Cephalosporins).

Fungi

Systemic fungal infections in horses can be difficult to treat because of the lack of availability of affordable treatments and the difficulty involved in culturing and identifying the organisms. However, some generalizations about susceptibilities can be made. Many of the yeast and yeastlike infections in horses have good susceptibility to the triazole antifungals—fluconazole, itraconazole, and voriconazole—including the organisms that cause candidiasis, histoplasmosis, blastomycosis, and coccidioidomycosis. Fluconazole is a rational treatment for these pathogens because it has excellent oral bioavailability and produces sustained plasma and tissue concentrations.[15] This drug is now available in a generic human formulation, which has decreased its cost for effective therapy. Some *Candida* spp. have developed resistance to fluconazole however, and alternative therapies may be necessary. *Aspergillus* spp. are typically sensitive to itraconazole and voriconazole, but not to fluconazole. *Fusarium* spp. present a very difficult treatment dilemma in that they are resistant to many of the available drugs. Only voriconazole and amphotericin B demonstrate significant in vitro antifungal activity against *Fusarium* spp. If systemic treatment for dermatophytosis is required, griseofulvin has been used because it is labeled for use in the horse.

BACTERIAL SUSCEPTIBILITY TESTING

Agar Disk Diffusion Test

When bacterial resistance is likely, a susceptibility test is recommended. Bacterial susceptibility to drugs has traditionally been tested with the agar disk diffusion (ADD) test, also known as the Kirby-Bauer test. With this test, paper disks impregnated with the drug are placed on an agar plate and the drug diffuses into the agar. The zone of inhibition around the disk is correlated to the bactericidal or bacteriostatic activity of the drug against the bacteria. The ADD must be performed according to strict procedural standards for inoculation size, depth of agar, and incubation time set by the Clinical and Laboratory Standards Institute (CLSI), formerly known as the National Committee for Clinical Laboratory Standards (NCCLS).[16,17] The ADD test results are qualitative and determine only resistance or sensitivity for the bacteria tested. If this test is performed using standardized procedures, it is valuable; at times, however, it may overestimate the degree of susceptibility.

Minimum Inhibitory Concentration Determination

Laboratories typically measure the minimum inhibitory concentration (MIC) of an organism directly with an antimicrobial dilution test. The test is most often performed by inoculating the wells of a plate with the bacterial culture and adding multiple dilutions of antibiotics across the rows of the plate. The MIC is recorded by observing the lowest concentration required to inhibit bacterial growth. In some laboratories, other methods to measure the MIC are being used, such as the E-test (epsilometer test) by AB Biodisk. The E-test is a quantitative technique that identifies the MIC by direct measurement of bacterial growth along a concentration gradient of the antibiotic contained in a test strip.

When the MIC is measured, resistance and susceptibility are determined by comparing the organism's MIC to the drug's breakpoint, as standardized by CLSI.[16-18] If bacteria have an MIC equal to or below the "susceptible" breakpoint, treatment with this drug should produce a cure unless there are other factors independent of the drug's activity. An MIC equal to or above the "resistant" breakpoint indicates that the organism is resistant regardless of the dose administered or location of the infection. An MIC in the "intermediate" range means that the organism is resistant to the drug unless dosing modifications are used, or unless the drug concentrates at the site of infection, as with topical treatment, or in the lower urinary tract for drugs excreted via the kidney.

Even though we believe that an MIC determination is valuable to guide therapy, some limitations exist. One important limitation for interpreting susceptibility information for pathogens infecting horses is that interpretive criteria to establish susceptibility breakpoints are available for only a small number of drugs used in horses (ceftiofur, gentamicn) (See Tables 1 and 2 in the CLSI M-31 document under Group A.[18]) For other drugs, human interpretive criteria are used.

PHARMACOKINETIC-PHARMACODYNAMIC OPTIMIZATION OF DOSES

To achieve a cure, the drug concentration at the site of the infection should be maintained above the MIC, or some multiple of the MIC, for at least a portion of the dose interval. Antibacterial dosage regimens are based on this assumption. (See Appendix C.) However, drugs vary with respect to the magnitude of the peak concentration and the time above the MIC that is needed for a clinical cure. Pharmacokinetic-pharmacodynamic (PK-PD) relationships of antibiotics attempt to describe how these factors can correlate with clinical outcome.[19,20] Parameters that describe the plasma concentration versus time profile may be used as pharmacokinetic factors to predict antibiotic cures (Fig. 71-1). The "C_{max}" is simply the maximum plasma concentration attained during a dosing interval. The C_{max} is related to the MIC by the C_{max}/MIC ratio. The "AUC" is the total area under the curve. The AUC for a 24-hour period is related to the MIC value by the AUC_{24}/MIC ratio. (Some authors refer to this as the "AUIC," but this term has other meanings, and AUIC should not be used.) The duration of effective plasma concentrations is determined by the time above MIC measured in hours (T>MIC, or $T_{>MIC}$), or reported as the percent of the time above the MIC during a 24-hour dosing interval.[33]

Antibiotics can be bactericidal, bacteriostatic, or both, depending on the drug and the organism. For a drug that is bactericidal, its action may be either concentration dependent or time dependent. If concentration dependent, the clinician should administer a high enough dose to maximize the C_{max}/MIC ratio or the AUC_{24}/MIC ratio. If time dependent, the drug should be administered frequently enough to maximize the T>MIC. For bacteriostatic drugs, the drug concentration should be kept above the MIC at the site of action for as long as possible during the dosing interval. Examples of how these relationships affect drug regimens for some drugs used in horses are described next.

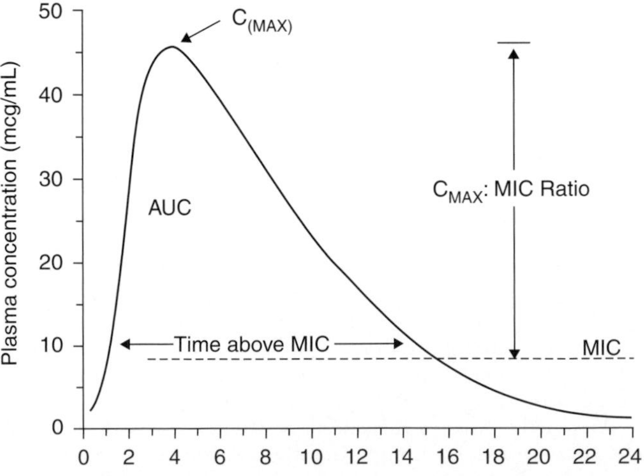

Fig. 71-1 Plasma concentration versus time profile and minimum inhibitory concentration *(MIC)*. Relationship between MIC and pharmacokinetic terms are shown; see text. Maximum (peak) plasma concentration, C_{MAX}/MIC ratio; Time above MIC (T>MIC), *AUC*, area under the curve.

Aminoglycosides

Aminoglycosides are concentration-dependent bactericidal drugs; therefore, the higher the drug concentration, the greater the bactericidal effect. An optimal bactericidal effect occurs if a high enough dose is administered to produce a peak of 8 to 10 times the MIC. This can be accomplished by administering a single IV dose once daily, because a significant postantibiotic effect has been demonstrated. This regimen is at least as effective, and perhaps less nephrotoxic, than lower doses administered more frequently.[21,22] Current dosing regimens in horses employ this strategy. The single daily dose is related to the drug's volume of distribution (Vd) using the equation Dose = $C_{max} \times Vd$. A once-daily dose for gentamicin in adult horses using these guidelines is 4 to 6.8 mg/kg.[23] The efficacy of these regimens has not been tested for conditions encountered in veterinary medicine, but the relationships are supported by studies in experimental animals. These regimens assume some competency of the immune system. If the animal is severely immunocompromised, the clinician may consider a more frequent interval for administration and synergistic combinations with β-lactam antibiotics.

Fluoroquinolones

Fluoroquinolone antibiotics are rapidly bactericidal and exhibit a significant postantibiotic effect. As reviewed in several papers,[19,24-26] either the C_{max}/MIC ratio or the AUC_{24}/MIC ratio may predict clinical cure in studies of laboratory animals and in a limited number of human clinical studies. There are no published studies involving horses (or dogs and cats) to indicate which of these parameters will better predict clinical cure or what the respective target ratios might be. However, studies in experimental animals have demonstrated that a C_{max}/MIC ratio of 8 to 10 or an AUC_{24}/MIC ratio greater than 100 to 125 has been associated with a cure. The cited AUC/MIC ratio above 125 refers to administration to critically ill, neutropenic human patients. In other patients the ratio to achieve a cure may not be that high. Wright et al.[25] presented evidence that AUC_{24}/MIC ratios as low as 30 to 55 are associated with a clinical cure. This difference may reflect the severity of illness in the subjects of these investigations, but it also may be organism specific. With clinical doses used for many infections in veterinary medicine, the AUC/MIC ratios are often lower than 125, and clinical cures are still observed. An examination of the current use of the fluoroquinolones in veterinary medicine suggests that, in immunocompetent animals, AUC/MIC ratios of 50 to 60 are likely to be effective.[26]

Current guidelines recommend doses of fluoroquinolones to achieve C_{max}/MIC ratios above these threshold levels, which have been associated with a lower incidence of the development of resistance.[27] Sensitive bacteria from horses might be expected to have an MIC for enrofloxacin of 0.125 mg/mL or less based on available information.[28] Pharmacokinetic studies available from horses showed that to achieve desirable PK-PD indices administering enrofloxacin, IV doses of 5 mg/kg once daily or 7.5 to 10 mg/kg orally may be adequate.[29-32] We have monitored plasma concentrations in many clinical equine patients after oral and injectable administration of enrofloxacin (unpublished observations by the authors) and confirmed that these doses are adequate to achieve targeted plasma concentrations.

Beta-Lactam Antibiotics

Beta-lactam antibiotics such as penicillins, potentiated aminopenicillins, and cephalosporins are slowly bactericidal. Their concentration should be kept above the MIC throughout most of the dosing interval (long T>MIC) for the optimal bactericidal effect.[33] In general, the goal is to maintain plasma concentrations above the MIC for at least 50% of the dosing interval. For the treatment of some gram-negative bacteria, some regimens for penicillins and cephalosporins require administration three to four times per day to meet this target. Some of the third-generation cephalosporins have longer half-lives, and less frequent dosing intervals have been used for these drugs (e.g., cefotaxime, ceftiofur). Because the MICs are lower for gram-positive bacteria, and antibacterial effects occur at concentrations below the MIC (postantibiotic effect, PAE), longer dose intervals may be possible for infections caused by gram-positive compared with gram-negative bacteria.

Bacteriostatic Drugs

Drugs such as the tetracyclines, macrolides (erythromycin and derivatives), sulfonamides, and chloramphenicol derivatives act in a bacteriostatic manner against most bacteria. However, against susceptible gram-positive bacteria, the macrolides appear to be bactericidal and can demonstrate a postantibiotic effect. Chloramphenicol also can produce a bactericidal effect if the organism is very susceptible.

Bacteriostatic drugs are most effective when concentrations of the drug at the site of the infection are maintained above the MIC for the entire dosing interval. In this way, they act in a time-dependent manner. However, the most predictive PK-PD index for antibacterial success is the AUC/MIC ratio. Many of the bacteriostatic drugs must be administered frequently or demonstrate a long half-life to achieve this goal. A property of some of these drugs is that they persist in tissues for a prolonged time, allowing infrequent dosing intervals. The macrolide derivative azithromycin (Zithromax, Pfizer) has shown tissue half-lives as long as 70 to 90 hours in cats and dogs, permitting infrequent dosing. Accumulation and persistence of azithromycin in polymorphonuclear leukocytes (PMNs) and macrophages of foals has also been demonstrated.[34] Concentrations of clarithromycin can be maintained with twice-daily dosing in horses.[35] Tissue concentrations of TMS persist long enough to allow once-daily dosing for many infections, although a study in equine joint infections showed that twice daily was more effective.[36]

TISSUE PENETRATION OF DRUGS

For most tissues, antibiotic drug concentrations in the serum or plasma can predict the drug concentration in the extracellular space (interstitial fluid). This is because no physical barrier impedes drug diffusion from the vascular compartment to extracellular tissue fluid.[37] Pores (fenestrations) or microchannels in the endothelium of capillaries are large enough to allow drug molecules to penetrate. One important limitation involves drugs that are highly protein bound in the blood;[38] examples of drugs for which this may be important in equine medicine include doxycycline and itraconazole.

For most antimicrobial drugs, the plasma drug concentrations produce tissue fluid concentrations in lung, pleural space, skin, abdominal fluid, joint fluid, soft tissues, and bone that are similar to steady-state plasma drug concentrations. For example, gentamicin reached concentrations in lymph fluid of horses that closely paralleled plasma concentrations.[39] A study from our laboratory showed that ticarcillin diffuses into mare's tissues adequately when one accounts for the percentage of tissue occupied by extracellular water.[40] Although gentamicin and ticarcillin are not very lipophilic, they are able to diffuse from the plasma to extracellular fluid of these tissues easily. Rapid equilibration between the extracellular fluid and plasma is possible because of high surface area/volume ratio (high SA/V). That is, the surface area of the capillaries is high relative to the volume into which the drug diffuses.

Some caution is advised when interpreting tissue concentrations reported in pharmacokinetic papers. Tissue concentrations in homogenized tissues reflect the *total tissue content* (intracellular and extracellular drug concentration) rather than the drug concentration in interstitial fluid. Drug concentrations from homogenized tissues will also reflect both protein-bound and protein-unbound drug, as well as drug bound to the tissues. It is only the unbound form of the drug that is microbiologically active. Therefore, homogenized tissue drug concentrations often overestimate the actual drug at the site, or they may underestimate the drug concentrations in extracellular fluid if the drug has low lipophilicity.

Drug diffusion into an abscess or cavitated lesion may be delayed because the volume into which the drug must diffuse is higher, resulting in a lower SA/V, lower drug concentrations, and slower equilibrium between plasma and tissue. Therefore, observed slow equilibrium or a low peak drug concentration in this case is more a factor of the geometry of the tissue (low SA/V), than a physical barrier to diffusion. For an abscess or granuloma, penetration by antibiotics also is impaired because drug penetration relies on simple diffusion from the plasma compartment, and the site of infection may lack an adequate blood supply.

Tissues once assumed to present a barrier to drug diffusion actually attain adequate drug penetration. For example, it is a common misconception that drug penetration into synovial fluid of joints is impaired in horses. Penetration of ampicillin and gentamicin is adequate from the vascular compartment to synovial fluid in horses,[41] but equilibrium is often delayed because of the synovial volume (low SA/V). Ensink et al.[42] and Anderson et al.[39] also showed the ability of plasma concentrations to predict synovial fluid concentrations. In their studies of gentamicin and ampicillin, delayed equilibrium was caused by the lower SA/V ratio in joints, but after equilibrium was achieved, synovial fluid concentrations either paralleled plasma drug concentrations or declined more slowly. That these drugs penetrated joints is an important observation, because ampicillin and gentamicin are incapable of diffusing readily through lipid membranes and rely on diffusion through capillary pores. Beta-lactam antibiotics and aminoglycosides penetrated inflamed joints more rapidly and achieved higher concentrations than in healthy joints,[43] most likely from increased blood flow to the joint. However, penetration during chronic inflammation could be impeded by presence of pus and fibrosis.

When the SA/V ratio is small and the drug's elimination from the plasma is rapid, some drugs may not have sufficient time to diffuse adequately into infected sites. For example cefapirin diffuses poorly into infected tissue chambers in horses because (1) these tissue chambers have a different geometry (lower SA/V) than the tissue compartment predicted by a pharmacokinetic model, and (2) cefapirin is rapidly eliminated from plasma with a half-life of 19 minutes, which does not allow enough time for equilibrium between the tissue cage and serum.[44]

Impaired Diffusion into Tissues

Tissues that lack pores or channels may inhibit penetration of some drugs. In some tissues a lipid membrane (e.g., tight junctions in capillaries) presents a barrier to drug diffusion. In these cases a drug must be sufficiently lipid soluble or must be actively carried across the membrane to reach effective concentrations in tissues. These tissues include the central nervous system (CNS), eye, and prostate. Many clinicians believe that drug penetration across these barriers is not important when treating inflammatory diseases, because these barriers will be breached and drugs will be able to diffuse freely into the affected area. However, this is not always the case. In a study analyzing amikacin concentrations in the CSF of the horse, drug was not detected in any of the horses with a normal blood-brain barrier (BBB).[46] In one horse that developed septic meningitis during the study, drug was not detectable until 4 hours after the second injection and reached a peak of only 0.97 μg/mL, which did not occur until 8 hours after the fifth injection.

Box 71-1 summarizes drugs known to penetrate into the cerebrospinal fluid (CSF) and aqueous humor of horses. Also, a barrier exists between plasma and bronchial epithelium (blood-bronchus barrier).[45] This restricts penetration of some drugs in the bronchial secretions and epithelial fluid of the airways. However, disposition of drug into lung tissue not separated by the blood-bronchus barrier is not impaired (e.g., when treating pneumonia).

Lipophilic drugs (e.g., macrolides, fluoroquinolones, tetracyclines, trimethoprim, chloramphenicol) may be more likely to diffuse through lipid membranes for treating infections in these tissues. Depending on the susceptibility of the organism, these drugs have been used to treat infections of the CNS, respiratory tract, and eye.

Intracellular Drug Penetration

Most bacterial infections are located extracellularly, and a cure can be achieved with adequate drug concentrations in the extracellular (interstitial) space rather than intracellular space. Intracellular infections, however, present a different problem. For drugs to reach intracellular sites, they must either diffuse passively or utilize a transport process. One of the most important equine intracellular organisms is *Rhodococcus equi*. Drugs traditionally used for treatment of *R. equi* pneumonia in foals include erythromycin and rifampin because these drugs are known for their ability to achieve high concentrations intracellularly.[47] Treatment of rickettsial infections in horses also requires intracellular penetration. Infections caused by *Neorickettsia risticii* (formerly known as *Ehrlichia risticii*) and *Anaplasma phagocytophilium* (formerly known as *E. equi*) have been treated most often with tetracyclines because they are known to attain sufficient intracellular concentrations. Other intracellular organisms include *Chlamydia* and *Mycobacterium*. Staphylococci may become resistant to treatment in some cases because of intracellular survival.

Examples of drugs that accumulate in leukocytes, fibroblasts, macrophages, and other cells are fluoroquinolones, tetracyclines, macrolides (erythromycin, clarithromycin), and the azalides (azithromycin).[48] Beta-lactam antibiotics and aminoglycosides do not reach effective concentrations within cells. Doxycycline, despite high protein binding in horses, achieves leukocyte concentrations 17 times greater than maximum plasma concentrations.[49] This may explain why doxycycline is efficacious in the treatment of many bacterial infections, despite the low plasma concentrations. The erythromycin derivative azithromycin (Zithromax) achieves particularly high concentrations of active drug intracellularly. In equine studies the oral absorption of azithromycin in foals was 33%, and the concentrations achieved in phagocytes were 200 times the corresponding plasma concentrations.[34] Either clarithromycin or azithromycin may have potential for treating intracellular infections such as *R. equi* in foals. In a study comparing treatment with azithromycin and rifampin to clarithromycin and rifampin, the group that received clarithromycin at recommended doses[35] had a higher clinical success rate.[50] This difference might have resulted from higher activity for clarithromycin rather than a pharmacokinetic difference.[51]

Box • 71-1

Summary of Drugs Studied in Cerebrospinal Fluid (CSF) and Aqueous Humor in the Horse*

Drugs That Penetrate Intact Blood-Brain Barrier
Chloramphenicol (39%)
Ciprofloxacin (23%)
Enrofloxacin (25%)
Fluconazole (39%)
Metronidazole (31%)
Orbifloxacin (25%)
Streptomycin (4%)
Sulfamethoxazole (30%)
Trimethoprim (27%)

Drugs That Do Not Penetrate Intact Blood-Brain Barrier
Amikacin
Ceftiofur

Drugs That Penetrate Intact Blood-Aqueous Barrier
Chloramphenicol (16%)
Ciprofloxacin (4%)
Doxycycline (10.5%)
Fluconazole (37%)
Streptomycin (10%)
Voriconazole (41%)

Drugs That Do Not Penetrate Intact Blood-Aqueous Barrier
Cephalexin
Itraconazole

*The value in parentheses represents the percentage of drug found in the CSF or aqueous humor compared with that found in plasma or serum.

LOCAL FACTORS THAT AFFECT ANTIBIOTIC EFFECTIVENESS

Local tissue factors may decrease antimicrobial effectiveness. For example, pus and necrotic debris may bind and inactivate vancomycin or aminoglycoside antibiotics, causing them to be ineffective. Cellular material also can decrease the activity of topical agents such as polymyxin B. Foreign material in a wound, such as material surgically implanted, can protect bacteria from antibiotics and phagocytosis by forming a biofilm (glycocalyx) at the site of infection.[52,53] Cations can adversely affect the activity of antimicrobials at the site of infection. Two important drug groups diminished in activity by cations (e.g., Mg^{+2}, Al^{+3}, Ca^{+2}) at the site of infection are fluoroquinolones and aminoglycosides. (Cations such as magnesium, iron, and aluminum also can inhibit oral absorption of fluoroquinolones.)

The acidic environment of infected tissue may decrease the effectiveness of erythromycin, other macrolides, fluoroquinolones, and aminoglycosides. Penicillin and tetracycline activity is not affected as much by tissue pH, but hemoglobin at the site of infection will decrease the activity of these drugs. An anaerobic environment decreases the effectiveness of aminoglycosides because oxygen is necessary for drug penetration into bacteria. TMS combinations are sometimes not effective in vivo despite in vitro results that suggest susceptibility.[54] The impediment to successful TMS activity is the material in infected tissue that inhibits drug activity. In a study using experimental ponies, trimethoprim-sulfadiazine was administered at 30 mg/kg (combined) every 12 hours (q12h).[55] This dose produced drug concentrations above the MIC of the infecting pathogen, *Streptococcus equi* subsp. *equi*, in an infected tissue chamber model. However, trimethoprim-sulfadiazine was ineffective for eliminating the infection compared with injections of penicillin G. In a follow-up study the investigators showed that trimethoprim-sulfadiazine (30 mg/kg q12h) administered to ponies with experimentally infected tissue cages was also ineffective for preventing infection even if administered prophylactically.[56] The investigators of these studies propose that treatment failure with trimethoprim-sulfadiazine in ponies is cause by composition of the tissue fluid in the infected chamber. Tissues may contain thymidine and para-aminobenzoic acid (PABA), which are inhibitors of the action of trimethoprim and sulfonamides, respectively. On the other hand, penicillin, ampicillin, and ampicillin derivatives have been successful in these same *Streptococcus* tissue cage models and may be preferred for treatment of clinical cases.

As mentioned previously, an adequate blood flow is necessary to deliver an antibiotic to the site of infection. Effective antibacterial drug concentrations may not be attained in tissues that are poorly vascularized (e.g., extremities during shock, sequestered bone fragments, endocardial valves). An abscess rarely responds to antibiotic therapy alone because several factors hamper successful therapy: poor blood supply, material in tissue fluid and pus that may inactivate drugs, and a small SA/V ratio of the infected site.

ABSORPTION OF ANTIMICROBIALS IN HORSES

One of the challenges presented for antibiotic therapy in horses is actually delivering the drug into the animal. Injectable drugs can cause pain and irritation. Many oral drugs are poorly absorbed, which presents risks because unabsorbed drug in the intestine may disrupt the normal bacterial population and cause diarrhea and enteritis.

Injectable Drugs

Many injectable solutions can be administered intravenously (IV), which delivers high concentrations to tissues rapidly. Intramuscular (IM) administration also is suitable for some drugs, although pain and muscle injury from injection can be important drawbacks. The absorption rate from an IM injection usually is sufficient to achieve high concentrations rapidly, and absorption usually is complete. For some drugs, slow release of the drug from the IM injection may effectively prolong the dosing interval. Uboh et al.[57] showed that after IM administration of penicillin G potassium, the plasma penicillin concentrations 24 hours after administration were similar to concentrations after IM administration of procaine penicillin. Prior to that report, it was assumed that the sole reason for prolonged absorption of penicillin from procaine penicillin G was the presence of procaine and slow release from the injection site.[58] Apparently, however, IM injection of soluble salts (e.g., penicillin potassium) also will produce prolonged plasma concentrations.[57] The long half-life from IM injection of these solutions is probably caused by disruption of blood flow at the injection site after IM administration and slower uptake into the circulation. Because the rate of absorption determines the terminal half-life in these cases, half-life is prolonged. Pharmacokineticists refer to this as the "flip-flop effect." Systemic availability (% F) may be falsely overestimated in studies in which the flip-flop effect is observed.

As in cattle,[59] the site of IM injection also affects drug absorption. In studies comparing different IM sites, injections in the neck muscle of horses showed faster and more complete drug absorption compared with injections in the gluteal or hamstring muscles (semitendinosus).[58]

Oral Absorption

As reviewed by Baggot,[60] oral absorption is low for many drugs in horses. Drugs such as aminopenicillins (ampicillin, amoxicillin), cephalosporins, and macrolide antibiotics are not absorbed as rapidly or to as great an extent compared with administration of these drugs in small animals or humans. This limits the use of the oral route for many drugs in horses. For example, oral amoxicillin is absorbed well enough in humans, dogs, and cats to be a useful and practical route of administration. However, systemic availability of oral amoxicillin in adult horses is only 2% to 10%.[42,61] Ampicillin also is not a good option for oral administration in horses because of poor availability.[62] Even though oral absorption is poor for these drugs in adult horses, there may be an advantage for oral administration in foals because they appear to exhibit higher oral absorption. For example, compared with the poor absorption cited for adult horses, oral absorption of amoxicillin in foals is better, 36% to 42%.[63]

For cephalosporins, the same pattern is observed. Cefadroxil is absorbed better in the foal than in adult horses.[64,65] Oral absorption of cephalexin is low in horses (5%), but at 30 mg/kg orally q8h, concentrations can be maintained above the MIC of susceptible bacteria.[66]

Modification of some drugs has improved oral absorption in horses. The ester prodrugs of ampicillin, such as bacampicillin and pivampicillin, produce moderate systemic availability in horses after oral administration (35%-45%).[67] However, these prodrugs are no longer available as commercial products in the United States. Esters and salts of erythromycin also have improved oral absorption in horses. Erythromycin base administered to horses is rapidly degraded into inactive metabolites in the equine stomach and intestine, and systemic availability of erythromycin is poor.[68] However, if erythromycin is administered as an ester prodrug such as erythromycin estolate, it is absorbed as the intact ester and converted to the active drug after absorption. Oral absorption is also improved if erythromycin is administered as a phosphate salt, whereby it resists degradation in the stomach and intestine and is absorbed as active erythromycin.[69]

The use of an ester prodrug was recently demonstrated for cefpodoxime proxetil (Simplicef, Pfizer) in horses.[70] The clinical use of cefpodoxime is discussed in more detail later (see Cephalosporins).

The effect of food on the oral absorption of drugs in veterinary medicine is often overlooked. Most pharmacokinetic studies administer drugs to horses that have been fasted before and after drug administration. However, this may not be possible, or practical, in field conditions. Significantly decreased drug absorption has been demonstrated for several oral antibiotics in the horse when they are administered with feed. When healthy foals were given microencapsulated erythromycin base, they had decreased plasma concentrations and systemic bioavailability when they were allowed to eat hay up until the time of drug administration compared with those that were fasted.[68] Trimethoprim-sulfachlorpyridazine combinations were shown to bind to feed constituents and cecal contents in vitro.[71] In addition, systemic bioavailability was significantly decreased when the drug was administered as a topical dressing compared with nasogastric intubation.[72] Oral bioavailability of rifampin decreased from 68% when it was administered 1 hour before feeding to 26% when administered 1 hour after feeding.[60] Recent studies have also shown that the extent of oral absorption of doxycycline increased by approximately 50% when it was administered by nasogastric tube to a fasted horse versus a fed horse.[49] Whenever possible, feeding schedules should be taken into account when dosing with oral antibiotics.

Studies to predict oral absorption are underway. Oral absorption of some drugs in humans (and perhaps dogs) can be predicted from the Biopharmaceutics Classification System (BCS). The BCS is one of the most significant tools recently developed to facilitate product development and regulatory decisions. By understanding a compound's solubility and permeability characteristics, a mechanistic approach can be developed to predict oral drug absorption from the gastrointestinal (GI) tract. By understanding the relationship between a drug's in vivo absorption profile and the in vitro permeability and dissolution characteristics, it is possible to identify conditions under which the in vitro data could serve as a surrogate for in vivo bioequivalence testing.

Pharmaceutical compounds can be grouped into one of the following categories:

- Class I: High solubility, high permeability; generally very-well-absorbed compounds.
- Class II: Low solubility, high permeability; exhibit dissolution, rate-limited absorption.
- Class III: High solubility, low permeability; exhibits permeability-limited absorption.
- Class IV: Low solubility, low permeability; very poor oral bioavailability.

For class I drugs, oral absorption in horses likely will be good, even when compounded with various vehicles. Absorption of other classes, however, will depend on other factors. It may be possible for class III drugs to overcome some of the poor permeability problems with sufficiently high doses.

Local Drug Administration

Direct drug administration has been used to provide high concentrations of drugs in bones and joints of horses and decrease reliance on high systemic doses. Intraarticular administration of gentamicin to horses produces high synovial drug concentrations.[73,155] Because of the low SA/V ratio in joints and delayed equilibrium, drug clearance from joint fluid after this administration is slower than from the plasma and may provide effective concentrations for at least 24 hours. High concentrations in the limbs can also be achieved by regional limb perfusion.[156] In this technique an infected limb is perfused with an antibiotic, and the drug concentration is kept high by applying a temporary tourniquet to the limb proximal to the site of drug administration.[74] Regional limb perfusion of equine limbs allows high concentrations to be achieved in bone and joints of limbs without high doses and systemic exposure to the drug.

CONSIDERATIONS FOR ANTIMICROBIALS IN FOALS

In some cases, drug dosages for foals are similar to adults because of similarity in drug distribution and clearance. In other cases, doses should be modified because of differences in oral absorption, clearance, and distribution. When treating foals, equine practitioners should consult specific references to administer the safest and most effective dose.

Drug absorption and disposition in the foal are different than in the adult horse. In general, neonatal foals have a higher volume of distribution, a lower clearance, and a longer half-life than adult horses. Systemic bioavailability for some oral antibiotics is also often increased in neonatal foals, especially for the β-lactam antibiotics. A well-designed study on the absorption of cefadroxil in foals over 0.5 to 5 months showed that the oral absorption rate becomes faster with age, but bioavailability decreased from 99.6% at 0.5 months to 14.5% at 5 months.[64] Amoxicillin also is absorbed better in foals than adult horses.[42,63] The difference between foals and adults may be caused by an increased intestinal permeability in young foals, a change in gastric pH as the foal ages and the diet changes,[75] or a difference in intestinal transport carriers.

The horse's age also affects drug distribution. The difference is cause by a larger extracellular fluid compartment observed in young animals that leads to a larger volume of distribution of water-soluble drugs. A larger volume of distribution for neonatal foals may necessitate higher doses to achieve adequate plasma concentrations. The best example of this property is amikacin. In adult horses an appropriate dose for amikacin is 7.25 to 14.5 mg/kg once daily. However, because foals have a higher volume of distribution, a larger proportion of the administered dose is distributed to extracellular fluid. For example, the volume of distribution in foals has been measured at 0.5 to 0.7 L/kg[76,77] versus 0.17 and 0.26 L/kg in adults.[46,78] Therefore the dose of amikacin for foals should be increased to 20 to 25 mg/kg once daily. Gentamicin doses are also proportionately higher in foals than adults.

When treating foals, some antibiotics may also be more likely to distribute across diffusion barriers that they might not cross normally, such as the BBB. In foals less than 2 weeks of age, CSF protein concentrations are elevated compared with adults, which may be caused by a more permeable BBB.[79] Because the BBB may not be fully mature at birth, it may cause increased drug penetration into the CSF.[75]

Drug metabolism and elimination may be impaired in young foals because of a deficiency in hepatic drug metabolism capacity. This has been demonstrated in foals receiving chloramphenicol, which is extensively metabolized by the liver and is mostly excreted through the biliary system into the feces. When IV chloramphenicol was administered to foals at 1, 3, 7, 14, and 42 days of age, its clearance increased and elimination half-life decreased with increasing age.[80] Neonatal foals have a low capacity to metabolize enrofloxacin to ciprofloxacin, whereas in adult horses, ciprofloxacin concentrations are about 17% of the enrofloxacin concentrations.[81]

In some cases, drug dosages for foals are similar to adults because of similarity in drug distribution and clearance. In other cases, doses should be modified because of differences in oral absorption, clearance, and distribution. Equine practitioners should consult specific references when treating foals to administer the safest and most effective dose.

ADVERSE DRUG REACTIONS IN HORSES

Various adverse drug reactions caused by antimicrobials have been reported in the horse (Box 71-2). This section discusses the more severe reactions. Antimicrobial-associated diarrhea is the most frequently reported adverse effect of antibacterial drug administration to the horse. The mechanism is most likely related to a change in the GI and colonic microbial flora. The organisms most often associated with the disease are *Salmonella* and *Clostridium* spp. The lincosamides (clindamycin and lincomycin) should never be used in horses because they have been associated with a severe, often-fatal diarrhea. These antibiotics have even been used as an experimental model for colitis in the horse.[82] Other antibiotics associated with colitis are listed in Box 71-2.

The kidney is a frequent site for drug toxicity because many drugs are renally excreted and often become concentrated within the renal tubules. The aminoglycoside antibiotics are frequently associated with nephrotoxicity in many species, although the incidence has decreased with the implementation of once-daily dosing regimens. Aminoglycoside-induced nephrotoxicosis can be reversible with aggressive fluid therapy. Administration of IV calcium may also be beneficial.[83]

Cardiotoxicity is another often-fatal complication that has been associated with antimicrobial use in the horse. Intravenous doxycycline causes collapse and sudden death in horses when administered as a bolus or constant-rate infusion. Even at very low doses, doxycycline causes supraventricular tachycardia, systemic arterial hypertension, and clinical signs of discomfort.[84] Rapid IV administration of oxytetracycline may also cause collapse and death. This has historically been attributed to chelation of calcium and subsequent hypocalcemia or neuromuscular blockade, but it is more likely caused by a reaction to the drug vehicle.[85] Changes in serum calcium levels have not been observed with IV doxycycline, and no reaction occurs when the vehicle has been administered alone, so the mechanism of cardiotoxicity remains unclear.[84] The ionophore antibiotics are also cardiotoxic to horses, and extreme care should be taken whenever cattle or sheep being fed grain with these feed additives are on the premises. Tilmicosin, a macrolide antibiotic used in cattle and swine for the treatment of respiratory disease, is cardiotoxic to horses, as well as humans, and should not be used until safety data become available.

Drugs may induce injury to the articular cartilage and bone of foals. The most well-documented example is caused by the fluoroquinolone class of antimicrobials. Enrofloxacin and ciprofloxacin decrease cartilage and tendon cell proliferation and adherence in vitro at concentrations that are achieved in vivo.[86,87] Administration of enrofloxacin at 10 mg/kg/day for 7 days causes severe cartilage damage and lameness in foals.[81] Some musculoskeletal effects have also been observed in adult

Box • 71-2

Adverse Drug Reactions Associated with Antimicrobial Use in the Horse

Antibiotic-Associated Colitis

Severe or frequent
Clindamycin
Lincomycin
Neomycin
Oxytetracycline
Erythromycin (in adults)
Moxifloxacin
Florfenicol
Tylosin

Mild or infrequent
Trimethoprim-sulfanomide combinations
Penicillin
Doxycycline

Nephrotoxicity
Aminoglycosides
Polymixin B
Tetracyclines
Amphotericin B
Imipenem
Cephalosporins (rare)

Hepatotoxicity
Isoniazid

Cardiotoxicity
Doxycycline (intravenous)
Tetracycline (intravenous)
Tilmicosin
Monensin
Lasalocid sodium

Bone or Cartilage Effects in Growing Animals
Tetracyclines (not doxycycline)
Fluoroquinolones

Teratogenic Effects
Griseofulvin
Chloramphenicol
Sulfonamides
Pyrimethamine

Immune-Mediated Hemolytic Anemia
Penicillins
Cephalosporins
Trimethoprim-sulfamethoxazole

Neuromuscular Blockade
Aminoglycosides
Tetracyclines

Bone Marrow Suppression
Chloramphenicol
Trimethoprim-sulfa combinations
Pyrimethamine

horses, including inflammation of the tarsal plantar ligament, superficial digital flexor tendonitis, and tarsal sheath effusion.[88] These effects were observed, however, only with chronic administration of three to five times the recommended dose.

ALTERNATIVE USES OF ANTIMICROBIALS IN THE HORSE

Several antimicrobial agents have biologic activity unrelated to their effects on microbes. Tetracycline has been used frequently in foals for the treatment of flexural and angular limb deformities.[89,90] The proposed mechanism of action is chelation of intramuscular calcium, leading to relaxation of muscle tissue and tendons. However, differences were not detected in plasma calcium or ionized calcium concentrations after 50 to 67 mg/kg of oxytetracycline was administered to 4- or 5-day-old foals.[91] This is in the range of doses used for treatment of limb deformities in foals, typically 2 or 3 g per foal. The same study did not detect any deleterious effects on renal or hepatic parameters in healthy foals after two consecutive doses at this level, and drug clearance was not prolonged from such a large dose in the young foal.

Tetracyclines also have the ability to prevent neutrophil chemotaxis and apoptosis in vitro,[92,93] although the clinical relevance is questionable at drug concentrations achieved in vivo after oral administration.[94,95] Doxycycline decreases the production of proinflammatory cytokines, such as matrix metalloproteinases (MMP-8, MMP-9), interleukin-1 (IL-1), IL-6, and tumor necrosis factor alpha (TNF-α), from inflammatory cells.[96,97,98] Doxycycline inhibits MMPs from the horse[99] and has been successfully used for the treatment of melting corneal ulcers. It also inhibits staphylococcal exotoxin-induced cytokines and chemokines and improves the prognosis in a mouse model of endotoxemia.[100] This action by doxycycline is accomplished by attaining sufficiently high intracellular concentrations in leukocytes to interfere with intracellular processes.

Metronidazole reduces the clinical severity and GI inflammation in people with Crohn's disease.[101] It has been recommended for the treatment of colitis and other nonspecific causes of diarrhea in people, although no reports are available to demonstrate a similar effect in horses. Both metronidazole and ciprofloxacin decrease leukocyte migration through the intestinal cell wall and inhibit intestinal T-helper type 1 (Th1) cytokine production, thereby decreasing inflammation.[101]

Low doses of erythromycin are often used as a prokinetic drug in the horse. It acts by stimulating motilin receptors in the GI tract and promoting GI motility.[102] This may also contribute to the diarrhea seen with administration of erythromycin in adult horses and foals. This prokinetic property has not been attributed to other macrolides.

Polymyxin B is a cationic polypeptide antibiotic effective against gram-negative bacteria. Its use as an antibiotic has been limited because of its nephrotoxic effect at therapeutic doses. Polymyxin B is often used in equine medicine, however, as a treatment for endotoxemia. At doses below those needed for antibacterial effects, it binds to the lipid A moiety of the lipopolysaccharide and alters its structure so that it cannot interact with the horse's white blood cells and initiate the inflammatory cascade.[103,104] At doses of 1000 to 6000 IU/kg, IV polymyxin B significantly reduces fever, tachycardia, and serum TNF-α when administered before or 1 hour after challenge with endotoxin.[105] A more recent study[157] demonstrated that polymyxin B should be administered to horses at a dose of 6000 IU/kg (1 mg/kg) and repeated at 8-hour intervals for up to 5 treatments to treat endotoxemia. At this dosage regimen, it did not accumulate and was safe. Nevertheless, it is essential that the horse be well hydrated during therapy and that serum creatinine levels are monitored to prevent the development of acute renal failure.

UPDATE ON ANTIBIOTICS USED IN HORSES

Fluoroquinolone Antimicrobials

The fluoroquinolone antimicrobial drugs have been available for use in people and small animals for more than 10 years. The first drug in this group for veterinary use was enrofloxacin (Baytril, Bayer Corporation). Although none are registered for use in horses in the U.S., several pharmacokinetic studies have generated data for these drugs. These data, as well as clinical experience, have shown that this class of drugs can be valuable for treating infections in horses. Their important properties include (1) ability to administer by oral, IV, and IM routes, although only enrofloxacin is available in an injectable formulation in the United States, (2) spectrum of activity that includes staphylococci and gram-negative bacilli such as *Klebsiella pneumoniae, Escherichia coli,* and *Proteus* spp.; (3) spectrum of activity that does *not* include anaerobic bacteria, therefore posing little risk of disrupting bacteria in the GI tract; and (4) good safety profile in adult horses.

The spectrum of fluoroquinolone activity includes bacteria that may otherwise require treatment with injectable drugs or drugs that could carry a risk of adverse effects. It is important to recognize that the spectrum does not include *Streptococcus* or anaerobic bacteria, and the concentrations needed for activity against *Pseudomonas aeruginosa* may require doses that have not been tested for safety in horses.

Based on the studies cited, as well as clinical experience to date, an injectable dose of *enrofloxacin* at 2.5 to 5 mg/kg once daily or an oral dose of 7.5 to 10 mg/kg once daily is recommended. The higher oral dose is used to accommodate the decreased systemic availability from an oral dose. For orbifloxacin (Orbax, Schering-Plough), an oral dose of 5 mg/kg once daily is recommended.[106] These doses meet PK-PD criteria for susceptible bacteria discussed earlier in this chapter. For *marbofloxacin* (Zeniquin, Pfizer Animal Health), IV doses of 2 mg/kg q24h may be adequate for treatment of most gram-negative infections caused by *Enterobacteriaceae*.[107-109] However, this dose would not be adequate for many gram-positive bacteria, such as *Staphylococcus* spp., with MIC values of 0.25 μg/mL or higher. The breakpoint for susceptibility of small animal isolates is listed by CLSI[18] as 1.0 μg/mL or lower. The injectable formulation is not available in the United States; therefore, oral tablets would be required for administration. Marbofloxacin has systemic availability of approximately 62% in horses.[107] Oral dosing at 2 mg/kg may be adequate for susceptible *Enterobacteriaceae* with MIC values less than 0.2 μg/mL, but not for other bacteria. Doses higher than 2 mg/kg have not been studied in horses. *Ciprofloxacin* is not recommended because the oral absorption was poor in ponies and is assumed to also be low for adult horses.[14]

The method of administration for horses has been to (1) crush up tablets used in small animals, (2) administer the injectable solution (2.27% or 10%) IM (neck muscle) or IV, or (3) administer the concentrated 10% solution orally (Baytril-100 cattle formulation). All these methods appear to produce adequate plasma concentrations, except for the administration of the concentrated 10% solution (Baytril-100) orally. This solution has produced inconsistent and incomplete absorption in horses, possibly because of its insolubility in solutions of low pH.[110] In other studies, absorption of this solution was better when horses were fed.[111] This solution also has been associated with oral mucosal lesions in horses. Some clinicians have produced more consistent oral absorption and reduced mucosal irritation when the 100-mg/mL solution was compounded into a gel.[112]

Clinicians should be aware of possible interactions from oral administration of some drugs with fluoroquinolones. Oral administration of drugs that contain cations (Fe^{+3}, Mg^{+2}, Ca^{+2}, Al^{+3}) will significantly inhibit oral absorption. Compounds that may contain these cations include antacids, sucralfate (Carafate), and iron supplements. No significant interaction occurred when fluoroquinolones were mixed in our laboratory with molasses and iron-containing supplements such as Lixitinic (unpublished study by authors).

The newest generations of fluoroquinolones, which some authors call the "third-generation" fluoroquinolones, include trovafloxacin, grepafloxacin, gatifloxacin, gemifloxacin, and moxifloxacin. Two of these, trovafloxacin and grepafloxacin, have already been discontinued for use in people because of adverse effects (abnormal cardiac rhythms and hepatic injury). The new generation of fluoroquinolones, with substitutions at the C-8 position (e.g., C-8 methoxy) have the advantage of a broader spectrum of activity that includes anaerobic bacteria and gram-positive cocci. The difference in spectrum of activity is largely caused by increased activity against the DNA-gyrase of gram-positive bacteria, rather than activity against topoisomerase IV, which is the target in gram-positive bacteria for the older quinolones. Veterinary drugs of this group are being investigated, but none is currently registered. *Moxifloxacin* (Avelox) is a human drug of this group and has been used on a limited basis for treatment of infections in dogs and cats caused by bacteria that have been refractory to other drugs. When administered to horses, moxifloxacin had favorable pharmacokinetics that could make it suitable for oral use in horses.[113] However, oral administration also produced diarrhea in the experimental horses studied, and one of these horses tested positive for *Clostridium difficile* toxins A and B. The spectrum of activity of this drug may be broad enough to disrupt the normal flora. Until its safety can be established for horses, however, routine use of moxifloxacin is not recommended.

Macrolides and Derivatives

New macrolide antibiotics represent another class of drugs that are being considered for horses. The prototypic macrolide antibiotic is erythromycin. Oral absorption of erythromycin and its associated problems are discussed earlier in this chapter. Because of poor absorption and adverse effects (primarily diarrhea), new drugs have been developed that have better pharmacokinetic properties, improved spectrum of activity, and are better tolerated. The new macrolides and derivatives include clarithromycin (Biaxin), tulathromycin (Draxxin), tilmicosin (Micotil), and azalide azithromycin (Zithromax). As previously stated, tilmicosin, a cattle and swine antibiotic, should not be used in the horse until safety data become available. This caution should probably also be applied to tulathromycin.

The pharmacokinetics of *clarithromycin* have been investigated in foals and a dose of 7.5 mg/kg orally q12h is suggested for the treatment of *R. equi* pneumonia.[35] *Azithromycin* has been evaluated in foals in two independent pharmacokinetic studies.[34,114] Azithromycin has a half-life of 11 and 16 hours in foals after oral and IV dosing, respectively. The oral absorption is similar to people at 33%, and the volume of distribution is very high at 12 L/kg. One of the distinct advantages of azithromycin in horses is its ability to concentrate in leukocytes for extended periods. The concentration of azithromycin in neutrophils reached a level that was 200 times the plasma concentration and depleted with a half-life longer than 50 hours and was above a concentration of 5.68 μg/mL (above the MIC breakpoint) for 120 hours after administration.[34] Based on the pharmacokinetic data and the anecdotal clinical experience, veterinarians have used azithromycin in foals at a dose of 10 mg/kg once daily initially, followed by 10 mg/kg every other day, orally after clinical improvement is observed. Because of the difference in half-life, clarithromycin is recommended for twice-daily administration, whereas azithromycin can be administered once daily. Another difference is that clarithromycin exhibits time-dependent PK-PD characteristics, whereas azithromycin efficacy is determined by the AUC/MIC.[115] To maintain the duration of exposure for clarithromycin, twice-daily administration is needed.

Clinical experience with azithromycin and clarithromycin in the field has indicated that it has been safe for use in foals for the treatment of *R. equi* infections. Although each of these drugs has activity against gram-positive cocci, efficacy was only evaluated in one report of *R. equi* treatment. In people, these drugs are used to treat streptococcal respiratory infections. In a retrospective study, clarithromycin-rifampin combination was compared to erythromycin-rifampin and azithromycin-rifampin for the treatment of *R. equi* pneumonia. The foals treated with clarithromycin-rifampin had a higher overall short-term and long-term success rate and better radiographic improvement than foals treated with either of the other two combinations studied.[50] The only adverse effect reported was diarrhea in some foals.

Penicillins

The penicillin group of drugs includes penicillin G (also called benzyl penicillin) and the semisynthetic derivatives such as ampicillin, amoxicillin, and ticarcillin. These drugs, particularly penicillin G, have been used commonly in horses. Penicillin and the aminopenicillins (ampicillin and amoxicillin) have a limited spectrum of activity that includes streptococci, non-β-lactamase–producing strains of *Staphylococcus* spp., some gram-positive bacteria (e.g., *Actinomyces*), and some additional anaerobic bacteria. Many gram-negative anaerobic bacteria are less susceptible. The activity against most gram-negative bacteria, especially the *Enterobacteriaceae* (*E. coli*, *Klebsiella* spp., *Proteus* spp., *Enterobacter* spp.) is limited because these drugs are not resistant to the β-lactamase enzyme unless combined with a β-lactamase inhibitor such as sulbactam (e.g., ampicillin-sulbactam, Unasyn). At high doses, however, ampicillin may be administered to achieve sufficiently high concentrations for some of the *Enterobacteriaceae* (see dosing regimens next).

Dosing regimens for penicillin G have been studied in several reports. Pharmacokinetic studies are discussed earlier in this chapter.[57,58] Penicillin and potassium salts of penicillin G are administered IV, and occasionally IM, although IM injections can be painful and irritating. Procaine–penicillin G is designed to produce prolonged concentrations after IM injection because of slow absorption, although it may not be as prolonged as a similar regimen of potassium penicillin G.[57]

Details of pharmacokinetics and dosing regimens can be found in other references.[66,116-119] Formulations of ampicillin or amoxicillin include IV or IM ampicillin sodium aqueous solution, IM ampicillin trihydrate (e.g., Polyflex), and oral amoxicillin trihydrate. Some older formulations (e.g., amoxicillin injectable) are no longer available. The oral formulations are usually not administered to horses because of poor oral absorption. Although the absorption of ampicillin in dogs and cats has been reported to range from 30% to 40%, and for amoxicillin 64% to 68%, oral absorption of ampicillin in adult horses is only 2% to 3.5%.[62,67] Oral absorption of amoxicillin is somewhat higher in horses, 5.3% to 10.4%,[61] but is still too low to be practical for dosing. In foals, oral absorption of amoxicillin is 36.2% to 42.7%,[63] but this is a seldom-used route of administration.

Dosages are listed in Appendix C. Ampicillin trihydrate suspension (Polyflex) is administered IM, usually at a dose of 6.6 to 22 mg/kg q12 or q24h (most common). Ampicillin sodium is administered to horses IV at 10 to 20 mg/kg q6-8h and IM at 10 to 22 mg/kg q12h. Our laboratory performed computer simulations and Monte Carlo predictions (unpublished studies) to indicate that ampicillin sodium at a dose of either 22 mg/kg IM q12h or 22 mg/kg IV q8h achieves sufficient plasma concentrations to meet PK-PD criteria for MIC values of less than or equal to (≤) 2.0 μg/mL, which may be high enough for many *Enterobacteriaceae*. *Streptococcus* spp have a much lower MIC range (usually ≤ 0.25 μg/mL) and can be treated with much lower doses.

Cephalosporins

The cephalosporin antibiotics have many advantages in animals, including a broad spectrum of activity and a good safety profile. Cephalosporins studied in horses for clinical use include the first-generation cephalosporins cephalexin, cefazolin, cephapirin, and cefadroxil; the second-generation cephalosporin cefoxitin; and the third-generation cephalosporins ceftiofur and ceftriaxone.

Oral absorption of first-generation cephalosporins is somewhat limited, but this route can be used in some cases, as discussed earlier. First-generation cephalosporins have a spectrum that is limited to highly susceptible gram-negative bacilli *(Enterobacteriaceae)*, streptococci, and *Staphylococcus* spp. Cefazolin has somewhat better activity against gram-negative bacilli than first-generation cephalothin. Cefazolin is used occasionally in horses as a prophylaxis injection preoperatively or perioperatively. Pharmacokinetic studies are available to guide dosing.[120,121] Cefazolin has a slower terminal half-life from IM than IV administration. The IM injection is thought to have a longer half-life because of slower absorption (caused by a "flip-flop effect" discussed earlier). Subsequent doses of 10 to 20 mg/kg can be administered q8h IM or q6h IV.

Perhaps the most frequently used cephalosporin in horses is *ceftiofur*. Ceftiofur is metabolized quickly to an active metabolite, desfuroylceftiofur (and other metabolites). The metabolite has activity that resembles a third-generation cephalosporin in vitro. Ceftiofur was approved for use in horses for treatment of respiratory tract infections caused by *Streptococcus equi* subsp. *zooepidemicus* at a dose of 2.2 to 4.4 mg/kg q24h IM. Higher doses or more frequent intervals have been recommended for treating gram-negative organisms (e.g., *Klebsiella*, *Enterobacter*, *Salmonella*). Because these organisms are inherently more resistant, higher plasma concentrations are needed for efficacy. The susceptibility breakpoint for ceftiofur use in horses is very low (≤ 0.25 μg/mL) and organisms other than streptococci may be classified in vitro as resistant. Studies in foals indicated that a dose of 2.2 to 6.6 mg/kg could be given to foals IM or IV q12h for treatment of neonatal sepsis. Computerized simulations and Monte Carlo predictions by our laboratory (unpublished studies), using previously published pharmacokinetic data,[122] show that a dose of 4.4 mg/kg injected q12h will produce plasma concentrations above the MIC to meet the criteria for effective therapy. The simulation used an MIC value ≤ 1.0 μg/mL, which is typical for gram-negative bacteria *(E. coli, Klebsiella)* isolated from horses. Toxicity studies have shown that horses tolerate ceftiofur doses up to 11 mg/kg/day IM, with pain at the injection site and decreased feed consumption as the most common adverse effect at the highest dose.

An ester formulation of cefpodoxime, *cefpodoxime proxetil*, has been examined for use in horses.[70] This third-generation cephalosporin was recently registered for use in dogs (Simplicef, Pfizer). Cefpodoxime has higher activity against gram-negative bacteria than first-generation cephalosporins and is more active than many other third-generation cephalosporins against *Staphylococcus*. However, it is not active against *Pseudomonas aeruginosa*, enterococci, or MRSA. In a study in horses, oral absorption was good enough that a dose of 10 mg/kg q6-12h produced plasma concentrations that would potentially treat infections in horses.[70] When testing susceptibility for cefpodoxime, the breakpoint for susceptibility is lower than for other third-generation cephalosporins.[18] Therefore a bacterial isolate may be reported as sensitive to cefotaxime or ceftazidime, which has a breakpoint of ≤8 μg/mL, but resistant to cefpodoxime, which has a breakpoint of ≤2 μg/mL.[18] Specific disks are suggested for testing bacterial isolates, rather than relying on the results from other cephalosporins.

The newest development in the cephalosporin class is the fourth-generation drugs, represented by cefepime (Maxipime, Bristol-Myers Squibb). Cefepime has increased spectrum of activity compared with other cephalosporins and is broad enough to include both gram-positive and gram-negative bacteria. Cefepime is active against *P. aeruginosa* as well as *Klebsiella pneumoniae* and *E. coli* that are resistant to other drugs. Cefepime pharmacokinetics have been studied in foals and mares. Although clearance is rapid, this drug possibly could be used for infections resistant to other drugs. A dose for foals of 11 mg/kg IV q8h and for adults of 2.2 mg/kg IV q8h[123,124] is recommended. When cefepime was administered to horses orally, signs of colic were observed.[123]

Aminoglycosides

The aminoglycosides include gentamicin, tobramycin, amikacin, and kanamycin. Among these, gentamicin and amikacin are used most often in horses, with amikacin often preferred in neonates. Aminoglycosides are effective against gram-negative aerobes but poorly active against gram-positive aerobes, with the exception of coagulase-positive *Staphylococcus* spp. Obligate anaerobes and facultative anaerobes under anaerobic conditions are resistant to aminoglycosides. Amikacin is more active against a broader range of gram-negative bacteria than gentamicin and has lower susceptibility to enzymes involved in plasmid-mediated resistance, the most common mechanism for bacterial resistance to aminoglycosides.

Gentamicin or amikacin are often used in combination with a β-lactam antibiotic (e.g., penicillin, ampicillin) to produce a synergistic broad-spectrum bactericidal effect. The β-lactam–associated inhibition of bacterial cell wall synthesis enhances the uptake of aminoglycosides into bacteria, accounting for the synergy of this combination. Note, however, that these drugs should not be mixed in the same vial or syringe before dosing, because admixing these drugs produces in vitro inactivation of the aminoglycoside.

The activity and PK-PD characteristics of the aminoglycosides were discussed earlier. The aminoglycoside dosing regimens are designed to achieve high peak plasma concentrations of the drug (C_{max}) and, more specifically, a high C_{max}/MIC ratio.[22] These goals can be achieved by use of once-daily dosing, and current dosage regimens for adults and foals take into account these principles.[23,76,77,125] The longer interval between doses may lessen the risk of nephrotoxicity compared with more conventional aminoglycoside dosing (e.g., total daily dose divided equally into three doses and administered at 8-hour intervals). Aminoglycoside-induced renal toxicity results from accumulation of these agents in the renal cortex. After filtration at the glomerulus, aminoglycoside antibiotics bind to phospholipids on the brush border of proximal tubular cells and are subsequently reabsorbed. Accumulation of aminoglycosides in proximal tubular cells interferes with lysosomal, mitochondrial, and Na^+/K^+/ATPase function. Importantly, the uptake process is saturable; thus, sustained exposure of proximal tubular cells to the drug, as may occur with multiple daily-dosing regimens (or prolonged use of the drug), results in greater accumulation of the drug and increased risk of nephrotoxicity. Conversely, animal studies have demonstrated that administration of the daily dose of gentamicin as a single dose, thereby creating one high daily peak concentration of the drug, results in less renal injury than administration of the same total daily dose divided into three doses per day or by continuous infusion.

Among other factors, aminoglycoside toxicity is related to persistently high plasma trough concentrations of the drug (*trough concentration* is measured immediately before the next administered dose.) With once-daily dosing, the 24-hour interval between doses allows adequate time for drug clearance, thus limiting the exposure of the renal tubules to drug concentrations and decreasing the risk of nephrotoxicosis. Regardless of the frequency of treatment, aminoglycoside therapy still carries risk of renal injury when renal clearance is compromised because of a preexisting condition. To prevent aminoglycoside nephrotoxicosis and identify which animals may be at increased risk, close clinical monitoring is required, particularly in critically ill patients (e.g., hemodynamically unstable foals).

Measurement of serum or plasma aminoglycoside drug concentrations, termed *therapeutic drug monitoring* (TDM), has been used in foals and horses receiving aminoglycoside treatment to individualize the dose. In equine patients, TDM can be useful because drug disposition may vary widely among sick patients, especially in critically ill neonates.[77,126] Therefore, TDM can identify those patients with parameters that do not represent the average. TDM is employed to determine whether the target peak concentration (C_{max}) is achieved and if there is adequate clearance of the drug to prevent toxicity. Usually, at least three blood samples are collected and analyzed to determine the elimination half-life and estimate the drug clearance and distribution. Modifications of the dosage regimen can be made from these parameters. Geor and Papich[127] provide details on performing TDM in horses.

When selecting an aminoglycoside dosing regimen, attention must be paid to the site of infection, susceptibility of the pathogen, severity of illness, and patient's renal function. For example, the aminoglycoside antibiotics are poorly distributed to the lung and may not be the most appropriate antimicrobial selection for treatment of pulmonary infections. In a pyogenic infection, especially in an abscess, aminoglycosides may be inactivated by cellular debris.

Trimethoprim-Sulfonamides

Trimethoprim is most frequently combined with sulfadiazine or sulfamethoxazole for administration to horses. Ormetoprim is similar to trimethoprim, in terms of action, and has been combined with sulfadimethoxine. The effectiveness of these combinations is attributed to their synergistic effect in inhibiting folic acid metabolism in bacteria. Sulfonamides are competitive inhibitors of dihydrofolate synthesis. Trimethoprim inhibits the enzyme dihydrofolate reductase. Complete reviews are available on these combinations, with some specifically for use in horses.[54]

Tissue concentrations of TMS persist long enough to allow once-daily or twice-daily dosing for many infections. Studies performed in cattle and horses appear to support a T>MIC parameter as being the most important for clinical success.[128-131] In these studies, drug concentrations (of the combination) associated with clinical success persisted in plasma or tissue fluids for the duration of the dose interval. Most published dosage regimens for TMS are designed to take these pharmacokinetic properties into account (see Appendix C).

A susceptibility test should always measure inhibition of the combination, not the individual drugs. The spectrum of activity is broad. TMS combinations are active against many pathogens that infect horses, including *Pasteurella* spp., *Proteus,* and *Salmonella* spp. Occasionally, staphylococci, *Corynebacterium, Klebsiella, E. coli,* and streptococci are susceptible. *Pseudomonas, Enterococcus* spp., and *Bacteroides* are usually resistant. The activity of TMS against anaerobic bacteria can be variable. When measured in vitro, trimethoprim-sulfonamide has good activity against anaerobic bacteria in vitro, but clinical results are not as good because thymidine and PABA (inhibitors of trimethoprim-sulfonamide activity) may be present in anaerobic infections.

Sulfonamides in combination with trimethoprim that are used in horses include trimethoprim plus sulfadiazine (e.g., Tribrissen, Di-Trim) and trimethoprim plus sulfamethoxazole (Bactrim, Septra, generic). These preparations come in oral dosage forms, which include tablets for small animals and people and paste for horses. Veterinary formulations of injectable suspensions or solutions are no longer available in the United States. There are some injectable formulations for human medicine, but they are expensive.

Sulfonamides are used in horses for a variety of infections, including pleuritis, pneumonia, and abdominal and joint infections. It is significant that the activity of this combination is diminished in certain infected environments (see Local Factors that Affect Antibiotic Effectiveness). Their use for treating protozoa and potential adverse effects are discussed later (see Antiprotozoal Drugs).

ANTIFUNGAL DRUGS

Azoles

The azole antifungals can be divided into two main groups, the imidazoles and the triazoles, according to the number of nitrogen molecules on the azole ring. They are fungistatic, and their mechanism of action involves inhibition of fungal cytochrome P-450, which results in an inhibition of ergosterol in the fungal cell wall. The specificity of these drugs for fungal versus animal cytochrome P-450 is highly variable. The imidazoles tend to be less specific, whereas the newer triazoles are more specific, for fungal enzymes.

Imidazoles

The imidazoles are a group of broad-spectrum antifungal drugs that include miconazole and ketoconazole. *Miconazole* is only available as a topical cream and is frequently compounded for ophthalmic use. *Ketoconazole* is not absorbed after oral administration in the horse unless it is first dissolved in 1N hydrochloric acid and dosed intragastrically.[132]

Triazoles

The triazole group includes fluconazole, itraconazole, and the newest drug, voriconazole. All three drugs have been studied in horses, and their pharmacokinetic properties vary widely. *Fluconazole* is a highly water-soluble drug that has almost 100% bioavailability in the horse.[15] It has excellent tissue penetration and reaches therapeutic concentrations in the plasma, CSF, synovial fluid, aqueous humor, and urine for the treatment of susceptible yeasts and fungi. The half-life after oral administration is approximately 38 hours, and a loading dose of 14 mg/kg orally followed by 5 mg/kg orally once a day is recommended. Fluconazole has recently become available in generic formulations and is now less expensive than other antifungal drugs. Unfortunately, the spectrum of activity of fluconazole is narrower than for the other azole antifungals. It is active against the organisms that cause histoplasmosis, blastomycosis, coccidioidomycosis, and conidiobolomycosis.[15,133] It is active against yeasts, including some *Candida* sp., although resistance may be increasing. Fluconazole has virtually no in vitro activity against filamentous fungi such as *Aspergillus* and *Fusarium* spp.

Itraconazole has a similar spectrum of activity to fluconazole, but it is active against some *Aspergillus* spp. Most *Fusarium* strains, however, are still resistant.[134] Itraconazole is effective in horses for the treatment of mycotic rhinitis, osteomyelitis, and guttural pouch mycosis. [135-137] It also has been used to treat coccidioidomycosis.[136] It has been used safely for up to 6 months in the horse. The pharmacokinetics of itraconazole in horses are much less favorable than for fluconazole.[134] There are three formulations of itraconazole currently marketed: an oral capsule, an oral solution, and an IV solution. Bioavailability of the oral capsules is approximately 12%, and its absorption is highly variable because its dissolution relies on the acid environment of the stomach. The oral solution has better bioavailability, approximately 60%, but at the recommended dose of 5 mg/kg, 250 mL of solution is needed per dose for an adult horse because of the low concentration of the drug in the formulation. The IV formulation is prohibitively expensive. Itraconazole is practically insoluble in water and is only soluble and stable at a low pH. Compounded forms of itraconazole are available, but they are often unstable and have even poorer absorption than the marketed formulations. The compounded formulations should not be used in horses.

Voriconazole is the newest triazole antifungal. It has improved activity against *Aspergillus* and *Fusarium* spp. compared with other triazoles and an excellent safety profile in people. Preliminary pharmacokinetic data on voriconazole in the horse shows excellent bioavailability and a long elimination half-life.[138] The drug penetrates well into the aqueous humor after systemic administration as well as after topical administration of the IV formulation. A dose of 4 mg/kg q24-48h produces plasma concentrations that may be therapeutic for *Fusarium* spp. Lower doses or longer dosing intervals may be required for treating infections caused by yeast or *Aspergillus* spp.

Polyenes

The polyene antifungals include nystatin and amphotericin B. They have the advantage of being fungicidal by binding to ergosterol in the fungal cell wall, creating pores in the membrane. *Nystatin* is too toxic to administer parenterally and is not absorbed orally. Its main use in veterinary medicine is a topical ophthalmic preparation for the treatment of fungal keratitis.

Amphotericin B is used only sporadically in equine medicine. It has the broadest spectrum of activity of all the antifungal drugs, including against many *Candida* spp., *Aspergillus* spp., *Histoplasma* spp., *Blastomyces* spp., and *Coccidioides immitis*. It is also frequently used to treat *Fusarium* spp. in humans. No pharmacokinetic data are available on amphotericin B in the horse, but it has been given as an IV infusion at doses of 0.38 to 1.4 mg/kg.[139,140] Its use is often limited by its toxicity. Infusion reactions and nephrotoxicity are common.

Griseofulvin

Griseofulvin is a fungistatic drug with a limited spectrum of activity. It is used almost solely for the treatment of dermatophytosis. Its action depends on incorporation into skin and keratin, so it requires a long duration of therapy. It should not be used in pregnant mares; teratogenic effects have been reported in a mare treated in the second month of gestation.[141]

Lufenuron

There have been unsubstantiated anecdotal accounts of successful treatment of horses with lufenuron, a chitin inhibitor used in small animals for flea control (Program, Novartis Animal Health). However, lufenuron has poor oral absorption in horses, and no evidence indicates activity against important fungi that infect horses.[142]

ANTIVIRAL DRUGS

Unfortunately, there is little information on antiviral drugs to guide therapy in horses. A small number of pharmacokinetic and pharmacodynamic studies have been recently published regarding the use of clinically available antiviral drugs in the horse, and these studies are summarized here.

Cyclic Amines

Amantadine and rimantadine are cyclic amines used in the treatment of influenza virus infection. The mechanism of action of these drugs involves inhibiting the uncoating of viral ribonucleic acid (RNA) in infected cells and thus effectively preventing viral replication. In vitro testing suggests that amantadine suppresses viral replication at concentrations of 300 ng/mL, whereas rimantadine is more potent and has activity at concentrations as low as 30 ng/mL.[143,144]

Intravenous *amantadine* at a dose of 15 mg/kg may produce fatal seizures with few premonitory signs. Doses of 10 mg/kg were better tolerated but may still cause serious adverse effects in horses with lowered seizure thresholds. The bioavailability of oral amantadine was too variable to determine a dosing regimen that would be adequate for treatment in the majority of horses because of large interindividual variation.[143] The safety and efficacy of amantadine should be further investigated before its clinical use is recommended.

Rimantadine shows greater promise as an antiviral drug in horses. Rimantadine is available in a generic form as a 100-mg tablet. A multidose study examining the effects of oral rimantadine at a dose of 30 mg/kg q12h showed adequate absorption of the drug, with plasma concentrations maintained above the estimated effective concentration (30 ng/mL) throughout the dosing interval. No adverse effects were reported. In addition, in challenge studies using influenza virus A2, prophylactic rimantadine administration was associated with a significant decrease in rectal temperature and lung sounds.[144]

Nucleoside Analogs

Acyclovir is an acyclic guanosine derivative that has been used clinically in the horse for the treatment of equine herpesvirus type 1 (EHV-1) myeloencephalopathy. [145,146] IV acyclovir is the treatment of choice for herpes simplex encephalitis in humans, possibly because it crosses the BBB, with CSF concentrations approximately 50% of serum concentrations. Even though the oral form is now generic and inexpensive, oral absorption in horses is low and variable.[147,148] In vitro efficacy of acyclovir against EHV-1 strains has also been documented, but susceptibility varies with the strain of virus tested. Based on the results of simulated multiple IV doses, twice-daily (q12h) IV infusions of acyclovir (10 mg/kg) would result in plasma concentrations greater than 0.3 μg/mL for the entire treatment interval.[144] This study demonstrated that IV infusion of acyclovir results in plasma concentrations exceeding the concentration that inhibits plaque formation in vitro, suggesting clinical applicability for this drug in cases of EHV-1 infection in horses. However a single dose of 20 mg/kg of acyclovir administered orally did not result in concentrations greater than the lower limit of detection.

The analogs of acyclovir, such as famciclovir (penciclovir),[149] which are better absorbed than acyclovir in people, have not been examined in horses. *Famciclovir* in particular is a prodrug, metabolized to penciclovir, with much better oral absorption in people than acyclovir (70% vs. 20%). However, these drugs are many times more expensive than acyclovir and may be too costly to use in horses.

Interferons

Interferons are endogenously produced proteins with various immunomodulatory, antiproliferative and antiviral effects. Data on the use of these preparations in the horse is limited. Natural human interferon-α has been administered orally to horses with inflammatory airway disease with a significant decrease in total protein, immunoglobulin G (IgG), and IgA in bronchalveolar lavage fluid, suggesting adequate oral absorption; however, no actual drug concentrations were determined.[150] The antiviral effects of these drugs require further investigation.

Topical Antiviral Drugs

Topical application of antiviral drugs has been recommended for the treatment of herpes keratitis in the horse. The most frequently used drugs include trifluridine 1% solution and idoxuridine 0.5% solution. Their efficacy and activity against EHV-2 is unknown.

ANTIPROTOZOAL DRUGS

Treatment of Equine Protozoal Myeloencephalitis

The number of antiprotozoal drugs available for use in the horse has increased greatly over the past decade, mainly because of the increasing prevalence of equine protozoal myeloencephalitis (EPM). Folate synthesis inhibitors such as pyrimethamine; trimethoprim and sulfonamides; the triazine derivatives diclazuril, toltrazuril, and ponazuril; and the newly approved nitazoxanide (NTZ) have been considered for treatment in horses.

Folate Synthesis Inhibitors

Trimethoprim, sulfonamides, and pyrimethamine were the first drugs used to treat EPM. Each drug prevents protozoal synthesis of folic acid, however they act at different levels and on different enzyme substrates. Sulfonamides inhibit dihydrofolate synthesis through competitive inhibition of PABA, whereas trimethoprim and pyrimethamine inhibit dihydrofolate reductase. Because pyrimethamine and trimethoprim inhibit the same enzyme in the pathway, the use of both drugs is not necessary, and pyrimethamine is often chosen over trimethoprim because of its more potent effects on protozoa than bacteria. Pyrimethamine is coccidiocidal at concentrations of 1 μg/mL, whereas trimethoprim requires concentrations of 5 μg/mL for coccidiocidal activity. Sulfonamides have very little antiprotozoal action when used alone, but synergism occurs when they are used in combination with either trimethoprim or pyrimethamine.[151]

These drugs are inexpensive and generally safe. A disadvantage of pyrimethamine-sulfonamide combinations for treatment of EPM is that they require longer treatment periods than the triazine derivatives and NTZ, and clinical signs may return if therapy is discontinued too early. Few adverse effects have been associated with long-term treatment with these drugs, although anemia and pancytopenia may result from folate deficiency.[152] Congenital defects, including weakness, recumbency, and skin lesions, have been reported in foals born to mares being treated for EPM with sulfonamides, pyrimethamine, and folic acid.[153]

Triazine Derivatives

The triazene-derivative antiprotozoals include diclazuril (Clinacox), toltrazuril (Baycox), and ponazuril (Marquis). *Ponazuril* was the first drug approved for use in horses for the treatment of EPM in the United States and is the only member of this group that is commercially available in the U.S. It is an active metabolite of toltrazuril (toltrazuril sulfone). Ponazuril comes in a convenient paste formulation and is recommended for treatment at a dose of 2.5 mg/kg once daily for 28 days; however, dosing may be extended for another 28 days or until maximal improvement has been noted. Ponazuril is 90% effective at blocking merozoite production in vitro at concentrations of 1 μg/mL and is more than 95% effective at concentrations of 5 μg/mL.[151] *Diclazuril* demonstrated similar effectiveness in vitro and reaches therapeutic concentrations in the CSF after oral administration;[154] however, because of the limited oral absorption and large administration volume (500 g/horse) of diclazuril, many veterinarians prefer administration of ponazuril.

Nitazoxanide

Nitazoxanide (NTZ) is available as Navigator 32% paste (IDEXX Laboratories, Greensboro, NC). It is the newest drug to be approved for the treatment of EPM in the horse. It has a mechanism of action that involves intracellular reduction of the nitro group on the drug to a toxic free radical that interferes with cellular respiration in the protozoa. The in vitro concentration that inhibited merozoite production by 50% (IC_{50}) was 0.52 μg/mL. Field trials with NTZ have shown a 57% to 81% success rate, defined as an improvement in neurologic signs and/or conversion to a negative result on Western blot analysis of the CSF. This included a 78% success rate for horses that had previously been treated with other drugs for EPM. Adverse effects, reported from the administration of NTZ to horses, include diarrhea and fever. Some veterinarians reserve its use for horses that do not respond to other treatments.

Treatment of Other Protozoal Diseases

Other protozoal diseases occur infrequently in the horse. Equine piroplasmosis is rare but has been reported in the southeastern United States. Treatment involves administration of *imidocarb diproprionate* (2.2 mg/kg IM q24h for two doses). This regimen is reasonably effective for treatment of *Babesia caballi*, but higher doses for longer periods may be necessary to treat *Babesia equi*.[158] Adverse effects of imidocarb at higher doses include colic, hypersalivation, diarrhea, and death. Imidocarb should not be administered to donkeys because they tend to have severe reactions to the drug. Addition of parvaquone or buparvaquone may help with therapy but, when given alone, may cause treated horses to become carriers. *Giardia* is an infrequent cause of diarrhea in foals and should respond to treatment with metronidazole.

REFERENCES

See the CD-ROM for a list of references linked to the abstract in PubMed.

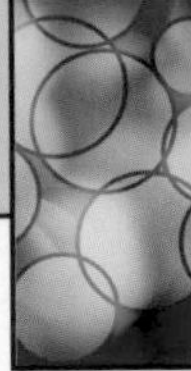

CHAPTER • 72

Immunotherapy

Maria Julia Bevilaqua Felippe Flaminio

As our understanding of immune responses and the pathogenesis of infectious disease has increased over the last two decades, there has been a concomitant increased interest in immunotherapeutics. *Immunomodulators* are substances that enhance or suppress immune responses (Table 72-1). This diverse group of therapeutic agents includes both nonspecific immunomodulators and drugs with highly selective targets within the immune system. For treatment of horses, recommendations are difficult because of the limited number of studies evaluating their efficacy in that species.

IMMUNOSTIMULANTS

Induction of Nonspecific Immune Responses

Many immunostimulants activate innate immunity and promote release of endogenous immune mediators (e.g., cytokines) as an aid in the treatment of immunodeficiency conditions, chronic infections, or cancer. In the 1890s, Dr. William Coley, a surgeon at New York Memorial Hospital, used killed *Streptococcus pyogenes* and *Serratia marcescens* (Coley's vaccine) to treat sarcomas, carcinomas, lymphomas, melanomas, and myelomas in his patients.[1] This treatment originated from the observation that tumors regressed when spontaneous acute infections occurred, especially with high fever. Coley and others initially used live bacteria to induce infection and fever; however, fatal infections eventually led to the use of an inactivated organism.

Immunostimulants induce a nonspecific activation of the immune system, unless they are associated with antigens (e.g., adjuvants in vaccines), and may amplify different effectors of the immune response, including phagocytosis and intracellular killing of organisms, antigen presentation, cytotoxic and antiviral activity, cytokine release, and antibody production.[2] Immunomodulators predominantly activate macrophages and dendritic cells in the liver, spleen, skin, and lungs.[3] The route of administration is designed to bring the drug into contact with *antigen-presenting cells* (APCs). In the horse, pulmonary intravascular macrophages are likely important for recognition of foreign antigens in circulation.[4,5] These large, mature, permanent resident macrophages of the pulmonary capillary

Table • 72-1

Immunomodulators

COMPONENT	ORIGIN	MECHANISM OF ACTION	IMMUNOLOGIC EFFECT
Immunostimulants			
Bacterial derivatives			
Propionibacterium acnes	Inactivated *P. acnes* extract	TLR2 receptor—mediated activation of NF-κB on monocytes and macrophages Th1-type response of lymphocytes	Cytotoxic, antitumoral, and antiviral effects Promotes neutrophil and macrophage attraction and activity
Mycobacterium spp.	Deproteinated *Mycobacterium* spp. cell wall extract	TLR2 and TLR4 receptor—mediated activation of NF-κB on macrophages and dendritic cells increase expression of co-stimulatory molecules on APCs.	NK-cell cytotoxic and antitumoral activities Promotes neutrophil and macrophage attraction and activity
Exogenous cytokines			
Interferon-alpha (IFN-α)	Human recombinant molecule Human natural purified molecule	Increase expression of antiviral components (PKR, Mx) Increase in MHC class I expression on infected cells Inhibits gene transcription	Potent antiviral effect Inhibits cell proliferation Proapoptosis effect Promote IFN-α secretion
Granulocyte colony-stimulating factor (G-CSF)	Canine recombinant molecule Human recombinant molecule	Myeloid stimulation factor	Promotes myeloid cell production and maturation of macrophages and dendritic cells

Table • 72-1

Immunomodulators—cont'd

COMPONENT	ORIGIN	MECHANISM OF ACTION	IMMUNOLOGIC EFFECT
Viral derivatives			
Parapoxvirus ovis	Chemically inactivated *Parapoxvirus ovis* strain D 1701	CD14-mediated inflammatory response of APCs	Promotes cytokine secretion NK-cell cytotoxicity Antiviral and phagocytic activity
Other immunostimulants			
Levamisole	Synthetic anthelmintic	Unknown	Phagocytic activity Antibody production
Caprine serum fraction	Purified serum protein fraction	Unknown	Unknown
Immunosuppressants			
Inhibitors of gene expression			
Glucocorticoids	Synthetic molecules	Binding to cytosolic glucocorticoid receptor promotes its translocation into nucleus to bind to glucocorticoid responsive elements. Binding to and neutralization of proinflammatory transcription factors (NF-κB, AP-1, CREB)	Potent antiinflammatory effect Antiphagocytic activity Inhibit APC maturation and activation Inhibit T-cell activation Inhibit antibody production
Kinase and phosphatase inhibitors			
Cyclosporine A	Fungal polypeptide	Binding to cyclophilin inhibits phosphorylation of NFAT and its translocation to the nucleus.	Inhibits T-cell activation and proliferation
Inhibitors of nucleotide synthesis			
Azathioprine	Purine analog precursor	Inhibits de novo pathway of purine synthesis; inhibits synthesis of DNA and RNA	Inhibits cell proliferation Inhibits T-cell activation
Alkylating agents			
Cyclophosphamide	Metabolite of nitrogen mustard	Alkylate DNA bases	Mutagenic, cytotoxic, antiproliferative, and chemotherapeutic effects
Chlorambucil	Metabolite of nitrogen mustard	Alkylate DNA bases	
Vinca alkaloids			
Vincristine	Vinca alkaloid	Binding to tubulin in the mitotic spindle prevents purine synthesis	Inhibit cell proliferation Thrombopoietic effect
Passive Immunotherapy			
Regular plasma	Pooled alloimmune plasma from horse donors	Passive transfer of immunoglobulins Binding of donor immunoglobulin to the Fc receptors of phagocytes in liver and spleen Saturation of endosome receptors involved in immunoglobulin degradation	Increases opsonization capacity Inhibits removal of antibody-bound red cells or platelets by phagocytes Accelerates catabolism of autoantibodies
Hyperimmune plasma	Pooled alloimmune plasma from antigen-specific vaccinated horses	Binding of immunoglobulins to organism's antigenic targets	Neutralizes the effects of and toxins
Antiserum-antitoxin	Serum concentrate of antigen-specific immunoglobulins	Binding of immunoglobulins to antigenic targets	Neutralizes the effects of toxins

TLR, Toll-like receptor; *NF-κB*, nuclear factor kappa B; *APCs*, antigen-presenting cells; *Th1*, T-helper cell type 1; *MHC*, major histocompatibility complex; *NK*, natural killer; *AP*, activator protein, *CREB*, cAMP response element–binding protein; *NFAT*, nuclear factor of activated T lymphocyte.

lumen phagocytose particulate material in the circulation, including bacteria, endotoxins, fibrin, and leukocytes. These cells likely secrete inflammatory mediators that result in alterations in systemic vascular resistance and permeability, are chemoattractants for neutrophil margination into the pulmonary vascular system, and produce additional proinflammatory mediators.

The innate immune response is a nonspecific recognition of and subsequent response to pathogens. Signal transduction pathways activate oxidative burst activity and the production of cytokines and chemokines. These responses initiate microbial defenses and inflammation. *Toll-like receptors* (TLRs) are type I transmembrane proteins expressed in cells responsible for this first encounter with a pathogen and the presentation of processed peptide to lymphocytes: macrophages, dendritic cells, and in some species, mucosal epithelial cells and dermal epithelial cells. Therefore, activation of TLRs may be induced in conditions in which an immune response is desired (e.g., vaccination). Blocking of TLR pathways may be beneficial to prevent life-threatening inflammation (e.g., sepsis).[10] In addition to TLRs, other important receptors, including mannose and complement receptors, are expressed on APCs.

The contribution of TLRs to the immune response was first observed with *Aspergillus fumigatus* infection of *Drosophila*.[7,8] Since then, as many as 12 TLRs have been identified in most mammals.[9] Each TLR recognizes a different *pathogen-associated molecular pattern* (PAMP); therefore, together they can mediate response to a wide range of organisms (Figure 72-1). In addition, TLRs may recognize low-molecular-weight synthetic molecules.

After antigen processing of an immunostimulant, intracellular signaling pathways for expression of proinflammatory genes and endogenous cytokines (IL-1, IL-6, TNF-α, and IFN-α) are activated (Figure 72-2). These mediators, while promoting the desirable immune responses, exert adverse systemic effects, including transient fever, lethargy, and decreased appetite.[6] Toxic effects of these crude or live bacterial products include increased vascular permeability, hypotension, pulmonary edema, diarrhea, hypersensitivity reactions with infiltrative/granulomatous cell reaction, autoantibody production, and collapse.

The use of immunostimulants in equine medicine is promoted for the preventive or adjunctive therapy of respiratory diseases and other infectious diseases, acquired immunosuppression secondary to stress (transportation, training, weaning), immunosuppressive treatment, infiltrative diseases, metabolic/endocrine diseases, malnutrition, or any condition that has reduced the ability of the immune system to fight against opportunistic and pathogenic organisms. Immunostimulants are also recommended for antitumor treatment (e.g., sarcoids) in the horse.

Bacterial Particles

Propionibacterium acnes

Propionibacterium acnes is a gram-positive bacterium studied since the 1950s (when it was known as *Corynebacterium parvum*)

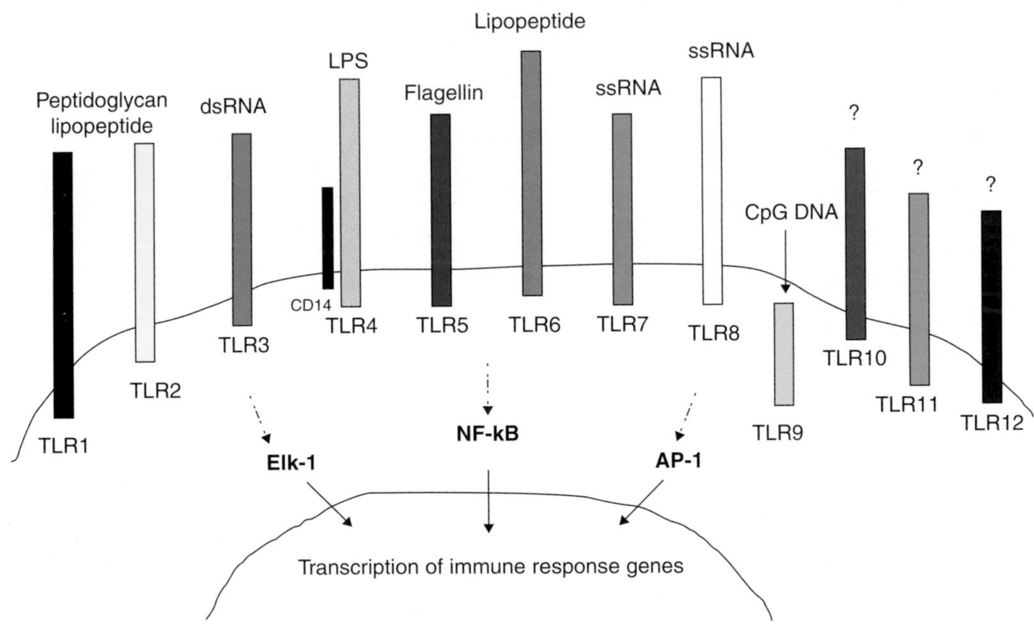

Fig. 72-1 Toll-like receptors. Each toll-like receptor *(TLR)* recognizes a different pathogen-associated molecular pattern (PAMP); together, therefore, they can identify a wide range of organisms, including gram-positive and gram-negative bacteria, viruses, fungi, and parasites. The binding to a TLR results in activation of signaling pathway cascades and the translocation of transcriptional factors (NF-κB, Elk-1, AP-1) into the nucleus, with subsequent cell activation and inflammatory cytokine expression. Immunomodulators may mimic the natural activation of antigen-presenting cells (APCs) through TLR receptor and consequently promote the availability of proinflammatory signals. *LPS*, Lipopolysaccharide; *dsRNA*, double-strand ribonucleic acid; *ss*, single-strand; *CpG*, cytosine-phosphate-guanosine; *NF*, nuclear factor; *AP*, activator protein.

for its antitumoral and antiviral properties. Immunostimulatory activity has been demonstrated in vitro and in vivo in humans and mice. These actions include (1) stimulation of monocytes and macrophages with production of inflammatory cytokines (IL-1, IL-6, and TNF-α), chemokine production (IL-8), phagocytosis and reactive oxygen species activity; (2) activation of CD8+ T cells (CTLs, cytotoxic T cells), natural killer (NK) cells, and lymphokine-activated killer (LAK) cells with interleukin-2 (IL-2) and interferon-alpha (IFN-α)–dependent cytotoxicity; (3) increase in resistance to intracellular bacteria and viruses in mice; (4) in vivo antitumoral effect; and (5) potential adjuvant with antigens.[11-14] The recognition of *P. acnes* PAMP is mediated by the TLR2 and TLR9 on monocytes and macrophages. Activation results in nuclear factor kappa B (NF-κB) activation and expression of interleukin-6 (IL-6), interleukin-8 (IL-8), and interleukin-1 (IL-1), leading to a T-helper cell type 1 (Th1) immune response.[15,16,16a]

Propionobacterium acnes (Eqstim, Neogen Corp., Lexington, Kentucky) is licensed for adjunctive therapy in the treatment of viral and bacterial infections of the respiratory tract of the horse in association with other conventional therapy. In healthy young horses, a series of three intravenous (IV) injections of *P. acnes* extract resulted in immunomodulatory responses.[17] It is suspected that the bacterial extract is rapidly taken up by the intravascular pulmonary macrophages, which in turn produce inflammatory cytokines and clinical effects (indicated by mild fever). In peripheral blood, nonopsonized phagocytosis is increased. In bronchoalveolar lavage (BAL) fluid, there is a decrease in total leukocyte counts, especially lymphocytes, with a proportional increase in macrophages. The CD4+/CD8+ T-lymphocyte ratio and LAK cell activity are increased in peripheral blood and BAL fluid after 3 days of administration of this immunostimulant. Peripheral blood mononuclear cells exhibit an increase in interferon-gamma (IFN-γ) and the NK-lysin antimicrobial peptide for up to 7 days after treatment.[18]

An open, randomized clinical trial demonstrated that administration of two doses of *P. acnes* before shipping reduced the incidence of transport-stress–induced respiratory disease by more than 60% compared with horses in a placebo-treated group.[19] In two blinded, randomized clinical studies of horses with naturally occurring respiratory disease treated with conventional therapy, 79% and 96% of the horses that received *P. acnes* recovered within 14 days of treatment, compared with 47% and 35%, respectively, of the horses from the placebo group.[20]

Bacille Calmette-Guérin Vaccine and Mycobacterium Cell Wall Extracts

Microbiologists Calmette and Guérin from the Pasteur Institute took 13 years to attenuate a strain of *Mycobacterium*

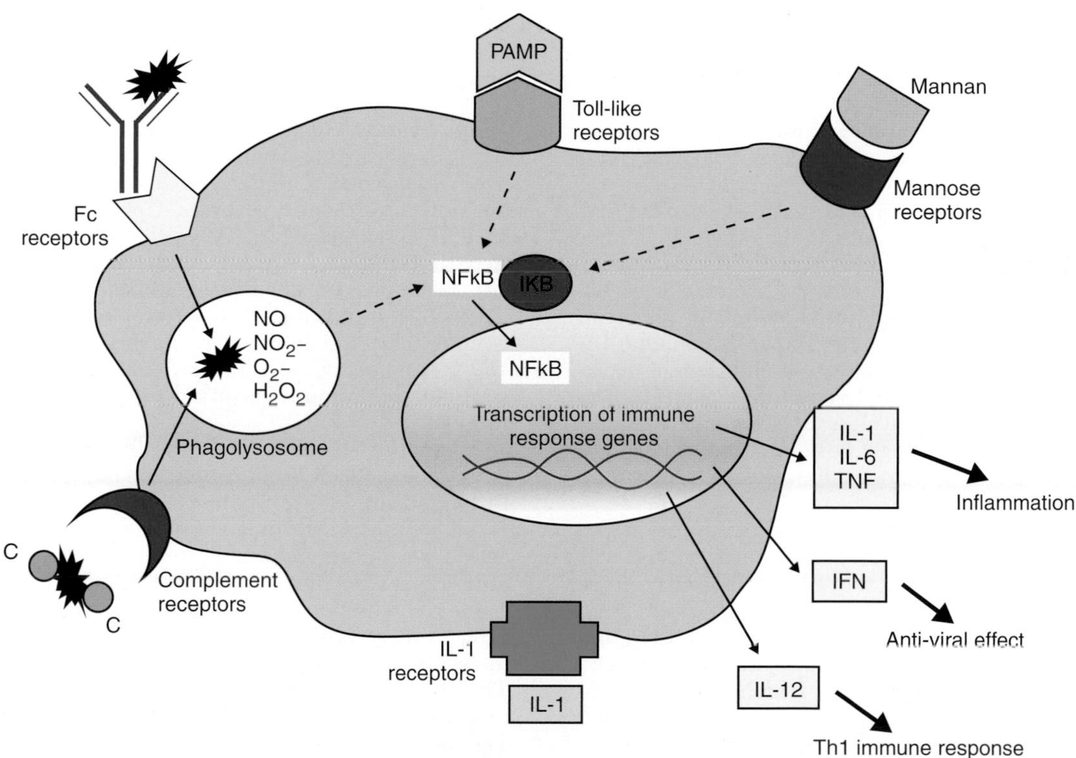

Fig. 72-2 Innate immunity. Antigen-presenting cells (APCs) display different mechanisms to detect antigens and pathogens at first encounter: Fcγ and complement receptors facilitate the phagocytosis of antibody-bound and complement (C)–bound organisms, respectively; on phagocytosis, reactive nitrogen and oxygen species (NO, NO_2–, O_2–, H_2O_2) are produced for the killing of the pathogen; toll-like receptors (TLRs) recognize specific pathogen-associated molecular patterns (*PAMPs*); mannose receptors bind to mannan on fungal and bacterial organisms; and the interleukin-1 *(IL-1)* receptor recognizes the IL-1 cytokine, which is released by activated inflammatory and epithelial cells to signal for "danger." Activation of APCs by these mechanisms results in translocation of nuclear factor kappa B *(NFκB)* into the nucleus, with subsequent signaling for the transcription of proinflammatory cytokines, including IL-1, IL-6, tumor necrosis factor alpha *(TNFα)*, interferon-alpha *(IFNα)*, and IL-12. *Th1*, T-helper cell type 1.

bovis by 230 serial passages in culture. This resulted in a loss of virulence without loss of immunogenic properties in the attenuated strain. Since then, genetic drift has resulted in different strains of bacille Calmette-Guérin (BCG), which induce the distinct immunogenic and therapeutic effects observed at present.[21] BCG was originally created for use as a vaccine against *Mycobacterium tuberculosis* in humans. Use as a nonspecific immunomodulator began in the 1970s for treatment of superficial bladder cancer.[22,23] Currently, BCG cell wall fractions and recombinant BCG (rBCG) combined with foreign antigens (viral, bacterial, or parasitic particles) or cytokines (e.g., human IFN-α gene) are available for clinical use and research.[24] The recombinant forms are studied for their application as adjuvants in specific immune responses.

Low-dose BCG vaccine and inactivated *Mycobacterium* preparations have a potent immunomodulatory effect on macrophages and dendritic cells primarily via TLR2 and TLR4.[25,26] In addition to enhanced production of the cytokines IL-12, IL-1, and tumor necrosis factor alpha (TNF-α), BCG-stimulated dendritic cells promote the upregulation of CD80, CD86, and CD40, which are important co-stimulatory molecules for T-cell activation. BCG vaccine–stimulated monocytes and macrophages induce Th1-type CD4+ T-cell proliferation in vitro.[27] BCG vaccine stimulates NK cell cytotoxicity and IFN-γ production via monocyte and macrophage IL-12 secretion. A comparable direct effect of BCG vaccine on NK cells in the absence of APCs has also been demonstrated in vitro.[28,29] In addition, BCG vaccine stimulates the expression of integrins, IL-1α and IL1β, IL-8, macrophage inflammatory protein 1α and 1β (MIP-1α, MIP-1β) and resistance to apoptosis in neutrophils.[30] Together, the immunostimulatory effects promote neutrophil and macrophage attraction and activation, which subsequently induces Th1-type CD4+ T-cell activation and NK-cell cytotoxic response.

Although the mechanisms of action of BCG vaccine have been widely studied in other species, to date there are limited in vitro or in vivo data describing the effects of this immunomodulator in the horse. Different components of the mycobacterial cell wall act as potent macrophage stimulants, including muramyl dipeptide and lipoarabinomannan. Equimune I.V. (Bioniche Animal Health Research) is an emulsion of deproteinized *Mycobacterium* cell wall fraction that claims to have reduced toxic effects without loss of immunostimulatory activity. It is indicated as a single-dose immunostimulant for the treatment of equine respiratory disease complex resulting from viral or bacterial infection.

A randomized, double-blind clinical study in horses with naturally occurring respiratory disease and treated with conventional therapy suggested that 83% of horses receiving one IV dose of purified *Mycobacterium* spp. cell wall extract recovered from respiratory clinical signs in a shorter time (7 days) than the placebo group (36%).[31] Live BCG vaccine or preparations of BCG cell wall fraction (Regressin-V, Bioniche Animal Health) have been used with quantifiable success (about 60%-70%) for intratumoral treatment of sarcoids in horses.[32] This therapy is more efficacious for treatment of facial lesions and in horses with a positive delayed hypersensitivity reaction to purified protein derivative before treatment and leukocytosis after the first injection.[33] Nonresponsive cases are associated with lesions elsewhere on the body (limbs, body wall), large size, or the presence of multiple sarcoid lesions.

Adverse reactions to BCG vaccine (attenuated form of mycobacterium) are more common in children. These reactions may include persistent local abscess at the site of injection and regional suppurative lymphadenopathy.[34] Adverse reactions to intravesical instillation of BCG vaccine for the treatment of superficial bladder carcinoma in human patients include disseminated BCG infection in distant organs: granulomatous hepatitis, miliary pulmonary disease, pulmonary granulomas, renal abscess, and retroperitoneal lymphadenopathy.[35] In addition, sepsis and hypersensitivity reactions (fever, pancytopenia, anaphylaxis, hepatitis, renal insufficiency) have been reported.[36] Pulmonary toxicity could be septic and secondary to mycobacteremia, which induces sensitization before a second BCG exposure. Hypersensitivity reactions a few weeks after immunotherapy may be observed in patients with disseminated pulmonary and hepatic granulomas, characterized by noncaseating epithelioid granuloma with Langhans-type giant cells and lymphocytes. In these cases, cultures for mycobacteria from blood and affected tissues are negative.[35,37]

In horses, adverse effects after immunotherapy with mycobacterial preparations include reaction at the injection site, fever, lethargy, and decreased appetite, likely related to the induced endogenous cytokine release. An acute reaction with pancytopenia, fever, hypotension, tachycardia, and tachypnea has been observed in a horse treated intralesionally for a sarcoid lesion (Flaminio, unpublished data). This horse had been previously treated with a BCG formula several months before this reaction. Four horses with a history of cough developed severe inflammatory reaction in the respiratory tract after immunomodulator administration. These horses had interstitial pneumonia, multifocal pulmonary granulomas, and bronchiolitis, with subsequent development of lung fibrosis despite glucocorticoid therapy.[38] Because of these types of adverse reactions, veterinary mycobacterium compounds have been removed from the market in some countries.

Unmethylated Cytosine-Phosphate-Guanosine Motifs

Cytosine-phosphate-guanosine (CpG) motifs are unmethylated dinucleotides present in high frequency in bacterial but not in vertebrate genomes. CpG motifs are recognized by TLR-9 expressed in APCs.[39] Synthetic oligodeoxynucleotide (ODN) motifs can mimic natural CpGs and stimulate macrophages, dendritic cells, and B cells. In general, CpG-ODN motifs induce a Th1-type immune response, with both cellular and humoral components.[40] Therefore, CpG-ODNs can be potentially used as immunomodulators for treatment of immune-mediated disorders or as adjuvants in vaccines.[41-43]

In murine B cells, CpG motifs induce robust T-cell–independent B-cell proliferation; enhance production of IL-6, IL-10, and antibodies; promote isotype switching; and prevent B-cell apoptosis.[44] In monocytes, macrophages, and dendritic cells, CpG motifs induce the production of large quantities of IL-12, and smaller quantities of IFN-α, TNF-α, and IL-6.[45] There is maturation of dendritic cells with upregulation of cell surface major histocompatibility complex class II (MHC II) molecule and co-stimulatory molecules, including CD86.[46] Therefore, these APCs become more capable of presenting processed antigen to T cells and promoting their activation. The increased production of IL-12 by APCs results in potent stimulation of NK cells and T cells, with subsequent IFN-γ release.

There is species specificity in the recognition of CpG motifs, and certain CpG motifs may have dissimilar effects on immune cells according to their sequence.[47] CpG-ODN–induced proliferation in vitro correlates well with in vivo responses, and this method is used to screen different motifs for clinical application.[48] Other synthetic products that contain a bicyclic heterobase in which the C in CpG is replaced by R (rybofuranosyl, RpG) are currently under investigation.[49]

As with many other immunomodulating agents, CpG motifs may be toxic and promote an undesirable, exacerbated immune response. Toxic responses to CpG motif have been demonstrated in mice after repeated administration of high doses of CpG motifs. A lethal synergism is observed when CpG motif administration is followed by endotoxin (lipopolysaccharide, LPS) challenge.[50] Despite promoting B-cell activity, CpG does not induce an anti-DNA antibody response or accelerate autoimmune disease. Further studies of the use of this immunomodulatory agent are necessary to identify CpG sequences with biologic effect, the type of response generated, potential clinical applications, and safety in the horse.

Exogenous Cytokines

Cytokines are proteins or glycoproteins secreted by immune cells and other cells in direct contact with microorganisms. Their effect is primarily autocrine or paracrine, and they function as messengers or mediators of the immune system.[70] Interleukins and other cytokines may be administered as immunomodulating agents to stimulate enhanced immune activity in the treatment of infectious, neoplastic and autoimmune diseases.

Interferon-α

Endogenous interferons (IFNs) are multifunctional proteins that play important roles in antiviral defense and cell proliferation/viability by binding to cell surface receptors on virus-infected cells and inducing transcription of specific genes. High IFN levels can control the rate of virus replication in early infection.[51] Type I IFNs are produced primarily by the innate immune system leukocytes (e.g., IFN-α) or fibroblasts (e.g., IFN-α and IFN-β) after viral infection.[52] Viral binding to extracellular receptors or the presence of viral products (dsRNA) bound to cytoplasmic receptors can induce expression of type I IFNs. Type II IFNs (IFN-γ) are produced by NK cells and T cells (in response to cytokines IL-12 and IL-18). Both types of IFN promote an "antiviral state" by interfering with the mechanisms of cell proliferation, translation, and subsequently, viral replication. In addition, IFNs make infected cells more susceptible to apoptosis (procaspase activity) and to recognition by CD8+ cytotoxic T cells by enhancing the expression of major histocompatibility complex class I (MHC I) on infected cells.

One of the most important antiviral activities of IFNs is induction of proteins that prevent proliferation or promote destruction of ribonucleic acid (RNA) molecules in the cell. These include the dsRNA-dependent protein kinase R, which controls transcription and translation of other genes with antiviral effect (e.g., NF-κB). The gene 2′-5′-oligoadenylate synthetase inhibits protein synthesis by promoting RNase activity. The Mx proteins interfere with virus polymerase and upregulate adenosine deaminase (ADAR), which is important for RNA editing, effectively inhibiting viral multiplication. Caspase proteins promote apoptosis.[53] IFNs are so important in the control of viral infection and replication that many viruses have developed mechanisms to inhibit the IFNs.[54]

Besides the potent direct antiviral effects of IFN-α, this cytokine promotes cell-mediated immunity. It enhances the cytotoxic effects of NK cells and LAK cells by increasing levels of perforins and granzymes (apoptotic effect), production of IFN-γ, and cell proliferation. Once IFN-γ secretion is enhanced, this stimulation is self-sustained with cell-to-cell contact for a time, even in the absence of additional IFN-α.[55] IFN-γ induces activation and maturation of APCs, potentiated even further by IL-12 and IL-15. IL-12 drives CD4+ T cells into a Th1-type response, resulting in additional IFN-γ production. Interleukin-15 supports the survival and proliferation of activated and memory T cells.[56] In addition, IFN-γ induces the production of reactive oxygen (O_2^-, superoxide; OH^-, hydroxyl; H_2O_2, hydrogen peroxide; $HClO^-$, hypochlorite) and reactive nitrogen (NO, nitric oxide; NO_2, nitrogen dioxide; HN_2, nitrous acid) products in phagocytes for effective microbial killing.[57]

Commercially available IFN-α is found in natural (in vitro purified human IFN-α with multiple subtypes) and recombinant forms (*Escherichia coli* clone expressing human IFN-α-2a subtype DNA). The natural form of IFN-α may provide broader biologic function compared with the single recombinant subtype. Low-dose IFN-α therapy is more efficient in antiviral activity than high doses, which may induce an excessive inflammatory response, downregulation of IFN receptors, and production of neutralizing antibodies. Studies using IFN-α as an adjuvant for influenza peptide vaccines in mice revealed a potential benefit in the induction of cytotoxic T lymphocyte (CTL) activity.[58]

IFN-α has been used therapeutically via oral or parenteral (subcutaneous, intramuscular) routes in people and horses for its antiviral and antiproliferative (antitumoral) activities. Parenteral high-dose human IFN-α-2a has been used to treat human patients with chronic hepatitis C, West Nile virus (WNV) infection, hairy cell leukemia, chronic myelogenous leukemia, and AIDS-related Kaposi's sarcoma.[59-62] Adverse effects associated with parenteral high-dose IFN-α-2a treatment include fever, fatigue, and myalgia. Contrasting results of in vitro experiments question the susceptibility of WNV to IFN-α. There is evidence of both resistance and susceptibility of the virus to the cytokine.[63,64] Nevertheless, human patients infected with WNV treated with high parenteral doses of IFN-α had rapid recovery and fewer sequelae. Additional clinical trials are underway.[65]

Oral IFN-α acts directly on oropharyngeal-associated lymphoid tissues by activating the antiviral state in those cells.[66] In horses, low-dose oral administration of natural human IFN-α has been used for the treatment of inflammatory airway disease and viral respiratory diseases.[67] In a double-blind, randomized, block-design study of horses with inflammatory airway disease (characterized by poor performance and exudate in the upper and lower airway), natural human IFN-α given orally reduced airway inflammation, pharyngeal lymphoid hyperplasia, nasal discharge, and cough compared with horses receiving placebo. The cytokine profile of BAL fluid cells returned to normal in horses that received oral IFN-α. A commercially available recombinant IFN-α-2a, which contains only one subtype of IFN-α, failed to reduce virus shedding and respiratory disease in experimental herpesvirus type 1 infection in horses.[68] A double-blind, randomized clinical trial testing the effect of oral treatment with natural or recombinant human IFN-α on inflammatory airway disease revealed that both IFN-α forms decreased the time to recovery and number of relapses compared with placebo.[69] In horses, IFN-α has been used parenterally for the treatment of WNV; however, to date, randomized, placebo-controlled trials have not been completed.

Other Cytokines: the Present and the Future

The two most common cytokines used in cancer immunotherapy in human patients (e.g., renal cell carcinoma) are IL-2 and IFN-α, which can be used independently (high doses) or in combination (lower doses).[71] Because only a small percentage of patients respond to cytokine therapy alone, this mode of treatment is often combined with traditional chemotherapy.[72] Effective response and toxicity are both dose dependent with this cytokine; therefore, to minimize systemic effect, peripheral blood or tumoral infiltrating lymphocytes (TILs) can be activated and expanded with cytokines (IL-2) in vitro and returned to the patient for a potentiated effect against tumor cells.[73] Hyporesponsive lymphocytes from the malignant effusion of lung cancer patients can be reactivated into CTLs when treated in vitro with IL-2 (or IL-15) and anti-CD3 antibodies.[74]

The use of cytokines in combination with conventional antibiotic therapy or as vaccine adjuvants has been beneficial in the treatment and prevention of infection with intracellular bacteria. The use of IL-12 alone has limited clinical application, but it has promising adjunctive properties to induce Th1-type immune response when paired with peptides in vaccines. In murine models, intranasal administration of IL-12 in combination with an antibiotic or antifungal medication improves survival and clearance of *Mycobacterium avium*, *Francisella tularensis*, influenza virus, or cryptococcal infection.[75-78] In human patients with asthma, treatment with IL-12 with the objective to inhibit Th2-type and promote Th1-type responses failed to improve airway hyperreactivity. Work with a cytokine fusion protein consisting of allergen (or allergen cDNA) fused to IL-12 or IL-18, or allergen cDNA fused with IL-18 cDNA, reveals redirection of immune responses into a Th1 type and reduction of airway hyperreactivity in a mouse model.[79,80]

Plasmid DNA coding for human IL-12 has been injected directly into equine melanoma tumors and promoted tumor regression with no adverse effects.[81] The antitumor effect of the plasmid DNA encoding IL-12 has been observed in murine tumor models; however, many of these therapies failed when applied to human patients with cancer.

The use of other cytokines to induce Th1-type immune response in clinical patients has had limited effect. Administration of IFN-γ to prevent *Pseudomonas aeruginosa* infection in a stress mouse model revealed recovery of IL-12 secretion but did not improve bacterial clearance or reduce mortality.[82]

Neonatal mice treated with fms-like tyrosine kinase 3 (Flt-3) ligand, a hematopoietic growth factor for dendritic cells, B cells, and NK cells, demonstrated a 100-fold increase in the innate resistance to herpes simplex virus type 1 and *Listeria monocytogenes*.[83] The dendritic cell induction was independent of mature T and B cells and their cytokines. This finding has important implications in neonatal immune defense because the adaptive immune system is not well developed.

Granulocyte-macrophage colony-stimulating factor (GM-CSF) is a cytokine used to reconstitute myeloid cells in the bone marrow and promote macrophage and dendritic cell development. This cytokine has also been evaluated as an adjuvant in vaccines or in combination with other cytokines (IFN-γ) to promote dendritic cell maturation for use in cancer immunotherapy. In the horse, subcutaneous administration of recombinant human granulocyte colony-stimulating factor (G-CSF) stimulates in vitro bone marrow cells from Standardbred horses with familial neutropenia and accelerates bone marrow production of neutrophils in foals with alloimmune neonatal neutropenia.[84,85] Response to G-CSF is immediate, and in the presence of normal myeloid precursors in the bone marrow, neutrophil counts may be within normal reference ranges within 48 hours of administration.

Other Immunomodulators

Parapoxvirus ovis

The use of poxvirus as an immunostimulant originated from observations related to the smallpox eradication program, in which vaccinated human patients had improvement in viral diseases and tumors. In vitro studies using murine, human, bovine, ovine, and swine cells suggest that the *Parapoxvirus* envelope contains proteins that promote the activation of NK cells, enhance phagocytic activity, and increase the release of INF-α, IL-2, TNF-α, and GM-CSF.[86] The mechanism of stimulation of APCs involves the CD14 molecule, with production of antiinflammatory IL-10 and Th2-type IL-4 cytokines.[87] Pretreatment with *Parapoxvirus ovis* protected mice in a dose-dependent manner from lethal vesicular stomatitis virus and herpes simplex virus type 1 infections.[88]

Administration of *Parapoxvirus ovis* (ecthyma virus or Orf virus) strain D 1701 is indicated for the prophylaxis of stress-induced respiratory diseases caused by transportation, hospitalization, and weaning; for the metaphylaxis and therapy of infectious diseases; and to enhance immunization response. In the horse, a blinded field study suggested that prophylactic administration of Baypamun (Bayer, Germany) to foals 6 and 4 days before weaning, and at 5 days thereafter, assisted in preventing and reducing the incidence of respiratory disease from 24% to 7.9%.[89] In a controlled field trial, Thoroughbred foals from the same farm received three doses of the immunotherapeutic drug or placebo immediately after birth and 24 or 48 hours later. These foals were monitored for 4 weeks, and 20% to 30% of the foals from the placebo group developed respiratory infections, whereas the foals in the groups receiving the immunomodulator did not. *Parapoxvirus ovis* was suggested to minimize but not to prevent respiratory clinical signs (based on nasal exudate scores) in horses naturally challenged by contact with virulent equine herpesvirus type1 or type 4 (EHV-1 or EHV-4). Young horses under stress induced by weaning, transportation, and commingling that were treated with this immunomodulating agent were more resistant to EHV-1 and EHV-4 infection, as well as development of respiratory clinical signs, when receiving *Parapoxvirus ovis*, compared with horses receiving placebo.

Levamisole Phosphate

Levamisole phosphate is a synthetic anthelmintic with reported immunomodulatory properties that have been rarely observed and poorly characterized in vitro and in vivo. In horses the effect of levamisole was tested in pregnant mares with weekly injections starting 4 to 6 weeks before parturition. Colostrum of mares receiving the immunostimulant had greater immunoglobulin G (IgG) and IgG(T) concentrations than did colostrum from control mares.[90] In sick foals, levamisole has been administered in the attempt to improve cell-mediated responses and phagocytic activity.

Caprine Serum Fraction

Caprine serum fraction is a sterile, filtered, purified, and standardized fraction of goat serum preserved in phenol and thimerosal (Pulmo-Clear, Colorado Serum Co., Denver). It is recommended as an immunomodulator for adjunctive therapy of lower respiratory tract disease in horses. A clinical efficacy trial in horses with unspecified lower respiratory tract disease suggested improvement in airway inflammation, as evaluated by endoscopic examination score after two doses of the immunomodulator.[91] Phenotypic analysis of leukocyte subpopulations, phagocytosis, and oxidative burst activity; LAK cell activity; and IL-2 receptor (IL-2R) expression were evaluated in peripheral blood and BAL fluid leukocytes after administration of two intramuscular (IM) injections of placebo or caprine serum fraction to six healthy yearling fillies. The results suggested immunomodulatory activity with an increase in CD4+/CD8+ T-lymphocyte ratio in peripheral blood. The cellularity of BAL fluid, especially B lymphocytes and macrophages, was reduced after administration of the immunomodulator. Other immune function tests, including

LAK cell activity, phagocytosis, and oxidative burst activity and IL-2R expression, were unchanged.

Acemannan

Acemannan immunostimulant consists of long-chain mannan polymers interspersed with acetyl groups and is derived from the pulp of the *Aloe vera* plant. In vitro studies have demonstrated immunostimulatory effects on macrophages (increased secretion of IL-1α, IL-6, TNF-α, nitric oxide, phagocytosis) and the stimulation of CTLs.[92,93] Commercially available products for topical use in veterinary medicine are indicated for wound healing.

Echinacea angustifolia

Standardized *Echinacea angustifolia* has been evaluated as an immunomodulator in horses. Findings suggest increased phagocytic capacity of neutrophils and increased numbers of lymphocytes, red cells, and hemoglobin in the peripheral blood compared with placebo groups.[94]

VACCINATION

The objective of a vaccine is to stimulate a protective immune response to an infectious organism (Figure 72-3). Often, protection requires both mucosal and circulatory humoral and cellular immune responses. Long-term protection with immunologic memory is fundamental.

Types of Vaccines

Vaccines come in a variety of types, including inactivated whole pathogen, protein vaccines, recombinant subunit vaccines, deoxyribonucleic acid (DNA) vaccines, modified live vaccines, and recombinant vector vaccines.[95] Different vaccine types elicit different levels of humoral and cellular immune response (Figure 72-4). The choice of vaccine depends on the type of desired immune response, accessible technology, and costs of production. In veterinary medicine the majority of commercially available vaccines lack scientific evidence of efficacy in disease prevention. Limited information from clinical trials and

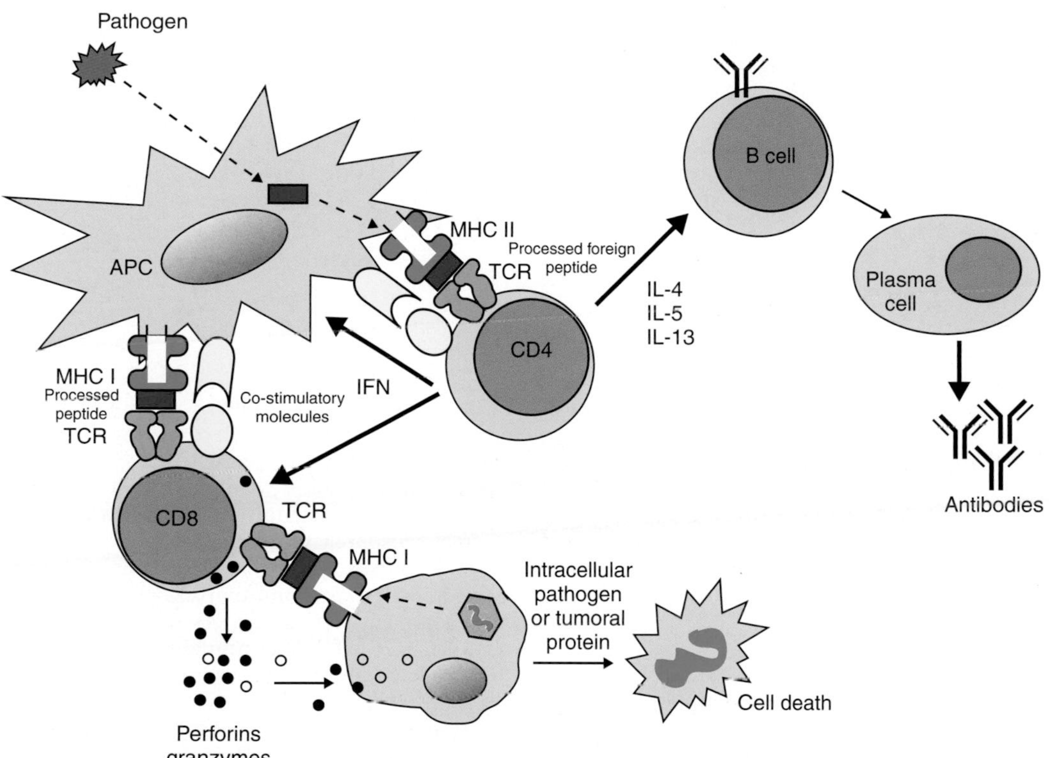

Fig. 72-3 Adaptive immunity. Immature dendritic cells phagocytose pathogens in the periphery and become activated with upregulation of major histocompatibility complex class II *(MHC II)* and co-stimulatory molecules (CD86, CD40). They migrate to the regional lymph node and present the processed pathogen to CD4+ T cells via MHC II (signal 1); the binding of co-stimulatory molecules with its ligands (CD86 with CD28, and CD40 with CD40 ligand) confirms T-cell activation (signal 2). According to the antigen-presenting cell *(APC)* activation status, CD4+ T cells differentiate into Th1-type or Th2-type immune cells. Th1 CD4+ T cells secrete interferon-gamma *(IFNγ)* and promote the activation of CD8+ T cells into cytotoxic T cells (CTLs). The CD8+ T cells can also be activated by APCs via MHC class I antigen presentation of processed antigen (cross-presentation); this process is required for immunity against intracellular pathogens and tumoral cells and for response to vaccines. Th2 CD4+ T cells secrete cytokines (IL-4, IL-5, IL-13) that promote B-cell differentiation into plasma cells, with subsequent antibody secretion. Therefore, activation of APCs is essential for the development of acquired immunity, and immunomodulators may be used to augment (e.g., adjuvants) or diminish (e.g., glucocorticoids) this process. *TCR*, T-cell receptor.

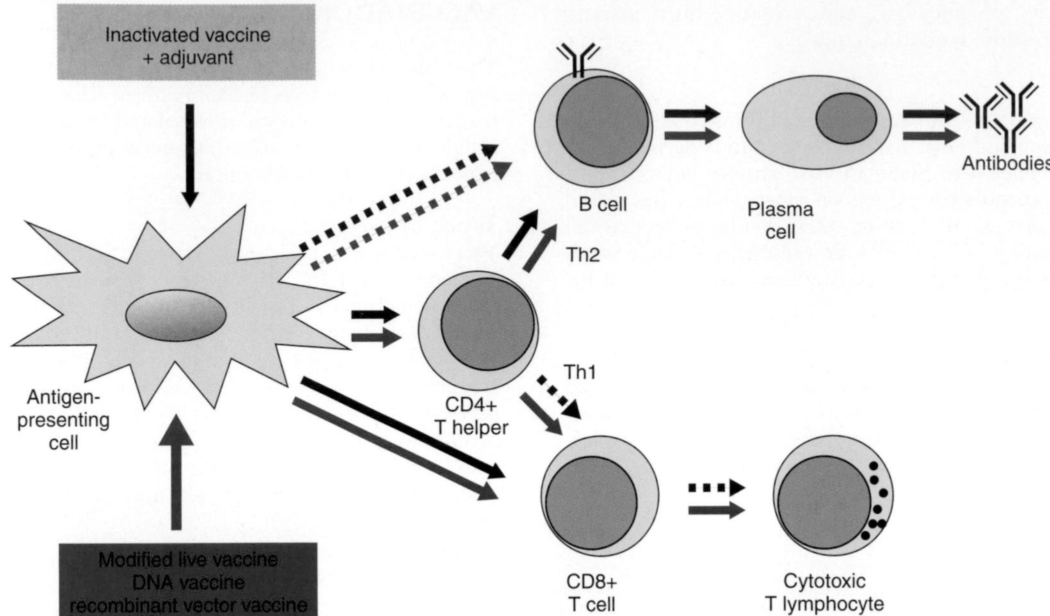

Fig. 72-4 Immune response to vaccines. Different vaccine types elicit different levels of humoral and cellular immune response. Inactivated vaccines *(black arrows)* are known to induce high levels of antibodies and depend on the activation of the immune cells by adjuvants. Modified live vaccines, DNA vaccines, and recombinant vector vaccines *(red arrows)* have been shown to induce both antibody production and, importantly, cellular immunity with activation of antigen-specific cytotoxic T lymphocytes (CTLs) that recognize infected cells. The development of CTLs with the use of inactivated vaccines is questionable *(dotted lines)* and may depend on the type of adjuvant.

clinical observations support the use of many of these vaccines. Seroconversion, measured as a clinical response, only indicates vaccine antigen recognition and humoral response and does not necessarily equate with protective immunity. Limited information on marketed vaccines is available regarding the type of immune response induced by a specific vaccine, the actual efficacy and duration of immunity induced when using products from different companies, the efficacy of multivalent vaccines, and proper vaccination schedules for different age and risk groups.

Vaccine Adjuvants

An *adjuvant* is a substance used to increase the immunogenicity of purified peptides or carbohydrates, improve antigen presentation in lymphoid tissues by inducing the expression of major histocompatibility molecules and co-stimulatory molecules, modulate antigen-specific immune response toward a Th1-type or Th2-type response, and decrease the dose of antigen and frequency of administration necessary to achieve vaccine efficacy.[96] Importantly, in the absence of an adjuvant, purified antigens may induce tolerance.

In veterinary medicine, many adjuvants have been used in commercially available vaccines.[97] Aluminum salts *(alum)* are safe, widely used adjuvants that induce primarily short-lived Th2-type humoral responses.[98] Bacterial structures provide important source of adjuvants, and they are recognized by toll-like receptors (TLRs) in APCs.[99] *Freund's complete adjuvant* (killed mycobacterium mixed with water-in-oil emulsion) induces strong Th1-type cellular immune responses with potential adverse effects. In contrast, *Freund's incomplete adjuvant* (water-in-oil emulsion without the killed mycobacterium) has a weaker effect on the immune response with a faint cytokine response. However, it induces stronger Th2-type responses than alum and releases antigen slower that oil-in-water emulsions. Water-in-oil emulsion adjuvants often cause reactions at the injection site. Cholera toxin and *E. coli* exotoxin are promising adjuvants for transcutaneous or mucosal immunizations, with potential to induce humoral and cell-mediated responses. Synthetic unmethylated CpG-ODNs that mimic bacterial CpG are being widely studied as adjuvants in vaccines to induce a Th1-type immune response.

Liposomes and archaeosomes are lipid vesicles that can be combined with antigens and incorporated in endosomes of APCs to induce both Th1-type and Th-2 type immune responses.[100] *Microparticle adjuvants* are made of nontoxic polymers, and they may be used for long-term release of antigens in an adverse environment (gastrointestinal tract, nasal passages).[101] When associated with immunomodulators, they can induce both humoral and cell-mediated immune responses. Protein carriers (toxoids, KLH) can be linked to antigens that are poorly immunogenic or cannot be recognized by the immune system.[102] *Saponins* are adjuvants originating from plants (Quil A, QS21, and other purified fractions) that can induce both Th1-type and Th2-type responses. Saponins can be associated with cholesterol and phospholipids and form immune-stimulating complexes (ISCOMs), which induce robust Th1-type immune responses.[103]

Neonatal Vaccination

The equine fetus is capable of responding to foreign antigens in utero. However, the naive immune system of the equine neonate takes approximately 2 to 3 months to expand its lymphocyte population in lymphoid tissues, peripheral blood, and organs.[104] During this period, maternal antibodies absorbed from colostrum passively immunize against a large number of pathogens that can be neutralized by humoral mechanisms. Control of intracellular pathogens may be a challenge to the neonate and young foal. Neutralizing antibodies alone may not be sufficient to eliminate or control infection.

Herd management on breeding farms include vaccination of mares 4 to 6 weeks before foaling with killed vaccines to increase the concentration of specific antibodies in colostrum. Paradoxically, there is evidence that maternal antibodies absorbed from colostrum, despite their crucial role in neonatal protection, interfere with the foal's humoral response to vaccine antigens (maternal antibody interference).[105] Questions about the effect of circulating maternal antibodies in the foal's immune response include (1) the potential effect of maternal antibodies on the equine neonatal cellular immune response and response to pathogens during natural exposure, (2) intrinsic limitations of the equine neonate in recognition of certain vaccine compounds versus others, (3) response to inactivated versus recombinant vector vaccination in foals, and (4) differences in half-lives of maternal antibodies that may affect vaccination schedules. Ideally, a vaccine should induce a rapid immune response that mimics the protective, long-term response that results from natural infection; should bypass maternal antibody interference; and should be immunogenic in the neonate.

Molecular Vaccines

A vaccine containing DNA is usually composed of naked or plasmid DNA that is directly injected into the target cell. Recombinant vaccines often include a viral vector that promotes endogenous production of a putative protective antigen. These vaccines have developed into several subtypes, one of which involves splicing together genetic material from more than one organism *(chimera)*. Advances in the use of DNA vaccines or recombinant vector vaccines will likely contribute to safe and successful immunization strategies for diseases that require cellular immunity and protection at the point of pathogen encounter (i.e., mucosal vaccines).[106-108]

Cancer Vaccines

Many challenges must be overcome before vaccines can be designed to successfully induce a specific immune response that reverses the progression of tumors.[109] Some cancer vaccines include a cancer-associated antigen and an adjuvant to enhance immune response.[110] For horses, vaccines made from the crude purification of tumor cells have been used as immunotherapy for melanomas, sarcoids, and papillomas, with variable results. Other examples of cancer vaccines studied in human and veterinary medicine include *idiotype vaccines* (monoclonal antibodies against immunoglobulin expressed on B-cell lymphoma), *DNA vaccines* (DNA from cancer cells inserted in plasmids that are injected in the patient), *heat shock protein-peptide vaccines* (cancer antigens associated with heat shock proteins), *vector vaccines* (virus vectors that encode antigens similar to cancer antigens), *genetically altered tumor cells* (tumor cells transfected with genes encoding cytokines that activate CTLs or the expression of co-stimulatory molecules), and *dendritic cell vaccines* (fusion of tumor cells from the patient with APCs).[111-115]

Immunotherapy for Hyposensitization

Immunotherapy may be used in treatment of immunoglobulin E (IgE)–mediated allergies to induce long-term tolerance by the administration of small but increasing concentrations of the known allergen at regular intervals over months to years.[116] The mechanisms involved in successful immunotherapy are not completely understood but may include redirection from a Th2 response to a Th1 immune response. Th2-type cytokines (IL-4, IL-13) favor the production of IgE, whereas IFN-γ inhibits the production of those cytokines and promotes the secretion of allergen-specific IgG.[109] Alternatively, immunotherapy increases the secretion of IL-10 by regulatory CD4+/CD25+ cells.[117] In horses, immunotherapy has been used to treat atopy or skin hypersensitivity, with variable results (50%-80% response).[118] Although immunotherapy may be an efficient method to minimize clinical signs of hypersensitivity, its future in equine medicine will depend on the development of improved testing for the identification of relevant allergens. DNA vaccines containing vectors encoding specific antigens may substitute protein allergen vaccines. Novel adjuvants that induce Th1-type responses may also be used.[119]

PASSIVE IMMUNITY

Passive immunity is the transfer of preformed antibodies from the immunized individual (donor) to a recipient (patient). Plasma containing polyvalent immunoglobulins may be used therapeutically to replace deficits of endogenous immunoglobulin production (failure of transfer of immunoglobulins through colostrum in neonates, humoral immunodeficiencies) or to transfer large amounts of specific immunoglobulins from donors immunized with relevant antigens (hyperimmune plasma). Immunoglobulin replacement may prevent and help to fight infections or the effects of toxins.

Transfer of Nonspecific Antibodies

Intravenous plasma transfusion with normal plasma is routine practice in neonatal foals with failure of transfer of passive immunity from colostrum and in foals with sepsis. Plasma transfusion increases total serum IgG levels and opsonization capacity in foals.[120,121] In general, serum IgG protective levels are greater than 400 to 500 mg/dL; however, in foals, the goal is to reach concentrations greater than 800 mg/dL because of the high exposure to pathogens in the environment (antibody consumption), short half-life of donor immunoglobulin, and time necessary for endogenous production of immunoglobulins by the foal (4-5 weeks).[96,122,123]

Circulating antibodies participate in immune defense by neutralizing antigens, facilitating phagocytosis (opsonization), and promoting antibody-dependent cell cytotoxicity (ADCC) by NK cells (Figure 72-5). Phagocytosis is an essential component of the innate immune system, and it is facilitated by the presence of opsonins, which may function through C3 receptors (for complement) or Fcγ receptors (for immunoglobulins) on phagocytes. Complement activity in presuckle foals is approximately 13% of adult activity, increasing to 64% by 1 month of age and 85% by 5 months.[121] In foals with sepsis, plasma transfusion is essential to improve opsonization capacity. Recent studies have demonstrated significant individual variation in the opsonic capacity of plasma from different adult horses.[124] This variability is independent of IgG concentrations. The use of pooled plasma from different donors may decrease this variability in the total opsonization capacity.

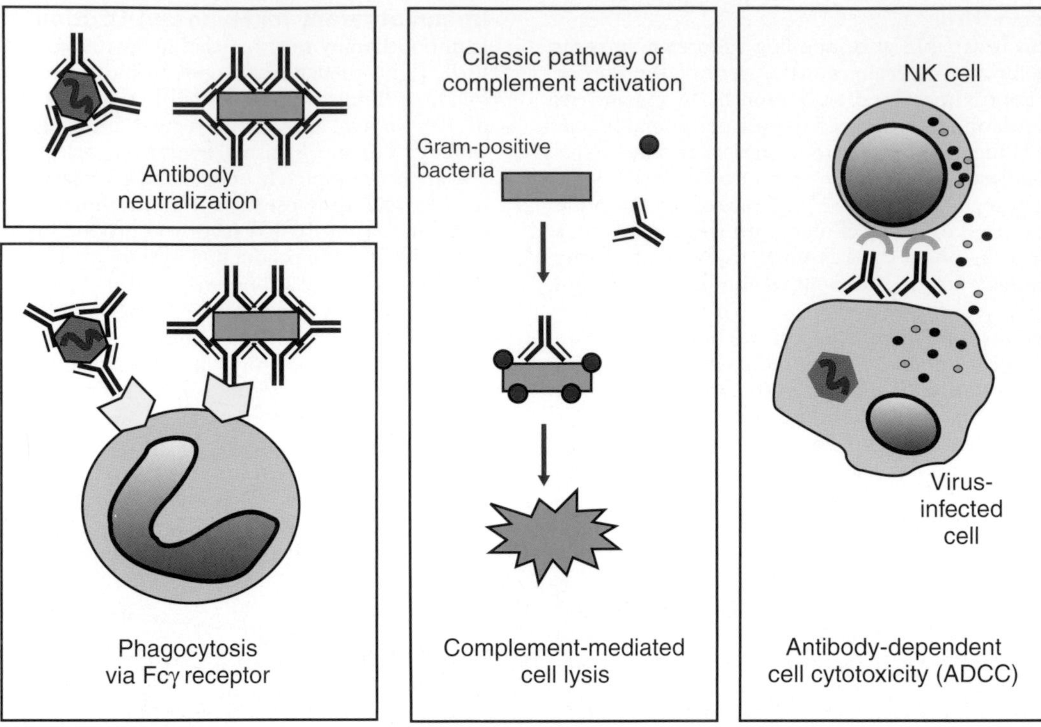

Fig. 72-5 Mechanisms of antibody protection. Antibodies can neutralize pathogens by direct binding. They also facilitate phagocytosis (opsonization), and antibody-bound pathogen is phagocytosed via the Fcγ receptor on the cell membrane of neutrophils and macrophages. Antibodies can also activate complement via the classic pathway, which results in cell destruction. In addition, antibody-bound infected cells can be recognized by Fcγ receptors on natural killer *(NK)* cells and activate antibody-dependent cell cytotoxicity (ADCC) using perforins and granzymes for target cell destruction.

Transfer of Antigen-Specific Antibodies

Rhodococcus equi

Intravenous administration of commercially available *Rhodococcus equi* hyperimmune plasma obtained from donors vaccinated with *R. equi* antigens increases specific antibody levels against *R. equi* in the serum of foals for 60 days after transfusion.[25] Hyperimmune plasma transfusion provides some benefits in the control of disease on enzootic farms. However, it is not known if the positive effects are obtained from nonspecific (opsonins) or specific (antibodies) elements in plasma[126] (see Chapter 32).

West Nile Virus

Antibodies against West Nile virus are commercially available for horses in the form of hyperimmune plasma. A trial in hamsters has been performed to test for efficacy of passive transfer against viral challenge in a dose-dependent manner. Plasma transfusion before and 1 day after challenge neutralized the inoculated virus efficiently. A plaque reduction neutralization test (PRNT) using serum from horses that received IV plasma transfusion indicated that 2 mL of plasma/kg body weight provides a titer of 30, which is higher than protective levels obtained after vaccination (PRNT titer of 5). Additional studies are necessary to validate the efficacy of hyperimmune plasma transfusion for treatment of horses with WNV encephalitis (see Chapter 21).

Endotoxemia

In the adult horse with colitis and endotoxemia, the benefit of hyperimmune plasma to the lipopolysaccharide core antigen of *Escherichia coli,* obtained from horses vaccinated with the J5 *E. coli* vaccine, in survival and clinical outcome is controversial. Although plasma transfusion may be beneficial in treatment of endotoxemia, other plasma factors may play a role in this positive effect (see Chapter 37).

Clostridium botulinum

Plasma with high concentrations (>5000 IU and >20,000 IU) of *Clostridium botulinum* type B antitoxin is commercially available for treatment of horses with botulism. In addition, polyvalent hyperimmune plasma is available at the University of Pennsylvania, New Bolton Center.[127] Intravenous administration of botulinum antitoxin is most efficient in the initial phase of disease to neutralize neurotoxins before they bind to the presynaptic membranes at the neuromuscular junctions (see Chapter 46).

Clostridium tetani

Tetanus antitoxin is commercially available for the treatment of tetanus or prevention of disease in nonvaccinated foals and horses with an unknown history of vaccination (see Chapter 47). Combined active-passive method (tetanus toxoid vaccine and tetanus toxoid antiserum) for simultaneous protection and immunization is efficient for prevention of tetanus in the horse.[128] Administration of tetanus antitoxin at high doses intravenously or into the subarachnoid space may be efficacious to block neurotoxins before they bind to gangliosides at the presynaptic inhibitory motor nerve endings.[129] In adult horses, there is a risk of hepatitis secondary to antitoxin administration (serum hepatitis); such a response has not been observed in foals.[130]

Snake Venoms

Snake antivenin for IV use is more often accessible in areas where encounters with poisonous snakes are likely; in general, polyvalent antivenin contains antibodies against toxins of local snakes. The neutralizing ability of the antiserum results primarily from IgG(T).[131] The relatively small amount of venom injected during the bite rarely causes death of a large horse, and local swelling and secondary bacterial infection can be treated with conventional therapy. However, an incident involving a foal or pony may be life-threatening, and early administration of antivenin is recommended.

Transfusion-Induced Immunomodulation

In addition to providing immunoglobulins for protection, antibodies may modulate immune responses by neutralizing circulating foreign antigens in the recipient. At high doses, plasma IgG may compete for Fc receptor binding on phagocytic cells, resulting in decreased phagocytic function.[132] This effect is desired in the control of inflammatory responses and in the prevention of removal of erythrocytes or platelets with autoantibodies on their surface. Plasma transfusion has been used in horses for this effect in the treatment of immune-mediated anemia or thrombocytopenia.

Plasma transfusion with high concentrations of immunoglobulins accelerates the catabolism and elimination of autoantibodies and is therapeutic in humoral-mediated autoimmune diseases.[133] The clearance of IgG depends on plasma concentrations, and low concentrations may increase plasma half-life up to 10 times. During IgG degradation by endocytosis, immunoglobulins that do not bind endosome receptors are degraded; immunoglobulins that are bound to receptors are protected from degradation and return to circulation (recycled). If there is excess IgG, receptors become saturated, and a large number of IgG molecules are not protected from degradation. Therefore, a single dose of plasma with high concentration of IgG induces the accelerated degradation of antibodies.

Transfusion-induced immunomodulation has been studied in human patients who receive whole-blood transfusion. The donor-blood immune cells and antigens (foreign) may be able to modulate the immune system of the recipient in a very complex form.[134] In general, blood transfusion promotes immunotolerance, which can be clinically observed by prolonged graft survival, increased tumor recurrence, and increased susceptibility to infections. Studies in mice and people indicate decreased macrophage function, IL-2 secretion, NK-cell activity, and peripheral blood CD4/CD8 T-cell ratio. Nevertheless, antigens expressed on cells and proteins (antibodies) of the blood donor stimulated antibody production by the recipient's immune system.[135] Antiidiotype antibodies may be produced after whole-blood or plasma transfusion. The recipient may build a humoral and cellular response against the donor antigens. The variable region (idiotype) of the new antibodies becomes antigenic, which then induces antiidiotype antibody production.

Whole-blood transfusion-associated graft-versus-host disease is also a concern. Lymphocytes from the donor may not be recognized and may be destroyed by the recipient's immune system (patients with immunosuppression, neonates) and become engrafted.[136] When activated, donor cells may recognize the recipient cells as foreign and build a T-cell–mediated and NK-cell–mediated immune response against the recipient's cells. Tissue destruction at many levels occurs in the recipient: liver, bone marrow, gastrointestinal tract, and skin. In response to the inflammatory process, the recipient's own cytokines amplify the engrafted-cell effect.[137] Clinical signs associated with this type of response are observed 1 to 3 weeks after blood transfusion and may include fever, pancytopenia, hepatitis, diarrhea, skin rash, hemorrhage, and death.

IMMUNOSUPPRESSANTS

Immunosuppressive therapy is important in treatment of autoimmune disorders mediated by autoreactive B lymphocytes or T lymphocytes (CD4+ or CD8+ cells). Production of autoantibodies or reactive T lymphocytes can result from molecular mimicry of microbes and self-epitopes, failure of the antiidiotype control mechanism, or development of new epitopes on self-proteins from tissue injury caused by viruses, bacterial exotoxins, or antibiotics.

The ideal immunosuppressant drug would induce long-term, specific inflammatory or immune nonresponsiveness with short-term administration; maintain competent immune response to infectious organisms; and induce minimal adverse systemic effects. Therapeutic use of monoclonal antibodies directed against specific targets of the immune response may eventually allow design of these ideal drugs. The mechanism of action of immunosuppressant drugs has become more specific, largely because of advances in management of organ transplantation patients, with the development of drugs that target defined molecules or response pathways. The combination of drugs to target different sites of cellular metabolism has increased the success of immunosuppressive therapy.

Based on their primary mechanism of action, immunosuppressants may be classified as (1) inhibitors of gene expression or transcription (glucocorticoids), (2) phosphatase (cyclosporine, tacrolimus, rapamycin) and kinase (leflunomide) inhibitors, (3) inhibitors of nucleotide synthesis (azathioprine), (4) alkylating agents (cyclophosphamide, chlorambucil), and (5) monoclonal antibodies (against T-cell receptor, IL-2R).[138,139]

Inhibitors of Gene Expression or Transcription

Glucocorticoids

Glucocorticoids are potent antiinflammatory and immunosuppressant medications that are frequently used to treat inflammatory, allergic, autoimmune, and neoplastic (lymphoma, lymphosarcoma) diseases and to prevent allograft rejection in transplantation. Their effect, duration, and intensity depend on individual pharmokinetic and pharmacodynamic parameters.[140] Frequently used glucocorticoids in horses include hydrocortisone, dexamethasone, prednisolone, methylprednisolone, isoflupredone, triamcinolone, beclomethasone, and fluticasone.[141-143] In addition to applications in antiinflammatory therapy, glucocorticoids in horses have been used for the treatment of a broad range of diseases that directly involve the immune system: atopy or skin hypersensitivity reactions, contact dermatitis, recurrent airway disease, immune-mediated hemolytic anemia, immune-mediated thrombocytopenia, immune-mediated myositis, uveitis, purpura hemorrhagica, vasculopathy, pemphigus foliaceus, and lymphomas or lymphosarcomas.[144-147]

Glucocorticoids should be used judiciously in the treatment of primary infectious processes (e.g., bacterial, viral, or protozoal meningitis) and in neonates because of their immunosuppressive effect. Chronic treatment with glucocorticoids may lead to susceptibility to infection, hypokalemia, adrenal suppression, hyperglycemia, gastrointestinal ulceration, delayed wound healing, growth suppression, osteoporosis, myopathy, and hypertension. Therefore, many studies focus on identifying strategies to inhibit the proinflammatory mediators selectively and treat inflammation or autoimmune diseases without adverse effects.

Glucocorticoids are lipophilic and pass freely through cell membranes. They bind to a cytosolic glucocorticoid receptor (GR), a transcription factor that subsequently translocates to the nucleus and regulates gene transcription by binding to glucocorticoid-responsive elements.[148] Importantly, glucocorticoids bind to and inhibit proinflammatory transcription factors NF-κB, activator protein-1 (AP-1), and cyclic adenosine monophosphate (cAMP) response element–binding protein (CREB). In certain cell types, glucocorticoids can increase the synthesis and function of the NF-κB inhibitory protein (iκB-alpha), which prevents NF-κB translocation into the nucleus. This results in repression of transcription and protein synthesis of cytokines, chemokines, inflammatory enzymes, and adhesion molecules[149] (Box 72-1).

Phosphatase and Kinase Inhibitors

Cyclosporine

Cyclosporine is a cyclic polypeptide with immunosuppressive effects. It binds to the cytoplasmic receptor cyclophilin and subsequently to the catalytic domain of the cytoplasmic phosphatase calcineurin.[150] This binding results in the inhibition of dephosphorylation of transcription factors, importantly the nuclear factor of activated T lymphocyte (NFAT), which prevents its translocation to the nucleus. Therefore the production of key elements of T-cell activation and proliferation (IL-2, IL-4, CD40L, TNF-α, IFN-γ, c-myc) is suppressed. Cyclosporine has been used in the horse for intravitreal treatment of recurrent uveitis. Potential adverse effects of cyclosporine include vasoconstriction, hypertension, nephrotoxicity, and hepatotoxicity. Significant bone marrow suppression is not usually observed.

Box • 72-1

Effects of Glucocorticoid Suppressor Mechanisms

- *Migration of inflammatory cells to the site of inflammation:* Reduce the expression of chemotactic proteins and adhesion molecules: macrophage chemotactic protein (MCP-1), intercellular adhesion molecule (ICAM-1), vascular cellular adhesion molecule (VCAM-1), E-selectin, and migration inhibition factor (MIF).
- *Neutrophils, monocytes, and macrophages:* Inhibit phagocytosis, expression of complement and immunoglobulin receptors, bactericidal and fungicidal activity, chemotactic response, and secretion of cytokines (IL-1, IL-6, IL-8, IL-12, IFN-β, TNF-α) and other products (prostaglandins, nitric oxide).
- *T cells:* Suppress proliferative response, IL-2 secretion, and the upregulated expression of the co-stimulatory molecule CD40L ligand on activated CD4+ T cells. Although glucocorticoids decrease cytokine secretion in general, the reduced production of IL-12 and resistant production of IL-10 by monocytes and macrophages result in decreased secretion of IFN-γ and increased production of IL-4, favoring a Th2-type response. In addition, glucocorticoids inhibit early T-cell receptor (TCR) signaling and the transcription of protease granzymes in cytotoxic T cells.
- *Antibodies:* Suppress production of new antibodies.
- *Dendritic cells:* Impair T-cell—mediated terminal maturation of dendritic cells and consequently decrease dendritic cell secretion of IL-1β, IL-6, and TNF-α and expression of co-stimulatory molecule CD86.
- *Eosinophils:* Promote apoptosis.

Tacrolimus

Tacrolimus is a macrolide antibiotic that binds to the cytoplasmic FK-binding protein (FK-BP), and the resultant protein complex inhibits calcineurin. The NF-AT transcription factor is inhibited, and transcription of IL-2, IL-2R, IL-3, IL-4, IL-5, IFN-γ, TNF-α, and GM-CSF is impaired. Tacrolimus is considered to be a more powerful immunosuppressive drug than cyclosporine.

Rapamycin (or Sirolimus)

Rapamycin is a macrolide antibiotic that binds to FK-BP and blocks translation of mRNA into proteins required for progression through G1 phase of the cell cycle. Therefore, rapamycin inhibits the proliferative signal generated by IL-2R (late T-cell function inhibitor) and induces cell cycle arrest or apoptosis.

Mycophenolate Mofetil

Mycophenolate mofetil (MMF) is a prodrug of mycophenolic acid that inhibits an important enzyme (IMPDH, inosine monophosphate dehydrogenase) involved in the de novo biosynthesis of guanosine. This drug is a very specific T- and B-lymphocyte proliferation inhibitor.[151] The most significant adverse effects are diarrhea and gastric ulceration.

Leflunomide

Leflunomide is a synthetic isoxazole prodrug of malononitriloamide, which inhibits a critical tyrosine kinase (DHODH) involved in de novo biosynthesis of pyrimidine. Therefore, it inhibits cell proliferation, importantly of T and B cells.

Inhibitors of Nucleotide Synthesis

Azathioprine

Azathioprine is a prodrug of 6-mercaptopurine, a purine analog that is incorporated into the DNA of lymphocytes and inhibits the de novo pathway of purine synthesis. Therefore, it inhibits the synthesis of DNA and RNA and consequently, lymphocyte activation and proliferation. Azathioprine has been used in horse for the treatment of immune-mediated anemia, immune-mediated thrombocytopenia, vasculopathy, and pemphigus foliaceus.[152,153] The use of azathioprine allows reduction in glucocorticoid dose when the two are combined in therapy. Because proliferation of many cell types can also be inhibited, adverse effects associated with azathioprine treatment include leukopenia, alopecia, and hepatotoxicity.

Alkylating Agents

Cyclophosphamide and Chlorambucil

The metabolites of the nitrogen mustard derivatives, cyclophosphamide (phosphoramide and acrolein) and chlorambucil (phenylacetic acid mustard), alkylate DNA bases. The results are mutagenic, cytotoxic, antiproliferative, and chemotherapeutic effects. The mutagenic effect increases the risk of development of secondary malignancies. Cyclophosphamide has a greater effect on B cells and therefore is used in the treatment of autoantibody-mediated diseases. In horses, these drugs have been used for the treatment of lymphosarcoma.[154]

Adverse effects associated with cyclophosphomide and chlorambucil therapy include anemia, leukopenia, and alopecia.

Vinca Alkaloids

Vincristine

Vincristine is a vinca alkaloid with antitumor, immunosuppressive, and thrombocytopoietic effects. It binds to tubulin in the mitotic spindle and prevents purine synthesis by inhibiting glutamic acid utilization; thus it inhibits cell proliferation. In horses, vincristine has been used for the treatment of immune-mediated thrombocytopenia and lymphosarcoma.[155] Mild neurologic adverse effects (proprioceptive deficits, ileus) may occur.

Monoclonal Antibodies

The development of species-specific monoclonal antibodies (mAbs) and the identification of appropriate antigenic targets have contributed to the advance in the use of mAbs in medicine.[156] The great advantage of mAbs is the specificity of response, which may minimize adverse effects. Examples of mAbs used in the treatment of human cancer are rituximab (targets CD20 on non-Hodgkin's lymphoma), trastuzumab (targets HER2/neu on breast cancer), and daclizumab (targets IL-2Rα on cutaneous T-cell lymphoma and hairy B-cell leukemia). The use of mAbs linked to cytotoxic drugs or radioisotopes is currently being investigated. These antibodies would deliver toxins to specific cancer cell targets and minimize systemic exposure (e.g., gemtuzumab for treatment of myelogenous leukemia).[157]

In autoimmune disorders (e.g., T-cell–mediated psoriases), IV single-dose injection of anti–IL-12 mAbs is well tolerated and induces concentration-dependent improvement of psoriatic lesions.[158] The anti–IFN-γ (infliximab), which blocks this crucial inflammatory mediator in its early signaling, has been approved for the treatment of human rheumatoid arthritis, Crohn's disease, ankylosing spondylitis, and vasculitis.[159]

REFERENCES

See the CD-ROM for a list of references linked to the abstract in PubMed.

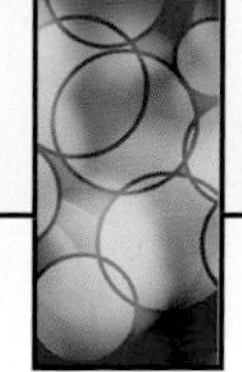

APPENDIX A

Infectious Disease Rule-Outs for Medical Problems*

Debra C. Sellon

RESPIRATORY PROBLEMS

Cough
Pleuropneumonia (1)
Pharyngeal or laryngeal abscess (1)
Pulmonary abscess (1)
Guttural pouch empyema or mycosis (1, 28)
Bacterial pneumonia (1, 28)
Equine influenza (12)
Equine herpesvirus (13)
Equine viral arteritis (14)
African horse sickness (15)
Equine rhinovirus (16)
Equine adenovirus (16)
Hendra virus (16)
Strangles (28)
Nocardiosis (30)
Rhodococcus equi (32)
Tuberculosis (33)
Glanders (39)
Pneumocystosis (50)
Pneumocystis carinii infection (50)
Coccidioidomycosis (51)
Pythiosis, zygomycosis (55)
Pulmonary aspergillosis (56)
Cryptococcosis (57)
Parascaris equorum larval migration (62)
Lungworms (62)

Nasal Discharge
Lymphoid pharyngeal hyperplasia (1)
Bacterial pneumonia (1)
Pleuropneumonia (1)
Guttural pouch mycosis (1)
Lung abscess (1)
Guttural pouch empyema, chondroids (1, 28)
Equine influenza (12)
Equine herpesvirus (13)
Equine viral arteritis (14)
African horse sickness (15)
Equine adenovirus (16)
Equine rhinovirus (16)
Hendra virus (16)
Strangles (28)
Nocardiosis (30)
Rhodococcus equi (32)
Tuberculosis (33)
Glanders (39)
Coccidioidomycosis (51)
Ascarid migration (62)
Nasal fungal infection (55, 56)
Pulmonary aspergillosis (56)
Cryptococcosis (57)
Surra *(Trypanosoma evansi)* (61)
Dourine *(Trypanosoma equinum)* (61)
Besnoitiosis (61)
Ascarid migration (62)
Lungworm infection (62)

Respiratory Noise
Arytenoid chondritis (1)
Guttural pouch empyema (1)
Guttural pouch mycosis (1)
Strangles (28)
Conidiobolomycosis (55)

Rhinitis, Sinusitis
Glanders (39)
Conidiobolomycosis (55)
Aspergillosis (56)

Pleural Effusion
Pleuropneumonia (1)
African horse sickness (15)

Lower Respiratory Tract Inflammation
Pneumonia (1)
Pleuropneumonia (1)
Aspiration pneumonia (1)
Interstitial pneumonia (1)
Endocarditis (2)
Myocarditis (2)
Neonatal septicemia (6)
Influenza (12)
Equine herpesviruses (13)
Adenovirus (16)
Hendra virus (16)
Rhinovirus (16)
Streptococcal diseases (28)
Corynebacterium pseudotuberculosis (30)
Rhodococcus equi (32)
Mycobacteria (33)
Glanders (39)
Anaerobic infection (48)
Pneumocystosis (50)
Pulmonary aspergillosis (56)
Pulmonary habronemiasis (62)

*Numbers in parentheses refer to chapters in which diseases are discussed.

Lungworms (62)
Ascarid migration (62)

GASTROINTESTINAL PROBLEMS

Diarrhea in Adult Horses

Aeromonas spp. (3)
Mycobacterial infections (33)
Endotoxemia (37)
Salmonellosis (38)
Potomac horse fever (43)
Enteric clostridiosis (44)
Histoplasmosis (57)
Cryptosporidiosis (61)
Giardiasis (61)
Parasitism (62)
Cyathostomiasis (62)
Cestodes (63)

Diarrhea in Foals

Aeromonas spp. (3)
Neonatal septicemia (6)
Rotavirus (17)
Coronavirus (18)
Rhodococcus equi (32)
Lawsonia intracellularis (36)
Endotoxemia (37)
Salmonellosis (38)
Clostridium perfringens type A, B, or C (44)
Clostridium difficile (44)
Tyzzer's disease (45)
Cryptosporidiosis (61)
Giardiasis (61)
Gastrointestinal parasites (61, 62)
Strongyloidosis (62)

Adominal Pain

Peritonitis (3)
Abdominal abscess (3)
Neonatal septicemia (6)
Oophoritis (8)
Equine viral arteritis (14)
African horse sickness (15)
Rabies (19)
West Nile virus (21)
Purpura hemorrhagica (*Streptococcus zooepidemicus* subsp. *equi*) (28)
Corynebacterium pseudotuberulosis (30)
Anthrax (30)
Rhodococcus equi (32)
Lawsonia intracellularis (36)
Endotoxemia (37)
Salmonellosis (38)
Potomac horse fever (43)
Enteric clostridiosis (44)
Botulism (46)
Tetanus (47)
Pythiosis (55)
Piroplasmosis (60)
Ascarid impaction (62)
Strongylosis (62)
Cestodes (63)

Dysphagia

Guttural pouch mycosis (1)
Guttural pouch empyema (1, 28)
Pharyngeal or laryngeal infection or abscess (1)
Oral infection (3)
Bacterial meningitis or encephalitis (4)
Rabies (19)
Alphaviruses (20)
West Nile virus infection (21)
Strangles (28)
Botulism (46)
Tetanus (47)
Equine protozoal myeloencephalitis (59)
Sarcocystosis (61)
Tick paralysis (64)

Icterus

Cholangiohepatitis, cholangitis (3)
Hepatic abscess (3, 28,30)
Equine viral arteritis (14)
Equine infectious anemia (23)
Leptospirosis (34)
Ehrlichiosis (42)
Tyzzer's disease (45)
Piroplasmosis (60)
Surra (61)
Dourine (61)
Ascarids (62)

Oral Ulcerations or Vesicles

Equine herpesvirus (13)
Equine viral arteritis (14)
Vesicular stomatitis (24)
Jamestown Canyon virus (26)
Mycobacterial infections (33)

Hepatomegaly, Hepatic Inflammation

Equine infectious anemia (23)
Rhodococcus equi (32)
Mycobacterial infections (33)
Leptospirosis (34)
Endotoxemia (37)
Tyzzer's disease (45)
Echinococcosis (61)

Abdominal Mass

Abdominal abscess (3)
Strangles (28)
Corynebacterium pseudotuberculosis (30)
Rhodococcus equi (32)
Mycobacterium spp. (33)
Echinococcus infection (61)

Abdominal Effusion

Abdominal abscess (3)
Peritonitis (3)
Streptococcal infections (28)
Rhodococcus equi (32)
Coccidioidomycosis (51)
Verminous arteritis (62)
Corynebacterium pseudotuberculosis (30)

CENTRAL NERVOUS SYSTEM PROBLEMS

Cortical Signs

Parasite migration (4, 61)
Brain abscess, meningitis (4, 28)
Neonatal septicemia (6)
Equine herpesvirus type 1 (13)
Rabies (19)
Eastern equine encephalitis (20)

Western equine encephalitis (20)
Venezuelan equine encephalitis (20)
Japanese encephalitis virus (21)
West Nile virus (21)
Borna disease (22)
Main Drain virus (26)
Snowshoe hare virus (26)
Jamestown Canyon virus (26)
Equine encephalosis (26)
Glanders (39)
Candidiasis (53)
Aflatoxicosis (56)
Cryptococcus neoformans (57)
Equine protozoal myeloencephalitis (59)
Piroplasmosis (60)

Brain Stem Signs

Temporohyoid osteoarthropathy (1)
Guttural pouch mycosis or empyema (1, 28)
Parasite migration (4, 61)
Brain stem abscess (4, 28)
Equine herpesvirus type 1 (13)
Rabies (19)
West Nile virus (21)
Borna disease (22)
Equine protozoal myeloencephalitis (59)

Spinal Cord or Peripheral Nerve Signs

Vertebral body abscess (4)
Discospondylitis (4)
Equine herpesvirus type 1 (13)
Rabies (19)
West Nile virus (21)
Borna disease (22)
Equine infectious anemia (23)
Rhodococcus equi (32)
Lyme disease (35)
Granulocytic ehrlichiosis (42)
Botulism (46)
Tetanus (47)
Equine protozoal myeloencephalitis (59)
Dourine (61)
Surra (61)
Tick paralysis (64)

URINARY TRACT PROBLEMS

Dysuria, Stranguria, Pollakiuria

Cystitis (9)
Urethritis (9)
Pyelonephritis (9)
Urinary calculi (9)
Habronemiasis (62)

Incontinence

Parasite migration (4, 62)
Equine herpesvirus type 1 (13)
Rabies (19)
Equine protozoal myeloencephalitis (59)

Hematuria

Seminal vesiculitis (8)
Cystitis (9)
Urinary tract infection (9)
Urolithiasis (9)
Corynebacterium pseudotuberculosis (30)
Leptospirosis (34)
Endotoxemia (37)
Salmonellosis (38)
Enteric clostridiosis (44)
Habronemiasis (62)

Renal Failure

Pyelonephritis (9)
Urolithiasis (9)
Leptospirosis (34)
Endotoxemia, sepsis (37)
Piroplasmosis (60)

MUSCULOSKELETAL PROBLEMS

Myositis, Increased Muscle Enzyme Activity

Sarcocystosis (5, 61)
Equine influenza (12)
Equine herpesviruses (13)
African horse sickness (15)
Strangles (28)
Streptococcal infections (28)
Clostridial myonecrosis (45)
Anaerobic bacterial infections (48)
Surra (61)

Lameness, Stiffness, Arthritis

Aortoiliac thrombosis (2)
Septic arthritis (5)
Osteomyelitis (5)
Bacterial tenosynovitis (5)
Neonatal septicemia (6)
Rabies (19)
West Nile virus (21)
Borna disease (22)
Purpura hemorrhagica (strangles) (28)
Streptococcal infections (28)
Staphylococcal infections (29)
Corynebacterium pseudotuberculosis (30)
Rhodococcus equi (32)
Lyme disease (35)
Endotoxemia (37)
Brucellosis (40)
Potomac horse fever (43)
Clostridial myonecrosis (45)
Tetanus (47)
Coccidioidomycosis (51)
Candidiasis (53)
Equine protozoal myeloencephalitis (59)

Muscle Fasciculations

Rabies (19)
West Nile virus (21)
Borna disease (22)
Anthrax (30)
Endotoxemia (37)
Botulism (46)
Tetanus (47)

CARDIOVASCULAR PROBLEMS

Cardiomyopathy, Myocarditis, Endocarditis

Bacterial endocarditis (2)
Inflammatory valvulitis (2)
Equine influenza (12)
Equine herpesvirus (13)
African horse sickness (15)

Streptococcal infections (28)
Rhodococcus equi (32)
Granulocytic ehrlichiosis (42)

REPRODUCTIVE PROBLEMS

Abortion, Infertility, Early Embryonic Loss, Birth of Weak Foals

Endometritis (8)
Pyometra (8)
Oophoritis (8)
Salpingitis (8)
Neosporosis (8)
Nocardioform placentitis (8)
Aeromonas hydrophila (8)
Chlamydiosis (8)
Mycoplasma infection (8)
Bacterial placentitis (8)
Fungal placentitis (8)
Equine herpesvirus type 1 (13)
Equine viral arteritis (14)
Equine infectious anemia (23)
Streptococcal infections (28)
Rhodococcus equi (32)
Mycobacterial infections (33)
Leptospirosis (34)
Salmonellosis (38)
Brucellosis (40)
Contagious equine metritis (41)
Potomac horse fever (43)
Coccidioidomycosis (51)
Candidiasis (53)
Aspergillosis (56)
Piroplasmosis (60)
African animal trypanosomiasis (61)
Surra (61)
Dourine (61)

Scrotal/Preputial Enlargement

Epididymitis (8)
Equine herpesvirus type 3 (8)
Orchitis (8)
Streptococcal infections (28)
Corynebacterium pseudotuberculosis (30)
Glanders (39)
Dourine (61)
Habronemiasis (62)
Onchocerciasis (62)

HEMOLYMPHATIC PROBLEMS

Enlarged Lymph Nodes

Upper respiratory tract infection (1)
Equine influenza (12)
Equine herpesviruses (13)
Equine rhinovirus (16)
Equine adenovirus (16)
Strangles (28)
Corynebacterium pseudotuberculosis (30)
Rhodococcus equi (32)
Mycobacterial infections (33)
Glanders (39)
Pythiosis (55)
Histoplasmosis (57)
Cryptococcosis (57)
Blastomycosis (57)
Epizootic lymphangitis (57)

Lymphangitis

Corynebacterium pseudotuberculosis (30)
Rhodococcus equi (32)
Glanders (39)
Sporotrichosis (52)

Anemia

Equine infectious anemia (23)
Chronic infections (28)
Streptococcal infection (28)
Corynebacterium pseudotuberculosis (30)
Granulocytic ehrlichiosis (42)
Clostridial myonecrosis (45)
Piroplasmosis (babesiosis) (60)
Dourine (61)
Surra (61)
African animal trypanosomiasis (61)
Gastrointestinal parasitism (61, 62, 63)

Petechial Hemorrhages

Neonatal septicemia (6)
Equine viral arteritis (14)
Equine infectious anemia (23)
Purpura hemorrhagica (strangles) (28)
Endotoxemia, septicemia, bacteremia (37)
Salmonellosis (38)
Granulocytic ehrlichiosis (42)
Potomac horse fever (43)
Piroplasmosis (60)
African animal trypanosomiasis (61)
Surra (61)

Ventral Abdominal or Limb Edema

Pleuritis, pleuropneumonia (1)
Pericarditis (2)
Thrombophlebitis (2)
Bacterial endocarditis (2)
Equine herpesvirus (13)
Equine viral arteritis (14)
Equine infectious anemia (23)
Purpura hemorrhagica (strangles) (28)
Corynebacterium pseudotuberculosis (30)
Anthrax (30)
Mycobacterial infections (33)
Endotoxemia (37)
Granulocytic ehrlichiosis (42)
Monocytic ehrlichiosis (43)
Piroplasmosis (60)
Dourine (61)
Surra (61)
African animal trypanosomiasis (61)
Gastrointestinal parasitism (62)

Hypoalbuminemia

Mycobacterial infections (33)
Equine infectious anemia (36)
Lawsonia intracellularis (36)
Salmonellosis (38)
Enteric clostridiosis (44)
Gastrointestinal parasitism (61, 62, 63)
Cyathostomiasis (62)

Immunodeficiency
Equine herpesvirus type 2 (13)
African animal trypanosomiasis (61)

Thrombocytopenia
Equine viral enteritis (14)
African horse sickness (15)
Equine infectious anemia (23)
Endotoxemia (37)
Salmonellosis (38)
Granulocytic ehrlichiosis (42)
Potomac horse fever (43)
Enteric clostridiosis (44)
Babesiosis (60)
Trypanosomiasis (61)

OCULAR PROBLEMS

Uveitis
Neonatal septicemia (6)
Viral infection (10)
Setaria infection (10)
Verminous migration (10)
Uveitis (10, 34)
Streptococcal infections (28)
Rhodococcus equi (32)
Leptospirosis (34)
Lyme disease (35)
Granulocytic ehrlichiosis (42)
Onchocerciasis (62)

Keratitis
Temporohyoid osteoarthropathy (1)
Neonatal septicemia (6)
Bacterial keratitis (10)
Fungal keratitis (10, 56)
Equine herpesviruses (13)
Dourine (61)
Onchocerciasis (62)

Conjunctivitis
Chlamydiosis (10)
Thelazia (10)
Equine influenza (12)
Equine herpesviruses (13)
Equine viral arteritis (14)
African horse sickness (15)
Equine adenovirus (16)
Streptococcal infections (28)
Lyme disease (35)
Blastomycosis (57)
Epizootic lymphangitis (57)
Piroplasmosis (60)
Surra (61)
Dourine (61)
Besnoitiosis (61)
Onchocerciasis (62)
Habronemiasis (62)

Corneal Edema
Equine herpesvirus type 2 (13)
Leptospirosis (34)
Aspergillosis (56)
Onchocerciasis (62)

Blindness
Guttural pouch empyema (1)
Brain abscess (4)
Meningitis (4)
Toxoplasmosis (10)
Echinococcosis (10, 61)
Equine leukoencephalomalacia (10)
Rabies (19)
Alphavirus encephalitides (20)
Japanese encephalitis (21)
West Nile virus (21)
Aspergillosis (56)
Equine protozoal myeloencephalitis (59)

INTEGUMENTARY PROBLEMS

Hair Loss
Dermatophilosis (31)
Dermatophytosis (54)
Besnoitiosis (61)
Pinworms (62)
Onchocerciasis (62)
Lice (64)
Mite infestation (64)
Culicoides hypersensitivity (64)

Pruritus
Malassezia infection (7)
Folliculitis (7)
Besnoitiosis (7, 61)
Rabies (19)
Dermatophilosis (31)
Dermatophytosis (54)
Onchocerciasis (62)
Pinworms (62)
Culicoides hypersensitivity (64)
Pediculosis (64)
Lice (64)
Mites (64)

Crusting, Scaling
Bacterial folliculitis (7)
Malassezia infection (7)
Poxvirus (7)
Besnoitiosis (7, 61)
Dermatophilosis (31)
Dermatophytosis (54)
Onchocerciasis (62)
Culicoides hypersensitivity (64)
Mite infestation (64)

Ulcers, Fistulas, Granulomatous Lesions
Leishmaniasis (7)
Equine sarcoid (25)
Staphylococcal infections (29)
Corynebacterium pseudotuberculosis (30)
Nocardiosis (30)
Mycobacterial infections (33)
Glanders (39)
Brucellosis (40)
Sporotrichosis (52)
Pythiosis (55)
Basidiobolomycosis (55)
Mucormycosis (55)
Habronemiasis (62)
Myiasis (64)

Papulonodular Lesions
Bacterial furunculosis (7)
Molluscum contagiosum (7)
Leishmaniasis (7)
Papillomatosis (25)
Dermatophytosis (54)
Fly or tick bites (64)
Warbles (64)
Straw itch mites (64)

Large Nodular Dermatoses or Abscesses
Equine sarcoid (25)
Streptococcal infections (28)
Staphylococcal infections (29)
Corynebacterium pseudotuberculosis (30)
Nocardiosis (30)
Rhodococcus equi (32)
Mycobacterial infections (33)
Glanders (39)
Coccidioidomycosis (51)
Sporotrichosis (52)
Zygomycosis (55)
Pythiosis (55)

SUDDEN DEATH

Collapse and Sudden Death
Guttural pouch mycosis (acute hemorrhage) (1)
Septic thromboembolism (2)
Ruptured pulmonary or abdominal abscess (3)
Neonatal septicemia (6)
Hendra virus (16)
Anthrax (30)
Salmonellosis (38)
Potomac horse fever (43)
Enteric clostridiosis (44)
Clostridial myonecrosis (45)
Tyzzer's disease (foals) (45)
Botulism (46)

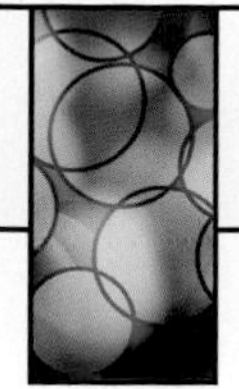

APPENDIX B

Vaccination Guidelines for Horses in North America

DISEASE/ VACCINE	FOALS/WEANLINGS	YEARLINGS	PERFORMANCE HORSES	PLEASURE HORSES	BROODMARES*	COMMENTS
Tetanus (inactivated toxoid) Core vaccine: all horses	*Foal of vaccinated mare:* First dose: 6 months Second dose: 7 mo Third dose[†]: 9-10 mo *Foal of nonvaccinated mare:* First dose: 3-4 mo Second dose: 4-5 mo Third dose[†]: 6-8 mo	Annual	Annual	Annual	Annual, 4-8 wk before foaling	Booster at time of penetrating injury or surgery if last dose of tetanus toxoid was not administered within past 6 mo.
Encephalomyelitis (EEE, WEE inactivated vaccine) Core vaccine: all horses	**WEE, EEE: (in low-risk areas)** *Foal of vaccinated mare:* First dose: 6 months Second dose: 7 months Third dose[†]: 9-10 mo *Foal of nonvaccinated mare:* First dose: 3-4 mo Second dose: 4-5 mo Third dose[†]: 6-8 mo	Annual, spring	Annual, spring	Annual, spring	Annual, 4-8 wk before foaling	For VEE, follow same protocol as for WEE/EEE if indicated by threat of exposure or requirements for interstate or international transportation. VEE may be available only as a combination vaccine with EEE and WEE.
	EEE: (in high-risk areas) First dose: 3-4 mo Second dose: 4-5 mo Third dose[†]: 6-8 mo	Annual, spring	Annual, spring	Annual, spring	Annual, 4-8 wk before foaling	In high-risk areas for EEE, booster EEE and WEE every 6 mo. A series of at least three doses is recommended for primary immunization of foals.
West Nile virus (WNV) (inactivated or canarypox-vectored recombinant vaccine) Core vaccine: all horses	*Foal of vaccinated mare:* First dose: 3-4 mo Second dose: 4-5 mo Third dose[†]: 6-8 mo *Foal of nonvaccinated nonexposed mare:* First dose: ≤3 mo Second dose: 1 mo later For the inactivated vaccine, administration of third dose, 2-3 mo	Semiannual (twice annually) or annual depending on regional duration of season for challenge by WNV-infected mosquitoes.	Semiannual or annual depending on regional duration of season for challenge by WNV-infected mosquitoes.	Semiannual or annual depending on regional duration of season for challenge by WNV-infected mosquitoes.	Semiannual or annual; time one booster 4-8 wk before foaling. Avoid administration to mares during the first 60 days of gestation if possible.	Peak seasonal exposure to WNV is in summer and fall. In areas with prolonged season for WNV-infected mosquitoes, time one booster in early spring to precede local mosquito activity and second booster in middle to late summer to precede expected peak local incidence of disease. Mosquito control is important for effective WNV prevention in both

DRUG	BRAND NAME	DOSING INFORMATION
Antibiotics—cont'd		
Oxytetracycline	LA-200, other forms	*Ehrlichiosis:* 3.5 mg/kg IV q12h, or up to 10 mg/kg IV or IM, q24h (give IV slowly) *Foals* (flexural limb deformities): As much as 44 and up to 70 mg/kg IV (2-3 g per foal), with two doses 24 hr apart, has been used.
Penicillin G	Generic	Sodium or potassium penicillin: 22,000 U/kg IV q6-8h Procaine penicillin: 22,000 U/kg IM q12h Doses up to 44,000 U/kg q6h have been used for refractory cases.
Rifampin	Rifadin	10 mg/kg PO q24h For *Rhodococcus equi:* 5-10 mg/kg PO, q12h; always use in combination with a macrolide or azalide.
Sulfonamides	Generic	See Trimethoprim-sulfonamides.
Ticarcillin	Ticar	44 mg/kg IV or IM, q6-8h Ticarcillin also is used intrauterine in mares.
Tilmicosin	Micotil	Do not use in horses until more safety data become available.
Trimethoprim-sulfadiazine or trimethoprim-sulfamethoxazole	Tribrissen, Uniprim, Bactrim	15 mg/kg IV q12h, or 20-30 mg/kg PO q12-24h; formulations contain a sulfonamide/trimethoprim ratio of 5:1.
Vancomycin	Vancocin	4.3-7.5 mg/kg as IV infusion q8h
Antifungals		
Amphotericin B	Fungizone	0.1-0.6 mg/kg as IV infusion q24h; start at low doses and increase gradually.
Fluconazole	Diflucan, generic	Loading dose of 14 mg/kg PO, followed by 5 mg/kg PO q24h; liver enzymes should be monitored.
Griseofulvin	Fulvicin U/F	5 mg/kg PO q24h
Itraconazole	Sporanox	Oral solution: 5 mg/kg PO q24h Oral capsules: 7.5-10 mg/kg PO q24h; absorption is low and variable. IV solution: 1.5 mg/kg IV q24h
Voriconazole	Vfend	2-4 mg/kg PO q24h, or 1 mg/kg IV q24h; use higher doses for *Fusarium* spp.
Antiprotozoals		
Pyrimethamine	Daraprim	1 mg/kg PO q24h; used in combination with a sulfonamide for the treatment of EPM.
Trimethoprim-sulfonamide combinations	Tribrissen, Uniprim, Bactrim	See under Antibiotics.
Ponazuril	Marquis	5 mg/kg PO q24h; treatment recommended for a minimum of 28 days for EPM.
Diclazuril	Clinacox	5 mg/kg (500 g of Clincacox) PO q24h; treatment recommended for a minimum of 28 days for EPM.
Nitazoxanide	Navigator	Starting dose of 25 mg/kg (11.36 mg/lb) PO q24h for 5 days, followed by 50 mg/kg (22.72 mg/lb) PO q24h for 23 days for EPM; monitor for possible gastrointestinal complications.

IM, Intramuscularly; *IV,* intravenously; *PO,* orally; *SC,* subcutaneously; *q24h,* every 24 hours; *EPM,* equine protozoal myeloencephalitis.

Index

Greek Characters

A

Page numbers followed by b indicate boxes; f, figures; t, tables.

E

I

J

K

L

M

O

Q

R

S

T

U